Diagnosis and Treatment
of Voice Disorders

2nd edition

Diagnosis and Treatment

of Voice Disorders

2nd edition

John S. Rubin, MD, FACS, FRCS
Consultant Otolaryngologist
Royal National Throat, Nose, and Ear
  Hospital
Division of the Royal Free N.H.S. Trust
and
Honorary Consultant Otolaryngologist
St. Bartholomew's Hospital
London, England
and
Honorary Senior Lecturer
Institute of Laryngology and Otology
University College of London
and
Visiting Associate Professor
Department of Otolaryngology
Albert Einstein College of Medicine
Bronx, New York

Robert T. Sataloff, MD, DMA, FACS
Professor, Department of
  Otolaryngology—
  Head and Neck Surgery
Jefferson Medical College
Thomas Jefferson University
and
Chairman, Department of
  Otolaryngology—
  Head and Neck Surgery
Graduate Hospital
and
Adjunct Professor
Department of Otorhinolaryngology—
  Head and Neck Surgery
University of Pennsylvania
Philadelphia, Pennsylvania
and
Adjunct Professor
Department of Otolaryngology—
  Head and Neck Surgery
Georgetown University
Washington, DC

Gwen S. Korovin, MD, FACS
Clinical Assistant Professor
Department of Otolaryngology
New York University School of Medicine
and
Consulting Otolaryngologist
Ames Vocal Dynamics Laboratory
Lenox Hill Hospital
and
Attending Physician
Department of Otolaryngology
Manhattan Eye, Ear, and Throat
  Hospital
and
Attending Physician
Department of Otolaryngology
Lenox Hill Hospital
New York, New York

THOMSON

DELMAR LEARNING™

Australia Canada Mexico Singapore Spain United Kingdom United States

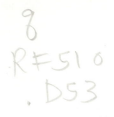
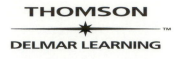

THOMSON
DELMAR LEARNING

Diagnosis and Treatment of Voice Disorders, 2nd edition

John S. Rubin, MD, FACS, FRCS
Robert T. Sataloff, MD, DMA, FACS
Gwen S. Korovin, MD, FACS

Health Care Publishing Director:
William Brottmiller

Executive Editor:
Cathy L. Esperti

Acquisitions Editor:
Candice Janco

Senior Developmental Editor:
Elisabeth F. Williams

Executive Marketing Manager:
Dawn F. Gerrain

Production Coordinator:
Catherine Ciardullo

Project Editor:
Bryan Viggiani

Art/Design Coordinator:
Connie Lundberg-Watkins

Editorial Assistant:
Maria D'Angelico

For permission to use material from this text or product, contact us by
Tel (800) 730-2214
Fax (800) 730-2215
www.thomsonrights.com

Library of Congress Cataloging-in-Publication Data

Diagnosis and treatment of voice disorders / [edited by] John S. Rubin, Robert T. Sataloff, Gwen S. Korovin.-- 2nd ed.
    p. ; cm
Includes bibliographical references and index.
    ISBN 0-7693-0135-5 (alk. paper)
    1.   Voice disorders.
    [DNLM: 1. Laryngeal Diseases--diagnosis. 2. Voice Disorders--therapy. 3. Laryngeal Diseases--surgery. 4. Larynx. 5. Voice. WV 500 D536 2003] I. Rubin, John S. (John Stephen) II. Sataloff, Robert Thayer. III. Korovin, Gwen S.
    RF510 .D53 2003
    616.85'5--dc21

                                        2002073669

Notice to the Reader

The publisher does not warrant or guarantee any of the products described herein or perform any independent analysis in connection with any of the product information contained herein. The publisher does not assume, and expressly disclaims, any obligation to obtain and include information other than that provided to it by the manufacturer.

The reader is expressly warned to consider and adopt all safety precautions that might be indicated by the activities herein and to avoid all potential hazards. By following the instructions contained herein, the reader willingly assumes all risks in connection with such instructions.

The publisher makes no representation or warranties of any kind, including but not limited to, the warranties of fitness for particular purpose or merchantability, nor are any such representations implied with respect to the material set forth herein, and the publisher takes no responsibility with respect to such material. The publisher shall not be liable for any special, consequential, or exemplary damages resulting, in whole or part, from the readers' use of, or reliance upon, this material.

Dedication

It has been seven years since the untimely death of Wilbur James Gould. We wish to again dedicate this book to his memory. Dr. Gould was a true master of laryngology, a giant in the field of voice disorders, and a personal mentor to all the authors.

One of the authors (JSR) wrote a brief poem about Jim, shortly following his death, which is included below and which we feel at the distance of the intervening years still encompasses our feelings about this remarkable man.

The authors

to Wilbur James Gould
in memoriam

We are a special club,
those of us whose lives he changed.
We are select
but not so few,
for he threw his net widely
and he chose wisely.

We are a special club—
we had the audacious luck
to learn from him,
to be taught by him,
to be with him
as his brain hatched up
idea after idea,
project after project.

He pushed us,
or he cajoled us,
or he talked us
into the lab,
into learning voice,
into loving laryngology.
He did whatever he felt it took—

and he did it time and again,
until it worked.

And then there are his patients,
for almost 50 years
the tens of thousands whom he touched,
whom he was always willing to see,
whom he healed
as much by caring
as by treating.

He is Wilbur James Gould
I doubt that there will ever be another
such as he.
We are his legacy,
and now we must, each of us,
fufill it.

TABLE OF CONTENTS

UNIT 3: MANGEMENT

CONTRIBUTORS

Jean Abitbol, MD
Ancien Chef de Clinique
Faculté de Médecine de Paris
and
Oto-Rhino-Laryngologiste
Phoniatre-Chirurgie Laser
Paris, France
Chapters 17, 23

Patrick Abitbol, MD
Oto–Rhino–Laryngologiste
Interne Des Hopitaux de Paris
Paris, France
Chapters 17, 23

Milan Amin, MD
Assistant Professor
Department of Otolaryngology—
    Head and Neck Surgery
MCP Hahnemann University
Philadelphia, Pennsylvania
Chapter 24

R. J. Baken, PhD
Professor and Director of Laryngology
    Research
Department of Otolaryngology
New York Eye and Ear Infirmary
New York, New York
Chapter 9

Michael S. Benninger, MD
Chairman
Department of Otolaryngology—
    Head and Neck Surgery
Henry Ford Hospital
Detroit, Michigan
Chapters 8, 18, 27

Andrew Blitzer, MD, DDS
Professor of Clinical Otolaryngology
College of Physicians and Surgeons
Columbia University
Director
New York Center for Voice and Swallowing
    Disorders
Medical Director
New York Center for Clinical Research
New York, New York
Chapter 15

Linda M. Carroll, PhD, CCC-SLP
Assistant Professor
Department of Otolaryngology
Mount Sinai School of Medicine
Mount Sinai Medical Center
New York, New York
Chapter 32

Albert Castro, MD
Radiologue
Directeur du Centre d'Imagerie Médicale
    Numérisée Monceau
Paris, France
Chapter 17

Raymond H. Colton, PhD
Professor of Otolaryngology and
   Communication Disorders
Professor
Research Laboratories
Department of Otolaryngology
SUNY Health Science Center at Syracuse
Syracuse, New York
Chapter 14

Mark S. Courey, MD
Associate Professor
Department of Otolaryngology
Medical Director
Vanderbilt Voice Center
The Village at Vanderbilt
and
Acting Director
Department of Otolaryngology
Head and Neck Surgery Associates
Saint Thomas Hospital
Nashville, Tennessee
Chapter 36

Carole M. Dean, MD, FRCS (C)
Instructor
Department of Otolaryngology
Thomas Jefferson University
Philadelphia, Pennsylvania
Chapter 39

Brian P. Driscoll, MD, FACS
Attending Physician
Greater Baltimore Medical Center
Baltimore, Maryland
Chapter 16

Ruth Epstein, PhD, MRCSLT
Lead Principal Speech and
Language Therapist
Royal National Throat, Nose, and Ear Hospital
Royal Free NHS Trust
London, England
Chapter 34

Ramon A. Franco, Jr., MD
Instructor and Laryngology Fellow
Department of Otology and Laryngology
Harvard Medical School
Division of Laryngology
Massachusetts Eye and Ear Infirmary
Boston, Massachusetts
Chapters 37, 40

Adrian Fourcin, PhD
Emeritus Professor of Experimental
   Phonetics and Linguistics
University College London
London, England
Chapter 33

Glendon M. Gardner, MD
Regional Coordinator for Otolaryngology
Department of Otolaryngology—
   Head and Neck Surgery
Henry Ford Hospital
Detroit, Michigan
Chapters 8, 18, 27

George S. Goding, Jr., MD
Associate Professor
Department of Otolaryngology
University of Minnesota School of Medicine
and
Department of Otolaryngology
Hennepin County Medical Center
Minneapolis, Minnesota
Chapter 35

Rodolphe Gombergh, MD
Radiologue
Directeur du Centre d'Imagerie Médicale
    Numérisée Monceau
Paris, France
Chapter 17

Thomas M. Harris, FRCS
Consultant
Ear, Nose, and Throat Surgeon
University Hospital Lewisham
and
Director, Voice Disorders Unit
Queen Mary's Hospital
Sidcup, Kent, England
Chapters 30, 33

Mary J. Hawkshaw, RN, BSN, CORLN
Executive Director
American Institute for Voice and Ear
    Research
Philadelphia, Pennsylvania
Chapters 11, 20

Gerald B. Healy, MD
Professor of Otology and Laryngology
Harvard Medical School
and
Otolaryngologist-in-Chief
Children's Hospital
Boston, Massachusetts
Chapter 22

Yolanda D. Heman-Ackah, MD
Assistant Professor
Laryngology and Professional Voice Care
Director
The Voice Center
University of Illinois at Chicago
Chicago, Illinois
Chapter 35

David H. Henick, MD
Clinical Assistant Professor
Department of Otolaryngology
Albert Einstein College of Medicine
Bronx, New York
Chapter 2

Reinhart J. Heuer, PhD
Senior Research Scientist
American Institute for Voice and Ear
    Research
and
Professor
Department of Communication Sciences
Temple University
Philadelphia, Pennsylvania
Chapter 29

Young-Ho Kim, MD, PhD
Section of Otolaryngology
Department of Surgery
Yale University School of Medicine
New Haven, Connecticut
Chapter 3

Gwen S. Korovin, MD, FACS
Clinical Assistant Professor
Department of Otolaryngology
New York University School of Medicine
and
Consulting Otolaryngologist
Ames Vocal Dynamics Laboratory
Lenox Hill Hospital
and
Attending Physician
Department of Otolaryngology
Manhattan Eye, Ear, and Throat Hospital
and
Attending Physician
Department of Otolaryngology
Lenox Hill Hospital
New York, New York
Chapters 13, 34

James A. Koufman, MD
Director, Center for Voice Disorders
and
Professor of Otolaryngology
Wake Forest University School of Medicine
Winston-Salem, North Carolina
Chapters 12, 24

Jeffrey T. Laitman, PhD
Professor of Cell Biology and Anatomy
Department of Otolaryngology
Director of Anatomy and
    Functional Morphology
Professor of Otolaryngology
Mount Sinai School of Medicine
and
Research Associate
Department of Anthropology
American Museum of Natural History
New York, New York
Chapter 1

Robert S. Lebovics, MD, FACS
Chief, Division of Otolaryngology—
    Head and Neck Surgery
Cabrini Hospital and Medical Center
New York, New York
Chapter 25

Steven H. Levy, MD
Medical Director, Psych Arts
Research Associate
American Institute for Voice and
    Ear Research
Philadelphia, Pennsylvania
Chapter 29

Jacob Lieberman, DO, MA
Registered Osteopath and Psychotherapist
and
Team Member
The Voice Research Laboratory
Queen Mary's Hospital
Sidcup, Kent, England
and
Former Research Fellow
British School of Osteopathy
London, England
Chapter 33

Christy L. Ludlow, PhD, CCC-Speech
Chief, Laryngeal and Speech Section
National Institute of Neurological Disorders
    and Stroke
National Institutes of Health
Bethesda, Maryland
Chapter 28

Eric A. Mann, MD, PhD
Staff Otolaryngologist
Laryngeal and Speech Section
National Institute of Neurological Disorders
    and Stroke
National Institutes of Health
Bethesda, Maryland
Chapter 28

Thomas Murry, PhD
Professor
Department of Otolaryngology
University of Pittsburgh
Pittsburgh, Pennsylvania
Chapter 31

H. Bryan Neel III, MD, PhD
Professor and Past Chair
Department of Otorhinolaryngology—
    Head and Neck Surgery
Mayo Medical School
Rochester, Minnesota
and
Member
Board of Regents of the University of
    Minnesota
Minneapolis, Minnesota
Chapter 25

Drew M. Noden, PhD
Professor
Department of Biomedical Sciences
New York State College of Veterinary Medicine
Cornell University
Ithaca, New York
Chapter 1

Robert H. Ossoff, DMD, MD
Associate Vice Chancellor for Health Affairs
Director
Vanderbilt Bill Wilkerson Center for
    Otolaryngology and Communication Sciences
Guy M. Maness Professor and Chairman
Department of Otolaryngology
Vanderbilt University Medical Center
Nashville, Tennessee
Chapter 36

Reza Rahbar, DMD, MD, FACS
Department of Otolaryngology
Children's Hospital
and
Assistant Professor of Otology and
    Laryngology
Department of Otology and Laryngology
Harvard Medical School
Boston, Massachusetts
Chapter 22

Lorraine Olson Ramig, PhD
Professor
Department of Speech-Language
    Hearing Science
University of Colorado—Boulder
and
Research Associate
Wilbur James Gould Voice Center
The Denver Center for the Performing Arts
Denver, Colorado
Chapter 26

Vijay Rao, MD
Professor
Department of Radiology
Jefferson Medical College
Thomas Jefferson University
Philadelphia, Pennsylvania
Chapter 35

Clark A. Rosen, MD, FACS
Director
University of Pittsburgh Voice Center
and
Associate Professor
Department of Otolaryngology
University of Pittsburgh School of Medicine
Department of Communication Science
    and Disorders
University of Pittsburgh School of Health
    and Rehabilitation Sciences
Pittsburgh, Pennsylvania
Chapter 31

Deborah Caputo Rosen, RN, PhD
Medical Psychologist
Bala Cynwyd, Pennsylvania
Chapter 29

John S. Rubin, MD, FACS, FRCS
Consultant Otolaryngologist
Royal National Throat, Nose, and Ear Hospital
Division of the Royal Free N.H.S. Trust
and
Honorary Consultant Otolaryngologist
St. Bartholomew's Hospital
London, England
and
Honorary Senior Lecturer
Institute of Laryngology and Otology
University College of London
and
Visiting Associate Professor
Department of Otolaryngology
Albert Einstein College of Medicine
Bronx, New York
Chapters 6, 13, 30, 33, 34

Ira Sanders, MD
Associate Professor
Department of Otolaryngology
Director of Research
Grabscheid Voice Center
Mount Sinai School of Medicine
New York, New York
Chapter 5

Clarence T. Sasaki, MD
Ohse Professor of Surgery and Chairman
Section of Otolaryngology
Yale University School of Medicine
New Haven, Connecticut
Chapter 3

Robert Thayer Sataloff, MD, DMA, FACS
Professor, Department of Otolaryngology—
   Head and Neck Surgery
Jefferson Medical College
Thomas Jefferson University
and
Chairman, Department of Otolaryngology—
   Head and Neck Surgery
Graduate Hospital
and
Adjunct Professor
Department of Otorhinolaryngology—
   Head and Neck Surgery
University of Pennsylvania
Philadelphia, Pennsylvania
and
Adjunct Professor
Department of Otoloaryngology—
   Head and Neck Surgery
Georgetown University
Washington, DC
Chapters 11, 19, 20, 29, 39

Kiminori Sato, MD, PhD
Clinical Professor
Department of Otolaryngology—
   Head and Neck Surgery
Kurume University School of Medicine
Kurume, Japan
Chapter 4

Ronald C. Scherer, PhD
Professor
Department of Communication Disorders
Bowling Green State University
Bowling Green, Ohio
Chapter 7

Craig Schwimmer, MD
Private Practice
Dallas, Texas
Chapter 8

H. Steven Sims, MD
Assistant Professor of Otolaryngology
University of Nebraska College of Medicine
Omaha, Nebraska
Chapter 16

Marshall E. Smith, MD
Associate Professor
Division of Otolaryngology—
    Head and Neck Surgery
University of Utah Medical Center
Salt Lake City, Utah
and
Research Associate
Wilbur James Gould Voice Center
The Denver Center for the Performing Arts
Denver, Colorado
Chapter 26

Steven E. Sobol, MD
Senior Resident
Department of Otolaryngology
McGill University
Montreal, Quebec, Canada
Chapter 21

Joseph R. Spiegel, MD, FACS
Associate Professor of Otolaryngology—Head
    and Neck Surgery
Thomas Jefferson University
and
Vice Chairman
Department of Otolaryngology—
    Head and Neck Surgery
Graduate Hospital
Philadelphia, Pennsylvania
Chapters 11, 20, 39

Lucian Sulica, MD
Director
Center for Voice Disorders
Department of Otolaryngology
New York Eye & Ear Infirmary/Beth Israel
    Medical Center
New York, New York
and
Assistant Professor
Department of Otolaryngology
New York Medical College
and
Assistant Professor
Department of Otolaryngology
Albert Einstein College of Medicine
Bronx, New York
Chapter 15

Ted L. Tewfik, MD, FRCSC
Professor of Otolaryngology
McGill University
and
Director of Otolaryngology
Montreal Children's Hospital
Montreal, Quebec, Canada
Chapter 21

Harvey M. Tucker, MD, FACS
Professor of Otolaryngology—
    Head and Neck Surgery
Case Western Reserve University School
    of Medicine
Cleveland, Ohio
Chapter 38

Thomas R. Van De Water, PhD
Director
Cochlear Implant Research Program
University of Miami Ear Institute
Professor
Department of Otolaryngology
Miami, Florida
Chapter 1

Gayle E. Woodson, MD
Professor of Otolaryngology
University of Florida at Gainesville
Gainesville, Florida
Chapter 10

Peak Woo, MD
Director
The Grabscheid Center
The Mount Sinai Medical Center
Department of Otolaryngology
New York, New York
Chapters 14, 41

Eiji Yanagisawa, MD, FACS
Clinical Professor of Otolaryngology
Yale University School of Medicine
and
Attending Otolaryngologist
Yale-New Haven Hospital
and
Attending Otolaryngologist
Hospital of Saint Raphael
New Haven, Connecticut
Chapters 6, 16

Steven M. Zeitels, MD, FACS
Director
Division of Laryngology
Massachusetts Eye and Ear Infirmary
and
Associate Professor
Department of Otology and Laryngology
Harvard Medical School
Boston, Massachusetts
Chapters 37, 40

PREFACE

In the years since the first edition of *Diagnosis and Treatment of Voice Disorders*, there have been many exciting advances in the field of voice. In preparing the second edition, we have tried to amplify the classic information that was presented in the first edition, integrating the latest discoveries and concepts without diluting the "basics." In some cases, chapters have been replaced; in others, major rewriting was necessary; and in a few cases, the original chapters were retained with only minimal alterations. We hope that this book will serve not only as a compendium of laryngology, but also as a useful clinical text and reference.

The chapters on "Formation of the Larynx: From Homeobox Genes to Critical Periods" and "Laryngeal Development" required only limited revision. They stand as erudite, definitive discussions of laryngeal development. The chapters on "Anatomy of the Human Larynx" and "Functional Fine Structures of the Human Vocal Fold Mucosa" have been updated substantially, mirroring the interest in research in these areas. Their concise reviews of the latest discoveries in understanding the structure of the larynx should be invaluable to anyone working with the human voice, and especially to clinicians. "Microanatomy of the Vocal Fold Musculature" presents the newest and latest concepts, many of which differ from traditional understanding of the anatomy of the laryngeal muscles. The chapter on "Benign Vocal Fold Pathology Through the Eyes of the Laryngologist" has been rewritten extensively and offers practical insight into not only our current understanding of vocal fold pathology, but also the clinical applications of that understanding. Scherer's chapter on "Laryngeal Function During Phonation" has been rewritten and expanded; it is an extraordinary synthesis of laryngeal physiology. "Laryngeal Neurophysiology" is a new chapter that provides a practical overview of the basic information that underlies neurolaryngology, an area of particular and growing clinical importance. Baken's chapter "Dynamic Disorders of the Voice: A Chaotic Perspective on Vocal Irregularities" is truly a classic contribution to the literature. It offers a remarkably accessible window into the world of non-linear dynamics, and the application of chaos theory to understanding voice function. Woodson's revised chapter on "Research in Laryngology" provides a current perspec-

tive on where the field has been going recently, and directions it is likely to follow in the future.

"History and Physical Examination in Patients With Voice Disorders" has been expanded and updated, and provides practical insights into the latest concepts in history taking and physical examinations of professionals and nonprofessionals with voice complaints. "Evaluation of Biomechanics by Fiberoptic Laryngoscopy" has been revised and stresses the important dynamic information that can be obtained through informed observation of the larynx during phonation. "Introduction to the Laboratory Diagnosis of Choice Disorders" and "Measuring Vocal Fold Function" have been revised and expanded to include the most current information, such as high-speed analysis of vocal fold motion and videokymography. "Laryngeal Electromyography" and "Laryngeal Photography and Videography" have also been updated and continue to be particularly practical chapters, containing information that is useful to both beginners and the experienced laryngologist.

"3D Laryngeal CT Scan for Voice Disorders" is a unique, new chapter. It describes techniques that have not been published previously in English and includes three-dimensional images that are almost shocking in their beauty and anatomic depiction of laryngeal detail. It also describes practical techniques for virtual video endoscopy, introducing the concept of the "vocal scan." Benninger's chapter on "The Evaluation of Voice Outcomes and Quality of Life" explains techniques for outcomes assessment; and the new chapter "Voice Impairment, Disability, Handicap and Medical/Legal Evaluation" provides further explanations of timely concepts, and practical applications for the laryngologist. "Common Medical Diagnoses and Treatment of Patients With Voice Disorders" contains information on most of the diagnoses encountered in professional and nonprofessional voice patients, including not only the most common entities, but also many obscure diagnoses.

Tewfik's "Congenital Anomalies of the Larynx" is a new chapter that covers this complex topic in a concise manner, and includes particularly useful tables. It complements the new chapter on "Voice Disorders in the Pediatric Population," which reviews the most common and most serious disorders encountered by the pediatric otolaryngologist.

Abitbol's new chapter "The Larynx: A Hormonal Target" is replete with new information about laryngeal effects from activity throughout the endocrine system, with particular emphasis on the sex hormones and their effect on the voices of women. Koufman's revised chapter on "Laryngopharyngeal Reflux and Voice Disorders" provides a dynamic discussion of this extremely common disorder and its clinical importance. "Infectious and Inflammatory Disorders of the Larynx" is effectively a new chapter that provides information on essentially all clinically relevant disorders in this complex area.

"Neurologic Disorders of the voice" has been revised extensively. It reviews the most current thinking in neurolaryngologic abnormalities, and complements the chapters on vocal fold paralysis and spasmodic dysphonia. Gardner's chapter on "Vocal Fold Paralysis" explores not only diagnosis, but also the most advanced concepts in surgical treatment. Ludlow's chapter on "Management of Spasmodic Dysphonias" offers exceptional scholarly insight and clinical experience in describing the diagnosis and treatment of this challenging group of disorders.

"Psychologic Aspects of Voice Disorders" has been extensively revised and expanded to include new treatment concepts, and to update information about psychotropic medications. Harris' chapter on "Medications and the Voice" is a new addition to the book and is designed to provide an overview of commonly used medications and their effects on voice function. The chapters on "The Role of the Speech-Language Pathologist in the Treatment of Voice Disorders" and "The Role of the Voice Specialist in the Non-medical Management of Benign Voice Disorders" are detailed, practical chapters that convey guidelines for management and specific approaches to voice therapy and training.

The chapter on "Laryngeal Manipulation" is new both to the text and to the field of Laryngology. Co-authored by an osteopathic physician, two experienced laryngologists, and an acoustic scientist, it offers insights into the value of laryngeal manipulation in the clinical management of voice disorders. "Special Considerations for the Professional Voice User" has been revised extensively and addresses special issues relative to singers, actors, and other voice professionals not covered elsewhere in the text. The chapter on "Laryngotracheal Trauma" is new, elegantly written, and provides details, radiologic images, and surgical approaches for patients with laryngeal injury.

The revised chapter on "Surgical Management of Benign Voice Disorders" synthesizes the most current surgical approaches for treatment of structural lesions that do not respond to voice therapy. The chapter on "Laryngeal Framework Surgery" reviews Isshiki's landmark contributions and incorporates the most recent advances in phonosurgery of the laryngeal skeleton. Tucker's chapter on "Laryngeal Reinnervation" presents not only a review of his noteworthy contribution, but also a comprehensive discussion on a variety of current approaches, including a brief discussion of laryngeal transplantation. The chapter on "Premalignant Lesions of the Larynx" is new. It provides useful photographs in addition to a systemic discussion of these complex problems and their management. The chapter "Surgery for Laryngeal Cancer" is also new and condenses an extraordinary amount of information on this expansive topic. It discusses everything from staging to traditional approaches to laryngeal cancer surgery, to the latest concepts in limited resection of vocal fold malignancies. Woo's chapter on "Diagnosis and Management of Postoperative Dysphonia" remains an important and practical guide for helping patients with less-than-optimal vocal quality following laryngeal surgery.

This 2nd edition of *Diagnosis and Treatment of Voice Disorders* provides an accessible, practical text and reference for laryngologists, speech-language pathologists, singing and acting voice specialists, nurses, and other professionals entrusted with the care of patients with voice disorders.

John S. Rubin, MD, FACS, FRCS
Robert T. Sataloff, MD, DMA, FACS
Gwen S. Korvin, MD, FACS

UNIT 1

Basic Science

CHAPTER 1

Formation of the Larynx: From Homeobox Genes to Critical Periods

Jeffrey T. Laitman, PhD

Drew M. Noden, PhD

Thomas R. Van De Water, PhD

The human larynx is a complex structure that must serve respiratory, protective, and vocalization functions. Although there have been detailed descriptions of some of the major histologic and morphologic events of the laryngeal development of the human embryo[1] and of both embryonic and fetal mice,[2] much still remains to be uncovered and insights gained into the mechanisms and critical periods of laryngeal development, especially during the fetal and postnatal periods. This chapter addresses two areas of laryngeal development in which our knowledge base is incomplete, areas that are important to our understanding of the structure-function relationship of this unique organ.

This chapter is divided into two basic themes: First we address early embryologic events, including tissue primordia and tissue interactions that contribute to the establishment of the laryngeal primordium and the role that genetic analysis may play in determining if homeobox genes participate in the formation and patterning of the larynx. Second, we address the identification and significance of critical periods in prenatal and postnatal laryngeal development in humans.

ESTABLISHING LARYNGEAL PRIMORDIA

Common Developmental Themes

Laryngeal morphogenesis occurs normally only if cell and tissue movements bring about a convergence of epithelial, connective tissue, myogenic, endothelial, and neuronal precursors beneath the caudal region of the pharynx. These precursors have greatly varied embryonic histories, and each cell lineage undergoes developmental programming that prepares its members to participate as chondrocytes and myocytes in laryngeal morphogenesis.

Achieving this programming is an *epigenetic* process for each precursor population. This means that cells engage in a progressive series of interactions involving others cells and the extracellular milieu that alters the function of specific genes. Some interactions are common to many laryngeal precursor populations; others are unique to one subpopulation.

Tissue interactions affect rates of cell proliferation; pathways and speeds of cell migration; and both the commitment to and the expression of specific cell phenotypes. Clearly, these processes must be temporally and spatially coordinated in order for so many disparate progenitors to achieve an integrated outcome.

Most laryngeal precursors have sites of origin and exhibit patterns of movements that are evolutionarily conserved. A key feature of this conserved plan is the presence in all vertebrate embryos of a *segmental organization* within many developing tissues. This is manifest especially in hindbrain-branchial arch and trunk axial regions. While the larynx is not generally viewed as a segmentally organized set of structures, tissues developing nearby, many formed from common progenitors, do exhibit a segmental organization during their development.

The expression patterns of several members of gene families that are involved in lineage delineation and spatial programming of head and neck tissues similarly show a segmental organization. Abnormal expression of some of these genes, either as a result of germ line mutations in humans or experimental gene manipulation in transgenic mice, also results in disruptions of hindbrain, branchial, otic, and laryngeal morphogenesis.

The first objective of this section is to identify the origins of laryngeal precursors and document their movements to the site of laryngeal morphogenesis. The second goal is to identify when and where each of these populations become programmed to form tissues of the types and shapes appropriate to their final location, including the genetic bases for their decisions. The reader should be warned that laryngeal development has received little attention by experimental biologists. Thus, many of the hypotheses regarding laryngeal development presented here are by inference, based on properties of neighboring structures.

Origins of Laryngeal Precursors

The larynx develops at the boundary between "head" and "trunk" regions of the embryo. Rostrally, the pharynx forms a set of segmentally arranged endodermal outpocketings, the *pharyngeal pouches*, between which are located *branchial arches* (also called pharyngeal or visceral arches). Some vertebrates establish a large number of branchial arches, retaining many as gills, but birds and mammals form only three or four recognizable swellings on each side of the head (Figure 1-1). (The development, indeed existence, of the fifth and sixth

branchial arches in higher vertebrates remains controversial and will not be considered in this chapter). Most of the cells that fill branchial arches do not arise locally, but rather migrate into the arches from the dorsal margin of the brain. These are *neural crest cells* (Figure 1-2). The structure from which they arise, the hindbrain, also manifests a partially segmental organization, and the crest cells that fill each branchial arch can be traced to a specific segment.

To the caudal side of the developing larynx, segmental organization is largely restricted to the dorsal axial region. *Somites* are transient structures that reside immediately adjacent to the caudal hindbrain and spinal cord. The first somite forms immediately caudal to the primordium of the inner ear (otic vesicle). After a short epithelial stage, each somite segregates into myogenic, skeletogenic, angiogenic, and connective tissue-forming subpopulations, many of which move laterally and ventrally and contribute to the formation of peripheral structures, including the larynx. Paraxial mesoderm located beneath and rostral to the ear primordium does not form recognizable somites, but does give rise to all the same lineages and also contributes to intramembranous osteocytes of the parietal and frontal bones.

The larynx receives contributions from precursors that originate on both sides of this arbitrary head-trunk boundary. Relating the quite distinct organization of developing head and trunk structures to the larynx is a special challenge. Described next are the specific origins and patterns of migration of each lineage.

Pharyngeal Endoderm

The epithelial lining of the pharynx, from which the laryngeal groove and tracheal diverticulum arise, is

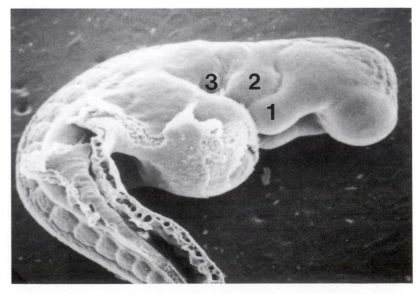

FIGURE 1-1. *Scanning electron micrograph showing the swelling of the first and second branchial arches (1, 2), which indicates that neural crest cells have already completed their ventral migrations. Note the location of the cardiac loop; this structure will shift caudally as the future laryngeal region of the pharynx closes. The specimen is a 16-day, 22-somite domestic cat embryo. 1, 2, and 3 refer to the numbering of the branchial arches.*

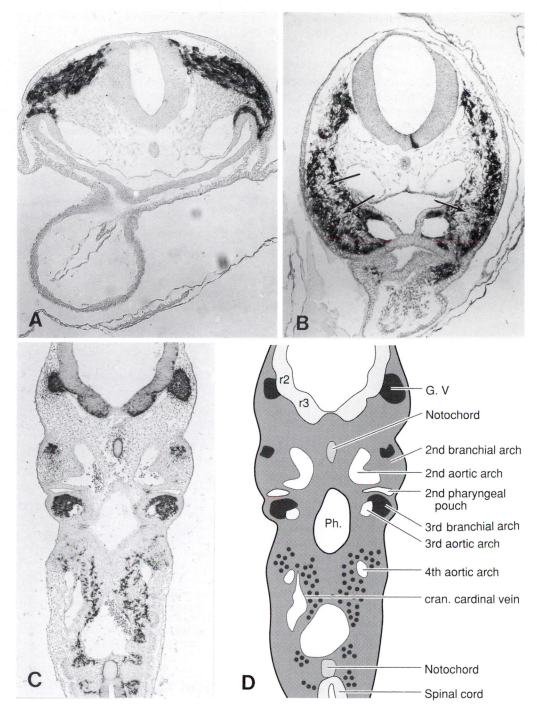

FIGURE 1-2. *Sections stained with antibodies to chick neural crest cells. (A) Neural crest cells migrating from the hindbrain roof at the level of rhombomere 4 and contacting the margin of the first pharyngeal pouch. (B) A later stage, by which time the full ventral expansion of the first arch neural crest population is completed. The arrows indicate branchial muscle precursors that have been surrounded by migrating crest cells. Some second arch crest cells are present in the future distal outflow tract. (C) A longitudinal section through a 4-day embryo, with landmarks indicated in sketch. (D) Note that crest cells have fully populated the third and fourth branchial arches. Cells from the caudal hindbrain penetrate occipital somites and are approaching the roof of the caudal pharynx. Most of these are precursors of the enteric nervous system. r2 and r3 = rhombomeres 2 and 3; Ph. = pharynx; G.V. = trigeminal (5th) sensory ganglion.*

formed along with the endodermal lining of the gut during the early gastrulation stage. Cells within the epiblast, which is the superficial layer of the embryonic disc (inner cell mass), move internally through the rostral margin of the primitive streak and establish a new epithelial layer, the endoderm.[3] While this is occurring, cells in the previously formed internal layer, the hypoblast, are displaced peripherally and become extraembryonic. Once internalized, the endodermal cells proliferate rapidly and the sheet expands to form the entire intraembryonic endodermal primordium. Shortly thereafter, the positional identities of most endodermal structures (eg, thyroid, thymus, lung, stomach, pancreas) are established. However, to date, it is not known when or how the laryngeal regions of the pharynx are spatially delineated.

Lateral Mesoderm

The next set of epiblast cells to ingress following formation of the endoderm become mesenchymal and migrate away from the midline, between the epiblast and endodermal layers, to establish mesoderm. In human embryos this process occurs during the third week of gestation and results in the formation of definitive mesoderm-endoderm relations.

Fate-mapping studies in avian embryos have identified lateral mesoderm located beside the first somite as the source of laryngeal connective tissues, including the arytenoid and cricoid cartilages (Figure 1-3A).[4] These data contradict earlier assertions that all skeletal elements associated with the larynx are homologous to gill-associated structures in anamniotes and therefore are derived from the neural crest. Birds do not have a structure homologous to the thyroid cartilage. Therefore, the embryonic origin of the thyroid cartilage has not been positively identified, although, based on its relation to other structures, an origin from the neural crest is likely.

Lateral mesoderm located caudal to the laryngeal primordium forms the tracheal cartilages and associated connective tissues. Lateral mesoderm located rostral to the laryngeal primordium is exclusively angiogenic and cardiogenic. Angiogenic precursors are a unique population. They are one of the earliest progenitor populations to be delineated,[5] and many endothelial precursors execute extensive, apparently undirected, migrations.[6] Angioblasts formed in mesoderm throughout the developing head invade presumptive laryngeal mesoderm, and precursors arising beside the caudal pharynx may seed distant parts of the head and the heart (Figure 1-3B).[7]

Paraxial Mesoderm

All striated voluntary muscles in the body arise within paraxial mesoderm, in either somites or unsegment-

ed head mesoderm. Myogenic cells originating within the first two somites migrate ventrally and come to reside beside the caudal pharynx.[8] These laryngeal muscle precursors appear to move in concert with a larger population of myogenic cells derived from somites 2 to 5 that are destined to form tongue and laryngeal muscles (Figure 1-4).[9] As this column of migrating myoblasts reaches the level of the pharynx, laryngeal precursors break away while glossal precursors contin-

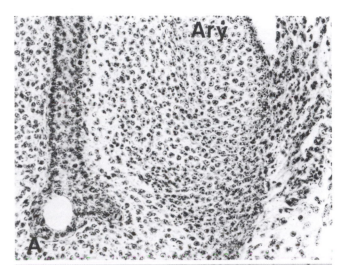

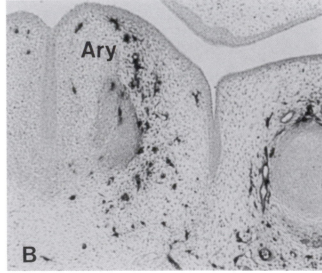

FIGURE 1-3. *(A) The embryonic larynx from a chick embryo that had previously received a transplant of lateral mesoderm from a quail embryo. Quail cells, recognized by the presence of a distinct nuclear marker, have formed the arytenoid cartilage. (B) Section from an embryo that received a similar transplant, but the section is stained with an antibody that only recognizes quail endothelial cells. Following the transplantation, angioblasts moved invasively in all directions.*

ue moving beneath the pharynx and then rostrally. Myoblasts arising in paraxial mesoderm located rostral to the somites form branchial muscles innervated by somatic components of cranial motor nerves V, VII, and IX and extraocular muscles innervated by cranial nerves III, IV, and VI.[8,10,11]

In contrast to many jaw muscles, the intrinsic laryngeal musculature does not show overt signs of muscle organization, such as alignment of primary myocytes,

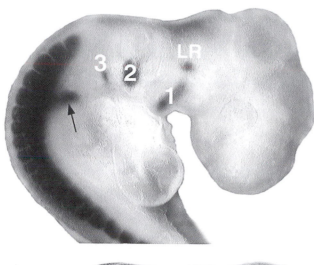

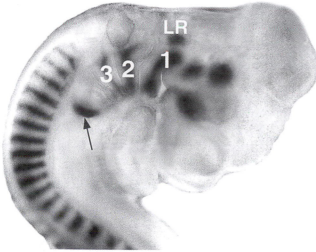

FIGURE 1-4. *Chick embryos at 2.5 (top) and 3.5 days of incubation treated to reveal the sites of expression of myf-5 mRNA, which is produced only in early differentiating skeletal muscle cells. Arrows show the hypoglossal cord, which contains myoblasts that form initially in the lateral margin of somites and migrate ventrally to become tongue and laryngeal muscles. 1, 2, 3 indicate myoblasts in the branchial arches; LR is the primordium of the lateral rectus. Precursors of other extra-ocular muscles are evident in the 3.5-day specimen.*

until after adjacent cartilagenous structures have begun to condense. However, examination of this population for the expression of muscle-specific regulatory genes (Figure 1-4) reveals that commitment to the myogenic lineage occurs much earlier,[12] prior to the onset of myoblast migration.

Hindbrain and Neural Crest Cells

Shortly after the neural tube closes, a series of circumferential indentations demarcates different regions of the brain. Within the hindbrain, additional delineations define a segmented pattern of hyperplastic neuroepithelial compartments called *rhombomeres*. Motor neurons that project to branchial and laryngeal muscles within each branchial arch and the larynx arise within specific sets of rhombomeres (Figure 1-5). Motor neurons associated with cranial nerve X (including the so-called "cranial root" of cranial nerve XI) arise over an extended length of the hindbrain that includes the most caudal rhombomere.

Neural crest cells form within neural folds or the roof of the neural tube along most of its length. Rostrally, these cells envelop the prosencephalon, but in the rest of the head and trunk they migrate laterally away from their dorsal origins. Neural crest cells are the source of all peripheral autonomic neurons and pigment cells, and most peripheral sensory and glial cells.[13] Additionally within the head, neural crest cells are a major source of skeletal and other connective tissues of the midfacial and branchial regions (Figure 1-6) reviewed in 1988 by Noden.[14] The hyobranchial skeleton is of neural crest origin, as likely is the thyroid cartilage.

Neural crest cells are the primary source of loose connective tissues, including dermis, smooth muscle, fascia, and tendons in the facial and branchial regions. Thus, tendinous connective tissues of muscles attaching to any jaw or hyobranchial skeletal structures are of neural crest origin. This includes suprahyoid and some infrahyoid (eg, thyrohyoid) muscles. Those muscles that are fully intrinsic to the larynx or that extend caudally from its cartilages derive their connective tissue elements from lateral mesoderm.

Analyses of Spatial Organization

Cellular Interactions

Early in its development, each cell lineage undergoes a series of progressive commitments resulting in the expression of *phenotypic properties* appropriate to its history and location. For example, only those epithelial cells located in the dorsomedial and ventrolateral margins of each somite become myoblasts. Their neighbors become a variety of dense and loose connective tissues.

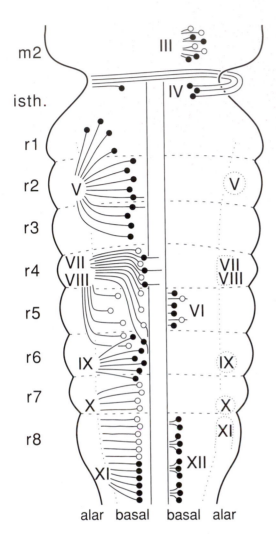

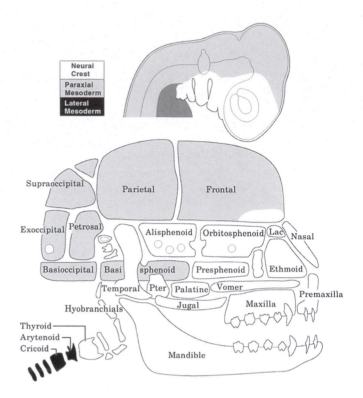

FIGURE 1-6. *Schematic representation of the mammalian skull indicating the origins of each skeletal element. The distribution pattern in skeletal tissues reflects segregations of neural crest, lateral mesoderm, and paraxial mesoderm that are established early in development as a result of migratory patterns.*

FIGURE 1-5. *Schematic representation of the distribution of primary motor neurons in a mammalian embryo. Note the clear segregation of most, but not all, motor nuclei. Some neurons in nuclei III and VI will later undergo transmedian migrations.*

Similarly, neural crest cells emigrating from the roof of the hindbrain are heterogeneous. In vivo and in vitro clonal analyses indicate that a small number of newly formed crest cells are committed to neuronal or melanogenic lineages, but most are multipotent and become committed in response to signals emanating either from tissues adjacent to their migratory routes or from other neural crest cells.[15,16] However, neither of the preceding examples explains how progenitor populations become committed to form a specific muscle (eg, cricothyroid) or skeletal element (eg, cricoid cartilage).

Establishing *spatial organization* within embryonic tissues is an obligate multicellular activity. The structures formed by each cell population must have the three-dimensional shape appropriate for the location in which they form. Extensive cellular and genetic analyses indicate that *the processes of phenotypic commitment and spatial organization involve different and distinct mechanisms.*

Clues regarding possible mechanisms of spatial organization within the many populations that move into each branchial arch come from comparisons of lineage data for each component (Figure 1-7). Early in their migration neural crest cells emigrating from a particular region of the hindbrain become associated with mesodermal myoblast cells from the same axial level (Figure 1-2B), and both populations move in concert into the nearest branchial arch. Furthermore, they subsequently become innervated by motor and sensory axons from the corresponding region of the hindbrain. Thus, all branchial arch constituents (except angioblasts) arise and maintain a strict *registration* from their time of origin to their terminal differentiation. At issue now is whether this close registration among different lineages defines a necessary precondition for the normal morphogenesis of peripheral musculoskeletal structures, including the larynx.

Transplantation experiments have indeed shown that interactions among these embryonic constituents are critical for normal morphogenesis, although maintaining registration throughout the migratory phase is only one possible means of ensuring that these interactions occur. Precursors of trunk muscles can be transplanted in place of head muscle precursors in the avian embryo, with donor cells labeled so as to be recognizable at later stages. The results of these experiments, and comparable analyses of limb muscles, are consistent: grafted precursors often are able to form muscles that are structurally and, as far as is known, functionally normal for their new location.[17,18] Thus, despite having a different place of birth, grafted embryonic muscle precur-

sors receive and recognize cues from surrounding tissues that instruct them where to move and to stop, what orientation of primary myocyte alignment to initiate, and which skeletal elements are appropriate for establishing tendinous attachments.

The implication of defining a subordinate population, in this case myoblasts, is that there must be an ordinate population, one in which spatial organization is established and used as a template by other tissues. In fact, there is; and in all situations analyzed it has been shown that *connective tissue precursors impose spatial organization* on surrounding tissues.

As described above, cells derived from the neural crest form all connective tissues in branchial arches. Neural crest cells originating at the level of rhombomere 2 (presumptive mandibular arch cells) will, if trans-

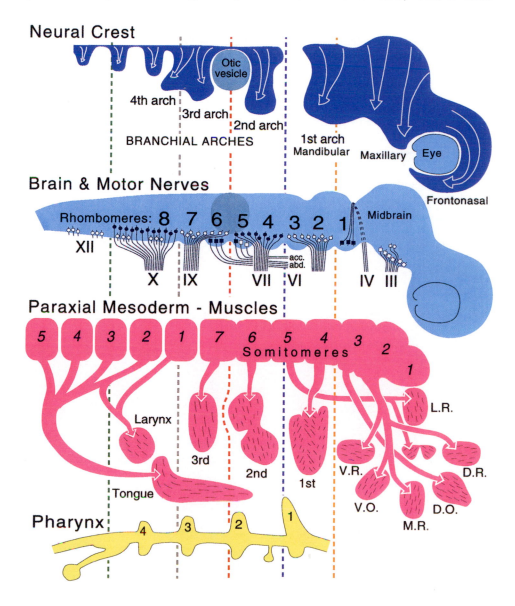

FIGURE 1-7. *Schematic staggered view of craniofacial precursor locations. Sites of origin of neural crest and mesodermal cells as well as the locations of epithelial structures in the brain and pharynx are illustrated. Structures are aligned to reflect their actual relative positions. The progenitors of many peripheral structures, especially branchial arches, trace their ancestry to common axial levels. VR is the central rectus; VO, the ventral oblique; MR, the medial rectus; DO, the dorsal oblique; DR, the dorsal rectus; and LR, the lateral rectus muscles of the eye.*

planted in place of rhombomere 4 or 6 (presumptive second or third branchial arch) crest precursors, migrate into an inappropriate branchial arch and therein generate a normal jaw skeleton.[19] Moreover, this population will impose a first arch organization on the overlying epidermis and the angioblasts and myoblasts that come into contact with the ectopic neural crest tissues. Thus, while individual cells within the primordium of the neural crest are not committed to specific phenotypes, the population is spatially specified based on its original axial location. The same is true for rhombomeres and for the sclerotomal parts of somites, both of which usually maintain their original positional identity after transplantation to a different axial level.

These data established a hierarchy of spatial organizing influences in which connective tissues, including those formed by neural crest in the head and mesoderm in the body axis and limbs, are pattern-generating populations. Developing muscles, blood vessels, and epidermal structures depend on interactions with these primary pattern-generating tissues to establish their final pattern of differentiation. In the case of the neural crest, precursors acquire this commitment while still part of an intact neural tube or neural plate, which takes the timetable for spatial organization of peripheral head tissues back to events occurring during or before the neurula stage. While no experiments have specifically analyzed precursors of laryngeal connective tissues, every other musculoskeletal system examined operates according to the same hierarchic basis for spatial organization.

Genetic Analyses: Homeobox Genes

Until recently, our understanding of mechanisms underlying spatial organization were limited to the cellular, and largely phenomenologic, analyses presented above. This is rapidly changing with the discovery of genes that, when mutated, cause a change of spatial organization in very specific parts of the body. These changes are called homeotic transformations, and the genes are collectively called *homeotic genes* (reviewed by McGinnis and Krumlauf[20] and Duboule and Morata[21]). Homeotic genes all share a highly conserved 180-base pair sequence called the homeobox; this sequence encodes for a DNA binding peptide. Members of this family are found in nearly every multicellular animal and many plants. All produce transcriptional regulatory peptides, so that the primary function of each gene is to activate or repress other genes.

During invertebrate evolution, clusters of homeotic genes arose with the novel feature that the relative position of each gene on a chromosome corresponds to the relative position along the body axis in which they exert a strong influence (Figure 1-8). Early in chordate evolution a series of partial chromosomal duplications produced four nearly complete copies of this set of homeo-tic genes, which in mammals are called *Hox* genes. The significance of these duplications is that for each mammalian *Hox* gene, there are one, two, or even three very similar genes, and it is known that partial redundancy of function is a critical aspect of their organization. Many *Hox* genes are transiently active immediately prior to or during the initial delineation of the hindbrain and are

FIGURE 1-8. *Expression sites of* Hox *genes of the* b *series in the hindbrain of mammalian embryos. The expression boundaries correspond to specific rhombomeric junctions, and this pattern is highly conserved. The boundaries of gene expression in paraxial mesoderm would be shifted caudally to the cervical and thoracic regions. Hox genes of the* a *series have a similar expression pattern, but paralogous genes of the* c *and* d *series are only weakly or not expressed in the head region. The rostral boundaries of expression of two of the four sets of* Hox *genes found in mammalian embryos are indicated for the hindbrain.*

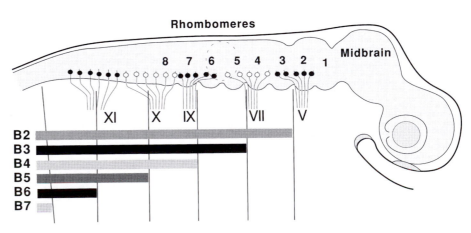

expressed in migrating cephalic neural crest cells;[20] other members of the family are expressed in key transitional zones of axial skeletal primordia, for example, somites that form the occipital-atlantal-axial skeleton, and in limb buds and many parts of the digestive and reproductive tracts. At least one, *Hox-a-2*, has been detected in the embryonic laryngeal mesenchyme.[22]

With the use of transgenic techniques in mice, it is possible to delete or spatially misdirect the patterns of expression of specific *Hox* genes. The loss of a functional *Hox d-3* gene, whose expression boundary is in somites at the occipital-cervical junction, results in a frame shift such that the first cervical vertebra develops with characteristics of the occipital bone.[23] While these skeletal tissues are spatially disrupted, laryngeal muscles derived from the same somites are normal, as would be expected if the spatial organization of myoblasts was imposed by mesoderm surrounding the pharynx.

Transgenic mice with loss of *Hox a-2* function develop with rhombomeres 4 to 5 now having no *Hox* genes of the *a* series expressed, which is the normal situation in rhombomeres 2 to 3. In these animals, neural crest cells migrating from rhombomere 4 enter the second branchial arch, but therein establish a first branchial arch skeleton,[24,25] similar to the results described above following neural crest transplantation. Thus, gene knockout experiments corroborate the results of transplantation analyses and link *Hox* gene activity with spatial organization of somites, hindbrain, and cephalic neural crest populations.

As yet, there is no causal link between specific *Hox* gene function and laryngeal morphogenesis, and there is no way of predicting whether these skeletal tissues, whose early development is intimately linked to pharyngeal endoderm, require expression of a specific *Hox* or other spatial organizing gene for their morphogenesis. Nor is it yet known whether the loss of *Hox* gene function or other disruption of cell-cell interactions is antecedent to congenital anomalies of laryngeal structures.[26] However, with methods for performing cell lineage analyses, tissue recombination experiments, and gene gain or loss of function experiments now available, the resolution to these problems is at hand.

CRITICAL PERIODS IN THE DEVELOPMENT OF THE FETAL AND POSTNATAL LARYNX

Although the foundations for laryngeal morphology are established during the period of organogenesis, recent studies have shown that significant aspects of maturation also occur in critical periods of both fetal (8

weeks to birth) and postnatal development. Of particular importance during this time are maturational events concerning changes in laryngeal position relative to contiguous aerodigestive tract structures.

Basic Mammalian Pattern of Laryngeal Position

In order to appreciate fully the development of the fetal larynx, it is necessary to review briefly the nature of laryngeal position in mammals. In most mammals, at all stages of postnatal development, the larynx during normal respiration is situated relatively "high" in the neck.[27] Its position, measured from the cranial aspect of the epiglottis to the caudal border of the cricoid cartilage, corresponds to the level of the basiocciput or first cervical vertebra (C1) to the third or fourth cervical vertebra (C3 or C4) in most terrestrial mammals. This laryngeal position corresponds to high positions for the hyoid bone, tongue, and pharyngeal constrictors. For example, the tongue at rest lies almost entirely within the oral cavity, with no portion of it forming part of the anterior pharyngeal wall. Accordingly, the supralaryngeal region of the pharynx is noticeably small, with little or no oral portion.

A major corollary of high laryngeal position is that the epiglottis abuts, or direct overlaps, the soft palate. The epiglottis can thus pass up behind the soft palate and allow the larynx to open directly into the nasopharynx, creating what is often called the *intranarial* larynx. This configuration provides a direct air channel from the external nares through the nasal cavities, nasopharynx, larynx, and trachea to the lungs. Liquids, and in some species even chewed or solid material, can pass on either side of the interlocked larynx and nasopharynx via the isthmus faucium, through the piriform sinuses to the esophagus, following the so-called lateral food channels. This anatomic configuration may permit the patency of the laryngeal airway in some species while streams of liquid or semisolid food are transmitted around each side of the larynx during swallowing. In essence, two largely separate pathways are created: a respiratory tract from the nose to the lungs, and a digestive tract from the oral cavity to the esophagus (see References 27-32). The importance of this dual pathway system for many mammals has often been noted (see particularly References 28-30).

Development of Laryngeal Position in the Human Fetus

The position of the larynx relative to contiguous structures in human newborns and young infants closely resembles the basic mammalian pattern described above. While the high position of the infant larynx has been noted in many studies (eg, Crelin[28] and

Laitman[29]), only recently have investigations begun to pinpoint the late fetal period as the crucial time for the establishment of laryngeal position sufficient to allow epiglottic-soft palate overlapping.[33,34] Indeed, recent studies have shown that fetal life is a critical period for the development of *both* structure and future functions of the upper respiratory and digestive pathways.[33-35]

The second trimester (13 to 26 weeks of gestation), in particular, has been shown to be a period of intense developmental activity. Studies have shown that by week 15 of development, earlier than previously reported, the epiglottis is already present, indicating that the epiglottic primordium may appear earlier in development than classically believed (Figure 1-9A).[33] Throughout this period the larynx is found high in the neck, generally corresponding (from epiglottic tip to inferior border of the cricoid) to the level of the basioccipital bone to the third cervical vertebra. By week 21 the epiglottis is found to be almost in apposition to the uvula of the soft palate. Between weeks 23 and 25 the epiglottis and soft palate are found to overlap for the first time, thus providing the anatomic "interlocking" of the larynx into the nasopharynx characteristic of most mammals (Figure 1-9B).

A major maturational horizon in the aerodigestive region is accomplished with the attainment of larynx-nasopharynx interlocking. Establishment of this anatomic relationship allows the creation of essentially separate respiratory and digestive routes that will function as such in the newborn infant. Recent ultrasound investigations have shown upper respiratory activity patterns strongly suggestive of an operational "two-tube" system beginning to function even prenatally, that is, the larynx remains highly positioned and intranarial during fetal swallowing movements.[34]

A developmental Rubicon may thus be achieved between weeks 23 and 25. Indeed, this period may reflect a critical time in the development of the entire upper respiratory region. Not only is the larynx attaining a position that for the first time can accomplish an intranarial larynx, but contiguous portions of the skull base, the de facto roof of the upper respiratory tract, also appear to be undergoing considerable remodeling.[33,36] This may be quite significant, as the shape of the basicranium has been shown both comparatively and experimentally to bear a direct relationship to the location of the larynx in the neck.[37,38] What may be beginning at this time is a remodeling and refinement of the positional anatomy of the entire upper respiratory region in order to provide the anatomic framework for the newborn upper respiratory and digestive tracts. Aspects of soft tissue structures such as the larynx, and

skeletal framework such as the skull base, are assuming both the morphology and positional relationships that will be required to sustain life postnatally.

The upper respiratory region is thus an area undergoing intense developmental activity at this time. While laryngeal and basicranial modifications are occurring during this stage of fetal life in the *upper* respiratory region, concomitant changes are also occurring in the *lower* respiratory tract. For example, the period of 23 to 25 weeks corresponds to the maturation of the pulmonary glandular epithelium.[28,39] This alveolar epithelium is responsible for the production of surfactant in the fetal lung, a substance that has been shown to be essential for independent respiratory function. The contemporaneous occurrence of the anatomic development of the fetal larynx to permit soft palate-epiglottic overlap with increasing levels of lung surfactant suggests that the timing of upper and the timing of lower respiratory tract maturation are closely related. Indeed, it appears that proper fetal maturation of the larynx may well be a major factor in determining the beginnings of respiratory independence in particular, and fetal viability overall. Understanding with increasing precision the attainment of these horizons, or factors that may alter them, can be of considerable importance in planning measures for the intervention and treatment of premature births.

Postnatal Changes in the Human Larynx

The newborn and young infant period is more accurately seen as an extension of the pattern established during the late second and early third trimester in upper respiratory and digestive tract anatomy rather than as a distinct stage. Indeed, newborns and young infants until approximately 1 1/2 to 2 years of age continue to maintain a larynx situated high in the neck (Figure 1-9C to 1-9E). The larynx corresponds to the basiocciput-C1 and extends to the superior border of C4 in newborn infants, and descends slightly to the level between C2 and C5 by about 2 years of age. As exhibited in the late fetal period, the tongue at rest is found entirely within the oral cavity, with no portion of it forming the upper anterior wall of the pharynx.

The maintenance of high laryngeal position in newborns and young infants enables the existence of largely separate respiratory and digestive pathways similar to those described in other terrestrial mammals. These essentially separate pathways prevent the mixing of most ingested food and inhaled air. These routes may also enable the baby to breathe and swallow some liquids almost simultaneously in a manner similar to that shown in nonhuman primates.[28,29,31,32,40-42] Because

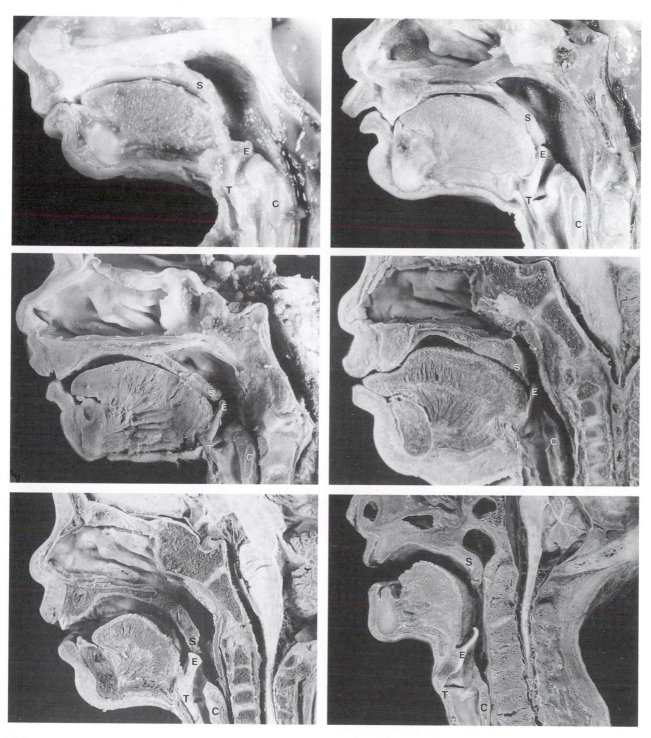

FIGURE 1-9. *Midsagittal sections through the head and neck of a developmental series of humans. (A) 15-week fetus, (B) 24-week fetus, (C) newborn, (D) 7 months, (E) 15 months, (F) adult. (C = cricoid cartilage; E = epiglottic cartilage; S = soft palate; T = thyroid cartilage.) The larynx is not fully developed at 15 weeks, and the epiglottis is not able to approximate the soft palate. By 24 weeks, the epiglottis is able to overlap the soft palate. Notice the high position of the larynx in all except the adult. (From Laitman and Reidenberg.*[49]*)*

of this high laryngeal position, newborns appear to be essentially, if not as classically believed obligatory,[43] nose breathers. As with nonhuman primates, the connection between the epiglottis and the soft palate is constant except for interruptions that may occur during the swallowing of a particularly large or dense bolus of food or liquid, during vocalization, during crying, or when disease is present. Indeed, developmental abnormalities that cause the epiglottis to be dislodged from its normal position have been shown to relate directly to concomitant feeding disorders.[44]

From a linguistic point of view, the high position of the larynx in a human newborn or young infant strongly affects the ability to modify sounds. Although high laryngeal position effectuates the dual pathway system, it severely limits the array of sounds babies produce. Many studies (eg, Laitman[45] and Lieberman[46]) have shown that the high position of the larynx greatly restricts the supralaryngeal portion of the pharynx available to modify the initial, or fundamental, sounds produced at the vocal folds. Thus, an individual with a larynx situated high in the neck, such as is found in a newborn human or monkey, would have a more restricted range of vocalizations available than would individuals with larynges placed lower in the neck. The linguistic analyses by Lieberman,[46,47] in particular, have identified the quantal vowels [i], [u], and [a] as sounds that human infants or nonhuman primates cannot produce. As these vowels are the limiting articulations of a vowel triangle that is language-universal, their absence considerably restricts an individual's speech capabilities.

While the larynx remains high in the neck until around the second year, functional changes, such as the first occasional instances of oral respiration, have been noted to occur considerably earlier, indeed within the first half year of life.[40] The period between 4 and 6 months, in particular, may represent a crucial stage in aerodigestive tract activity. At this time, neuromuscular control mechanisms of the larynx and pharynx are beginning to change even before true structural "descent" of the larynx has occurred. This changeover period may also indicate a time of potential respiratory instability owing to the transition from one respiratory pattern to another. It should be remembered that this is also a time of considerable maturational change within the central nervous system itself. The combination of nervous system maturation and developmental change in respiratory patterns may predispose the infant to a number of developmentally related problems. The occurrence of the sudden infant death syndrome (SIDS or crib death), for example, may be related to these first upper respiratory changes and to the subtle changes in laryngeal position or central and peripheral neuromotor con-

trol of the larynx.[48] The precise time of shifts that occur in breathing patterns, concomitant changes in digestive tract coordination, or the neurophysiologic mechanisms that would accompany them, remain poorly understood and warrant detailed study.

While the focus of this chapter has been on the prenatal development of the larynx, it is important to note that major maturational shifts in laryngeal position and function continue as development continues during the postnatal period.[49,50] The path of human laryngeal development is as much one of postnatal change as it is of prenatal formation and modification. Humans undergo a substantial postnatal reorganization of both laryngeal position and associated functions, dramatically more so than that found in other mammals.

The postnatal descent of the larynx into the neck is one of the most distinctive aspects of human ontogeny.[27,49,51] Whereas the purpose of the fetal period appears to be to establish those positional arrangements commensurate with the requirements of the infantile (ie, mammalian) pattern of laryngeal interlocking, the postnatal descent of the human larynx appears as a uniquely human occurrence. Permanent laryngeal descent, which seems to commence during the second year, eventually results in a larynx with a position corresponding to the level between the upper border of C3 and the lower border of C5 in a 7-year-old child, and lying opposite of the lower border of C3 and the upper part of C4 to the upper border of C7 by adulthood (Figure 1-9F).[48] This positional change of the larynx dramatically alters our patterns of breathing and swallowing, as by necessity these routes must now intersect. The permanently lowered larynx also produces an enlarged supralaryngeal aspect of the pharynx. This resultant pharyngeal expansion, in turn, allows greater modification of sounds produced at the vocal folds than that possible for infant humans or other mammals. The descent of the larynx has thus provided the anatomic ability to produce fully articulate speech.

REFERENCES

1. Zaw-Tun HA, Burdi AR. Re-examination of the origin and early development of the human larynx. *Acta Anat (Base 1)*. 1985;122:163-184.

2. Henick DH. Three-dimensional analysis of murine laryngeal development. *Ann Otol Rhinol Laryngol*. 1993;102(suppl 159):1-24.

3. Garcia-Martinez V, Alverez IS, Schoenwolf GC. Locations of the ectodermal and nonectodermal subdivisions of the epiblast at stages 3 and 4 of

avian gastrulation and neurulation. *J Exp Zool.* 1993;267:431-446.

4. Noden DM. The use of chimeras in analyses of craniofacial development. In: Le Douarin N, McLaren A, eds. *Chimeras in Developmental Biology.* London, England: Academic; 1984:241-280.

5. von Kirschhofer K, Grim M, Christ B, et al. Emergence of myogenic and endothelial cell lineages in avian embryos. *Dev Biol.* 1994;163:270-278.

6. Noden DM. Embryonic origins and assembly of blood vessels. *Am Rev Respir Dis.* 1989;140:1097-1103.

7. Noden DM. Origins and patterning of avian outflow tract endocardium. *Development.* 1991;111:867-876.

8. Noden DM. The embryonic origins of avian craniofacial muscles and associated connective tissues. *Am J Anat.* 1983;168:257-276.

9. Noden DM, Marcucio RM, Borycki A-G, Emerson CP. Differentiation of avian craniofacial muscles. I. Patterns of early regulatory gene expression and myosin heavy chain synthesis. *Dev Dynamics.* 1999;216:96-112.

10. Wahl CM, Noden DM, Baker R. Developmental relations between VIth nerve motor neurons and their targets in the chick embryo. *Dev Dynamics.* 1994;201:191-202.

11. Trainor PA, Tan S-S, Tam PPL. Cranial paraxial mesoderm: Regionalization of cell fate and impact on craniofacial development in mouse embryos. *Development.* 1994;120:2397-2408.

12. Marcucio RM, Noden DM. Myotube heterogeneity in developing chick craniofacial skeletal muscles. *Dev Dynamics.* 1999;214:178-194.

13. Noden DM. Spatial integration among cells forming the cranial peripheral nervous system. *J Neurobiol.* 1993;24:248-261.

14. Noden DM. Interactions and fates of craniofacial mesenchyme. *Development.* 1988;103:121-140.

15. Fraser SE, Bronner-Fraser M: Migrating neural crest cells in the trunk of the avian embryo are multipotent. *Development.* 1991;112:913-920.

16. Sieber-Blum M, Ito K, Richardson MK, et al. Distribution of pluripotent neural crest cells in the embryo and the role of brain-derived neurotrophic factor in the commitment to the primary sensory neuron lineage. *J Neurobiol.* 1993;24:173-184.

17. Noden DM. Patterning of avian craniofacial muscles. *Dev Biol.* 1986;116:347-356.

18. Hacker A, Guthrie S. A distinct developmental programme for the cranial paraxial mesoderm in the chick embryo. *Development.* 1998;125:3461-3472.

19. Noden DM. The role of the neural crest in patterning avian cranial skeletal, connective and muscle tissues. *Dev Biol.* 1983;96:144-165.

20. McGinnis W, Krumlauf R. Homeobox genes and axial patterning. *Cell.* 1992;68:283-302.

21. Duboule D, Morata G. Colinearity and functional hierarchy among genes of the homeotic complexes. *Trends Genet.* 1994;10:358-364.

22. Tan DP, Ferrante J, Nazarali A. Murine *HOX 1.11* homeobox gene structure and expression. *Proc Natl Acad Sci.* 1992;89:6280-6284.

23. Condie BG, Capecchi MR. Mice homozygous for a targeted disruption of *Hoxd-3* (*Hox-4.1*) exhibit anterior transformations of the first and second cervical vertebrae, the atlas and the axis. *Development.* 1993;119:579-595.

24. Gendron-Maguire M, Mallo M, Zhang M, et al. *Hoxa-2* mutant mice exhibit homeotic transformation of skeletal elements derived from cranial neural crest. *Cell.* 1993;75:1317-1331.

25. Rijii FM, Mark M, Lakkaraju S, et al. A homeotic transformation is generated in the rostral branchial region of the head by disruption of *Hox-2*, which acts as a selector gene. *Cell.* 1993;75:1331-1349.

26. Chen JC, Holinger LD. Congenital laryngeal lesions: Pathology study using serial macrosections and review of the literature. *Pediatr Res.* 1994;14:301-325.

27. Laitman JT, Reidenberg JS. Specializations of the human upper respiratory and upper digestive systems as seen through comparative and developmental anatomy. *Dysphagia.* 1993;8:318-325.

28. Crelin ES. Development of the upper respiratory system. *Ciba Clin Symp.* 1976;28(3):3-26.

29. Laitman JT. *The Ontogenetic and Phylogenetic Development of the Upper Respiratory System and Basicranium in Man.* (Ph.D. dissertation. Yale University). Ann Arbor, MI: University Microfilms; 1977.

30. Negus VE. *The Comparative Anatomy and Physiology of the Larynx.* New York, NY: Grune & Stratton; 1949.

31. Laitman JT, Crelin ES, Conlogue GJ. The function of the epiglottis in monkey and man. *Yale J Biol Med.* 1977;50:43-49.

32. German RZ, Crompton AW. Integration of swallowing and respiration in infant macaques (Macaca fascicularis). *Am J Phys Anthropol.* 1993;16(suppl):94.

33. Magriples U, Laitman JT. Developmental change in the position of the fetal human larynx. *Am J Phys Anthropol.* 1987;72:463-472.

34. Wolfson VP, Laitman JT. Ultrasound investigation of fetal human upper respiratory anatomy. *Anat Rec.* 1990;227:363-372.

35. Isaacson G, Birnholz JC. Human fetal upper respiratory tract function as revealed by ultrasonography. *Ann Otol Rhinol Laryngol.* 1991;100:743-747.

36. Moore SL, Laitman JT. A critical period in fetal human cranial base development. *Anat Rec.* 1991;229:61A.

37. Laitman JT, Heimbuch RC, Crelin ES. Developmental change in a basicranial line and its relationship to the upper respiratory system in living primates. *Am J Anat.* 1978;152:467-483.

38. Reidenberg JS, Laitman JT. Effect of basicranial flexion on larynx and hyoid position in rats: an experimental study of skull and soft tissue interactions. *Anat Rec.* 1991;220:557-569.

39. Liggins GC, Schellenberg JL. Aspects of fetal lung development. In: Jones CT, Nathanielsz PW, eds. *The Physiological Development of the Fetus and Newborn.* London, England: Academic Press; 1985:178-189.

40. Sasaki CT, Levine PA, Laitman JT, et al. Postnatal descent of the epiglottis in man: a preliminary report. *Arch Otolaryngol.* 1977;103:169-171.

41. Polgar G, Weng TR. The functional development of the respiratory system: from the period of gestation to adulthood. *Am Rev Respir Dis.* 1979;120:625-695.

42. Harding R. Function of the larynx in the fetus and newborn. *Ann Rev Physiol.* 1984;46:645-659.

43. Moss ML. The veloepiglottic sphincter and obligate nose breathing in the neonate. *J Pediatr.* 1965;67:330-331.

44. Mukai S, Mukai C, Asaoka K. Ankyloglossia with deviation of the epiglottis and larynx. *Ann Otol Rhinol Laryngol.* 1991;100:3-20.

45. Laitman JT. The evolution of the hominid upper respiratory system and implications for the origins of speech. In: de Grolier E, ed. *Glossogenetics: The Origin and Evolution of Language.* Paris, France: Harwood Academic; 1983:63-90.

46. Lieberman P. *The Biology and Evolution of Language.* Cambridge, MA: Harvard University Press; 1984.

47. Lieberman P, Laitman JT, Reidenberg JS, et al. The anatomy, physiology, acoustics and perception of speech: essential elements in analysis of the evolution of human speech. *J Hum Evol.* 1992;23:447-467.

48. Laitman JT, Crelin ES. Developmental change in the upper respiratory system of human infants. *Perinatol Neonatol.* 1980;4:15-22.

49. Laitman JT, Reidenberg JS. Comparative and developmental anatomy of laryngeal position. In: Bailey B, ed. *Head and Neck Surgery-Otolaryngology.* Philadelphia, PA: Lippincott; 1993:36-43.

50. Roche AF, Barkla DH. The level of the larynx during childhood. *Ann Otol Rhinol Laryngol.* 1965;74:645-654.

51. Laitman JT, Crelin ES. Postnatal development of the basicranium and vocal tract region in man. In: Bosma JF, ed. *Symposium on Development of the Basicranium.* Washington, DC. US Government Printing Office; 1976:206-220.

CHAPTER 2

Laryngeal Development

David H. Henick, MD

The critical stages in the prenatal development of the human larynx provide valuable insight into the anatomy and clinical malformations of the mature larynx. Earlier theories of laryngeal development espoused the concept of a tracheoesophageal septum. Observations of laryngeal development over the past decade challenge the validity of these earlier theories. Computer-generated solid-model three-dimensional reconstructions have allowed for a more precise analysis of embryologic events than the wax-model reconstructions used over the past century. Furthermore, the computer image has allowed the observer to understand complex anatomic changes over both space and time. The development of clinical laryngeal malformations presented in this chapter can be correlated with arrested stages of normal laryngeal development.

DEVELOPMENT OF THE LARYNGEOPHARYNGEAL REGION

Before discussing the history of laryngeal development, it is helpful to consider Figure 2-1, a dorsal view of the developing laryngopharyngeal region taken from a popular embryologic textbook. It provides a perspective of the developing larynx as one would view a larynx endoscopically. Imagine if the dorsal wall of the foregut were removed, and one was now viewing the epithelium of the ventral foregut floor. The limitation of this illus-tration, however, is that it provides only one perspective of laryngeal development. It fails to portray the complex anatomic changes occurring in both the sagittal and the coronal planes of the developing larynx.

As a reference point, this illustration views the level of the pharyngeal floor *(PhF)*, which is equivalent to the level of the fourth pharyngeal pouch *(4PP)*. The sagittal slit seen in the pharyngeal floor (labeled as *Laryngeal orifice*) has been interpreted by many authors as mean-ing different anatomic locations. For example, some authors believe that it represents the opening to the infraglottic region,[1] or the glottic region,[2,3] and finally, more recent observations support evidence that it rep-resents the opening to the supraglottic region.[4]

This confusion in the literature can be attributed to several factors. (1) Previous authors have labeled vari-ous anatomic sites inconsistently. (2) Wax models, which are created from postmortem human fetal histo-logic sections, have been the mainstay of our current understanding of laryngeal development. Observations that are made on these models are subject to individual interpretation. (3) Prior to the existence of the Carnegie collection, there was no centralization of the specimens and wax-model reconstructions. This has presented each subsequent scientist with the need to analyze and compare new findings and updated information from earlier studies.

FIGURE 2-1. *Development of the human larynx, as seen by unroofing the embryo to show floor of the pharyngeal cavity. (A) At 5 mm; (B) at 9 mm; (C) at 12 mm; (D) at 16 mm; (E) at 40 mm (x7); (F) sagittal hemisection, at birth (x1.5). In A-E, His[2] assumed the "ascending notch" reached the level of the pharyngeal floor, and the tracheoesophageal separation would be at the level shown. Hence, according to His, figures A-E would represent the cephalic end of the trachea. According to Zaw-Tun, figures A-E represent the entrance to the primitive laryngopharynx, which eventually becomes the supraglottis. (From Arey LB. Developmental Anatomy, 7th ed. Philadelphia, PA: WB Saunders; 1954. Used by permission.)*

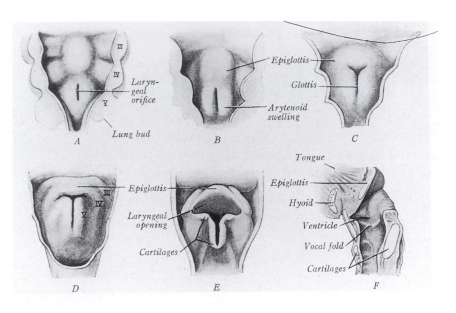

RESEARCH STUDIES

There have been several landmark studies on the origin and development of the larynx. Probably the most influential work, performed in the late 19th century, was contributed by His.[2] In his description of the developing gastrointestinal tract and pharyngeal arches, His[2] proposed that the respiratory primordium *(RP)* appears as an outpouching from the cephalic portion of the pharynx by the third week of gestation. His[2] described an ascending tracheoesophageal septum, identified as a groove behind the respiratory primordium, which would ascend to the level of the fourth pharyngeal pouch. This would divide the foregut into a ventral trachea and a dorsal esophagus. This theory implied that the distance between the fourth pharyngeal pouch, or pharyngeal floor, and the separation of the trachea and esophagus would gradually decrease over time.

Several investigators subsequently accepted His's[2] theory of an ascending tracheoesophageal septum, and added their own novel interpretations. In Figure 2-2, schematic drawings represent developmental theories of the larynx according to Kallius, Frazer, and Walander. Each author demonstrated the presence of the ascending tracheoesophageal septum (the striped line,) which separates the trachea and esophagus up to the level of the fourth pharyngeal pouch or pharyngeal floor. Although these authors agreed that the trachea and the esophagus are separated by an ascending tracheoesophageal septum, they disagreed about the site of the obliteration of the pharynx, otherwise known as the epithelial lamina *(EL).* Kallius thought it occurred above

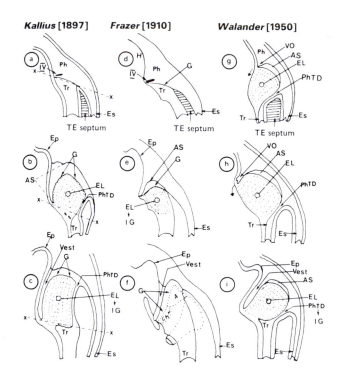

FIGURE 2-2. *Historical concepts of development of laryngeal cavity. Kallius (A-C), Frazer (D-F), and Walander (G-I) accepted concept of tracheoesophageal septum originally proposed by His, Zaw-Tun and Burdi (Figs. 2-2 to 2-6, 2-9 to 2-11 from Henick DH. Three-dimensional analysis of murine laryngeal development. In* Annals of Otology, Rhinology and Laryngology. *102:(suppl 159), 1993. Reproduced with permission.)*

the pharyngeal floor, Frazer thought it occurred below the pharyngeal floor, and Walander thought it occurred precisely at the level of the pharyngeal floor.[1,3,5]

In contrast to the foregoing hypothesis, Zaw-Tun[4] demonstrated that no such tracheoesophageal septum exists, even as a transitory structure during normal laryngeal development. To review, His demonstrated an ascending tracheoesophageal septum, which begins at the level of the respiratory primordium, dividing the foregut to form the trachea ventrally and the esophagus dorsally. This theory suggests that the distance between tracheoesophageal separation point and the level of the fourth pharyngeal pouch would decrease over time, as indicated by the stippled box.[2] Zaw-Tun, however, found that the respiratory primordium continues as a ventro-caudal outgrowth of the foregut lumen, which ultimately gives rise to the entire upper and lower respiratory system. Zaw-Tun demonstrated that the separation of the esophagus and trachea was not the result of an ascending tracheoesophageal septum, but was caused by the descending outgrowth of the respiratory primordium.

In contrast to His, Zaw-Tun found that the foregut segment which separates the original site of the respiratory primordium from the pharyngeal floor does not change over time. Zaw-Tun classified this foregut segment as the primitive laryngopharynx *(PLPh)*. The primitive laryngopharynx would eventually give rise to the supraglottic larynx.[4,6]

SCIENTIFIC ANALYSIS

The computer has enabled the scientist to analyze complex anatomic relationships as they change over space and time. A recent study[7] utilized computer-generated three-dimensional solid-model reconstructions to portray the critical stages in the development of the murine larynx. The mouse was chosen as an animal model because (1) laryngeal development is essentially uniform in all mammals, (2) the genetic analysis of murine development is well defined, and (3) embryos of a predetermined age can be easily and accurately staged. The results of this developmental study were in close correlation with the findings of Zaw-Tun and will be described in further detail.

Serial histologic sections of the laryngopharyngeal region of mice embryos were obtained from day 9 of gestation to day 18. STERECON, a computer graphics system designed to allow three-dimensional tracings of structural contours from two-dimensional images, was used to generate the three-dimensional models.[8,9] Photographic transparencies of each histologic section were then projected onto a screen that was the same size as a high-resolution computer monitor. By means of a digitizing tablet, color-coded lines were drawn on the monitor, outlining the structures of interest, for example, the epithelial lining of the foregut, foregut lumen, muscles, cartilages, and arteries. The resulting contours were stored in a database and used to form wire-frame models. Wire-frame models were then transferred to a Silicon Graphics workstation and rendered as solid, shaded reconstructions with Wavefront Technologies software. This allowed anatomic structures to be viewed in continuity, in any desired orientation, and in relation to any other given structure. In addition, internal structures could be visualized by sectioning the models in various planes.

HUMAN DEVELOPMENT

Human development is divided into an embryonic period, or the first 8 weeks of human gestation, and the subsequent fetal period.[10] The embryonic period has a total of 23 stages of development according to the Carnegie staging system. Each stage has a characteristic feature not seen in a previous stage. Laryngeal development is first seen at stage 11 (approximately 4 weeks of human gestation, and 9 days of murine gestation).

Figure 2-3 is a lateral view of a three-dimensional reconstruction of the epithelial lining of the developing laryngopharyngeal region. The first sign of the respiratory system is seen as an epithelial thickening along the ventral aspect of the foregut known as the respiratory primordium *(RP)*. The respiratory primordium is separated from the hepatic primordium *(HP)* by the septum transversum *(ST)*, a structure that will eventually develop into the central tendon of the diaphragm.

Figure 2-4 is a schematic representation of the laryngopharyngeal regions of a stage 12 embryo in comparison with the mature fetal larynx in a midsagittal plane. The respiratory diverticulum *(RD)* is a ventral outpocketing of foregut lumen that extends into the respiratory primordium. The site of origin of the respiratory diverticulum is called the primitive pharyngeal floor *(PPhF)* and eventually develops into the glottic region of the adult larynx. The cephalic portion of the respiratory diverticulum eventually develops into the infraglottic *(IG)* region of adult larynx. The primate pharyngeal floor is separated from the pharyngeal floor *(PhF)*, or the level of the fourth pharyngeal pouch *(4PP)*, by a segment of foregut originally classified by Zaw-Tun as the primitive laryngopharynx *(PLPh)*;[4,6] this will eventually become the adult supraglottic larynx.

Figure 2-4B is a ventral view of a three-dimensional reconstruction of the epithelial lining of the laryngopharyngeal region of a stage 12 embryo. The respiratory diverticulum has given rise to bilateral projections called bronchopulmonary buds *(BPB)*; these will even-

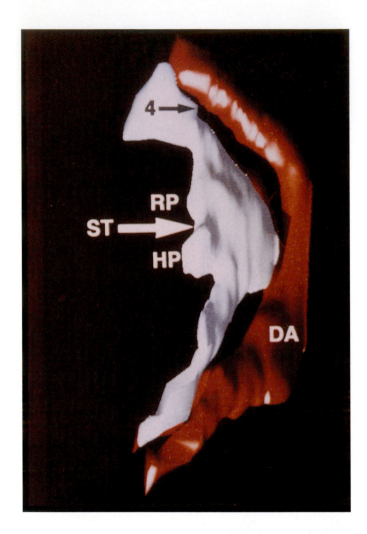

FIGURE 2-3. *Stage 11 (17-somite mouse embryo, E9.5). Lateral view of 3-D reconstruction of epithelial lining of foregut. First evidence of respiratory system is indicated by epithelial thickening along ventral aspect of foregut called respiratory primordium (RP). Respiratory primordium is separated from hepatic primordium (HP) by septum transversum (ST), which is indicated by solid white arrow. Septum transversum will eventually develop into central tendon of developing diaphragm. 4—site of developing fourth pharyngeal pouch, DA—dorsal aorta.*

FIGURE 2-4. *Stage 12 (22-somite mouse embryo, E10). (A) Schematic representation of midsagittal section through laryngopharyngeal region. Respiratory diverticulum (RD) is ventral outpocketing of foregut lumen that extends into respiratory primordium (RP). Similarly, hepatic diverticulum (HD) results from extension of foregut lumen into hepatic primordium (HP). Cephalic portion of RD will eventually develop into infraglottic region of adult larynx. Site of origin of RD is called primitive pharyngeal floor (PPhF); it will eventually develop into glottic region of adult larynx. Esophagus (Es) separates from RD at level of PPhF. Primitive pharyngeal floor is separated from fourth pharyngeal pouch (4PP) by segment of foregut called primitive laryngopharynx (PLPh). Pharyngeal floor (PhF) is at same level as 4PP. Primitive laryngopharynx will eventually develop into supraglottic region of adult larynx. Ht—heart, ST—septum transversum. (B) Ventral view of 3-D reconstruction of epithelial lining of laryngopharyngeal region. Respiratory diverticulum has given rise to bilateral projections called bronchopulmonary buds (BPB); they will eventually develop into lung parenchyma. DA—dorsal aorta, 4—fourth pharyngeal pouch.*

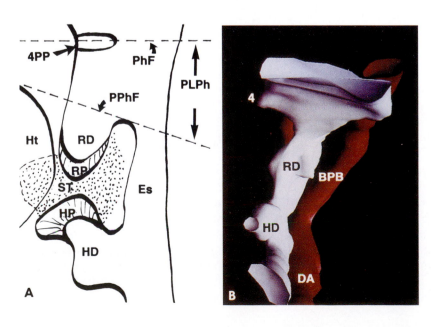

tually develop into the lower respiratory tract. The bronchopulmonary buds are tethered to the superior aspect of the septum transversum.

Dynamic changes to the developing foregut region are occurring at this and subsequent stages. For example, the heart (*Ht*) and the hepatic primordium are proliferating at a rapid rate on opposing surfaces of the septum transversum. These differential forces are exerted upon the adjacent foregut region, which leads to a dramatic lengthening of the foregut in a cephalocaudal plane. The result can be seen as the distance between the respiratory primordium and the hepatic primordium increases over time.

In stage 13 (Figure 2-5), the bronchopulmonary buds are drawn caudally and inferiorly because they are tethered to the septum transversum and the cephalic aspect of the foregut, and the respiratory diverticulum migrates superiorly. As a result, (1) two primary main-stem bronchi develop and (2) the carina is seen as a distinct region that develops from the caudal aspect of the respiratory diverticulum, and it is the site of origin of the two primary bronchi.

Figure 2-6 shows the distance between the carina and the respiratory diverticulum by two white solid arrows in a stage 14 embryo. The lengthening of this foregut segment will eventually give rise to the developing trachea.

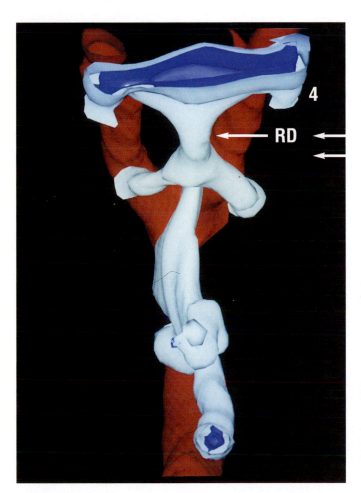

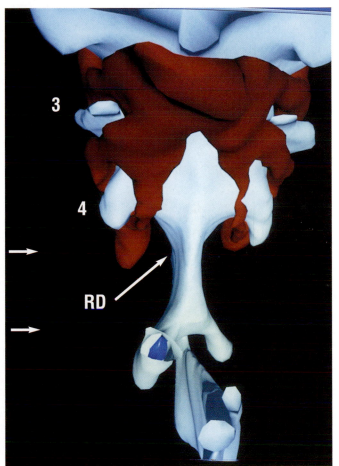

FIGURE 2-5. *Stage 13 (28-somite mouse embryo, E10.5). Ventral view of epithelial lining of foregut. Bronchopulmonary buds have continued to be drawn dorsocaudally from carina (Ca) because of cephalic rotation of embryo and because bronchopulmonary buds are tethered to septum transversum. Carina (Ca) develops from caudal aspect of respiratory diverticulum (RD). Two white solid arrows indicate distance between RD and Ca. HD—hepatic diverticulum.*

FIGURE 2-6. *Stage 14 (35-somite mouse embryo, E11). Ventral view of 3-D reconstruction of epithelial lining of laryngopharyngeal region. Compared with Figure 2-6, lengthening of Ca from RD is demonstrated with two white solid arrows. Lengthening of this foregut segment will eventually give rise, in part, to developing trachea. Carina (Ca) continues to descend from site of respiratory diverticulum (RD). Numerals 3 and 4—third and fourth pharyngeal pouches.*

At this point in development, dramatic lengthening of the trachea and esophagus occurs. Anatomically, the esophagus is in close proximity to the region of the carina. Vascular compromise to the developing esophagus may give rise to esophageal atresia, or the spectrum of tracheoesophageal anomalies seen in Figure 2-7.

Esophageal atresia in a newborn infant usually presents clinically with increased salivation requiring frequent suctioning, with the pulmonary triad of coughing, choking, and cyanosis. These symptoms are the result of saliva pooling in the blind proximal esophageal pouch with the subsequent overflow into the infant's airway. Aspiration is greater in infants who have a direct airway connection because of an associated tracheoesophageal fistula.

Tracheoesophageal fistula with a proximal esophageal pouch and distal tracheoesophageal fistula occurs in 80% to 85% of affected patients and results in gastric distention caused by air ingested with each breath. The stomach distention associated with increased gastric acid production results in respiratory symptoms caused by (1) direct tracheal aspiration of the mixture of refluxed air or gastric acid and (2) decreased diaphragmatic excursion. If the diagnosis is delayed or missed and feeding is begun, choking episodes occur, with the potential for further airway soilage.

Vascular compromise to the developing trachea at this stage of development may give rise to complete tracheal agenesis, or tracheal stenosis with complete tracheal rings (Figure 2-8). Classically, both these anomalies are associated with normal laryngeal and pulmonary development as the insult is limited to the region of the developing trachea.

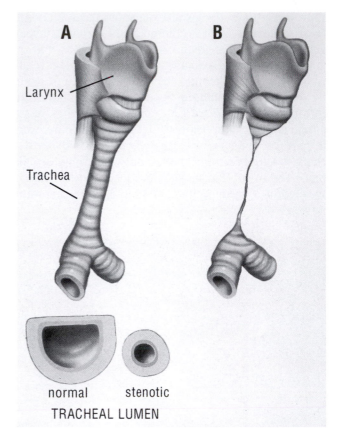

FIGURE 2-8. *Tracheal anomalies. (A) Tracheal stenosis. Axial sections demonstrate the concentric circular tracheal cartilage with the loss of the membranous trachea posteriorly. (B) Tracheal atresia. Relatively normal laryngeal and pulmonary development is seen in both of these anomalies.*

FIGURE 2-7. *Esophageal atresia and spectrum of tracheo-esophageal fistulae. (A) Esophageal atresia, proximal tracheoesophageal fistula (<1%). (B) Tracheoesophageal H-Fistula, no atresia (4%). (C) Esophageal atresia, distal tracheoesophageal fistulae (87%). (D) Esophageal atresia, proximal and distal tracheoesophageal fistulae (<1%).*

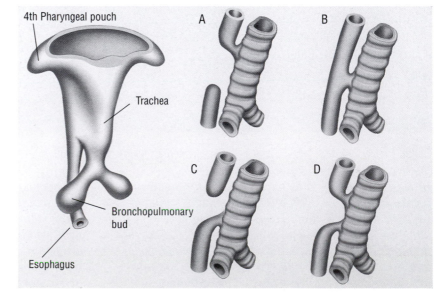

Figure 2-9 demonstrates a coronal reconstruction of a late stage 14 embryo. The infraglottis *(IG)*, which is the most cephalic portion of the respiratory diverticulum, has the characteristic shape of an upright triangle when sectioned in coronal plane; this is characteristic of the adult conus elasticus. The primitive laryngopharynx, which extends from the infraglottis to the level of the fourth pharyngeal pouch, has become compressed bilaterally along its ventral aspect, called the epithelial lamina *(EL)*. This compression is caused by forces exerted by the proliferating triangular-shaped, laryngeal meso-dermal anlage *(LMA)* and branchial arch arteries. The laryngeal mesodermal anlage eventually develops into the laryngeal cartilages and muscles. An elevation of median pharyngeal floor gives rise to the arytenoid swellings. This occurs at the same level as the fourth pharyngeal pouch. The trachea *(Tr)* is seen as the uniformly circular lumen separating the infraglottis from the carina *(Ca)*.

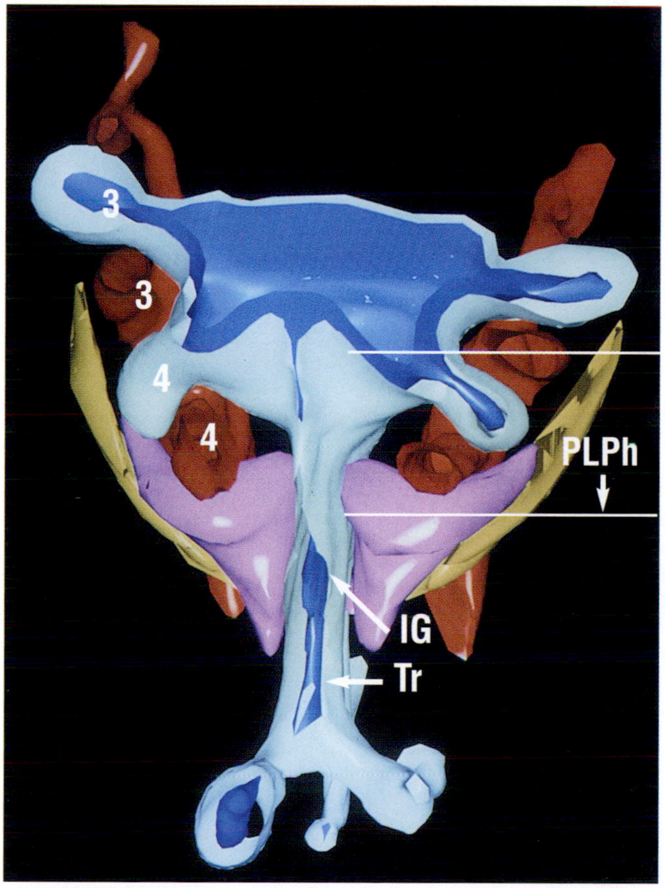

In stage 15, the epithelial lamina continues to obliterate the primitive laryngopharynx from a ventral to dorsal direction until obliteration is essentially complete by stage 16. Figure 2-10 is a lateral view of a three-dimensional reconstruction of the laryngopharyngeal region of a stage 16 embryo. A glass simulation is used to represent the epithelial lining of the foregut so that the internal changes to the lumen (blue) can be seen. The primitive laryngopharynx is seen as the segment of the foregut between the infraglottis, which was a characteristic shape of an inverted triangle when sectioned in the sagittal plane, and the arytenoid swellings (yellow). Complete obliteration of the primitive laryngopharynx is seen except for a ventral laryngeal cecum *(LC)*, and a dorsal pharyngoglottic duct *(PhGD)*. The dorsal pharyngoglottis is the last remnant of patent communication between the hypopharynx and the infraglottis.

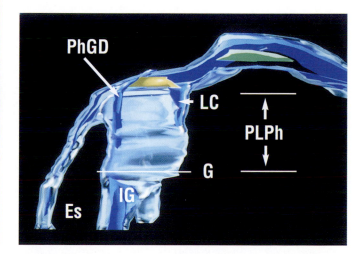

FIGURE 2-9. *Stage 14 (36-somite mouse embryo, E11.5). Coronal section of a 3-D reconstructed embryo. Region of primitive laryngopharynx (PLPh) has become compressed bilaterally, likely because of forces exerted by the (purple) laryngeal mesodermal anlage and fourth branchial artery (4, red). Infraglottis (IG) has characteristic shape of upright triangle when sectioned in this coronal plane. Infraglottis is separated from carina by ovoid-circular lumen of trachea. Also, at level of fourth pharyngeal pouch (4), elevation of median pharyngeal floor will give rise to developing arytenoid swellings.*

FIGURE 2-10. *Stage 16 (50-somite mouse embryo E12 to E12.5) Lateral view of 3-D reconstruction of foregut epithelial lining. Glass simulation was used so that internal (blue) luminal anatomy could be visualized. Primitive laryngopharynx (PLPh) extends from floor of pharynx (level of AS; yellow) to infraglottic region below (IG; previously cephalic end of respiratory diverticulum). Glottis (G) is just cephalic to IG. Primitive laryngopharynx is completely obliterated except for narrow pharyngoglottic duct (PhGD) dorsally and developing laryngeal cecum (LC) ventrally.*

The laryngeal cecum originates as a triangular-shaped lumen along the ventral aspect of the arytenoid swellings and progresses caudally along the ventral aspect of the primitive laryngopharynx until it reaches the level of the glottis in stage 18 (Figure 2-11). In stage 19, the epithelial lamina begins to recanalize from a dorsocephalad to a ventrocaudal direction. In the process, communication is reestablished between the ventral laryngeal cecum and the dorsal pharyngoglottis. The last portion of the primitive laryngopharynx to recanalize is at the glottic level, as indicated by the white broken line in Figure 2-12. It is the incomplete recanalization of the epithelial lamina that can give rise to the full spectrum of supraglottic and glottic atresias seen clinically. In stage 21, the laryngeal cecum gives rise bilaterally to the laryngeal ventricles.

Figure 2-13 is a schematic representation of a stage 18 embryo prior to the recanalization of the epithelial lamina. Complete failure of the epithelial lamina to recanalize would give rise to a type 1 atresia (Figure 2-13D). Complete recanalization of the epithelial lamina except at the glottic level would give rise to a type 3 atresia, or a glottic web (Figure 2-13F). Partial recanalization of the epithelial lamina would give rise to a type 2 atresia (Figure 2-13E). In types 1 and 2 atresia, there is an associated subglottic stenosis as the insult in development occurred at an earlier point in development, preventing the complete development of the infraglottic region. In addition, there are no signs of laryngeal ventricles, as this is one of the last structures to normally develop.

Development of the laryngeal cartilages and muscles is first seen in a stage 14 embryo, seen initially as the triangular-shaped laryngeal mesodermal anlage adjacent to the primitive laryngopharynx (Figure 2-9). Eventually, the laryngeal mesodermal anlage consolidates into two distinct regions, a hyoid and a thyrocricoid anlage. Fusion of the laryngeal mesodermal anlage occurs dorsally in the cricoid region by stage 18. Chondrification begins along the ventral aspect of the cricoid in stage 17 and progresses dorsally until fusion

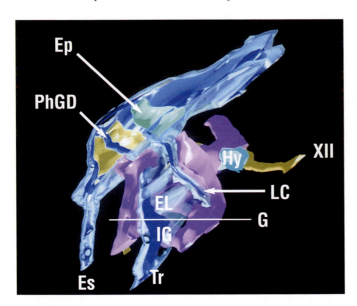

FIGURE 2-11. *Stages 17 and 18 (62-somite mouse embryo, E14). Lateral view of 3-D reconstruction of foregut epithelial lining of laryngopharyngeal region with its surrounding laryngeal mesodermal anlagen (purple). Glass simulation was used to enhance visualization of internal luminal anatomy (blue). Compared to Figure 2-10 (stage 16), primitive laryngopharynx is still obliterated except for pharyngoglottic duct (PhGD) dorsally and laryngeal cecum (LC) ventrally, which has, at this stage, descended to glottic (G) region (white line). Eventually, recanalization of epithelial lamina (EL) will bring dorsal PhGD into communication with ventral LC to give rise to laryngeal vestibule, or supraglottic larynx. Ep—epiglottis anlage, Hy—hyoid anlage, XII—12th cranial nerve, Tr—trachea, Es—esophagus.*

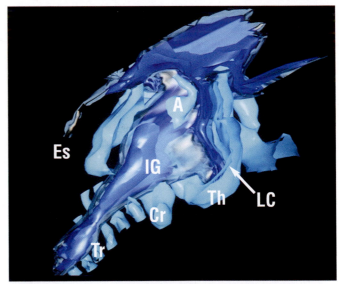

FIGURE 2-12. *Stages 19 through 23 (E16 mouse embryo). 3-D reconstruction of laryngopharyngeal region, sectioned in midsagittal plane exposing right medial aspect of embryo. Glass simulation is used to view luminal (dark blue) anatomy. White broken lines indicate area in which epithelial lamina has not completely recanalized. It has been suggested that incomplete recanalization of epithelial lamina can give rise to full spectrum of supraglottic stenosis and glottic webs seen clinically. Es—esophagus, A—arytenoid cartilage, Th—thyroid cartilage, Cr—cricoid cartilage, Tr—trachea, IG—infraglottis, LC—laryngeal cecum.*

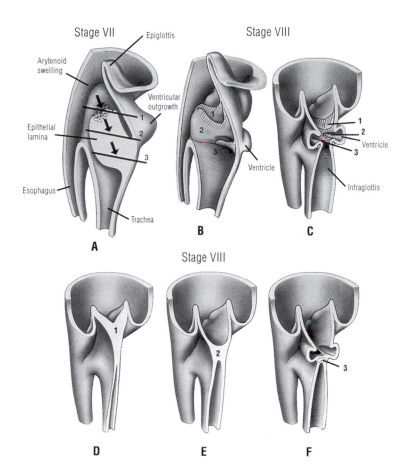

FIGURE 2-13. *Stage 18 embryo prior to the recanalization of the epithelial lamina. (A-C) Normal development. (D) Type I atresia results in a complete supraglottic stenosis. (E) Type II atresia results in partial supraglottic stenosis. Communication between supraglottis and infraglottis is usually maintained through a patent pharyngoglottic duct. (F) Type III atresia corresponds to formation of a glottic web.*

occurs along the posterior cricoid lamina by stage 20. It is the incomplete fusion dorsally of the laryngeal mesodermal anlage or the chondrification process that can give rise to the full spectrum of laryngotracheal clefts seen clinically.

Four types of clefts have been described in a classification system proposed by Benjamin[11]: type 1, interarytenoid area; type 2, partial cricoid; type 3, total cricoid: remains above the thoracic inlet; type 4, laryngotracheoesophageal cleft. Chapter 21 will review these anomalies in greater detail.

REFERENCES

1. Frazer JE. The development of the larynx. *J Anat Physiol.* 1910;44:156-191.

2. His W. Anatomic Menschlicher Embryonen. III: Zur Geschichte der Organe. Leipzig: Vogel; 1885:12-19.

3. Kallius E. Beitrage zur Entwicklungsgeschichte des Kehlkopfes. *Anat Hefte Wiesbadan.* 1897;9:303-363.

4. Zaw-Tun HA. The tracheo-esophageal septum—Fact or fantasy? Origin and development of the respiratory primordium and esophagus. *Acta Anat (Basel).* 1982;114:1-21.

5. Walander A. Prenatal development of the epithelial primordium of the larynx in the rat. *Acta Anat (Basel).* 1950;10(suppl 13).

6. Zaw-Tun HA, Burdi AR. Re-examination of the origin and early development of the human larynx. *Acta Anat (Basel).* 1985;122:163-184.

7. Henick DH. Three-dimensional analysis of murine laryngeal development. *Ann Otol Rhinol Laryngol.* 1993;102(suppl 159):1-24.

8. Marko M, Leith A, Parsons D. 3-Dimensional reconstructions of cells from serial sections and whole cell mounts using multi-level contouring of stereomicrographs. *J Electron Microsc Tech.* 1988;9:395-411.

9. Leith A, Marko M, Parsons D. Computer graphics for cellular reconstructions. *IEEE Comput Graphics Applicat.* 1989;9:16-23.

10. O'Rahilly R, Muller F. Respiratory and alimentary relations in staged human embryos. New embryological data and congenital anomalies. *Ann Otol Rhinol Laryngol.* 1984;93:421-429.

11. Benjamin B, Inglis A. Minor congenital laryngeal clefts: Diagnosis and classification. *Ann Otol Rhinol Laryngol.* 1989;98:417-420.

CHAPTER 3

Anatomy of the Human Larynx

Clarence T. Sasaki, MD

Young-Ho Kim, MD, PhD

The human larynx functions as a complex sphincter that directs both airflow and bolus transport at the junction of the digestive and lower respiratory tracts. The larynx has evolved to fulfill three obligations.[1] First, the larynx protects the airway during swallowing. Second, the phasic contraction and relaxation of laryngeal muscles during inspiration and expiration modulate airflow to the lungs. Last, the larynx plays a central role in phonation. Laryngeal anatomy reflects the specialization required by these multiple roles.

INTRODUCTION

Conceptually, the larynx consists of a cartilaginous, bony, and membranous framework, over which a mucosal lining is draped.[2] The laryngeal muscles control the relative positions of individual components of the framework during the various laryngeal actions of swallowing, respiration, and phonation.

Laryngeal Framework

The thyroid, the cricoid, the epiglottic, and the paired arytenoid cartilages constitute the major framework of the larynx (Figures 3-1 through 3-3). The corniculate and cuneiform cartilages, which are also both paired structures, are of considerably less importance. The quadrangular and the triangular membranes are connected to the laryngeal cartilages and comprise the underlying structure for the vocal folds.

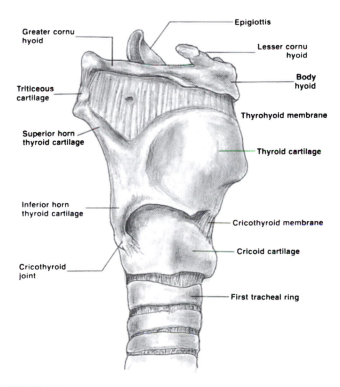

FIGURE 3-1. *Laryngeal framework, lateral view.*

Hyoid Bone

Because the hyoglossus, geniohyoid, and mylohyoid muscles attach to the hyoid bone, this bone has been

27

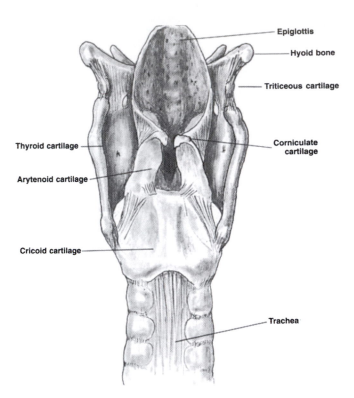

FIGURE 3-2. *Laryngeal framework, posterior view.*

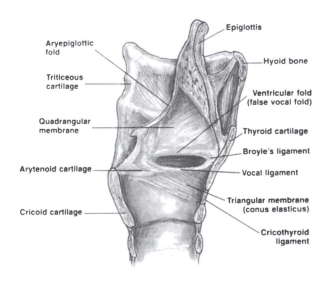

FIGURE 3-3. *Laryngeal framework, sagittal section.*

called a lingual bone. Nonetheless, the hyoid serves as an important place of attachment for the larynx; consequently, this bone also can be considered to be a part of the larynx. The hyoid bone is a U-shaped bone that consists of a body centrally and the greater and lesser cornua laterally (Figure 3-1). On each side, the greater cornu is inferior to the lesser cornu. The thyrohyoid membrane connects the thyroid cartilage with the hyoid bone.

The hyoid bone is only partially ossified at birth. Its ossification is usually complete by the age of 2 years.

Thyroid Cartilage

The thyroid cartilage consists of two pentagonal plates, or laminae, that meet anteriorly in the midline. The angle between the plates in the male larynx is 90°, while in the female larynx, this angle is 120°. This angle is more prominent in men than women and is colloquially known as the Adam's apple. The overall shape and positioning of the laminae also differ between men and women; that is, the thyroid cartilage assumes a funnel-type configuration in the male larynx, while the female thyroid cartilage has a more cylindrical shape. Anteriorly, the superior edges of the laminae meet to form the V-shaped thyroid notch. Extending superiorly and inferiorly from the posterior edge of the laminae are the superior and inferior horns. The lateral thyrohyoid ligament connects the superior horn to the hyoid bone. The inferior horn articulates with the cricoid cartilage in the cricothyroid joint, a true synovial joint.

The thyroid cartilage is composed of hyaline-type cartilage, which can undergo calcification and even ossification with aging.[3,4] In general, this ossification, which commences at approximately 20 years of age, starts in the posterior laminae and the inferior horns. The central portions of the laminae tend not to undergo these changes, and usually remain relatively radiolucent until well into old age. These changes occur earlier in men, and the extent of the changes is also greater in men. Because the ossified cartilage is radiodense, these areas can be mistaken for intraluminal foreign bodies on plain radiographs.

The thyroid cartilage is covered by a thick perichondrium on its external surfaces, and its perichondrium is thinner on its internal surface. A small prominence on the internal surface lacks a perichondrial cover; this area corresponds to the attachment point for the anterior commissure of the vocal folds.

Cricoid Cartilage

The cricoid cartilage is classically described as a signet ring, with a thin anterior arch and a broader posterior lamina about 20-30 mm in height (Figures 3-1 and 3-2). The cricothyroid membrane connects the thyroid and cricoid cartilages anteriorly. In the midline, this membrane is thickened and forms the cricothyroid ligament. The inferior cornua of the thyroid cartilage articulate posterolaterally with the cricoid cartilage. The inferior edge of the cricoid cartilage is firmly attached to the first tracheal ring. Along the superior aspect of the cricoid lamina, facets for the articulation with the arytenoid cartilages are present.

Like the thyroid cartilage, the cricoid cartilage is composed of hyaline cartilage. The cricoid ossifies first posteriorly in the cricoid lamina, and the cricoid arch undergoes these changes later as the process sweeps anteriorly. Ossification of the cricoid cartilage starts slightly after this process begins in the thyroid cartilage. Similar in appearance to ossified thyroid cartilage, these radiodense areas can mimic intraluminal foreign bodies on soft tissue radiographs.[3,4]

Epiglottic Cartilage

The epiglottic cartilage is shaped as a leaf and defines the anterior border of the laryngeal inlet (Figures 3-2 and 3-3). Its anterior surface projects above the thyroid cartilage and faces the base of tongue and lingual tonsils. The epiglottic cartilage's inferior portion is considerably narrower than its broader, rounder superior part. The petiole, or the stem-like inferior extension of the epiglottic cartilage, is connected to the thyroid cartilage just below the thyroid notch by the thyroepiglottic ligament. The hyoepiglottic ligament runs from the lingual surface of the epiglottic cartilage to the posterior surface of the hyoid. Along the inferior aspect of the laryngeal surface of the petiole, the epiglottic tubercle partially overhangs the anterior commissure.

This cartilage consists of fibroelastic cartilage and does not calcify or ossify. It is considerably thinner than the cricoid and thyroid cartilages. The epiglottic perichondrium is more tightly bound to the underlying cartilage on the laryngeal surface of the epiglottis than on its lingual surface. Consequently, acute inflammatory processes often produce more marked mucosal edema on the lingual surface of the epiglottis, rather than on its laryngeal surface. This distribution of edema results in posterior displacement of the epiglottis into the laryngeal airway during acute epiglottitis. Mucous glands extend into tiny indentations within the cartilage on both surfaces, although more glands are present on the laryngeal surface.

Arytenoid Cartilages

The arytenoid cartilages are paired pyramidal-shaped cartilages that rest upon the superior edge of the cricoid lamina (Figures 3-2 and 3-3). Each arytenoid consists of two processes, an apex and a base. The vocal ligament attaches to the vocal process, and the intrinsic laryngeal muscles insert upon the muscular process and elsewhere. The base has a concave contour, and it articulates with the cricoid cartilage in a synovial joint. The motion of this joint is very complex and involves more than just simple rotation of the arytenoid around its vertical axis.

The apices of these cartilages and the vocal process are composed of elastic cartilage, while the remainder is mainly hyaline cartilage. The arytenoid cartilages also ossify, beginning at approximately age 30 years.[3,4]

Minor Cartilages

The corniculate cartilages, also known as the cartilages of Santorini, are located just above the arytenoid apices (Figure 3-2). They consist of fibroelastic cartilage. The cuneiform cartilages, also known as the cartilages of Wrisberg, are found within the superior aspect of the aryepiglottic folds, just lateral to the corniculate cartilages. Even though the cuneiform cartilages are composed of hyaline cartilage, they do not appear to ossify.[3,4] These cartilages provide rigidity to the aryepiglottic folds (described below), which function as ramparts that guide the food bolus away from the laryngeal inlet posterolaterally toward the piriform sinuses.

The triticeal cartilages are embedded in the lateral thyrohyoid ligaments. These cartilages are composed of hyaline cartilage, and they also may be absent in the human larynx. The triticeal cartilages commonly calcify and should not be mistaken for a foreign body on cervical radiographs.[3,4] The adjacent lateral thyrohyoid ligaments also ossify, but less frequently.

Thyrohyoid Membrane

The thyrohyoid membrane connects the posterosuperior edge of the hyoid bone and the superior edge of the thyroid cartilage (Figure 3-1). It is thickened medially and laterally, giving rise to the medial thyrohyoid ligament and the paired lateral thyrohyoid ligaments. Posterior to the lateral thyrohyoid ligaments, the internal branch of the superior laryngeal nerve and vessels pierce the thyrohyoid membrane to enter the larynx.

Quadrangular Membrane

On each side of the larynx, the quadrangular membrane extends from the lateral edge of the epiglottis to arytenoid cartilage posteriorly (Figure 3-3). The superior border of each quadrangular membrane is a free edge that extends posterioinferiorly from the epiglottis to the corniculate cartilages. The aryepiglottic fold corresponds to this free border. Each quadrangular membrane's inferior edge is also free; it extends from the inferior epiglottis to the vocal process of the arytenoid. This portion of the quadrangular membrane corresponds to the false vocal folds, also known as the ventricular or vestibular folds. Because of this arrangement, the anterior vertical height of this membrane is considerably greater than its corresponding posterior vertical dimension. The superior and inferior edges of this membrane are thickened, giving rise to the aryepiglottic ligament and the vestibular ligament, respectively.

Triangular Membrane

The triangular membrane is a paired fibroelastic structure (Figure 3-3). Its inferior edge is firmly attached to the cricoid cartilage. Its base is located anteriorly, at attachments to both the cricoid and thyroid cartilages. Each triangular membrane's apex inserts upon the vocal process of the arytenoid cartilage. The free superior edge of this membrane is thickened and forms the vocal ligament. The attachment of the vocal ligament to the thyroid cartilage is known as Broyle's ligament. Both triangular membranes together constitute the conus elasticus. Anteriorly, the thick part of the anterior conus elasticus forms the cricothyroid ligament.

LARYNGEAL MUCOSA

The laryngeal mucosa is draped over the laryngeal skeleton. The resulting relationships are best appreciated in a coronal section of the larynx (Figure 3-4). Following the internal contour of the larynx in a superior to inferior direction, the mucosa lines the thyrohyoid membrane and a portion of the thyroid cartilage. The mucosa then extends superiorly covering the lateral aspect of the quadrangular membrane. The space between the quadrangular membrane and thyroid cartilage is the piriform sinus or recess, which has a pear shape. The lining comes over the superior edge of the quadrangular membrane, creating the aryepiglottic fold, and descends along the medial aspect of this membrane, creating the false vocal fold. That portion of the airway that is located between the aryepiglottic folds is known as the laryngeal vestibule. The mucosa then proceeds laterally forming a pouch, known as the laryngeal ventricle, or the ventricle of Morgagni. The superior aspect of the ventricle is called the laryngeal saccule, or the saccule of Hilton. Along the floor of the ventricle, the mucosa continues medially to the triangular membrane and vocal ligament. The mucosa covers the vocal ligament and the inferior aspect of the triangular membrane, and is continuous with the tracheal mucosa.

The mucosa is also reflected over the lingual surface of the epiglottis. This arrangement creates two pouches between the base of the tongue and the epiglottis. These valleculae are bounded laterally by the glossoepiglottic folds. The median glossoepiglottic fold corresponds to the hyoepiglottic ligament and separates the two valleculae.

Both pseudostratified ciliated columnar epithelium (also known as respiratory epithelium) and stratified squamous epithelium comprise the laryngeal mucosa. Stratified squamous epithelium covers the piriform sinus, the lingual surface of the epiglottis, the superior half of the laryngeal surface of the epiglottis, the supe-

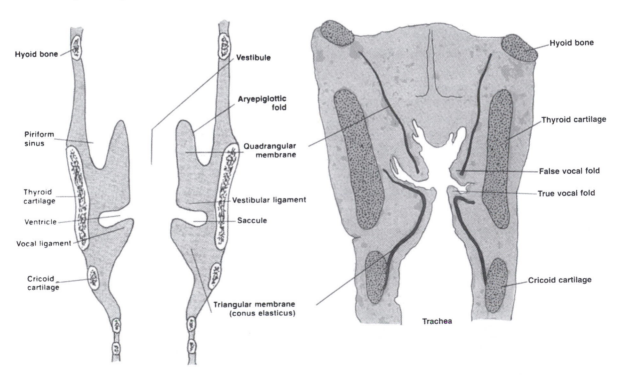

FIGURE 3-4. *Human larynx, coronal view.*

rior surface of the false vocal folds, true vocal folds, and the undersurface of the true vocal folds. Respiratory epithelium lines the subglottic area, the laryngeal ventricle, the laryngeal vestibule, and the inferior half of the laryngeal surface of the epiglottis. Mucus-secreting goblet cells are found within this respiratory epithelium and are prominent within the mucosa of the false vocal folds. Beneath the respiratory epithelium, numerous seromucous tubuloalveolar glands are present, especially in the medial part of the aryepiglottic fold, the laryngeal saccule, and the posterior surface of the epiglottis. These glands and goblet cells help lubricate the surface of the larynx; such secretions are essential for normal laryngeal function, particularly vocal fold vibration. In addition, lysozyme and other antibacterial proteins and glycoproteins in the secretions of these glands and goblet cells serve to protect the larynx against bacterial infections. Inflammatory cells are also located within the stroma deep to the epithelium. These cells may be organized into germinal centers. The squamous epithelium is nonkeratinizing, although it may keratinize in certain pathologic conditions. Furthermore, the respiratory epithelium may undergo metaplastic changes with chronic irritation and become a keratinizing or nonkeratinizing stratified squamous epithelium.

This arrangement of the true vocal folds inferiorly and the ventricular folds superiorly enhances the ability of the larynx to act as a valve for airflow into and from the lungs. In the absence of active muscular contraction, the adducted true vocal folds block the flow of air into the lungs at a pressure head greater than 140 mm Hg.[1] Yet, they offer minimal resistance to flow in the opposite direction. Thus, it is essential that the glottis be actively opened for airflow to pass through the larynx and into the lung during each inspiration. Similarly, the ventricular folds passively resist egress of air at subglottic pressure of up to 30 mm Hg, but they do not significantly impede the entry of air into the lungs. It is believed that the ventricular folds are involved in the production of an adequate cough.

LARYNGEAL MUSCLES

The laryngeal muscles can be divided into three groups: intrinsic, extrinsic, and accessory. The intrinsic muscles directly act upon the arytenoids. The only extrinsic muscle is the cricothyroid muscle. The accessory muscles either elevate or depress the larynx.

Other classifications of the laryngeal muscles have been proposed. A common alternative approach places the cricothyroid muscle with the intrinsic muscles and considers all the remaining elevators and depressors of the larynx as extrinsic laryngeal muscles.

This discussion will describe intrinsic, extrinsic, and accessory laryngeal muscles, as outlined above.

Intrinsic Muscles

The articulation between the cricoid and arytenoid cartilages is a complex one, involving a sliding of the arytenoid across the cricoid cartilage, not just a rotation of the arytenoid about its vertical axis. This motion reflects the saddle-shaped contour of each surface of the cricoarytenoid joint. During adduction of the vocal processes of the arytenoid cartilages, each vocal process moves medially, inferiorly, and posteriorly, while during abduction, each vocal process moves laterally, superiorly, and posteriorly.[5] This pattern of movement occurs as each arytenoid cartilage rocks around the long axis of the cricoarytenoid joint facets. Discussion of the intrinsic muscles of the larynx often oversimplifies this joint in two ways. First, the joint is assumed to purely permit rotation of the arytenoid on the cricoid. Second, each intrinsic laryngeal muscle is assumed to act alone. In reality, arytenoid movement is the composite of all the actions of the intrinsic muscles acting together. Nonetheless, consideration of the actions of the intrinsic muscles is traditionally facilitated by making these two assumptions.

The intrinsic laryngeal muscles consist of the muscles of the quadrangular membrane and the muscles of the arytenoid cartilage.[2] The first group includes the thyroepiglottic, thyroarytenoid, and aryepiglottic muscles (Figure 3-5). The second set is composed of the interarytenoid, posterior cricoarytenoid, and lateral cricoarytenoid muscles (Figures 3-5 through 3-7).

The muscles of the quadrangular membranes consist of a nearly continuous sheet of muscles that originate from the posterior midportion of the thyroid cartilage. The thyroarytenoid muscle is made up of both horizontal and more vertically oriented fibers. The thyroarytenoid muscle inserts upon the vocal process of the arytenoid. Its deep portion constitutes the vocalis muscle. The aryepiglottic muscles run along each quadrangular membrane parallel to its free edge from the epiglottis to the arytenoid cartilages. These muscles extend posteriorly and are at least partially continuous with the oblique arytenoid muscles.

The origins of the posterior and lateral cricoarytenoid muscles are the posterior and lateral aspects of the cricoid cartilage, respectively. The posterior cricoarytenoid muscle inserts upon the posteromedial surface of the muscular process of the arytenoid cartilage, while the lateral cricoarytenoid muscle inserts upon the anterolateral surface of the muscular process of the arytenoid cartilage. The interarytenoid muscle, also known as the transverse arytenoid muscle, con-

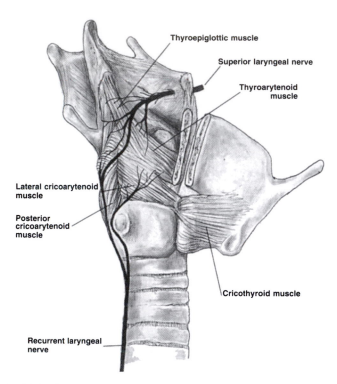

FIGURE 3-5. *Laryngeal intrinsic muscles, lateral view. Innervation is also depicted.*

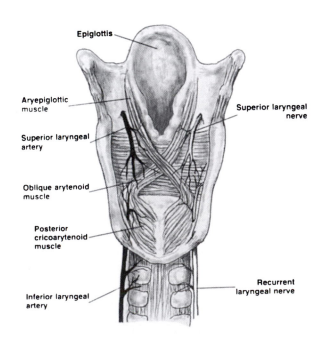

FIGURE 3-6. *Laryngeal intrinsic muscles, posterior view. Innervation and blood supply are also depicted.*

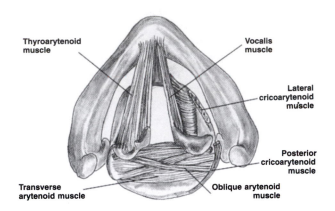

FIGURE 3-7. *Laryngeal intrinsic muscles, arytenoid group, superior view.*

nects the posterior parts of the arytenoid cartilages. The oblique arytenoid muscles run superficially across the interarytenoid muscles and the arytenoid cartilages. Each oblique arytenoid muscle diagonally crosses its contralateral counterpart.

The intrinsic laryngeal muscles are not merely abductors and adductors of the vocal folds. While vocal fold abduction and adduction are essential functions of these muscles, the intrinsic laryngeal muscles also determine the vibratory characteristics (ie, tension, mass per unit length) and cross-sectional contour of the vocal folds. The primary abductors of the vocal folds are the posterior cricoarytenoid muscles, which rotate the vocal process of the arytenoid laterally by pulling its muscular process medially (Figure 3-8A). Contraction of the posterior cricoarytenoid muscles expands the glottis in the horizontal dimension during forced inspiratory efforts. The posterior cricoarytenoid muscles lengthen and stiffen the vocal folds. As this happens, the vocal folds become thinner and their edges become rounder. These muscles are found to contain three distinct neuromuscular compartments: vertical, oblique, and horizontal bellies. The vertical and oblique bellies rock the arytenoid backwards while sliding it laterally, thus causing a maximal dilation of the airway. The horizontal belly causes a swiveling motion of the arytenoid. It is proposed that the vertical and oblique bellies normally cause vocal fold abduction during respiration, while the horizontal belly primarily is used to adjust the position of the vocal process during phonation.[6,7] The lateral cricoarytenoid muscles draw the muscular processes of the arytenoid cartilages laterally, thereby adducting the vocal folds and narrowing the glottic opening (Figure 3-8B). This movement of the arytenoid cartilages lowers the position of the vocal folds. The lateral cricoarytenoid muscles also thin the free edge of each vocal fold by increasing its length. The interarytenoid and oblique arytenoid muscles directly pull the arytenoid cartilages together, also adducting the vocal folds (Figure 3-8C). Because of the complexity of the cricoarytenoid joint, these muscles act primarily to stabilize the arytenoid cartilages on the cricoid cartilage during vocal fold adduction. The interarytenoid and oblique arytenoid muscles do not alter the vibratory characteristics of the vocal folds significantly.

The thyroarytenoid muscles are adductors of the vocal folds (Figure 3-8D). These muscles also shorten and tense the true vocal folds. In addition, contraction and relaxation of the vocalis muscles change the vibratory characteristics of the vocal folds by altering their mass and the tension of the vocal ligament. The vocalis muscles act to shorten and thicken the vocal folds. The aryepiglottic muscles help close the laryngeal inlet by folding the epiglottis posteriorly.

The intrinsic laryngeal muscles function to shut the larynx at three levels. Most inferiorly, forced adduction of the vocal folds by contraction of the thyroarytenoid, lateral cricothyroid, interarytenoid, and oblique arytenoid muscles closes the glottis tightly. Medial rotation of the vocal processes of the arytenoid cartilages also tightly closes the false vocal folds. Most superiorly, the epiglottis is drawn posteriorly by the aryepiglottic muscles. These three tiers of closure represent a most effective mechanism of protection of the airway against aspiration.[1]

Extrinsic Muscles

The only extrinsic muscles of the larynx are the paired cricothyroid muscles. These muscles, which are located on the exterior surface of the larynx, each consist of two parts. Their anterior portion arises from the superior edge of the cricoid arch and inserts upon the posterolateral border of the thyroid cartilage, while the oblique portion extends from the lateral surface of the cricoid cartilage to the inferior edge of the thyroid cartilage. In canine cricothyroid muscles, three distinct muscle bellies (rectus, oblique, and horizontal) have been identified, each separated by distinct connective tissue planes. Differences in their electrical activity patterns suggest these three bellies probably play separate roles in the complex function of this muscle.[8]

The cricothyroid muscle tilts the larynx by approximating the cricoid and thyroid anteriorly utilizing the cricothyroid joint (Figure 3-8E). By doing so, the cricothyroid muscle lengthens the vocal fold by up to one-third of its original length and lowers the relative position of the vocal fold within the larynx. This action effectively expands the glottis in its anteroposterior dimension during expiration and inspiration. The cricothyroid muscle also is a weak adductor of the true vocal folds. At the

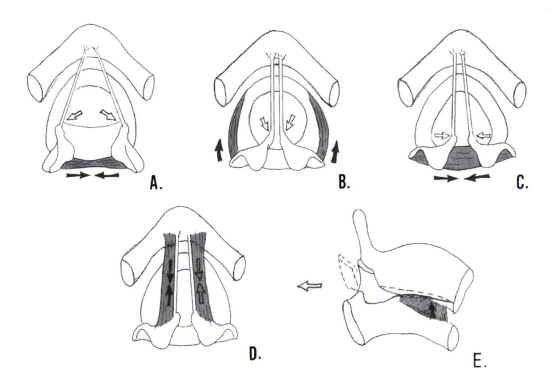

FIGURE 3-8. *Actions of the intrinsic and extrinsic laryngeal muscles. (A to D) Superior view; (E) lateral view.*

same time, contraction of the cricothyroid muscle augments the tension of the vocal fold while decreasing its mass per unit length during pitch elevation. Because the cricothyroid muscle stretches the vocal fold, this muscle thins the vocal fold and sharpens its edge. These characteristic changes produced by the cricothyroid muscles in the vocal folds indicate that the cricothyroid muscles are an important determinant of the pitch of the acoustic signal of the vibrating vocal folds.

Accessory Muscles

The accessory muscles can be divided into elevator and depressor groups (Figure 3-9). The first group includes the digastric (both bellies), the stylohyoid, the geniohyoid, and the mylohyoid muscles, all of which act to pull the larynx superiorly. Additionally, contraction of the hyoglossus muscle elevates the larynx if the remainder of the tongue musculature remains fixed. The anterior belly of the digastric, the geniohyoid, and the mylohyoid muscles also move the larynx under the base of tongue, an important maneuver in the prevention of aspiration during deglutition. Such action plays a vital role in deglutition by expanding the hypopharynx and thus easing the passage of the bolus inferiorly. This movement also serves to protect the airway against aspiration as the anterosuperior displacement of the tongue pulls the laryngohyoid complex away from the bolus path. The depressor muscles include the sternohyoid, sternothyroid, and omohyoid muscles, which all pull the larynx inferiorly. The thyrohyoid muscle pulls the hyoid bone and thyroid cartilage together.

The pharyngeal constrictor muscles are also closely related to the larynx. The middle and inferior constrictor muscles insert upon the greater cornua of the hyoid and the thyroid lamina, respectively. Their contraction draws the larynx posterosuperiorly. The cricopharyngeus muscle, located inferior to the inferior constrictors, arises from the cricoid cartilage and encircles the esophageal inlet. This muscle functions as an upper esophageal sphincter by maintaining a tonic state of contraction. During swallowing, the constrictor muscles propel the bolus into the esophagus, while the cricopharyngeus muscle relaxes as the bolus enters the esophagus.

LARYNGEAL INNERVATION

The main somatic innervation to the larynx is from the vagus nerve through the superior and recurrent laryngeal nerves (Figure 3-10). The superior laryngeal nerve passes between the external and internal carotid arteries at about the level of the crossing of the hypoglossal nerve. This nerve then travels inferiorly to the tip of the hyoid, where it divides into external and internal branches. The external branch descends with superior thyroid vessels on the surface of the inferior

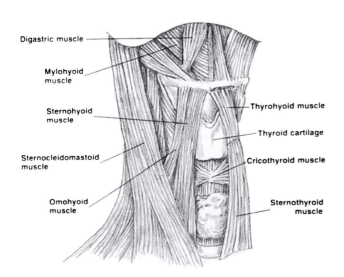

FIGURE 3-9. *Laryngeal accessory muscles, anterior view.*

Digastric muscle

Mylohyoid muscle

Sternohyoid muscle

Sternocleidomastoid muscle

Omohyoid muscle

Thyrohyoid muscle

Thyroid cartilage

Cricothyroid muscle

Sternothyroid muscle

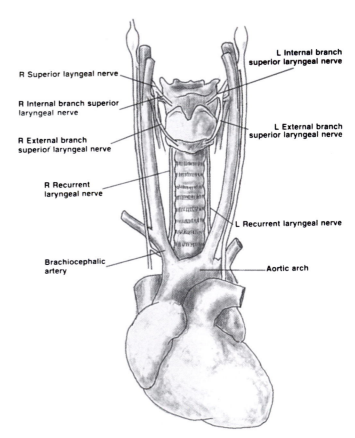

FIGURE 3-10. *Paths of the recurrent and superior laryngeal nerves.*

R Superior layngeal nerve

R Internal branch superior laryngeal nerve

R External branch superior laryngeal nerve

R Recurrent laryngeal nerve

Brachiocephalic artery

L Internal branch superior laryngeal nerve

L External branch superior laryngeal nerve

L Recurrent laryngeal nerve

Aortic arch

constrictor muscle. The internal branch pierces the thyrohyoid membrane to enter the interior larynx. The recurrent laryngeal nerves, also known as the inferior laryngeal nerves, take a longer route to the larynx. On the right side, the recurrent laryngeal nerve branches from the vagus at the subclavian artery. This recurrent laryngeal nerve then loops around the subclavian artery and proceeds superiorly in the tracheoesophageal groove to enter the larynx between the cricopharyngeus and the esophagus. On the left side, the route of the recurrent laryngeal nerve is similar, except that the nerve passes around the aortic arch distal to the ligamentum arteriosum.

The course of the recurrent laryngeal nerve reflects the embryologic branchial arch system, whose further development and partial involution influence the positioning of the recurrent laryngeal nerve. In a small percentage of individuals, the right inferior laryngeal nerve does not pass around the subclavian artery.[9] This nonrecurrent laryngeal nerve descends directly to the larynx. Invariably associated with this anomaly is a right retroesophageal subclavian artery that arises from the aorta distal to the ligamentum arteriosum.

All the intrinsic muscles of the larynx are innervated by the corresponding ipsilateral recurrent laryngeal nerve (Figures 3-5 and 3-6). Only the interarytenoid muscle receives bilateral innervation. Sensory information from the muscle spindles of the intrinsic muscles is conveyed by the recurrent laryngeal nerve. The cricothyroid muscle is supplied by the external branch of the superior laryngeal nerve. The somatic motor nucleus for the recurrent laryngeal nerve and the external branch of the superior laryngeal nerve is the nucleus ambiguus.

Somatic sensory innervation for the mucosa above the glottis is carried by the internal branch of the ipsilateral superior laryngeal nerve, which is divided into three divisions. The superior division mainly supplies the mucosa of the laryngeal surface of the epiglottis; the middle division supplies the mucosa of the true and false vocal folds and the aryepiglottic fold; and the inferior division supplies the mucosa of the arytenoid, subglottis, anterior wall of hypopharynx, and upper esophageal sphincter.[10] The corresponding innervation for the remaining major portions of the subglottis is from the ipsilateral recurrent laryngeal nerve (Figures 3-5 and 3-6). The thyroepiglottic joint and the cricothyroid joint are both innervated by the internal branch of the ipsilateral superior laryngeal nerve. The cricothyroid joint also receives sensory innervation from the external branch of the ipsilateral superior laryngeal nerve. The external branch of the superior laryngeal nerve also conveys sensory information from the anterior midline portion of the subglottis, as demonstrated in a cat model[11]; a similar pattern of innervation is probably true in the human larynx as well. These sensory nerves project to the ipsilateral nucleus solitarius, and their corresponding sensory ganglion is the nodose ganglion.

The somatic sensory receptors of the larynx are distributed in a well-characterized pattern. The true vocal folds have fewer mucosal surface receptors than the laryngeal surface of the epiglottis, which has the greatest density of receptors in the larynx.[12] In addition, the distribution of chemoreceptors is limited to the supraglottic mucosa.

Histologic examination has revealed the presence of free nerve endings, Merkel's cells, Meissner's corpuscles, and taste buds scattered in the larynx. Mechanoreceptors are located either in the superficial mucosa or in the muscles and laryngeal joints. Some of them are spontaneously active whereas others are silent until stimulated. A large number of taste buds populate the laryngeal surface of the epiglottis and extend caudally along the aryepiglottic folds, reaching peak density at the caudal extreme of the folds. These respond to a number of chemical stimuli and to water. Taste buds of the larynx tend to be stimulated by the pH and tonicity of the stimulating solution. Chemoreceptors of the larynx are adapted to detect chemicals that are not saline-like in composition and can play an important role in modifying reflexes involved in the maintenance of upper airway patency.[13,14]

The recurrent laryngeal and internal branch of the superior laryngeal nerves carry parasympathetic innervation from the dorsal motor nucleus to the subglottic and supraglottic regions, respectively. The sympathetic innervation is from the superior cervical ganglion.

The nerve of Galen, which is also known as the ramus communicans, connects the superior laryngeal nerve and the recurrent laryngeal nerve. It provides visceral motor input to the tracheal and esophageal mucosa as well as to the tracheal smooth muscle. The baroreceptors and chemoreceptors of the aortic arch are also innervated by the nerve of Galen, which relays this sensory information to the solitary nucleus.

LARYNGEAL BLOOD SUPPLY

Each side of the larynx has a dual blood supply from the inferior and superior laryngeal arteries. The inferior laryngeal artery is a branch of the inferior thyroid artery, which travels from the thyrocervical trunk superiorly to the inferior pole of the thyroid gland. Of note, the thyrocervical trunk is a constant feature on the right side, but on the left, the trunk may be so short that its branches, the inferior thyroid artery, the suprascapular artery, and the transverse cervical artery, arise directly from the subclavian artery. The inferior laryngeal artery enters the larynx with the recurrent laryngeal nerve and supplies the arytenoids, the false folds, and the laryngeal ventricle (Figure 3-6). The superior laryngeal artery is a branch from the superior thyroid artery, itself a branch of the external carotid artery. The superior laryngeal artery travels with the superior laryngeal nerve and enters the larynx with this nerve's internal branch to supply the piriform sinus and the quadrangular membrane (Figure 3-6).

The venous drainage parallels the larynx's arterial supply. The superior laryngeal vein empties into the internal jugular vein, while the inferior laryngeal vein empties into the thyrocervical trunk, a tributary of the subclavian vein.

LARYNGEAL LYMPHATIC DRAINAGE

Two systems of lymphatics drain the larynx. The superficial system is intramucosal only, and there is free communication between the left and right sides. Its contribution is relatively minor. The deep system drains the ipsilateral tissues only and is located submucosally.

The lymphatic flow from the larynx travels inferiorly and superiorly. The subglottic lymphatics drain via the middle pedicle and the paired posterolateral pedicles. The middle pedicle pierces the cricothyroid membrane and travels to the pretracheal and Delphian lymph nodes, which in turn, drain to the deep cervical lymph nodes. The posterolateral pedicle follows the inferior thyroid artery to ultimately reach the inferior deep lateral cervical, the subclavian, the paratracheal, and the tracheoesophageal lymph nodes. The supraglottic lymphatic vessels form a pedicle that exits the larynx with the superior laryngeal and superior thyroid vessels. This lymph drainage travels to the superior deep cervical lymph nodes associated with the internal jugular vein. In addition, lymph from the laryngeal ventricle flows through the cricothyroid membrane and ipsilateral thyroid gland to reach the prelaryngeal, paratracheal, prethyroid, supraclavicular, and pretracheal lymph nodes. The true vocal folds themselves lack significant lymphatic drainage.

CLINICAL SUBDIVISIONS

For clinical assessments, the larynx is divided into the supraglottis, glottis, and subglottis. The supraglottis, which surrounds the laryngeal vestibule, extends from the tip of the epiglottis to the junction between respiratory and squamous epithelium in the floor of the laryngeal ventricle. From a practical viewpoint, however, this inferior boundary is considered to be at the junction of the floor and lateral wall of the ventricle, so that the entire floor of the ventricle is considered to be part of the glottic larynx. Strictly speaking, the glottic larynx consists of the true vocal folds, the anterior commissure and the so-called posterior commissure. Because the vocal folds do not join posteriorly, there is no true posterior commissure. Instead, it is more appropriate to describe a posterior part of the glottic larynx, consisting of the arytenoid cartilages and the superior edge of the cricoid lamina.[15] The subglottis extends inferiorly from the area on the undersurface of the vocal folds where the squamous epithelium becomes a respiratory epithelium. Operationally, this margin is defined as occurring 5 millimeters below the free edge of the vocal folds. The inferior edge of the subglottis is the inferior border of the cricoid cartilage.

The term *epilarynx* describes the epiglottis and aryepiglottic folds above the hyoid bone. Here, malignant disease more closely resembles hypopharyngeal carcinomas, but this region is considered to be part of the anatomic larynx.

The valleculae, piriform sinuses, and the posterior cricoid esophageal inlet regions are all extralaryngeal. They are parts of the oropharynx and hypopharynx.

LARYNGEAL SPACES

A variety of compartments in the larynx are created by the arrangement of the various laryngeal membranes and mucosal reflections. The paraglottic space is found lateral to the laryngeal ventricle. This area is bounded by the thyroid lamina, the conus elasticus, and the quadrangular membrane. The paraglottic space communicates with the gap between the cricoid and thyroid cartilages, creating an important passageway for the spread of carcinoma arising in the ventricle. The preepiglottic space is bounded by the vallecular mucosa superiorly, the thyrohyoid membrane and thyroid cartilage anteriorly, and the epiglottis posteriorly and inferiorly. This space contains areolar tissue, lymphatic channels, and blood vessels.

VOCAL FOLD HISTOLOGY

The glottis consists of an anterior, or intermembranous, part and a posterior, or intercartilaginous, part. The true vocal fold extends from the tip of the vocal process of the arytenoid cartilage anteriorly to the anterior commissure. The cartilage of the vocal process does not participate in the vibratory actions of the true vocal fold and is not considered to be a part of the vocal fold.

The true vocal fold is a laminated structure composed of mucosa and muscle (Figure 3-11).[16-18] The overlying epithelium, as previously described, is of a nonkeratinizing, stratified squamous type. The lamina propria beneath this epithelium contains three layers: the superficial, intermediate, and deep layers. The superficial layer corresponds to Reinke's space and is made of mostly amorphous material. Elastic and collagenous fibers comprise the intermediate and deep layers, which together form the vocal ligament. The vocalis muscle is deep to the vocal ligament. The anterior macula flava is a thickening of the intermediate layer of the anterior vocal fold. The collagenous anterior commissure tendon extends from the anterior macula flava and the vocal fold deep layer to the thyroid cartilage. The posterior macula flava resembles the anterior macula flava. A transitional area of chondrocytes and fibroblasts lies between the posterior macula flava and the arytenoid vocal process, which is composed of elastic cartilage.

From a mechanical viewpoint, this histologic arrangement is actually three layers. The squamous epithelium and the superficial layer of the lamina propria form the cover, the intermediate and deep layers of the lamina propria form the transitional zone, and the vocalis muscle forms the body. This simplification is known as the cover-body concept and helps describe the vibratory characteristics of the vocal folds in health and disease.

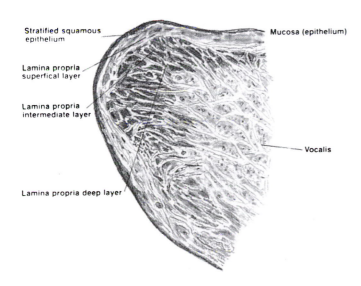

Stratified squamous epithelium

Lamina propria superficial layer

Lamina propria intermediate layer

Lamina propria deep layer

Mucosa (epithelium)

Vocalis

FIGURE 3-11. *Schematic illustration of vocal histologic structure.*

THE PEDIATRIC LARYNX

The adult and pediatric larynges are not identical. Major differences include the position of the larynx, as well as the configuration and relative sizes of the laryngeal cartilages. Lastly, the histologic structure of the vocal fold differs in the pediatric population.

Position

At birth, the cricoid is approximately at the level of the fourth cervical vertebra, and the epiglottis may be visualized over the dorsum of the tongue. The larynx descends slightly so that the cricoid is at the level of the fourth and/or fifth vertebra by age 2 years. During puberty, there is a rapid descent of the larynx so that it acquires its adult position in the neck. The cricoid cartilage is anterior to the seventh and sixth cervical vertebrae in men and women, respectively.

In the neonate, the epiglottis is in close apposition to the uvula and soft palate. This placement probably accounts for the observation that the neonate is an obligate nasal breather. The epiglottis descends between the ages of 4 and 6 months to a more mature placement.[19]

Framework Configuration and Size

The infantile epiglottis has an omega shape that provides less support for the aryepiglottic folds. The angle between the thyroid laminae in the newborn is approximately 110-120°. In the fully developed larynx, the epiglottis has a leaf-like appearance, and the angle between the thyroid laminae is 90° and 120° in men and women, respectively.

The infantile larynx is smaller relative to body size compared to the adult counterpart. In addition, the subglottic region is the narrowest part of the child's larynx, while the glottis forms the narrowest point of the adult larynx. Rapid growth from birth until age 6 and again during adolescence occurs as the larynx assumes its more mature configuration.

Histology

The pediatric vocal fold is considerably different from its adult counterpart.[17] The ratio between the cartilaginous and the membranous portions of the vocal fold is 1:1 in the neonate and 2:3 in the adult. The lamina propria of the vocal fold lacks clearly defined layers and is relatively thick in the neonatal larynx. Between the ages of 1 and 4 years, the vocal ligament, which is absent in the neonate, develops. Two layers appear in the lamina propria between the ages of 6 and 12 years. The fully mature lamina propria, consisting of superficial, intermediate, and deep layers, is only apparent by the conclusion of adolescence.

THE GERIATRIC LARYNX

The vocal fold also undergoes considerable sex-specific changes with aging.[20] In the female larynx, both the mucosa and vocal fold cover thicken with aging. In addition, the superficial layer of the lamina propria loses density as it becomes more edematous. The intermediate layer of the lamina propria tends to atrophy only in men. The deep layer of the lamina propria of the male vocal fold thickens because of increased collagen deposition. The vocalis muscle atrophies in both men and women.

The aging process also alters the histologic appearance of the false vocal folds.[21] Within the submucosa of the respiratory epithelium of the larynx, the seromucous glands become less prominent with increasing age. These changes are more pronounced for the mucous components of these glands compared with their serous portions.

As these glands atrophy, fatty infiltration increases. Additionally, the connective tissues of the false vocal folds fragment and become less dense in the geriatric larynx. These observations may account for age-related changes in laryngeal function.

THE VOCAL TRACT CONCEPT

Two general theories have been proposed to explain human voice production. The neuromuscular hypothesis stated that contractions of the intrinsic laryngeal muscles encoded by neural input directly initiate the vocal fold vibrations. This idea has been disproven. Even the larynx with bilateral recurrent laryngeal nerve palsies is capable of voice production. According to the myoelastic-aerodynamic theory, the release of subglottic pressure through the medialized vocal folds opens the glottis. As this pressure is released, the intrinsic elastic tension of the vocal folds draws the glottis closed again. The Bernoulli effect, in which flow produces decreased pressure, also tends to bring the vocal folds together. This cycle is repeated many times. In this way, the vocal folds are caused to vibrate. The sound waves created by the balance between subglottic pressure and vocal fold tension and the Bernoulli effect is then further modified by the resonance chambers of the hypopharynx, oropharynx, nasopharynx, nasal cavity, and oral cavity.

The vocal tract then includes not only the larynx, but also the lower respiratory and upper aerodigestive tracts. The pulmonary system, including the trachea, bronchi, lungs, thorax, and the related muscles of respiration, functions as an activator for phonation by providing the airflow and subglottic pressure. The larynx houses the vibrator source (ie, the true vocal folds). The muscles of the upper aerodigestive tract alter the dimensions and shape of the superior vocal tract and in doing so change the resultant resonant frequencies. Components of the initial sound signal are thus enhanced. By relatively rapid changes in the configuration (ie, volume, cross-sectional area, etc) of the upper vocal tract, a wide range of speech sounds can be produced. In this way, the specific sounds of human speech result from this complex interaction.

Initial studies of the contribution of the upper aerodigestive tract to human voice production utilized two-dimensional plain radiographs to assess the positioning of soft tissues. Computed tomography (CT) scans have also been applied for this purpose. Most recently, magnetic resonance imaging (MRI), which has multiplanar imaging capacity, has provided information about the three-dimensional shape of the upper vocal tract during phonation.[22] In particular, the positioning of the tongue within the oral cavity is well visualized with this technique (Figure 3-12).

Consideration of the anatomy of the activator and resonator components of the vocal tract is beyond the scope of this discussion of laryngeal anatomy.

REFERENCES

1. Sasaki CT, Isaacson G. Dynamic anatomy of the larynx. *Problems in Anesthesia.* 1988;2:163-174.

2. Graney DO, Flint FW. Larynx and hypopharynx: Anatomy. In: Cummings CW, Frederickson JM, Harker LA, Krause CJ, Schuller DE, eds. *Otolaryngology–Head and Neck Surgery.* 3rd ed. St. Louis, MO: Mosby Year Book; 1993:1693-1703.

3. Hately W, Evison E, Samuel E. The pattern of ossification in the laryngeal cartilages: a radiological study. *Br J Radiol.* 1965;38:585-591.

4. Chamberlain WE, Young BR. Ossification (so-called "calcification") of normal laryngeal cartilages mistaken for foreign body. *Am J Roentgenology and Radium Therapy.* 1935;33:441-450.

5. Hirano M, Yoshida T, Kurita S, et al. Anatomy and behavior of the vocal process. In: Baer T, Sasaki C, Harris KS, eds. *Laryngeal Function in Phonation and Respiration.* Boston, MA: Little Brown and Company; 1987:3-13.

6. Sanders I, Jacobs I, Wu BL, et al. The three bellies of the canine posterior cricoarytenoid muscle: implications for understanding laryngeal function. *Laryngoscope.* 1993;103:171-177.

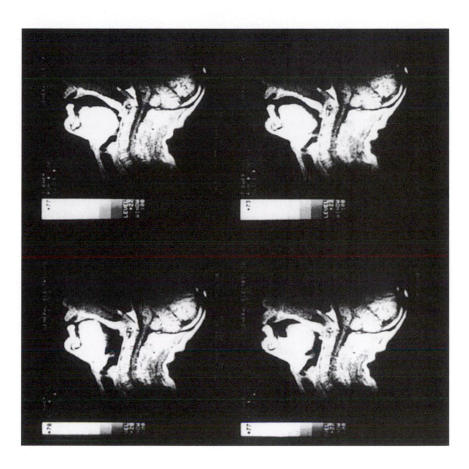

FIGURE 3-12. *MRI of upper vocal tract, sagittal section.*

7. Sanders I, Rao F, Biller HF. Arytenoid motion evoked by regional electrical stimulation of the canine posterior cricoarytenoid muscle. *Laryngoscope.* 1994;104:456-462.

8. Zaretsky LS, Sanders I. The three bellies of the canine cricothyroid muscle. *Ann Otol Rhinol Laryngol.* 1992;156(suppl):3-16.

9. Work WP. Unusual position of the right recurrent laryngeal nerve. *Ann Otol Rhinol Laryngol.* 1941;50:769-775.

10. Sanders I, Mu L. Anatomy of human internal superior laryngeal nerve. *Anat Rec.* 1998;252:646-656.

11. Suzuki M, Kirchner JA. Afferent nerve fibers in the external branch of the superior laryngeal nerve in cat. *Ann Otol Rhinol Laryngol.* 1968;77:1059-1070.

12. Shin T, Watanabe S, Wada S, et al. Sensory nerve endings in the mucosa of the epiglottis—morphologic investigations with silver impregnation, immunohistochemistry, and electron microscopy. *Otolaryngol Head Neck Surg.* 1987;96:55-62.

13. Anderson JW, Sant'Ambrogio FB, Mathew OP, et al. Water-responsive laryngeal receptors in the dog are not specialized endings. *Resp Physiol.* 1990;79:33-43.

14. Bradley RM. Sensory receptors of the larynx. *Am J Med.* 2000;108(suppl 4a):47-50.

15. Hirano M, Kurita S, Kiyokawa K, et al. Posterior glottis: morphological study in excised human larynges. *Ann Otol Rhinol Laryngol.* 1986;95:576-581.

16. Hirano M. Phonosurgical anatomy of the larynx. In: Ford CN, Bless DM, eds. *Phonosurgery: Assessment and Surgical Management of Voice Disorders.* New York, NY: Raven Press; 1991:25-41.

17. Hirano M, Kurita S. Histological structure of the vocal fold and its normal and pathological variations. In: Kirchner JA, ed. *Vocal Fold Histopathology—A Symposium.* San Diego, CA: College-Hill Press; 1986:17-24.

18. Hirano M, Sato K, eds. *Histological Color Atlas of the Human Larynx.* San Diego, CA: Singular Publishing Group, Inc; 1993.

19. Sasaki CT, Levine PA, Laitman JT, et al. Postnasal descent of the epiglottis in man. *Arch Otolaryngol.* 1977;103:169-171.

20. Hirano M, Kurita S, Sakaguchi S. Aging of the vibratory tissue of human vocal folds. *Acta Otolaryngol.* 1989;107:428-433.

21. Gracco C, Kahane JC. Age-related changes in the vestibular folds of the human larynx: a histomorphometric study. *J Voice.* 1989;3(3):204-212.

22. Baer T, Gore JC, Gracco LC, et al. Analysis of vocal tract shape and dimensions using magnetic resonance imaging: vowels. *J Acoust Soc Am.* 1991;90(2) (pt 1):799-828.

CHAPTER 4

Functional Fine Structures of the Human Vocal Fold Mucosa

Kiminori Sato, MD, PhD

Viscoelastic properties of the lamina propria of human vocal fold mucosa determine vibratory behavior and depend on extracellular matrices, such as collagenous fibers, reticular fibers, elastic fibers, glycoproteins, and glycosaminoglycan. Three-dimensional structures of these extracellular matrices are indispensable to the viscoelastic properties of the vocal fold mucosa. Fine structures of the vocal fold mucosa influence vibrating behavior and voice quality.

This chapter discusses functional fine structures of human adult vocal fold mucosa as vibrating tissue with viscoelasticity.

HISTOANATOMY OF THE GLOTTIS

The glottis (Figure 4-1) is composed of an intermembranous portion or anterior glottis and intercartilaginous portion or posterior glottis.[1,2] Their borders are defined by a line between the tips of the bilateral vocal processes.[1,2] The anterior glottis is required for phonation and the posterior glottis, primarily for respiration.[2] Thus, voice disorders are usually caused by lesions of the anterior glottis.

The vibratory portion of the vocal fold is connected to the thyroid cartilage anteriorly via the intervening anterior macula flava and anterior commissure tendon. Posteriorly, this portion is joined to the vocal process of

arytenoid cartilage via the intervening posterior macula flava. Thus, there are gradual changes in stiffness between the pliable vocal fold and hard cartilage.[1,3,4] The vocal processes form a firm framework of the glottis and are more pliable toward the tip.[4] Elastic cartilage is found not only at the tip of the vocal process but also at the superior portion of the arytenoid cartilage from the vocal process to the apex.[3] The vocal process bends at the elastic cartilage portion during adduction and abduction.[3,5]

Adult vocal folds have a layered structure consisting of epithelium; superficial, intermediate, and deep layers of the lamina propria; and vocalis muscle.[1,6] These layers may be grouped as three sections: a cover, consisting of the epithelium and superficial layer of the lamina propria; a transition zone, consisting of the intermediate and deep layers of the lamina propria; and a body, consisting of the vocalis muscle.[1,6] This layered structure is very important for vibration. The intermediate and deep layers of the lamina propria form the vocal ligament. Vocal ligaments run between the anterior and posterior maculae flavae.[1]

At birth, there is no structure corresponding to the vocal ligament and layered structure in adult vocal folds.[1,7,8] Development of the vocal ligament and layered structure of the vocal fold is complete at the end of adolescence.[7]

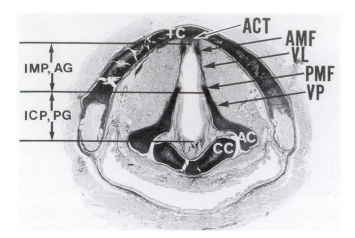

Figure 4-1. *Horizontal section of human female larynx at the level of glottis (Elastica van-Gieson stain). IMP: intermembranous portion, AG: anterior glottis, ICP: intercartilaginous portion, PG: posterior glottis, TC: thyroid cartilage, AC: arytenoid cartilage, CC: cricoid cartilage, ACT: anterior commissure tendon, AMF: anterior macula flava, VL: vocal ligament, PMF: posterior macula flava, VP: vocal process of arytenoid cartilage.*

FINE STRUCTURES OF THE HUMAN ADULT VOCAL FOLD MUCOSA

Epithelium

The free edge of the membranous vocal fold (anterior glottis) is covered with stratified squamous epithelium. The mucosa has pseudostratified ciliated epithelium in the posterior glottis.[1,2,9]

On the surface of epithelial cells, microridges and microvilli are present (Figure 4-2A). Lubrication of the vocal folds is essential for normal phonation. Microridges and microvilli facilitate the spreading and retention of a mucous coat on the epithelium.[10]

The epithelium consist of 6-7 layers of squamous cells. The cells of basal layers are columnar or polyhedral. Many desmosomes at the junction of two adjacent epithelial cells make firm intercellular adhesion (Figure 4-2B). Near the surface, the number of desmosomes decreases and the cells are more flattened. The superficial layers are composed of thin squamous cells (Figure 4-2A).

Basal Lamina (Basement Membrane)

At the boundary between epithelium and underlying lamina propria, a supporting structure, the basal lamina, is present (Figure 4-3). Basal lamina of the vocal

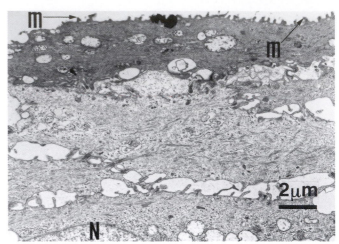

FIGURE 4-2A. *Superficial layers of stratified squamous epithelium of the vocal fold (Transmission electron micrograph [TEM]). m: microridge and microvilli, N: Nucleus.*

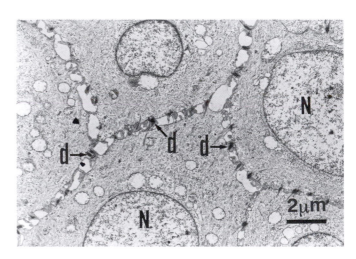

FIGURE 4-2B. *Intermediate layers of stratified squamous epithelium of the vocal fold (TEM). d: desmosome, N: Nucleus.*

fold is composed of two zones, lamina lucida and lamina densa. The lamina lucida is a low density clear zone adjacent to the cell membrane. Lamina densa is a greater density area of filaments adjacent to the lamina propria. Lamina densa contains type IV collagen.

Hemidesmosomes bind basal cells to the basal lamina. Anchoring fibrils tether the basal lamina to underlying connective tissue, the lamina propria of the vocal fold mucosa.[11,12]

The basal lamina mainly provides physical support to the epithelium[13] and is essential for repair of the epithelium.[14]

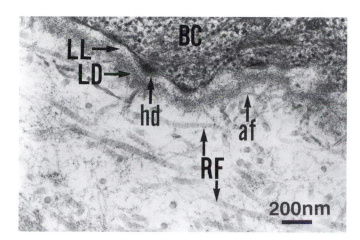

FIGURE 4-3. *Basal lamina of the vocal fold (TEM). BC: basal cell of the stratified squamous epithelium, LL: lamina lucida, LD: lamina densa, af: anchoring fibril, hd: hemidesmosome, RF: reticular fiber.*

Superficial Layer of the Lamina Propria (SLLP)

This layer, referred to as Reinke's space, is a superficial layer that vibrates a good deal during phonation. The viscoelasticity of the lamina propria of the vocal fold mucosa, especially the superficial layer, is a major determinant of the vibratory behavior of the structure.

Supportive functions and viscoelasticity of connective tissue depend largely on extracellular matrices. The main extracellular matrices of the vocal fold mucosa are reticular, collagenous and elastic fibers, glycoprotein and glycosaminoglycan.[15]

Extracellular Matrices of SLLP (Reinke's Space)

As fibrillar proteins, collagenous and reticular fibers (Figure 4-4A) are required for structural maintenance. They are responsible for tensile strength and resilience and serve as stabilizing scaffolds in extracellular matrices. The predominant collagen in the superficial layer of the lamina propria of the vocal fold mucosa is type III,[11] a major constituent of slender, 50 nm or less fibers traditionally called reticular fibers.

Reticular fibers (type III collagen) have a function of structural maintenance in expansible organs.[13] Reticular fibers are present in superficial and intermediate layers of the lamina propria of the vocal fold mucosa. They are most abundant around the vocal fold edge, then decrease in areas near the superior and inferior portions of the vocal folds. Reticular fibers are located in the portion of the vocal fold mucosa that undergoes the greatest vibration.[15] Slender fibrils of the reticular fibers do not form bundles but rather branches and anastomoses (Figure 4-4B). The delicate three-

dimensional structures of reticular fibers contribute to structural maintenance of the vocal fold mucosa during vibration without disturbing vibration.[15]

Elastic fibers are also fibrillar proteins (Figure 4-4B). They stretch by small force and return to their original dimensions when the force is removed.[13] In SLLP of the vocal fold mucosa, elastic fibers are slender, run in various directions, branch and anastomose to form loose networks (Figure 4-4B).

Ground substances of the vocal fold mucosa consist of glycosaminoglycan (acid mucopolysaccharide) and glycoprotein. One glycosaminoglycan in the vocal fold mucosa is hyaluronic acid,[16] which has very high viscosity in aqueous solution and thus is largely responsible for the consistency of ground substances.[13]

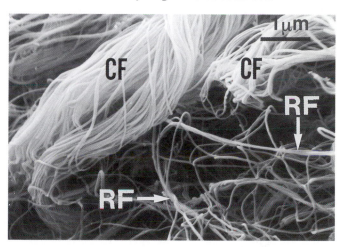

FIGURE 4-4A. *Reticular and collagenous fibers in SLLP of vocal fold mucosa (Scanning electron micrograph [SEM], NaOH maceration method). RF: reticular fibers, CF: collagenous fibers.*

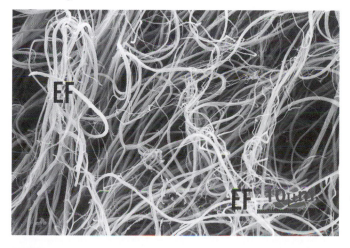

FIGURE 4-4B. *Elastic fibers in SLLP of vocal fold mucosa (SEM, NaOH maceration method). EF: elastic fibers.*

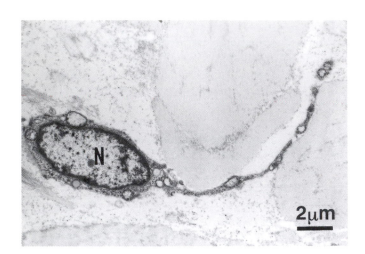

FIGURE 4-4C. *Fibroblasts in SLLP of vocal fold mucosa (TEM). N: nucleus.*

The reticular fibers which form delicate three-dimensional networks and spaces among the fibers are relatively large and there are innumerable potential spaces. The extracellular interstitial spaces are minute chambers or compartments occupied by other extracellular matrices, that is, elastic fibers and glycosaminoglycan (hyaluronic acid), which provide viscoelasticity to the tissue.[15] The three-dimensional structures of reticular fibers and other extracellular matrices are key components for structural maintenance and viscoelasticity of SLLP of vocal fold mucosa as vibrating tissue.

Fibroblasts in SLLP (Reinke's Space)

Fibroblasts are one of the interstitial cells that produce collagenous fibers and other extracellular matrices. Some fibroblasts are present throughout the human adult vocal fold mucosa (Figure 4-4C). Fibroblasts are spindle-shaped and the nuclei, elliptic. The nucleus-cytoplasm ratio is large with poorly developed rough endoplasmic reticulum and Golgi apparatus. Fibroblasts in SLLP (Reinke's space) synthesize few extracellular matrices;[17] they are inactive and at rest under normal conditions.[17]

Intermediate and Deep Layers of the Lamina Propria

The intermediate layer is primarily made up of elastic fibers, the deep layer, of collagenous fibers.[6] Both layers comprise the vocal ligament (Figures 4-1 and 4-5).

FINE STRUCTURES OF MACULA FLAVA OF THE HUMAN ADULT VOCAL FOLD

Maculae flavae are located at the anterior and posterior ends of both membranous vocal folds[1,18] and make conspicuous mucosal bulges. When analyzed through the mucosa, they appear as a white-yellow mass. The macula flava is elliptical in shape, about 1.5 × 1.5 × 1 mm in size, and composed of fibroblasts, elastic and collagenous fibers, and ground substance.[18]

Extracellular Matrices of the Macula Flava

The maculae flavae are dense masses of fibrous tissue (Figure 4-6A)[18] containing many fibrillar proteins such as collagenous, reticular and elastic fibers, and ground substances such as glycosaminoglycan (hyaluronic acid).[19]

Fibroblasts in Macula Flava

The distribution of fibroblasts differs according to the site within the vocal fold mucosa.[17] Cell density is greater in maculae flavae (Figure 4-6B) and sparse in Reinke's space.[17] In the macula flava there are numerous spindle-shaped fibroblasts and non-conventional fibroblasts stellate in shape.[19]

Stellate cells (non-conventional fibroblasts) (Figure 4-6C) are present in human adult maculae flavae but absent in Reinke's space.[19] Some morphologic and functional differences are apparent in these cells that differentiate them from conventional fibroblasts. Stellate cells are irregular and stellate in shape and possess slender cytoplasmic processes.[19] Lipid droplets are present in the cytoplasm.[19] Stellate cells have a small nucleus-cytoplasm ratio and well-developed rough endoplasmic reticulum and Golgi apparatus, suggesting active protein synthesis.[19] Stellate cells actively synthesize collagenous fibers, including reticular fibers, and other extracellular matrices such as elastic fibers and

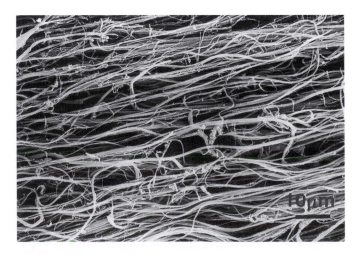

FIGURE 4-5. *Vocal ligament of vocal fold mucosa (SEM, NaOH maceration method). Fibers run roughly parallel to the vocal fold edge.*

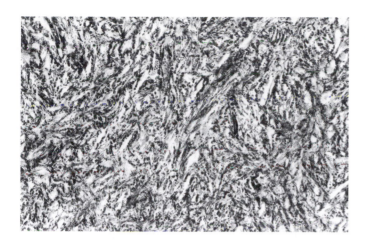

FIGURE 4-6A. *Macula flava of the vocal fold mucosa (Elastica van-Gieson stain, original X 200). Fibers are dense in the macula flava.*

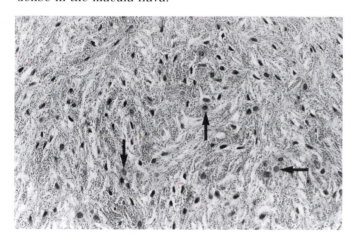

FIGURE 4-6B. *Macula flava of the vocal fold mucosa (hematoxylin and eosin stain, original X 200). Cells (arrows) are dense in the macula flava.*

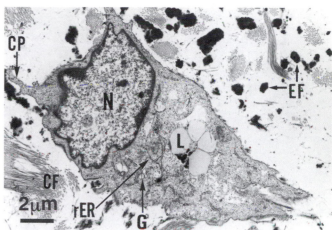

FIGURE 4-6C. *Stellate cell (non-conventional fibroblast) in macula flava (TEM, tannic acid stain). N: nucleus, rER: rough endoplasmic reticulum, G: Golgi apparatus, L: lipid droplet, CP: cytoplasmic process, CF: collagenous fibers, EF: elastic fibers.*

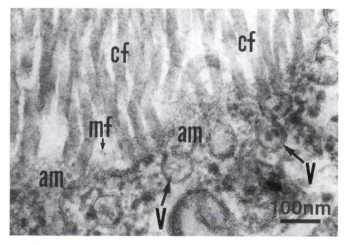

FIGURE 4-6D. *Synthesis of collagenous fibers by stellate cell (TEM, tannic acid stain). V: vesicle, am: amorphous materials, mf: microfibril, cf: collagenous fibril.*

glycosaminoglycan (hyaluronic acid) under normal conditions.[19] Stellate cells are involved in the metabolism of extracellular matrices essential for the viscoelasticity of the lamina propria of the human adult vocal fold mucosa as vibrating tissue. Whether stellate cells belong to a new category of cells remains unclear. They may be transformed fibroblasts.

Stellate cells actively synthesize collagenous, reticular and elastic fibers in human adult macula flava (Figures 4-6D and 4-6E).[19] There are many vesicles at the periphery of the cytoplasm and newly released amorphous materials are present on the cell surface of stellate cells. Microfibrils 10 to 15 nm in width are situated around this amorphous material. Collagenous fibrils are found near microfibrils. Microfibrils assemble and elastin is deposited on them. The amorphous sub-

stance of elastic fibers is produced by the fusion of microfibrils. Stellate cells actively synthesize glycosaminoglycan. Much glycosaminoglycan, especially hyaluronic acid, is found around stellate cells in the human adult macula flava.[19]

The macula flava in newborn vocal folds is important for the growth and development of the vocal ligament and layered structure.[20] Age-related changes in the macula flava influence fibrous components in the vocal folds and are one of the causes of aging of the voice.[21,22]

Maculae flavae are also present at the anterior and posterior ends of animal vocal folds; there is no struc-

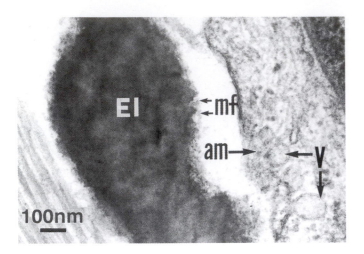

FIGURE 4-6E. *Synthesis of elastic fibers by stellate cell (TEM, tannic acid stain). V: vesicle, am: amorphous materials, mf: microfibril, El: elastin.*

ture equivalent to the human vocal ligament or layered structure.[23] Fine structures and functions of human adult maculae flavae differ from those of animal maculae flavae.[24]

RELATIONSHIP BETWEEN VOICE DISORDERS AND FINE THREE-DIMENSIONAL STRUCTURES OF EXTRACELLULAR MATRICES OF THE VOCAL FOLD MUCOSA

As mentioned above, three-dimensional structures of extracellular matrices are essential for structural maintenance and viscoelasticity of the human vocal fold mucosa. Macula flava of the human adult vocal fold mucosa may possibly be required for metabolism of extracellular matrices of the vocal fold mucosa under normal conditions.

For normal phonation, the layered structure of the vocal fold, and normal stiffness, mass, and homogeneity of the vocal fold mucosa are necessary. Not only changes in the three-dimensional structure of extracellular matrices but also qualitative and quantitative changes of each extracellular matrix influence the viscoelasticity necessary for normal phonation and may cause voice disorders.[25-28]

OTHER FINE STRUCTURES OF THE HUMAN ADULT VOCAL FOLD MUCOSA

Vessels

Blood vessels are unique in the mucosa of the vocal fold edge, where only small vessels such as arterioles, venules, and capillaries (Figure 4-7A) are present.[1,29] These vessels enter the vocal fold edge from the anterior or posterior end of the membranous vocal fold and run roughly parallel to the edge.[29] Blood vessels in the mucosa at the free edge are clearly distinct from those in the mucosa of the upper and lower surfaces of the vocal fold, as well as those in the vocalis muscle. The structures of the vessels in the vocal fold mucosa are suited for vibration.[29]

Many pericytes (Figure 4-7A) are present around capillaries, arterial capillaries and venous capillaries, in the vocal fold mucosa.[30] Pericytes encircle the capil-

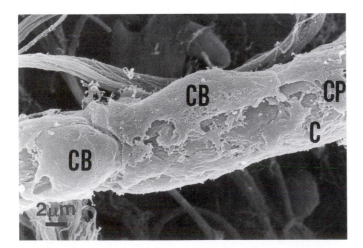

FIGURE 4-7A. *Capillary in SLLP of vocal fold mucosa (SEM, NaOH maceration method). The cell body (CB) and cytoplasmic processes (CP) encircle the capillary (C).*

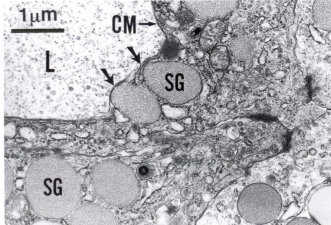

FIGURE 4-7B. *Laryngeal gland (TEM). Acinar lumen with expelled secretory material of serous cell. L: acinar lumen, CM: cell membrane, SG: secretory granule.*

lary walls. Processes of pericytes form tight intercellular junctions with endothelial cells.[30] The vessels in the vocal fold mucosa, the vibrating portion of the vocal folds, do not rupture easily, even during frequent and strong vibration. Pericytes in the vocal fold mucosa provide mechanical support and protection to capillary walls, particularly during phonation.[30]

Vessels in the vocal fold mucosa are related to voice disorders. Fragility of and alteration in the permeability of the vessels are causes of edema of SLLP (Reinke's space), which may become Reinke's edema.[31] Hemorrhage of vessels is one etiology of vocal fold polyps.[32]

Laryngeal Glands

Many mixed seromucinous type glands are present in the human larynx (Figure 4-7B). The location of the glands that form the lubrication is characteristic[1,9] and reviewed in the chapter by Sasaki (Chapter 3). No glands or glandular duct openings may be found at the free edge of the membranous portion of the vocal folds in most cases.[1,9] The vocal folds are lubricated by secretions from glands and lubrication of the vocal folds is required for normal phonation. The amount and quality, especially viscosity, of secretions influence phonation.

Functional disorders of the laryngeal glands, for example, age-related changes, partially alter vocal fold functions. Age-related morphologic changes in the laryngeal glands influence not only the amount but also quality of the secretions and diminish lubrication of the vocal folds, thus explaining one component of vocal aging.[33]

SUMMARY

Substantial advances in understanding the fine structure of the vocal folds has shed new light on phonatory function. Familiarity with the latest and most sophisticated insights into vocal fold structure is invaluable to physicians and surgeons striving to provide their patients with the most meticulous and effective interventions.

REFERENCES

1. Hirano M, Sato K. *Histological Color Atlas of the Human Larynx.* San Diego, CA: Singular Publishing Group, Inc; 1993.

2. Hirano M, Kurita S, Kiyokawa K, Sato K. Posterior glottis. Morphological study in excised human larynges. *Ann Otol Rhinol Laryngol.* 1986;95:576-581.

3. Sato K, Kurita S, Hirano M, Kiyokawa K. Distribution of elastic cartilage in the arytenoids and its physiologic significance. *Ann Otol Rhinol Laryngol.* 1990;99:363-368.

4. Sato K, Hirano M, Nakashima T. Ultrastructure of the vocal process of the arytenoid cartilage. *Ann Otol Rhinol Laryngol.* 2000;109:650-653.

5. Hirano M, Yoshida T, Kurita S, Kiyokawa K, Sato K, Tateishi O: Anatomy and behavior of the vocal process. In: Baer T, Sasaki C, Harris K, eds. *Laryngeal Function in Phonation and Respiration.* San Diego, CA: Singular Publishing Group Inc; 1991:3-13.

6. Hirano M. Phonosurgery. Basic and clinical investigations. *Otologia Fukuoka.* 1975;21(suppl 1):239-298.

7. Hirano M, Kurita S, Nakashima T. Growth, development and aging of human vocal folds. In: Bless DM, Abbs JH, eds. *Vocal Fold Physiology.* San Diego, CA: College-Hill Press; 1983:22-43.

8. Sato K, Kashiwagi S, Hirano M. Ultrastructure of the mucous membrane of the human newborn vocal folds. *J Otolaryngol Jpn.* 1997;100:479-483.

9. Sato K. Three dimensional anatomy of the larynx. Investigation by whole organ sections. *Otologia Fukuoka.* 1987;33(suppl 1):153-182.

10. Tillmann E, Pietzsch-Rohrschneider I, Huenges H. The human vocal cord surface. *Cell Tiss Res.* 1977;185:279-283.

11. Gray SD, Hirano M, Sato K. Molecular and cellular structure of vocal fold tissue. In: Titze IR, ed. *Vocal Fold Physiology.* San Diego, CA: Singular Publishing Group, Inc; 1993:1-35.

12. Gray SD, Pignatari SSN, Harding P. Morphologic ultrastructure of anchoring fibers in normal vocal fold basement membrane zone. *J Voice.* 1994;8:48-52.

13. Fawcett DW. *A Textbook of Histology.* Philadelphia, PA: W.B. Saunders Co; 1986.

14. Fawcett DW. *The Cell.* Philadelphia, PA: W.B. Saunders Co; 1981.

15. Sato K. Reticular fibers in the vocal fold mucosa. *Ann Otol Rhinol Laryngol.* 1998;107:1023-1028.

16. Matsuo K, Watanabe S, Hirano M, Kamimura M, Tanaka Y, Takazono I. Acid mucopolysaccharide and glycoprotein in the vocal fold. Alterations with aging. *Pract Otol Kyoto.* 1984;77:817-822.

17. Hirano M, Sato K, Nakashima T. Fibroblasts in human vocal fold mucosa. *Acta Otolaryngol (Stockh).* 1999;119:271-276.

18. Sato K, Hirano M. Histologic investigation of the macula flava of the human vocal fold. *Ann Otol Rhinol Laryngol.* 1995;104:138-143.

19. Sato K, Hirano M, Nakashima T. Stellate cells in the human vocal fold (in preparation).

20. Sato K, Hirano M. Histologic investigation of the macula flava of the human newborn vocal fold. Ann *Otol Rhinol Laryngol.* 1995;104:556-562.

21. Sato K, Hirano M. Age-related changes of the macula flava of the human vocal fold. *Ann Otol Rhinol Laryngol.* 1995;104:839-844.

22. Hirano M, Sato K, Nakashima T. Fibroblasts in geriatric vocal fold mucosa. *Acta Otolaryngol.* 2000;120:336-340.

23. Kurita S, Nagata K, Hirano M. Comparative histology of mammalian vocal folds. In: Kirchner JA, ed. *Vocal Fold Histopathology. A Symposium.* San Diego, CA: College-Hill Press, 1986:1-10.

24. Sato K, Hirano M, Nakashima T. Comparative histology of the maculae flavae of the vocal folds. *Ann Otol Rhinol Laryngol.* 2000;109:136-140.

25. Hirano M, Kurita S, Sakaguchi S. Ageing of the vibratory tissue of human vocal folds. *Acta Otolaryngol (Stockh).* 1989;107:428-433.

26. Sato K, Sakaguchi S, Kurita S, Hirano M. A morphological study of aged larynges. *Larynx Jpn.* 1992;4:84-94.

27. Sato K, Hirano M. Age-related changes of elastic fibers in the superficial layer of the lamina propria of vocal folds. *Ann Otol Rhinol Laryngol.* 1997;106:44-48.

28. Sato K, Hirano M. Electron microscopic investigation of sulcus vocalis. *Ann Otol Rhinol Laryngol.* 1998;107:56-60.

29. Mihashi S, Okada M, Kurita S, et al. Vascular network of the vocal fold. In: Stevens KN, Hirano M, eds. *Vocal Fold Physiology.* Tokyo, Japan: University of Tokyo Press; 1981:45-59.

30. Sato K, Hirano M. Fine three-dimensional structure of pericytes in the vocal fold mucosa. *Ann Otol Rhinol Laryngol.* 1997;106:490-494.

31. Sato K, Hirano M, Nakashima T. Electron microscopic and immunohistochemical investigation of Reinke's edema. *Ann Otol Rhinol Laryngol.* 1999;108:1068-1072.

32. Koike Y. A clinical and histopathological study on the laryngeal polyp. *Otologia Fukuoka.* 1968;14(suppl 2):279-305.

33. Sato K, Hirano M. Age-related changes in the human laryngeal glands. *Ann Otol Rhinol Laryngol.* 1998;107:525-529.

CHAPTER 5

The Microanatomy of the Vocal Fold Musculature

Ira Sanders, MD

The object of this chapter is to describe the neuro-muscular organization of the larynx, especially as it relates to voice production. The initial part of the chapter will review the course of the main laryngeal nerves and the innervation and function of each muscle. The second part will present a hypothetical overview of voice production based on what is being learned about the anatomy of the laryngeal muscles. The descriptions depicted here are based on the author's review of the literature and original research in humans and animals and differs from generally described laryngeal anatomy and physiology in the following key areas:

1. In the human larynx there are a number of connections between the superior and recurrent laryngeal nerves. These connections may allow the superior laryngeal nerve to supply motor innervation to the intrinsic laryngeal muscles. The most consistent connection is present in the interarytenoid muscle. In this location both recurrent laryngeal nerves as well as both internal superior laryngeal nerves combine in a neural plexus. In about half of the population, another connection is present in the area of the pyriform sinus. This connection, which we have termed the communicating nerve, is an extension of the external superior laryngeal nerve. The communicating nerve arises from the inner surface of the cricothyroid muscle and passes across the pyriform sinus to enter into the thyroarytenoid muscle. The communicating nerve is especially interesting as it appears to supply motor and sensory innervation to the area around the vocal process of the arytenoid and therefore may be of importance to phonation.

2. The thyroarytenoid muscle in both the human and the dog appears to be composed of at least two different bellies. Instead of bellies, muscle physiologists prefer the term *compartments*, and this term will be used in this chapter. The medial compartment of the thyroaytenoid muscle, the vocalis, contains a high proportion of slow-twitch muscle fibers. The lateral compartment of the thyroarytenoid, the muscularis, has a high percentage of fast-twitch muscle fibers and appears to be specialized to produce fast dynamic movements. It is hypothesized that the vocalis is responsible for controlling the tension of the vocal fold for phonation while the muscularis is specialized for adducting the vocal cord. The histologic specializations seen in the vocalis and the muscularis are seen in other laryngeal muscles. Together these areas may function as physically separate phonatory and articulatory subsystems.

3. The vocalis itself is composed of two compartments, an inferior and a superior. It is hypothe-

sized that these structures may correspond to the different masses in the two-mass model of vocal fold vibration. The inferior vocalis appears to control the tension in the subglottic aspect of the vocal fold. The inferior vocalis may be the area of the vocal fold responsible for determining the fundamental frequency of vocal fold vibration. In addition, it may also be responsible for controlling phonation onset. The superior vocalis is only well developed in the adult human. It is hypothesized that it has evolved to contribute to voice quality, especially the formant frequencies. In addition, the peculiar anatomy and vibratory dynamics of the superior vocalis suggest that it may operate by controlling sound production at the time of superior vocal fold closure.

LARYNGEAL NEUROMUSCULAR ANATOMY

The larynx is innervated by two main branches of the vagus nerve: the superior and recurrent laryngeal nerves (Figure 5-1).[1] The superior laryngeal nerve (SLN) branches off the vagus high in the neck at the inferior end of the nodose ganglion and bifurcates into two nerves: the internal and the external. The internal enters into the larynx at the thyrohyoid foramen and is believed to supply the sensory innervation to the entire mucosa of the larynx above the vocal folds. As will be shown below, there is reason to believe that the internal SLN also may supply some motor innervation to laryngeal muscles. The external SLN passes down the front of the larynx to supply motor innervation to the cricothyroid muscle. An extension of this nerve passes inside the larynx and may supply motor and sensory innervation to the vocal folds.

The RLNs are the main source of motor innervation to the larynx. The RLNs have an unusual course. They travel with the vagus nerve into the chest before branching. On the left the RLN usually loops under the aorta and on the right under the branchiocephalic artery. The RLNs then turn superiorly to enter into the larynx. Upon entering the larynx the RLN proceeds to supply motor innervation to the laryngeal muscles in the following sequence: posterior cricoarytenoid, interarytenoid, lateral cricoarytenoid, thyroarytenoid.

The Posterior Cricoarytenoid Muscle

The sole abductor of the vocal folds is the posterior cricoarytenoid (PCA). This muscle originates from the back of the cricoid cartilage and inserts into the muscular process of the arytenoid cartilage. The PCA of the

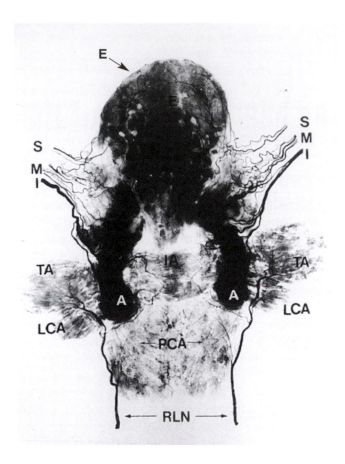

FIGURE 5-1. *The nerve supply of the human larynx. An entire human larynx was processed with Sihler's stain, a technique that renders soft tissue translucent while counterstaining nerves. The larynx was then dissected to isolate the superior (SMI) and recurrent laryngeal nerves (RLN) as well as all laryngeal muscles and the arytenoid (A) and epiglottic (E) cartilages.*

The RLNs are seen entering the larynx from the inferior direction. The first muscle to be innervated by the RLN is the posterior cricoarytenoid muscle (PCA). The second RLN branch travels beneath the PCA to innervate the interarytenoid muscle (IA). Finally, the RLN gives off a branch to innervate the lateral cricoarytenoid muscle (LCA) before terminating in the thyroarytenoid muscle (TA).

The superior laryngeal nerves enter the larynx from the superior direction. They travel down the lateral sides of the larynx and give off branches that pass medially to supply sensory innervation to the laryngeal mucosa. The superior laryngeal nerve usually divides into three main branches: a superior branch (S) innervates the epiglottis (E); a middle branch (M) innervates the false vocal fold; and an inferior branch (I) innervates the arytenoid (A) and postcricoid area.

human is composed of at least two compartments (Figure 5-2).[2-4] On its lateral side is the vertical compartment, which inserts onto the lateral aspect of the muscular process of the arytenoid. On the medial side of the PCA is the horizontal compartment, which inserts onto the medial aspect of the muscular process of the arytenoid cartilage. In the human each of these compartments usually receives its own nerve branch from the RLN. This nerve branch innervates only one compartment with little overlap between them. Anatomically, these compartments can almost be considered separate muscles. The vertical and horizontal compartments of the PCA may have different functions.

The role of the whole PCA during phonation is controversial. Speech consists of voiced and unvoiced segments in rapid succession. It is widely accepted that the PCA pulls the vocal folds apart after voicing.[5-8] In this way it can be thought of as participating in the articulation of the vocal folds that occurs during speech. However, the role of the PCA during voicing is less clear. Human electromyography shows that at high intensities and high pitches, the PCA is noticeably active. It is believed that under these conditions the PCA activity counterbalances the anterior pull of the thyroarytenoid and cricothyroid muscles.[9-11]

Although the functions of the compartments of the human PCA are unknown, a variety of experiments have been performed in the dog in attempt to clarify the association between PCA anatomy and function.[12-14] The canine PCA is composed of three grossly distinct compartments: the vertical, oblique, and horizontal. The orientation of these compartments differs by 20° to one another so that the entire muscle spans a 60° arc. Each of these compartments has a different insertion on the muscular process of the arytenoid cartilage, and this potentially allows the compartments to move the arytenoid in different ways. Indeed the cricoarytenoid joint is believed to have three arcs of motion.[15-19] The cricoid side of this joint is shaped like a cylinder upon which sits the concave bottom of the cricoid cartilage. The arytenoid cartilage can slide laterally along the cylindrical facet of the cricoid. This motion is seen during quiet respiration when the glottic opening appears triangular. During forceful inspiration a second abducting motion occurs. This is a backward rocking of the arytenoid cartilage. This rocking causes the vocal process of the arytenoid cartilage to swing laterally. This motion maximally opens the glottis and gives it the appearance of a pentagon. The third abducting motion of the arytenoid cartilage is a swiveling motion. This motion consists of the arytenoid's rotating like a gate without any of the sliding or rocking motions. The exis-

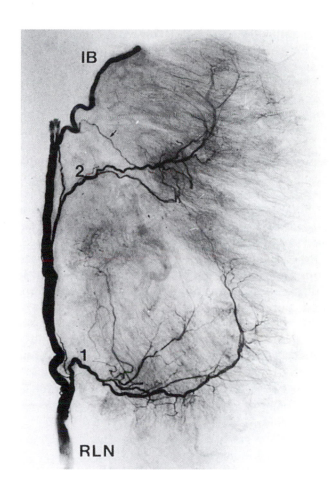

FIGURE 5-2. *The PCA muscle processed by Sihler's stain. The initial branch of the RLN is to this muscle. Upon entering the larynx, the RLN passes superiorly along the lateral edge of the PCA muscle. In two-thirds of the specimens, two branches came off separately from the RLN to innervate two different areas of the muscle. The first branch innervates the lateral half of the muscle (the vertical) while the second branch innervates the medial half (the horizontal compartment). The clear separation of the nerve supplies to the two compartments suggests that they may be independently controlled by the nervous system. The small arrow points to one of the communicating nerve branches that connect the nerves to the PCA and interarytenoid muscles. Numerals 1 and 2 mark the two separate RLN nerve branches to the two compartments of the PCA muscle. (IB = nerve branch to interarytenoid muscle.)*

tence and possible function of this third motion are controversial.

When electrical stimulation is applied to each of the compartments of the dog PCA, the stimuli do move the arytenoid in different ways.[13] Specifically, the vertical and oblique compartments slide the arytenoid laterally and rock it backward, the motions that can be seen during inspiration. In contrast, stimulating the horizontal compartment results in what appears to be a swiveling of the arytenoid. This causes an abduction of the vocal process with little displacement of the body of the arytenoid. When and how the swiveling action is used during vocal fold motion is obscure. It is possible that the swiveling motion is used during phonation to help position the vocal process. It is also conceivable that the horizontal compartment is not an abductor at all. Instead it may act as an adductor, just like the interarytenoid, and bring the posterior ends of the arytenoid together.

The actual role of the PCA compartments in the dog has not been tested by electromyography. However, the basic activity can be inferred by examining certain histologic indicators. Perhaps the most useful of these indicators is the distribution of fast- and slow-twitch muscle fibers. Muscle fibers can be divided into fast and slow on the basis of their reaction to myofibrillar ATPase stain.[20] Fast muscle fibers tend to contract more rapidly and develop more force than slow-twitch fibers. It has long been recognized that some whole muscles are mostly composed of either slow or fast fibers and are therefore specialized for either tonic or dynamic motions. Recently it has become clear that within the same muscle there can be regions that have differing proportions of the two fiber types. These regions, which are called compartments, have different activity patterns.[21]

Examination of the PCA of the dog shows that this muscle contains compartments with different proportions of fast- and slow-twitch muscle fibers. The proportion of slow-twitch muscle fibers in the horizontal compartment (41%) is almost twice that of the oblique compartment (23%).[12] These results suggest that the activity pattern of the horizontal compartment differs from that of the oblique. As will be shown below in the thyroarytenoid muscle, slow-twitch muscle fibers within a laryngeal muscle compartment appear to indicate that the compartment is involved with phonation. Whether this is true for the horizontal compartment of the PCA awaits confirmation through electromyography.

The Interarytenoid Muscle

The interarytenoid muscle is an unpaired muscle that originates from the back of each arytenoid cartilage. It is sometimes referred to as the transverse interarytenoid to differentiate it from the oblique interarytenoids, which are actually continuations of the aryepiglottic musculature.[21] When contracting, the interarytenoid muscle approximates the posterior ends of the arytenoid cartilages, thereby playing an important role in both the phonatory and the sphincteric mechanisms of the larynx.

In 1882, Mandelstamm reported that the interarytenoid muscle appeared to be innervated by both RLNs.[22] This was subsequently supported by dissections of human and animal laryngeal nerves and is now the accepted view in modern anatomy texts.[23-25] A more controversial idea is that the interarytenoid muscle is also innervated by the internal SLN. Anatomic dissections and histologic studies support the possibility that internal SLN innervates the interarytenoid muscle.[1,26,27] However, because electrical stimulation of the internal SLN does not cause vocal fold motion and sectioning of the nerve does not affect normal motion, it is generally assumed that the internal SLN branches pass through the muscle to supply sensation to the mucosa.[13,25,28]

When the interarytenoid muscle is examined in human larynges that have been processed by Sihler's stain, the four main laryngeal nerves are seen to contribute to a complicated plexus (Figure 5-3).[29] In addition, in almost every case, some axons from the internal SLN can be seen terminating among muscle fibers. It is not known whether the internal SLN axons that terminate within the muscle are contributing motor innervation to the interarytenoid muscle fibers or sensory innervation to the proprioceptive elements within the muscle. As for the internal SLN axons that join the plexus, they may pass through this plexus to travel into the RLN and then enter into the intrinsic laryngeal muscles. There is evidence that some axons travel downward from the interarytenoid muscle to innervate the PCA.[30] The interarytenoid nerve plexus has connections from side to side, and these may contain axons that travel from either the SLN or the RLN to the contralateral side of the larynx.

The Lateral Cricoarytenoid Muscle

The lateral cricoarytenoid muscle originates from the cricoid arch and inserts onto the muscular process of the arytenoid cartilage.[4] Contraction of the muscle adducts the vocal folds, and this adduction is important for phonation and reflex glottic closure.[31] A minority of investigators have also claimed an abductor function for the lateral cricoarytenoid muscle.[32] The most lateral fibers of the muscle are almost in line with the long axis of the cricoarytenoid joint so that their contraction may pull the arytenoid laterally. Zemlin has pointed out that both actions of the lateral cricoarytenoid are seen during whispering. Specifically, the tips of the arytenoids

The lateral cricoarytenoid muscle is innervated by a single branch from the RLN (Figure 5-4).[34] Upon entering the muscle, the nerve forms a neural plexus within the center of the muscle. There does not appear to be any difference in the neural branching pattern in the medial or lateral sides of the muscle. In general the nerve supply to the lateral cricoarytenoid muscle appears to be the simplest and most consistent of all the laryngeal muscles.

The Thyroarytenoid Muscle

The thyroarytenoid muscle (TA) is clearly the most important muscle for phonation. There have been many attempts to characterize this muscle as being composed of two basic compartments: a medial part, the vocalis, which is more involved in phonation; and a lateral part, the muscularis, which is more involved with adduction.[35] Some anatomists have claimed that the organization of the muscle fibers in the vocalis is different from that of the muscularis. However, in 1960, Sonensson reviewed this topic and concluded that there

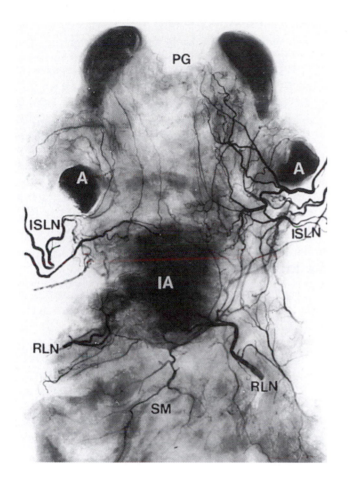

FIGURE 5-3. *The interarytenoid muscle processed by Sihler's stain. The interarytenoid muscle is innervated by nerve branches from both RLNs as well as both SLNs. The nerve branches combine within the muscle to form a complicated plexus. This arrangement allows axons to transfer between each of the main laryngeal nerves. It is possible that superior laryngeal axons transfer to the RLN to supply innervation to the intrinsic laryngeal muscles. In addition, axons from the SLN often terminate within the interarytenoid muscle and appear to be innervating muscle fibers. However, whether these axons actually control the muscle fibers is unknown. The interarytenoid innervation pattern is one of the most variable of the laryngeal muscles. (A = arytenoid cartilage; ISLN = internal SLN; and SM = subglottic mucosa.)*

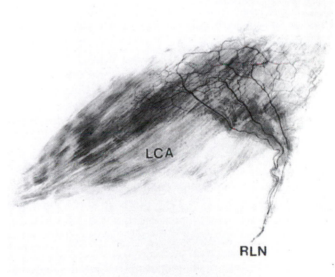

FIGURE 5-4. *The lateral cricoarytenoid muscle processed by Sihler's stain. The innervation of the lateral cricoarytenoid muscle is fairly consistent between specimens. A single branch from the RLN enters the muscle near its insertion on the arytenoid cartilage. The intramuscular nerve pattern consists of a plexus that is limited to the superior half of the muscle. Note that the plexus appears to be organized around muscle fascicles. (LCA = lateral cricoarytenoid.)*

are adducted toward the midline while the bodies of the arytenoid are pulled apart. These actions result in a small triangular chink in the posterior glottis through which the air stream passes.[33]

is no anatomic or histologic evidence to support the idea of a separate vocalis and muscularis.[36] Since Sonensson, various new histologic methods have been developed to study muscle. The most helpful of these is the myofibrillar ATPase reaction, which, as described above, basically divides muscle fibers into a fast and slow type. Numerous studies have applied this stain to the human TA, but none has reported any local concentrations of fast- or slow-twitch fibers.[37-39] Very recently, work has been performed to show that in the human TA there are indeed histologic differences suggesting separate vocalis and muscularis compartments.[40] However, as these compartments are more clearly seen in the canine TA, it will be discussed first.

So that the compartments of the canine TA could be studied, the muscle was totally sectioned from anterior to posterior and stained for ATPase.[41] Areas within the muscle were then followed in serial sections from their origins to insertions and the proportion of slow- and fast-twitch muscle fibers was calculated for each of these areas. It was found that the canine TA was divided into three basic compartments (Figure 5-5). Laterally is the muscularis; it originates from the muscular process of the arytenoid cartilage and inserts anteriorly into the thyroid cartilage. The muscularis is composed of about 100% fast muscle fibers. Medially is the vocalis, which is composed of almost 50% slow-twitch muscle fibers. The vocalis originates from the vocal process and the medial edge of the arytenoid and inserts into the subglottic mucosa and conus elasticus. In between the muscularis and the vocalis, another compartment can be discerned, the canine TA. This compartment is termed the centralis; it originates from the fossa oblongata of the arytenoid (the flat anterior surface of the arytenoid body) and inserts anteriorly into dense connective tissue continuous with the cricothyroid membrane.

The physical arrangement of these three compartments gives each of them a mechanical advantage in performing specific tasks. The attachment of the muscularis on the muscular process of the arytenoid gives this compartment a mechanical advantage in adducting the vocal fold. The centralis seems positioned to shorten the vocal fold in the anterior-posterior direction. In contrast, the direct insertion of the vocalis onto the mucosa suggests that this compartment can only be involved with controlling the tension of the mucosa to affect vibration.

It was found that the vocalis in the dog is itself composed of two distinct compartments. The superior compartment is the smaller of the two and is composed of small groups of muscle fascicles. It originates from the vocal process and terminates directly into the mucosa at the midpoint of the vocal fold. The inferior vocalis is a large densely packed muscle fascicle. It originates from the medial edge of the arytenoid and passes anteriorly to insert into the conus elasticus. It should be noted that in the dog the conus elasticus extends only halfway to the vocal fold edge. The dog has no vocal ligament, and except for the small superior vocalis muscle, the area of the free edge of the vocal fold is composed of soft tissue.

The human TA has certain obvious differences compared with the dog TA. First, the conus elasticus extends all the way to the free edge of the vocal fold, where its edge forms the vocal ligament. Second, the area around the vocal ligament, which is primarily soft tissue in the dog, is filled in with muscle fibers in the human. This appears to be a tremendous expansion of the small superior vocalis that is seen in the dog. Third, the proportion of slow to fast muscle fibers has doubled or tripled throughout the human TA compared with the dog. These slow fibers are arranged in a gradient with the medial edge of the muscle approaching 100% slow-twitch and gradually changing into almost 100% fast-twitch at the lateral edge (Figure 5-6). Somewhere in the middle of the muscle can be seen a line of transition that appears to demarcate the vocalis from the muscularis. Fourth, the human TA does not appear to have a compartment analogous to the dog centralis. Fifth, the subglottic area that contains the inferior vocalis in the dog cannot be clearly demarcated in the human. Instead, the same region often contains a very high local concentration of slow-twitch muscle fibers. Finally, the nerve supply of the human TA also appears to have separate terminal branches for both the muscularis and the vocalis (Figure 5-7). However, the vocalis nerve supply has dramatically increased its size and complexity in the human. This appears partly caused by the expansion of the superior vocalis in the human.

The External SLN

The external SLN passes along the front of the larynx and terminates in the cricothyroid muscle (Figure 5-8).[41] Upon entering the cricothyroid muscle, the nerve usually bifurcates to supply the rectus and oblique compartments. The external SLN does not only innervate the cricothyroid muscle. In humans, about 50% of the time an extension of the SLN passes out of the medial aspect of the muscle to enter into the TA (Figure 5-9). This nerve is referred to as the communicating nerve.[42] The communicating nerve usually bifurcates into two discernible branches. One either anastomoses with the RLN or terminates directly on muscle fibers. This branch is presumed to be motor. The second branch terminates in the subglottic mucosa and around the vocal process

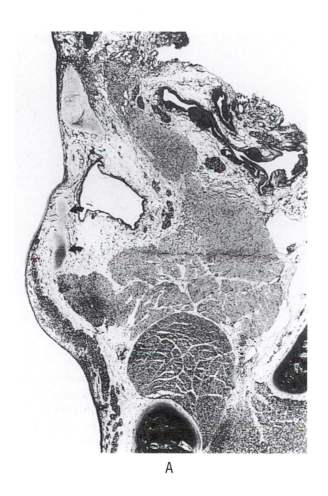
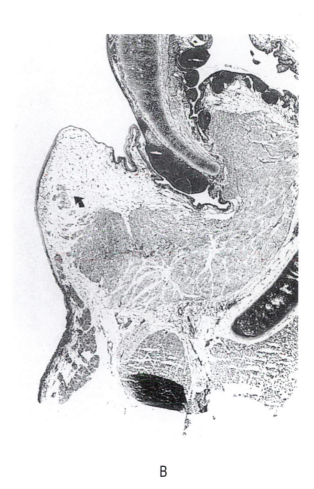

A   B

FIGURE 5-5. *(A-D) Serial cross sections of the canine vocal fold stained for myofibrillar ATPase. (E) The approximate location of each section. By determining the origin and insertion of each part of the thyroarytenoid muscle, one can divide the muscle into compartments. The lateral half of the muscle constitutes the muscularis. This compartment originates from the muscular process of the arytenoid cartilage and inserts anteriorly into the thyroid cartilage. In the middle of the canine thyroarytenoid muscle is the centralis compartment. The centralis originates from the body of the arytenoid cartilage and largely inserts into connective tissue continuous with the cricothyroid membrane. Finally, the medial one-sixth of the thyroarytenoid muscle is the vocalis compartment. The vocalis can be discerned in the muscle sections because it has a higher proportion of slow-twitch muscle fibers than the other compartments. The vocalis is itself composed of two identifiable subcompartments, the superior and inferior. The superior vocalis originates from the vocal process of the arytenoid cartilage and inserts into mucosa at the mid-vocal cord. The inferior vocalis originates from the medial edge of the arytenoid cartilage and inserts anteriorly into the conus elasticus. It is hypothesized that during phonation the vocalis controls the tension along the medial edge of the vocal fold. In addition, the inferior and superior subcompartments may function independently. The inferior vocalis may control the fundamental frequency of phonation, while the superior vocalis may control the higher frequencies, which determine phonation quality.*

(A) This section is 2 mm posterior to the tip of the vocal process of the arytenoid cartilage. The arrow points to the vocal process. (B) A section just in front of the vocal process. Note that where there was cartilage in the previous slide there now is a series of muscle fascicles that originated from the vocal process. These muscle fascicles constitute the superior vocalis.

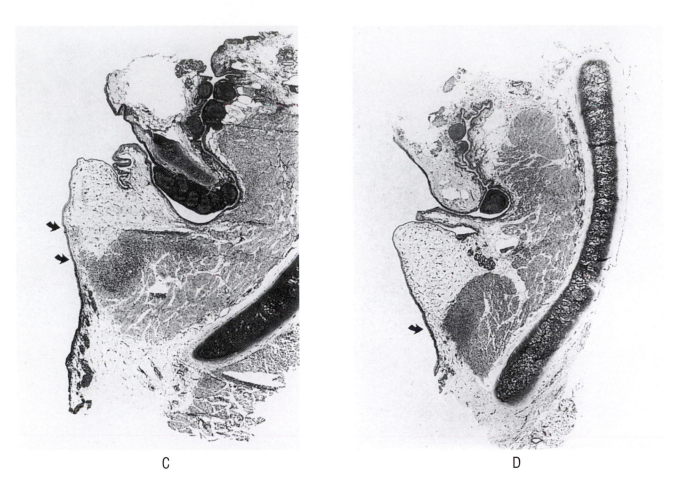

C   D

FIGURE 5-5 *(Continued). (C) A section through the middle of the vocal fold. Note that the superior vocalis has migrated toward the mucosal surface where it inserts. (D) A section through the anterior third of the vocal fold. Note that all the superior vocalis has inserted into the mucosa and is no longer present in the section. Also note that the inferior vocalis now inserts into the conus elasticus.*

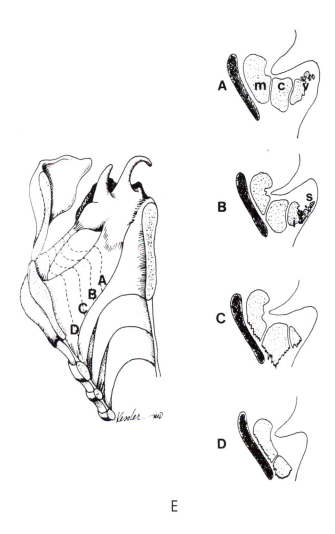

E

FIGURE 5-5 *(Continued). (E) Left, drawing of canine vocal fold showing the approximate locations of sections A-D; right, drawings of sections A-D outlining the muscle compartments within the thyroarytenoid muscle. In section A the compartments are labeled as follows:* M = *muscularis;* C = *centralis;* V = *vocalis. In section B the inferior* (I) *and superior* (S) *vocalis are marked.*

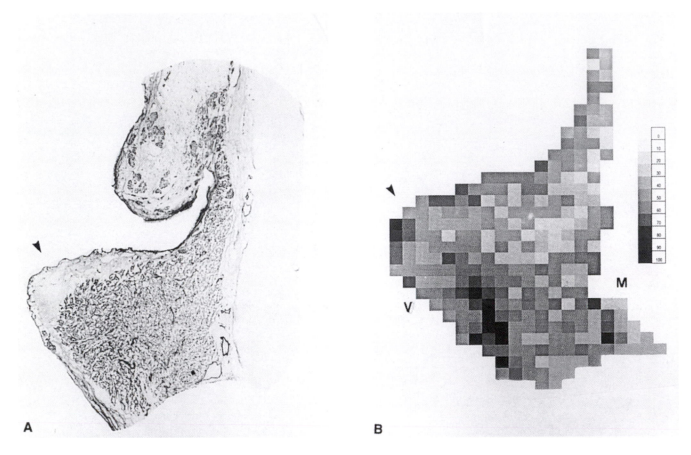

FIGURE 5-6. *(A) Cross section of the human thyroarytenoid muscle stained for fast- and slow-twitch muscle fibers. Fast-twitch fibers are light; slow-twitch fibers are dark. Slow-twitch fibers are concentrated in the medial half of the muscle. This slow medial half of the human thyroarytenoid muscle is believed to constitute the vocalis. Another obvious difference between the human and the dog is that the superior vocalis has expanded in the human to fill the whole superior vocal fold (arrowhead points to the vocal ligament). In contrast, in the dog this area is mostly soft tissue and contains a comparatively small superior vocalis muscle. (B) Graphic display of slow-twitch fiber proportions from Figure 5-6A. The proportions of slow-twitch muscle fibers in small regions of the thyroarytenoid muscle have been computed and converted into a gray scale. White areas are 100% fast-twitch; black areas are 100% slow-twitch. The presentation of the data in this form makes it easier to appreciate how the slow-twitch muscle fibers are concentrated in the medial half of the muscle. Note that small areas alongside the subglottic mucosa are 100% slow-twitch. It is hypothesized that the concentration of slow-twitch muscle fibers along the subglottic mucosa of the human vocal fold is homologous to the inferior vocalis of the dog (arrowhead points to the vocal ligament).*

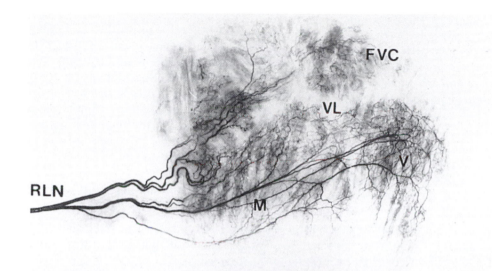

A

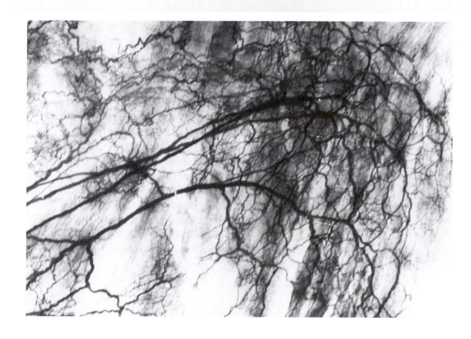

B

FIGURE 5-7. *(A) Human thyroarytenoid muscle processed with Sihler's stain, which clears the muscle while counter-staining nerve. The recurrent laryngeal nerve terminates in the thyroarytenoid muscle. Some nerve branches pass superiorly to innervate the aryepiglottic muscles in the false vocal fold. The main branches pass through the thyroarytenoid muscle to terminate in the medial side of the muscle, the area that is believed to be the vocalis. The vocalis innervation is much denser than that in the lateral half of the muscle, the muscularis (M). In most cases the vocalis is innervated by a single separate branch from the recurrent laryngeal nerve (arrow). The heavy inner-vation of the vocalis may indicate that to perform its phonatory role it requires very fine neural control. (FVC = false vocal fold (cord); VL = area of vocal ligament.) (B) Magnification of the area of the vocalis seen in part A. The organization of the terminal nerve branching pattern of the vocalis is very complex. The axons form a dense plexus around very small groups of muscle fibers. This suggests that the motor units in this area are very small.*

and is presumed to be sensory. The nature and purpose of the communicating nerve are unknown. However, whenever it is present it innervates structures that are critical for phonation. There is currently no explanation of why it is present only half the time, and what nerve fulfills its role when the communicating nerve is absent.

The Cricothyroid Muscle

The cricothyroid muscle originates from the bottom of the thyroid alae and inserts into the top of the cricoid cartilage. In the 16th century, Vesalius noted that the muscle is composed of two gross compartments now known as the rectus and the oblique.[43] Recently, the cricothyroid muscle of the dog was found to have a third compartment, the horizontal.[44] Cricothyroid contraction causes elevation of the anterior cricoid ring by rotation at the cricothyroid joint. This action elongates the glottis by increasing the distance between the arytenoid and the thyroid cartilage.[4,33] A second action of the muscle is anterior-to-posterior sliding of the thyroid cartilage over the cricoid,[19,45] although some investigators claim that the cricothyroid joint is incapable of this motion.[46]

The cricothyroid muscle has important functions during both phonation and respiration. During phonation the cricothyroid lengthens the vocal folds. This lengthening and thinning of the vocal folds decreases its vibrating mass and is believed to play a major role in increasing phonatory pitch.[47] The cricothyroid also varies the anteroposterior dimension of the larynx during respiration. Simultaneous contractions of the PCA muscle and the cricothyroid make the airway larger than during PCA contraction alone.[48,49]

SPECULATIONS OF PHONATORY CONTROL

Anatomic evidence can only suggest function; therefore, any description of laryngeal function based on anatomy must be speculative. On the other hand, the purpose of research is to uncover new directions to be pursued, and they require hypotheses that can be tested. In this section the anatomic data presented above will be interpreted to describe a hypothesis of how phonation is controlled.

The Lower Vocalis and the Control of Fundamental Frequency

In 1940, Farnsworth published photographs of the vocal folds of the human that were taken with an ultra-high-speed movie camera.[50] The most striking finding from this study was that the lower part of the vocal fold vibrates slightly out of phase from the upper part. During vocal fold closure the lower part can be seen as a sharp ledge while the upper part lags in a more lateral position. These observations led directly to the two-mass model,[51] the most commonly cited theory of how the vocal folds vibrate. The presence of a ledge similar to that seen by Farnsworth has subsequently been reported in a variety of different experiments. For example, Matsushita viewed excised human and dog larynges from below and noted that a ledge was seen in the subglottic area.[52] This ledge served as the initiation line of the mucosal wave so that it was given the descriptive, albeit unwieldy, name of *the mucosal upheaval*. Berke et al have reported a similar configuration in the canine larynx when it is artificially made to phonate in vivo.[53]

FIGURE 5-8. *The cricothyroid muscle processed by Sihler's stain. The external SLN enters the cricothyroid muscle near the division between the rectus and the oblique compartment. After an initial rearrangement it divides into two main branches that supply the two compartments. Note that in both compartments, but especially in the oblique, the secondary nerve branches appear to extend into the origin and insertions of the muscle fibers. (CT = cricothyroid muscle; ESLN = external SLN; O = oblique belly of cricothyroid; R = rectus belly of cricothyroid.)*

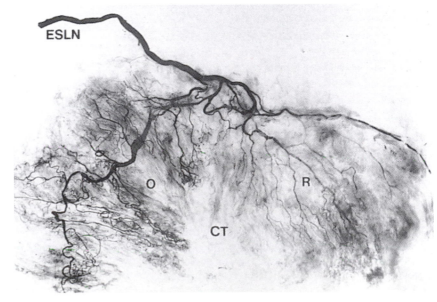

FIGURE 5-9. *The communicating nerve branch is shown processed by Sihler's stain. A neural communication is often found between the SLN and the RLN in the region of the piriform fossa (arrow). The communication is a continuation of the external SLN through the cricothyroid muscle. In its most common form the communicating nerve divides into two parts. One part is presumed to be motor and either joins the RLN or terminates in the TA muscle (1). A second part is sensory and terminates around the vocal process of the arytenoid (2). The structures innervated by the communicating nerve are heavily involved in phonation; however, the exact function of this nerve has yet to be determined. (CT = cricothyroid muscle; ESLN = external SLN.)*

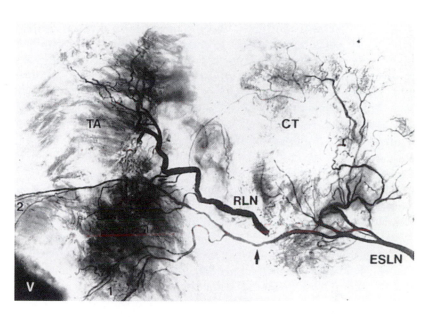

Finally, Hirano et al have reported the presence of the mucosal upheaval in humans when the vibrating folds are viewed from below, although the ledge is not as sharply defined as in excised larynges.[54] The existence of a line from which the mucosal wave begins has therefore been documented in vivo when human larynges are viewed from both above and below, in experimental canine larynges, and in excised human and canine larynges when artificially vibrated and viewed from below. It may be that the line seen in these different experiments is the same phenomenon and relates to a basic structure of the vocal fold.

The structure that corresponds to the mucosal upheaval is suggested by a recent experiment by Yumoto et al.[55] Excised canine larynges were viewed from below and artificially set into vibration. The mucosal upheaval was marked on the mucosa, and the larynx was then sectioned. The area of the mucosal upheaval was seen to begin at the point where the TA muscle approaches the subglottic mucosa. To be more specific, the mucosal upheaval is exactly at the juncture between what has been described earlier in this chapter as the inferior and the superior vocalis. Tying these observations together, it appears that the upper and lower masses of the two-mass model may correspond to concrete structures within the TA, the superior and the inferior vocalis.

In the human, the inferior vocalis is less well-defined than in the dog. One reason for this is that the human TA has expanded to form a large superior vocalis so that the gross appearance of the entire medial part of the TA appears to be that of a continuous muscle. However, with muscle fiber typing the inferior vocalis appears to correspond to a collection of slow-twitch fibers directly adjacent to the subglottic mucosa.

The question now arises as to the function of the inferior vocalis. It is hypothesized that the inferior vocalis is primarily responsible for the control of fundamental frequency. This area leads the rest of the vocal fold during vibration and has a much lower amplitude of vibration.[56] The appearance of this area during vibration is that it is the generator of the vocal fold oscillation and that the mucosal wave is generated from its motion. Once the mucosal wave begins, it will complete its motion upward and across the remainder of the vocal fold surface. Tension changes above the inferior area would be expected to have no effect on the frequency of vibration. The tension in the inferior vocalis may therefore be controlled separately from that of surrounding TA muscle. It is even possible that during the initiation of vibration, the actual start of oscillation is dependent on the inferior vocalis's achieving a set tension.

The Superior Vocalis and the Control of Quality

The human superior vocalis is a unique structure. In the adult human the area is packed with muscle fibers innervated by an extremely complex nerve supply. In contrast, in the dog, the chimpanzee, and even the newborn human, the area is mostly composed of soft tissue. These differences suggest that the superior vocalis has evolved to perform a key role for human speech.

Observations of vocal fold vibration suggest that the superior vocalis itself contains smaller subcompartments that can be independently controlled by the nervous system. For example, to raise pitch during falsetto, the vibrating edge of the vocal folds is progressively shortened.[57] This shortening begins posteriorly by bringing the vocal folds together to dampen vibration. At higher pitches more and more of the vocal folds are brought together until the vibrating edge is confined to a few millimeters in the very anterior aspect of the vocal fold. This phenomenon can be explained as the progressive damping of vocal fold vibration by the recruitment of small bundles of muscle fibers in the superior part of the vocalis. During modal speech the same independent control of muscle fiber groups may be occurring. Instead of dampening vibration, the nervous system could control tension in discrete areas of the superior vocalis so as to mold the vibration of the vocal fold.

Why would the shape of the superior edge of the vocal fold be important? The answer is suggested by studies that examine vocal fold shape during phonation. For example, cross-sectional radiographs of the vocal folds (tomograms) have been made of individuals phonating different vowels at the same pitch and intensity.[58,59] In these experiments the shape of the vocal folds varies dramatically. It can be speculated that one role of superior vocalis muscle groups is to mold the shape of the vocal fold during the phonation of different vowels. Vowels are characterized by their first and second formants, and because fundamental frequency was held constant during these experiments, it suggests that the superior vocalis molds the shape of the vocal fold to enhance the production of the speech formants, along with the greater effect of tongue shape. In support of this is one of the first inverse filter studies of voicing by Miller.[60] He found that individuals could vary the relative amounts of acoustic energy in different formants by more than 20-fold. This control of the higher formants appeared to be independent of the control of fundamental frequency.

A final speculation on the superior vocalis regards the mechanism by which its action produces changes in sound. Usually the actual sound produced by the vocal folds is believed to be produced in the open phase of the vibration cycle. However, there have been occasional reports that claim that the higher frequencies are actually produced during the instant of vocal fold contact at the beginning of the closure phase. These reports begin with Helmholtz, who compared his perception of the human speaking voice with that of multiple acoustic experiments.[61] Another example is that of Miller,[60] who found that the production of the higher frequencies of sound evidently occurs at vocal fold closure. Other investigators have also reported that the highest acoustic energies are produced around the instant of vocal fold closure.[62] Recent experiments that have measured the actual forces within the glottis report that

peak intraglottal pressure occurs at the time of vocal fold closure, these closure pressures being much higher than at any point of the open cycle. These observations suggest that some part of the sound production occurs during vocal fold closure.

Furthermore the unusual dynamics of the vocal fold during closure suggest a unique mechanism of sound production. As mentioned above, the movement of the vocal folds is such that the inferior and superior aspects of the vocal fold are out of phase. During closure, the inferior vocalis area contacts first, and this is rapidly followed by closure of the superior vocalis area. Therefore, the subglottic area is first sealed and then the small volume of air between the rapidly closing superior vocalis areas must be displaced superiorly at high acceleration. This acceleration may be sufficient to produce sound.

Most recently, additional information has been obtained regarding the unique nature of the human thyroarytenoid (TA) muscle, and especially the superior vocalis compartment (SV). The superior vocalis has certain microstructural and molecular characteristics which make it an unusual if not unique type of mammalian muscle (Figure 5-10). Within the human TA the SV compartment appears to contain the most specializations, including rare muscle fiber types and high concentrations of muscle spindles.[63] Histologic examination shows that the SV is also remarkable for its high proportion of extremely short muscle fibers and unusual intramuscular connection system.[64] In teased SV samples, about 70% muscle fibers could be micro-dissected intact. Ninety-five percent of the microdissected muscle fibers were less than 5 mm in length and more than half were less than 2 mm. As the average TA muscle is at least 2 cm in length the majority of muscle fibers within the SV must originate and insert within the muscle without directly connecting to either the thyroid or arytenoid cartilages.

The high proportion of short muscle fibers is reflected in the many types of connections seen in the SV. Muscle fibers often are connected in series by thin tendons. In addition these tendons also merged into the endomysium of the larger diameter muscle fibers. The shapes of muscle fibers is also variable. Thin cylindrical muscle fibers with tapered ends are most common; however, short bulbous muscle fibers are also common. Variably shaped muscle fibers were often found in the same microdissected preparation, suggesting that these unusual shapes were not an artifact but did represent the in vivo condition. The SV subcompartment also contained many muscle fibers that were seen to divide into two or more smaller fibers. These branches often connected to other muscle fibers to form netlike arrays.

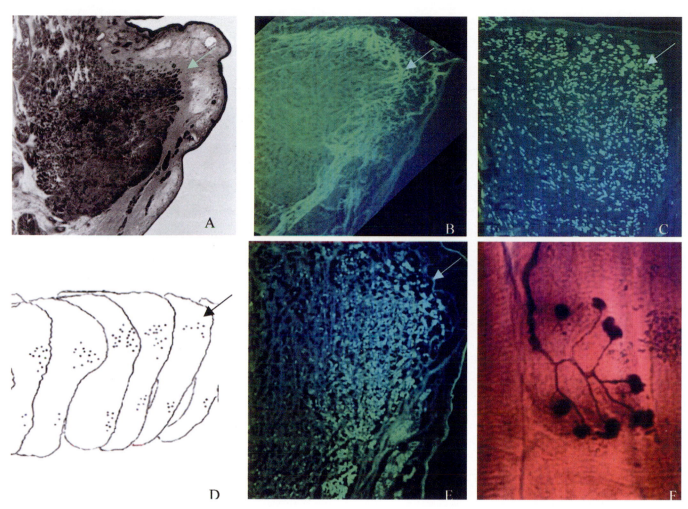

FIGURE 5-10. *Specializations of the human vocalis compartment of the thyroarytenoid muscle. (A) Frontal section of human mid-vocal fold. Medial (right) side of the thyroarytenoid muscle is the vocalis compartment; arrow points to the superior vocalis in the region of the vocal ligament. (B) Immunoreaction for elastin, an elastic type of connective tissue that is uncommon in most muscles. A thick band of elastin is seen along the whole perimeter of the vocalis. It infiltrates into the muscle just below the vocal ligament. (C) Immunoreaction for alpha cardiac myosin, a rare type of myosin found in the muscle fibers of the atria of the heart, the extra-ocular muscles and, now, the human vocalis. (D) Location of slow tonic muscle fibers. Drawing of frontal sections taken from intervals along the vocal fold where slow tonic muscle fibers were found and mapped from sections such as photomicrograph. Note that the largest concentration of slow tonic muscle fibers is found just next to the vocal ligament. A smaller group is present in the inferior vocalis. (E) Immunoreaction for slow tonic myosin. Although some reaction is present throughout the vocalis, the reaction is greatest in the superior vocalis. Note that the muscularis compartment of the thyroarytenoid muscle (the lateral side) contains no slow tonic myosin reaction. (F) An en grappe motor endplate from a muscle fiber in the superior vocalis. These unusual motor endplates are found only on slow tonic muscle fibers.*

Similar branching muscle fibers have been described in the extra-ocular muscles and a few other muscles. It is believed that the branching muscle fibers and dense connecting network reflects a special way of distributing force within the muscle.

Using antibodies to different types of the contractile protein myosin, it has been shown that the superior vocalis contains muscle fibers with very rare types of myosin, such as alpha cardiac, slow tonic, and developmental myosins. The most interesting of these is undoubtedly the slow tonic muscle fibers (STMF), as they have a different anatomy and physiology than normal twitch muscle fibers. STMF have multiple motor endplates with the characteristic *en grappe* shape.[65,66] Each motor endplate controls the contraction of the part of the muscle fiber in its area, as the STMF membrane does not propagate an action potential. Instead of contracting with a twitch, STMF exhibit slow and prolonged contractions, much like smooth muscle.

Although rare in mammals, STMF are relatively common in birds and amphibians. What is known about their physiology comes mostly from observing the function of muscles containing large amounts of STMF. In birds, shoulder muscles which connect the wings to the trunk contain a high proportion of STMF; these muscles are believed to keep the wings locked in place,[67] especially during soaring or gliding activities when the wings are relatively immobile. In contrast, the dynamic flight muscles of the wings are composed of almost entirely fast-twitch muscle fibers. One muscle that has been extensively studied is the anterior latissimus dorsi muscle. This muscle contains nearly 100% STMF and acts to stabilize the wing in the shoulder joint for extended periods, such as when a bird is soaring. As such, it serves to maintain continual tone because of its high resistance to fatigue. In other muscles they seem to be intermixed with large numbers of muscle spindles, the receptor that senses the length of a muscle. This association of STMF and muscle spindles is believed to act as a large sensory unit, the STMF somehow allowing the muscle spindles to do their job better.

In mammals STMF have been found in two muscle groups. All species appear to contain the STMF in their extra-ocular muscles. In humans the stable contraction of STMF are believed to allow for gaze fixation and slow pursuit movements. The only other muscles known to contain STMF are the middle ear muscles of certain social carnivores such as the cats, but not in other species such as some nonhuman primates. Under experimental conditions it has been shown that mild contraction of the STMFs serves to stiffen the middle ear ossicles and results in the filtering of certain frequencies.[68] If this mechanism is used in vivo it may be a way that animals filter out extraneous frequencies other than those from their *con specifics* (same species).

The presence of STMF in the human vocal fold is, then, a bit of a surprise. This is only the second area in the human that is known to contain these special fibers. The area where the STMF are at highest concentrations, the superior vocalis, is just beneath the vibrating edge of the vocal fold. The highest numbers of muscle fibers were found in the center of the membranous vocal fold, and decreased both anteriorly and posteriorly. This

region is the most mobile during vocal fold vibration and changes in muscle stiffness would be expected to greatly affect this vibration, and thereby change the acoustic output. Therefore, it may be that the STMF have evolved to allow some control of the vocal fold edge that is important for human speech. This is supported by the fact that the entire superior vocalis does not appear to exist in other species, including other primates such as the chimpanzee. Instead, the same area contains only soft tissue. Interestingly, neonatal human vocal folds also only contain soft tissue in this area.

If it is hypothesized that a special system has evolved to produce critical aspects of human speech, it would follow that speech disorders affect this system. Certainly there is much to learn before we can make any conclusions; however, preliminary evidence suggests that this may be true. For example, idiopathic Parkinson's disease is a neurologic disorder in which the voice is affected. Patients adopt a weak breathy speaking voice and, upon examination, the vocal folds are bowed. Comparison of vocal folds from patients with IPD with those of normals shows that the IPD have a dramatic decrease in the amount of STMF and other associated specializations normally seen in the SV area (Figure 5-11). Whether the bowing of the vocal folds seen in these cases is secondary to volume loss in the SV compartment is not known. However, the example shows how the understanding of the basic science of voice production may be relevant to the pathologic condition.

Whatever the exact mechanism may be for sound production during vocal fold closure, the superior vocalis may play a critical role. Through independent control of superior vocalis tension, the nervous system can strongly affect the amplitude and strength of vibration at the area of the vocal ligament. These changes may control the overtones produced at the vocal folds, which are interpreted perceptually as changes in quality of the voice.

The Muscularis and Centralis Compartments of the TA

The vocalis takes up only a small percentage of the TA. In the canine larynx, two other distinct compartments can be appreciated on the basis of their positions within the muscle and the course of their muscle fibers. The most lateral fibers of the TA in both the human and the dog originate from the muscular process of the arytenoid cartilage and insert into the thyroid cartilage. This compartment, which we have termed the muscularis, is composed of almost 100% fast-twitch muscle fibers. The architecture of the muscularis gives it a mechanical advantage in adducting the arytenoid cartilage. It may be inferred that this area may be a separate

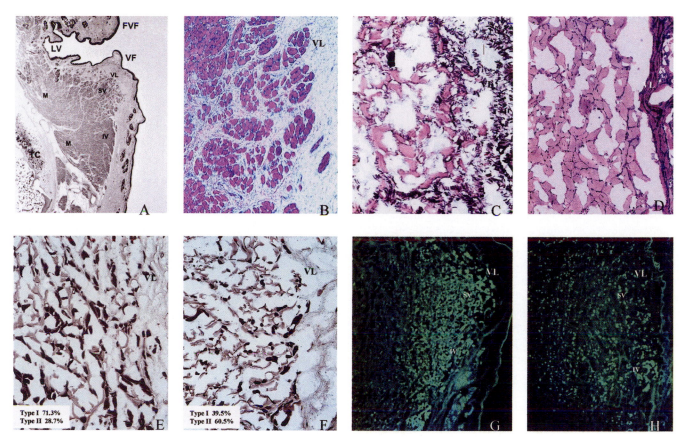

FIGURE 5-11. *Loss of vocalis specialized structure in Idiopathic Parkinson's Disease (IPD).*
(A&B are from a normal individual without IPD; C/D, E/F, G/H are all comparisons of normal/IPD.)
The specialized qualities seen in the human vocalis appear to be related to human speech, and may be preferentially affected by certain neurologic disorders. For example, preliminary results in patients with IPD suggest that these specialized characteristics are preferentially lost in this disease, a possible explanation for the bowed appearance of the vocal folds in this disease. (A) Frontal section of normal human vocal fold showing the various compartments. (B) High power view of normal superior vocalis compartment and its distinctive separate fascicles with muscle fibers of variable diameters (10x). (C) Stained for elastin (dark purple) shows that the muscle fibers of the normal superior vocalis are surrounded by elastic fibers. (D) A specimen from the same area of superior vocalis in an age-matched subject with IPD shows that the elastin is almost completely missing. (E) ATPase staining of normal superior vocalis shows that a majority of muscle fibers are slow-twitch (dark). (F) A specimen from the IPD patient shows that the ratio has shifted to one of predominantly fast muscle fibers. (G) Immuno-fluorescence for slow tonic myosin in a normal patient shows reaction throughout the vocalis with most concentrated in the superior vocalis area. (H) In the IPD patient the amount of slow tonic myosin is dramatically less and the concentration in the superior vocalis is lost.

functional compartment that is mostly active during reflex glottic closure and adduction into the phonatory position.

A third compartment, the centralis, can be appreciated in the dog TA. The centralis originates from the flat anterior face of the body of the arytenoid cartilage and passes anteriorly to insert into connective tissue of the cricothyroid membrane. The centralis appears to have a mechanical advantage in pulling the whole arytenoid forward. An intriguing aspect of the canine centralis is that it appears to be innervated by the communicating nerve and not the RLN. As mentioned above, the communicating nerve is present about 50% of the time and is an extension of the external SLN. Glycogen depletion and degeneration experiments in the dog suggest that the centralis receives its motor innervation from the communicating nerve. The arrangement suggests that the centralis may be evolutionarily related to the cricothyroid muscle. Possibly the relationship is functional, with both the centralis and cricothyroid cooperating to control the intrinsic tension of the vocal fold. There are many unanswered questions regarding both the centralis and the communicating nerve, and this will be a fertile area for future research.

Phonatory Subsystems

In the vocalis, slow-twitch muscle fibers appear to be associated with phonation and fast-twitch muscle fibers with adduction. As concentrations of slow-twitch muscle fibers occur within other laryngeal muscles, it is possible that these areas are also directly involved in phonation. The areas of slow-twitch muscle fiber concentrations may function together as a phonatory subsystem within the larynx. The organization of a hypothetical phonatory subsystem can be summarized as follows: Once the vocal folds are adducted into position for phonation, only small parts of the laryngeal muscles are highly active. The candidates for a phonatory subsystem include the vocalis compartment of the TA, the horizontal compartment of the posterior cricoarytenoid muscle, the transverse interarytenoid muscle (but not the oblique interarytenoid), and a poorly defined part of the cricothyroid muscle. It is interesting that anatomic studies of the human larynx have demonstrated that muscle spindles, a proprioceptive element involved in fine control of muscle tension, are only found in those four locations.

Just as phonation is associated with slow-twitch muscle fibers, articulation of the vocal folds may be associated with fast-twitch muscle fibers. The muscle fibers of the lateral compartment of the TA (the muscularis) are almost 100% fast-twitch in both humans and dogs. It is possible that this specialization for rapid motion in the muscularis is to perform the adduction required in reflex glottic closure. High concentrations of fast-twitch muscle fibers are also found in the false vocal fold and in the lateral cricoarytenoid. Together these areas form a sheet of muscle on the outside of the larynx that cooperates to rapidly adduct the vocal folds.

REFERENCES

1. Dilworth TFM. The nerves of the human larynx. *J Anat.* 1922;56:48-52.

2. Sanders I, Wu BL, Mu L, et al. The innervation of the human posterior cricoarytenoid muscle: evidence for at least two neuromuscular compartments. *Laryngoscope.* 1994;104:880-884.

3. Zemlin WR, Davis P, Gaza C. Fine morphology of the posterior cricoarytenoid muscle. *Folia Phoniatr (Basel).* 1984;36:233-240.

4. Negus VE. *The Comparative Anatomy and Physiology of the Larynx.* New York, NY: Grune & Stratton; 1949.

5. Faaborg-Andersen K. Electromyographic investigation of intrinsic laryngeal muscles in humans. *Acta Physiol Scand.* 1957;41(suppl 140).

6. Ishizaka K, Flanagan JF. Synthesis of voice sounds from a two mass model of the vocal cords. *Bell Sys Tech J.* 1972;51:1233-1267.

7. Hirano M, Ohala J. Use of hooked wire electrodes for electromyography of the intrinsic laryngeal muscles. *JSHR.* 1969;12:362-373.

8. Hirose H, Gay T. The activity of the intrinsic laryngeal muscles in voicing control—an electromyographic study. *Phonetica.* 1972;25:140-164.

9. Dedo HH. The paralyzed larynx: an electromyographic study in dogs and humans. *Laryngoscope.* 1970;80:1455-1517.

10. Kotby MN, Haugen LK. Critical evaluation of the action of the posterior cricoarytenoid muscle, utilizing direct EMG study. *Acta Otolaryngol (Stockh).* 1970;70:260-268.

11. Gay T, Hirose H, Strome M, et al. Electromyography of the intrinsic laryngeal muscles during phonation. *Ann Otol Rhinol Laryngol.* 1972;81:401-409.

12. Sanders I, Jacobs I, Wu BL, et al. The three bellies of the canine posterior cricoarytenoid muscle: implications for understanding laryngeal function. *Laryngoscope.* 1993;103:171-177.

13. Sanders I, Rao F, Biller HF. Arytenoid motion evoked by regional electrical stimulation of the canine posterior cricoarytenoid muscle. *Laryngoscope.* 1994;104:458-462.

14. Drake W, Li Y, Rothschild MA, et al. A technique for displaying the entire nerve branching pattern of a whole muscle: results in ten canine posterior cricoarytenoid muscles. *Laryngoscope.* 1993;103:141-148.

15. Willis R. On the mechanism of the larynx. *Trans Cambridge Philosoph Soc.* 1933;4:323-352.

16. Sonesson B. Die funktionelle Anatomie des Cricoarytenoid-gelenkes. *Z Anat Entwick Lungsgesch.* 121:292-303.

17. Von Leden H, Moore P. The mechanics of the cricoarytenoid joint. *Arch Otolaryngol.* 1961;73:541-550.

18. Frable MA. Computation of motion at the cricoarytenoid joint. *Arch Otol.* 1961;73:551-555.

19. Ardran GM, Kemp FH. The mechanism of the larynx. Part I: The movements of the arytenoid and cricoid cartilages. *Br J Radiol.* 1966;39:641-654.

20. Guth L, Samaha FJ. Procedure for the histochemical demonstration of actomyosin ATPase. *Exp Neurol.* 1970;28:365-367.

21. Williams PL, Warwick R, Dyson M, et al. *Gray's Anatomy.* 37th ed. Edinburgh: Churchill Livingstone; 1989:1117,1256,1258.

22. Windhorst U, Hamm TM, Stuart DG. On the function of muscle and reflex partitioning. *Behav Brain Sci.* 1989;12:629-681.

23. Lemere F. Innervation of the larynx. I: Innervation of laryngeal muscles. *Am J Anat.* 1932;51:417-438.

24. King BT, Gregg RL. An anatomical reason for the various behaviors of paralyzed vocal cords. *Ann Otol Rhinol Laryngol.* 1948;57:925-944.

25. Rueger RS. The superior laryngeal nerve and the interarytenoid muscle in humans: an anatomical study. *Laryngoscope.* 1972; 82:2008-2031.

26. Pressman JJ. Sphincter action of the larynx. *Arch Otolaryngol.* 1941;33:351-377.

27. Vogel PH. The innervation of the larynx of man and the dog. *Am J Anat.* 1952;90:427-447.

28. Ogura JH, Lam RL. Anatomical and physiological correlations on stimulating the human superior laryngeal nerve. *Laryngoscope.* 1953;63:947-959.

29. Mu L, Sanders I, Wu BL, et al. The intramuscular innervation pattern of the human interarytenoid muscle. *Laryngoscope.* 1994;104:33-39.

30. Li Y, Sanders I, Biller HF. Axons enter the human posterior cricoarytenoid muscle from the superior direction. *Arch Otolaryngol-Head Neck Surg.* 1995;121(7):754-757.

31. Hirano M, Ohala J, Vennard W. The function of the laryngeal muscles in regulating fundamental frequency and intensity of phonation. *J Speech Hear Res.* 1969;12:616-628.

32. Stroud MH, Zwiefach E. Mechanism of the larynx and recurrent nerve palsy. *J Laryngol Otol.* 1956;70:86-96.

33. Zemlin WR. *Speech and Hearing Science: Anatomy and Physiology.* Englewood Cliffs, NJ: Prentice-Hall; 1968.

34. Sanders I, Mu L, Wu BL, et al. The intramuscular nerve supply of the human lateral cricoarytenoid muscle. *Acta Otolaryngol (Stockh).* 1993;113:679-682.

35. Wustrow F. Bau und funktion des menschlichlen Musculus vocalis. *Z Anat Entwick Lungsgesch.* 1952;116:506-552.

36. Sonesson B. On the anatomy and vibratory pattern of the human vocal folds. *Acta Otolaryngol.* 1960;(suppl 156).

37. Tieg E, Dahl HA, Thorkelson H. Actinomyosin ATPase activity of human laryngeal muscles. *Acta Otolaryngol.* 1978;85:272-281.

38. Sahgal V, Hast MH. Histochemistry of primate laryngeal muscles. *Acta Otolaryngol.* 1974; 78:277-281.

39. Kersing W. *De stembandmusculatur een histologische en histochemische studie* [Thesis]. University of Utrecht, Utrecht, Holland. 1983.

40. Sanders I, Wu BL, Biller HF. Phonatory specializations of human laryngeal muscles. *Ann Otol Laryngol.* In press.

41. Sanders I, Han Y, Biller HF. *Evidence that the tension of the vocal cord mucosa is under the direct control of vocalis muscle fibers.* Presented at the 23rd Annual Symposium of The Voice Foundation; June 6-11, 1994; Philadelphia, PA.

42. Wu BL, Sanders I, Biller FH. The human communicating nerve: an extension of the external superior laryngeal nerve which innervates the vocal cord. *Arch Otolaryngol.* 1994;120:1321-1328.

43. Vesalius A. *De corporis humani fabrica,* 1545.

44. Zaretsky L, Sanders I. The three bellies of the canine cricothyroid muscle. *Ann Otol Laryngol.* 1992; 156(suppl):2.

45. Vilkman EA, Pitkanen R, Suominen H. Observations on the structure and the biomechanics of the cricothyroid articulation. *Acta Otol (Stockh).* 1987;103:117-126.

46. Stone RE, Nuttal AL. Relative movements of the thyroid and cricoid cartilages assessed by neural stimulation in dogs. *Acta Otolaryngol (Stockh).* 1974;78:135-140.

47. Ferrein A. *De la formation de la voix de l'homme. Mem Acad R Sci (Paris).* 1741;51:409-430.

48. Suzuki M, Kirschner JA, Murakami Y. The cricothyroid as a respiratory muscle. Its characteristics in bilateral recurrent laryngeal nerve paralysis. *Ann Otol Rhinol Laryngol.* 1970;79.

49. Konrad HR, Rattenborg CC. Combined action of laryngeal muscles. *Acta Otolaryngol (Stockh).* 1969;67:646-649.

50. Farnsworth DW. High speed motion pictures of the human vocal cords. *Bell Lab Record.* 1940;18:203-208.

51. Hiroto I, Hirano M, et al. Electromyographic investigation of the intrinsic laryngeal muscles related to speech sounds. *Ann Otol Rhinol Laryngol.* 1967;76:861-872.

52. Matsushita H. The vibratory mode of the vocal folds in the excised larynx. *Folia Phoniatr (Basel).* 1975;27:7-18.

53. Berke GS, Moore DM, Hantke DR, et al. Laryngeal modeling: theoretical, in vitro, in vivo. *Laryngoscope.* 1987;97:871-881.

54. Hirano M, Yoshida Y, Tanaka S. Vibratory behaviour of human vocal cords viewed from below. In: Gauffin J, Hammarberg B, eds. *Vocal Fold Physiology.* San Diego, CA: Singular; 1991:chap 1.

55. Yumoto E, Kadota Y, Kurokawah H. Infraglottic aspect of canine vocal fold vibration: affect of increase of mean air flow rate and lengthening of vocal fold. *J Voice.* 1993;7(4):311-318.

56. Baer T. Measurement of vibration patterns of excised larynges. *J Acoust Soc Am.* 1983;54:318.

57. Pressman JJ. Physiology of the vocal cords in phonation and respiration. *Arch Otolaryngol.* 1942;35:355-398.

58. Van Den Berg J. On the role of the laryngeal ventricle in voice production. *Folia Phoniatr (Basel).* 1955;7:57-69.

59. Van Den Berg J. Myoelastic-aerodynamic theory of voice production. *Speech Hear Res.* 1958;1(3):227-243.

60. Miller RL. Nature of the vocal cord wave. *J Acoust Soc Am.* 1959;31(6):667-677.

61. Helmholtz H. *On the Sensations of Tone as a Physiologic Basis for the Theory of Music.* New York, NY: Dover; 1954.

62. Jiang JJ, Titze IR. Measurement of vocal fold intra-glottal pressure and impact stress. *J Voice.* 1994;8:132-144.

63. Sanders I, Han Y, Wang J, Biller HF. Muscle spindles are concentrated in the superior vocalis subcompartment of the human thyroarytenoid muscle. *J Voice.* 1998;12:7-16.

64. Wang J, Han Y, Sanders I. The superior vocalis of the human thyroarytenoid muscle contains a specialized and possibly unique muscle fiber architecture. *Bull Am Acad Otolaryngol Head Neck Surg.* 1998;17:49.

65. Morgan DL, Proske U. Vertebrate slow muscle: I structure, pattern of innervation and mechanical properties. *Physiol Reviews.* 1984;64:103-168.

66. Hess A. Vertebrate slow muscle fibers. *Physiol Reviews.* 1970;50:40-62.

67. Simpson S. The distribution of tonic and twitch muscle fibers in the avian wing. *Am Zoologist.* 1979;19:925 (Abstract).

68. Fernand VSV, Hess A. The occurrence, structure and innervation of slow and twitch muscle fibers in the tensor tympani and stapedius of the cat. *J Physiol.* 1969;200:547-554.

CHAPTER 6

Benign Vocal Fold Pathology Through the Eyes of the Laryngologist

John S. Rubin, MD, FACS, FRCS

Eiji Yanagisawa, MD, FACS

There are numerous causes of benign vocal fold pathology. Because the laryngeal tract can only respond in certain ways, the symptoms produced are limited, and the resultant degree of clinical dysphonia depends more on the degree of air-wasting, amount of contact of the vocal folds, and alteration of vocal fold stiffness/mass effect, than on the specific disorder.

While the entire body must be looked upon as the vocal organ, this chapter will limit itself to benign processes directly affecting the vocal folds. It is being written by the laryngologist for the laryngologist. Thus, the primary focus will be on processes brought about by vocal misuse and abuse, eg, polyps, nodules, granulomas, cysts, Reinke's edema.

Some of the confusion regarding etiology and pathogenesis of vocal abuse related processes is the result of failure of the pathologist to make crisp distinctions. Often, H&E stains of nodules and polyps look alike.[1] Some of the blame must also be laid on the laryngologist for not giving adequate anatomic orientation of the lesion or clinical expectation. The pathologist and the laryngologist need to consider themselves a team. Much as with cancer specimens, the laryngologist should develop the habit of reviewing and orienting each specimen with the pathologist.

A representative series of benign pathology excised from the vocal folds is taken from Bouchayer (Table 6-1).[2]

Specimen	Percentage of Total
nodule	24%
cyst	17%
(14% epidermoid, 3% retention)	
sulcus	12%
polyp	11%
other	7%
pseudocyst	6%
Reinke's	6%
polypoid nodule	5%
chronic laryngitis	4%
postoperative scarring	3%
microweb	3%
granuloma	1%
papillomatosis	<1%
Total	**1283 lesions**

TABLE 6-1. *Example of Pathologic Epecimens Removed at Surgery for Benign Vocal Fold Lesions. From Bouchayer M and Cornut G. Microsurgery for benign lesions of the vocal folds.* Ear Nose Throat J. *1988;67:446-466.*

RELEVANT ANATOMY OF THE VOCAL FOLD

The key to a reasoned approach to management of these lesions is a detailed understanding of the relevant anatomy of the vocal fold and, in particular, of the laryngeal "cover," as most of the pathology is found there. In previous chapters, Sasaki and Sato have already extensively described anatomic aspects relating to the vocal fold edge. Nonetheless, for orientation to the remainder of this chapter, certain anatomic aspects will be emphasized. Much of the following is attributable to Hirano and/or Gray.

The notion of cover and body fit well with studies of vocal fold vibration showing not only medial-lateral motion but also vertical motion.[3,4] The mucosal wave is caused by a mucosal upheaval, which starts low on the vocal fold and travels superiorly. The concept is that medial and superficial tissue glide over a more rigid body.[5]

The cover consists of the epithelium and superficial layer of the lamina propria (SLLP). The middle (MLLP) and deep (DLLP) layers of the lamina propria make up the vocal ligament. Whereas the SLLP is reasonably well-defined, the vocal ligament is not; at its depths, some collagenous fibers insert into the underlying vocalis muscle (Figure 6-1).[6,7] The MLLP and the DLLP constitute the transition and the muscle makes up the body.

Considerable work has detailed the lamina propria in humans to be composed of cells, mostly fibroblasts, and matrix substances excreted by these cells, including interstitial proteins (glycosaminoglycans and proteoglycans) and fibrous proteins (especially collagen and elastin).[8,9] Capillaries, veins, and macrophages are also found there.[8]

Gray points out that the vast majority of the "cover" is extracellular and of the body, cellular. He considers the fibrous proteins to be scaffolding and the interstitial proteins to be "filling" by virtue of their location in the spaces between. In his view, the former are designed to handle stress and the latter to control tissue viscosity and water content.[10]

The larynx changes throughout life. There is, for example, a steady increase in elastin content of the lamina propria as we age, with a decrease in its distensibility caused by cross-branching.[11] There is also a thinning of the SLLP in the elderly.[11] Yet, as pointed out by

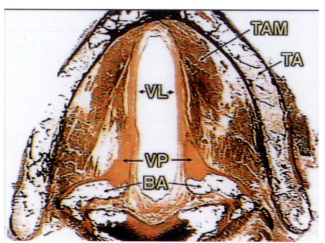 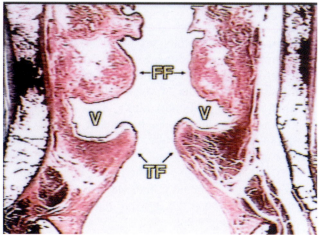

FIGURE 6-1. *The whole organ sections of the mid larynx.*

Left: Transverse section (stained for elastic tissues)
    VL   = vocal ligament
    VP   = vocal process of the arytenoid cartilage (the vocal process never ossifies)
    BA   = body of the arytenoid cartilage (the body usually ossifies)
    TAM = thyroarytenoid muscle
    TA   = thyroid ala

Right: Coronal section (hematoxylin and eosin)
    FF   = false fold
    V   = ventricle
    TF   = true fold

(Courtesy of John A. Kirchner, MD, Yale University, New Haven, CT)

Woo,[12] the vast majority of elderly patients with voice disorders have disease processes associated with aging rather than physiologic aging alone. Only 4% have bowing and breathiness consistent with presbylarynges.

In the normal adult male vocal fold, the mucosa is approximately 1.1 mm in thickness, and the length of the membranous segment is approximately 15 mm.[13] The vocal fold is classically described as being two-thirds membranous and one-third cartilaginous, although Hirano reports that the membranous to cartilaginous ratio is 3 to 2.[13] At the anterior and posterior ends of the membranous vocal fold, the intermediate layer condenses to form the anterior and posterior macula flava, connecting the vocal fold to the anterior commissure tendon and to the vocal process of the arytenoid, respectively. Hirano postulates that they serve as cushions against the trauma of vocal fold vibration.[6]

Epithelium

On coronal section of the membranous vocal fold, the most superficial layer encountered is stratified squamous epithelium. This layer is thin but stiff. Whereas most of the laryngopharynx consists of respiratory pseudostratified ciliated columnar epithelium, only the anterior surface of the epiglottis, superior margin of the aryepiglottic folds, and margins of the vocal folds are covered with stratified squamous epithelium.[14] This in itself affects distribution of neoplasms; for example, squamous papilloma have a predilection for stratified squamous epithelium (Figure 6-2).

The epithelium is 5-25 cell thickness deep and multilayered. Cells are mitotically formed in the basal layer, and attached to the basement membrane by hemidesmosomes. Their nuclei are euchromatic denoting intense metabolic activity.[15] As they mature and migrate out, they are known as "pickle" cells. The most superficial layer consists of 1-3 flattened cells with small condensed nuclei; they are generally lost by surface abrasion.

The epithelium is mucus-coated derived not only from glands in the ventricles but also from special mucin-producing cells embedded in the epithelium.[16] Langerhan's cells, which are immunologically active, are found in the epithelium.[17]

Basement Membrane Zone

Gray has studied the basement membrane zone (BMZ), which mechanically links the epidermis and the SLLP.[18] He identified a chain-link fence arrangement of anchoring fibers which provide increased structural integrity and which he postulates allow for tissue compression and bending. Of interest, the population density of anchoring fibers is greatest in the mid-membranous region, an area subject to most stress.[18]

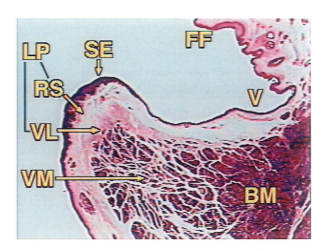

FIGURE 6-2. *Enlarged view of coronal section of vocal fold.*

SE = *squamous epithelium*
LP = *lamina propria*
RS = *Reinke's space (superficial layer of lamina propria)*
VL = *vocal ligament (formed by intermediate and deep layers of lamina propria)*
VM = *vocalis muscle*
BM = *body of thyroarytenoid muscle*
V   = *ventricle*
FF = *false fold*

(Courtesy of John A. Kirchner, MD, Yale University, New Haven, CT)

SLLP (Reinke's Space)

Just deep to the BMZ is the SLLP (Reinke's space). This layer contains loose tissue with sparse collagenous or mature elastin fibers, and few to no capillaries, seromucinous glands, or lymphatics. It does contain elastin precursors (elaunin and oxytalan) and a ground substance network of mucopolysaccharides, decorin and hyaluronic acid[8,11,18] allowing for a pliable consistency.[19]

Macrophages and myofibroblasts have also been found in about one-third of specimens studied by Catten et al. In that review, women had significantly more macrophages than men, suggesting an inflammatory response of the SLLP to trauma, the macrophages being involved in immunologic "mop-up" activities.[20] Similarly, fibroblasts are activated following trauma.[21]

Fibronectin is found in normal nondamaged vocal folds, maximally in the SLLP. It may be one determinant of tissue deformability in the SLLP.[1] Of interest, it is known to be deposited as a result of tissue injury.

The SLLP is sharply delimited by dense fibrous tissue in the anterior commissure, along the vocal process of the arytenoid and beneath the free margin of the vocal fold. The upper limit is not as well defined and may vary considerably in size, usually reaching to the inferior aspect of the ventricle and occasionally to the inferior surface of the ventricular fold. Use of the ventricular folds has been postulated to force fluid within Reinke's space towards the free edge of the vocal fold.[22]

Middle Layer of the Lamina Propria (MLLP)

The MLLP consists predominantly of longitudinally oriented, mature elastin fibers. Other proteins also responsible for its mechanical properties include hyaluronic acid and fibromodulin.[11] Hyaluronic acid is found in greater quantities in the MLLP than elsewhere in the lamina propria. Hyaluronic acid molecules are hydrophilic because of their inherent negative electrical charge. They are relatively inflexible molecules, and may act both as a space filler and as a "shock absorber," particularly in men in whom they are found to be more abundant than women.[8]

Deep Layer of the Lamina Propria (DLLP)

The DLLP consists primarily of collagenous fibers that are arrayed in a longitudinal pattern, parallel to both the vocal fold edge and the vocalis muscle. Fibroblasts are more abundant in this layer than other areas of the lamina propria.[20]

INJURY (GENERAL)

The cause of vocal fold injury and the pathologic response to that injury have been debated for years. Concepts of injury have included the following:

1. Microtrauma from excessive force during phonation causing vascular changes with interruption of the microcirculation. The temporary ischemia may be followed by disruption of capillaries and increased permeability, possibly with microhematomae, followed by rapid organization and then a fibrous mass. Once edema accumulates, it is difficult to dissipate as the lymphatic drainage of the vocal folds is so poor.[23]

2. Voice misuse. Examples might include prolonged use of intensity changes, rather than frequency changes for emphasis, use of a monotone, affectation of a low fundamental frequency. All of these could cause edema of the lamina propria.[24]

3. Direct compression on the vocal fold surface by the hammering effect of forceful vibrations during phonation, causing mucosal changes with a tendency toward parakeratosis, acanthosis, and development of rete ridges, especially in long-standing polyps and nodules. Hyaline changes seen therein may represent further degeneration in certain types of polyps and nodules.

Epidermoid cysts may represent a form of implantation dermoid cyst because of the microtrauma, sending islets of squamous epithelium into the lamina propria.[25]

4. Effects of systemic/external factors. These are multifactorial and might include smoking, gastroesophageal reflux, environmental irritants, musculoskeletal issues, endocrine disorders, and allergy.

Inhalatory or nutritional allergy has been postulated to make the laryngeal mucosa more susceptible to all the above-mentioned factors.[26] Dixon has stated that nutritional allergy and chemical sensitivity are particularly common causes of laryngeal signs, including mild swelling and irritation of the vocal folds and increased mucus production.[27]

Any number of systemic illnesses, ranging from viral laryngitis to AIDS, can cause a state of increased capillary fragility and/or decreased platelet function. Similarly, systemic use of such medications as corticosteroids, aspirin or nonsteroidal anti-inflammatory drugs (NSAIDS), or hormonal changes surrounding menstruation could also contribute. See the chapters by Rubin et al on "Special Considerations for the Professional Voice User," or by Harris and Rubin on "Medications and the Voice" for further insights.

It should be recalled that the locus of vocal fold trauma, the junction of the anterior one-third and posterior two-thirds of the vocal fold, actually represents the midpoint of the membranous vocal fold, ie, the site of highest trauma on phonation.

Histopathologic Injury

Recently Gray et al have presented theories of injury patterns from electron microscopic and immunohistochemical investigations of benign vocal fold pathology. Their research can be summarized as follows:

1. One type of injury pattern found included BMZ and SLLP disruption. The BMZ was characterized by marked thickening with disorientation and disarray of the anchoring fibers. The SLLP was characterized by abnormally increased deposition of fibronectin (an early response to injury). This injury pattern is rarely seen in other body tissues, and is suggestive of repetitive injury.[1,18] This pattern was commonly seen in vocal fold nodules and in some vocal fold polyps.

2. Another type of injury pattern demonstrated the BMZ to be reasonably intact, but with a relative absence of structural glycoproteins and fibrous proteins in the SLLP. This led to a propensity to increased deformability, or a "jelly-like" state, and was seen in some polyps and Reinke's edema/polypoid corditis.[1]

NONSPECIFIC LARYNGITIS

Acute Nonspecific Laryngitis

Acute nonspecific laryngitis is an extremely common ailment, only rarely coming to the attention of the laryngologist. It can result from many causes: voice abuse, menses, a viral exanthem or bacterial infection, laryngeal irritation from smoke or chemicals, and others.

Clinical Presentation and Vocal Dynamics

The patient complains of a painful throat, often with the feeling of pain upon initiation of swallow. Progressive hoarseness is noted, occasionally even complete aphonia. The voice tends to improve somewhat after swallowing, gently clearing the throat or initiating speaking, and then worsens after prolonged speaking.

Usually, laryngoscopy demonstrates vocal fold edema to some degree. Erythema, especially along the vibratory aspects of the folds, and dilated mucosal blood vessels may be noted.

Treatment

Management is judicious voice rest, increased fluid intake, and humidification. Generally acute nonspecific laryngitis is self-limited and will resolve in a few days unless it is bacterial in etiology, in which case antibiotics may be indicated.

Chronic Nonspecific Laryngitis

Whereas the causes of this process are somewhat similar to acute laryngitis, the process is long-standing, with diffuse mucosal edema and occasionally with epithelial hyperplasia. Smoking is often an underlying etiology. Mucosal changes may be irreversible.[28]

Clinical Presentation and Vocal Dynamics

The patient presents with chronic hoarseness and pain; laryngoscopy reveals thickened and dull vocal folds, usually with mild generalized edema. The mucosa may be redundant in association with areas of leuko-plakia and hyperkeratosis. It may appear quite similar to early Reinke's edema.

Treatment

Management includes voice rest, humidification, and elimination of any irritant. Biopsy may be necessary to rule out a laryngeal malignancy. Kleinsasser recommends that surgery, when deemed necessary, be performed on one side first and then the other, with at least a 3-week interval between procedures to allow for adequate healing.[29]

LARYNGITIS ASSOCIATED WITH GASTROESOPHAGEAL REFLUX DISEASE (GERD): MORE RECENTLY TERMED LARYNGOPHARYNGEAL REFLUX

This subject is extensively described in the chapter by Koufman.

GERD was initially associated with laryngeal pathology by Chevalier Jackson.[30] The popularity of this concept among otolaryngologists waxed and waned until GERD was nearly forgotten. In 1968, Cherry and Margulies revived interest in it.[31] In the 1980s, it became more apparent to laryngologists that GERD plays an important role in patients with voice disorders. In fact, laryngopharyngeal manifestations of GERD represent laryngopharyngeal reflux, also called extra-esophageal reflux.

Clinical Presentation and Vocal Dynamics

Symptoms can be plebeian. The patient may complain of hoarseness, local irritation, cough or catarrh, throat clearing, pain upon initiation of swallow, and/or a lump in the throat.[32] In performers there may be no symptoms as the patient is inured to the process. Heartburn and bilious taste in the mouth are classically described but uncommon to obtain in the history. Male predominance has been reported.

Physical findings most commonly are inflammation and edema of arytenoids and postcricoid mucosa.

Treatment

Management includes a change in eating and drinking habits, head of bed elevation, and a trial of H2-blockers or proton pump inhibitors. With the advent of laparoscopic surgery there may be more of a role in the future for surgical restoration of the sphincter. See the section on granuloma, Dr. Koufman's chapter on GERD, and Dr. Sataloff's chapter on medical management of benign voice disorders for further insights.

COMMON DISCRETE LARYNGEAL LESIONS SEEN BY THE VOICE SPECIALIST

Vocal Fold Polyp

Whereas vocal fold nodules have the greater overall prevalence, vocal fold polyps appear to be the more common benign surgical lesion removed.

In Kleinsasser's review of 900 cases of vocal fold polyps, he found that 76% of patients were males. The mean age was 40 years in males and 38 years in females. Ten percent of polyps were bilateral and 5% were both multiple and unilateral. Eighty to 90% of patients smoked cigarettes. Other contributing factors included inhaled allergens and irritants. All polyps occurred at the anterior one-third of the vocal fold.[33] In general, polyps develop on the free edge of the musculomembranous portion of the vocal fold, as this is the location of maximal aerodynamic and muscular forces (Figure 6-3).

Pathogenesis and Histology

Phonotrauma with mechanical stress causing localized subepithelial edema, the development and subsequent abrupt reduction of high subglottic pressure, and increased hyperemia of the vocal fold with vasodilation have all been linked to polyp formation.[33-35] Increased permeability of vessel walls then allows extravasation of edematous fluid, fibrin, and erythrocytes. Subsequently, labyrinthine thin-walled vascular spaces form. These are not vasoformative neoplasms, but reactive endothelial cells similar to a thrombus.[35,36]

Ultrastructural studies have demonstrated the BMZ to be more or less unaltered. Large clusters of angiomatous appearing vessels frequently disrupted the laminar pattern; fibronectin deposition clustered around these clusters. There was a relative decrease of Collagen type IV in the surface epithelium and one author felt that perhaps this predisposed to polyp formation.[37] Another researcher found an 11-fold increase of Langerhans' cells in polyps compared to normal controls, suggesting a marked immune response, perhaps to the underlying injury.[38]

Polyps represent one extreme of a chronic edematous swelling of the vocal fold.[39] The gross appearance varies: it may be reddish or white, large or small, sessile or pedunculated. Most are small and sessile, however. Polyps are associated with other vocal fold lesions in 15% of cases.[40] As polyps become more advanced, there appear grape-like convolutions of blood vessels which become progressively pedunculated.[33]

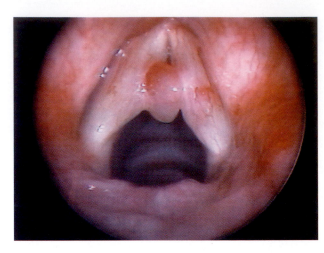

FIGURE 6-3. *Pedunculated polyp arising from the midportion of the left true vocal fold (telescopic view).*

On H&E, histology varies. There are 2 distinct subtypes and 1 combined group by light microscopy (Figure 6-4):

1. Gelatinous polyps: These have very loose edematous stroma, and sparse collagen fibers, between which lie small blood vessels, a few fibrocytes, histiocytes, and mast cells.

2. Telangiectatic polyps: These have homogeneous eosinophilic deposits and fibrin collections in the stroma. Characteristic are labyrinthine sinus-like channels lying between the homogeneous deposits or within the fibrin.[36]

3. Mixed type polyps: These have features of gelatinous and telangiectatic polyps. Polyps of mixed or transitional type are the most common type of polyp seen and contain a nucleus of tortuous vessels embedded in a gelatin substance and covered by squamous epithelium.[36]

Clinical Presentation and Vocal Dynamics

Vocal analysis of patients with vocal fold polyps have demonstrated: 1) the size of the polyp is negatively correlated to fundamental frequency; 2) the size of the polyp is positively correlated to the roughness of voice, the asymmetry and irregularity of vocal fold vibration, and the pitch and amplitude perturbation quotient; and 3) the glottic gap is negatively correlated to maximum phonation time and sound pressure level, but positively correlated to mean airflow rate.[41]

Clinically, initial symptoms are hoarseness and breathiness with reduced dynamic range and decreased

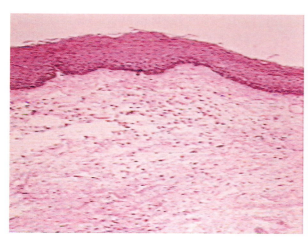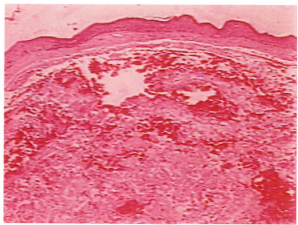

FIGURE 6-4 *Histologic section showing two types of laryngeal polyps: (1) gelatinous polyp (left) and (2) telangiectatic polyp (right). (Courtesy of Romeo A. Vidone, MD, Hospital of St. Raphael, New Haven, CT)*

vocal intensity. The lesion interferes with glottic closure causing decreased flexibility and elasticity of the free edge. It also interferes with vibratory movement of the contralateral fold.

The stiffness varies depending on the histologic type of polyp; stiffness increases when the main feature is hyaline degeneration and thrombosis, but decreases when the main feature is edema.[6] Increased mass of cover causes disturbance of periodicity and synchrony of vibration.[24]

A unilateral polyp may cause diplophonia because of the differing vibratory frequencies of the two folds.[42] Large polyps may cause dyspnea, intermittent dysphagia, and even airway embarrassment. They may rest on the subglottis and may cause a ball-valve effect during labored breathing.[43] Laryngoscopy is usually rapidly diagnostic; the typical polyp appears smooth, soft, and translucent with a broad base.

Treatment

Surgery is frequently required; voice therapy is less likely to be curative than for laryngeal nodules. Nonetheless, initial management with a course of voice therapy is warranted, in association with cessation of cigarette smoking and general removal of environmental irritants. Under these circumstances it is possible that resolution of underlying edema will occur and surgery may be avoided.

Surgical management depends on the size of the polyp. The base of the polyp, which often infiltrates the lamina propria, should generally be removed, preserving as much SLLP as possible and avoiding injury to the vocal ligament. Such an excision may leave a cavity. Often this is not a problem and will fill in without a notch.[40]

Chronic generalized polyps are treated like Reinke's edema with a lateral incision. Staged removal may be required in this setting. More discrete polyps are removed by grasping medially and excising (or lasering). In cases in which fibrous or hyaline infiltration has occurred, voice results will not be ideal. Postoperative voice therapy will be necessary.[39]

Vocal Fold Nodule

Vocal nodules are generally believed to be the most common discrete vocal fold lesion in both children and adults. The etiology is vocal abuse: in children screaming may produce nodules; in adults vocal misuse results from excessive muscle tension which may be related to anxiety, need for a loud voice, and so forth,[44,45] or just from excessive vocalizing. They are rarely seen in introverted bashful individuals. Other postulated etiologies include the use of an unnaturally low fundamental frequency. Men may adopt such fundamental frequency to give themselves an air of authority; women to make the voice more appealing or authoritative; and children may emulate their elders.[24]

When discussing vocal fold nodules, it must be remembered that many older series of vocal fold "nodules" were diagnosed without the benefit of the stroboscope. In fact "nodules" may well be much less common findings than previously believed.

Vocal nodules occur around the free edge of the vocal fold at the anteroposterior midpoint of the membranous fold. They typically are whitish, small, sessile, generally bilateral, and often symmetric (Figure 6-5).

All Kleinsasser's patients were female, between ages 20 and 40. Nearly all were schoolteachers, young mothers, amateur singers, or pop singers. None had studied singing.[46] He states that he has never seen a true

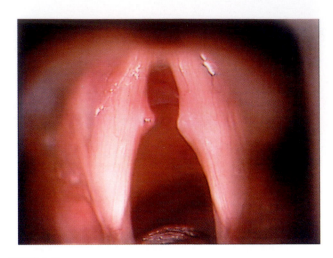

FIGURE 6-5. *Laryngeal nodules (direct microlaryngoscopic view).*

singer's nodule in a man. In our experience nodules may occur in well-trained singers if they oversing or sing when they are ill, or if they misuse/abuse their voices while speaking. Nodules may occur in males as well as females. Nevertheless, we agree with Kleinsasser's basic premises.

Pathogenesis and Histology

Vocal nodules begin as edema and vasodilatation; depending on the chronicity of injury, the edema may differentiate into a hyalinized fibrous nodule.[24,39] Kambic hypothesizes that if the condition persists as generalized edema and does not result in a nodule, it may degenerate into a polyp.[35] The nodule is confined to the superficial layer of the lamina propria.

Grossly, smaller nodules appear glassy-transparent and soft; larger nodules are more solid, conical and usually asymmetric as they enlarge. This evolution represents stages in a process. Singers nodules have been likened to epithelial callus from phonotrauma.[46]

Histologically, nodules demonstrate:

1. The stratified squamous epithelium is hyperkeratotic and sometimes slightly acanthotic. There may also be parakeratosis. An increase in depth of rete ridges with a markedly thickened basement membrane is evident.

2. The subepithelial layer and core are infiltrated with dense irregularly arranged collagen fibers and abundant fibroblasts. It is only minimally vascularized and there are scarcely any inflammatory cells.

3. Edema is present in the connective tissue core; it may be subtle or be a dramatic finding.

4. No fibers in Reinke's space connect to or fix the epithelium to the muscular body of the vocal fold.[7,19,25,46]

Ultrastructural studies have demonstrated the BMZ to be up to three times normal in thickness. The fibronectin pattern was disordered with loss of laminar pattern and more dense than normal. It was seen throughout the lamina propria (rather than mostly in the SLLP as is seen in normals).[37]

Clinical Presentation and Vocal Dynamics

Nodules frequently interfere with complete closure of the glottis during phonation. Mass and stiffness of the cover are increased slightly, but the body is unaffected. The lesion may interfere slightly with the vibratory function of the contralateral fold. On stroboscopic evaluation, pronounced vibration of the anterior segment of the folds extending back to the nodules is seen. A small posterior glottic deficiency of closure is often noted. The clinical findings are hoarseness and breathiness. In singers, loss of frequency range is noted, especially loss of the higher frequencies.[6,24,46]

Treatment

The management of vocal fold nodules is nonsurgical, at least initially. The etiology of the vocal abuse should be carefully investigated and addressed. Voice therapy is the mainstay of therapy; at least 90% of vocal fold nodules will respond to appropriate treatment.

If surgery is eventually required, it should be recalled that this process is strictly superficial. The goal of surgery is a straight edge across the vibratory surface of the vocal fold with minimal disruption of the SLLP.

Reinke's Edema

Reinke's edema is also known as polypoid degeneration, chronic polypoid corditis, chronic edematous hypertrophy, and chronic hypertrophic laryngitis. There has been considerable interest in its pathogenesis and histology in recent years. Reinke's edema is an inflammatory process being the end result of chronic irritation by vocal abuse; it has been postulated that it may begin as polyps or nodules and then evolve with continued trauma.[42]

Pathogenesis and Histology

Etiologic agents have been investigated extensively. In general, smoking appears to be the major etiologic factor identified. In their series of patients with Reinke's edema, Fritzell found 98% of men and 94% of women studied to be smokers, and cessation of smoking improved the larynx, while neither surgery nor voice therapy helped if the patient continued smoking. They found no evidence for allergic disposition in their patients.[47] Other "caustic" exposures to the glottis considered have included gastroesophageal reflux and voice abuse.[48]

Abnormally high subglottic pressure has been noted in Reinke's edema (and certain other functional voice disorders). It has been postulated that this increased pressure together with the other caustic exposures may contribute to the superior distension of the SLLP and increased vascular permeability.[48]

Attempts to correlate thyroid dysfunction as a possible etiology for Reinke's edema have had varied success. Of three studies reviewed, two have not demonstrated any relationship[49,50] while one has.[51]

In general, Reinke's edema is an accumulation of fluid in the superior aspect of the SLLP along the entire length of the membranous fold. It remains localized because of dense anterior and posterior fibrous tissue connections and the poor lymphatic supply. It is almost always bilateral, but may be asymmetric (Figure 6-6).

Histologically, Vecerina-Volic et al have characterized two types of findings: "pale" (transparent) and "livid" (marked subepithelial vascularization.[52] In both types the lamina propria is very loose and edematous, filled with lakes of mucoid fluid interweaved with sheets or masses of immature young elastic fibers.[6,25,29,53]

Authors vary regarding the relative thickness of the basement membrane. Some find it to be thickened[46,52] and the number of anchoring fibers increased.[54] Others differ.[1,37]

In the "pale" type (perhaps just early cases) a limited, fusiform, glazed swelling is noted. The epithelium is thin and the collection of clear watery fluid visible.

In the "livid" (advanced) type, the edematous masses increase, the color changes to yellow-gray, and the fluid thickens to glue-like consistency (Figure 6-6).[46]

Tillmann's studies[55,56] contradict earlier-held beliefs of distended lymphatics in the advanced type. His findings suggest that Reinke's edema has "hollow places" most lined by a layer of mesothelial fibroblast-like cell which develop like neobursae from mechanical strain.

Ultrastructurally and cytologically, studies have demonstrated few structural proteins and little fibronectin in the extracellular matrix.[1] The "pale" type demonstrates stromal cells with numerous intracytoplasmic granules, indicating high metabolic activity. The "livid" type has multiple dilated and irregularly spread vessels.[52] The endothelium has been characterized as having many fenestrae and vesicles, and to exude plasma. Vascular endothelial growth factor is also present.[52] All these features predispose to edema formation in Reinke's space.

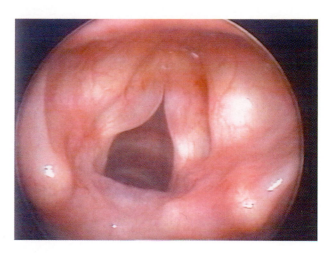

FIGURE 6-6. *Reinke's edema of both vocal folds (telescopic view).*

Clinical Presentation and Vocal Dynamics

There is increased mass of cover but decreased stiffness. The body is not affected but the lesion interferes with the contralateral fold.[9] The glottis does usually close completely during phonation. On laryngoscopy, diffuse irregular vocal folds are noted with a ballooned appearance.

Clinically, the most common sign is lowering of pitch. The vocal quality is hoarse, harsh, gravelly, and breathy. The voice can also be diplophonic. Phonatory characteristics include: 1) an abnormally low mean speaking fundamental frequency; 2) severely reduced dynamic range affecting upper and lower extremes, 3) the highest sustainable tone at least one octave below normals.[57]

Treatment

Speech therapy is necessary to treat the underlying voice disorder. In early stages, and in association with cessation of cigarette smoking, aggressive nonsurgical therapy may be adequate. Most advanced cases will require surgery, however. A decision to operate is based on symptomatology and not the appearance of the folds.

When operating, the free margin must be respected and mucosa should be resected conservatively, if at all. The incision should be, if possible, placed superiorly and laterally, well away from the vibratory surface. The myxoid fluid can generally be bluntly eliminated while respecting the vocal ligament. The mucosa is redraped and excess mucosa trimmed. The patient must not smoke postoperatively.[39,40,58] Two recent studies, one with "cold" instruments and one with the laser have demonstrated a marked improvement in fundamental frequency, to near normal following surgery in most patients. In Zeitels' cases the average fundamental frequency in women rose from 123 to 154 Hz. There were failures, however, particularly in individuals who did not stop smoking.[48,59]

Vocal Fold Cyst

Intracordal cysts of the vocal fold are either mucus retention or epidermoid cysts. Hypotheses explaining pathogenesis include: 1) occlusion of one or a few mucus gland ducts of the inferior part of the vocal fold. The pressure of the secretions would then promote squamous metaplasia; 2) ingrowth of squamous elements from the free edge of the membranous vocal fold caused by microtrauma from vocal abuse; or 3) congenital anomaly.

Cysts occur equally in both sexes. They are located in the SLLP. Occasionally they will open into the laryngeal lumen or partly insert on the vocal ligament (Figure 6-7).[6,7]

Clinical Presentation and Vocal Dynamics

Milutinovic studied a series of patients with cysts and found functional hyperkinetic vocal abuse patterns, with increased muscular activity during phonation.[60] Colton has identified increased mass as well as stiffness of cover.[7]

Clinically the patient presents with hoarseness. On stroboscopy, unilateral submucosal swelling is noted with rigidity of the involved vocal fold and an asynchronous wave. Frequently edema of the contralateral fold is observed.[39]

Treatment

Cysts do not respond to nonsurgical management. The object of surgery is resection of the lesion with min-

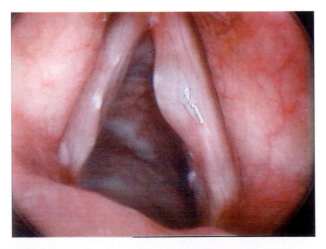

FIGURE 6-7. *Laryngeal cyst involving the midportion of the right true vocal fold (telescopic view).*

imal injury to underlying tissue. Hirano suggests a technique whereby the incision is placed immediately posterior to the cyst at the mediolateral midpoint of the cyst. He emphasizes the difficulty of elevation of covering epithelium mucosa.[61]

Epidermoid Cysts

Epidermoid cysts are whitish structures, which tend to bulge out on the superior and medial aspect of the middle of the musculomembranous vocal fold. They are limited by a cyst wall in the superficial lamina propria and may be attached to connective tissue elements.

Grossly they contain pearly white epithelial debris. Histologically the cavity is bordered by a thin layer of keratinizing stratified squamous epithelium. The debris contains desquamated keratin and cholesterol crystals. The mass expands in a centripetal fashion. Dilated capillaries are sometimes noted converging toward the lesion on the superior aspect of the vocal fold.[40] There is usually no evidence of inflammation.[25]

Clinically it is not always easy to diagnose cysts by examination. In Bouchayer's series only 10% were obviously cysts. Another 55% were suspected to be cysts because of subtle fullness and dilated converging capillaries and stroboscopy showing absent or reduced vibratory pattern; however, 35% were only diagnosed at surgery.[62]

Mucus Retention Cysts

These present quite similarly to the epidermoid cyst; they are yellow cystic masses with mucoid contents caused by obstruction of a gland. They are also usually located in the middle of the musculomembranous vocal fold. As the free edge of the fold is typically devoid of glands, they tend to occur on the inferior aspect. The fold is distorted by the cyst and exhibits loss of vibration. The contralateral fold often develops a nodule.

Histologically in young cysts, the epithelium tends to be columnar and similar to terminal ducts of the small subglottic seromucous glands.[46]

Surgery involves meticulous dissection of the cyst wall from the underlying tissues. The membrane is delicate and often ruptures during removal. All cyst remnants must be removed and the mucous membrane repositioned, ideally without any resection of overlying epithelium.

Postoperatively there is usually no depression visible and the vocal fold returns to normal. Vocal quality is generally much improved but there may be residual huskiness with loss of resonance in the low frequencies.[2]

Other Types of Cysts and Pseudocysts

Other types of cysts and pseudocysts involving the larynx include pseudocysts, posthemorrhagic cysts, ventricular and saccular cysts, and epiglottic cysts. Relatively little has been written about pseudocysts or posthemorrhagic cysts, yet both are not infrequently seen in the busy voice clinic. In Bouchayer's surgical series, he noted a 6% incidence of pseudocysts (as compared with a 3% incidence of epidermoid cysts).[2] In the authors' experience, neither pseudocysts nor posthemorrhagic cysts represent true cysts, in that they do not have a true capsule. Rather they represent a localized area of polypoid degeneration. We have occasionally identified a small scar just below pseudocysts and have posited a relationship thereto (Tom Harris, FRCS, personal communication, 2000). We have been able to identify some pseudocysts as well as some mucus retention cysts of the true vocal fold with the use of ultrasound (Lee et al, unpublished data, 2000).

Ventricular cysts, saccular cysts, and epiglottic cysts are all true cysts of the larynx. As these do not directly involve the true vocal folds they will not be discussed further here. That said, as ventricular cysts and saccular cysts enlarge, they can have an effect both on the voice and on the glottal airway.

Sulcus Vergeture and Sulcus Vocalis

Sulcus Vergeture and Sulcus Vocalis are uncommon clinical conditions. Greisen reports 15 patients with sulcus out of a series of 1,400 referred with voice disorders.[63] Nakayama, however, identified shallow sulci in 4 of 20 larynges removed from random autopsy samples.[64] Thus subclinical sulcus may be more common than expected.

Bouchayer and Cornut distinguish sulcus vergeture from vocalis in the following manner: They consider sulcus vergeture to be a linear depression along the medial margin of the vocal fold which does not extend to the vocal ligament. They consider sulcus vocalis to be a focal invagination of the epithelium, attaching deeply to or through the vocal ligament.[40] Ford distinguishes sulcus into three types, 1 through 3, in which type 1 is a physiologic sulcus with preserved vibratory activity and anatomic layers of the lamina propria. He calls vergeture type 2 and sulcus vocalis type 3.[65] Lindestad and Hertegard do not distinguish them separately (Figure 6-8).[66]

Pathogenesis

Bouchayer has proposed a congenital basis of sulcus vocalis, resulting from faulty development of the 4th and 6th branchial arches. He has also suggested the possible occurrence of rupture of an epidermoid cyst.[62] In support of this concept, Bouchayer has noted a small opening into the lumen in some cases.[2] Most patients with sulcus vocalis can trace their dysphonia to childhood.

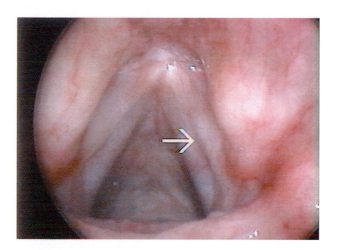

FIGURE 6-8. *Sulcus vergeture. This is an atrophic depression along the free margin of the vocal fold (arrow) (telescopic view) and may be considered a variant of sulcus vocalis.*

The possibility of acquired sulcus has been raised by Nakayama et al,[64] who have identified sulcus deformities on the true folds, adjacent to cancer on 48% of their laryngeal specimens.

Histology

Sulcus vocalis is located in the region of the superficial layer of the lamina propria. From a histologic standpoint the sulcus creates a blind sac; the epithelial walls are thickened stratified squamous epithelium. Hyperkeratosis is a feature, particularly in the deeper aspect of the pit. Collagenous fibers are increased and capillaries decreased throughout.[2,7] The sulcus extends through the level of the superficial lamina propria (which is absent in the area of the sulcus) to adhere to the vocal ligament, the extent depending probably on the inflammatory reaction.

In Ford's series[65] of 20 cases of vergeture or sulcus, all were associated with bilateral abnormalities. In 10 of the cases of sulcus either an epidermoid cyst was identified (n = 9) or an open epidermoid pit was found (n = 1).

Clinical Presentation and Vocal Dynamics

Mechanically, the mass of cover is reduced while the stiffness is increased. The body is not affected.[7] At stroboscopy, a spindle-shaped closure defect may be seen, together with a medial furrow during inhalation, markedly impaired vibration, and frequently supraventricular hyperfunction.[40,63,65] (By contrast, on mirror laryngoscopy the larynx may actually look relatively normal.) Because of the compensatory hyperfunction, the condition is easy to overlook or confuse with the overlying vocal-abuse related pathology.

Clinically, the patient complains of a severely hoarse voice and vocal fatigue. The voice tends to be breathy and aesthenic, especially in males. It is typically effortful. Phonation time is invariably short.[63]

Treatment

Treatment is difficult. Voice therapy has limited success but is essential as an adjunct. Surgical intervention has included injection of teflon[67]; excision of the sulcus with microscissors,[2] or CO_2 laser[68]; incision with undermining, with or without steroid injection[2]; bioimplant[69-71]; medialization thyroplasty[72]; slicing, to break up linear tension.[65,73] Recently there has been considerable interest in fat implantation.[71] Rubin has begun using a deep-ithelialization technique with promising early results. The ideal surgical goal is replacement of the sulcus with normal tissue; currently no such procedure exists.[6] Consequently surgical procedures must be conservative.

Vocal Fold Scarring

Scarring can occur at any site along the vocal fold. The etiology may be trauma, intubation, inflammation, burn, or surgery. It can also occur in any layer.

Pathogenesis

Bouchayer notes 4 typical scar patterns as a result of excessive surgery. These are notches, webs, fibrous scars, and vocal fold rigidity, the latter especially after laser.[2,40]

Clinical Presentation and Vocal Dynamics

Postoperative vocal fold scarring poses a great therapeutic challenge. In essence, one must differentiate between dysphonia caused by the scarring versus that caused by the underlying pathology. Scar tissue, which is dense collagen, is much stiffer than normal tissue. This stiffness will be increased in the layer involved. Mass will vary depending on the amount and extent of injury.[7] Stroboscopy or high-speed photography is extremely important to assess vocal fold vibration. Scarring is likely to cause areas of adynamism and stiffness, interfere with or even obliterate the layered structure and the mucosal wave, and thereby alter phonation. It may also cause dysphonia by mechanical restriction, either of vocal fold vibration or of closure. This is particularly so in cases of dense web or fibrosis.[74]

Objective aerodynamic and acoustic assessment are valuable to diagnosis and documentation, therapy, and to evaluation of efficacy. (See the chapter by Korovin and Rubin, "Introduction to the Laboratory Diagnosis of Vocal Disorders" for further details.)

Treatment

The patient must understand the limitations of treatment. Similarly, before undertaking surgery, the voice team needs to understand the pathology, the vocal needs of the patient, and his or her motivation.

The speech-langauge pathologist must be involved before and after any surgical manipulation. Much as with sulcus vocalis, the patient will have developed compensatory voicing behaviors, which are usually hyperfunctional and counterproductive. The speech-language pathologist will need to work with the patient in an attempt to rid him or her of these behavioral patterns prior to consideration of any surgical intervention.

In general, surgical correction must be approached warily because the ideal procedure, that of replacement of the scarred area with normal tissue, does not yet exist. Procedures to restore the mucosal wave have included the following: steroid injection into the scar or vibratory margin; elevation of a microflap with or without steroid injection; injection of autologous fat into the underlying muscle; injection of collagen into the vocal ligament; and autologous fat implantation. Webs have been treated with excision, z-plasty, and stenting (Harvey Tucker, M.D, personal observation, 2000).[74-77]

Refer to the chapter by Woo for more insights into this problem.

Granuloma of the Larynx

A useful initial approach to vocal granuloma is a review of a study by Lehmann, who identified 61 cases out of 1,300 patients with voice disorders. Twenty-nine were post-traumatic (most caused by intubation), 28 were contact granuloma, and 4 were of unknown etiology. The mean age was 44. Forty-two out of 61 were unilateral, and 51 occurred on the vocal process of the arytenoid. Of the patients with contact granuloma 27 were male.[78] A third major etiology for granuloma is laryngopharyngeal reflux.[6]

Symptoms are mainly moderate or intermittent dysphonia, vocal fatigue, and decreased dynamic range. Less common symptoms include throat-clearing, laryngeal pain, and a dry cough.

Contact Granuloma

These occur mainly in men of a certain vocal pattern and personality. Characteristics frequently noted include: 1) vocal abuse, especially seen in men trying to assume an unnaturally low fundamental frequency. This and laryngopharyngeal reflux are the most commonly accepted causative factors; 2) "en coups de glotte" attack, the achievement of high vocal intensity in a very brief period resulting in the clashing of arytenoids; and

3) a psychologic profile consisting of an aggressive personality, introversion, depression, emotional tension, and cancerophobia.[46]

Pathogenesis and Histology

Contact granuloma occur on the arytenoid process. They are unilateral and have a "2-lipped" form, fitting the vocal process of the contralateral side, which in turn develops slight epithelial hyperplasia.[46]

Histologically there is diversity. Lehmann noted 11 with simple pachydermia, 7 with surface ulceration, 10 with ulcerated granulation tissue.[78] Snow noted the base to be shaggy or granular with the healing process leading perhaps to a nonspecific granuloma.[24] Mossallam found dense connective tissue core with abundant collagen and fibroblasts, excessive vascularity but no edema or inflammation.[25]

Clinical Presentation and Vocal Dynamics

Clinically, the initial complaint is varying degrees of hoarseness and a low-pitched pressed quality to the voice, as well as frequent need to cough and clear the throat.[42] Stroboscopically the anterior folds do not close fully but the cartilaginous portions hammer together.

Treatment

Therapy is voice rest, voice therapy, and reflux treatment as discussed below. Surgery is only required if there is concern of malignancy, but it may be recommended in cases where the granuloma has not improved following several months of conventional therapy. There may also, particularly in recalcitrant cases, be a role for direct injection of steroid into the granuloma or of a dilute solution of botulinum toxin into the ipsilateral thyroarytenoid or lateral cricoarytenoid muscles.[79]

Granuloma From Laryngopharyngeal Reflux

Some controversy exists as to the role of laryngopharyngeal reflux in "contact granuloma." Ohman found 74% of patients with vocal fold granuloma to have esophageal dysmotility versus 30% in the general population.[80] Lehmann, on the other hand, only identified reflux in 1/32 patients with contact granulomas.[78] Feder postulates that both hyperfunctional and hyperacidic granuloma have vocal abuse as the primary etiologic factor.[81] This controversy notwithstanding, laryngopharyngeal reflux most likely represents a separate etiology for granuloma. We believe that antireflux therapy is an appropriate management plan in this group of patients. (See Koufman's chapter for further insights into this subject.)

Intubation Granuloma

The incidence of intubation granuloma is low, varying from 1:100 to 1:20,000 procedures. There is no direct correlation between duration of intubation and occurrence; it has been postulated that an overly large tube, excessive motion of tube or patient, and secondary infection in a debilitated patient are all etiologic factors,[28] and many laryngologists believe that reflux is usually a factor. Unlike contact granuloma, the incidence of intubation granuloma incidence is similar in women and men (women represented 4% of patients with contact granuloma but 44% of patients with intubation granuloma in Lehmann's series were women) (Figure 6-9).[78]

Histology

Histologic studies have demonstrated: 1) the epithelial covering is often eroded with a thick fibrin layer; 2) the connective tissue stroma is filled with abundant fibroblast and collagen fibers; 3) the stroma is much more vascular (hemangioma-like) than the stroma of contact granuloma.[25,46] The lesion is initially broad-based and then develops a mushroom-like configuration. Symptoms are similar to those of other laryngeal granulomata.

Treatment

Some authors[28,63] suggest surgical removal followed by voice therapy; others, including us, suggest medical and/or voice therapy primarily. It should be recalled that these granulomata not infrequently resolve on their own, without referral to any medical personnel.

Nonspecific and Other Granulomatous Conditions

There are a variety of other conditions characterized by granuloma which can affect the larynx.

Postsurgical Granuloma

These have to a large extent been described in the post-trauma section. It should be noted, however, that

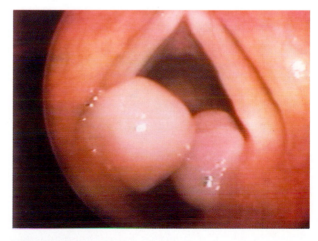

FIGURE 6-9. *Bilateral postintubation granuloma (telescopic view).*

granulomatous changes can occur on the larynx in locations other than the arytenoid processes when excessive tissue, especially including muscle, has been removed, or for other reasons (such as reflux) that have not always been identified. This was the case in 6 patients with granulomata in Lehmann's series.[78]

Postinjection Granuloma

As more experience has accrued with long-term results from endolaryngeal teflon injection, so has more experience with teflon granuloma. Teflon paste injection causes early, brief-onset inflammatory reaction. On a longer-term basis, a foreign body granuloma forms around the teflon. Usually this is self-limited and the short- and long-term results of injection are satisfactory. If the injection is too superficial or too extensive, a foreign body granuloma can cause severe dysphonia with increase in both mass and stiffness (Figure 6-10). Granulomas may occur even when technique has been perfect. Sometimes they develop many years after initially successful teflon injection, which is one of the reasons why this substance has been largely abandoned since the latter 1980s.

Surgical removal is extremely difficult, and the post-surgical voice result is unpredictable.[82] Endoscopic or external techniques may be used.

Inflammatory Arthritis

The cricoarytenoid joint is a synovial joint; hence, it can become involved by a variety of inflammatory processes, including rheumatoid arthritis, gouty arthritis, mumps, tuberculosis, syphilis, gonorrhea, Tietze's syndrome, lupus erythematosus, and so forth.[28] The most common of these etiologies is rheumatoid arthritis, which will be described.

Clinical

Symptoms include hoarseness (most commonly), a feeling of a lump in the throat, odynophagia, dysphonia, and pharyngeal fullness. The patient may complain of difficulty swallowing pills. Physical examination reveals acute inflammation and edema of the mucosa overlying the arytenoid cartilage. There is usually some motion, but frequently the mobility is severely diminished. The arytenoid process is tender to palpation. CT demonstrates subluxation of the cricoarytenoid joint.

Treatment

Therapy is aimed at the underlying condition. If the airway is compromised, an arytenoidopexy or arytenoidectomy might be indicated, or even tracheotomy.

Sarcoidosis

Laryngeal involvement is uncommon but can occur. A large series identified it in 1.3% of cases.[83] The lesion is usually supraglottic, sparing the vocal fold. It can also occur in the subglottic larynx. In Neel's series, the appearance of the larynx was strikingly similar in all patients with supraglottic involvement. The supraglottic larynx was chronically edematous and pale pink. The rim of the epiglottis had a turban-like thickening. When the true vocal folds were involved, it was a reflection of the more extensive subglottic disease. Vocal fold mobility was intact in this series.[84]

Diagnosis is made by biopsy, demonstrating epithelioid tubercles and noncaseating granuloma with giant

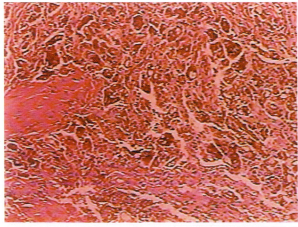
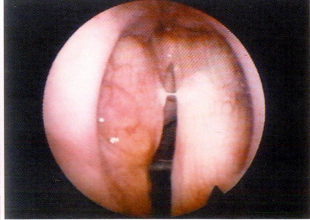

FIGURE 6-10. *Post-teflon injection granuloma involving the left true vocal fold. (Left) telescopic view; (Right) histologic section of teflon granuloma showing multiple foreign bodies. (Courtesy of Richard N. Eisen MD, Yale University, New Haven, CT and Greenwich Hospital, Greenwich CT)*

cells and macrophages. The angiotensin-converting enzyme level frequently is elevated and there may be hyperglobulinemia and hypercalcemia.[85]

Sarcoidosis can also cause vocal fold palsy by mediastinal compression of the left recurrent laryngeal nerve[86,87] or by cranial neuropathy.[28]

Symptoms are frequently mild but progressive airway obstruction can occur, either by diffuse edema or exophytic masses, especially if there is subglottic involvement.[88]

Autoimmune Processes

Systemic lupus erythematosus (SLE) is associated with mucous membrane lesions in 16% of patients and occasionally may involve the larynx. SLE may cause a multitude of processes, including: arthritis of the cricoarytenoid joint, vocal fold hyperplasia, mucosal nodularity, ulceration, inflammation, edema, as well as necrotizing vasculitis with airway obstruction. These latter lesions may mimic acute epiglottitis. Teitel et al have recently reviewed 4 personal cases and 97 cases reported in the literature. They note 28% with laryngeal edema and 11% with vocal fold palsy. The majority of symptoms in patients, including hoarseness, dyspnea, and even vocal fold palsy, resolved following therapy with corticosteroids.[89]

Another uncommon autoimmune disease entity that can affect the larynx is relapsing polychondritis. This disorder involves cartilaginous structures, the most common being the ear (which is affected in 75% of patients), followed by the nose. What is frequently not appreciated is that at some time during the course of the disease process the larynx and trachea can be affected in up to 50% of patients.[90] Involvement is manifested by progressive upper airway obstruction. Symptoms are pain and hoarseness and the findings are erythema and edema.

Laryngotracheal involvement is the most serious consequence of relapsing polychondritis. Airway obstruction may be caused by either destruction of the cartilaginous support or encroachment on the lumen by granulation tissue. This is not an easy diagnosis to make and generally is not made until more than two sites containing cartilage are affected. Two patients in McCaffrey's series of 29 had airway obstruction as their initial presention caused by subglottic involvement and requiring tracheotomy.[28,90]

Idiopathic Granulomata

Idiopathic granulomata and their involvement of the larynx, eg, Wegener's granulomatosis, polymorphic reticulosis, and idiopathic midline granuloma are all covered well by Lebovics in his chapter.

SUMMARY

This chapter has limited itself to benign non-neoplastic processes affecting the vocal folds. It has mainly investigated processes which are commonly seen by the laryngologist specializing in care of voice disorders. In this fashion, an attempt has been made to outline laryngeal pathology from the viewpoint of the laryngologist.

It is clear that the majority of processes seen by the laryngologist relate to the basement membrane zone and to the superficial layer of the lamina propria, and tend to either be self-induced or caused by local irritants.

The vocal dynamics vary depending on the mass and stiffness of the underlying process, as well as the degree of air-wasting caused by the process. Treatment tends to be conservative; management of the underlying self-abusive pattern or irritant is as important as surgical therapy, or even more important.

Goals of surgery in this group of patients are minimal disturbance of underlying tissues and replacement of tissue with tissue which is as near to normal as possible; as has been shown, in some processes the ideal treatment is still not available.

REFERENCES

1. Gray SD, Hammond E, Hanson DF. Benign pathologic responses of the larynx. *Ann Otol Rhinol Laryngol.* 1995;104:13-18.

2. Bouchayer M, Cornut G: Microsurgery for benign lesions of the vocal folds. *Ear Nose Throat J.* 1988;67:446-466.

3. Hirano M. Phonosurgery: basic and clinical investigations. *Otol Fukuoka.* 1975;21:239-242.

4. Sato S. Phonosurgery: basic study on the mechanism of phonation and endolaryngeal microsurgery. *Otol Fukuoka.* 1977;23:171-184.

5. Hirano M, Yoshida T, Tanaka S. Vibratory behavior of human vocal folds viewed from below. In: Gauffin J, Hammarberb B, eds. *Vocal Fold Physiology.* San Diego, CA: Singular Publishing; 1991:1-6.

6. Hirano M. Phonosurgical anatomy of the larynx. In: Ford CN, Bless DM, eds. *Phonosurgery: Assessment and Surgical Management of Voice Disorders.* New York, NY: Raven Press; 1991:25-41.

7. Colton RH, Casper JK. Understanding voice problems. A physiological perspective for diagnosis and treatment. Baltimore, MD: Williams & Wilkins; 1990:51-69.

8. Hammond TH, Zhou R, Hammond EH, Pawlak A, Gray SD. The intermediate layer: a morphologic study of the elastin and hyaluronic acid constituents of normal vocal folds. *J Voice*. 1997;11:59-66.

9. Hirano M. Structure of the vocal fold in normal and disease states: Anatomical and physical studies. In: Ludlow C, ed. *Proceedings of the Conference on the Assessment of Vocal Pathology*. ASHA Report # 11; 1981.

10. Gray SD, Titze IR, Alipour F, Hammond TH. Biomechanical and histologic observations of vocal fold fibrous proteins. *Ann Rhinol Laryngol*. 2000;109:77-85.

11. Hammond TH, Gray SD, Butler J, Zhou R, Hammond E. Age and gender-related elastin distribution changes in human vocal folds. *Otolaryngol Head Neck Surg*. 1998;119:314-322.

12. Woo P, Casper J, Colton R, Brewer D. Dysphonia in the aging: physiology versus disease. *Laryngoscope*. 1992;102:139-144.

13. Kurita S, Nagata K, Hirano M. Comparative histology of mammalian vocal folds. In: Kirchner JA, ed. *Vocal Fold Histopathology: A Symposium*. San Diego, CA: College-Hill Press; 1986:1-10.

14. Meller SM. Functional anatomy of the larynx. In: Fried MP, ed. *Otolaryngol Clin North Am*. 1984;17:3-12.

15. Stiblar-Martincic D. Histology of laryngeal mucosa. *Acta Otolaryngol (Stockh)*. 1997;527 (suppl):138-141.

16. Gipson IK, Spurr-Michaud SJ, Tisdale AS. Stratified squamous epithelia produce mucin-like glycoproteins. *Tissue Cell*. 1995;27:397-405.

17. Thompson AC, Griffin NR. Langerhan cells in normal and pathological vocal cord mucosa. *Acta Otolaryngol (Stockh)*. 1995;115:830-832.

18. Gray SD, Pignatari SSN, Harding P. Morphologic ultrastructure of anchoring fibers in normal vocal fold basement zone. *J Voice*. 1994;8:48-52.

19. Hirano M, Kurita S. Histological structure of the vocal fold and its normal and pathological variations. In: Kirchner JA, ed. *Vocal Fold Histopathology: A Symposium*. San Diego, CA: College-Hill Press; 1986:17-24.

20. Catten M, Gray SD, Hammond TH, Zhou R, Hammond E. Analysis of cellular location and concentration in vocal fold lamina propria. *Otolaryngol Head Neck Surg*. 1998;118:663-667.

21. Hirano M, Sato K, Nakashima T. Fibroblasts in human vocal fold mucosa. *Acta Otolaryngol*. 1999;119:271-276.

22. Kambic V, Gale N, Radsel Z. Anatomical markers of Reinke's space and the etiopathogenesis of Reinke edema. *Laryngo-Rhino-Otologie*. 1989;68(4):231-235.

23. Hiroto J. The etiology of polyp and polypoid degeneration of the vocal fold. *IALP Congress Proceedings. Special paedagogisk Forlag*. Copenhagen; 1977.

24. Snow JB. Surgical therapy for vocal dysfunction. *Otolaryngol Clin North Am*. 1984;17:91-100.

25. Mossallam I, Kotby MN, Ghaly AF, et al. Histopathological aspects of benign vocal fold lesions associated with dysphonia. In: Kirchner JA, ed. *Vocal Fold Histopathology: A Symposium*. San Diego, CA: College-Hill Press; 1986:65-80.

26. Hocevar-Boltezar I, Radsel Z, Zargi M. The role of allergy in the etiopathogenesis of laryngeal mucosal lesions. *Acta Otolaryngol (Stockh)*. 1997;527 (suppl):134-137.

27. Dixon HS. Allergy and laryngeal disease. *Otolaryngol Clin North Am*. 1992;25:239-250.

28. Fried MP, Shapiro J. Acute and chronic laryngeal infections. In: Paparella MM, Shumrick DA, Gluckman JL, et al, eds. *Otolaryngology*. 3rd ed. Philadelphia, PA: WB Saunders; 1991:2245-2256.

29. Kleinsasser O. *Microlaryngoscopy and Endolaryngeal Microsurgery*. Philadelphia, PA: WB Saunders; 1968.

30. Jackson C: Contact ulcer of the larynx. *Ann Otol Rhinol Laryngol*. 1928;37:227-230.

31. Cherry J, Margulies SI. Contact ulcer of the larynx. *Laryngoscope*. 1968;73:1937-1940.

32. Sataloff RT, Castell DO, Katz PO, Sataloff DM. *Reflux Laryngitis and Related Disorders*. San Diego, CA: Singular Publishing Group; 1999.

33. Kleinsasser O. Pathogenesis of vocal cord polyps. *Ann Otol Rhinol Laryngol*. 1982;91:378-381.

34. Roch JB, Cornut G, Bouchayer M. Modes of appearance of vocal cord polyps. *Rev Laryngol Otol Rhinol (Bord)*. 1989;110:389-390.

35. Kambic V, Radsel Z, Zargi M, et al. Vocal cord polyps: incidence, histology and pathogenesis. *J Laryngol Otol*. 1981;95:609-618.

36. Frenzel H. Fine structural and immunohistological studies on polyps of human vocal folds. In: Kirchner JA, ed. *Vocal Fold Histopathology: A*

Symposium. San Diego, CA: College-Hill Press; 1986:39-50.

37. Courey MS, Shohet JA, Scott MA, Ossoff RH. Immunohistochemical characterization of benign laryngeal lesions. *Ann Otol Rhinol Laryngol.* 1996;105:525-531.

38. Melgarejo-Moreno P, Helin-Meseguer D. Estudio mediante anticuerpos policlonales S-100 de las células de Langerhans en los polipos de cuerda vocal. *Acta Otorrinolaringol Esp.* 1999;50:203-204.

39. Werkhaven J, Ossoff RH. Surgery for benign lesions of the glottis. In: Koufman JA, Isaacson G, eds. *Otolaryngol Clin North Am.* 1991;24:1179-1199.

40. Bouchayer M, Cornut G. Instrumental microscopy of benign lesions of the vocal folds. In: Ford CN, Bless DM, eds. *Phonosurgery: Assessment and Surgical Management of Voice Disorders.* New York, NY: Raven Press; 1991:143-165.

41. Sanada T, Tanaka S, Hibi S, et al. Relationship between the degree of lesion and that of vocal dysfunction in vocal cord polyp. *Nippon Jibiinkoka Gakkai Kaiho.* 1990;93:388-392.

42. Stringer SP, Schaefer SD. Disorders of laryngeal function. In: Paparella MM, Shumrick DA, Gluckman JL, et al, eds. *Otolaryngology.* 3rd ed. Philadelphia, PA: WB Saunders; 1991:2257-2272.

43. Yanagisawa E, Hausfeld JN, Pensak ML. Sudden airway obstruction due to pedunculated laryngeal polyps. *Ann Otol Rhinol Laryngol.* 1983;92:340-343.

44. McFarlane SC. Treatment of benign laryngeal disorders with traditional methods and techniques of voice therapy. *Ear Nose Throat J.* 1988;67:425-435.

45. Kauffmann I, Lina-Granade G, Truy E, et al. Chronic hoarseness in children. Evaluation based on personal series of 64 cases. *Pediatrics.* 1992;47:313-319.

46. Kleinsasser O. Microlaryngoscopic and histologic appearances of polyps, nodules, cysts, Reinke's edema, and granulomas of the vocal cords. In: Kirchner JA, ed. *Vocal Fold Histopathology: A Symposium.* San Diego, CA: College-Hill Press; 1986:51-55.

47. Fritzell B, Hertegard S. A retrospective study of treatment for vocal fold edema: A preliminary report. In: Kirchner JA, ed. *Vocal Fold Histopath-ology: A Symposium.* San Diego, CA: College-Hill Press; 1986:57-61.

48. Zeitels SM, Hillman RE, Bunting GW, Vaughn T. Reinke's edema: phonatory mechanisms and management strategies. *Ann Otol Rhinol Laryngol.* 1997;106:533-543.

49. White A, Sim DW, Maran AGD. Reinke's oedema and thyroid function. *J Laryngol Otol.* 1991; 105:291-292.

50. Wedrychowicz B, Nijander D, Betkowski A, Jastrzebski J. Obrzek reinkego a niedoczynnosec tarczycy. *Otolaryngol Pol.* 1992;46:538-542.

51. Benfari G, Carluccio F, Murgiano S, Lentini A. Test di stimolazione della ghiandola tiroide nell'edema di Reinke. Studio in 28 pazienti. *An Clinica Otorrinolaringol Ibero Am.* 1992;19:485-491.

52. Vecerina-Volic S, Kirincic N, Markov D. Some morphological, histological, cytological and histochemical aspects of Reinke's oedema. *Acta Otolaryngol.* 1996;116:322-324.

53. Remenar E, Elo J, Frint T. The morphologic basis for development of Reinke's oedema. *Acta Otolaryngol (Stockh).* 1984;97:169-176.

54. Knobber D. Die basalmembran bei erkrankungen der stimmlippen: elektronenmikroskopische und immunmorphologische befunde. *Laryngorhino-otologie.* 1994;73:642-646.

55. Tillmann B, Rudert H. Licht und elektronen-mikroskopische untersuchungen zum reinkeodem. *HNO.* 1982;30:280-284.

56. Tillmann B, Rudert H, Schunke M, Werner JA. Morphological studies on the pathogenesis of Reinke's edema. *Eur Arch Otorhinolaryngol.* 1995;252:469-474.

57. Bennett S, Bishop S, Lumpkin SMM. Phonatory characteristics associated with bilateral diffuse polypoid degeneration. *Laryngoscope.* 1987;97: 446-450.

58. Bouchayer M, Cornut G. Microsurgical treatment of benign vocal fold lesions: indications, technique, results. *Folia Phoniatr.* 1992;44:155-184.

59. Murry T, Abitbol J, Hersan R. Quantitative assessment of voice quality following laser surgery for Reinke's edema. *J Voice.* 1999;13:257-264.

60. Milutinovic Z, Vasiljevic J. Contribution to the understanding of the etiology of vocal fold cysts: a functional and histologic study. *Laryngoscope.* 1992;102:568-571.

61. Hirano M, Yoshida T, Hirade Y, et al. Improved surgical technique for epidermoid cysts of the vocal fold. *Ann Otol Rhinol Laryngol.* 1989;98:791-795.

62. Bouchayer M, Cornut G, Witzig E, et al. Epidermoid cysts, sulci and mucosal bridges of the true vocal cord: a report of 157 cases. *Laryngoscope.* 1985;95:1087-1094.

63. Greisen O. Vocal cord sulcus. *J Laryngol Otol.* 1984;98:293-296.

64. Nakayama M, Ford CN, Brandenburg JH, Bless DM. Sulcus vocalis in laryngeal cancer: a histopathologic study. *Laryngoscope.* 1994;104:16-24.

65. Ford CN, Inagi K, Bless D, Khidr A, Gilchrist KW. Sulcus vocalis: a rational analytical approach to diagnosis and management. *Ann Otol Rhinol Laryngol.* 1996;105:189-200.

66. Lindestad PA, Hertegard S. Spindle-shaped glottal insufficiency with and without sulcus vocalis: a retrospective study. *Ann Otol Rhinol Laryngol.* 1994;103:547-553.

67. Lee ST, Niimi S: Vocal fold sulcus. *J Laryngol Otol.* 1990;104:876-878.

68. Remacle M, Declaye X, Hamoir M, et al. CO_2 laser treatment of the glottic sulcus and of epidermoid cyst. Technic and results. *Acta Otorhino-laryngol Belg.* 1989;43:343-350.

69. Cornut G, Bouchayer M. Phonosurgery for singers. *J Voice.* 1989;3:269-276.

70. Ford CN, Bless DM. Selected problems treated by vocal fold injections of collagen. *Am J Otolaryngol.* 1993;14:257-261.

71. Sataloff RT. *Professional Voice: The Science and Art of Clinical Care.* 2nd ed. San Diego, CA: Singular Publishing Group; 1997:627-628.

72. Sataloff RT. Vocal fold scar. In: Sataloff RT. *The Science and Art of Clinical Care.* 2nd ed. San Diego, CA: Singular Publishing Group; 1997:555-559.

73. Ford CN, Bless DM, Prehn RB. Thyroplasty as primary and adjunctive treatment of glottic insufficiency. *J Voice.* 1992;6:277-285.

74. Pontes P, Behlau M. Treatment of sulcus vocalis: auditory perceptual and acoustic analysis of the slicing mucosa surgical technique. *J Voice.* 1993;7:365-376.

75. Mikaelian D, Lowry LD, Sataloff RT. Lipoinjection for unilateral vocal cord paralysis. *Laryngoscope.* 1991;101:465-468.

76. Ford CN, Bless DM. Selected problems treated by vocal fold injection of collagen. *Am J Otolaryngol.* 1993;14:257-261.

77. Sataloff RT, Spiegel JR, Hawkshaw M, Rosen DC, Heuer RJ. Autologous fat implantation for vocal fold scar: a preliminary report. *J Voice.* 1997;11:238-246.

78. Lehmann W, Widman JJ. Nonspecific granulomas of the larynx. In: Kirchner JA, ed. *Vocal Fold Histopathology: A Symposium.* San Diego, CA: College-Hill Press; 1986:97-107.

79. Sataloff RT, Castell DO, Katz PO, Sataloff DM. *Reflux Laryngitis and Related Disorders.* San Diego, CA: Singular Publishing Group; 1999:48-49.

80. Ohman L, Oloffson J, Tibbling L, et al. Esophageal dysfunction in patients with contact ulcer of the larynx. *Ann Otol Rhinol Laryngol.* 1983;92:228-230.

81. Feder RJ, Mitchell MJ. Hyperfunctional hyperacidic and intubation granulomas. *Arch Otolaryngol.* 1984;110:582-584.

82. Benjamin B, Robb P, Clifford A, et al. Giant teflon granuloma of the larynx. *Head Neck.* 1991;13:453-456.

83. Carasso B. Sarcoidosis of the larynx causing airway obstruction. *Chest.* 1974;65:693-695.

84. Neel HB Jr, McDonald TJ. Laryngeal sarcoidosis report of 13 patients. *Ann Otol Rhinol Laryngol.* 1982;91:359-362.

85. Kirchner, JA. Nonepithelial benign tumors of the larynx. In: Kirchner JA, ed. *Vocal Fold Histopathology: A Symposium.* San Diego, CA: College-Hill Press; 1986:81-91.

86. Povedano Rodriguez V, Seco Pinero MI, Jaramillo Perez J. Sarcoidosis as a cause of paralysis of the recurrent laryngeal nerve. Presentation of a case. *An Otorrinolaringol Ibero Am.* 1992;19:443-448.

87. Abramowicz MJ, Ninane V, Depierreux M, et al. Tumour-like presentation of pulmonary sarcoidosis. *Eur Respir J.* 1992;5:1286-1287.

88. Weisman RA, Canalis RF, Powell WJ. Laryngeal sarcoidosis with airway obstruction. *Ann Otol Rhinol Laryngol.* 1980;89:58-61.

89. Teitel AD, MacKenzie CR, Stern R, et al. Laryngeal involvement in systemic lupus erythematosus. *Semin Arthritis Rheum.* 1992;22:203-214.

90. McCaffrey TV, McDonald TJ, McCaffrey LA. Head and neck manifestations of relapsing polychondritis: review of 29 cases. *Otolaryngology.* 1978;86:473-478.

CHAPTER 7

Laryngeal Function During Phonation

Ronald C. Scherer, PhD

The larynx performs many functions to aid communication and allow life. As an open flow valve, it permits breathing, blowing, and sucking, as well as yawning, voiceless consonant production, and musical instrument playing. As a transient closed valve, it produces coughing and throat clearing. As a prolonged closed valve, it participates in swallowing and effortful behaviors such as lifting and defecation. As a voiceless repetitive articulator, it valves airflow to produce staccato whistling. As a voiced repetitive articulator, it produces laughter, the singing ornament trillo, and repetitive glottalization of vowels such as the admonition with rising pitch and intensity "a-a-a-ah!" As an incompletely closed voiceless valve, it produces whisper. As a partially or completely closed voicing valve, the larynx produces vowels and prolonged voiced consonants, and as a speech coarticulator, it participates in the production of consonant-vowel strings. For example, the word "seat" begins with an open glottis for the /s/, the glottis acting as an open flow valve allowing airflow under lung pressure to travel through the glottis and through the anterior oral constriction. This is followed by vocal fold approximation for the /i/ vowel, the larynx acting as a partially or completely closed voicing valve. Finally, the glottis opens as an open flow valve to permit the impoundment of air pressure behind the anterior oral /t/-occlusion with the subsequent release of air, creating the characteristic aspiration.

The purpose of this chapter is to describe the larynx as a partially or completely closed voicing valve, that is, as the organ that produces phonation. Neuromuscular, biomechanic, and aeroacoustic characteristics determine phonation duration, pitch, loudness, quality, register, and vocal fold motion, through control of or changes in vocal fold length, mass and tension, vocal fold contour, arytenoid and vocal fold adduction, subglottal pressure, and vocal tract size and shape. This chapter emphasizes the reasonable hypothesis that effective interventions to help people with voice concerns (whether these involve prevention, rehabilitation, surgery, pharmacology, or training) can be improved by an understanding of basic vocal function.[1,2]

OVERVIEW OF BASIC CHARACTERISTICS OF PHONATION

The basic perceptual characteristics of phonation are the presence and change of duration, pitch, register, loudness, and quality. Each of these has one or two primary biomechanical control variables. These will be discussed briefly in this section, followed by discussions of selected topics in greater detail.

Duration of phonation refers to the length of time the vocal folds oscillate during the creation of sound. In the normal larynx, adduction is one of two main control variables for duration; the vocal folds must be sufficiently close to permit oscillation. Subglottal air pressure is also necessary to provide sufficient force to move the vocal folds at the beginning of each vibratory cycle. After phonation commences, to then cease phonation, the arytenoid cartilages can be moved apart (abducted), or moved further together (more highly adducted), both ceasing phonation if the degree of abduction or adduction is great enough. Additional ways to cause phonation to cease are to lower subglottal air pressure, or impound air pressure in the vocal tract above the glottis, until the pressure drop across the glottis is too low to sustain vocal fold vibration.

The perception of pitch, corresponding to the physical measure of fundamental frequency, and vocal register (the very low pitches of vocal fry, the conversational pitches of chest or modal register, and the very high pitches of falsetto), are highly dependent on vocal fold length[3,4] and the associated tension of the vocal fold mucosal cover. The string model for frequency,[5-8]

$$(\text{Equation 1}), \quad F^o = \left(\frac{1}{2L}\right) = \left(\frac{T}{\rho}\right)0.5$$

where T is the tension of the vocal fold mucosal cover, ρ is the density of the tissue, and L is the length of the vibrating vocal folds, is an explanatory model suggesting that tension of the vocal fold cover governs the fundamental frequency (tension T increases faster than vocal fold length L when the vocal folds are lengthened, and ρ is essentially constant regardless of phonatory condition.[8,9]

The loudness of sounds is related to their acoustic intensity, and phonation during speech is primarily dependent upon subglottal pressure. An increase in subglottal pressure changes the characteristics of the airflow that exits the glottis (the glottal volume velocity) during vocal fold vibration, creating an increase in acoustic intensity (see below).

At the glottal level, vocal quality variation, governed primarily by the closeness of the vocal folds, ie, by adduction (separate from tissue or neurologic abnormalities), is related primarily to the perception of normal, breathy, and pressed qualities. Breathiness occurs when the vocal folds are slightly abducted such that they do not close completely during each cycle, allowing some of the glottal volume flow to be unmodulated and turbulent.[10] A breathy voice also can be created by full vocal fold closure (anterior to the vocal processes) but with the posterior glottis open, allowing turbulent air to flow between the arytenoid cartilages. If there is hyperadduction of the vocal folds, but with a significant opening of the posterior glottis, a pressed-breathy (or pressed-leakage) quality can result.[11,12] Pressed or constricted voice quality without breathiness results

from full glottal adduction, and little air flows through the glottis.[13]

Intervention strategies to improve voice production require an appreciation of the basic mechanics of phonation. The remainder of this chapter offers a more thorough discussion of basic control characteristics of voice production.

DURATION OF PHONATION

Figure 7-1 illustrates the adductory range of phonation and the corresponding distances between the vocal processes of the arytenoid cartilages, the ventricular folds, and the superomedial eminences of the arytenoid cartilage apexes. Phonation takes place over only a small range of adduction (the *phonatory adductory range*) permitted by movement of the arytenoid cartilages (approximately 14% of the adductory range as shown in the single-subject example of Figure 7-1). From an adductory standpoint, therefore, duration of phonation depends on the potential for the vocal folds to be placed within the phonatory adductory range, and the length of time the vocal folds are actually placed within that range. To discontinue phonation, the arytenoid cartilages can be configured to produce sufficient overcompression of the vocal folds or, alternatively, sufficient abduction.

Phonation requires a certain minimal amount of subglottal air pressure to set the vocal folds into vibration (the *phonatory threshold pressure*[14]) and then to maintain phonation. If the vocal folds are placed in the phonatory adductory range, the subglottal pressure must coordinate with the tissue characteristics of the vocal folds (stiffness, mass, and damping) to cause them to move to begin the first cycle.[14] Lucero[15] suggests, using a theoretical approach, that the pressure threshold should reduce as the vocal folds are brought closer to each other, and as the glottal angle between the vocal folds comes closer to zero or slightly divergent, consistent with Titze[14] and Chan, Titze, and Titze.[16] The threshold pressure typically varies with fundamental frequency, ranging from about 3 cm H_2O (0.3 kPa) for lower pitches to about 6 cm H_2O (0.6 kPa) for higher pitches[17] because of greater tension of the vocal fold cover with vocal fold lengthening. The amount of subglottal pressure at phonation offset is less than the onset pressure, not to exceed about half the onset pressure.[18-22] Because the phonatory threshold pressure is an important measure for glottal efficiency and clinical diagnostics, it is important that it be measured with care.[23]

There also may be an upper limit of subglottal pressure beyond which phonation is prevented or becomes unstable.[14] This upper limit may correspond to the upper limits of the *phonetogram*, a graph of the intensity range versus the fundamental frequency range of phonation for a particular person[24-28] (the recommendation of the term *voice range profile* for the phonetrogram was accepted by the Voice Committee of the International Association of Logopedics and Phoniatrics[29]). Subglottal pressures have been measured as high as 30-50 cm H_2O in loud phonation[30] (singing loudly at high pitches may produce even greater subglottal pressures[13]), but typically are below 10 cm H_2O for conversational speech.[30,31]

Intervention in voice surgery, therapy, and training often attempts to regain normal thresholds or to lower existing thresholds, the latter possibly creating less effortful phonation (relative to the employed forces of the respiratory system). Establishment of lower phonation thresholds may correspond to more physiologically efficient phonation and less voice fatigue.

The discussion directly above refers to the dependence that phonation has on subglottal pressure. More appropriately, phonation is dependent upon the *transla-*

ryngeal pressure, defined as the subglottal air pressure minus the supraglottal air pressure for phonation on exhalation. Note that the translaryngeal pressure is the difference between the subglottal and supraglottal pressures acting on the inferior and superior surfaces of the vocal folds, respectively, as well as the pressure difference that drives the air through the glottis. If the translaryngeal air pressure were zero, the pressure would be equal on all surfaces of the vocal folds, air would not pass, and phonation would not occur. This can be approached, for example, with overly prolonged voiced consonants such as /b/, /d/, and /g/ during the complete occlusion of the vocal tract. Prolonging the voicing of these consonants creates buildup of supralaryngeal air pressure until that pressure nearly equals the subglottal pressure, causing cessation of phonation as the translaryngeal pressure drops below the minimum sustaining pressure difference.

Thus, the creation and duration of phonation depend upon how close the vocal folds are to each other and the amount of translaryngeal air pressure (disregarding tis-

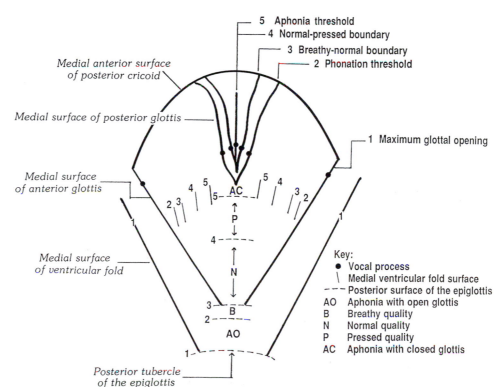

FIGURE 7-1. *Adductory range of the larynx. This figure is a composite from photographs of glottal adductory positions obtained from a single adult male subject using rigid videolaryngoscopy. Positions of the medial surface of the anterior (membranous) glottis, posterior glottis, ventricular folds, and the posterior tubercle of the epiglottis are shown. Stages of glottal positioning include maximum glottal opening (position 1) to full adduction when phonation is not possible (position 5). The other positions (2, 3, and 4) are the position for adductory phonatory threshold and boundary locations between breathy, normal, and pressed voice qualities in this subject, perceptually judged and checked against electroglottograph (EGG) recordings. The adductory phonation range is only about 14% of the entire adductory range (see text).*

5 Aphonia threshold
4 Normal-pressed boundary
3 Breathy-normal boundary
2 Phonation threshold
1 Maximum glottal opening

Medial anterior surface of posterior cricoid

Medial surface of posterior glottis

Medial surface of anterior glottis

Medial surface of ventricular fold

Posterior tubercle of the epiglottis

Key:
● Vocal process
\ Medial ventricular fold surface
--- Posterior surface of the epiglottis
AO Aphonia with open glottis
B   Breathy quality
N   Normal quality
P   Pressed quality
AC Aphonia with closed glottis

sue abnormality). To cease phonation, the vocal folds can be over-adducted or over-abducted, or the translaryngeal pressure can be lowered by decreasing the subglottal pressure or by increasing supraglottal pressure through supraglottal occlusion. All four methods most likely are used in normal speech production, and the ability of a patient to demonstrate all four methods is relevant diagnostically. These mechanisms for phonation cessation potentially can be compromised by arytenoidal, respiratory, or articulatory dysfunction, or by abnormal adductory configuration caused by vocal fold tissue change.

FUNDAMENTAL FREQUENCY OF PHONATION

Perceived pitch corresponds (nonlinearly) to the physical measure of fundamental frequency F_0,[32] which in turn corresponds to the number of cycles per second of the glottal motion during phonation. For normal phonation, the motion of the vocal folds is similar from cycle to cycle, giving rise to nearly equal periods of time between glottal closures.

Each phonatory cycle releases time-varying glottal flow (also called the glottal volume velocity) that generates sound. For normal phonation, acoustic excitation is created throughout the varying flow cycle, with a primary location giving the greatest excitation. Figure 7-2 shows two glottal volume velocity cycles of human phonation (top trace). The cycle period is T, which is 10 ms (and thus $F_0 = 1/T = 100$ Hz). The glottal volume velocity (usually given in liters per second, L/s, or cubic centimeters per second, cm³/s) begins to exit the glottis gradually, rises to a peak, and then "shuts off" relatively abruptly. Air exits the glottis from time A to time B during the lateral then medial motion of the membranous vocal folds. The glottis is closed, or nearly so, from B to C. The amount of airflow during the interval B to C (seen as the offset from the horizontal baseline in Figure 7-2) corresponds to air "leakage" when the arytenoid cartilages are separated to some degree.

The lower trace of Figure 7-2 is the time derivative of the volume velocity signal of the upper trace. At any moment in time, the value on the lower trace equals the slope of the volume velocity signal at that moment. The fastest change of the volume velocity in the figure is at time D, and corresponds to the point M on the derivative waveform. The point M corresponds to the moment of time at which the greatest acoustic excitation is created.[33,34]

Perceptual judgments of an unclear voice (rather than confusion of pitch per se) occur when the more prominent moments of acoustic excitation during each cycle are not consistent from one cycle to the next (for

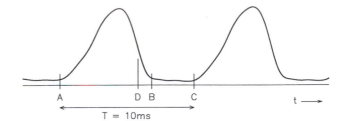

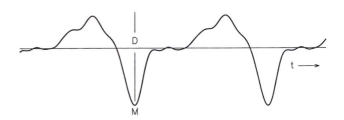

FIGURE 7-2. *Glottal volume velocity waveforms and their derivatives. The top trace is a glottal volume velocity signal, and the bottom trace is the derivative of the top trace, showing the instantaneous slopes of the top trace. Cycle period is T (from time A to time C). "Open" glottis time is from A to B, and "closed" glottis time is from B to C. The moment of the maximum flow shutoff rate, or the maximum negative derivative of the glottal volume velocity signal, occurs at time D and corresponds to point M.*

a review of cyclic instabilities, see References 32, 35, 36). The time between primary acoustic excitations from one cycle to the next varies a small amount during normal phonation, helping to create a natural voice quality. However, the variation of periods can increase if there are tissue abnormalities such as swelling, nodules, polyps, unilateral stiffness, and so forth, causing kinematic (vocal fold motion) and glottal flow inconsistencies from cycle to cycle. Consecutively varying periods of primary acoustic excitations also can be created by turbulent airflow through the glottis (as in breathy voice), creating added noise to the acoustic signal. Aperiodicities can be measured by jitter, one definition being the average cycle-to-cycle difference in period or equivalent frequency, with large values of jitter corresponding to a sense of vocal roughness.[32] Figure 7-3 illustrates quasi-periodic cycles of the acoustic output of a prolonged vowel with a calculation of the segment's jitter value.

Jitter may be caused by or related to neuromuscular innervation abnormalities[37-40] as well as the structural and turbulence causes given above. Because tension of the vocal folds is highly dependent on the passive lengthening of the vocal fold cover, as suggested by

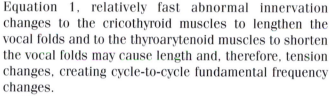

FIGURE 7-3. *Aperiodicity of a microphone signal for a prolonged vowel. The periods of the microphone signal are indicated using the instants of the minimum values, and the calculation of the corresponding jitter is given. This is an example of a measure of voicing perturbation.*

Microphone Signal

$p_1 = 6.60 \rightarrow F_o = 151.52$ Hz
$p_2 = 6.55 \rightarrow F_o = 152.67$ Hz
$\vdots$
$p_{12} = 6.50 \rightarrow F_o = 153.85$ Hz

$N = 12$

Jitter :

$$J = \frac{100 \sum\limits_{i=2}^{N} |Fo_i - Fo_{i-1}|}{(N-1)\overline{Fo}}$$

$$= 0.82$$

Equation 1, relatively fast abnormal innervation changes to the cricothyroid muscles to lengthen the vocal folds and to the thyroarytenoid muscles to shorten the vocal folds may cause length and, therefore, tension changes, creating cycle-to-cycle fundamental frequency changes.

Pitch and vocal quality are also affected by changes that occur over longer time lengths than a phonatory cycle. Diplophonia (the existence of two pitches simultaneously[41]) and subharmonics (integer subdivisions of the fundamental frequency) come from multicycle length modulations of the volume velocity signal. These give rise to primary acoustic excitations at varying time intervals as well as about twice (or more) the primary phonatory period.[42-49] Figure 7-4 shows an example of the presence of cycle clustering in the glottal volume velocity signal of a spasmodic dysphonia patient. The cause of this dysfunction appears to be related to hyperadduction or asymmetry of laryngeal muscle function.

In vocal fry and "creaky" voice, pitch may be extremely low and the voice may have varied roughness qualities, depending on the complexity of the low fre-

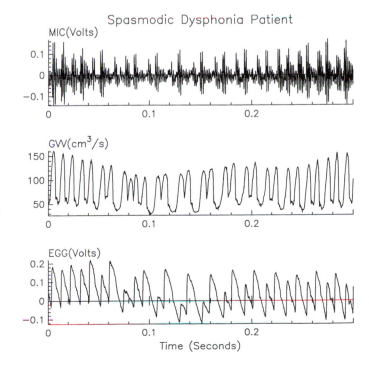

FIGURE 7-4. *Voicing period alterations in a spasmodic dysphonia patient. Microphone, glottal volume velocity, and EGG signals are given, top to bottom. Notice the change from essentially single cycles to cycle clustering of two (and one case of three) cycles. The clustering of two cycles can be seen in all three signals: apparent motion variation of vocal fold contact, double flow pulsing, and double acoustic excitation seen in the microphone signal. (Data courtesy of Dr. Kimberly Fisher)*

quency periodicities combined with higher frequency periodicities.[50-54] Figure 7-5 illustrates three different examples of vocal fry[53] (in Reference 53, 11 different types of vocal fry and creaky voice are illustrated). For each case, the microphone signal and the electroglottograph signal are displayed. These samples were created intentionally by a single normal adult male subject. The electroglottographic (EGG) signal may correspond to the contact area between the vocal folds when they touch each other during each cycle.[32,55] Figure 7-5A illustrates vocal fry of low and specific pitch. Each cycle shows a single primary acoustic excitation. This excitation corresponds to the fast upward movement of the

EGG signal which corresponds to glottal closure and, therefore, to the glottal volume velocity "shutoff." Figure 7-5B illustrates the typical bimodal electroglottograph signal for vocal fry, with corresponding double acoustic excitations during each (low pitch) cycle. Figure 7-5C illustrates an extreme case of multiple cyclic motions of the vocal folds during each relatively long cycle, with corresponding acoustic excitations.

Pitch can be altered by fluid engorgement (edema). The usual explanation for pitch drop in edema cases is that greater mass creates lower natural frequencies. For example, computer modeling of phonation using biomechanical characteristics of tissue mass, stiffness, and damping relate fundamental frequency to the inverse of the vocal fold mass.[56] Figure 7-6 shows the results of increasing vocal fold mass (only) in a two-mass model of vocal fold function adapted from Ishizaka and Flanagan[57] by Smith.[58] Figure 7-6 shows a decrease in frequency by approximately 5.6 semitones for a doubling of the mass of the vocal folds. For example, for a subglottal pressure of 8 cm H_2O, the change in fundamental frequency for a doubling of the mass is approximately 134 Hz to 97 Hz in the figure.

Subglottal pressure plays a significant role in the control of pitch. Figure 7-6 suggests that an increase in subglottal pressure for a constant vocal fold mass will increase the fundamental frequency. The F_0 changes from 120 Hz to 156 Hz for a mass "M" and subglottal pressure from 4 to 16 cm H_2O for the conditions of Figure 7-6. The literature suggests that a change of 1 cm H_2O subglottal pressure results in a fundamental frequency change of 3-6 Hz.[59-62] The air pressure pushing against the undersurface of the vocal folds moves the vocal fold laterally and somewhat upwardly.[19,63-66] The extent of the lateral excursion is dependent upon the amount of the subglottal pressure and the length of the vocal folds.[6,67,68] Thus, for a constant anterior-posterior length of the glottis, a greater subglottal pressure will literally push the vocal folds to a greater lateral extent, creating a greater maximum *stretch* than for a lower subglottal pressure. Greater maximum stretch creates higher effective tension and thus a higher fundamental frequency.[6] Intonational (pitch) changes during conversational speech appear to be caused by a significant combination of the passive vocal fold stretch by both the cricothyroid muscles and the subglottal pressure[69,70] (refer especially to the general discussion at the end of Reference 70).

Tension of the vocal fold cover may be changed (and therefore fundamental frequency changes) by external adjustments affecting the length of the vocal folds. Anterior pull of the hyoid bone by suprahyoid muscles may help tilt the thyroid cartilage forward to position its

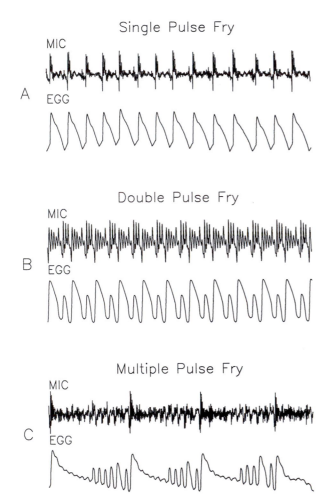

FIGURE 7-5. *Three vocal fry examples. (A) Single glottal pulses at 30 Hz; (B) double glottal pulses at 62 Hz for the period combining the two pulses; and (C) a multiple pulse case with a low frequency of 7.5 Hz and a higher frequency of 93 Hz. In each grouping, the upper trace is the microphone signal and the lower trace is the electroglottograph signal. The examples were produced by a single adult male subject. See Reference 53.*

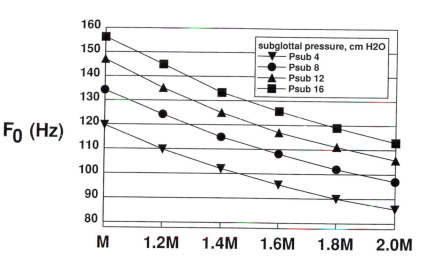

FIGURE 7-6. *Vocal fold mass effect on fundamental frequency. As the amount of mass of the vocal fold in vibration increases, the fundamental frequency decreases. The abscissa ranges from a value of* M = 0.16 g *to twice that. The figure also indicates that fundamental frequency is dependent upon subglottal pressure. (Figure courtesy of Dr. Marshall Smith, who used an adaptation of the Ishizaka and Flanagan simulation.[57,58])*

inferior border closer to the superior border of the anterior cricoid cartilage (similar to the function of the cricothyroid muscle), thus increasing vocal fold length and raising the fundamental frequency, as shown by Honda.[71] Alternatively, a suggestion is put forward by Sundberg et al[72] that the cricoid cartilage may be tilted down posteriorly, shortening the vocal fold length, by an inferior tracheal pull. This would come about by lowering the diaphragm with higher lung volume levels (or by coactivation of the diaphragm during phonation), inducing a pitch drop unless compensated for by increased cricothyroid muscle activity.

The above discussion emphasizes the contribution to pitch control through tension change of the vocal fold cover through passive stretch or by increasing subglottal pressure. The fundamental frequency is also dependent upon the activity of the vocalis (thyroarytenoid) muscle.[73,74] The vocalis muscle acts antagonistically to the cricothyroid muscle relative to length change of the cover.[73,75,76] Thus, if only the cover is vibrating, as in soft, high-pitch phonation, increase in vocalis contraction should shorten and reduce the tension of the mucosal cover, and thereby lower the fundamental frequency. However, if the vocalis muscle participates in the motion of the vocal fold to a significant degree, as in loud, low-pitch phonation, increase in vocalis muscle contraction will increase the effective tension of the entire tissue in motion as a primary effect, and thereby raise the fundamental frequency. The effect on F_0 change related to vocalis muscle involvement conceptually depends on the relative amount of vocalis muscle participating in the vibratory mass, the tension within the vocalis muscle portion of the mass in motion, and the relative activity level of the vocalis muscle, as Titze, Jiang, and Drucker[73] analytically describe. In general then, pitch is controlled by many combinations of

cricothyroid muscle contraction (to passively stretch the tissue in motion), vocalis muscle contraction (to passively shorten the cover and actively increase the tension of the vibratory vocalis portion), and subglottal pressure increase (to increase the amount of vocal fold mass placed into vibratory motion and passively stretch the tissue in motion). As a general rule, fundamental frequency would be expected to rise if there is greater tension (passive plus active) of the tissue in motion or less mass of the tissue in motion. Intervention strategies dealing with pitch alteration need to take into consideration these physiologic and aerodynamic bases.

As a segue to the next section on loudness and vocal quality, it is noted that various combinations of cricothyroid and vocalis muscle contraction, with adduction, may change vocal quality, especially relative to the medial shaping of the vocal fold. Greater vocalis muscle contraction tends to round (or medialize) the medial contour of the vocal fold,[74,77,78] potentially decreasing the vibratory threshold pressure[14] and creating a relatively longer closed time of the vocal folds each cycle,[79] which may change the voice spectra to reflect a brighter, louder sound.

LOUDNESS AND QUALITY OF PHONATION

Loudness and quality of phonation are perceptual correlates to the physical measures of intensity and acoustic spectra, respectively.[13,32,80,81] Both perceptions depend upon the glottal volume velocity waveform characteristics and vocal tract resonance structure. We will emphasize the glottal volume velocity here.

Figure 7-7 illustrates a typical glottal volume velocity waveform in modal register with corresponding schematized glottal motion. The general shape of the glottal volume velocity waveform shows that the flow

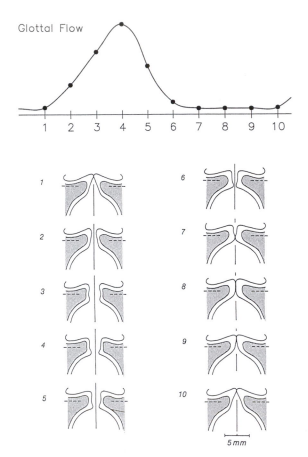

FIGURE 7-7. *Glottal volume velocity waveform and corresponding glottal motion. The specific phases of the glottal cycle shown in the motion schematic are indicated on the glottal volume velocity waveform. (Adapted with permission from Hirano, M. Clinical Examination of Voice. Copyright 1981, Springer-Verlag.[30])*

typically begins more gradually than when it is shut off, and the flow maximum is produced after the time when the maximum of the glottal area occurs. This flow delay characteristic (or *skewing* to the right relative to the glottal area) is related to the inertance of the airway, glottal wall motion, and glottal shape. The inertive effect[82,83] refers to the fact that the air within the vocal tract has mass. When the glottis just opens, the air (being driven by the translaryngeal air pressure) moves through the glottis to meet the column of air of the vocal tract. The air coming through the glottis must literally move other air already within the vocal tract, and this requirement slows the motion of the air as it first comes out of the glottis.[2,84] Corresponding to this event is the increase in air pressure just above the glottis as air moves through the glottis into the air above, thus typically reducing the translaryngeal pressure drop.[2,85-89] If

the vocal tract were modeled as a uniform tube, greater glottal airflow skewing would be created from greater inertance by elongating the vocal tract (through larynx lowering or lip protrusion) or by narrowing the cross-sectional vocal tract area.[89,90] Fant[86] showed analytically that skewing increases not only with an increase of the vocal tract inertance (which changes with certain vowels and is higher with a constriction at the false fold level), but also with an increase in the maximum glottal excursion during the phonatory cycle, a faster glottal closing time, a lower subglottal pressure, and a smaller glottal kinetic flow factor *k* (the latter is derived in detail in References 91 and 92), concepts fruitful for clinical and training considerations. After the moment of maximum flow, the airflow will reduce to zero or to its minimum value as the two vocal folds come together at the end of glottal closing.

Skewing of the glottal volume velocity is related to the motion of the vocal folds according to a numerical model by Alipour and Scherer.[93] The lower margin of the vibrating vocal fold may have a different amplitude of motion than the upper margin, and the two margins may vary in their relative phase during the cycle. Skewing of the glottal volume flow appears to increase as the amplitude of the lower margin increases relative to the upper margin, and decreases as the phase lead of the lower margin increases relative to the upper margin. This suggests that there may be an optimal compromise between amplitude and phase differences between the lower and upper glottal margins to maximize the skewing of the glottal volume velocity.

As Figure 7-7 shows, the glottis takes on a number of shapes during the vibratory cycle. A duct that expands in shape (a diffuser shape as suggested in steps 4, 5, and 6 of Figure 7-7) can have less resistance to flow than one of the same but constant (uniform) diameter.[91,92,94,95] The minimum flow resistance may occur when the glottis creates a diffuser shape of small angle (estimated to be between 5° and 10°[96-97]), which would most likely occur just past the time of the maximum glottal area. Therefore, when the glottis takes on the shape of a small-angled diffuser, the flow resistance may be less than at maximum glottal opening, and greater flow may then exit the glottis, to help skew the flow to the right relative to glottal area.

In general, then, if greater skewing of the glottal volume velocity is desired (as would be the case for any clinical or training condition needing greater energy in higher harmonic frequencies, see below), physiologic maneuvers should be considered to bring about the following: increase in the inertance of the vocal tract, increase in the lateral excursion of the vocal folds, decrease in the phase lead of the lower margin relative to the upper margin, and increase in the speed of glottal closure. These maneuvers would depend upon adjustments of the vocal tract shaping and length, level of glottal adduction (see below), level of subglottal pressure, and alteration in differential thyroarytenoid muscle contraction. These coordinations for optimal shaping and sizing of the glottal volume velocity waveform are central themes of needed research.

The qualities of the voice depend upon the glottal volume velocity waveform. Figure 7-8 shows an example of breathy (hypoadducted), normal, and pressed (hyperadducted) phonations in a normal adult male. The figure demonstrates typical variations of the glottal flow, the spectrum of the glottal flow, and the electroglottograph (EGG) waveforms for these qualities (the signals are not exactly time aligned). A Glottal Enterprises wide-band pneumotach system was used to acquire the inverse filtered (glottal) flow, and a Synchrovoice Laryngograph was used to obtain the EGG signal. Breathy voice is characterized by a more sinusoidal flow waveform than for normal phonation, with a significant flow bias. The flow bias is seen as a shift of the waveform away from the zero-flow baseline, indicating that there is always some flow exiting the glottis because of nonclosure throughout the cycle (the bias is also called the *DC*

flow). In pressed phonation, the peaks of the flow arc significantly smaller than for normal phonation, and the amount of time within the cycle during which the air exits the glottis is relatively short. Spectrally, the breathy quality example has energy primarily in the first two partials, whereas greater energy is distributed to higher harmonic frequencies in the normal and pressed quality examples. Up to 1000 Hz, the spectral slope is relatively steep at -17.3 dB/octave for breathy voice, less steep at -14.4 dB/octave for normal, and flattest at -10.8 dB/octave for the pressed condition for the examples in Figure 7-8. Notice the relative reduction in the level of the fundamental frequency compared to the first overtone from breathy to normal to pressed. The EGG waveforms suggest that there was a relatively large change of contact area between the surfaces of the two vocal folds during the breathy voicing, as seen by the relatively large amplitude (note that the greater the extent of the EGG waveform, the more vocal fold contact area change there is presumed to be[55]). However, the time during which the glottis was open, shown by the baseline length of the waveform, was relatively long in the breathy phonation compared to the other two qualities. The height of the pressed quality EGG waveform is shortest, suggesting relatively less dynamic contact of the vocal

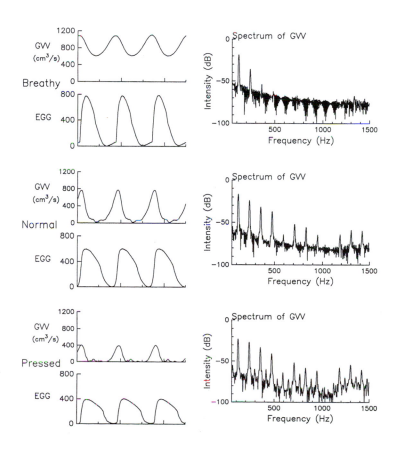

FIGURE 7-8. *Breathy, normal, and pressed voice qualities. Glottal volume velocity and EGG waveforms are shown, as well as the spectrum of the glottal volume velocity waveforms. The subject was a normal adult male.*

fold surfaces. This was explained by viewing the subject's larynx with stroboscopy; in pressed voice, the compression allowed only a restricted anterior glottal region to vibrate, thus resulting in the relatively short amplitudes because less of the total medial vocal fold surface participated in the vibration.

The overall intensity or sound pressure level (SPL) of the output sound may increase with increase in the maximum rate of change of the glottal volume velocity "shutoff" (the value M shown in Figure 7-2).[12,98-100] The maximum rate of change of the glottal flow is also the maximum negative slope, or *the maximum flow declination rate.* Greater maximum slope has the spectral effect of raising the energy of the partials primarily within the region of the first formant,[101] usually the most important spectral portion for overall SPL. This is like "turning [up] the volume control"[12(p.562)] (see also Reference 102). A doubling of the maximum negative slope corresponds empirically to an approximate increase of 5-9 dB in overall SPL.[12] Increased skewing of the glottal flow (discussed above) through increased vocal tract inertance and greater vocal fold motion should raise the overall SPL. For example, in their numerical study, Alipour and Scherer[93] found that increasing the amplitude of the lower glottal margin alone by 50% produced an increase in closing slope of more than 50%. These suggestions of acoustic (inertance) and kinematic (vocal fold motion) aides to enhance the desired characteristics of the glottal volume velocity need to be explored with human subject studies to eventually improve treatment and training of people with voice concerns.

It is of importance to note some other spectral effects of differences in the glottal volume velocity waveform. The amount of time the waveform shows air exiting the glottis (time A to time B in Figure 7-2) divided by the period of the cycle (time A to time C in Figure 7-2) is called the *open quotient*. The open quotient typically decreases when changing adduction from a more breathy to a more normal quality voice, and with increase in loudness.[14] When the open quotient decreases, there may be a minor reduction (a few dB) of the intensity of the fundamental frequency and possibly a minor boost (a few dB) of the intensity of the first overtone (an octave above the fundamental frequency).[102,103] Also, the greater the amplitude of the volume velocity waveform (or the greater the area under the volume velocity waveform), the greater is the amplitude of the fundamental frequency.[12,101,104] A doubling of the amplitude of the waveform corresponds to an increase of approximately 3-7 dB in the spectral level of the fundamental frequency. When the flow has nearly completely shut off, that is, when the flow has nearly

reached the baseline just before glottal closure, there is a "shutoff corner." The sharpness of this corner is related to the energy generated in the overtones of the voice, according to the modeling by Fant and his colleagues.[101-103] A change from a well-rounded corner to a very sharp corner can cause the intensity of the overtones to increase by up to 10-20 dB, undoubtedly affecting the quality of the sound[102,103] (changing glottal adduction from a breathy voice quality to a normal quality would sharpen this flow shutoff corner considerably). This concept needs exploration relative to how the vocal folds come together and to the perception of vocal quality, especially taken in the context of clinical intervention and vocal performance instruction.

The intensity and spectra of the glottal airflow are dependent on subglottal air pressure and fundamental frequency. As subglottal air pressure increases for a constant level of glottal adduction, the maximum (peak) airflow through the glottis increases. This follows from the greater maximum glottal width that is created when subglottal air pressure increases (see discussion above) and the greater driving pressure across the larger opening (see, eg, Reference 105). As the maximum value of the volume velocity waveform increases, the intensity level of the fundamental frequency increases, as discussed above.[12] Also, if the peak flow increases, the maximum flow derivative should typically increase as the flow must reduce to zero (or near zero) from a greater value if the time during which the flow decreases remains the same.[100] An increase in the maximum flow derivative will increase the overall SPL and augment the spectrum, as indicated above. In addition, the increase in subglottal pressure may cause the vocal folds to come back together faster (or perhaps alter their dynamic phasing) after their larger maximum excursion, creating a sharper flow shutoff corner near the baseline, raising the overall spectrum of the overtones. Therefore, greater subglottal pressure may contribute to increasing the flow peak, increasing the maximum flow derivative, and sharpening the baseline flow shutoff corner. These effects change the flow spectrum shape by increasing the intensity level of the fundamental frequency and increasing the intensity of the overtones, thus raising the overall intensity of the voice. Titze and Sundberg[99] show explicitly how a doubling of subglottal pressure (more precisely, a doubling of the difference between subglottal pressure and threshold pressure) raises source acoustic power by 6 dB. Fant[86] broke down the intensity increase relative to the contributions of increased air velocity, increased maximum glottal area during the cycle, reduced time the glottis is open, faster glottal closing, and an increased flow derivative, totaling approximately 6 dB in intensity gain for a doubling of subglottal pressure. The early literature showed that voice intensity is strongly associated with subglottal pressure,[106-110] and this discussion has attempted to offer what has been suggested as an explanation as to how the subglottal pressure increase affects the sound source volume velocity waveform and the resultant increase of intensity.

Intensity is affected strongly by the fundamental frequency of voice production. Titze and Sundberg[99] show that the glottal power output will increase by 6 dB for an octave rise in fundamental frequency (all else the same), caused by the increase in the maximum flow derivative as the fundamental frequency rises (the same waveform shape with a shorter cycle period has a larger maximum flow derivative). At this point, one might ask why females, who speak at about 9-10 semitones above the fundamental frequency of men,[32] typically do not sound louder than men, and indeed do not differ substantially from men in intensity.[111] The just-mentioned effect of the higher frequency for women (about a ratio of 1.7 to 1) is potentially offset by a larger amplitude of glottal volume velocity for males (a ratio of about 2 to 1) so that the SPL for females is only 1-2 dB lower than for males.[99,111] In possible contradiction, it is noted that Sapienza and Stathopoulos[112] found that the maximum flow derivative was essentially the same between men and women when they produced the same SPL values. Furthermore, Sulter and Wit[113] found that at normal and loud levels, the maximum flow derivative for untrained men was approximately double that for untrained women at comparable SPL levels. These conflicting data suggest that this area of study is unresolved.

Because vocal sound is created by the glottal volume velocity, intervention strategies should attempt to improve the glottal airflow waveform, as mentioned above. There may be combinations of voicing variables that produce optimally efficient voice production from acoustic and physiologic orientations. Titze[114] has reported maximal intensity production in excised dog larynges for vocal processes that are placed very near each other, with less intensity (ranging to a few dB) for greater and less adduction. Sundberg[13] (also see Reference 104) has proposed the term *flow mode,* a type of phonation in which the glottal volume velocity amplitude is relatively large with high efficiency of laryngeal function. This is further emphasized, perhaps diagnostically, by examining the value of the flow amplitude divided by the subglottal pressure (the *glottal permittance*[100]). This ratio allows a clear separation between a pressed (constricted) voice versus normal and "flow"

phonations (for a limited number of subjects[100]) because of the greater flow amplitudes for the same subglottal pressure in the normal and "flow" types. It is of considerable importance (theoretically and clinically) that professional (classically trained) male singers may produce voiced sounds at higher intensity levels than male nonsingers for the same subglottal pressures, caused primarily by greater glottal flow amplitudes (from adjusted flow impedance).[14,99] In addition, performance training strategies have emphasized vocal tract adjustments to match lower voicing partials with the first formant[115] or to create an enhanced higher formant region[116,117] by clustering formants numbers 3, 4 and 5, strategies that boost the output energy of certain partials of the voice, creating a "bright" or "carrying" voice with desirable performance qualities. These tactics are not dissimilar to strategies employed in voice pathology (eg, References 118 and 119).

VOCAL FOLD MOTION DURING PHONATION

Although it is important to realize that the creation of the sound of voicing is within the airflow exiting the glottis, and not in the motion of the vocal folds per se, the motion of the vocal folds helps to determine the characteristics of the airflow.

Basic kinematic (motion) aspects of normal vocal folds include the effects of increased subglottal pressure, vocal fold elongation, and glottal adduction. Increased subglottal pressure produces increased lateral pressures on the medial surfaces and vertical pressures on the undersurface of the vocal folds, creating greater maximum excursion during the vibratory cycle (as discussed above). Elongation of the vocal folds by increased contraction of the cricothyroid muscles and/or decreased contraction of the thyroarytenoid muscles modifies the cross-sectional shape of the vocal fold (with no change of total vocal fold mass) to form a reduced vocal fold thickness (measured in the vertical direction),[120-123] giving rise to potentially less vocal fold tissue contact during vocal fold closure. For the same subglottal pressure and glottal adduction, vocal fold lengthening would affect the glottal volume velocity waveform by increasing the open quotient and decreasing the maximum flow derivative. Increased adduction will affect the motion of the vocal folds by creating more contact between the vocal folds and a longer glottal closed time within each cycle.[48,124-128] Any abnormality of tissue morphology (swelling, stiffness, or growth along the vocal fold), unilaterally or bilaterally, may alter the vibratory motion to create different glottal volume velocity waveforms from cycle to cycle, or from cycle group to cycle group (refer to the earlier discussion on perturbation). Severe laryngitis associated with extreme edema creates the well-known response of aphonia (inability to phonate or absence of phonation), which may be explained by the mass being too great to permit vibration, and the rounded glottal shaping causing less-effective intraglottal pressures during phonation.[129] Refer to Hirano and Bless[130] for photographs of vibratory patterns for a number of vocal pathologies including nodules, polyps, cysts, and others.

These kinds of structural changes to the vocal folds lead to the question: How is the vibration of the vocal folds maintained? That is, what allows them to remain in oscillation? A response to this question will now be explored.

The mechanical phonatory motion of the vocal folds depends upon the folds being driven by air pressures within the glottis,[91,96,131-136] such air pressure forces working with the biomechanical characteristics of the vocal folds (mass, stiffness, damping) to overcome the damping losses within the tissue.[22,57,66,137-142] The *intraglottal pressures* are extremely important, then, in the maintenance of vocal fold oscillation.[2,8,142] If the intraglottal pressures are positive, they act to push the vocal folds away from each other. If the intraglottal pressures are negative, they pull the vocal folds toward each other. The polarity (positive or negative) of the intraglottal pressure depends upon both the dynamic air pressures directly above and below the glottis and the shape of the glottal airway, as will now be discussed (see References 2 and 90).

The acoustic air pressure just above the glottis may be important for maintaining vocal fold oscillation. As the glottis nears closure during a normal vibratory cycle, the airflow through the glottis decreases relatively quickly. The air that has already passed through the glottis continues to travel up the vocal tract, creating greater distance between itself (the air) and the glottis. This air momentum produces a negative rarefaction pressure directly above the glottis as the particles of air separate more and more from each other. Negative pressure at the glottal exit location would create pressures that are negative within the glottis (at least within the glottal duct near the exit) if the glottis has not closed at the lower glottal edge. The intraglottal negative pressure, located at least near the glottal exit, thus should facilitate the final closing of the glottis by pulling the two folds together (aided by the closing momentum of the tissue itself). The amount of the negative intraglottal pressure would depend upon the value of the maximum negative supraglottal pressure.

As the glottis opens during a vibratory cycle, the airflow through the glottis meets the mass of air directly above it, creating compression of the air and positive air pressure. The positive air pressure directly above the glottis creates positive air pressure within the glottis, at least near the glottal exit. The intraglottal positive pressure caused by the positive supraglottal pressure would therefore facilitate glottal opening by pushing on the vocal folds to help separate them. Thus, during opening, supraglottal positive pressure aids glottal opening, and during closing, supraglottal negative pressure aids glottal closing.

The glottis takes on two primary shapes during (exhalatory) phonation, *convergent* and *divergent* (see Figure 7-9).[18,143-145] During glottal opening, the convergent glottal shape is produced with a wider opening at glottal entrance and a narrower opening at glottal exit (Figure 7-7). Because of the convergent shape, a pressure drop (from a higher value to a lower value, Figure 7-9) is created from the positive tracheal pressure to the

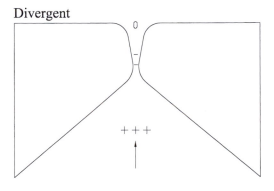

Divergent

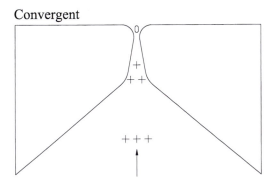

Convergent

FIGURE 7-9. *Pressures within the glottis relative to glottal shape. In the convergent glottis (lower sketch), the air pressures are positive in the entrance of the glottis and decrease to zero (or to the pressure just above the glottis). In the divergent glottis (upper sketch), the air pressures are negative in the entrance of the glottis and increase to zero (or to the pressure just above the glottis).*

pressure existing at the glottal exit location,[96] which may be close to positive (as discussed above) or near atmospheric. Thus, the glottal convergent shape (itself) creates a positive pressure within the glottis, and this positive pressure pushes on the vocal folds, facilitating glottal opening. This pressure decrease within the converging glottis follows directly from the Bernoulli equation (for steady flow).

During glottal closing, the divergent glottal shape may be most prominent; the configuration has a narrower opening at glottal entrance than at glottal exit (Figure 7-9). Divergent glottal duct shapes are similar to mechanical diffusers in that the expanding area allows pressures within the duct to increase between the upstream inlet and the downstream outlet.[94,96,97] The pressure at glottal entry is, therefore, lower than at exit, and is negative within the glottis if the glottal exit pressure is atmospheric (zero) or negative (per the discussion above on glottal closing). This negative pressure is caused by the divergent shape of the glottis, with the minimal duct diameter formed at entry, creating the lowest pressure there (at entry) essentially in accordance with the Bernoulli equation. The negative intraglottal pressure would pull on the vocal fold surfaces, facilitating glottal closure.

The "Bernoulli effect" refers to the existence of negative pressure in a narrowed location of a duct through which air (fluid) is flowing. This is the result of the trade-off (described by the Bernoulli equation) between air pressure and air particle velocity for different size sections of the duct (lower pressure and higher velocity exist in a narrower section). The Bernoulli effect has been used historically to help "explain" phonation (Tonndorf was an important early proponent of this concept for the maintenance of vocal fold oscillation, see Reference 146). That is, as the air particles speed up as they enter the glottis from the trachea, the air pressure supposedly would become negative throughout the glottis because it would constitute a smaller opening than the trachea, and then the negative pressure would suck the folds toward each other regardless of the glottal shape. This explanation is incomplete. During glottal opening, when the glottis has a convergent shape and the minimal glottal diameter is at the glottal exit, the Bernoulli energy equation does help to explain the pressure *reduction* from the glottal entrance to the glottal exit, but the intraglottal pressure is positive, not negative, despite the glottis being smaller than the trachea, because the pressure lowers from the positive tracheal value to the positive or near zero value at glottal exit. During glottal closing when the glottis forms a divergent (diffuser) shape, the pressure reduction from the tra-

chea to glottal entry may follow the Bernoulli equation for the most part, but the application of the Bernoulli equation within the glottis would essentially apply only in the special case of no flow separation from the glottal walls. *Flow separation,* in which the air flows away from the glottal wall rather than staying close to the wall, occurs when there is a sufficient pressure rise in the diverging glottal duct. This creates a condition where the Bernoulli equation no longer applies beyond the flow separation point.[96,132,133,147] The pressure will increase from a negative value at the entrance to the glottis to a rather constant value (equal to the air pressure just downstream of the glottis) a short distance past the air separation location for these divergent glottis conditions.[147] These concepts are based on steady (constant) flow modeling with static glottal shapes of many angles.[97]

The pressure on the medial vocal folds during vibration is more complex than indicated above. During phonation the glottis viewed superiorly is rather elliptical in shape, with greatest amplitude of motion near the middle of the membranous glottis. Pressures appear to vary the most during the cycle within the glottis at the location of the maximum motion, with cyclic pressure variations decreasing anteriorly and posteriorly to this location.[136] These dynamic glottal pressure changes are called *bidirectional pressure gradients.*[136]

Another interesting complexity of glottal pressures is that, even when the glottis forms a symmetric convergent or divergent duct, the pressures on the two vocal folds may not be identical because of flow separation only on one side of the glottis and not the other side, or because the flow bends to one side downstream of the glottis.[97,147] However, there may not be time to develop these glottal wall pressure differences during phonation because the geometry changes so quickly.[148-150] When the glottal duct is slanted to one side, as can be seen in some normal and abnormal phonations in which the two vocal folds vibrate out of phase with each other,[151-153] the pressures on the two sides of the glottis may be substantially different.[147] These pressure differences may promote the out-of-phase motion of the two vocal folds.

The actual interdependence among dynamic (time-varying) glottal shaping, translaryngeal pressures, and intraglottal pressures, and the application of equations of mechanics, require precise empirical measurement of glottal shaping, flows, and pressures during phonation, research yet to be adequately performed. In addition, the relationship among these aspects, the particle velocities that make up the glottal flow, and the resulting acoustic signal[33,154-164] extend this matter to the necessary and interfacing aeroacoustic level of phonation.

SUMMARY

This chapter has reviewed basic aspects of laryngeal function during phonation. The concepts underlying the understanding of duration, frequency, intensity, spectra, and vocal fold motion during phonation are the bases with which to make effective intervention decisions for laryngeal and voice change. These underlying concepts are applicable to both clinical and training practices.

ACKNOWLEDGMENTS

The author is grateful to and would like to thank Chwen Guo and Daoud Shinwari for their help with the figures, Kimberly Fisher for the use of her spasmodic dysphonia data, Marshall Smith for his figure dealing with vocal mass and fundamental frequency change, Tamara Field for help in preparing Figure 7-1, and David Kuehn for an anatomical discussion. This project was prepared with support from NIDCD grants P60 DC00976 RTC and R01 DC0357, and is dedicated to the memory and mentorship of Dr. Wilbur James Gould.

REFERENCES

1. Scherer RC. Aerodynamic assessment in voice production. In: Cooper JA, ed. *Assessment of Speech and Voice Production: Research and Clinical Applications*. NIDCD Monograph Vol 1-1991. Bethesda, MD: National Institute on Deafness and Other Communication Disorders, NIH; 1991:112-123.

2. Scherer RC. Physiology of phonation: A review of basic mechanics. In: Ford CN, Bless DM, eds. *Phonosurgery: Assessment and Surgical Management of Voice Disorders*. New York, NY: Raven Press; 1991:77-93.

3. Hollien H, Moore GP. Measurement of the vocal folds during changes in pitch. *J Speech Hear Res.* 1960;3:157-165.

4. Nishizawa N, Sawashima M, Yonemoto K. In: Fujimura O, ed. *Vocal Physiology: Voice Production, Mechanisms, and Function*. New York, NY: Raven Press; 1988:75-82.

5. Backus J. *The Acoustical Foundations of Music*. 2nd ed. New York, NY: WW Norton & Co; 1977.

6. Titze IR, Durham PL. Passive mechanisms influencing fundamental frequency control. In: Baer T, Sasaki C, Harris KS, eds. *Laryngeal Function in Phonation and Respiration*. San Diego, CA: College-Hill Press; 1987:304-319.

7. Colton RH. Physiological mechanisms of vocal frequency control: the role of tension. *J Voice.* 1988;2(3):208-220.

8. Titze IR. *Principles of Voice Production*. Englewood Cliffs, NJ: Prentice Hall; 1994.

9. Perlman AL, Titze IR. Development of an in vitro technique for measuring elastic properties of vocal fold tissue. *J Speech Hear Res.* 1988;31/2:288-289.

10. Colton RH, Casper JK. *Understanding Voice Problems*. Baltimore, MD: Williams & Wilkins; 1990.

11. Hammarberg B, Fritzell B, Gauffin J, Sundberg J. *Acoustic glottogram, subglottic pressure, and voice quality during insufficient vocal fold closure phonation*: *Proceedings of the International Conference on Voice, Kurume, Japan*. 1986:28-35.

12. Gauffin J, Sundberg J. Spectral correlates of glottal voice source waveform characteristics. *J Speech Hear Res.* 1989;32:556-565.

13. Sundberg J. *The Science of the Singing Voice*. Dekalb, IL: Northern Illinois University Press; 1987.

14. Titze IR. Phonation threshold pressure: a missing link in glottal aerodynamics. *J Acoust Soc Am.* 1992;91(5):2926-2935.

15. Lucero JC. Optimal glottal configuration for ease of phonation. *J Voice.* 1998;12:151-158.

16. Chan RW, Titze IR, Titze MR. Further studies of phonation threshold pressure in a physical model of the vocal fold mucosa. *J Acoust Soc Am.* 1997;101:3722-3727.

17. Verdolini-Marston K, Titze I, Druker D. Changes in phonation threshold pressure with induced conditions of hydration. *J Voice.* 1990;4(2):142-151.

18. Baer T. *Investigation of Phonation Using Excised Larynges* [dissertation]. Cambridge, MA: Massachusetts Institute of Technology; 1975.

19. Baer T. Observation of vocal fold vibration: Measurement of excised larynges. In: Stevens KN, Hirano M, eds. *Vocal Fold Physiology*. Tokyo, Japan: University of Tokyo Press; 1981:119-133.

20. Draper MH, Ladefoged P, Whitteridge D. Expiratory pressures and air flow during speech. *British Med J.* 1960;18:1837-1843.

21. Berry DA, Herzel H, Titze IR, Story BH. Bifurcation in excised larynx experiments. *J Voice.* 1996;10:129-138.

22. Lucero JC. A theoretical study of the hysteresis phenomenon at vocal fold oscillation onset-offset. *J Acoust Soc Am.* 1999;105:423-431.

23. Fisher KV, Swank PR. Estimating phonation threshold pressure. *J Speech Hear Res.* 1997;40:1122-1129.

24. Coleman RF, Mabis JH, Hinson JK. Fundamental frequency-sound pressure level profiles of adult male and female voices. *J Speech Hear Res.* 1977;20:197-204.

25. Klingholz F, Martin F. Die quantitative Auswertung der Stimmfeldmessung. *Sprache-Stimme-Gehor.* 1983;7:106-110.

26. Titze IR. Acoustic interpretation of the voice range profile (phonetogram). *J Speech Hear Res.* 1992;35:21-34.

27. Coleman RF. Sources of variation in phonetograms. *J Voice.* 1993;7(1):1-14.

28. Gramming P. *The Phonetogram: An Experimental and Clinical Study.* Malmo, Sweden: Department of Otolaryngology, University of Lund; 1988.

29. Bless DM, Baken RJ, Hacki T, et al. International Association of Logopedics and Phoniatrics (IALP) Voice Committee discussion of assessment topics. *J Voice.* 1992;6(2):194-210.

30. Hirano M. *Clinical Examination of Voice.* New York, NY: Springer-Verlag; 1981.

31. Hirose H, Niimi S. The relationship between glottal opening and the transglottal pressure differences during consonant production. In: Baer T, Sasaki C, Harris KS, eds. *Laryngeal Function in Phonation and Respiration.* San Diego, CA: College-Hill Press; 1987:381-390.

32. Baken RJ. Clinical *Measurement of Speech and Voice.* Boston, MA: College-Hill Press, Little, Brown & Co; 1987.

33. Kakita Y. Simultaneous observation of the vibratory pattern, sound pressure, and airflow signals using a physical model of the vocal folds. In: Fujimura O, ed. *Vocal Physiology: Voice Production, Mechanisms, and Function.* New York, NY: Raven Press Ltd.; 1988:207-218.

34. Fant G. Some problems in voice source analysis. *Speech Commun.* 1993;13:7-22.

35. Kiritani S, Hirose H, Imagawa H. High-speed digital image analysis of vocal cord vibration in diplophonia. *Speech Commun.* 1993;13:23-32.

36. Pinto NB, Titze IR. Unification of perturbation measures in speech signals. *J Acoust Soc Am.* 1990;87(3):1278-1289.

37. Larson C, Kempster G, Kistler M. Changes in voice fundamental frequency following discharge of single motor units in cricothyroid and thyroarytenoid muscles. *J Speech Hear Res.* 1987;30:552-558.

38. Kempster GB, Larson CR, Kistler MK. Effects of electrical stimulation of cricothyroid and thyroarytenoid muscles on voice fundamental frequency. *J Voice.* 1988;2(3):221-229.

39. Titze IR. A model for neurologic sources of aperiodicity in vocal fold vibration. *J Speech Hear Res.* 1991;34(3):460-472.

40. Baer T. Vocal jitter: A neuromuscular explanation. In: Lawrence V, Weinberg B, eds. *Transcripts of the Eighth Symposium on Care of the Professional Voice.* New York, NY: The Voice Foundation; 1979:19-22.

41. Cavalli L, Hirson A. Diplophonia reappraised. *J Voice.* 1999;13:542-556.

42. Isshiki N, Ishizaka K. Computer simulation of pathological vocal cord vibration. *J Acoust Soc Am.* 1976;60:1193-1198.

43. Moon FC. *Chaotic Vibrations.* New York, NY: John Wiley & Sons; 1987.

44. Gerratt BR, Precoda K, Hanson D, Berke GS. Source characteristics of diplophonia. *J Acoust Soc Am.* 1988;83:S66.

45. Wong D, Ito MR, Cox NB, Titze IR. Observation of perturbations in a lumped-element model of the vocal folds with application to some pathological cases. *J Acoust Soc Am.* 1991;89:383-394.

46. Berke GS, Gerratt BR. Laryngeal biomechanics: an overview of mucosal wave mechanics. *J Voice.* 1993;7(2):123-128.

47. Titze IR, Baken RJ, Herzel H. Evidence of chaos in vocal fold vibration. In: Titze IR, ed. *Vocal Fold Physiology: Frontiers in Basic Science.* San Diego, CA: Singular Publishing Group; 1993:143-188.

48. Scherer R, Gould WJ, Titze I, Meyers A, Sataloff R. Preliminary evaluation of selected acoustic and glottographic measures for clinical phonatory function analysis. *J Voice.* 1988;2:230-244.

49. Omori K, Kojima H, Kakani R, Slavit DH, Blaugrund SM. Acoustic characteristics of rough voice: subharmonics. *J Voice.* 1997;1:40-47.

50. Hollien H, Moore P, Wendahl RW, Michel JF. On the nature of vocal fry. *J Speech Hear Res.* 1966;9:245-247.

51. Keidar A. *Vocal Register Change: An Investigation of Perceptual and Acoustic Isomorphism* [dissertation]. Iowa City: The University of Iowa; 1986.

52. Titze IR. A framework for the study of vocal registers. *J Voice.* 1988:2(3):183-194.

53. Scherer RC. Physiology of creaky voice and vocal fry. *J Acoust Soc Am.* 1989;86(S1):S25(A).

54. Blomgren M, Chen Y, Ng ML, Gilbert HR. Acoustic, aerodynamic, physiologic, and perceptual properties of modal and vocal fry registers. *J Acoust Soc Am.* 1998;103:2649-2658.

55. Scherer RC, Druker DG, Titze IR. Electroglottography and direct measurement of vocal fold contact area. In: Fujimura O, ed. *Vocal Physiology: Voice Production, Mechanisms, and Function.* New York, NY: Raven Press, Ltd; 1988:279-291.

56. Ishizaka K, Matsudaira M. Analysis of the vibration of the vocal cords. *J Acoust Soc Jap.* 1968;24:311-312.

57. Ishizaka K, Flanagan JL. Synthesis of voiced sounds from a two-mass model of the vocal cords. *Bell Sys Tech J.* 1972;51(6):1233-1268.

58. Smith ME, Berke GS, Gerratt BR, Kreiman J. Laryngeal paralysis: theoretical considerations and effects on laryngeal vibration. *J Speech Hear Res.* 1992;35:545-554.

59. Rothenberg M, Mahshie J. Induced transglottal pressure variations during voicing. *Speech Commun.* 1986;14(3)-4:365-371.

60. Baer T. Reflex activation of laryngeal muscles by sudden induced subglottal pressure changes. *J Acoust Soc Am.* 1979:65:1271-1275.

61. Cheng YM, Guerin B. Control parameters in male and female glottal sources. In: Baer T, Sasaki C, Harris KS, eds. *Laryngeal Function in Phonation and Respiration.* San Diego, CA: College-Hill Press; 1987:219-238.

62. Baken RJ, Orlikoff RF. Phonatory response to step-function changes in supraglottal pressure. In: Baer T, Sasaki C, Harris KS, eds. *Laryngeal Function in Phonation and Respiration.* San Diego, CA: College-Hill Press; 1987:273-290.

63. Saito S, Fukuda H, Isogai Y, Ono H. X-ray stroboscopy. In: Stevens KN, Hirano M, eds. *Vocal Fold Physiology.* Tokyo, Japan: University of Tokyo Press; 1981:95-106.

64. Saito S, Fukuda H, Kitahara S, et al. Pellet tracking in the vocal fold while phonating—experimental study using canine larynges with muscle activity. In: Titze IR, Scherer RC, eds. *Vocal Fold Physiology: Biomechanics, Acoustics and Phonatory Control.* Denver, CO: The Denver Center for the Performing Arts; 1985:169-182.

65. Fukuda H, Saito S, Kitahara S, et al. Vocal fold vibration in excised larynges viewed with an x-ray stroboscope and an ultra-high-speed camera. In: Bless DM, Abbs JH, eds. *Vocal Fold Physiology, Contemporary Research and Clinical Issues.* San Diego, CA: College-Hill Press; 1983:238-252.

66. Alipour-Haghighi F, Titze IR. Simulation of particle trajectories of vocal fold tissue during phonation. In: Titze IR, Scherer RC, eds. *Vocal Fold Physiology: Biomechanics, Acoustics and Phonatory Control.* Denver, CO: The Denver Center for the Performing Arts; 1985:183-190.

67. Muta H, Fukuda H. Pressure-flow relationship in the experimental phonation of excised canine larynges. In: Fujimura O, ed. *Vocal Physiology: Voice Production, Mechanisms, and Function.* New York, NY: Raven Press, Ltd; 1988:239-247.

68. Titze IR, Luschei ES, Hirano M. Role of the thyroarytenoid muscle in regulation of fundamental frequency. *J Voice.* 1989;3(3):213-224.

69. Gelfer CE, Harris KS, Collier R, Baer T. Is declination actively controlled? In: Titze IR, Scherer RC, eds. *Vocal Fold Physiology: Biomechanics, Acoustics and Phonatory Control.* Denver, CO: The Denver Center for the Performing Arts; 1985:113-126.

70. Gelfer CE, Harris KS, Baer T. Controlled variables in sentence intonation. In: Baer T, Sasaki C, Harris KS, eds. *Laryngeal Function in Phonation and Respiration.* San Diego, CA: College-Hill Press; 1987:422-435.

71. Honda K. Relationship between pitch control and vowel articulation. In: Bless DM, Abbs JH, eds. *Vocal Fold Physiology, Contemporary Research and Clinical Issues.* San Diego, CA: College-Hill Press; 1983:286-297.

72. Sundberg J, Leanderson R, von Euler C. Activity relationship between diaphragm and cricothyroid muscles. *J Voice.* 1989;3(3):225-232.

73. Titze IR, Jiang J, Drucker DG. Preliminaries to the body-cover theory of pitch control. *J Voice.* 1988;1(4):314-319.

74. Choi HS, Berke GS, Ye M, Kreiman J. Function of the thyroarytenoid muscle in a canine laryngeal model. *Ann Otol Rhinol Laryngol.* 1993;102:769-776.

75. Arnold GE. Physiology and pathology of the cricothyroid muscle. *Laryngoscope.* 1961;71:687-753.

76. Fujimura O. Body-cover theory of the vocal fold and its phonetic implications. In: Stevens KN, Hirano M, eds. *Vocal Fold Physiology.* Tokyo, Japan: University of Tokyo Press; 1981:271-288.

77. Hirano M. Phonosurgery: Basic and clinical investigations. *Otologia (Fukuoka).* 1975;21:239-442.

78. Hirano M. The laryngeal muscles in singing. In: Hirano M, Kirchner JA, Bless DM, eds. *Neurolaryngology, Recent Advances.* Boston, MA: A College-Hill Publication, Little, Brown & Co; 1987:209-230.

79. Titze IR. A four-parameter model of the glottis and vocal fold contact area. *Speech Commun.* 1989;8:191-201.

80. Plomp R. *Aspects of Tone Sensation.* New York, NY: Academic Press; 1976.

81. Strong WJ, Plitnik GR. *Music Speech Audio.* Provo, UT: Soundprint; 1992.

82. Rothenberg M. Acoustic interaction between the glottal source and the vocal tract. In: Stevens KN, Hirano M,eds. *Vocal Fold Physiology.* Tokyo, Japan: University of Tokyo Press; 1981:305-328.

83. Rothenberg M. An interactive model for the voice source. In: Bless DM, Abbs JH, eds. *Vocal Fold Physiology, Contemporary Research and Clinical Issues.* San Diego, CA: College-Hill Press; 1983:155-165.

84. Titze IR. The physics of small-amplitude oscillation of the vocal folds. *J Acoust Soc Am.* 1988;83:1536-1552.

85. Kitzing P, Lofqvist A. Subglottal and oral pressures during phonation—preliminary investigation using a miniature transducer system. *Medical and Biological Eng.* 1975;13(5):644-648.

86. Fant G. Preliminaries to analysis of the human voice source. *STL-QPRS.* 1983;(4)1982:1-27.

87. Miller DG, Schutte HK. Characteristic patterns of sub- and supra-glottal pressure variations within the glottal cycle. In: Lawrence VL, ed. *Transcripts of the XIIIth Symposium: Care of the Professional Voice.* New York, NY: The Voice Foundation; 1984:70-75.

88. Cranen B, Boves L. A set-up for testing the validity of the two mass model of the vocal folds. In: Titze IR, Scherer RC, eds. *Vocal Fold Physiology: Biomechanics, Acoustics and Phonatory Control.* Denver, CO: The Denver Center for the Performing Arts; 1985:500-513.

89. Olson HF. *Solutions of Engineering Problems by Dynamical Analogies.* 2nd ed. New York, NY: D Van Nostrand Co; 1966.

90. Titze IR. Mean intraglottal pressure in vocal fold oscillation. *J Phonetics.* 1986;14:359-364.

91. Scherer RC, Guo CG. *Laryngeal modeling: translaryngeal pressure for a model with many glottal shapes. ICSLP Proceedings, 1990 International Conference on Spoken Language Processing.* Vol 1. The Acoustical Society of Japan, Japan; 1990:3.1.1-3.1.4.

92. Scherer RC, Guo CG. Generalized translaryngeal pressure coefficient for a wide range of laryngeal configurations. In: Gauffin J, Hammarberg B, eds. *Vocal Fold Physiology: Acoustic, Perceptual, and Physiological Aspects of Voice Mechanisms.* San Diego, CA: Singular Publishing Group; 1991:83-90.

93. Alipour F, Scherer RC. Pulsatile flow within an oscillating glottal model. *J Iran Mech Eng.* 1998;3;73-81.

94. Kline SJ. On the nature of stall. *ASME J Basic Eng.* 1959;81:305-320.

95. Miller DS. *Internal Flow, a Guide to Losses in Pipe and Duct Systems.* Cranfield, UK: British Hydromechanics Research Association; 1971.

96. Guo CG, Scherer RC. Finite element simulation of glottal flow and pressure. *J Acoust Soc Am.* 1993;94(2)(pt 1):688-700.

97. Scherer RC, Shinwari D. Glottal pressure profiles for a diameter of 0.04 cm. *J Acoust Soc Am.* 2000;107(5)(pt 2):2905.

98. Scherer R, Sundberg J, Titze I. Laryngeal adduction related to characteristics of the flow glottogram. *J Acoust Soc Am.* 1989;85(S1):S129(A).

99. Titze IR, Sundberg J. Vocal intensity in speakers and singers. *J Acoust Soc Am.* 1992;91:2936-2946.

100. Sundberg J, Titze I, Scherer R. Phonatory control in male singing: a study of the effects of subglottal pressure, fundamental frequency, and mode of phonation on the voice source. *J Voice.* 1993;7(1):15-29.

101. Fant G, Liljencrants J, Lin Q. A four-parameter model of glottal flow. *STL-QPSR.* 1985;(4)1985:1-13.

102. Gobl C, Karlsson I. Male and female voice source dynamics. In: Gauffin J, Hammarberg B, eds. *Vocal Fold Physiology: Acoustic, Perceptual, and Physiological Aspects of Voice Mechanisms.* San Diego, CA: Singular Publishing Group; 1991:121-128.

103. Fant G, and Lin Q. Comments on glottal flow modeling and analysis. In: Gauffin J, Hammarberg B, eds. *Vocal Fold Physiology: Acoustic, Perceptual, and Physiological Aspects of Voice Mechanisms.* San Diego, CA: Singular Publishing Group; 1991:47-56.

104. Sundberg J, Gauffin J. Waveform and spectrum of the glottal voice source. In: Lindblom B, Ohman S, eds. *Frontiers of Speech Communication Research.* New York, NY: Academic Press; 1979:301-322.

105. Scherer RC, Titze IR, Curtis JF. Pressure-flow relationships in two models of the larynx having rectangular glottal shapes. *J Acoust Soc Am.* 1983;73:668-676.

106. Ladefoged P, McKinney NP. Loudness, sound pressure, and subglottal pressure in speech. *J Acoust Soc Am.* 1963;35:454-460.

107. Isshiki N. Regulatory mechanism of voice intensity variations. *J Speech Hear Res.* 1964;7:17-29.

108. Isshiki N. Remarks on mechanism for vocal intensity variation. *J Speech Hear Res.* 1969;12:665-672.

109. Rubin HJ, LeCover M, Vennard W. Vocal intensity, subglottic pressure, and airflow relationships in singers. *Folia Phoniatr.* 1967;19:393-413.

110. Bouhuys A, Mead J, Proctor D, Stevens K. Pressure-flow events during singing. *Ann NY Acad Sci.* 1968;155:165-176.

111. Holmberg EB, Hillman RE, Perkell J. Glottal airflow and transglottal air pressure measurements for male and female speakers in soft, normal, and loud voice. *J Acoust Soc Am.* 1988;84:511-529.

112. Sapienza CM, Stathopoulos ET. Comparison of maximum flow declination rate: children versus adults. *J Voice.* 1994;8:240-247.

113. Sulter AM, Wit H. Glottal volume velocity waveform characteristics in subjects with and without vocal training, related to gender, sound intensity, fundamental frequency, and age. *J Acoust Soc Am.* 1996;100:3360-3373.

114. Titze IR. Regulation of vocal power and efficiency by subglottal pressure and glottal width. In: Fujimura O, ed. *Vocal Physiology: Voice Production, Mechanisms, and Function.* New York, NY: Raven Press, Ltd; 1988:227-238.

115. Raphael BN, Scherer RC. Voice modifications of stage actors: Acoustic analyses. *J Voice.* 1987;1:83-87.

116. Bartholomew WT. A physical definition of "good voice quality" in the male voice. *J Acoust Soc Am.* 1934;6:25-33.

117. Sundberg J. Articulatory interpretation of the "singing formant." *J Acoust Soc Am.* 1974;55:838-844.

118. Perkins WH. *Voice Disorders.* New York, NY: Thieme-Stratton Inc; 1983.

119. Verdolini K, Druker DG, Palmer PM, Samawi H. Laryngeal adduction in resonant voice. *J Voice.* 1998;12:315-327.

120. Hollien HF, Curtis JF. A laminagraphic study of vocal pitch. *J Speech Hear Res.* 1960;3:361-371.

121. Hollien HF. Vocal fold thickness and fundamental frequency of phonation. *J Speech Hear Res.* 1962;5(3):237-243.

122. Hollien HF, Colton RH. Four laminagraphic studies of vocal fold thickness. *Folia Phoniatr.* 1969;21:179-198.

123. Hollien HF, Coleman RF. Laryngeal correlates of frequency change: A STROL study. *J Speech Hear Res.* 1970;13(2):271-278.

124. Scherer RC, Vail VJ, Rockwell B. Examination of the laryngeal adduction measure EGGW. In: Bell-Berti F, Raphael LJ, eds: *Producing Speech: Contemporary Issues: A Festshrift for Katherine Safford Harris.* Woodbury, NY: American Institute of Physics; 1995:269-290.

125. Hess Mm, Verdolini K, Bierhals W, Mansmann U, Gross M. Endolaryngeal contact pressure. *J Voice.* 1998;12:50-67.

126. Verdolini K, Chan R, Titze IR, Hess M, Bierhals W. Correspondence of electroglottographic closed quotient to vocal fold impact stress in excised canine larynges. *J Voice.* 1998;12:415-423.

127. Verdolini K, Hess MH, Titze IR, Bierhals W, Gross M. Investigation of vocal fold impact stress in human subjects. *J Voice.* 1999;13:184-202.

128. Yamana T, Kitajima K. Laryngeal closure pressure during phonation in humans. *J Voice.* 2000;14:1-7.

129. Scherer RC, DeWitt K, Kucinschi BR. Effect of vocal radii on pressure distributions in the glottis. In review.

130. Hirano M, Bless DM. *Videostroboscopic Examination of the Larynx.* San Diego, CA: Singular Publishing Group; 1993.

131. Berg Jw van den, Zantema JT, Doornenbal P Jr. On the air resistance and the Bernoulli effect of the human larynx. *J Acoust Soc Am.* 1957;29:626-631.

132. Scherer RC. Pressure-flow relationships in a laryngeal airway model having a diverging glottal duct. *J Acoust Soc Am.* 1983;73(S1):S46(A).

133. Scherer RC, Titze IR. Pressure-flow relationships in a model of the laryngeal airway with a diverging glottis. In: Bless DM, Abbs JH, eds. *Vocal Fold Physiology, Contemporary Research and Clinical Issues.* San Diego, CA: College-Hill Press; 1983:179-193.

134. Gauffin J, Binh N, Ananthapadmanabha TV, Fant G. Glottal geometry and volume velocity waveform. In: Bless DM, Abbs JH, eds. *Vocal Fold Physiology: Contemporary Research and Clinical Issues.* San Diego, CA: College-Hill Press; 1983:194-201.

135. Ishizaka K. Air resistance and intraglottal pressure in a model of the larynx. In: Titze IR, Scherer RC. eds. *Vocal Fold Physiology: Biomechanics, Acoustics and Phonatory Control.* Denver, CO: The Denver Center for the Performing Arts; 1985:414-424.

136. Alipour R, Scherer RC. Dynamic glottal pressures in an excised hemilarynx model. *J Voice.* In press.

137. Ishizaka K, Matsudaira M. *Fluid mechanical considerations of vocal cord vibration.* SCRL Monograph No. 8, April 1972.

138. Titze IR. The human vocal cords: A mathematical model. Part I. *Phonetica.* 1973;28:129-170.

139. Titze IR. The human vocal cords: A mathematical model. Part II. *Phonetica.* 1974;29:1-21.

140. Titze IR. On the mechanics of vocal fold vibration. *J Acoust Soc Am.* 1976;60(6):136-1380.

141. Titze IR. Biomechanics and distributed-mass models of vocal fold vibration. In: Stevens KN, Hirano M, eds. *Vocal Fold Physiology.* Tokyo, Japan: University of Tokyo Press; 1981:245-270.

142. Alipour F, Titze IR. A finite element simulation of vocal fold vibration. In: *Proc. Fourteenth Annual Northeast Bioeng.* Conf. Durham; IEEE publications #88-CH2666-6; 1988:86-189.

143. Schonharl E. *Die Stroboskopie in der praktischen Laryngologie.* Stuttgart, Germany: Thieme; 1960.

144. Stevens KN, Klatt DH. Current models of sound sources for speech. In: Wyke B, ed. *Ventilatory and Phonatory Control Systems, an International Symposium.* New York, NY: Oxford University Press; 1974:279-292.

145. Hirano M. Structure and vibratory behavior of the vocal folds. In: Sawashima M, Cooper FS, eds. *Dynamic Aspects of Speech Production.* Tokyo, Japan: University of Tokyo Press; 1977:13-27.

146. Cooper DS. Voice: a historical perspective (Woldemar Tonndorf and the Bernoulli effect in voice production). *J Voice.* 1989;3(1):1-6.

147. Scherer RC, Shinwari D, DeWitt K, Zhang C, Kucinschi B, Afjeh A. Intraglottal pressure profiles for a symmetric and oblique glottis with a divergence angle of 10 degrees. *J Acoust Soc Am.* In press.

148. Pelorson X, Hirschberg A, van Hassel RR, Wijnands APJ. Theoretical and experimental study of quasisteady-flow separation within the glottis during phonation. Application to a modified two-mass model. *J Acoust Soc Am.* 1994;96:3416-3431.

149. Pelorson X, Hirschberg A, Wijnands APJ, Bailliet H. Description of the flow through in vitro models of the glottis during phonation. *Acta Acustica.* 1995;3:191-202.

150. Hofmans GCJ. *Vortex Sound in Confined Flows* [dissertation]. Eindhoven: CIP-Data Library Technische Universiteit Eindhoven; 1998.

151. von Leden H, Moore P, Timcke R. Laryngeal vibrations: measurements of the glottic wave. Part III: the pathologic larynx. *Arch Otolaryngol.* 1960;71:16-35.

152. Koike Y, Imaizumi S. Objective evaluation of laryngostroboscopic findings. In: Fujimura O, ed. *Vocal Physiology: Voice Production, Mechanisms and Functions.* New York, NY: Raven Press, Ltd; 1988:433-442.

153. Svec JG, Schutte HK. Videokymography: high-speed line scanning of vocal fold vibration. *J Voice.* 1996;10:201-205.

154. Kaiser J. Some observations on vocal tract operation from a fluid flow point of view. In: Titze IR, Scherer RC, eds. *Vocal Fold Physiology: Biomechanics, Acoustics and Phonatory Control.* Denver, CO: The Denver Center for the Performing Arts; 1985:358-386.

155. Teager H, Teager S. Active fluid dynamic voice production models, or there is a unicorn in the garden. In: Titze IR, Scherer RC, eds. *Vocal Fold Physiology: Biomechanics, Acoustics and Phonatory Control.* Denver, CO: The Denver Center for the Performing Arts; 1985:387-401.

156. McGowan RS. An aeroacoustic approach to phonation. *J Acoust Soc Am.* 1988;88:696-704.

157. McGowan RS. Phonation from a continuum mechanics point of view. In: Gauffin J, Hammarberg B, eds. *Vocal Fold Physiology: Acoustic, Perceptual, and Physiological Aspects of Voice Mechanisms.* San Diego, CA: Singular Publishing Group; 1991:65-72.

158. Berke GS, Moore DM, Monkewitz PA, Hanson DG, Gerratt BR. A preliminary study of particle velocity during phonation in an in vivo canine model. *J Voice.* 1989;3(4):306-313.

159. Shadle CH, Barney AM, Thomas DW. An investigation into the acoustic and aerodynamics of the larynx. In: Gauffin J, Hammarberg B, eds. *Vocal Fold Physiology: Acoustic, Perceptual, and Physiological Aspects of Voice Mechanisms.* San Diego: Singular Publishing Group; 1991:73-80.

160. Alipour F, Fan C. Pulsatile flow in a three-dimensional model of larynx. In: Biewener AA, Goel VK, eds. *Proceedings of 1993 ASB Meeting.* 1993:221-222.

161. Davies POAL, McGowan RS, Shadle CH. Practical flow duct acoustics applied to the vocal tract. In: Titze IR, ed. *Vocal Fold Physiology: Frontiers in Basic Science.* San Diego, CA: Singular Publishing Group; 1993:93-134.

162. Scherer R. Practical flow duct acoustics applied to the vocal tract: Response. In: Titze IR, ed. *Vocal Fold Physiology: Frontiers in Basic Science.* San Diego, CA: Singular Publication Group; 1993:134-142.

163. Alipour F, Scherer RC. Pulsatile airflow during phonation: an excised larynx model. *J Acoust Soc Am.* 1995;97:1241-1248.

164. Zhao W. *A Numerical Investigation of Sound Radiated From Subsonic Jet With Application to Human Phonation,* [dissertation]. West Lafayette, IN: Purdue University; 2000.

CHAPTER 8

Laryngeal Neurophysiology

Michael S. Benninger, MD

Glendon M. Gardner, MD

Craig Schwimmer, MD

The larynx provides the basic functions of airway protection, respiration, and voice. These are accomplished via a delicate balance of sensation, reflexes, and voluntary movement, all mediated through an intricate neurologic system. The ability to evaluate and treat a patient with neurologic dysfunction of the larynx requires an understanding of the complicated neuroanatomy of the larynx. Neurologic vocal fold immobility can result from insults which affect the motor input from the nucleus ambiguus to the final neuromuscular junction. Sensory disruption can effect the mechanical, tactile, thermal, pH, and other receptors necessary for the maintenance of reflexive pathways, resulting in alterations of normal laryngeal function.

This chapter describes the neuroanatomy and neurophysiology of the larynx and identifies key laryngeal reflexes.

NEUROANATOMY OF THE LARYNX

The vagus nerve (cranial nerve X), named for its wandering course, is the longest cranial nerve. It contains somatic sensory (skin near the ear and posterior external auditory canal), visceral afferent (from heart, pancreas, stomach, esophagus, and upper respiratory tract), somatic motor, autonomic afferent, and taste fibers.[1] The afferent fibers (visceral, taste, and somatic sensory) have cells which originate in the nodose and jugular ganglions, which are the sensory ganglia of the nerve. They enter the medulla and divide into descending and ascending branches.

Somatic motor fibers arise in the nucleus ambiguus to innervate the striated muscles of the larynx and a portion of the pharynx.[2] Intracranial or supranodose ganglion sectioning of the vagal nerve fibers results in degeneration of "large" and "intermediate" myelinated fibers of the recurrent laryngeal nerve, which consist of laryngeal motor axons originating in the nucleus ambiguus.[3] The nucleus ambiguus receives collaterals which control voluntary muscle movement of the larynx from the opposite pyramidal tract (Figure 8-1). Reflex pathways from terminal sensory nuclei are part of the reticular formation.

Taste fibers from the epiglottis and larynx pass in the vagus to join the tractus solitarius to terminate in the nucleus of the tractus solitarius, which contacts with the motor centers of the medulla oblongata, pons, and spinal cord for mastication and deglutition.

The superficial origin of the vagus is from eight to ten rootlets attached to the medulla oblongata (Figure 8-1). These lie in the groove between the olive and inferior peduncle with the roots of the glossopharyngeal nerve coursing superiorly and the spinal accessory nerve inferiorly. The rootlets unite to pass beneath the flocculus of the cerebellum. The vagus leaves the cranial vault through the jugular foramen along with the glossopha-

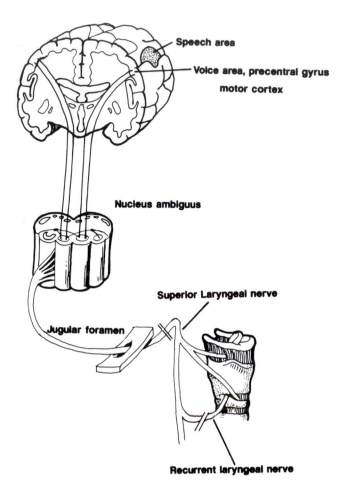

Speech area

Voice area, precentral gyrus
motor cortex

Nucleus ambiguus

Superior Laryngeal nerve

Jugular foramen

Recurrent laryngeal nerve

FIGURE 8-1. *Central neural schema of vagus nerve.*

ryngeal nerve, the jugular vein and the internal carotid artery, and near the hypoglossal nerve. It lies in the same dural sheath as the spinal accessory nerve but is separated from the glossopharyngeal nerve by a septum.[1]

The jugular ganglion or superior ganglion of the vagus nerve lies in the jugular foramen (Figure 8-2). These sensory ganglion cells enter the medulla just dorsal to the motor units. Some of the peripheral processes are distributed to the pharynx. The nodose ganglion or inferior ganglion lies just distal to the jugular foramen (Figure 8-2). The central processes of these cells pass through the jugular ganglion to enter the medulla along with the jugular cell rootlets. The peripheral processes of these ganglion cells make up the internal branch of the superior laryngeal nerves, other vagal branches to the larynx, trachea, esophagus, bronchi, and thoracic and abdominal viscera.

The cranial portion of the spinal accessory nerve joins the vagus near the nodose ganglion to supply motor branches of the vagus to the larynx and pharynx. The vagus nerve trunk passes within the carotid sheath

deep to, and between, the internal jugular vein and carotid artery as they descend in the neck. The left vagus nerve enters the thorax deep to the innominate vein between the subclavian and carotid arteries and passes between the aorta and the left pulmonary artery to give off the recurrent laryngeal nerve (RLN) branch as the vagus crosses the left side of the arch of the aorta (Figure 8-2). The RLN loops under the arch of the aorta just distal to the ligamentum arteriosum to pass on the side of the trachea to ascend deep to the carotid artery in the tracheoesophageal groove. It runs medial to the deep surface of the thyroid gland under the lower border of the inferior constrictor muscle to enter the larynx through the cricothyroid membrane behind the articulation of the inferior cornua of the thyroid cartilage with the cricoid cartilage. It supplies motor input to all the muscles of the larynx other than the cricothyroid muscle. The terminal branch of the RLN communicates with the fibers of the SLN and is called the ansa galeni.[4]

The right vagus nerve enters the thorax to cross superficial to the subclavian artery between the artery and the innominate vein. Here it loops under the subclavian, ascends behind it to lie in the tracheoesophageal groove. A rare nondescending right RLN occurs in less than 1% of humans. The intimate relation of the RLNs to the aorta, subclavian, thyroid, and cricothyroid joints allows for injury from surgery or neoplasms in these areas.

The diameter of the myelinated fibers has been found to be greater in the left RLN than the right.[5,6] This has led to the theory that the bundle-sized difference allows for almost simultaneous activation of the laryngeal muscles on the two sides, despite the left RLN being longer.[3] Nerve topographic studies have shown that nerve fiber content is divided between laryngeal and nonlaryngeal groups of nerve fibers in the RLN with laryngeal motor axons usually being found in the largest fascicles of the nerve.[3] Laryngeal motor axons have been found in the anterior position in the vagus superior to the hyoid bone and in the medial position inferior to the hyoid.[6]

The superior laryngeal nerve (SLN) arises from the vagus just caudal to the nodose ganglion and descends posteriorly to the internal carotid artery where it splits into internal and external branches near the greater cornua of the thyroid cartilage after communicating with a branch or the cervical sympathetics (Figure 8-2).

The internal branch, the larger of the two superior nerve branches, passes through the thyrohyoid membrane along with the superior laryngeal artery. This supplies parasympathetic secretory motor fibers to the glands of the larynx down to the level of true vocal fold, the aryepiglottic folds, epiglottis, and base of tongue. It supplies sensory fibers to these areas and terminates in a small branch that communicates with a branch of the RLN.[7] The internal branch of the SLN has also been found to send bilateral innervation to the interarytenoid muscles.[7,8] The communication between the SLN and RLN are also by nerve branches other than Galen's anastomosis.[9] The external branch of the SLN runs along the larynx to pass deep to the sternothyroid muscle to supply motor fibers to the cricothyroid muscle and a portion of the inferior constrictor. It supplies fibers to the pharyngeal plexus and has communication with the superior sympathetic cardiac nerve.[1]

Sensation from the supraglottic areas is transmitted via the SLN and from the glottic and subglottic areas via the RLN to the nodose ganglion and the tractus solitarius. Sensory and proprioreceptive nerve endings are more dense on the laryngeal surface of the epiglottis than on the true vocal folds and are greater at the posterior portion of the true vocal fold than the anterior commissure.[4,7]

LARYNGEAL CHEMOREFLEXES

The human larynx serves four basic functions: airway protection, respiration, phonation, and facilitating increases in intrathoracic pressure for lifting, coughing, defecating, and so forth.[10-13] Protective reflex closure of the human larynx has been described as its most basic and primitive function.[10] Simple, reflexive closure of the glottis during deglutition is referred to as the glottic closure reflex. In addition to local effects, chemical stimulation of the larynx elicits reflexive changes in the respiratory and cardiovascular systems. These effects include apnea, bradycardia, hypertension, bronchoconstriction, coughing, and changes in peripheral vascular resistance.[10-14] Such systemic responses to laryngeal stimulation are referred to as laryngeal chemoreflexes (LCR). Laryngospasm refers to reflexive muscular contraction that persists despite removal of the eliciting stimulus.

Anatomy and Physiology

A wide variety of receptor nerve endings, including subepithelial plexuses, intraepithelial nerve endings (myelinated and nonmyelinated), epiglottal taste bud-like structures, and others have been described in the hypopharynx and larynx.[12-18] Laryngeal receptors sensitive to decreases in temperature have been reported in dogs. These receptors have been localized to the mucosa

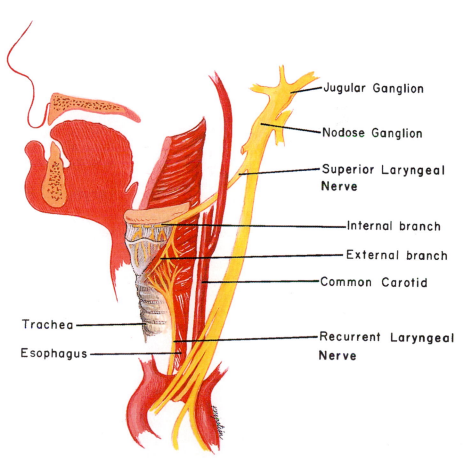

FIGURE 8-2. *Extracranial course of vagus, with superior and recurrent laryngeal nerves detailed.*

Jugular Ganglion

Nodose Ganglion

Superior Laryngeal Nerve

Internal branch

External branch

Common Carotid

Recurrent Laryngeal Nerve

Trachea

Esophagus

of the vocal folds in proximity to the vocal processes of the arytenoid cartilages. Their firing is rapidly blocked by topical application of lidocaine, suggesting a superficial location. Such receptors are specifically responsive to cold and are not responsive to mechanical changes such as transmural pressure, airflow, or local probing and are silent near body temperature.[16] The cooling effect of increased airflow, however, makes them indirectly sensitive to respiration. Laryngeal reflex effects can be reproduced by stimulation of the superior laryngeal nerves (SLN), and abolished by sectioning the SLN, suggesting that afferent stimuli are carried by the SLN.[10-12,14,16]

A wide variety of chemical substances have been studied across numerous species regarding elicitation of laryngeal chemoreflexes. The reflex effects caused by laryngeal instillation of water, milk, acidic substances, ammonia, cigarette smoke, graphite dust, capsaicin, glucose solutions, and others have been described, often with species-specific results.[12-16] For example, laryngeal cooling has been shown to result in increased lower airway resistance and bronchoconstriction in dogs,[16,19] as does mechanical stimulation of the larynx in cats.[20] Laryngeal instillation of water is known to cause bradycardia and to decrease the respiratory rate in dogs, piglets, lambs, and human infants.[21-25] It has been suggested that a common characteristic of apnea-inducing substances is a chloride concentration lower than that normally found in extracellular fluid, although this theory has recently been called into question.[23,25]

LARYNGEAL PROPRIORECEPTORS

In addition to chemo- and thermoreceptors, two classes of laryngeal proprioreceptors have been described. Low threshold, rapidly adapting mechanoreceptors are located in the capsules of all laryngeal joints. These receptors are responsible for transient adjustments in laryngeal muscle tone in response to joint movement (as in speech). Low threshold, slowly adapting mechanoreceptors are located within laryngeal muscles. These receptors adjust laryngeal muscle tone. Two opposing polysynaptic reflex arcs have been described: one inhibitory, which when elicited decreased the rate of motor unit discharge in cricothyroid, thyroarytenoid, and sternothyroid muscles; and one facilitatory, which, when elicited, increased the rate of motor unit discharge in cricothyroid and thyroarytenoid muscles.[17]

Slowly adapting mechanoreceptors, sensitive to changes in laryngeal transmural pressure (some positive, some negative, some both) have been identified. In one study in adult dogs, the majority of receptors were responsive only to collapsing pressure, with only 15% of receptors stimulated by distending pressure. This was thought to suggest a role in maintaining adequate laryngeal muscular tone during inspiration.[9,20]

Developmental Aspects of Laryngeal Chemoreflexes

Laryngeal chemoreflexes appear to be age-dependent. For instance, when adult canine larynges were perfused with agents that induce apnea in puppies, little or no effect on breathing was noted, but reflex coughing and swallowing did occur.[22] A study of piglets showed that stimulating SLN in animals younger than 1 month yielded only a slight decrease in respiratory rate and depth.[26] It has been noted that "In no species has a fatal or sustained apneic response been elicited in an adult animal or even an immature animal after a certain developmental period."[11]

It has been suggested that the maturation of central, antagonistic respiratory drive mechanisms prevents laryngeal chemostimulation from inducing apnea.[27] An anatomic basis for this supposition has been proposed. The superior laryngeal nerve, which carries the afferent arc of the laryngeal chemoreflex, terminates in the area of the solitary tract and dorsal nuclei. The motor fibers of vagus nerve responsible for the efferent reflex arc originate in the nucleus ambiguus and nucleus retroambigualus. These nuclei lie near the nuclei of the reticular system and could conceivably interact.[27,28]

Laryngeal Chemoreflexes and Sudden Infant Death Syndrome (SIDS)

SIDS is defined as the sudden death of any child or infant which is unexpected by history and in which a thorough postmortem examination fails to demonstrate an adequate cause for death. SIDS is the most common cause of death between 2 weeks and 1 year of age and has a peak incidence between the second and fourth months of life.[29]

Several lines of evidence suggest a link between LCR and SIDS. First, the LCR is an age-dependent reflex. Stimuli capable of producing fatal apneas in immature animals have been shown to elicit only reflexive swallowing in mature animals.[28,30,31] Second, a relationship has been shown between gastroesophageal reflux (GER) and infantile apneas. Infants who present with life-threatening apneas have a higher rate of significant GER events, longer periods of esophageal acidification, and increased risk for SIDS.[32] Additionally, apneic spells immediately following documented GER have been reported. It has recently been demonstrated that stimulation of distal esophageal sensory nerves in young puppies causes laryngospasm. This suggests that vagal pathways other than LCR might contribute to the relationship between GER and SIDS.[33]

Central Neuroanatomy

A comprehensive discussion of the central neuroanatomy and physiology of phonation is beyond the scope of this chapter. However, the reader should be aware that substantial advances have been made in our understanding of the importance of the cortex, subcortex, periaqueductal gray matter, and other areas in the phonatory process. The reader is encouraged to consult other sources. Much of this research is based on animal studies.[34,35]

SUMMARY

There are many factors involved in the physiology, reflexes, and pathology of neurolaryngeal disorders. Recent studies have advanced our understanding of the basic laryngeal neuroanatomic pathways, vocal fold proprioception, and laryngeal reflexes, and these concepts will likely play major roles in future investigation, assessment, and treatment of laryngeal neural dysfunction.

REFERENCES

1. *Gray's Anatomy of the Human Body.* Philadelphia, PA: Lea & Febiger; 1956:1012-1020.

2. Yoshida Y, Miyazaki T, Hirano M, et al. Arrangement of motorneurons innervating intrinsic laryngeal muscles of cats as demonstrated by horseradish peroxidase. *Acta Otolaryngol.* 1982;94:329-334.

3. Malmgren L, Gacek R. Peripheral motor innervation of the larynx. In: Blitzer A, ed. *Neurologic Disorders of the Larynx.* New York, NY: Thieme Medical; 1992:36-43.

4. Tucker H. *The Larynx.* 2nd ed. New York, NY: Thieme Medical; 1993:17.

5. Harrison D. Fibre size frequency in the recurrent laryngeal nerves of man and giraffe. *Acta Otolaryngol.* 1981;91:383-389.

6. Shin T, Rabuzzi D. Conduction studies of the canine recurrent laryngeal nerves. *Laryngoscope.* 1971;81:586-596.

7. Sasaki C, Isaacson G. Functional anatomy of the larynx. *Otolaryngol Clin North Am.* 1988;21:595-612.

8. Sanders I, Mu L. Anatomy of the human internal superior laryngeal nerve. *Anat Rec.* 1998;252:646-656.

9. Sanders I, Wu B, Liancai M, et al. The innervation of the human larynx. *Arch Otolaryngol Head Neck Surg.* 1993;119:934-939.

10. Sasaki C, Suzuki M. Laryngeal reflexes in cat, dog, and man. *Arch Otolaryngol Head Neck Surg.* 1976;102:400-402.

11. Cooper D, Lawson W. Laryngeal sensory receptors. In: Blitzer A, ed. *Neurologic Disorders of the Larynx.* New York, NY: Thieme Medical; 1992:16.

12. Boushey H, Richardson P, Widdicombe J, et al. The response of laryngeal afferent fibers to mechanical and chemical stimuli. *J Physiol.* 1974;240:153-175.

13. Matthew O, Sant'Ambrogio G, Fisher J, et al. Laryngeal pressure receptors. *Respir Physiol.* 1984;57:113-122.

14. Suzuki M, Kirchner J. Afferent nerve fibers in the external branch of the superior laryngeal nerve in the cat. *Ann Otol Rhinol Laryngol.* 1962;77:549-570.

15. Palecek F, Matthew O, Sant'Ambrogio F, et al: Cardiorespiratory responses to inhaled laryngeal irritants. *Inhalation Toxicol.* 1990;2:93-104.

16. Sant'Ambrogio G, Matthew O, Sant'Ambrogio F, et al. Characteristics of laryngeal and recurrent laryngeal cold receptors. *Respir Physiol.* 1988;71:287-298.

17. Abo-El-Enein M, Wyke B. Laryngeal myotactic reflexes. *Nature.* 1966;209:682-685.

18. Sant'Ambrogio F, Tsubone H, Matthew O, et al. Afferent activity in the external branch of the superior laryngeal and recurrent laryngeal nerves. *Ann Otol Rhinol Laryngol.* 1991;100:944-950.

19. James Y, Barthelemy P, Delpierre S. Respiratory effects of cold air breathing in anesthetized cats. *Respir Physiol.* 1983;54:41-54.

20. Tomori Z, Widdicomb J. Muscular, bronchomotor and cardiovascular reflexes elicited by mechanical stimulation of the respiratory tract. *J Physiol.* 1969;200:25-49.

21. Gooding G, Richardson M, Trachy R. Laryngeal chemoreflex: anatomic and physiologic study by use of the superior laryngeal nerve in the piglet. *Otolaryngol Head Neck Surg.* 1987;97:28-38.

22. Woodson G, Brauel G. Arterial chemoreceptor influences on the laryngeal chemoreflex. *Otolaryngol Head Neck Surg.* 1992;107:775-782.

23. Davies A, Koenig J, Thatch B. Upper airway chemoreflex responses to saline and water in

preterm infants. *J Appl Physiol.* 1988;64:1412-1420.

24. Davies A, Koenig J, Thatch B. Characteristics of upper airway chemoreflex prolonged apnea in human infants. *Am Rev Resp Dis.* 1989;139:668-673.

25. Boffs D, Bartlett D. Chemical specificity of a laryngeal apneic reflex in puppies. *J Appl Physiol.* 1982;53:455-462.

26. Lee J, Stoll B, Downing S. Properties of the laryngeal chemoreflex in neonatal piglets. *Am J Physiol.* 1977;233:30-37.

27. Van Vliet B, Uenishsi M. Antagonistic interaction of laryngeal and central chemoreceptor respiratory reflexes. *Am J Appl Physiol.* 1992;72:643-649.

28. Rimell F, Gooding G, Johnson K. Cholinergic agents in the laryngeal chemoreflex model of sudden infant death syndrome. *Laryngoscope.* 1993; 103:223-230.

29. Beers M, Berkow R, eds. *Merck Manual of Diagnosis and Therapy.* 17th ed. Whitehouse Station, NJ: Merck & Co Inc; 1999.

30. Sasaki C. Development of laryngeal function: etiologic significance in the sudden infant death syndrome. *Laryngoscope.* 1979;89:1964-1981.

31. Downing S, Lee J. Laryngeal chemosensitivity: a possible mechanism for sudden infant death. *Pediatrics.* 1975;55:640-648.

32. Kelly D, Shannon D. Sudden infant death syndrome and near sudden infant death syndrome: a review of the literature 1964-1982. *Pediatr Clin North Am.* 1982;19:1241.

33. Bauman N, Sanler A, Schmidt C. Reflex laryngospasm induced by stimulation of distal esophageal afferents. *Laryngoscope.* 1994;104:209-214.

34. Yoshida Y, Mitsumasu T, Miyazaki T, Hirano M, Kaneseki T. Distribution of mononeurons in the brain stem of monkeys, innervating the larynx. *Brain Res Bull.* 1984;13:413-419.

35. Fukuyama T, Umezaki T, Shin T. Origin of laryngeal sensory evoked potentials (LSEPs) in the cat. *Brain Res Bull.* 1993;31:381-392.

CHAPTER 9

Dynamical Disorders of Voice: A Chaotic Perspective on Vocal Irregularities

R. J. Baken, PhD

The modern era of voice research might fairly be said to have begun about 50 years ago, with the elaboration of a crucial understanding: phonation results from and is governed by the biomechanical characteristics of vocal fold tissue interacting with glottal aerodynamic properties. That insight was the heart of the myoelastic-aerodynamic theory of phonation,[1-3] a construct that physiologic observation of vocal fold behavior has amply validated. Numerous mathematical models of vocal fold function that were founded upon it[4-5] have generally had extraordinarily impressive predictive and explanatory power. As a result, the process of normal phonation is quite well understood.

Unfortunately, despite very serious efforts by many of our best researchers over a significant period of time, there are still large gaps in our comprehension of laryngeal phonatory behavior. Nowhere are these lacunae wider than in our understanding of many of the anomalies encountered in abnormal vocal function, and (when one actually looks for them) even in the normal voice.[6] The increase of frequency and amplitude perturbation that is so characteristic of dysphonia, for example, remains only poorly explained, despite several hypotheses of varying attractiveness.[7-13] The "pitch breaks" of the adolescent also lack a coherent explanatory model, as has the "biphonation" of the infant's cry.[14-15]

Even less well explained is the kind of situation illustrated in Figure 9-1A, which shows the fundamental frequency (F_0) of successive periods during a sustained vowel by an 81-year-old female with a diagnosis of spasmodic dysphonia. Her F_0 undergoes a relatively slow cyclic variation at a rate of about 4 cycles per second, most likely caused by tremor of the laryngeal muscles. There is also, however, a much faster frequency variation that is sometimes observable at the peaks of the slower oscillations. This is harder to explain. However, most striking are the outbreaks of "diplophonia"—more properly, subharmonic oscillation—that occur in the "valleys" of the F_0 pattern and that persist halfway up the next peak. We have had no easy explanation for this kind of behavior. Even less have we been able to offer coherent and parsimonious explanations for the more complex patterns of F_0 change, like that of Figure 9-1B, that are not uncommon in dysphonic voices. While we have developed a fairly clear picture of the mechanisms of the phonationally regular, we have not done nearly as well in elucidating the vocally complex or erratic.

The fact is, of course, that we have not done much worse in dealing with oscillatory misbehavior than most of the broader sciences of which we are a part. All have been impeded by a paucity of scientific tools for describing disorder, modeling instability, and characterizing capriciousness.

The outlook improved dramatically about 20 years ago with the recognition of the pivotal importance, broad applicability, and enormous explanatory power of

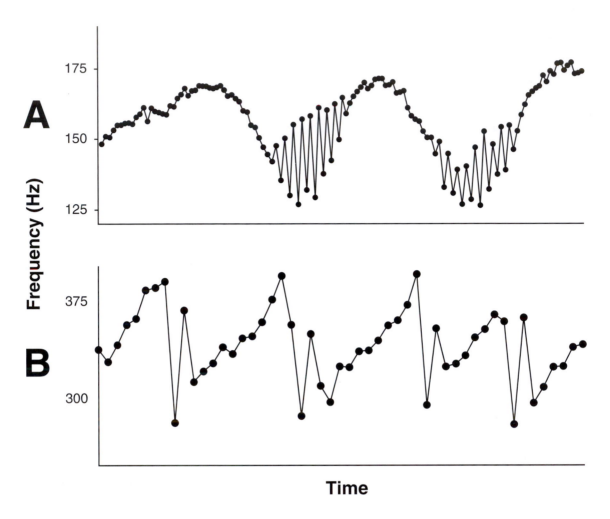

FIGURE 9-1. *Fundamental frequency of successive periods during sustained vowels. (A) An aged spasmodic dysphonic woman, showing subharmonic oscillation during the low parts of a tremor cycle; (B) very complex patterns of F_O change in the voice of a dysphonic patient.*

a radically different way of considering natural phenomena. The new discipline is formally known as the *theory of nonlinear dynamics,* but it is more popularly called *chaos theory.* It offers a different way of looking at life functions[16-18] that has begun to have a significant impact in the biomedical world. Cochlear function,[19] abnormal motor behavior,[20] cardiac electrical instability,[21-25] Cheyne-Stokes respiration,[26] cerebral electrophysiology,[27] and even menopausal hot flashes[28] have been explored with the new tools—both qualitative and quantitative—that it provides. The application of chaos theory to voice production is now well under way.[29-45] It holds the promise of important breakthroughs in understanding those erratic phenomena of voice, normal and disordered, that have thus far proved so intractable.

The purpose of this chapter is to consider a few of the most basic concepts of chaos theory, and to show how

they might profitably be applied to problems of vocal dysfunction. The theory itself is intensely mathematical, and the mathematics can be quite difficult and counterintuitive. It is, therefore, useful to take a very informal concept-oriented approach even though doing so greatly circumscribes the extent to which important areas can be developed. The purpose is not to provide a tutorial introduction to applied chaos theory so much as to suggest something of the flavor of this relatively new branch of the sciences and to suggest why it holds such promise. To do this, some conjectures will be proposed that might explain the sudden appearance of phonatory anomalies that are so characteristic of disordered voices. Insofar as possible, we will proceed in a completely non-mathematical (and consequently non-rigorous) way, because it seems likely that doing so will meet the needs of most readers who would like to understand the general tenor of what is involved, but who are unlikely to want to tackle nonlinear dynamical analyses themselves (at least not yet). Numerophiles and those who wish really to explore the area should consult a good general text.*

CHAOS DEFINED

The very term "chaos" has become trendy, a fashionable buzzword that is too often dropped into discussions as a synonym for "erratic," "unpredictable," or "very complex." But the word *chaos* has, in fact, a very specific definition. If it is to be a useful concept, it is important to specify exactly what "chaos" really means.

---

* The classic source of understanding for numerophobes is Gleick (1987),[46] a volume that appeared for many weeks on the best-seller lists. A very brief nontechnical presentation is Crutchfield, Farmer, et al (1986)[47] For those who can tolerate a minimal mathematical exposition, Abraham and Shaw[48-51] offer an excellent—and lighthearted—starting point that calls for no background at all. More mathematically rigorous introductions are provided by Rasband,[52] Baker and Golub,[53] Moon,[54] and Thompson and Stewart.[55] Eubank and Farmer (1990)[56] is a classic, and is surprisingly approachable. A good overview of chaos in several scientific disciplines is available in Cvitanovic (1984),[57] while Glass and Mackey[58] explore nonlinear dynamics of various biological systems, and West[59] concisely reviews nonlinear dynamics considered in pathophysiology.

Basically, behavior can be said to be chaotic **if and only if:**

- *It is the product of a deterministic system.* "Deterministic" means that the observed behavior is governed by a rule. We may not understand what that rule is but we must know that it does, in fact, exist and that it is controlling the system. *The fact that there is a governing nonlinear rule is the sine qua non of a chaotic system.*

- *The system is nonlinear.* In the simplest sense, a linear system is one whose function can be plotted as a straight line on a graph. Figure 9-2A is an example. All other things being equal, it shows that airflow through the vocal tract is directly and *linearly* proportional to the pressure in the lungs. A *nonlinear* function, on the other hand, is represented by a curved line (which can be quite complex). Figure 9-2B is illustrative. It shows the relationship that has been observed[60] between subglottal pressure and the intensity of the vocal signal.

- Despite the determinism (rule-based operation) of the generating system, the *output is nonetheless unpredictable.* This requirement needs to be understood carefully. It does, of course, imply that the behavior might be random-looking. But it also allows, for example, for the system to produce a number of different *patterns* of response (within each of which a succession of

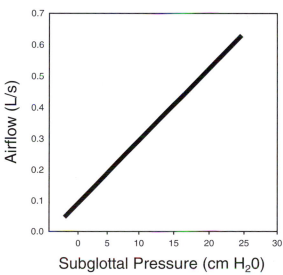
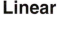
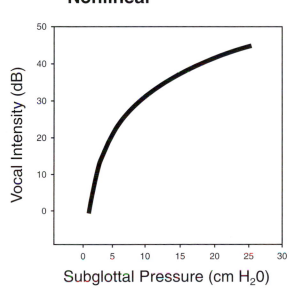

FIGURE 9-2. *Linear and nonlinear functions.*

output states might be completely predictable). If one is not able to specify, to any arbitrarily specified level of precision, which pattern will be produced at any given time, the system may validly be described as chaotic (provided, of course, that the other requirements are met).

- The system must have a relatively small number of parameters. That is, it must be controlled by only a few factors. Put another way, a chaotic system, however much it behaves in complex ways, must nonetheless be a fairly simple system. For reasons that will shortly become clear, it is described as a "low dimensional" system.

- *Finally, the behavior of the system must be "exquisitely sensitive to initial conditions."* What

this means is that extremely small differences in some controlling parameter can have dramatically large effects on the qualitative aspects of the system's behavior. Note, in Figure 9-3, how changing the coefficient *a* in the function $x_{n+1} = ax_n(1-x_n)$ by a mere 0.005, from *a* = 3.855 to *a* = 3.860, alters the qualitative nature of the output dramatically.**

** Known as the "logistic equation" this is a favorite example of a chaotic generator. Despite its extreme simplicity, its output can be astoundingly complex. Any of the texts cited in the previous footnote will provide more information about this "simple" system.

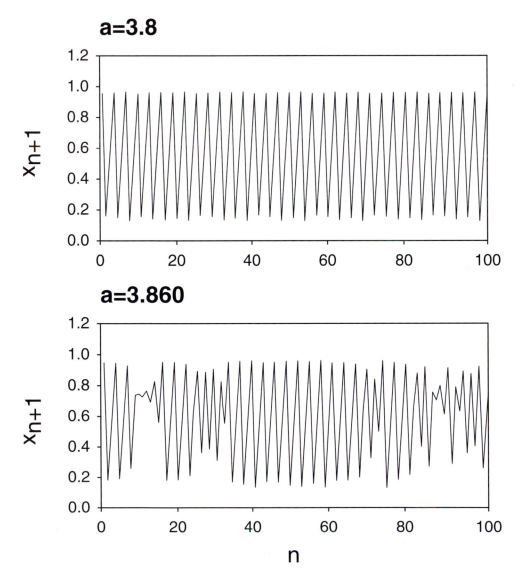

FIGURE 9-3. *Output of the "logistic equation" can be dramatically altered by tiny changes of its coefficient "a."*

In fact, radical shifts in the output of a chaotic system can be produced by changes that are *infinitesimally* small. "Infinitesimal" is used here in its literal, mathematical sense. Therefore, we can never have enough decimal places in our specification of the controlling variable to be able to predict the resultant behavior of the system with absolute certainty. Furthermore, an infinitesimally small difference is, from a practical point of view, a difference of zero. This implies that a chaotic system can change its behavior for no measurable reason at all.

DYNAMICS OF A SYSTEM

It is vital to understand that one cannot tell if a system is behaving in a chaotic manner just by looking at its output. Consider the two data sets plotted in Figure 9-4. One was produced by a chaotic system (that is, by a system that has the defining characteristics just discussed). The other, as best one can tell, is simply random. Which is the chaotic one? There are often ways to find out, but looking is not one of them. Not everything that looks random is chaotic.

Trajectories in State Space

How can one describe the dynamics (the behavior) of a system? One of the best ways is to plot its behavior in *state space* (often called *phase space*). It is easier to understand what this means from an example than from a definition, and the example will prove useful in developing some further concepts.

Consider a pendulum—like one that hangs from a clock, illustrated in Figure 9-5. Give it, for the sake of our example, the rather special property that it is not subject to friction, so that once started, it swings forever. It turns out that the dynamics of this extraordinarily simple (linear) system can be fully described in terms of the position and velocity of the pendulum. We can show their relationship graphically, as in Figure 9-6. The position of the pendulum (in degrees, θ) to the left or right of midline is plotted on the horizontal axis, while its speed (in degrees per second, toward the left or right) is plotted on the vertical axis. The (two-dimensional) space that these axes create is one example of a *state space* (also called a *phase space*). The ellipse that results is a *trajectory* that passes through all the points in this space that are possible for a simple pendulum. It, therefore, demarcates all the combinations of position and speed that this uncomplicated dynamic system can have. As it happens, the pendulum is so simple that a two-variable state space is enough to define its dynamics *completely*. That is, there is nothing else that we need to know (or would have to derive) about this system to understand all its operation.

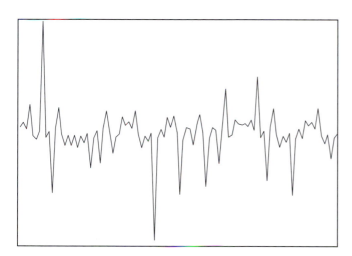

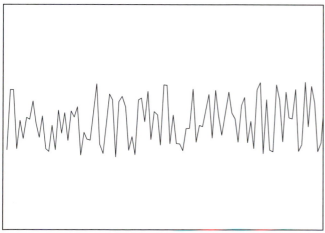

FIGURE 9-4. *Only one of these patterns was produced by a chaotic system. Which one?*

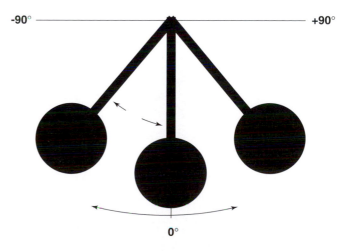

FIGURE 9-5. *Simple pendulum, swinging through an angle* θ.

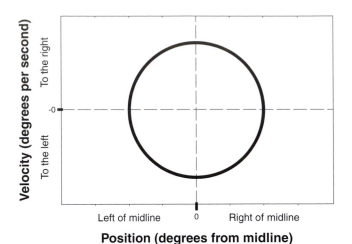

FIGURE 9-6. *Relationship of the position and velocity of the pendulum of Figure 9-5. The plane of the graph is the "state space" of the pendulum system.*

If the pendulum were free to swing not only from side to side, but also front-to-back (so that its motion described not an arc, but a circle) then we would need another axis to describe its motion in this direction, as in Figure 9-7. Adding an axis creates a three-dimensional space, which is the minimum necessary to describe this system. Hence, it could be called a three-dimensional dynamical system. "Dimension" is the way in which we specify the number of axes, each representing an independent variable, that is necessary to describe the dynamics of a system.

Attractors

Real pendulums, of course, are subject to friction. With each oscillation a little energy is lost and the width of the swing decreases, until finally the pendulum hangs at rest. To counter this, pendulum clocks have a mechanism that gives the pendulum a little "kick" when it passes a certain position in its swing cycle, adding back the energy that it lost during the previous oscillation. Because of the kick the trajectory of the pendulum system in state space has a little "glitch" in it, as in Figure 9-8.

Now, the amount of energy added by each kick is constant, and is just enough to keep the pendulum's arc at a given width. Suppose, therefore, that the pendulum is started by pulling it very far from the midline—to a position much further out than it would normally swing. Remembering that the once-per-cycle kick only provides enough energy for a swing of moderate width, it is clear that the amount of energy lost to friction on the initial huge swing will not be fully made up by the kick. Therefore, the next swing will be a little less energetic, and a little less wide. In fact, more energy is lost during each wider-than-normal swing than is restored by the kick, and so the swings will constantly become less wide until the arc is just the right size—the size at which the energy lost is exactly made up by the energy that the kick adds. Because, at this arc width, the energy loss and addition are exactly balanced, the pendulum will

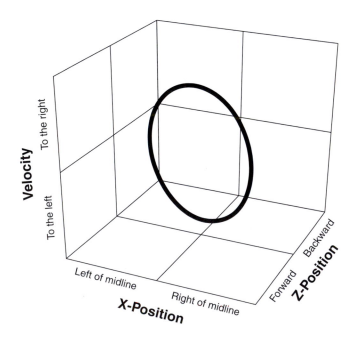

FIGURE 9-7. *A third axis is required to describe the movement of a pendulum that can swing not only side-to-side, but also front-to-back. The state space of such a pendulum is three-dimensional.*

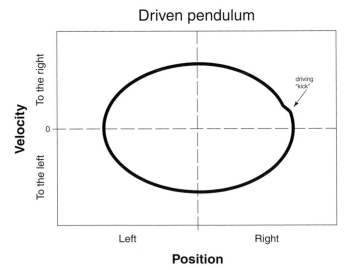

FIGURE 9-8. *A real pendulum needs a small "kick" during each swing to make up for frictional losses. The kick produces a glitch in the trajectory in phase space, but delivers the energy that keeps the system going.*

continue to oscillate in an arc of that width forever (or as long as the clock is kept wound up). The situation is illustrated in Figure 9-9A.

A similar situation prevails, in reverse, if we start the pendulum swinging from a position that is not as far out as it usually goes. Each swing, being smaller than usual, loses less energy than the standard-sized once-per-cycle kick delivers, so with each swing there is a net gain of energy, and each oscillation is a bit larger than the one before (Figure 9-9B). Finally, the swing is large enough that the energy lost equals the energy gained, and thereafter the pendulum follows the same trajectory in phase space "forever."

The final trajectory, then, has an important property. Starting the pendulum from almost anywhere in the state space—with however much displacement from the midline, and with however strong a push one might give it—it will always end up swinging with the same frequency and arc width. All paths seem to be compelled to head for the same final trajectory, which is therefore called an *attractor*.

Model Behavior

The human vocal system is extraordinarily complex and is largely inaccessible to direct observation.

Furthermore, there is a very limited number of ways in which one can manipulate it for experimental purposes. One means of getting around these problems is to use a mathematical model of the vocal folds (and sometimes of other elements of the vocal tract as well). A respectable number of models have been developed, each expressing its creator's conceptualization of the nature of the forces driving phonatory oscillation. One of the least complex and best known is the Ishizaka-Flanagan (1972)[61] model. It simplifies each vocal fold to an upper and a lower mass. They are more or less tightly coupled to each other but each is free to move toward or away from the glottis. The user chooses such important biomechanical and aerodynamic parameters as the size and stiffness of each mass, the length of the glottis, the subglottal pressure, and so on. Despite its very significant simplification of a complex system, it does provide a useful portrayal—validated by comparison to real phonation—of vocal fold oscillation under a wide range of physiologic conditions. Furthermore, its simplicity is ideal for present purposes, because it makes it possible to explore the potential for chaotic behavior in a "phonatory apparatus" that has only a few controlling variables, and hence in a system that should be easily understandable.

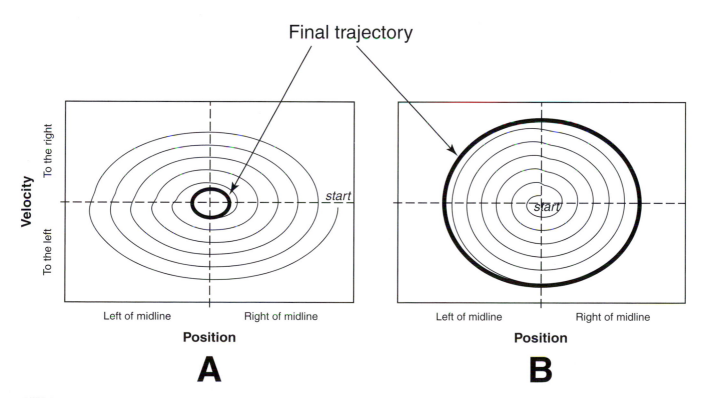

FIGURE 9-9. *The constant-sized kick provides just enough energy to keep the pendulum swinging with an arc of only a certain size—no bigger and no smaller. No matter how the pendulum is started, it will end up swinging with an arc of that certain size. The system is attracted to a special trajectory in state space.*

Model Phonation

If we set parameters for the two-mass model to some reasonable values—say moderate stiffness and subglottal pressure—and let it run, it oscillates quite well. Typical vibration is shown in Figure 9-10. The shaded area in the plot is the region where this vocal fold moves past the midline, and hence overlaps the opposite fold. Obviously, in real life this cannot happen. Instead, the vocal folds collide and deform each other. However, in the purely mathematical world of the model all things are possible, and the position trace has been allowed to extend into this realm of impossibility to provide some sense of how much deformation there would be.

Note that, as in the living larynx, there is a phase difference between the upper and lower lips of the vocal fold. Also, again as in nature, it takes a few oscillatory cycles for full vibratory amplitude to be achieved. The record of airflow through the modeled glottis shows a regular train of pulses, although their shape is not a precise representation of that of real voice.

One way to show the dynamics of the model's vocal fold in a state space is to plot the position of the upper mass of the vocal fold against the position of the lower mass, as in Figure 9-10. The trajectory of the system in this state space bears an obvious resemblance to the outward-spiraling trajectory of a simple pendulum shown in Figure 9-9B. That is, driven by the energy boost from the subglottal pressure, the trajectory spirals out from the starting condition until ultimately it reaches and is held by an attractor. The attractor itself is quite different, however. Instead of being a single line in state space, it appears to be "unstable" in that it is a *cluster* of lines. An enlargement of a small region of the attractor, shown on the right of Figure 9-11, reveals that the lines of the attractor show signs of being "bundled." In fact, although not shown here, each "bundle" of lines could be shown to be itself composed of bundles, and those bundles of still other bundles, and so on, ad infinitum. With a little mathematical trickery—the details of which are beyond our present discus-

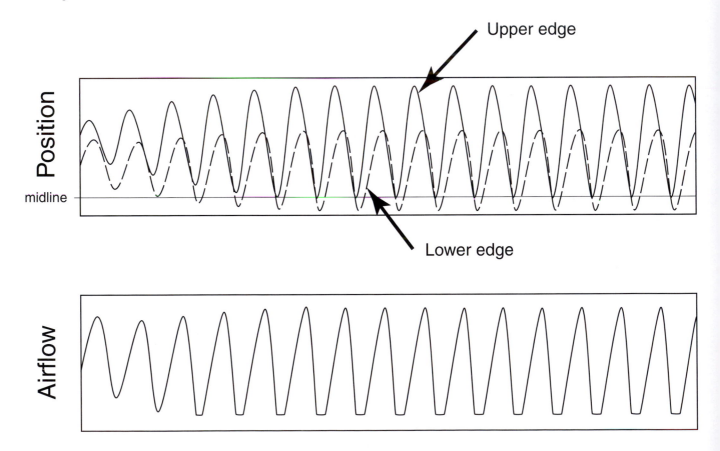

FIGURE 9-10. *Typical oscillation just after onset of the vocal folds in the two-mass model. Top: Position of the vocal fold's upper and lower edges. Bottom: Transglottal airflow.*

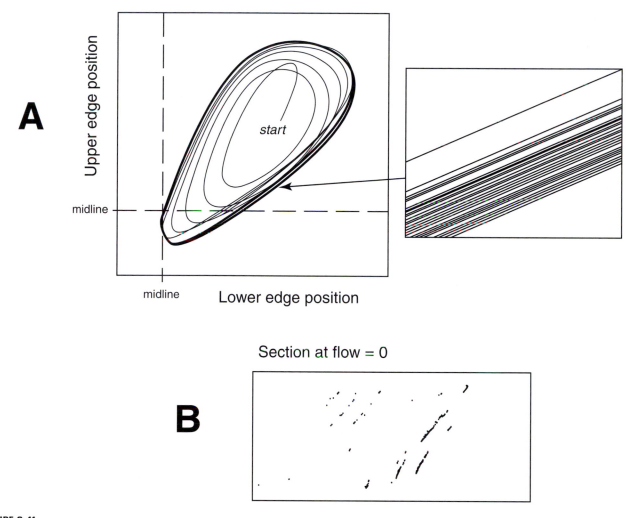

FIGURE 9-11. *Oscillation of the vocal fold of the two-mass model shown in an "Upper-edge/lower-edge" state space. (A) After start-up the system seems to be drawn to an attractor. However, magnifying that attractor shows that it is really a bundle of separate lines. Increasing the magnification would reveal ever-smaller bundles of lines. (B) Plotting a "cross section" of the attractor shows that the bundles of lines that compose it are arranged in layers. This is, therefore, a "strange attractor" that has fractal properties.*

sion[†]—it is possible to "cut" across these bundles, something like chopping across a fistful of spaghetti, and then to look at the cut surface. If we do this, as in Figure 9-11B, we find that not only are the lines "bundled," but the bundles are arranged in layers. As it happens, if we were to repeatedly enlarge each layer, we would see that each layer is itself composed of layers— layers within layers, ad infinitum. In short, the appearance of the attractor at every magnification would have very much the appearance of any other magnification. This property of any small part being a miniature version of the whole—technically referred to as "self-similarity at all scales"—makes the attractor a "fractal" structure.[‡] An attractor that is fractal is said—in the techni-

---

[†] Except, perhaps, to note that the result is termed as Poincaré section, and to suggest that the techniques for doing this and for interpreting the results are found in numerous introductory texts in the field of nonlinear dynamical systems theory.

[‡] Because fractal shapes are often surprisingly and intriguingly beautiful they have captured the imagination of many in recent years. Accordingly, there are many excellent books for neophytes who would like to learn more about them. The best known is by Mandelbrot (1977),[62] who founded the field of fractal geometry. A somewhat more useful text—complete with computer algorithms for generating fractal images—is Peitgen and Saupe, 1988.[63]

cal jargon of nonlinear dynamics—to be *strange*. Strange attractors are characteristic of chaotic systems.

The Ishizaka-Flanagan two-mass model, and other simple models of the vocal folds have, in fact, been shown to be chaotic systems,[30,37,64,65] and thus can serve us well in our present exploration of the role of chaos in vocal dysfunction.

A Moment's Consideration of an Important Bias

Although oscillation of the model's vocal folds is governed by an attractor, that attractor, by being fractal, allows each cycle—in fact, it *requires* each cycle—to be slightly different from every other one. That is worth thinking about for a moment, because the oscillation we are dealing with here is generated by an equation. An equation does not change while the model is running. An equation does not involve perturbing factors—variations in subglottal pressure, small alterations of muscle tension, minuscule shifts of mucus, or shifts of vocal tract posture. Despite this, the output shows observable perturbation.

Our bias is to believe that any effect—such as the radical shifts of F_0 of Figure 9-1—must have a proximate cause which is, in principle, identifiable. That bias accounts for several theories and speculations concerning the origins of, for example, frequency and amplitude perturbation. However, perturbation in the output of a mathematical model is a common observation (for example Wong, Ito, et al, 1991)[64] and can only be an inherent result of the equations that form it. It cannot, in a model, be the product of immediate outside causes. The question naturally arises: How much of the perturbation of the normal (real) vocal signal is caused by small pressure variations, little muscle twitches, and the like. How much is simply inherent in the vocal fold dynamics—as shown by a strange attractor? Similarly, the theory of nonlinear dynamics makes it clear that the behavior of a system can alter in the absence of any external influence. Effects do not necessarily have immediate causes.

Basin of Attraction: The Attractor's Realm

It is worthwhile to look at the dynamics of the pendulum once again. Recall that it gets a little push whenever it passes a given point in its swing, and this little boost is just sufficient to replace the energy lost to friction. Figure 9-12 recapitulates some things that were said about this system earlier. That is, if the pendulum is started from a position either more than or less than its usual displacement, oscillations either diminish or enlarge until their amplitude represents an equilibrium between the energy gain and loss. The final trajectory that represents this equilibrium state is an attractor,

because the dynamics of the system seem—in some metaphorical sense—to be drawn to it.

The plane of the state space of Figure 9-12 contains all the possible combinations of position and velocity that, in principle, a pendulum could have. A reasonable question is "Which starting combinations of position and velocity (that is, which starting positions in the state space) will produce a trajectory that ends up on the attractor? Are there any regions (starting combinations of position and velocity) that will *not* lead to the attractor?"

It might seem that all positions in the space are equally subject to the attractor's lure, but that is *not* the case. The reason is that the pendulum gets its absolutely essential little boost only when it swings past a given position in its arc. If its starting swing is not wide enough to pass this point it gets no push and, therefore, its lost energy will not be returned. Absent the restoration of frictional losses, the pendulum's swing grows ever more feeble. Rather than reach the attractor, it will end up hanging, absolutely still, at the 0 position/0 velocity locus in the state space. In fact, that point is itself a "point attractor" for all position-velocity combinations that do not take the pendulum past the boost-point in its swing. The gray shading marks the starting region from which the trajectory is attracted not to sustained oscillation but to hanging at rest.

The state space of Figure 9-12 is thus composed of two different regions that, so to speak, dictate different outcomes for the dynamics of the system. There is a zone (shaded gray) within which starting points lead to a "point attractor" (the rest position). There is also a zone that occupies all the rest of the plane, and within which all starting points lead ultimately to the oscillatory attractor. Each zone is the *basin of attraction* for its attractor.

Voice specialists have used the concept of a basin of attraction, even if unknowingly, for quite some time. The voice range profile (VRP, Figure 9-13) is considered an important evaluative tool. What it depicts is the region in a vocal intensity—vocal frequency "state space" in which (essentially) periodic oscillation of the vocal folds (that is, voice) is possible.[††] Outside the VRP's polygon,

---

[††] Purists would not be happy with this statement. For one thing, vocal intensity and vocal F_0 are not parameters that govern vocal fold oscillation—they are measures of some aspects of the results of oscillation—and, in fact, are not even independent. For another thing, the VRP boundary includes at least two different kinds of phonatory oscillation (modal and falsetto register, for instance), and each is likely to have its own attractor. Nonetheless, the analogy is a useful one—both from the pint of view of theory and from the perspective of clinical interpretation.

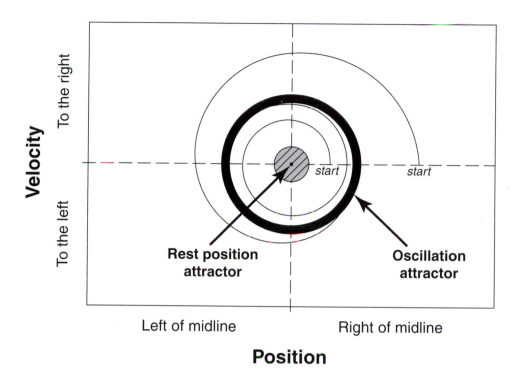

FIGURE 9-12. *The pendulum's state space really has two attractors. One—shown by a heavy line—is an oscillation, but the other—represented by a dot in the middle of the plane—is hanging motionless. Most starting points on the plane lead to the oscillation attractor, but some lead to the motionless condition. There are two "basins of attraction" in the state space.*

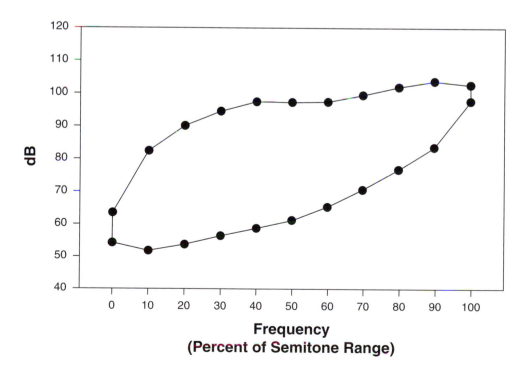

FIGURE 9-13. *A typical voice range profile.*

vocal fold motion (if there is any) is not periodic, and, hence, is not phonatory. The VRP polygon can, therefore, be considered to be the boundary of a "phonatory oscillation basin of attraction."

In the case of the pendulum the boundaries of the basins of attraction are neat and well defined. But this is not always—or even commonly—the case in more complex systems. In fact, it is not really the case for the VRP, because if the patient's voice were to be tested at *every* frequency (instead of at decibel intervals) of the phonatory frequency range, minor variations in maximal and minimal vocal intensity would make the boundary line much more jagged.

The structure of a basin of attraction can be very complex indeed, and its boundary can be exceedingly irregular. Those possibilities will be crucial to our consideration of voice irregularities and will be visited again later.

VOCAL IRREGULARITIES: THE CHAOTIC POINT OF VIEW

We are now ready to look at some different kinds of vocal irregularity from a nonlinear dynamics point of view.

Intermittent Aperiodicity: The Case of the Missing Vibration

The voice of the dysphonic patient is often characterized by significant increases of frequency and amplitude perturbation, and very brief failures of vocal fold oscillation are not uncommon. A traditional view of vocal fold physiology would likely hold that instability of muscular tension and/or subglottal air pressure is responsible for the increases in jitter and shimmer, while the transient failures are probably the product of "twitches"—brief alterations of muscle tension.

However, nonlinear dynamics theory offers a different possibility. Figure 9-14 shows the output (glottal flow pulses and state-space representation) when the two-mass model is set for conditions of low vocal fold tension and moderate subglottal pressure. The flow record shows what, at first glance, seems to be completely erratic glottal pulses. Yet, there are short regions of subharmonic oscillation ("diplophonia") and, interestingly enough, two instances (arrows) where phonatory oscillation is momentarily seriously impaired. It is clearly not possible for these aberrations to be the result of instabilities of muscular tension or driving pressure, much less muscle twitches, because the model includes no such phenomena.

The representation of the dynamics in the upper-mass/lower-mass state space shows a very complex

attractor‡‡ that roves over a large area of the plane that it occupies. The situation is similar to that of Figure 9-11, only greatly exaggerated. The complexity of the attractor forces each glottal cycle to be somewhat different from its neighbors and results in the bursts of pattern that are seen. Occasionally the attractor visits relatively extreme positions (arrows). Simultaneous observation of the development of the attractor and the glottal pulse record makes it clear that glottal pulses are "missed" at these instants. What nonlinear dynamics theory says is that vocal irregularities might not have their origins in physiologic instability.

Start-up Problems

Sometimes it is difficult to get the voice going. There may be a transient aphonia (a "frog in the throat," as the saying has it) or a bizarre "glitch" of vocal frequency—bane of the adolescent male. The fault is usually laid to mucus, or to a difficulty of tensional adjustment, or perhaps to poorly controlled vocal fold adduction. However, once again, nonlinear dynamics theory offers another and simpler possibility.

Figure 9-15 shows the glottal pulsing and associated dynamics for a different choice of parameters for the two-mass model. The records of transglottal flow show that oscillation is initially quite unstable but then converts to a more regular pattern. The state-space plots indicate that, for most of the time period shown, the vocal folds are "flopping" erratically, but, ultimately, their behavior is captured by the attractor, and stable phonation ensues. It is worth pointing out once again that no outside influence—such as a change of vocal fold tension, or an alteration of the subglottal pressure—has occurred to stabilize phonatory function. The model's parameters have not changed. Both types of behavior—irregular dysphonic vibration and stable phonatory oscillation—have been produced by the very same physiologic conditions. It has simply taken a while for the dynamics of the situation to find the attractor.

Swirling Around the Basin

It is not unusual for a dysphonic patient to have periods of relatively good voice interrupted by moderately long episodes of altered phonation or aphonia. While these might be the result of changes in the status of the vocal tract, they might also reflect switching of the

---

‡‡ Running the model for a long time with these parameters produces a trajectory (which, for the sake of clarity, is not reproduced here) that strongly suggests that this is, in fact, an attractor. Note that this level of complexity is not uncommon among strange attractors.

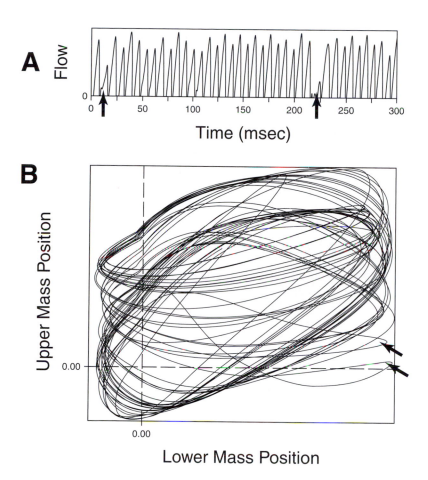

FIGURE 9-14. *Irregular phonation by the two-mass model. (A) Time-domain representation of airflow. (B) State-space representation.*

dynamics of the vocal system from one attractor to another.

To see why this might happen, we return to the concept of the basin of attraction. It was noted earlier that, unlike the smooth basin boundaries of Figures 9-12 and 9-13, the basin boundaries of chaotic attractors are exceedingly irregular. In fact, they are fractal. This means, let us recall, that they exhibit self-similarity at all scales, so that every time a region is magnified more detail appears.

The relevance of this to the problem of sudden shifts of vocal fold oscillation can be explored with Figure 9-16, which shows part of a (computed) basin of attraction and its boundary. Although the data of Figure 9-16 actually have no relationship to voice production,††† it will be useful to pretend that the figure shows a vocal-

fold tension/subglottal pressure state space. The white region is part of the basin of attraction for the attractor for stable vocal fold vibration; call it the "phonation basin." Tension/pressure combinations in the black zone are outside the phonation basin and will result in erratic (dysphonic or aphonic) behavior of the vocal folds. Call this the "dysphonia zone."

Even when viewed at low magnification (Figure 9-16A), the boundary of the phonation basin looks extremely irregular. Enlarging just the little bit of it in the rectangle shows more detail (Figure 9-16B), and demonstrates that the phonation basin is "invaded" by fine projections of the dysphonia zone that were not observable at the lower magnification. Enlarging a rectangular zone of Figure 9-16B shows even deeper extensions into the phonation basin. If one were to continue the process of enlargement one would discover (because the boundary is fractal) that there are ever-finer incursions of the dysphonia zone into the phonation basin. In fact, continuing the magnification to infinity would reveal that there are extensions that are *infinitesimally* wide.

---

††† Those with some prior experience in nonlinear dynamics theory or fractal geometry might recognize that part of the boundary of Mandelbrot set has been pressed into service for this illustration.

The numerous and ever-finer projections of the dysphonia region show that the phonation basin (the part of state space in which the dynamics of the system is drawn to a regular-phonation attractor) is, in actuality, infested with dysphonia regions—some of them only infinitesimally large. Those regions, although surrounded by the phonation basin, are actually *outside* it. From these minuscule or infinitesimal areas the dynamics is

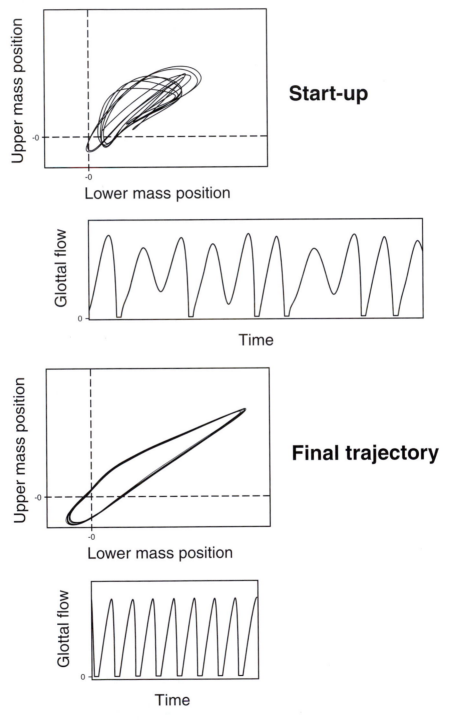

FIGURE 9-15. *When first started, the vocal folds of the model may "flop" irregularly (state-space and time-domain representation at top). Ultimately, however, the system may be captured by an attractor, and regular oscillation established (lower state-space and time-domain plots).*

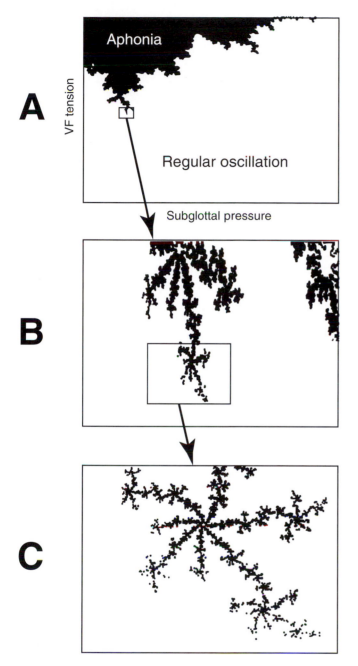

FIGURE 9-16. *A basin of attraction may be deeply penetrated by ever-finer fingers of a different basin. Therefore, what appears to be inside one basin may actually be part of another.*

not drawn to the phonation attractor. In exactly the same way, the phonation basin has projections that extend into the dysphonia zone, which is therefore also riddled with tiny regions that *will* lead to a stable attractor. The contamination of each zone with areas that "belong to" the other grows more severe as one approaches the boundary—which, in the common understanding of the word, is not so much a separation as a fuzzy region.

During oscillation, the subglottal pressure and vocal fold tension are constantly varying. Put another way, the location of the system in the pressure/tension state space is constantly changing. If the state of the system finds itself in one of those regions that belongs to the dysphonia zone it may be attracted away from the stable phonatory attractor, causing regular phonation to end. Similarly, during aphonic behavior, the trajectory may encounter a small region that may cause it to be drawn back to the phonatory attractor, re-establishing regular oscillation. It might seem that this is just a fancy way of saying that shifts of vocal function are caused by alterations of phonatory parameters. However, because the "misplaced" regions (phonation basin in the dysphonia zone; dysphonia zone embedded in phonation basin) may be infinitesimally small, it may require only an unmeasurably tiny alteration of control parameters to drive the dynamics into one of them. An "unmeasurably tiny" variation is, in practice, *no* variation. From the point of view of nonlinear dynamics theory, it is perfectly reasonable that phonation might undergo major qualitative changes in the absence of any observable cause.

The Misbehavior of Intact Systems

Basic concepts of nonlinear dynamics, then, offer alternative explanations for at least some of the aberrant behavior of the vocal system that commonly plague the dysphonic patient. Transient vocal "glitches," problems of voice initiation, and the intrusion of erratic or unusually patterned vibration can all easily be accommodated within the construct of chaos theory. A significant advantage accrues from this point of view: It becomes unnecessary to invoke the causative intervention of antecedent momentary events which have often been at best difficult, and quite commonly impossible, to detect in living patients.

It would be foolish in the extreme to propose that nonlinear dynamics theory is the appropriate explanatory model for all vocal dysfunctions.[‡‡‡] It could even be argued that it is not optimal for most disorders. However, it is ideally suited to the hitherto-inexplicable and odd phenomena that are frequent conundrums of routine clinical practice. Nonlinear dynamics theory suggests that some dysphonias—and perhaps many—may be the product of an *intact phonatory system.* The

---

[‡‡‡] The belief that aspects of the theory not considered here may offer a much better framework for the description of vocal function does not seem too far a stretch.

possibility is clear that at least some voice problems—and perhaps many—betray not structural or physiologic, but rather *dynamical* disorders.[66-68]

The future may be much more chaotic.

REFERENCES

1. van den Berg Jw. Subglottic pressures and vibrations of the vocal folds. *Folia Phoniatr.* 1957;9:65-71.

2. van den Berg Jw. Myoelastic-aerodynamic theory of voice production. *J Speech Hear Res.* 1958; 1:227-244.

3. van den Berg Jw, Zantema JT, Doornenbal P Jr. On the air resistance and the Bernoulli effect of the human larynx. *J Acoust Soc Am.* 1957;29:626-631.

4. Titze IR. The human vocal cords: a mathematical model. Part I. *Phonetica.* 1973;28:129-170.

5. Titze IR. The human vocal cords: a mathematical model. Part II. *Phonetica.* 1974;29:1-21.

6. Buder EH, Cannito MP, Dressler D, Woodson GE, Murry T. Phonatory analysis of spasmodic dysphonia: modulations, subharmonics, and Botox response. Presented at: Annual Meeting of the American Speech-Language-Hearing Association; 1999; San Antonio, TX.

7. Baer T. Vocal jitter: a neuromuscular explanation. In: Lawrence V, Weinberg B, eds. *Transcripts of the Eighth Symposium: Care of the Professional Voice.* New York, NY: Voice Foundation; 1980:19-24.

8. Larson CR, Kempster GB, Kistler MK. Changes in voice fundamental frequency following discharge of single motor units in cricothyroid muscles. *J Speech Hear Res.* 1987;30:552-558.

9. Titze IR. A model for neurologic sources of aperiodicity in vocal fold vibration. *J Speech Hear Res.* 1991;34:460-472.

10. Kaiser JF. Some observations on vocal tract operation from a fluid flow point of view. In: Titze IR, Scherer RC, eds. *Vocal Fold Physiology: Biomechanics, Acoustics, and Phonatory Control.* Denver, CO: Denver Center for the Performing Arts; 1983:359-386.

11. Teager HM, Teager SM. Active fluid dynamic voice production models, or: There is a unicorn in the garden. In: Titze IR, Scherer RC, eds. *Vocal Fold Physiology: Biomechanics, Acoustics, and Phonatory Control.* Denver, CO: Denver Center for the Performing Arts; 1983:386-401.

12. Liljencrants J. Numerical simulations of glottal flow. In: Gauffin J, Hammarberg B, eds. *Vocal Fold Physiology: Acoustic, Perceptual, and Physiological Aspects of Voice Mechanisms.* San Diego, CA: Singular Publishing; 1991:98-112.

13. Shadle CH, Barney AM, Thomas DW. An investigation into the acoustics and aerodynamics of the larynx. In: Gauffin J, Hammarberg B, eds. *Vocal Fold Physiology: Acoustic, Perceptual, and Physiological Aspects of Voice Mechanisms.* San Diego, CA: Singular Publishing; 1991:73-82.

14. Lind J, ed. *Newborn Infant Cry.* Uppsala, Sweden: Almqvist and Wiksells; 1965.

15. Wasz-Höckert O, Lind J, Vuorenkoski V, Partanen T, Valanne E. *The Infant Cry: A Spectrographic and Auditory Analysis.* London, England: Heinemann; 1968.

16. Glass L. Nonlinear dynamics of physiological function and control. *Chaos.* 1991;1:247-250.

17. Goldberger AL, Rigney DR, West BJ. Chaos and fractals in human physiology. *Sci Am.* 1990; 262(2):43-49.

18. Pool R. Is it healthy to be chaotic? *Science.* 1989;243:604-607.

19. Teich MC, Lowen SB, Turcott RG. On possible peripheral origins of the fractal auditory neural spike train. In: Lim DJ, ed. *Abstracts of the Fourteenth Midwinter Meeting: Association for Research in Otolaryngology;* 1991:50.

20. Beuter A, Labrie C, Vasilakos K. Transient dynamics in motor control of patients with Parkinson's disease. *Chaos.* 1991;1:279-286.

21. Goldberger AL. Cardiac chaos. *Science.* 1989;243: 1419.

22. Sheldon R, Riff K. Changes in heart rate variability during fainting. *Chaos.* 1991;1:257-264.

23. Kaplan DT, Talajic M. Dynamics of heart rate. *Chaos.* 1991;1:251-256.

24. Coumel P, Maison-Blanche P. Complex dynamics of cardiac arhythmias. *Chaos.* 1991;1:335-342.

25. Skinner JE, Goldberger AL, Mayer-Kress G. Chaos in the heart: implications for clinical cardiology. *Biotechnology.* 1990;8:1018-1024.

26. Kryger MH, Millar T. Cheyne-Stokes respiration: stability of interacting systems in heart failure. *Chaos.* 1991;1:265-269.

27. Rapp PE, Bashore TR, Martinerie JM, Albano AM, Zimmerman ID, Mees AI. *Brain Topogr.* 1989;2:99-118.

28. Kroenenberg F. Menopausal hot flashes: randomness or rhythmicity? *Chaos.* 1991;1:271-278.

29. Pickover CA, Khorsani A. Fractal characterization of speech waveform graphs. *Comput Graphics.* 1986;10:51-61.

30. Awrejcewicz J. Bifurcation portrait of the human vocal cord oscillations. *J Sound Vibration.* 1990;136:151-156.

31. Baken RJ. Irregularity of vocal period and amplitude: a first approach to the fractal analysis of voice. *J Voice.* 1990;4:185-197.

32. Mende W, Herzel H, Wermke K. Bifurcations and chaos in newborn cries. *Physics Lett A.* 1990;145:418-424.

33. Herzel H, Steinecke I, Mende W, Wermke K. Chaos and bifurcations in voiced speech. In: Mosekilde E. ed. *Complexity, Chaos, and Biological Evolution.* New York, NY: Plenum Press; 1991.

34. Titze IR, Baken RJ, Herzel H. Evidence of chaos in vocal fold vibration. In: Titze IR, ed. *Vocal Fold Physiology: Frontiers in Basic Science.* San Diego, CA: Singular Publishing; 1993:143-188.

35. Baken RJ. The aged voice: a new hypothesis. *Voice (Journal of the British Voice Association).* 1994;3:57-73.

36. Kakita Y, Okamoto H. Visualizing the characteristics of vocal fluctuation from the viewpoint of chaos: An attempt toward qualitative quantification. In: Fujimura O, Hirano M, eds. *Vocal Fold Physiology: Voice Quality Control.* San Diego, CA: Singular Publishing; 1994:235-348.

37. Steinecke I, Herzel H. Bifurcations in an asymmetric vocal-fold model. *J Acoust Soc Am.* 1995;97:1874-1884.

38. Herzel H, Berry D, Titze IR, Steinecke I. Nonlinear dynamics of the voice: signal analysis and biomechanical modeling. *Chaos.* 1995;5:30-34.

39. Berry DA, Herzel H, Titze IR, Story BH. Bifurcations in excised larynx experiments. *J Voice.* 1996:10;129-138.

40. Fletcher, NH. Nonlinearity, complexity, and control in vocal systems: In: Davis PJ, Fletcher NH, eds. *Vocal Fold Physiology: Controlling Complexity and Chaos.* San Diego, CA: Singular Publishing; 1996:3-16.

41. Herzel H. Possible mechanisms of vocal instabilities. In: Davis PJ, Fletcher NH, eds. *Vocal Fold Physiology: Controlling Complexity and Chaos.* San Diego, CA: Singular Publishing; 1996:63-75.

42. Kumar A, Mullick SK. Nonlinear dynamical analysis of speech. *J Acoust Soc Am.* 1996;100:615-629.

43. Behrman A, Baken RJ. Correlation dimension of electroglottographic data from healthy and pathologic subjects. *J Acoust Soc Am.* 1997;102:2371-2379.

44. Ouaknine M, Giovanni A, Guelfucci B, Teston B, Triglia JM. Nonlinear behavior of vocal fold vibration in an experimental model of asymmetric larynx: role of coupling between the two folds. *Revue de Laryngologie, Otologie, et Rhinologie.* 1998;119:249-252.

45. Behrman A. Global and local dimensions of vocal dynamics. *J Acoust Soc Am.* 1999;106:432-443.

46. Gleick J. *Chaos: Marking a New Science.* New York, NY: Viking Penguin; 1987.

47. Crutchfield JP, Farmer JD, Packard NH, Shaw RS. Chaos. *Sci Am.* December 1986;46-57.

48. Abraham RH, Shaw CD. *Dynamics—The Geometry of Behavior. Part One: Periodic Behavior.* The Visual Mathematics Library: VisMath Vol 1. Santa Cruz, CA: Aerial Press; 1982.

49. Abraham RH, Shaw, CD. *Dynamics—The Geometry of Behavior. Part Two: Chaotic Behavior.* The Visual Mathematics Library: VisMath Vol 2. Santa Cruz, CA: Aerial Press; 1983.

50. Abraham RH, Shaw CD. *Dynamics—The Geometry of Behavior. Part Three: Global Behavior.* The Visual Mathematics Library: VisMath Vol 3. Santa Cruz, CA: Aerial Press; 1985.

51. Abraham RH, Shaw CD. Dynamics—*The Geometry of Behavior. Part Four: Bifurcation Behavior.* The Visual Mathematics Library: VisMath Vol 4. Santa Cruz, CA: Aerial Press; 1982.

52. Rasband SN. *Chaotic Dynamics of Nonlinear Systems.* New York, NY: Wiley; 1990.

53. Baker GL, Golub JP. *Chaotic Dynamics: An Introduction.* New York, NY: Cambridge University Press; 1990.

54. Moon FC. *Chaotic Vibrations: An Introduction for Applied Scientists and Engineers.* New York, NY: Wiley; 1987.

55. Thompson JMT, Stewart HB. *Nonlinear Dynamics and Chaos: Geometrical Methods for Engineers and Scientists.* New York, NY: Wiley; 1986.

56. Eubank S, Farmer D. *An Introduction to Chaos and Randomness.* Boston, MA: Addison-Wesley; 1990.

57. Cvitanovic P, ed. *Universality in Chaos.* 2nd ed. New York, NY: Adam Hilger (IOP Publishing, Ltd.); 1984.

58. Glass L, Mackey MC. *From Clocks to Chaos.* Princeton, NJ: Princeton University Press; 1988.

59. West BJ. *Fractal Physiology and Chaos in Medicine.* Singapore: World Scientific; 1990.

60. Isshiki N. Regulatory mechanism of voice intensity variation. *J Speech Hear Res.* 1964;7:17-29.

61. Ishizaka K, Flanagan JL. Synthesis of voiced sounds from a two-mass model of the vocal cords. *Bell Sys Tech J.* 1972;51:1233-1268.

62. Mandelbrot BB. *The Fractal Geometry of Nature.* New York, NY: Freeman; 1977.

63. Peitgen H-O, Saupe D, eds. *The Science of Fractal Images.* New York, NY: Springer-Verlag; 1988.

64. Wong D, Ito M, Cox NB, Titze IR. Observation of perturbations in a lumped-element model of the vocal folds with application to some pathological cases. *J Acoust Soc Am.* 1991;89:383-394.

65. Lucero JC. Dynamics of the two-mass model of the vocal folds: Equilibria, bifurcations, and oscillation region. *J Acoust Soc Am.* 1993;94:3104-3111.

66. Mackey MC, Glass L. Oscillations and chaos in physiological control systems. *Science.* 1977;197:287-289.

67. Goldberger AL, West BJ. Chaos in physiology: Health or disease. In: Holton A, Olsen LF, eds. *Chaos in Biological Systems.* New York, NY: Plenum Press; 1987:1-5.

68. Mackey MC, Milton JC. Dynamical diseases. *Ann NY Acad Sci.* 1987;504;16-32.

CHAPTER 10

Research in Laryngology

Gayle E. Woodson, MD

The origins and development of laryngology have been driven largely by advances in the ability to visualize the larynx. The birth of laryngology as a specialty was enabled by the introduction of mirror laryngoscopy. In the latter twentieth century, the development of fiberoptics greatly enhanced the ability to observe the larynx, and this provided another surge of interest in laryngeal disorders. However, sustained, meaningful progress in laryngology, as in any medical specialty, results from "bridging" research: the collaborative efforts of clinicians who seek better ways to care for their patients, and of basic scientists who seek to understand structure and function. Some of the fruits of such research include sound principles of vocal hygiene, improved methods of voice therapy, and the emergence of phonosurgical techniques. However, there remain many important unsolved questions that could improve the care of laryngeal disorders. If properly harnessed, the current exponential increase in medical knowledge and technology could provide answers that would transform drastically the field in the coming years.

CRUCIAL RESEARCH ISSUES IN LARYNGOLOGY

The primary need is for information that would improve the management of serious clinical problems, such as disabling voice disorders, laryngeal airway impairment, and dysphagia. However, there are also many significant gaps in our fundamental knowledge of phonation, respiration, and deglutition, and these deficiencies limit clinical progress. The gross anatomy of the larynx has been described well for centuries, but the complexity of laryngeal motion and the importance of the microscopic architecture of the vocal fold have been appreciated only in recent years. Developments in experimental techniques and molecular biology may provide important tools for elucidating structure-function relationships, but are likely to raise new questions that will change the direction and focus of research interest. Thus, it is impossible to predict what future investigations will accomplish. This chapter reviews some important developments in laryngeal research and considers the implications of each for future research directions.

Hirano described the unique layered structure of connective tissue in the vocal fold cover, and pointed out the crucial role of this tissue in normal phonation.[1] Consequently, entirely new research questions arose. What factors are responsible for the development and maintenance of this layered structure? What biologic processes and factors are involved in laryngeal scarring? How can the normal structure be restored for a scarred vocal fold? Surgery is by far the most frequent cause of scarring that limits vocal fold mobility. What surgical techniques or medical therapy can be used to prevent scarring?

Laryngeal motion is more complex than previously recognized. The vocal folds do not merely open and close, lengthen and shorten. The cricoarytenoid joints, and hence the vocal folds, are capable of moving in three dimensions. Moreover, intrinsic laryngeal muscles appear to be divided into functional compartments with different functions. For example, the human posterior cricoarytenoid muscle has two bellies, with different vectors of force on the arytenoid cartilage and separate nerve branches.[2,3] The thyroarytenoid muscle can be divided into regions with different myosin composition.[4] The functional significance of compartmentalization and complex motion has not been established. Activation patterns may be significantly different for speech, deglutition, and respiratory tasks. Control of pitch and vocal quality undoubtedly requires precise adjustments in glottic configuration. Further research in vivo and in excised human larynges could address these issues.

Complexity in motor control could account for some of the difficulties in regaining normal motion after regeneration or repair of the recurrent laryngeal nerve. Lack of normal vocal fold motion, despite reinnervation, has been attributed to synkinesis, the simultaneous contraction of opposing muscles. Research in animals has confirmed the inappropriate reinnervation of laryngeal muscles after nerve injury.[5-7] However, immobility caused by synkinesis would require that opposing forces exactly cancel each other out. This implies precisely orthogonal vectors with exactly equal strength—not the most likely outcome of a random process. Therefore, other factors should be investigated, such as mechanical reduction of joint mobility, or irreversible muscle changes.

The first successful laryngeal transplant, performed in January of 1998, has generated more questions about reinnervation, because of some unexpected findings. Not only did the larynx survive, function was better than anticipated.[8] The patient, who received a transplant to replace a severely traumatized larynx, still requires a tracheotomy, because of deficient inspiratory abduction. However, he is able to eat normally and has a surprisingly functional voice. Despite the fact that only one recurrent laryngeal nerve was reanastomosed, both vocal folds have become reinnervated and have good muscle tone. The patient was initially unable to swallow, because of severe aspiration; however, months after the transplant, he regained laryngeal sensation and was able to swallow. If phonation involves complex motor control, then why has this patient recovered this much vocal function? Why are both vocal folds essentially equally reinnervated when the nerve was only reanastomosed on one side? This case does demonstrate that laryngeal transplantation is technically possible. Whether or not it is economically feasible remains to be seen.

The neural control of voice in speech is not well understood but is clearly complex. The spectrum of vocal dysfunction in patients with neurologic disorders is broad, implying the existence of various pathways susceptible to impairment. Patients with spasmodic dysphonia (SD) (presumably a midbrain disorder) have significant variation in symptom severity with task, implying differing levels of midbrain control, or perhaps different feedback mechanisms.[9] In fact, it is possible that impaired sensory feedback could be involved in the pathophysiology of SD. Research to elucidate the neural pathways involved in speech control could ultimately lead to effective interventions for patients with neurogenic dysphonia.

It is well recognized that phonation is only one component of voice production. Resonance of the vocal tract, including the pharynx, skull, and chest, is an important determinant of vocal quality. In fact, resonant characteristics may be key factors in determining vocal register and imbuing singers with an exceptional voice. Classical voice training focuses attention on resonant structures. However, the physical basis for source and tract interactions, and the potential for volitional modification of resonance, are not well understood. Information about these relationships could eventually empower interventions to improve vocal function, not only for performance, but also for everyday use.

Vocal function may be impaired by a variety of systemic illnesses. Therapeutic drugs can also affect the voice, although there is very little available objective information on such effects. The precise mechanism of impairment or site of lesion is not always apparent. For example, rheumatoid arthritis occasionally involves the cricoarytenoid joint. More often, hoarseness in patients with rheumatoid arthritis is caused by irritation by gastroesophageal reflux, promoted by steroid or anti-inflammatory medication. Medications that inhibit angiotensin-converting enzyme have been reported to cause an irritative cough, which can damage the larynx. The mechanism of this effect is not known. Studies of drug effects on the larynx may have relevance to mechanisms in patients with idiopathic chronic cough.

The larynx is an organ that differs profoundly with gender, apparently in response to changes in hormone status. The male larynx grows dramatically during puberty with the onset of increases in testosterone. With menopause, submucosal edema accumulates in the female larynx.[10] Thus it is not surprising that endocrine disorders can profoundly affect the larynx. Myxedema of hypothyroidism is manifested in the larynx. Masculinizing tumors, male hormone therapy, pregnancy, or menopause can deepen the voice. The vocal changes appear to be irreversible, but the mechanism is unknown. It could involve increases in connective tissue or muscle bulk. Research in frogs has indicated a sex-linked difference in laryngeal muscle myosin.[11] Research on hormonal effects could provide very useful information about laryngeal function.

Gastroesophageal reflux is extremely common and can have far reaching effects on the voice. It is one of the most common causes of chronic laryngitis. It is not clear why some patients with significant reflux develop laryngeal pathology and others do not. Abusive vocal habits have been implicated, but there are likely to be other cofactors. Research into the epidemiology and pathogenesis of reflux laryngitis could provide useful information not only for treating laryngitis, but also for potentially preventing more severe sequelae that have been attributed to reflux, such as cancer or laryngotracheal stenosis.

Laryngotracheal stenosis itself is a problem that merits careful study. Most often it is the result of endotracheal intubation and or tracheotomy; however, the majority of intubated patients are not so affected. Previously, excessive cuff pressure and prolonged intubation were identified as cofactors. Modification of the cuff, to reduce pressure, and changes in intubation practices have diminished, but not eliminated stenosis. Those patients who are affected may have some underlying impairment of wound healing, as surgery to correct the stenosis is plagued by high failure rates. Recent research has suggested that the use of topical mitomycin can reduce the rate of restenosis following corrective surgery.[12] This is encouraging evidence that therapeutic intervention could be effective in prevention and treatment of stenosis. Research is needed to identify the responsible mechanisms, to guide the development of effective therapy and prevention, and to permit prospective identification of patients at high risk for developing stenosis.

EFFICACY OF VOICE THERAPY

A major problem in caring for patients with voice disorders is the lack of data regarding the efficacy of treatment, and in particular, the efficacy of voice therapy. Wide clinical experience and numerous small studies support the efficacy of various voice therapy regimens for specific voice disorders. Extrapolations can also be made from the results of vocal pedagogy. It is well known that breath control is crucial in singing. Classical voice training has long focused on breath support, even before the myoelastic theory of phonation was developed. Nevertheless, the importance of breath support in conversational speech is grossly undervalued. In conversational speech, most humans use the larynx very inefficiently, converting less than 1% of the aerodynamic power of the lungs into sound. Although such an inefficient vocal mechanism may be adequate for minimal use situations, it is likely to fail in conditions of prolonged vocalization, noisy environment, and/or psychologic duress. Inadequate breath support is widely recognized as one of the most common causes of functional dysphonia. However, further research is required to elucidate the mechanisms involved, so that effective intervention can be developed.

Vocal training can greatly enhance vocal efficiency. It has been noted that the larynges of trained singers age less rapidly. Trained singers can also compensate for many variations in physiologic or environmental conditions, and can often produce a normal sounding voice in the presence of laryngeal pathology, such as edema or nodules. The study of vocal mechanism in gifted or exceptional singers or speakers can demonstrate the range of human capacity, and identify specific strategies to improve vocal efficiency in patients with inadequate phonation.

Although experience and logic support the value of voice therapy, definitive clinical trials are rare. Ironically, a major factor limiting progress in studying the efficacy of voice disorders is the very lack of outcomes data. Definitive data cannot be generated without funding; funding requires pilot data; and pilot data cannot be generated without some source of funding, either start-up funding, or third-party reimbursement for treatment. The Catch-22 situation is that third parties frequently do not pay for voice therapy, or significantly restrict indications. It is difficult to reverse this policy in the absence of hard data.

Another limitation to studying the efficacy of treatment is the lack of consensus regarding objective measures for documenting improvement. Despite decades of research, there is still no gold standard of vocal function measures analogous to the audiogram for hearing. Acoustic measures are relatively easy to obtain, but are not clinically reliable in severe voice disorders. Perceptual analyses are more valid across the spectrum of vocal function, yet such measures are inherently subjective and only semiquantitative. Furthermore, reliable perceptual analysis requires listener training, and ideally, blinded evaluation. Perceptual data are not practical for routine clinical use or large studies. Aerodynamic measures provide physiologic data that correlate with the effort of speaking; however, this data collection is more difficult and less widely used. A promising development is the use of a questionnaire, the *Vocal Handicap Index*. Research is urgently needed to establish standards and to acquire a database of normal and pathologic function. We also do not really know the limits to vocal performance in normal individuals. Normative acoustic and aerodynamic data are lacking for children across development. Carefully planned and well-supported studies are needed to collect this information.

In laryngology, there is no lack of questions significant to research. Where the next twenty years of research will take us is unknown. The only certainty is that thoughtful bridging research will continue to improve the care of patients with voice disorders.

REFERENCES

1. Hirano M. Phonosurgical anatomy of the larynx. In: Ford CN, Bless DM, eds. *Phonosurgery.* New York, NY: Raven Press; 1991.

2. Bryant NJ, Woodson GE, Kaufman K, et al. Human posterior cricoarytenoid muscle compartments: anatomy and mechanics. *Arch Otol.* 1996;122:1331-1336.

3. Sanders I, Wu BL, Mu L, et al. The innervation of the human larynx posterior cricoarytenoid muscle: evidence for at least two neuromuscular compartments. *Laryngoscope.* 1994;104:880-884.

4. Sanders I, Han Y, Wang J, Biller H. Muscle spindles are concentrated in the superior vocalis subcompartment of the human thyroarytenoid muscle. *J Voice.* 1998;12:7-16.

5. Nahm I, Shin T, Chiba T. Regeneration of the recurrent laryngeal nerve in the guinea pig: reorganization of motoneurons after freezing injury. *Am J Otoloryngol.* 1990;11:90-98.

6. Flint PW, Downs DH, Colterera M. Laryngeal synkinesis following reinnervation in the rat. *Ann Otol Rhinol Laryngol.* 1991;100:797-806.

7. Nahm I, Shin T, Watanabe H, Naeyama T. Misdirected regeneration of injured recurrent laryngeal nerve in the cat. *Am J Otolaryngol.* 1993;14:43-48.

8. Strome M. Presentation at the Annual Meeting of the American Laryngological Association; 1999.

9. Swenson M, Zwirner P, Murry T, Woodson GE. Medical evaluation of patients with spasmodic dysphonia. *J Voice.* 1992;6:320-324.

10. Close LG, Woodson GE. Common upper airway disorders in the elderly. *Geriatrics.* 1989;44:67-72.

11. Catz DS, Fischer LM, Moschella MC, Tobias ML, Kelley DB. Sexually dimorphic expression of a laryngeal-specific, androgen-regulated myosin heavy chain gene during *Xenopus laevis* development. *Dev Biol.* 1992;154:366-376.

12. Rahbar R, Valdez TA, Shapshay S. Preliminary results of intraoperative mitomycin-C in the treatment and prevention of glottic and subglottic stenosis. *J Voice.* 2000;14:282-286.

UNIT 2

Clinical Assessment

History and Physical Examination of Patients with Voice Disorders

Robert T. Sataloff, MD, DMA, FACS

Joseph R. Spiegel, MD, FACS

Mary J. Hawkshaw, RN, BSN, CORLN

A comprehensive history and physical examination usually reveals the cause of voice dysfunction. Effective history taking and physical examination depend upon a practical understanding of the anatomy and physiology of voice production.[1-4] Because dysfunction in virtually any body system may affect phonation, medical inquiry must be comprehensive. The current standard of care for all voice patients evolved from advances inspired by medical problems of voice professionals such as singers and actors. Even minor problems may be particularly symptomatic in singers and actors because of the extreme demands they place upon their voices. However, a great many other patients are voice professionals. They include teachers, salespeople, attorneys, clergy, physicians, politicians, telephone receptionists, and anyone else whose ability to earn a living is impaired in the presence of voice dysfunction. Because good voice quality is so important in our society, the majority of our patients are voice professionals, and all patients should be treated as such.

The scope of inquiry and examination for most patients is similar to that required for singers and actors, except that performing voice professionals have unique needs, which require additional history and examination. Questions must be added regarding performance commitments, professional status, and voice goals, the amount and nature of voice training, performance environment, rehearsal practices, abusive habits during speech and singing, and many other matters. Such supplementary information is essential to proper treatment selection and patient counseling in singers and actors. However, analogous factors must also be taken into account for stockbrokers, factory shop foremen, elementary schoolteachers, homemakers with several noisy children, and many others. Consequently, in order to provide a broad perspective and greater amount of practical information, this chapter includes a brief discussion of history taking and physical examination in professional voice users. Physicians familiar with the management of these challenging patients are well equipped to evaluate all patients with voice complaints. It should be recognized that this chapter, while comprehensive, is certainly not complete. Readers interested in additional information, particularly regarding professional voice performers, are encouraged to consult other sources, including those from which much of this chapter is derived.[1-3]

PATIENT HISTORY

Extensive historical background is necessary for thorough evaluation of the voice, and the otolaryngologist who sees voice patients (especially singers) only occasionally cannot reasonably be expected to remember all the pertinent questions. Although some laryngologists consider a lengthy inquisition helpful in estab-

lishing rapport, many of us who see a substantial number of voice patients each day within a busy practice need a thorough but less time-consuming alternative. A history questionnaire can be extremely helpful in documenting all the necessary information, in helping the patient sort out and articulate his or her problems, and in saving the clinician time recording information. The author (RTS) has developed a questionnaire[5,6] that has proven helpful (Appendix 11-1). The patient is asked to complete the relevant portions of the form at home or in the waiting room before seeing the doctor. A similar form has been developed for voice patients who are not singers.[6]

No history questionnaire is a substitute for direct, penetrating questioning by the physician. However, the direction of most useful inquiry can be determined from a glance at a questionnaire, obviating the need for extensive writing, which permits the physician greater eye contact with the patient and facilitates rapid establishment of the close rapport and confidence that are so important in treating voice patients. The physician is also able to supplement initial impressions and historical information from the questionnaire with seemingly leisurely conversation during the physical examination. The use of the history questionnaire has added substantially to the efficiency, consistent thoroughness, and ease of managing these delightful, but often complex, patients. A similar set of questions is also used with new patients by the speech-language pathologist, and many enlightened singing teachers when assessing new students.

How Old Are You?

Serious vocal endeavor may start in childhood and continue throughout a lifetime. As the vocal mechanism undergoes normal maturation, the voice changes. The optimal time to begin serious vocal training is controversial. For many years, most singing teachers advocated delay of vocal training and serious singing until near puberty in the female and after puberty and voice stabilization in the male. However, in a child with earnest vocal aspirations and potential, starting specialized training early in childhood is reasonable. Initial instruction should teach the child to vocalize without straining and to avoid all forms of voice abuse. It should not permit premature indulgence in operatic bravado. Most experts agree that taxing voice use and singing during puberty should be minimized or avoided altogether, particularly by the male. Voice maturation (attainment of stable adult vocal quality) may occur at any age from the early teenage period to the fourth decade of life. The dangerous tendency for young singers to attempt to

sound older than their vocal years frequently causes vocal dysfunction.

All components of voice production are subject to normal aging. Abdominal and general muscular tone frequently decrease, lungs lose elasticity, the thorax loses its distensibility, the mucosa of the vocal tract atrophies, mucous secretions change character, nerve endings are reduced in number, and psychoneurologic functions change. Moreover, the larynx itself loses muscle tone and bulk and may show depletion of submucosal ground substance in the vocal folds. The laryngeal cartilages ossify and the joints may become arthritic and stiff. Hormonal influence is altered. Vocal range, intensity, and quality all may be modified. Vocal fold atrophy may be the most striking alteration. The clinical effects of aging seem more pronounced in female singers, although vocal fold histologic changes may be more prominent in males. Excellent male singers occasionally extend their careers into their seventies or beyond.[7,8] However, some degree of breathiness, decreased range, and other evidence of aging should be expected in elderly voices. Nevertheless, many of the changes we typically associate with elderly singers (wobble, flat pitch) are caused by lack of conditioning, rather than inevitable changes of biologic aging. These aesthetically undesirable concomitants of aging can often be reversed.[3,9]

What Is Your Voice Problem?

Careful questioning as to the onset of vocal problems is needed to separate acute from chronic dysfunction. Often an upper respiratory tract infection will send a patient to the physician's office, but penetrating inquiry may reveal a chronic vocal problem that is the patient's real concern, especially in singers and actors. Identifying acute and chronic problems before beginning therapy is important so that both patient and physician may have realistic expectations and make optimal therapeutic selections.

The specific nature of the vocal complaint can provide a great deal of information. Just as dizzy patients rarely walk into the physician's office complaining of "rotary vertigo," voice patients may be unable to articulate their symptoms without guidance. They may use the term *hoarseness* to describe a variety of conditions that the physician must separate. Hoarseness is a coarse or scratchy sound most often associated with abnormalities of the leading edge of the vocal folds such as laryngitis or mass lesions. Breathiness is a vocal quality characterized by excessive loss of air during vocalization. In some cases, it is caused by improper technique. However, any condition that prevents full approximation of the vocal folds can be responsible. Such causes

include vocal fold paralysis, a mass lesion separating the leading edges of the vocal folds, arthritis of the cricoarytenoid joint, arytenoid dislocation, scarring of the vibratory margin, senile vocal fold atrophy (presbyphonia), psychogenic dysphonia, malingering, and other conditions.

Fatigue of the voice is inability to continue to speak or sing for extended periods without change in vocal quality and/or control. The voice may show fatigue by becoming hoarse, losing range, changing timbre, breaking into different registers, or exhibiting other uncontrolled aberrations. A well-trained singer should be able to sing for several hours without vocal fatigue. Fatigue is often caused by misuse of abdominal and neck musculature or "oversinging," singing too loudly, or too long. Vocal fatigue may also be a sign of general tiredness or serious illnesses such as myasthenia gravis.

Volume disturbance may manifest as inability to sing loudly or inability to sing softly. Each voice has its own dynamic range. Within the course of training, singers learn to sing more loudly by singing more efficiently. They also learn to sing softly, a more difficult task, through years of laborious practice. Actors and other trained speakers go through similar training. Most volume problems are secondary to intrinsic limitations of the voice or technical errors in voice use, although hormonal changes, aging, and neurologic disease are other causes. Superior laryngeal nerve paralysis impairs the ability to speak or sing loudly. This is a frequently unrecognized consequence of herpes infection ("cold sores"), or Lyme disease, and may be precipitated by any viral upper respiratory tract infection.

Most highly trained singers require only about ten minutes to half an hour to "warm up the voice." Prolonged warm-up time, especially in the morning, is most often caused by reflux laryngitis. Tickling or choking during singing is most often a symptom of an abnormality of the vocal fold's leading edge. The symptom of tickling or choking should contraindicate singing until the vocal folds have been examined. Pain while singing can indicate vocal fold lesions, laryngeal joint arthritis, infection, or gastric acid reflux irritation of the arytenoid region. However, pain is much more commonly caused by voice abuse with excessive muscular activity in the neck rather than an acute abnormality on the leading edge of a vocal fold. In the absence of other symptoms, these patients do not generally require immediate cessation of singing pending medical examination. However, sudden onset of pain (usually sharp pain) while singing may be associated with a mucosal tear or a vocal fold hemorrhage and warrants voice conservation pending laryngeal examination.

Do You Have Any Pressing Voice Commitments?

If a singer or professional speaker (eg, actor, politician) seeks treatment at the end of a busy performance season and has no pressing engagements, management of the voice problem should be relatively conservative and designed to ensure long-term protection of the larynx, the most delicate part of the vocal mechanism. However, the physician and patient rarely have this luxury. Most often, the voice professional needs treatment within a week of an important engagement, and sometimes within less than a day. Younger singers fall ill shortly before performances, not because of hypochondria or coincidence, but rather because of the immense physical and emotional stress of the preperformance period. The singer is frequently working harder and singing longer hours than usual. Moreover, he or she may be under particular pressure to learn new material and to perform well for a new audience. The singer may also be sleeping less than usual because of additional time spent rehearsing or because of the discomforts of a strange city. Seasoned professionals make their living by performing regularly, sometimes several times a week. Consequently, any time they get sick is likely to precede a performance. Caring for voice complaints in these situations requires highly skilled judgment and bold management.

Tell Me About Your Vocal Career, Long-Term Goals, and the Importance of Your Voice Quality and Upcoming Commitments.

To choose a treatment program, the physician must understand the importance of the patient's voice and his or her long-term career plans, the importance of the upcoming vocal commitment, and the consequences of canceling the engagement. Injudicious prescription of voice rest can be almost as damaging to a vocal career as injudicious performance. For example, although a singer's voice is usually his or her most important commodity, other factors distinguish the few successful artists from the multitude of less successful singers with equally good voices. These include musicianship, reliability, and "professionalism." Canceling a concert at the last minute may seriously damage a performer's reputation. Reliability is especially critical early in a singer's career. Moreover, an expert singer often can modify a performance to decrease the strain on his or her voice. No singer should be allowed to perform in a manner that will permit serious injury to the vocal folds, but in the frequent borderline cases, the condition of the larynx must be weighed against other factors affecting the singer as an artist.

How Much Voice Training Have You Had?

Establishing how long a singer or actor has been performing seriously is important, especially if his or her active performance career predates the beginning of vocal training. Active untrained singers and actors frequently develop undesirable techniques that are difficult to modify. Extensive voice use without training or premature training with inappropriate repertoire may underlie persistent vocal difficulties later in life. The number of years a performer has been training his or her voice may be a fair index of vocal proficiency. A person who has studied voice for one or two years is somewhat more likely to have gross technical difficulties than is someone who has been studying for twenty years. However, if training has been intermittent or discontinued, technical problems are common, especially among singers. In addition, methods of technical voice use vary among voice teachers. Hence, a student who has had many teachers in a relatively brief period of time commonly has numerous technical insecurities or deficiencies that may be responsible for vocal dysfunction. This is especially true if the singer has changed to a new teacher within the preceding year. The physician must be careful not to criticize the patient's current voice teacher in such circumstances. It often takes years of expert instruction to correct bad habits.

All people speak more often than they sing, yet most singers report little speech training. Even if a singer uses the voice flawlessly while practicing and performing, voice abuse at other times can cause damage that affects singing.

Under What Kinds of Conditions Do You Use Your Voice?

The Lombard effect is the tendency to increase vocal intensity in response to increased background noise. A well-trained singer learns to compensate for this tendency and to avoid singing at unsafe volumes. Singers of classical music usually have such training and frequently perform with only a piano, a situation in which the balance can be controlled well. However, singers performing in large halls, with orchestras, or in operas early in their careers tend to oversing and strain their voices. Similar problems occur during outdoor concerts because of the lack of auditory feedback. This phenomenon is seen even more among "pop" singers. Pop singers are in a uniquely difficult position; often, despite little vocal training, they enjoy great artistic and financial success and endure extremely stressful demands on their time and voices. They are required to sing in large halls or outdoor arenas, not designed for musical performance, amid smoke and other environmental irritants, accompanied by extremely loud background music. One frequently neglected key to survival for these singers is the proper use of monitor speakers. These direct the sound of the singer's voice toward the singer on the stage and provide auditory feedback. Determining whether the pop singer uses monitor speakers and whether they are loud enough for the singer to hear is important.

Amateur singers are often no less serious about their music than are professionals, but generally they have less ability to compensate technically for illness or other physical impairment. Rarely does an amateur suffer a great loss from postponing a performance or permitting someone to sing in his or her place. In most cases, the amateur singer's best interest is served through conservative management directed at long-term maintenance of good vocal health.

A great many singers who seek physicians' advice are primarily choral singers. They often are enthusiastic amateurs, untrained but dedicated to their musical recreation. They should be handled as amateur solo singers, educated specifically about the Lombard effect, and cautioned to avoid the excessive volume so common in a choral environment. One good way for a singer to monitor loudness is to cup a hand to his or her ear. This adds about 6 dB[10] to the singer's perception of his or her own voice and can be a very helpful guide in noisy surroundings. Young professional singers are often hired to augment amateur choruses. Feeling that the professional quartet has been hired to "lead" the rest of the choir, they often make the mistake of trying to accomplish that goal by singing louder than others in their sections. These singers should be advised to lead their section by singing each line as if they were soloists giving a voice lesson to the people standing next to them, and as if there were a microphone in front of them recording their choral performance for their voice teacher. This approach usually not only preserves the voice but also produces a better choral sound.

How Much Do You Practice and Exercise Your Voice? How, When, and Where Do You Use Your Voice?

Vocal exercise is as essential to the vocalist as exercise and conditioning of other muscle systems is to the athlete. Proper vocal practice incorporates scales and specific exercises designed to maintain and develop the vocal apparatus. Simply acting or singing songs and giving performances without routine studious concentration on vocal technique is not adequate for the vocal performer. The physician should know whether the vocalist practices daily, whether he or she practices at the same time daily, and how long the practice lasts.

Actors generally practice and warm up their voices for ten to thirty minutes daily, although more time is recommended. Most serious singers practice for at least one to two hours per day. If a singer routinely practices in the late afternoon or evening but frequently performs in the morning (religious services, school classes, teaching voice, choir rehearsals, etc.), one should inquire into the warm-up procedures preceding such performances as well as cool-down procedures after voice use. Singing "cold," especially early in the morning, may result in the use of minor muscular alterations to compensate for vocal insecurity produced by inadequate preparation. Such crutches can result in voice dysfunction. Similar problems may result from instances of voice use other than formal singing. Schoolteachers, telephone receptionists, salespeople, and others who speak extensively also often derive great benefit from five or ten minutes of vocalization of scales first thing in the morning. Although singers rarely practice their scales too long, they frequently perform or rehearse excessively. This is especially true immediately before a major concert or audition, when physicians are most likely to see acute problems. When a singer has hoarseness and vocal fatigue and has been practicing a new role for fourteen hours a day for the last three weeks, no simple prescription will solve the problem. However, a treatment regimen can usually be designed to carry the performer safely through his or her musical obligations.

The physician should be aware of common habits and environments that are often associated with abusive voice behavior and should ask about them routinely. Screaming at sports events and at children is among the most common. Extensive voice use in noisy environments also tends to be abusive. These include noisy rooms, cars, airplanes, sports facilities, and other locations where background noise or acoustic design impairs auditory feedback. Dry, dusty surroundings may alter vocal fold secretions through dehydration or contact irritation, altering voice function. Activities such as cheerleading, teaching, choral conducting, amateur singing, and frequent communication with hearing-impaired persons are likely to be associated with voice abuse, as is extensive professional voice use without formal training. The physician should inquire into the patient's routine voice use and should specifically ask about any activities that frequently lead to voice change such as hoarseness or discomfort in the neck or throat. Laryngologists should ask specifically about other activities that may be abusive to the vocal folds such as weight lifting, aerobics, and the playing of some wind instruments.

Are You Aware of Misusing or Abusing Your Voice During Singing?

A detailed discussion of vocal technique in singing is beyond the scope of this chapter. The reader is referred to other sources.[11-13] However, the most common technical errors involve excessive muscle tension in the tongue, neck, and larynx; inadequate abdominal support; and excessive volume. Inadequate preparation can be a devastating source of voice abuse and may result from limited practice, limited rehearsal of a difficult piece, or limited vocal training for a given role. The latter error is tragically common. In some situations, voice teachers are at fault and both the singer and teacher must resist the impulse to "show off" the voice in works that are either too difficult for the singer's level of training or simply not suited to the singer's voice. Singers are habitually unhappy with the limitations of their voices. At some time or another, most baritones wish they were tenors and walk around proving they can sing high Cs in *"Vesti la giubba."* Singers with other vocal ranges have similar fantasies. Attempts to make the voice something that it is not, or at least that it is not yet, are frequently harmful.

Are You Aware of Misusing or Abusing Your Voice During Speaking?

Common patterns of voice abuse and misuse will not be discussed in detail in this chapter. They are covered elsewhere in this book and in other literature.[14-16] Voice abuse and/or misuse should be suspected particularly in patients who complain of voice fatigue associated with voice use, whose voices are worse at the end of a working day or week, and in any patient who is chronically hoarse. Technical errors in voice use may be the primary etiology of a voice complaint, or it may develop secondarily because of a patient's effort to compensate for voice disturbance from another cause.

Dissociation of one's speaking and singing voices is probably the most common cause of voice abuse problems in excellent singers. Too frequently, all the expert training in support, muscle control, and projection is not applied to a singer's speaking voice. Unfortunately, the resultant voice strain affects the singing voice as well as the speaking voice. Such damage is especially likely to occur in noisy rooms and in cars, where the background noise is louder than it seems. Backstage greetings after a lengthy performance can be particularly devastating. The singer usually is exhausted and distracted; the environment is often dusty and dry; and generally a noisy crowd is present. Similar conditions prevail at postperformance parties, where smoking and alcohol worsen matters. These situations should be avoided by any singer with vocal problems and should be controlled through awareness at other times.

Three particularly abusive and potentially damaging vocal activities are worthy of note. *Cheerleading* requires extensive screaming under the worst possible physical and environmental circumstances. It is a highly undesirable activity for anyone considering serious vocal endeavor. This is a common conflict in younger singers because the teenager who is the high school choir soloist often is also student council president, yearbook editor, captain of the cheerleaders, and so on. *Conducting,* particularly choral conducting, can also be deleterious. An enthusiastic conductor, especially of an amateur group, frequently sings all four parts intermittently, at volumes louder than the entire choir, during lengthy rehearsals. Conducting is a common avocation among singers but must be done with expert technique and special precautions to prevent voice injury. Hoarseness or loss of soft voice control after conducting a rehearsal or concert suggests voice abuse during conducting. The patient should be instructed to record his or her voice throughout the vocal range singing long notes at dynamics from soft to loud to soft. Recordings should be made prior to rehearsal and following rehearsal. If the voice has lost range, control, or quality during the rehearsal, voice abuse has occurred. A similar test can be used for patients who sing in choirs, teach voice, or perform other potentially abusive vocal activities. Such problems in conductors can generally be managed by additional training in conducting techniques, and by voice training, including warm-up and cool-down exercises. *Teaching singing* may also be hazardous to vocal health. It can be done safely but requires skill and thought. Most teachers teach while seated at the piano. Late in a long, hard day, this posture is not conducive to maintenance of optimal abdominal and back support. Usually, teachers work with students continually positioned to the right or left of the keyboard. This may require the teacher to turn his or her neck at a particularly sharp angle, especially when teaching at an upright piano. Teachers also often demonstrate vocal works in their students' vocal ranges rather than their own, illustrating bad as well as good technique. If a singing teacher is hoarse or has neck discomfort, or his or her soft singing control deteriorates at the end of a teaching day (assuming that the teacher warms up before beginning to teach voice lessons), voice abuse should be suspected. Helpful modifications include teaching with a grand piano, sitting slightly sideways on the piano bench, or alternating student position to the right and left of the piano to facilitate better neck alignment. Retaining an accompanist so that the teacher can stand rather than teach from sitting behind a piano, and many other helpful modifications, are possible.

Do You Have Pain When You Talk or Sing?

Odynophonia, or pain caused by phonation, can be a disturbing symptom. It is not uncommon, but relatively little has been written or discussed on this subject. A detailed review of odynophonia is beyond the scope of this publication. However, laryngologists should be familiar with the diagnosis and treatment of a few of the most common causes, at least, as discussed in the chapter on "Common Diagnoses and Medical Treatments" in this book (Chapter 20) and elsewhere.[3]

What Kind of Physical Condition Are You In?

Phonation is an athletic activity that requires good conditioning and coordinated interaction of numerous physical functions. Maladies of any part of the body may be reflected in the voice. Failure to maintain good abdominal muscle tone and respiratory endurance through exercise, is particularly harmful in that deficiencies in these areas undermine the power source of the voice. Patients generally attempt to compensate for such weaknesses by using inappropriate muscle groups, particularly in the neck, causing vocal dysfunction. Similar problems may occur in the well-conditioned vocalist in states of fatigue. These are compounded by mucosal changes that accompany excessively long hours of hard work. Such problems may be seen even in the best singers shortly before important performances in the height of the concert season.

A popular but untrue myth holds that great opera singers must be obese. However, the vivacious, gregarious personality that often distinguishes the great performer seems to be accompanied frequently by a propensity for excess, especially culinary excess. This excess is as undesirable in the vocalist as it is in most other athletic artists, and it should be prevented from the start of one's vocal career. Appropriate and attractive body weight has always been valued in the pop music world and is becoming particularly important in the opera world as this formerly theater-based artform moves to television and film media. However, attempts at weight reduction in an established speaker or singer are a different matter. The vocal mechanism is a finely tuned, complex instrument and is exquisitely sensitive to minor changes. Substantial fluctuations in weight frequently cause deleterious alterations of the voice, although these are usually temporary. Weight reduction programs for people concerned about their voices must be monitored carefully and designed to reduce weight in small increments over long periods. A history of sudden recent weight change may be responsible for almost any vocal complaint.

Have You Noted Voice or Bodily Weakness, Tremor, Fatigue, or Loss of Control?

Even minor neurologic disorders may be extremely disruptive to vocal function. Specific questions should be asked to rule out neuromuscular and neurologic diseases such as myasthenia gravis, Parkinson's disease, tremors, other movement disorders, spasmodic dysphonia, multiple sclerosis, central nervous system neoplasm, and other serious maladies that may be present with voice complaints.[17,18]

Do You Have Allergy or Cold Symptoms?

Acute upper respiratory tract infection causes inflammation of the mucosa, alters mucosal secretions, and makes the mucosa more vulnerable to injury. Coughing and throat clearing are particularly traumatic vocal activities and may worsen or provoke hoarseness associated with a cold. Postnasal drip and allergy may produce the same response. Infectious sinusitis is associated with discharge and diffuse mucosal inflammation, resulting in similar problems, and may actually alter the sound of a voice, especially the patient's own perception of his or her voice. Futile attempts to compensate for disease of the supraglottic vocal tract in an effort to return the sound to normal frequently result in laryngeal strain. The expert singer or speaker should compensate by monitoring technique by tactile rather than by auditory feedback, or singing "by feel" rather than "by ear."

Do You Have Breathing Problems, Especially After Exercise?

Voice patients usually volunteer information about upper respiratory tract infections and "postnasal drip," but the relevance of other maladies may not be obvious to them. Consequently the physician must seek out pertinent history.

Respiratory problems are especially important in voice patients. Even mild respiratory dysfunction may adversely affect the power source of the voice.[19] Occult asthma may be particularly troublesome.[20] A complete respiratory history should be obtained in most patients with voice complaints, and pulmonary function testing is often advisable.

Have You Been Exposed to Environmental Irritants?

Any mucosal irritant can disrupt the delicate vocal mechanism. Allergies to dust and mold are aggravated commonly during rehearsals and performances in concert halls, especially older theaters and concert halls, because of numerous curtains, backstage trappings, and dressing room facilities that are rarely cleaned thoroughly. Nasal obstruction and erythematous conjunctivae suggest generalized mucosal irritation. The drying effects of cold air and dry heat may also affect mucosal secretions, leading to decreased lubrication, a "scratchy" voice, and tickling cough. These symptoms may be minimized by nasal breathing, which allows inspired air to be filtered, warmed, and humidified. Nasal breathing, whenever possible, rather than mouth breathing is proper vocal technique. While the performer is backstage between appearances or during rehearsals, inhalation of dust and other irritants may be controlled by wearing a protective mask such as those used by carpenters, or a surgical mask, that does not contain fiberglass. This is especially helpful when sets are being constructed in the rehearsal area.

A history of recent travel suggests other sources of mucosal irritation. The air in airplanes is extremely dry, and airplanes are noisy.[21] One must be careful to avoid talking loudly and to maintain good hydration and nasal breathing during air travel. Environmental changes can also be disruptive. Las Vegas is infamous for the mucosal irritation caused by its dry atmosphere and smoke-filled rooms. In fact, the resultant complex of hoarseness, vocal "tickle," and fatigue is referred to as "Las Vegas voice." A history of recent travel should also suggest jet lag and generalized fatigue, which may be potent detriments to good vocal function.

Environmental pollution is responsible for the presence of toxic substances and conditions encountered daily. Inhalation of toxic pollutants may affect the voice adversely by direct laryngeal injury, by causing pulmonary dysfunction that results in voice maladies, or through impairments elsewhere in the vocal tract. Ingested substances, especially those that have neurolaryngologic effects may also adversely affect the voice. Nonchemical environmental pollutants such as noise can cause voice abnormalities as well. Laryngologists should be familiar with the laryngologic effects of the numerous potentially irritating substances and conditions found in the environment.[22] We must also be familiar with special pollution problems encountered by performers. Numerous materials used by artists to create sculptures, drawings, and theatrical sets are toxic and have adverse voice effects. In addition, performers are routinely exposed to chemicals encountered through stage smoke, and pyrotechnic effects.[23-25] Although it is clear that some of the "special effects" result in serious laryngologic consequences, much additional study is needed to clarify the nature and scope of these occupational problems.

Do You Smoke, Live With a Smoker, or Work Around Smoke?

The deleterious effects of tobacco smoke on mucosa are indisputable. Anyone concerned about the health of his or her voice should not smoke. Smoking causes erythema, mild edema, and generalized inflammation throughout the vocal tract. Both smoke itself and the heat of the cigarette appear to be important. Marijuana produces a particularly irritating, unfiltered smoke that is inhaled directly, causing considerable mucosal response. Voice patients who refuse to stop smoking marijuana should at least be advised to use a water pipe to cool and partially filter the smoke. Some vocalists are required to perform in smoke-filled environments and may suffer the same effects as the smokers themselves. In some theaters, it is possible to place fans upstage or direct the ventilation system so as to create a gentle draft toward the audience, clearing the smoke away from the stage. "Smoke eaters" installed in some theaters are also helpful.

Do Any Foods Seem to Affect Your Voice?

Various foods are said to affect the voice. Traditionally, singers avoid milk and ice cream before performances. In many people, these foods seem to increase the amount and viscosity of mucosal secretions. Allergy and casein have been implicated, but no satisfactory explanation has been established. Restriction of these foods from the diet before a voice performance may be helpful in some cases. Chocolate may have the same effect and should be viewed similarly. Chocolate also contains caffeine, which may aggravate reflux or cause tremor. Voice patients should be asked about eating nuts. This is important not only because some people experience effects similar to those produced by milk products and chocolate, but also because they are extremely irritating if aspirated. The irritation produced by aspiration of even a small organic foreign body may be severe and impossible to correct rapidly enough to permit performance. Highly spiced foods may also cause mucosal irritation. In addition, they seem to aggravate reflux laryngitis. Coffee and other beverages containing caffeine also aggravate gastric reflux and may promote dehydration and/or alter secretions and necessitate frequent throat clearing in some people. Fad diets, especially rapid weight-reduc-

ing diets, are notorious for causing voice problems. Lemon juice and herbal teas are considered beneficial to the voice. Both may act as demulcents, thinning secretions, and may very well be helpful. Eating a full meal before a speaking or singing engagement may interfere with abdominal support or may aggravate upright reflux of gastric juice during abdominal muscle contraction.

Do You Have Morning Hoarseness, Bad Breath, Excessive Phlegm, a Lump in Your Throat, or Heartburn?

Reflux laryngitis is especially common among singers and trained speakers because of the high intra-abdominal pressure associated with proper support, and because of lifestyle. Singers frequently perform at night. Many vocalists refrain from eating before performances because a full stomach can compromise effective abdominal support. They typically compensate by eating heartily at postperformance gatherings late at night and then go to bed with a full stomach. Chronic irritation of arytenoid and vocal fold mucosa by reflux of gastric secretions may occasionally be associated with dyspepsia or pyrosis. However, the key features of this malady are bitter taste and halitosis on awakening in the morning, a dry or "coated" mouth, often a scratchy sore throat or a feeling of a "lump in the throat," hoarseness, and the need for prolonged vocal warm-up. The physician must be alert to these symptoms and ask about them routinely, otherwise the diagnosis will often be overlooked because people who have had this problem for many years or a lifetime do not even realize it is abnormal.

Do You Have Trouble With Your Bowels or Belly?

Any condition that alters abdominal function, such as muscle spasm, constipation, or diarrhea, interferes with support and may result in a voice complaint. These symptoms may accompany infection, anxiety, various gastroenterologic diseases, and other maladies.

Are You Under Particular Stress or in Therapy?

The human voice is an exquisitely sensitive messenger of emotion. Highly trained voice professionals learn to control the effects of anxiety and other emotional stress on their voices under ordinary circumstances. However, in some instances this training may break down or a performer may be inadequately prepared to control the voice under specific stressful conditions. Preperformance anxiety is the most common example, but insecurity, depression, and other emotional disturbances are also generally reflected in the voice. Anxiety reactions are mediated in part through the autonomic nervous system and result in a dry mouth, cold clammy skin, and thick secretions. These reactions are normal, and good vocal training coupled with assurance that no abnormality or disease is present generally overcomes them. However, long-term, poorly compensated emotional stress and exogenous stress (from agents, producers, teachers, parents, etc.) may cause substantial vocal dysfunction and may result in permanent limitations of the vocal apparatus. These conditions must be diagnosed and treated expertly. Hypochondriasis is uncommon among professional singers, despite popular opinion to the contrary.

Recent publications have highlighted the complexity and importance of psychologic factors associated with voice disorders.[26,27] A comprehensive discussion of this subject is also presented elsewhere in this book. It is important for the physician to recognize that psychologic problems may not only cause voice disorders, but they may also delay recovery from voice disorders that were entirely organic in etiology. Professional voice users, especially singers, have enormous psychologic investment and personality identifications associated with their voices. A condition that causes voice loss or permanent injury often evokes the same powerful psychologic responses seen following the death of a loved one. This process may be initiated even when physical recovery is complete, if an incident (injury or surgery) has made the vocalist realize that voice loss is possible. Such a "brush with death" can have profound emotional consequences in some patients. It is essential for laryngologists to be aware of these powerful factors and manage them properly if optimal therapeutic results are to be achieved expeditiously.

Do You Have Problems Controlling Your Weight? Are You Excessively Tired? Are You Cold When Other People are Warm?

Endocrine problems warrant special attention. The human voice is extremely sensitive to endocrinologic changes. Many of these are reflected in alterations of fluid content of the lamina propria just beneath the laryngeal mucosa. This causes alterations in the bulk and shape of the vocal folds and result in voice change. Hypothyroidism[28-32] is a well-recognized cause of such voice disorders, although the mechanism is not fully understood. Hoarseness, vocal fatigue, muffling of the voice, loss of range, and a sensation of a lump in the throat may be present even with mild hypothyroidism. Even when thyroid function tests results are within the low normal range, this diagnosis should be entertained, especially if thyroid-stimulating hormone levels are in the high normal range or are elevated. Thyrotoxicosis may result in similar voice disturbances.[29]

Do You Have Menstrual Irregularity, Cyclical Voice Changes Associated with Menses, Recent Menopause, or Other Hormonal Changes or Problems?

Voice changes associated with sex hormones are encountered commonly in clinical practice and have been investigated more thoroughly than have other hormonal changes.[33,34] Although a correlation appears to exist between sex hormone levels and depth of male voices (higher testosterone and lower estradiol levels in basses than in tenors),[28] the most important hormonal considerations in males occur during or related to puberty,[35,36] as discussed in the chapter on common diagnoses and treatments (Chapter 20). Voice problems related to sex hormones are more common in female singers.[37-53] They are also reviewed in the "common diagnoses" chapter.

Do You Have Jaw Joint or Other Dental Problems?

Dental disease, especially temporomandibular joint (TMJ) dysfunction, introduces muscle tension in the head and neck, which is transmitted to the larynx directly through the muscular attachments between the mandible and the hyoid bone, and indirectly as generalized increased muscle tension. These problems often result in decreased range, vocal fatigue, and change in the quality or placement of a voice. Such tension often is accompanied by excess tongue muscle activity, especially pulling of the tongue posteriorly. This hyperfunctional behavior acts through hyoid attachments to disrupt the balance between the intrinsic and extrinsic laryngeal musculature. TMJ problems are also problematic for wind instrumentalists and some string players, including violinists. In some cases, the problems may actually be caused by instrumental technique. The history should always include information about musical activities, including instruments other than the voice.

Do You or Your Blood Relatives Have Hearing Loss?

Hearing loss is often overlooked as a source of vocal problems. Auditory feedback is fundamental to speaking and singing. Interference with this control mechanism may result in altered vocal production, particularly if the person is unaware of the hearing loss. Distortion, particularly pitch distortion (diplacusis) may also pose serious problems for the singer. This appears to be caused not only by aesthetic difficulties in matching pitch, but also by vocal strain which accompanies pitch shifts.[54]

Have You Suffered Whiplash or Other Bodily Injury?

Various bodily injuries outside the confines of the vocal tract may have profound effects on the voice.

Whiplash, for example, commonly causes changes in technique, with consequent voice fatigue, loss of range, difficulty singing softly, and other problems. These problems derive from neck muscle spasm, abnormal neck posturing secondary to pain, and consequent hyperfunctional voice use. Lumbar, abdominal, head, chest, supraglottic, and extremity injuries may also affect vocal technique and be responsible for the dysphonia that prompted the voice patient to seek medical attention.

Did You Undergo Any Surgery Prior to the Onset of Your Voice Problems?

A history of laryngeal surgery in a voice patient is a matter of great concern. It is important to establish exactly why the surgery was done, by whom it was done, whether intubation was necessary, and whether voice therapy was instituted pre- or postoperatively if the lesion was associated with voice abuse (vocal nodules). If the vocal dysfunction that sent the patient to the physician's office dates from the immediate postoperative period, surgical or perisurgical trauma must be suspected.

Otolaryngologists frequently are asked about the effects of tonsillectomy on the voice. Singers especially may consult the physician after tonsillectomy and complain of vocal dysfunction. Certainly removal of tonsils can alter the voice.[55,56] Tonsillectomy changes the configuration of the supraglottic vocal tract. In addition, scarring alters pharyngeal muscle function, which is trained meticulously in the professional singer. Singers must be warned that they may have permanent voice changes after tonsillectomy; however, these can be minimized by dissecting in the proper plane to lessen scarring. The singer's voice generally requires three to six months to stabilize or return to normal after surgery, although it is generally safe to begin limited singing within two to four weeks following surgery. As with any procedure for which general anesthesia may be needed, the anesthesiologist should be advised preoperatively that the patient is a professional singer. Intubation and extubation should be performed with great care and the use of nonirritating plastic rather than rubber or ribbed metal endotracheal tubes is preferred. Use of a laryngeal mask may be advisable for selected procedures, but this device is often not ideal for tonsillectomy, for mechanical reasons.

Surgery of the neck, such as thyroidectomy, may result in permanent alterations in the vocal mechanism through scarring of the extrinsic laryngeal musculature. The cervical (strap) muscles are important in maintaining laryngeal position and stability of the laryngeal skeleton, and they should be retracted rather than divided whenever possible. A history of recurrent or superior laryngeal nerve injury may explain a hoarse, breathy, or weak voice. However, in rare cases even a singer can compensate for recurrent laryngeal nerve paralysis and have a nearly normal voice.

Thoracic and abdominal surgery interfere with respiratory and abdominal support. After these procedures, singing and projected speaking should be prohibited until pain has subsided and healing has occurred sufficiently to allow normal support. Abdominal exercises should be instituted before resumption of vocalizing. Singing and speaking without proper support are often worse for the voice than not using the voice for performance at all.

Other surgical procedures may be important factors if they necessitate intubation or if they affect the musculoskeletal system so that the person has to change stance or balance. For example, balancing on one foot after leg surgery may decrease the effectiveness of the support mechanism.

What Medications and Other Substances Do You Use?

A history of alcohol abuse suggests the probability of poor vocal technique. Intoxication results in incoordination and decreased awareness, which undermine vocal discipline designed to optimize and protect the voice. The effect of small amounts of alcohol is controversial. Although many experts oppose its use because of its vasodilatory effect and consequent mucosal alteration, many people do not seem to be adversely affected by small amounts of alcohol such as a glass of wine with a meal. However, some people have mild sensitivities to certain wines or beers. Patients who develop nasal congestion and rhinorrhea after drinking beer, for example, should be made aware that they probably have a mild allergy to that particular beverage and should avoid it before voice commitments.

Patients frequently acquire antihistamines to help control "postnasal drip" or other symptoms. The drying effect of antihistamines may result in decreased vocal fold lubrication, increased throat clearing, and irritability leading to frequent coughing. Antihistamines may be helpful to some voice patients, but they must be used with caution.

When a voice patient seeking the attention of a physician is already taking antibiotics, it is important to find out the dose and the prescribing physician, if any, as well as whether the patient frequently treats himself or herself with inadequate courses of antibiotics often supplied by colleagues. Singers, actors, and other speakers sometimes have a "sore throat" shortly before important vocal presentations and start themselves on inappropriate antibiotic therapy, which they generally discontinue after their performance.

Diuretics are also popular among some performers. They are often prescribed by gynecologists at the vocalist's request to help deplete excess water in the premenstrual period. They are not effective in this scenario because they cannot diurese the protein-bound water in the laryngeal ground substance. Unsupervised use of these drugs may cause dehydration and consequent mucosal dryness.

Hormone use, especially use of oral contraceptives, must be mentioned specifically during the physician's inquiry. Women frequently do not mention them routinely when asked whether they are taking any medication. Vitamins are also frequently not mentioned. Most vitamin therapy seems to have little effect on the voice. However, high-dose vitamin C (5 to 6 g/day), which some people use to prevent upper respiratory tract infections, seems to act as a mild diuretic and may lead to dehydration and xerophonia.[57]

Cocaine use is common, especially among pop musicians. This drug can be extremely irritating to the nasal mucosa, causes marked vasoconstriction, and may alter the sensorium, resulting in decreased voice control and a tendency toward vocal abuse.

Many pain medications (including aspirin and ibuprofen), psychotropic medications, and many others may be responsible for the voice complaint. Laryngologists must be familiar with the laryngologic effects of the many substances ingested medically and recreationally. These can be reviewed elsewhere in this book and in other literature.[58]

PHYSICAL EXAMINATION

A detailed history frequently reveals the cause of a voice problem even before a physical examination is performed. However, a comprehensive physical examination, often including objective assessment of voice function, is also essential.[1,3,59] Physical examination must include a thorough ear, nose, and throat evaluation, and assessment of general physical condition. A patient who is extremely obese or appears fatigued, agitated, emotionally stressed, or otherwise generally ill has increased potential for voice dysfunction. This could be caused by any number of factors: altered abdominal support, loss of fine motor control of laryngeal muscles, decreased bulk of the submucosal vocal fold ground substance, change in the character of mucosal secretions, or similar mechanisms. Any physical condition that impairs the normal function of the abdominal musculature is suspect as cause for dysphonia. Some conditions, such as pregnancy, are obvious; however, a sprained ankle or broken leg that requires the singer to balance

in an unaccustomed posture may distract him or her from maintaining good abdominal support and thereby result in voice dysfunction. A tremorous neurologic disorder, endocrine disturbances such as thyroid dysfunction or menopause, the aging process, and other systemic conditions also may alter the voice. The physician must remember that maladies of almost any body system may result in voice dysfunction, and the doctor must remain alert for conditions outside the head and neck. If the patient uses his or her voice professionally for singing, acting, or other vocally demanding professions, physical examination should also include assessment of the patient during typical professional vocal tasks. For example, a singer should be asked to sing. Evaluation techniques for assessing performance are described elsewhere.[3,59]

Complete Ear, Nose and Throat Examination

Examination of the ears must include assessment of hearing acuity. Even a relatively slight hearing loss may result in voice strain as a singer tries to balance his or her vocal intensity with that of associate performers. Similar effects are encountered among speakers, but they are less prominent in the early stages of hearing loss. This is especially true of hearing losses acquired after vocal training has been completed. The effect is most pronounced with sensorineural hearing loss. Diplacusis makes vocal strain even worse. With conductive hearing loss, singers tend to sing more softly than appropriate rather than too loudly, and this is less harmful.

During an ear, nose, and throat examination, the conjunctivae and sclerae should be observed routinely for erythema that suggests allergy or irritation, for pallor that suggests anemia, and for other abnormalities such as jaundice. These observations may reveal the problem reflected in the vocal tract even before the larynx is visualized.

The nose should be assessed for patency of the nasal airway, character of the nasal mucosa, and nature of secretions, if any. A patient who is unable to breathe through the nose because of anatomic obstruction is forced to breathe unfiltered, unhumidified air through the mouth. Pale gray allergic mucosa or swollen infected mucosa in the nose suggests abnormal mucosa elsewhere in the respiratory tract.

Examination of the oral cavity should include careful attention to the tonsils and lymphoid tissue in the posterior pharyngeal wall, as well as to the mucosa. Diffuse lymphoid hypertrophy associated with a complaint of "scratchy" voice and irritative cough may indicate infection. The amount and viscosity of mucosal and salivary secretions should also be noted. Xerostomia is particularly important. Dental examination should focus not only on oral hygiene but also on the presence of wear facets suggestive of bruxism. Bruxism is a clue to excessive tension and may be associated with dysfunction of the temporomandibular joints, which should also be assessed routinely. Thinning of the enamel of the central incisors in a normal or underweight patient may be a clue to bulimia. However, it may also result from excessive ingestion of lemons, which some singers eat to help thin their secretions.

The neck should be examined for masses, restriction of movement, excess muscle tension, and scars from prior neck surgery or trauma. Laryngeal vertical mobility is also important. For example, tilting of the larynx produced by partial fixation of cervical muscles cut during previous surgery may produce voice dysfunction, as may fixation of the trachea to overlying neck skin. Particular attention should be paid to the thyroid gland. Examination of posterior neck muscles and range of motion should not be neglected. The cranial nerves should also be examined. Diminished fifth nerve sensation, diminished gag reflex, palatal deviation, or other mild cranial nerve deficits may indicate cranial polyneuropathy. Postviral, infectious neuropathies may involve the superior laryngeal nerve and cause weakness, fatigability, and loss of range and projection in the voice. The recurrent laryngeal nerve is also affected in some cases. More serious neurologic disease may also be associated with such symptoms and signs.

Laryngeal Examination

The unique aspects of the examination directed toward the larynx are worthy of special attention. Examination of the larynx begins when the patient enters the physician's office. The range, ease, volume, and quality of the speaking voice should be noted. Technical voice classification is beyond the scope of most physicians. However, the physician should at least be able to discriminate substantial differences in range and timbre such as between bass and tenor, or alto and soprano. Although the correlation between speaking and singing voices is not perfect, a speaker with a low comfortable bass voice who reports that he is a tenor may be misclassified and singing inappropriate roles with consequent voice strain. This judgment should be deferred to an expert, but the observation should lead the physician to make the appropriate referral. Excessive volume or obvious strain during speaking clearly indicates that voice abuse or misuse is present and may be contributing to the patient's voice complaint.

Any patient with a voice problem should be examined by indirect laryngoscopy at least. Judging voice range, quality, or other vocal attributes by inspection of the vocal folds is not possible. However, the presence or absence of nodules, mass lesions, contact ulcers, hemorrhage, erythema, paralysis, arytenoid erythema, and other anatomic abnormalities must be established. Erythema of the laryngeal surface of the epiglottis is often associated with frequent coughing or clearing of the throat or with muscular tension dysphonia and is caused by direct trauma from the arytenoids during these maneuvers. A mirror or laryngeal telescope may provide a better view of the posterior portion of the vocal folds than is obtained with flexible endoscopy.

A laryngeal telescope may also be combined with a stroboscope to provide excellent visualization of the vocal folds and related structures. The author (RTS) usually uses a seventy degree laryngeal telescope, although ninety degree telescopes are preferable for some patients. The combination of a telescope and stroboscope provides optimal magnification and optical quality for assessment of vocal fold vibration. However, it is generally performed with the tongue in a fixed position; and the nature of the examination does not permit assessment of the larynx during normal phonatory gestures.

Flexible fiberoptic laryngoscopy can be performed as an office procedure and allows inspection of the vocal folds in patients whose vocal folds are difficult to visualize indirectly. In addition, it permits observation of the vocal mechanism in a more natural posture than does indirect laryngoscopy, permitting sophisticated dynamic voice assessment. In the hands of an experienced endoscopist, this method may provide a great deal of information about both speaking and singing techniques. The combination of a fiberoptic laryngoscope with a laryngeal stroboscope may be especially useful. This system permits magnification, photography, and detailed inspection of vocal fold motion. Sophisticated systems that permit flexible or rigid fiberoptic strobovideolaryngoscopy are currently available commercially. They are an invaluable asset for routine clinical use. The video system also provides a permanent record, permitting reassessment, comparison over time, and easy consultation. A refinement not currently available commercially is stereoscopic fiberoptic laryngoscopy, accomplished by placing a laryngoscope through each nostril, fastening the two together in the pharynx, and observing the larynx through the eyepieces.[60] This method allows visualization of laryngeal motion in three dimensions. However, it is used primarily in a research setting.

Rigid endoscopy with anesthesia may be reserved for the rare patient whose vocal folds cannot be assessed adequately by other means or for patients who need surgical procedures to remove or biopsy laryngeal lesions. In many cases this may be done with local anesthesia, avoiding the need for intubation and the traumatic coughing and vomiting that may occur even after general anesthesia administered by mask. Coughing after general anesthesia may be minimized by using topical anesthesia in the larynx and trachea. However, topical anesthetics may act as severe mucosal irritants in a small number of patients. They may also predispose the patient to aspiration in the postoperative period. If a patient has had difficulty with a topical anesthetic administered in the office, it should not be used in the operating room. When used in general anesthesia cases, topical anesthetics should usually be applied at the end of the procedure. Thus, if inflammation occurs, it will not interfere with performance of microsurgery. Postoperative duration of anesthesia is also optimized. The author has had the least difficulty with 4% Xylocaine.

OBJECTIVE TESTS

Reliable, valid, objective analysis of the voice is extremely important and is an essential part of a comprehensive physical examination. It is as valuable to the laryngologist as audiometry is to the otologist.[3,61,62] Familiarity with some of the measures and technologic advances currently available is helpful.

Strobovideolaryngoscopy

Integrity of the vibratory margin of the vocal fold is essential for the complex motion required to produce good vocal quality. Under continuous light, the vocal folds vibrate approximately 250 times per second while phonating at middle C. Naturally, the human eye cannot discern the necessary details during such rapid motion. The vibratory margin may be assessed through high-speed photography, strobovideolaryngoscopy, high-speech videokymography, electroglottography, or photoglottography. Strobovideolaryngoscopy provides the necessary clinical information in a practical fashion.

Strobovideolaryngoscopy is the single most important technologic advance in diagnostic laryngology with the possible exception of fiberoptic laryngoscopy. Stroboscopic light allows routine slow-motion evaluation of the mucosal cover layer of the leading edge of the vocal fold. This state-of-the-art physical examination permits detection of vibratory asymmetries, structural abnormalities, small masses, submucosal scars, and other conditions that are invisible under ordinary light.[3,63-65] For example, in a patient who has a poor voice after laryngeal surgery and a "normal-looking larynx," stroboscopic light often reveals adynamic seg-

ments that explain the problem even to an untrained observer (such as the patient). The stroboscope is also extremely sensitive in detecting changes caused by fixation from small laryngeal neoplasms in patients who are being followed for leukoplakia or after laryngeal irradiation. Documentation of the procedure by coupling stroboscopic light with the video camera allows later reevaluation by the laryngologist or other health care providers.

Stroboscopy does not provide a true slow-motion image, as obtained through high-speed photography (Figure 11-1). The stroboscope actually illuminates different points on consecutive vocal fold waves, each of which is retained on the retina for 0.2 second. The stroboscopically lighted portions of the successive waves are visually fused. The slow-motion effect is created by having the stroboscopic light desynchronized with the frequency of vocal fold vibration by approximately 2 Hz. When vocal fold vibration and the stroboscope are synchronized exactly, the vocal folds appear to stand still, rather than moving in slow motion (Figure 11-2). In most instances, this approximation of slow motion provides all the clinical information necessary.

Our routine stroboscopy protocol is described elsewhere.[64] We currently use a Kay Elemetrics digital stroboscope. In virtually all cases, we examine patients with both an Olympus flexible ENFL-3 laryngoscope and a rigid magnifying telescope. We have both 70° and 90° telescopes available, but we find the 70° telescope more useful in most cases. Examination with the flexible nasolaryngoscope is possible in virtually all cases, and this technique provides good information about vocal habits, vocal fold motion during speech and singing, and vibratory margin characteristics under stroboscopic light in

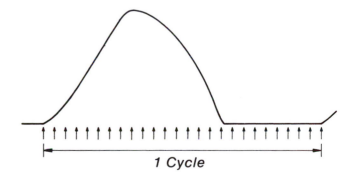

1 Cycle

FIGURE 11-1. *The principle of ultrahigh-speed photography. Numerous images are taken during each vibratory cycle. This technique is a true slow-motion representation of each vocal fold vibration.*

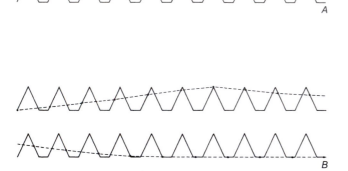

FIGURE 11-2. *The principle of stroboscopy. The stroboscopic light illuminates portions of successive cycles. The eye fuses the illuminated points into an illusion of slow motion. (A) If the stroboscope is synchronized with vocal fold vibration, a similar point is illuminated on each successive cycle and the vocal fold appears to stand still. (B) If the stroboscope is slightly desynchronized, each cycle is illuminated at a slightly different point, and the slow-motion effect is created.*

virtually every case. Examination with the telescope provides higher image quality and a larger image with a better light, and it occasionally reveals subtle abnormalities that are missed with the flexible laryngoscope.

We use a modification of the standardized method of subjective assessment of strobovideolaryngoscopic images, as proposed by Hirano et al.[65,66] Characteristics evaluated include the fundamental frequency, the symmetry of movements, periodicity, glottic closure, the amplitude of vibration, the mucosal wave, the presence of nonvibrating portions of the vocal fold, and other unusual findings. In addition, objective, frame-by-frame computer analysis is possible. However, this is now primarily of interest in research, and we are not using it on a routine clinical basis.

With practice, perceptual judgments of stroboscopic images provide a great deal of information. However, it is easy for the inexperienced observer to draw unwarranted conclusions because of normal variations in vibration. Vibrations depend upon fundamental frequency, intensity, and vocal register (Figure 11-3). For example, failure of glottic closure occurs normally in falsetto phonation. Consequently, it is important to note these characteristics and to examine each voice under a variety of conditions.

Fundamental frequency can be influenced by various vocal fold parameters. For example, fundamental frequency is increased with increasing vocal fold tension or

stiffness, increased subglottal pressure, or a shortened length of vibrating vocal fold. Fundamental frequency decreases as vocal fold mass increases.

Symmetry is assessed by observing both vocal folds simultaneously. In a trained voice, they are mirror images, opening with the same lateral excursions (symmetry of amplitude) and mirror-image waves (symmetry of phase). In untrained voices, phase asymmetry is common. Clinically significant asymmetries may be caused by differences between vocal folds in position, tension, elasticity, viscosity, shape, mass, or other mechanical properties.

Periodicity refers to the regularity of successive vibrations. Regular periodicity requires balanced control of expiratory force and the mechanical characteristics of the vocal folds. Irregular periodicity may be caused by an inability to maintain a steady expiratory stream of air, an inability to sustain steady laryngeal muscle contraction (as in neuromuscular disease), or marked differences in the mechanical properties of the vocal folds. Periodicity is assessed by locking the stroboscope in phase with vocal fold vibration. This should result in vocal folds that appear to stand still. If they move, vibration is aperiodic. Failure of glottic closure may be caused by vocal fold paresis or paralysis, an irregular vocal fold edge, a mass (or masses) separating the vocal fold edges, stiffness of a vibratory margin, cricoarytenoid joint dysfunction, falsetto singing, psychogenic dysphonia, and other causes. It is helpful to describe failures of glottic closure more specifically. They may be complete or incomplete, constant or intermittent, and may involve a posterior glottic chink, a specific small portion of the vocal folds, or as much as the entire vocal fold.

Amplitude of vibration and mucosal wave characteristics are assessed looking at the vocal folds one at a time. Small amplitude is associated with short vibrating segments of vocal fold, increased stiffness, increased mass, and vocal fold motion. Amplitude is increased by increasing subglottal pressure, such as that occurring with loud phonation. Amplitude is not generally affected very much by soft masses such as cysts and nodules.

The mucosal wave is affected by many factors. It is diminished by dryness, scar, mucosal stiffness or edema, epithelial hyperplasia, masses, dehydration, and falsetto phonation. It also varies with pitch. The mucosal wave is also increased with loud phonation (increased subglottal pressure) and altered by hypofunctional or hyperfunctional voice technique. If there is an area of stiffness on the vocal fold, this will impede the traveling mucosal wave. This situation is encountered with small scars, some mass lesions, and sulcus vocalis.

Nonvibrating segments (adynamic) are often signs of serious vocal fold injury involving scar that obliterates the complex anatomy of the lamina propria and mucosa. Adynamic segments are seen only under stroboscopic light or in high-speech motion pictures. They are found typically on vocal folds that have undergone previous surgery, hemorrhage, or other trauma. Often the vocal folds look normal under continuous light, but the voice is hoarse and breathy. The reason is obvious when the adynamic segment is revealed under stroboscopic light. Hypodynamic segments may also occur temporarily, as seen sometimes in acute vocal fold hemorrhage with submucosal hematoma.

Our strobovideolaryngoscopy system permits routine simultaneous imaging with three cameras. This allows visualization of the larynx; face, head, and neck; and a superimposed electroglottography (EGG) wave.

Other Techniques to Examine Vocal Fold Vibration

Other techniques to examine vocal fold vibration include ultrahigh-speed photography, electroglottography (EGG), photoelectroglottography and ultrasound glottography, and most recently videokymography[67] and high-speed video (digital or analog). Ultrahigh-speed photography provides images similar to those provided by strobovideolaryngoscopy but requires expensive, cumbersome equipment and delayed data processing. However, the images are true slow motion, rather than simulated. High-speed video offers similar advantages without most of the disadvantages of high-speed motion pictures, and may prove a useful adjunct to stroboscopy.

Electroglottography uses two electrodes on the skin of the neck above the thyroid laminae. A weak, high-frequency voltage is passed through the larynx from one electrode to the other. Opening and closing of the vocal folds varies the transverse electrical impedance, producing variation of the electrical current in phase with vocal fold vibration. The resultant tracing is called an electroglottogram. It traces the opening and closing of the glottis and can be compared with stroboscopic

images.[68] Electroglottography allows objective determination of the presence or absence of glottal vibrations and easy determination of the fundamental period of vibration and is reproducible. It reflects the glottal condition more accurately during its closed phase. Photoelectroglotto-graphy and ultrasound glottography are less useful clinically.[69]

Measures of Phonatory Ability

Objective measures of phonatory ability are among the easiest and most readily available to the laryngologist, helpful in treatment of professional vocalists with specific voice disorders, and are quite useful in assessing the results of surgical therapies. Maximum phonation time is measured with a stopwatch. The patient is instructed to sustain the vowel /a/ for as long as possible after deep inspiration, vocalizing at a comfortable frequency and intensity. The frequency and intensity may be determined and controlled by an inexpensive frequency analyzer and sound level meter. The test is repeated three times, and the greatest value is recorded. Normal values have been determined.[69] Frequency range of phonation is recorded in semitones and documents the vocal range from the lowest note in the modal register (excluding vocal fry) to the highest falsetto note. This is the physiologic frequency range of phonation and disregards quality. The musical frequency range of phonation measures lowest to highest notes of musically acceptable quality. Tests for maximum phonation time, frequency ranges, and many of the other parameters discussed later (including spectrographic analysis) may be preserved on a tape recorder or digitized and stored for analysis at a convenient future time and used for pretreatment and post-treatment comparisons. Recordings should be made in a standardized, consistent fashion.

Frequency limits of vocal register may also be measured. The registers are (from low to high) vocal fry, chest, mid, head, and falsetto. However, classification of registers is controversial, and many other classifications are used. Although the classification listed above is common among musicians, at present, most voice scientists prefer a scheme that classifies registers as pulse, modal, and loft. Overlap of frequency among registers occurs routinely.

Testing the speaking fundamental frequency often reveals excessively low pitch, an abnormality associated with chronic voice abuse and development of vocal nodules. This parameter may be followed objectively throughout a course of voice therapy. Intensity range of phonation (IRP) has proven a less useful measure than frequency range. It varies with fundamental frequency

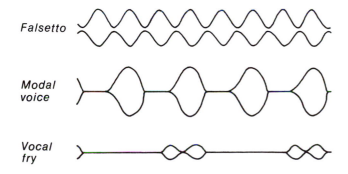

FIGURE 11-3. *The normal vibratory pattern of vocal folds.*

(which should be recorded) and is greatest in the middle frequency range. It is recorded in sound pressure level (SPL) re: 0.0002 microbar. For normal adults who are not professional vocalists, measuring at a single fundamental frequency, IRP averages 54.8 dB for males and 51 dB for females.[70] Alterations of intensity are common in voice disorders, although IRP is not the most sensitive test to detect them. Information from these tests may be combined in a fundamental frequency-intensity profile,[69] also called a phonetogram.

Glottal efficiency (ratio of the acoustic power at the level of the glottis to subglottal power) provides useful information but is not clinically practical because measuring acoustic power at the level of the glottis is difficult. Subglottic power is the product of subglottal pressure and airflow rate. These can be determined clinically. Various alternative measures of glottic efficiency have been proposed, including the ratio of radiated acoustic power to subglottal power,[71] airflow intensity profile[72] and ratio of the root mean square value of the AC component to the mean volume velocity (DC component).[73] Although glottal efficiency is of great interest, none of these tests is particularly helpful under routine clinical circumstances.

Aerodynamic Measures

Traditional pulmonary function testing provides the most readily accessible measure of respiratory function. The most common parameters measured include: (1) tidal volume, the volume of air that enters the lungs during inspiration and leaves during expiration in normal breathing; (2) functional residual capacity, the volume of air remaining in the lungs at the end of inspiration during normal breathing. It may be divided into expiratory reserve volume (maximal additional volume that can be exhaled) and residual volume (the volume of air remaining in the lungs at the end of maximal exhalation); (3) inspiratory capacity, the maximal volume of air that can be inhaled starting at the functional residual capacity; (4) total lung capacity, the volume of air in the lungs following maximal inspiration; (5) vital capacity, the maximal volume of air that can be exhaled from the lungs following maximal inspiration; (6) forced vital capacity, the rate of airflow with rapid, forceful expiration from total lung capacity to residual volume; (7) FEV1, the forced expiratory volume in 1 second; (8) FEV3, the forced expiratory volume in 3 seconds; (9) maximal mid-expiratory flow, the mean rate of airflow over the middle half of the forced vital capacity (between 25% and 75% of the forced vital capacity).

For singers and professional speakers with an abnormality caused by voice abuse, abnormal pulmonary function tests may confirm deficiencies in aerobic conditioning or reveal previously unrecognized asthma.[20] Flow glottography with computer inverse filtering is also a practical and valuable diagnostic test for assessing flow at the vocal fold level, evaluating the voice source, and imaging the results of the balance between adductory forces and subglottal pressure.[4,62] It also has therapeutic value as a biofeedback tool.

The spirometer, readily available for pulmonary function testing, can be used for measuring airflow during phonation. However, it does not allow simultaneous display of acoustic signals, and its frequency response is poor. A pneumotachograph consists of a laminar air resistor, a differential pressure transducer, and an amplifying and recording system. It allows measurement of airflow and simultaneous recording of other signals when coupled with a polygraph. A hot-wire anemometer allows determination of airflow velocity by measuring the electrical drop across the hot wire. Modern hot-wire anemometers containing electrical feedback circuitry that maintains the temperature of the hot wire provide a flat frequency response up to 1 KHz and are useful clinically.[73]

The four parameters traditionally measured in analyzing the aerodynamic performance of a voice are: subglottal pressure (P_{sub}), supraglottal pressure (P_{sup}), glottal impedance, and volume velocity of airflow at the glottis. These parameters and their rapid variations can be measured under laboratory circumstances. However, clinically their mean value is usually determined as follows:

$$P_{sub} - P_{sup} = MFR \times GR$$

where MFR is the mean (root mean square) flow rate and GR is the mean (root mean square) glottal resistance. When vocalizing the open vowel /a/, the supraglottic pressure equals the atmospheric pressure reducing the equation to:

$$P_{sub} = MFR \times GR$$

The mean flow rate is a useful clinical measure. While the patient vocalizes the vowel /a/, the mean flow rate is calculated by dividing the total volume of air used during phonation by the duration of phonation. The subject phonates at a comfortable pitch and loudness either over a determined period of time or for a maximum sustained period of phonation.

Air volume is measured by the use of a mask fitted tightly over the face or by phonating into a mouthpiece while wearing a noseclamp. Measurements may be made using a spirometer, pneumotachograph, or hot-wire anemometer. The normal values for mean flow rate under habitual phonation, with changes in intensity or register, and under various pathologic circumstances, were determined in the 1970s.[69] Normal values are available for both adults and children. Mean flow rate is a clinically useful parameter to follow during treatment for vocal nodules, recurrent laryngeal nerve paralysis, spasmodic dysphonia, and other conditions.

Glottal resistance cannot be measured directly, but it may be calculated from the mean flow rate and mean subglottal pressure. Normal glottal resistance is 20 to 100 dyne seconds/cm^5 at low and medium pitches and 150 dyne seconds/cm^5 at high pitches.[71] Subglottal pressure is less useful clinically because it requires an invasive procedure for accurate measurement. It may be determined by tracheal puncture, transglottal catheter, or measurement through a tracheostoma using a transducer. Subglottal pressure may be approximated using an esophageal balloon. Intratracheal pressure, which is roughly equal to subglottal pressure, is transmitted to the balloon through the trachea. However, measured changes in the esophageal balloon are affected by intraesophageal pressure, which is dependent upon lung volume. Therefore, estimates of subglottal pressure using this technique are valid only under specific, controlled circumstances. The normal values for subglottal pressure under various healthy and pathologic voice conditions have also been determined by numerous investigators.[69]

The phonation quotient is the vital capacity divided by the maximum phonation time. It has been shown to correlate closely with maximum flow rate[74] and is a more convenient measure. Normative data determined by various authors have been published.[69] The phonation quotient provides an objective measure of the effects of treatment and is particularly useful in cases of recurrent laryngeal nerve paralysis and mass lesions of the vocal folds, including nodules.

Acoustic Analysis

Acoustic analysis of voice signals is both promising and disappointing. The skilled laryngologist, speech-language pathologist, musician, or other trained listener frequently infers a great deal of valid information from the sound of a voice. However, clinically useful technology for analyzing and quantifying subtle acoustic differences is still not ideal. In many ways, the tape recorder (analog or digital, traditional or minidisc) is still one of the laryngologist's most valuable tools for acoustic analysis. Recording a patient's voice under controlled, repeatable circumstances before, during, and at the conclusion of treatment allows both the physician and the patient to make a qualitative, subjective acoustic

analysis. Objective analysis with instruments may also be made from recorded voice samples.

Acoustic analysis equipment can determine frequency, intensity, harmonic spectrum, cycle to cycle perturbations in frequency (jitter), cycle to cycle perturbations in amplitude (shimmer), harmonics/noise ratios, breathiness index, and many other parameters. The DSP SONA-GRAPH Model 5500 (Kay Elemetrics, Pine Brook, New Jersey) is an integrated voice analysis system. It is equipped for sound spectrography capabilities. Spectrography provides a visual record of the voice. The acoustic signal is depicted using time (x-axis), frequency (y-axis), and intensity (z-axis), shading of light versus dark. Using the band pass filters, generalizations about quality, pitch, and loudness can be made. These observations are used in formulating the voice therapy treatment plan. Formant structure and strength can be determined using the narrow-band filters, of which a variety of configurations are possible. In those clinical settings where singers and other professional voice users are routinely evaluated and treated, this feature is extremely valuable. A sophisticated voice analysis program (an optional program) may be combined with the Sona-Graph and is an especially valuable addition to the clinical laboratory. The voice analysis program (CSL, Kay Elemetrics) measures speaking fundamental frequency, frequency perturbation (jitter), amplitude perturbation (shimmer), harmonics-to-noise ratio, and provides a great number of other useful values. An electroglottograph (EGG) may be used in conjunction with the Sona-Graph to provide some of these voicing parameters. Examining the EGG waveform alone is possible with this setup, but its clinical usefulness has not yet been established. An important feature of the Sona-Graph is the long-term average (LTA) spectral capability, which allows for analyzing longer voice samples (30-90 seconds). The LTA analyzes only voiced speech segments, and may be useful in screening for hoarse or breathy voices. In addition, computer interface capabilities (also an optional program) have solved many data storage and file maintenance problems.

In analyzing acoustic signals, the microphone may be placed at the level of the mouth or may be positioned in or over the trachea, although intratracheal recordings are used for research purposes only. Position should be standardized in each office or laboratory.[75] Various techniques are being developed to improve the usefulness of acoustic analysis. Because of the enormous amount of information carried in the acoustic signal, further refinements in objective acoustic analysis should prove particularly valuable to the clinician.

Laryngeal Electromyography

Electromyography requires an electrode system, an amplifier, an oscilloscope, a loudspeaker, and a recording system.[76] Electrodes are placed transcutaneously into laryngeal muscles. It may be extremely valuable in confirming cases of vocal fold paresis, in differentiating paralysis from arytenoid dislocation, in distinguishing recurrent laryngeal nerve paralysis from combined recurrent and superior nerve paralysis, diagnosing other more subtle neurolaryngologic pathology, and in documenting functional voice disorders and malingering. It is also recommended for needle localization when using botulinum toxin for treatment of spasmodic dysphonia and other conditions.

PSYCHOACOUSTIC EVALUATION

Because the human ear and brain are the most sensitive and complex analyzers of sound currently available, many researchers have tried to standardize and quantify psychoacoustic evaluation. Unfortunately, even definitions of basic terms such as *hoarseness* and *breathiness* are still controversial. Psychoacoustic evaluation protocols and interpretations are not standardized. Consequently, although subjective psychoacoustic analysis of voice is of great value to the individual skilled clinician, it remains generally unsatisfactory for comparing research among laboratories or for reporting clinical results.

OUTCOMES ASSESSMENT

Measuring the impact of a voice disorder has always been challenging. However, recent advances have helped address this problem. Validated instruments such as the *Voice Handicap Index* (VHI)[77] are currently in clinical use, and are likely to be utilized widely in future years.

VOICE IMPAIRMENT AND DISABILITY

Quantifying voice impairment and assigning a disability rating (percentage of whole person) remain controversial. This subject is still not addressed comprehensively even in the most recent edition of the American Medical Association's *Guidelines for the Evaluation of Impairment and Disability (The Guides);* and *The Guides* still does not take into account the person's profession when calculating disability. Alternative approaches have been proposed[78] and advances in this complex arena are anticipated over the next few years. This subject is discussed in greater detail elsewhere in this book.

EVALUATION OF THE SINGING VOICE

The physician must be careful not to exceed the limits of his or her expertise, especially in caring for singers. However, if voice abuse or technical error is suspected, or if a difficult judgment must be reached on whether to allow a sick singer to perform, a brief observation of the patient's singing may provide invaluable information. This is accomplished best by asking the singer to stand and sing scales either in the examining room or in the soundproof audiology booth. Similar maneuvers may be used for professional speakers, including actors (who can vocalize and recite lines), clergy and politicians (who can deliver sermons and speeches), and virtually all other voice patients. The singer's stance should be balanced, with the weight slightly forward. The knees should be bent slightly and the shoulders, torso, and neck should be relaxed. The singer should inhale through the nose whenever possible allowing filtration, warming, and humidification of inspired air. In general, the chest should be expanded, but most of the active breathing is abdominal. The chest should not rise substantially with each inspiration, and the supraclavicular musculature should not be involved obviously in inspiration. Shoulders and neck muscles should not be tensed even with deep inspiration. Abdominal musculature should be contracted shortly before the initiation of the tone. This may be evaluated visually or by palpation. Muscles of the neck and face should be relaxed. Economy is a basic principle of all art forms. Wasted energy and motion and muscle tension are incorrect and usually deleterious.

The singer should be instructed to sing a scale (a five-note scale is usually sufficient) on the vowel /a/, beginning on any comfortable note. Technical errors are usually most obvious as contraction of muscles in the neck and chin, retraction of the lower lip, retraction of the tongue, or tightening of the muscles of mastication. The singer's mouth should be open widely but comfortably. When singing /a/, the singer's tongue should rest in a neutral position with the tip of the tongue lying against the back of the singer's mandibular incisors. If the tongue pulls back or demonstrates obvious muscular activity as the singer performs the scales, improper voice use can be confirmed on the basis of positive evidence. The position of the larynx should not vary substantially with pitch changes. Rising of the larynx with ascending pitch is evidence of technical dysfunction. This examination also gives the physician an opportunity to observe any dramatic differences between the qualities and ranges of the speaking voice and the singing voice.

Remembering the admonition not to exceed his or her expertise, the physician who examines many singers can often glean valuable information from a brief attempt to modify an obvious technical error. For example, deciding whether to allow a singer with mild or moderate laryngitis to perform is often difficult. On the one hand, an expert singer has technical skills that allow him or her to compensate safely. On the other hand, if a singer does not sing with correct technique and does not have the discipline to modify volume, technique, and repertoire as necessary, the risk of vocal injury may be increased substantially even by mild inflammation of the vocal folds. In borderline circumstances, observation of the singer's technique may greatly help the physician in making a judgment.

If the technique appears flawless, we may feel somewhat more secure in allowing the singer to proceed with performance commitments. More commonly, even good singers demonstrate technical errors when experiencing voice difficulties. In a vain effort to compensate for dysfunction at the vocal fold level, singers often modify their technique in the neck and supraglottic vocal tract. In the good singer, this usually means going from good technique to bad technique. The most common error involves pulling back the tongue and tightening the cervical muscles. Although this increased muscular activity gives the singer the illusion of making the voice more secure, this technical maladjustment undermines vocal efficiency and increases vocal strain. The physician may ask the singer to hold the top note of a five-note scale; while the note is being held, the singer may simply be told, "Relax your tongue." At the same time the physician points to the singer's abdominal musculature. Most good singers immediately correct to good technique. If they do, and if upcoming performances are particularly important, the singer may be able to perform with a reminder that meticulous technique is essential. The singer should be advised to "sing by feel rather than by ear," to consult his or her voice teacher, and conserve the voice except when it is absolutely necessary to use it. If a singer is unable to correct from bad technique to good technique promptly, especially if he or she uses excessive muscle tension in the neck and ineffective abdominal support, it is generally safer not to perform with even a mild vocal fold abnormality. With increased experience and training, the laryngologist may make other observations that aid in providing appropriate treatment recommendations for singer patients. Once these skills have been mastered for the care of singers, applying them to other patients is relatively easy, so long as the laryngologist takes the time to understand the demands of the individual's professional, avocational, and recreational vocal activities.

If treatment is to be instituted, at least a tape recording of the voice is advisable in most cases and essential before any surgical intervention. The author (RTS) routinely uses strobovideolaryngoscopy for diagnosis and documentation in virtually all cases as well as many of the objective measures discussed. Such testing is extremely helpful clinically and medicolegally.

ADDITIONAL EXAMINATIONS

A general physical examination should be performed whenever the patient's systemic health is questionable. Debilitating conditions such as mononucleosis may be noticed first by the singer as vocal fatigue. A neurologic assessment may be particularly revealing. The physician must be careful not to overlook dysarthrias and dysphonias characteristic of movement disorders and of serious neurologic disease. Dysarthria is a defect in rhythm, enunciation, and articulation that usually results from neuromuscular impairment or weakness such as may occur after a stroke. It may be seen with oral deformities or illness as well. Dysphonia is an abnormality of vocalization usually originating from problems at the laryngeal level.

Physicians should be familiar with the six types of dysarthria, their symptoms, and their importance.[79,80] Flaccid dysarthria occurs in lower motor neuron or primary muscle disorders such as myasthenia gravis and tumors or strokes involving the brain stem nuclei. Spastic dysarthria occurs in upper motor neuron disorders (pseudobulbar palsy) such as multiple strokes and cerebral palsy. Ataxic dysarthria is seen with cerebellar disease, alcohol intoxication, and multiple sclerosis. Hypokinetic dysarthria accompanies Parkinson's disease. Hyperkinetic dysarthria may be spasmodic, as in the Gilles de la Tourette's disease, or dystonic, as in chorea and cerebral palsy. Mixed dysarthria occurs in amyotrophic lateral sclerosis. The preceding classification actually combines dysphonic and dysarthric characteristics but is very useful clinically. The value of a comprehensive neurolaryngologic evaluation cannot be overstated.[81] More specific details of voice changes associated with neurologic dysfunction and their localizing value are available elsewhere.[3,16]

It is extremely valuable for the laryngologist to assemble an arts medicine team that includes not only a speech-language pathologist, singing voice specialist, acting voice specialist, and voice scientist, but also medical colleagues in other disciplines. Collaboration with an expert neurologist, pulmonologist, endocrinologist, psychologist, psychiatrist, internist, physiatrist, and others with special knowledge of, and interest in, voice disorders is invaluable in caring for patients with voice disorders. Such interdisciplinary teams have not only changed the standard of care in voice evaluation and treatment, but are also largely responsible for the rapid and productive growth of voice as a subspecialty.

REFERENCES

1. Sataloff RT. Professional singers: the science and art of clinical care. *Am J Otolaryngol.* 1981;2:251-266.

2. Sataloff RT. The human voice. *Sci Am.* 1992; 267:108-115.

3. Sataloff RT. *Professional Voice: The Science and Art of Clinical Care.* 2nd ed. San Diego, CA: Singular Publishing Group; 1997:1-1069.

4. Sundberg J. *The Science of the Singing Voice.* DeKalb, IL: Northern Illinois University Press; 1987:1-194.

5. Sataloff RT. Efficient history taking in professional singers. *Laryngoscope.* 1984;94:1111-1114.

6. Sataloff RT. *Professional Voice: Science and Art of Clinical Care.* 2nd ed. San Diego, CA: Singular Publishing Group; 1997:837-988.

7. Ackerman R, Pfan W. Gerotologische Untersuchungen zur Storunepanfalligkeit der Sprechstimme bei Berufssprechern. *Folia Phoniatr (Basel).* 1974;25:905-909.

8. von Leden H. Speech and hearing problems in the geriatric patient. *J Am Geriatr Soc.* 1977;25:422-426.

9. Sataloff RT, Spiegel JR, Rosen DC. The effects of age on the voice. In: Sataloff RT, ed. *Professional Voice: Science and Art of Clinical Care.* 2nd ed. San Diego, CA: Singular Publishing Group; 1997:259-267.

10. Schiff M. Comment at the Seventh Symposium on Care of the Professional Voice. The Juilliard School, New York, June 15 and 16, 1978.

11. Miller R. The singing teacher in the age of voice science. In: Sataloff RT, ed. *Professional Voice: Science and Art of Clinical Care.* 2nd ed. San Diego, CA: Singular Publishing Group; 1997:731-734.

12. Emerich KA, Baroody MM, Carroll LM, Sataloff RT. The singing voice specialist. In: Sataloff RT, ed. *Professional Voice: Science and Art of Clinical Care.* 2nd ed. San Diego, CA: Singular Publishing Group; 1997:735-754.

13. Miller, R. The singing teacher in the age of voice science. In: Sataloff RT, ed. *Vocal Health and Pedagogy.* San Diego, CA: Singular Publishing Group; 1998:297-300.

14. Wilder CN. Speech-language pathology and the professional voice user: an overview. In: Sataloff RT, ed. *Professional Voice: Science and Art of Clinical Care.* 2nd ed. San Diego, CA: Singular Publishing Group; 1997:695-698.

15. Rulnick RK, Heuer RJ, Perez KS, Emerich KA, Sataloff RT. Voice therapy. In: Sataloff RT, ed. *Professional Voice: Science and Art of Clinical Care.* 2nd ed. San Diego, CA: Singular Publishing Group; 1997:699-720.

16. Raphael BN, Sataloff RT. Increasing vocal effectiveness. In: Sataloff RT, ed. *Professional Voice: Science and Art of Clinical Care.* 2nd ed. San Diego, CA: Singular Publishing Group; 1997:721-730.

17. Aronson AE. *Clinical Voice Disorders.* 3rd ed. New York, NY: Thieme; 1990:70-193.

18. Sataloff RT, Mandel S, Rosen DC. Neurological disorders affecting the voice in performance. In: Sataloff RT, ed. *Professional Voice: Science and Art of Clinical Care.* 2nd ed. San Diego, CA: Singular Publishing Group; 1997:479-498.

19. Spiegel JR, Cohn JR, Sataloff RT, Fish JE, Kennedy K. Respiratory function in singers: medical assessment, diagnoses, treatments. *J Voice.* 1988;2:40-50.

20. Cohn JR, Sataloff RT, Spiegel JR, Fish JE, Kennedy K. Airway reactivity-induced asthma in singers (ARIAS). *J Voice.* 1991;5:332-337.

21. Feder RL. The professional voice and airline flight. *Otolaryngol Head Neck Surg.* 1984;92:251-254.

22. Herman H, Rossol M. Artificial fogs and smokes. In: Sataloff RT, ed. *Professional Voice: The Science and Art of Clinical Care.* 2nd ed. San Diego, CA: Singular Publishing Group; 1997:413-427.

23. Sataloff RT. The impact of pollution on the voice. *Otolaryngol Head Neck Surg.* 1992;106:701-705.

24. Opperman DA. Pyrotechnics in the entertainment industry: an overview. In: Sataloff RT, ed. *Professional Voice: The Science and Art of Clinical Care.* 2nd ed. San Diego, CA: Singular Publishing Group; 1997:393-407.

25. Rossol M. Pyrotechnics: health effects. In: Sataloff RT, ed. *Professional Voice: The Science and Art of Clinical Care.* 2nd ed. San Diego, CA: Singular Publishing Group; 1997:407-413.

26. Rosen DC, Sataloff RT. Psychological aspects of voice disorders. In: Rubin J, Korovin G, Sataloff RT, Gould WJ, eds. *Diagnosis and Treatment of Voice*

Disorders. New York, NY: Igaku-Shoin Medical Publishers; 1995:491-501.

27. Rosen DC, Sataloff RT. *Psychology of Voice Disorders.* San Diego, CA: Singular Publishing Group; 1997:1-261.

28. Gupta OP, Bhatia PL, Agarwal MK, Mehrotra ML, Mishr SK. Nasal pharyngeal and laryngeal manifestations of hypothyroidism. *Ear Nose Throat J.* 1977;56:10-21.

29. Malinsky M, Chevrie-Muller, Cerceau N. Etude clinique et electrophysiologique des alterations de la voix au cours des thyrotoxioses. *Ann Endocrinol (Paris).* 1977;38:171-172.

30. Michelsson K, Sirvio P. Cry analysis in congenital hypothyroidism. *Folia Phoniatr (Basel).* 1976;28:40-47.

31. Ritter FN. The effect of hypothyroidism on the larynx of the rat. *Ann Otol Rhinol Laryngol.* 1964;67:404-416.

32. Ritter FN. Endocrinology in Otolaryngology. Vol I. Paparella M, Shumrick D, eds. Philadelphia, PA: Saunders Publishing; 1973:727-734.

33. Meuser W, Nieschlag E. Sexual hormone und Stimmlage des Mannes. *Dtsch Med Wochenschr.* 1977;102:261-264.

34. Schiff M. The influence of estrogens on connective tissue. In: Asboe-Hansen G, ed. *Hormones and Connective Tissue.* Copenhagen, Denmark: Munksgaard Press; 1967:282-341.

35. Brodnitz F. The age of the castrato voice. *J Speech Hear Disord.* 1975;40:291-295.

36. Brodnitz F. Hormones and the human voice. *Bull NY Acad Med.* 1971;47:183-191.

37. Carroll C. Arizona State University at Tempe: Personal communication with Dr. Hans von Leden. September 1992.

38. von Gelder L. Psychosomatic aspects of endocrine disorders of the voice. *J Commun Disord.* 1974;7:257-262.

39. Lacina V. Der Einfluss der Menstruation auf die Stimme der Sangerinnen. *Folia Phoniatr (Basel).* 1968;20:13-24.

40. Wendler J. Zyklusabhangige Leistungsschwankungen der Stimme und ihre Beeinflussung durch Ovulationshemmer. *Folia Phoniatr (Basel).* 1972;24:259-277.

41. Brodnitz F. Medical care preventive therapy (panel). In: Lawrence VL, ed. *Transcripts of the Seventh Annual Symposium. Care of the*

Professional Voice. New York, NY: The Voice Foundation; 1978;3:86.

42. Dordain M. Etude Statistique de l'influence des contraceptifs hormonaux sur la voix. *Folia Phoniatr (Basel).* 1972:24:86-96.

43. Pahn V, Goretzlehner G. Stimmstorungen durch hormonale Kontrazeptiva. *Zentralbl Gynakol.* 1978;100:341-346.

44. Schiff M. "The pill" in otolaryngology. *Trans Am Acad Ophthalmol Otolaryngol.* 1968;72:76-84.

45. Deuster CV. Irreversible Stimmstorung in der Schwangerscheft. *HNO.* 1977;25:430-432.

46. Flach M, Schwickardi H, Simen R. Welchen Einfluss haben Menstruation and Schwangerschaft auf die augsgebildete Gesangsstimme? *Folia Phoniatr (Basel).* 1968;21:199-210.

47. Arndt HJ. Stimmstorungen nach Behandlung mit Androgenen und anabolen Hormonen. *Munch Med Wochenschr.* 1974;116:1715-1720.

48. Bourdial J. Les troubles de la voix provoques par la therapeutique hormonale androgene. *Ann Otolaryngol Chir Cervicofac.* 1970;87:725-734.

49. Damste PH. Virilization of the voice due to anabolic steroids. *Folia Phoniatr (Basel).* 1964;16:10-18.

50. Damste PH. Voice changes in adult women caused by virilizing agents. *J Speech Hear Disord.* 1967;32:126-132.

51. Saez S, Francoise S. Recepteurs d'androgenes: mise en evidence dans la fraction cytosolique de muqueuse normale et d'epitheliomas pharyngolarynges humains. *C R Acad Sci III.* 1975;280:935-938.

52. Vuorenkoski V, Lenko HL, Tjernlund P, Vuorenkoski L, Perheentupa J. Fundamental voice frequency during normal and abnormal growth, and after androgen treatment. *Arch Dis Child.* 1978;53:201-209.

53. Imre V. Hormonell bedingte Stimmstorungen. *Folia Phoniatr (Basel).* 1968;20:394-404.

54. Sundberg J, Prame E, Iwarsson J. Replicability and accuracey of pitch patterns in professional singers. In: Davis PJ, Fletcher NH, eds. *Vocal Fold Physiology: Controlling Chaos and Complexity.* San Diego, CA: Singular Publishing Group; 1996;291-306.

55. Gould WJ, Alberti PW, Brodnitz F, Hirano M. Medical care preventive therapy (panel). In: Lawrence VL, ed. *Transcripts of the Seventh Annual Symposium. Care of the Professional Voice.*

New York, NY: The Voice Foundation; 1978;3:74-76.

56. Wallner LJ, Hill BJ, Waldrop W. Voice changes following adenotonsillectomy. *Laryngoscope.* 1968;78:1410-1418.

57. Lawrence VL. Medical care for professional voice (panel). In: Lawrence VL, ed. *Transcripts of the Seventh Annual Symposium. Care of the Professional Voice.* New York, NY: The Voice Foundation; 1978;3:17-18.

58. Sataloff RT, Hawkshaw M, Rosen DC. Medications: effects and side-effects in professional voice users. In: Sataloff RT, ed. *Professional Voice: The Science and Art of Clinical Care,* 2nd ed. San Diego, CA: Singular Publishing Group; 1997:457- 471.

59. Sataloff RT. The professional voice: part II, physical examination. *J Voice.* 1987;1:191-201.

60. Fujimura O. Stero-fiberoptic laryngeal observation. *J Acoust Soc Am.* 1979;65:70-72.

61. Sataloff RT, Spiegel JR, Carroll LM, Darby KS, Hawkshaw MJ, Rulnick RK. The clinical voice laboratory: practical design and clinical application. *J Voice.* 1990;4:264-279.

62. Sataloff RT, Heuer RH, Emerich KA, Baroody MM, Rulnick RK, Hawkshaw, MJ. The clinical voice laboratory. In: Sataloff RT, ed. *Professional Voice: Science and Art of Clinical Care.* 2nd ed. San Diego, CA: Singular Publishing Group; 1997:215-243.

63. Sataloff RT, Spiegel JR, Carroll LM, Schiebel BR, Darby KS, Rulnick RK. Strobovideolaryngoscopy in professional voice users: results and clinical value. *J Voice.* 1988;1:359-364.

64. Sataloff RT, Spiegel JR, Hawkshaw MJ. Strobovideolaryngoscopy: results and clinical value. *Ann Otol Rhinol Laryngol.* 1991;100:725-727.

65. Bless D, Hirano M, Feder RJ. Video stroboscopic evaluation of the larynx. *Ear Nose Throat J.* 1987;66:289-296.

66. Hirano M. Phonosurgery: basic and clinical investigations. *Otologia (Fukuoka).* 1975;21:239-442.

67. Svec J, Shutte H. Videokymography: high-speed line scanning of vocal fold vibration. *J Voice.* 1996;10:201-205.

68. Leclure FLE, Brocaar ME, Verscheeure J. Electroglottography and its relation to glottal activity. F*olia Phoniatr (Basel).* 1975;27:215-224.

69. Hirano M. *Clinical Examination of the Voice.* New York, NY: Springer-Verlag; 1981:1-98.

70. Coleman RJ, Mabis JH, Hinson JK. Fundamental frequency sound pressure level profiles of adult male and female voices. *J Speech Hear Res.* 1977;20:197-204.

71. Isshiki N. Regulatory mechanism of voice intensity variation. *J Speech Hear Res.* 1964;7:17-29.

72. Saito S. Phonosurgery, basic study on the mechanisms of phonation and endolaryngeal microsurgery. *Otologia (Fukuoka).* 1977;23:171-384.

73. Isshiki N. *Functional Surgery of the Larynx.* Report of the 78th Annual Convention of the Oto-Rhino-Laryngological Society of Japan, Kyoto University, Fukuoka; 1977.

74. Hirano M, Koike Y, von Leden H. Maximum phonation time and air usage during phonation. *Folia Phoniatr (Basel).* 1968;20:185-201.

75. Price DB, Sataloff RT. A simple technique for consistent microphone placement in voice recording. *J Voice.* 1988;2:206-207.

76. Espaillat RM, Mandel S, Sataloff RT. Laryngeal electromyography. In: Sataloff RT, ed. *Professional Voice: The Science and Art of Clinical Care.* 2nd ed. San Diego, CA: Singular Publishing Group; 1997:245-255.

77. Benninger MS, Gardner GM, Jacobson BH, Grywalski C. New dimensions in measuring voice treatment outcomes. In: Sataloff RT, ed. *Professional Voice: The Science and Art of Clinical Care.* 2nd ed. San Diego, CA: Singular Publishing Group; 1997:789-794.

78. Sataloff RT. Voice and speech impairment and disability. In: Sataloff RT, ed. *Professional Voice: The Science and Art of Clinical Care.* 2nd ed. San Diego, CA: Singular Publishing Group; 1997:795-801.

79. Darley F, Aronson AE, Brown JR. Differential diagnosis of patterns of dysarthria. *J Speech Hear Res.* 1969;12:246-249.

80. Darley F, Aronson AE, Brown JR. Clusters of deviant speech dimensions in the dysarthrias. *J Speech Hear Res.* 1969;12:462-496.

81. Rosenfield DB. Neurolaryngology. *Ear Nose Throat J.* 1987;66:323-326.

APPENDIX 11-1

Patient History Form for Professional Voice Users

Name _____ **Age** _____ **Sex** _____ **Race** _____

Height _____ **Weight** _____ **Date** _____

How long have you had your present voice problem?

Who noticed it?

Do you know what caused it?   Yes   No

If so, what?

Did it come on slowly or suddenly?   Slowly   Suddenly

Is it getting: Worse,   Better,   Same?

Which symptoms do you have? (Please check all that apply)

Hoarseness (coarse or scratchy sound)

Fatigue (voice tires or changes quality after speaking for a short period of time)

Volume disturbance: (trouble speaking) softly,   loudly

Loss of range: high,   low

Prolonged warm-up time (over 1/2 hr to warm up voice)

Breathiness

Tickling or choking sensation while speaking

Pain in throat while speaking

Other (Please specify):

Have you ever had training for your singing voice?

   Yes   No

Have there been periods of months or years without lessons in that time?

   Yes   No

How long have you studied with your present teacher?

   Teacher's name:

   Teacher's address:

   Teacher's telephone number:

Please list previous teachers and years during which you studied with them:

In what capacity do you use your voice professionally?

   Actor

   Announcer (television/radio/sports arena)

   Attorney

   Clergy

   Politician

   Salesperson

   Teacher

   Telephone operator or receptionist

Other (Please specify):

Do you have an important performance soon?

Yes   No

Date(s):

Do you do regular voice exercises?

Yes   No

If yes, describe:

Do you play a musical instrument?

Yes   No

If yes, please check all that apply:

Keyboard (Piano, Organ, Harpsichord, Other _____)

Violin, Viola, Cello

Bass

Plucked Strings (Guitar, Harp, Other _____)

Brass

Wind with single reed

Wind with double reed

Flute, Piccolo

Percussion

Bagpipe

Accordion

Other (Please specify):

Do you warm up your voice before practice or performance?

    Yes   No

Do you warm-down after using it?

    Yes   No

How much are you speaking at present (average hours per day)?

    Rehearsal   Performance   Other

Please check all that apply to you:

    Voice worse in the morning

    Voice worse later in the day, after it has been used

    Sing performances or rehearsals in the morning

    Speak extensively (teacher, clergy, attorney, telephone, work, etc.)

    Cheerleader

    Speak extensively backstage or at postperformance parties

    Choral conductor

    Frequently clear your throat

    Frequent sore throat

    Jaw joint problems

    Bitter or acid taste; bad breath or hoarseness first thing in the morning

    Frequent "heartburn" or hiatal hernia

    Frequent yelling or loud talking

    Frequent whispering

    Chronic fatigue (insomnia)

    Work around extreme dryness

    Frequent exercise (weight lifting, aerobics, etc.)

    Frequently thirsty, dehydrated

    Hoarseness first thing in the morning

Chest cough

Eat late at night

Ever use antacids

Under particular stress at present (personal or professional)

Frequent bad breath

Live, work, or perform around smoke or fumes

Traveled recently:

    When:

    Where:

Your family doctor's name, address, and telephone number:

Your laryngologist's name, address, and telephone number:

Recent cold?

    Yes   No

Current cold?

    Yes   No

Have you been evaluated by an allergist?

    Yes   No

    If yes, what allergies do you have?

    [none, dust, mold, trees, cats, dog, foods, other]

    If yes, give name and address of allergist:

    Are you allergic to any medications?   Yes   No

    If yes, please list:

How many packs of cigarettes do you smoke per day?

Smoking history:

Never

Quit. When?

Smoked about_____packs per day for_____years.

Smoked_____packs per day. Have smoked for_____years.

Do you work in a smoky environment?

Yes   No

How much alcohol do you drink?

none,   rarely,   a few times per week,   daily

If daily, or few times per week, on the average, how much do you consume?

1, 2, 3, 4, 5, 6, 7, 8, 9, 10, more glasses per day,   week of beer,   wine,   liquor

Did you use to drink more heavily?

Yes   No

How many cups of coffee, tea, cola, or other caffeine-containing drinks do you drink per day?

List other recreational drugs you use:

[marijuana, cocaine, amphetamines, barbiturates, heroin, other_____]

Have you noticed any of the following? (Check all that apply)

Hypersensitivity to heat or cold

Excessive sweating

Change in weight: gained/lost_____lb. In_____weeks/_____months

Change in your voice

Change in skin or hair

Palpitation (fluttering) of the heart

Emotional lability (swings of mood)

Double vision

Numbness of the face or extremities

Tingling around the mouth or face

Blurred vision or blindness

Weakness or paralysis of the face

Clumsiness in arms or legs

Confusion or loss of consciousness

Difficulty with speech

Difficulty with swallowing

Seizure (epileptic fit)

Pain in the neck or shoulder

Shaking or tremors

Memory change

Personality change

For females:

Are you pregnant?   Yes   No

Are your menstrual periods regular?   Yes   No

Have you undergone hysterectomy?   Yes   No

Were your ovaries removed?   Yes   No

At what age did you reach puberty?

Have you gone through menopause?   Yes   No

Have you ever consulted a psychologist or psychiatrist?

Yes   No

Are you currently under treatment?

Yes   No

Have you injured your head or neck (whiplash, etc.)?

Yes   No

Describe any serious accidents related to this visit:

Are you involved in legal action involving problems with your voice?

Yes   No

List names of spouse and children:

Brief summary of ENT problems, some of which may not be related to your present complaint.

Hearing loss

Ear pain

Ear noises

Facial pain

Lump in face or head

Lump in neck

Dizziness

Stiff neck

Facial paralysis

Nasal obstruction

Nasal deformity

Nosebleeds

Mouth sores

Trouble swallowing

Trouble breathing

Eye problem

Excess eye skin

Excess facial skin

Jaw joint problem

Other (Please specify):

Do you have or have you ever had:

  Diabetes

  Seizures

  Hypoglycemia

  Psychologic therapy or counseling

  Thyroid problems

  Frequent bad headaches

  Syphilis

  Ulcers

  Gonorrhea

  Kidney disease

  Herpes

  Urinary problems

  Cold sores (fever blisters)

  Arthritis or skeletal

  High blood pressure problems

  Severe low blood pressure

  Cleft palate

  Intravenous antibiotics or diuretics

  Asthma, lung or breathing problems

  Heart attack

  Angina

  Irregular heartbeat

  Rheumatic fever

Other heart problems

Unexplained weight loss

Cancer of _____

Other tumor _____

Blood transfusions

Hepatitis

Tuberculosis

AIDS

Glaucoma

Meningitis

Multiple sclerosis

Other illnesses (Please specify):

Do any blood relatives have:

Diabetes

Hypoglycemia

Cancer

Heart disease

Other major medical problems such as those listed above.

Please specify:

Describe serious accidents unless directly related to your doctor's visit here.

None

Occurred with head injury, loss of consciousness, or whiplash

Occurred without head injury, loss of consciousness, or whiplash

Describe:

List all current medications and doses (include birth control pills and vitamins).

   None

   Aspirin

   Codeine

   Medication for allergies

   Novocaine

   Penicillin

   Sulfamides

   Tetracycline

   Erythromycin

   Keflex/Ceclor/Ceftin

   Iodine

   X-ray dyes

   Adhesive tape

   Other: (Please specify)

List operations:

   Tonsillectomy   (age_____)

   Adenoidectomy (age_____)

   Appendectomy   (age_____)

   Heart surgery   (age_____)

   Other: (Please specify)

List toxic drugs or chemicals to which you have been exposed:

   Streptomycin, Neomycin, Kanamycin

   Lead

Mercury

Other: (Please list)

Have you had x-ray treatments to your head or neck (including treatments for acne or ear problems as a child), treatments for cancer, etc.?

Yes   No

Describe serious health problems of your spouse or children

CHAPTER 12

Evaluation of Laryngeal Biomechanics by Fiberoptic Laryngoscopy

James A. Koufman, MD

Biomechanical analysis of the performance of athletes has become relatively common. It is accomplished by linking a video system to a computer system so that movement can be evaluated critically in ultra-slow motion, frame-by-frame. With this approach, patterns of movement can be identified that are, at one extreme, optimally efficient and, at the other extreme, maladaptive, or even abusive. Using similar methods, laryngeal biomechanics also can be studied.

Like injured athletes, people with voice disorders often demonstrate patterns of abnormal biomechanics (abnormal laryngeal muscle tension), which voice clinicians can identify during laryngeal examination by transnasal fiberoptic laryngoscopy (TFL).[1,2] However, these same patterns sometimes are observed in people who have no problems with their voices; for example, they may be seen transiently in singers working at the limits of the voice in terms of loudness and/or pitch.[3]

What are the abnormal muscle tension patterns? How much laryngeal muscle tension is physiologic, ie, what's normal? When do observed muscle tension patterns indicate a functional (nonorganic) voice disorder? When do they indicate compensation for an organic condition?

TFL is the first and single most important laryngeal examination for patients with laryngeal and voice disorders because assessment of laryngeal biomechanics holds the key to understanding the underlying glottal condition. Most dysfunctional states are associated with hyperkinetic laryngeal biomechanics, eg, supraglottic contraction; however, used properly, TFL distinguishes compensatory from intrinsic laryngeal behaviors. In the author's practice, the TFL findings often determine the type of diagnostic work-up and the initial approach to management.

LARYNGEAL EXAMINATION METHODS

For over a hundred years, indirect *mirror laryngoscopy* (ML) was the standard method for performing a laryngeal examination, but although clinicians could visualize the larynx using that technique, they could not visually assess (examine) vocal function. Approximately two decades ago, *telescopic laryngoscopy* (TL), *transnasal fiberoptic laryngoscopy* (TFL), and *videostroboscopy*, became available in the United States, and for the first time, laryngeal biomechanics could be evaluated effectively in a clinical setting. Since then, a great deal has been learned about laryngeal function and the biomechanics of patients with voice disorders. Although each voice clinician may have preferred examination methods, there are specific indications for, and advantages and disadvantages of, each technique (ML, TL, and TFL); these are summarized in Table 12-1.

The technique of TL is similar to ML, but instead of a mirror, a rigid optical instrument is used. To perform

I. Mirror laryngoscopy
   A. Advantages
      1. Quick overview
      2. Prognostic for telescopic laryngoscopy
   B. Disadvantages
      1. Poorly tolerated (gagging)
      2. Can only assess sustained vowel sounds, eg, /i/
      3. Alters laryngeal biomechanics
II. Telescopic laryngoscopy
   A. Advantages
      1. Excellent optics; best for photography
      2. Magnification; best for videostroboscopic evaluation of free-edge lesions
   B. Disadvantages
      1. Poorly tolerated (gagging)
      2. Alters laryngeal biomechanics
      3. Can only assess vowel sounds, eg, /i/
      4. Cannot assess the entire vocal tract
      5. Cannot assess connected speech or singing
III. Transnasal fiberoptic laryngoscopy
   A. Advantages
      1. Best way to assess laryngeal biomechanics
      2. Can assess the entire vocal tract
      3. Well tolerated by almost all patients
      4. Can assess the voice across the dynamic and pitch ranges of the voice during connected speech and singing
      5. Good for videostroboscopy
   B. Disadvantages
      1. Magnification and optics inferior to that of the telescopic instruments

TABLE 12-1. *Advantages and Disadvantages of Laryngeal Examination Methods*

TL, the examiner grasps the subject's tongue, pulls it forward, and inserts the telescope into the oropharynx. This method (as well as ML) limits the phonatory repertoire of the patient to producing a sustained vowel, eg, /a/ or /i/; connected speech and singing cannot be evaluated. In other words, grasping the tongue and inserting the instrument during TL significantly alters laryngeal biomechanics. In addition, TL may cause gagging, so that the technique is sometimes limited by subject intolerance, unless effective prior laryngopharyngeal topical anesthesia is established.

On the other hand, TFL is well tolerated by virtually all patients, alters laryngeal biomechanics very little, if at all, and provides essential diagnostic information in the vast majority of cases. TFL (with or without stroboscopy) is recommended at the first examination for all patients with voice disorders and TL with stroboscopy at the second, the latter for patients with specific vocal fold lesions for which enhanced optics (magnification) is needed. However, TFL with videostroboscopy will suffice in many patients.

These recommendations are based upon use of state-of-the-art TFL systems. While the optics (resolution and magnification) of currently available TFL systems are still not quite as good as those of TL systems, the gap has narrowed in recent years. Theoretically, when TFL optics improve to the level of current TL optics, the latter examination will become obsolete, because the TFL is more physiologic and permits a comprehensive examination of laryngeal function.

Technique of Transnasal Fiberoptic Laryngoscopy (TFL)

TFL is usually performed by spraying a topical anesthetic into one, or both, of the nasal passages; most patients have a best side based upon the presence of some nasal septal abnormality, such as a spur. A standard anesthetic such as xylocaine may be used, but as an alternative, 2% cocaine with 1% ephedrine may be used. Although many subjects can tolerate TFL without any anesthetic, topical anesthesia is recommended.

There are many types of fiberscopes available, and, in general, the larger the external diameter, the better the light and optics; unfortunately, a fiberscope with an external diameter of 3.7 mm is the largest instrument that can be used in the vast majority of patients without producing nasal discomfort. Fiberscopes with external diameters of up to 4.2 mm are acceptable, but the time needed for vasoconstriction may be somewhat longer.

The fiberscope may be introduced along the floor of the nose, or between the middle and the inferior turbinates. The latter is the preferable route in most patients because the mucosa of the turbinates "gives" to accommodate the instrument, whereas the mucosa of the septum and floor of the nose do not. Not only is the upper route between the turbinates more comfortable for the patient, this higher path seems to accommodate the curve of the fiberscope better than the lower route, so that optimal laryngeal examination (without gagging) is more likely. Thus, the examiner's first choice should be between the turbinates, but if a significant septal abnormality is encountered, then the path along the floor of the nose may be used.

The fiberscope is then positioned above the larynx. It may be placed high in the pharynx, behind the palate, to gain an overview, or within millimeters of the vocal folds for stroboscopy. As TFL only minimally alters laryngeal biomechanics, most patients are able to speak and sing during the examination.

Both connected speech and sustained vowel tasks across the dynamic and pitch ranges of the voice should be used during this examination. For the diagnosis of subtle movement disorders such as tremors, phonation of a sustained vowel tends to be most revealing.

In addition, the hardness of the glottal attack should be manipulated during examination. Having the patient phonate using a soft aspirate glottal attack usually removes supraglottic compensatory vocal behaviors, and enables the clinician to estimate the relative contribution of compensatory laryngeal behaviors that may be a significant component of the abnormal biomechanical findings.

Vocal fry can be used as a voice probe to see what happens when the patient attempts to relax the vocal folds. The absence of vocal fold lesions and an inability of the patient to produce a glottal fry imply neuromuscular dysfunction, eg, excessive laryngeal muscle tension or paresis.

For evaluating paresis—specifically, limited vocal fold abduction—the task that best elicits full abduction is the sniff. Sniffing (a short inhalation) through the nose with flaring of the nostrils produces an abduction that is brisker and more complete than that observed when a patient is asked to "take a deep breath." When evaluating a patient for vocal fold paresis or paralysis, the best (task) sequence is to ask the patient to alternately say /i/ and to sniff, in rapid, continuous succession. We call this the "/i/sniff" maneuver. Subsequent frame-by-frame review of the videotape of this segment of the examination provides the clinician with the best opportunity to assess vocal fold mobility.

If a patient complains of pitch-specific abnormalities, such as "my voice cracks in my passaggio (the transition to the high range), the clinician may examine this phenomenon by asking the patient to sing and demonstrate the problem. Thus, problem areas of the voice can be assessed visually. In singers, it frequently is useful to assess biomechanics for both speech and singing tasks, both before and after a period of warm-up, because both the laryngeal biomechanics and the appearance of the vocal folds may change after singing. Observed muscle tension may increase the ability to see vocal fold changes; for example, the free edges may become erythematous, and abnormalities (such as prenodules) that were not seen initially may become apparent.

To perform stroboscopy using the fiberscope, the instrument must be very close to the vocal folds themselves. This is best accomplished by having the patient take a deep breath and then sustain a long, relatively high-pitched vowel, while the fiberscope is advanced to within 2-3 mm of the folds. The fiberscope must then be withdrawn, back to the starting position, before the patient stops phonating. With this maneuver, the laryngeal position and configuration are stable usually for several seconds, long enough to allow the examiner a close stroboscopic examination of the vocal folds. The recommended technique of TFL is summarized in Table 12-2.

Videostroboscopy

Videostroboscopy is actually two separate functions, videoendoscopy and stroboscopy. Although often performed simultaneously, the two components actually provide different information. Stroboscopy itself is most

A. Preparing the patient
  1. Explain the procedure
  2. Examine the nasal passage with a speculum to select the more-open side
  3. Topically anesthetize and vasoconstrict the mucosa
  4. Position the patient in the extreme sniffing position (seated, leaning forward from the waist, elbows resting on lap, chin up, shoulders down)
B. Introducing the fiberscope
  1. Between the turbinates
  2. Second choice, along the floor of the nose
C. Vocal tasks
  1. Sustained vowels, eg, /i/, /A/
  2. Connected speech
     ("The cake is great, and the rainbow is beautiful")
  3. Pitch range and glissando
  4. Singing
  5. Yawning and sighing
  6. Vocal fry
  7. Whistling
  8. Sniffing
  9. Reproducing the problem
D. Stroboscopy
  1. Move in and out during phonation to avoid stimulating cough
  2. For certain lesions:
     a. Vocal fold cysts
     b. Leukoplakia and erythroplasia
     c. Postoperatively

TABLE 12-2. *Technique of Transnasal Fiberoptic Laryngoscopy*

useful for examining the vocal folds when the vocal fold lesions are present; videorecording allows playback (including slow-motion review) of the examination for purposes of documentation, analysis, consultation, and in order to obtain still photographs.

The laryngeal examination can be videotaped in virtually all patients, but there are many limitations to optimal stroboscopic examination. Stroboscopy is an "invaluable" (essential) diagnostic tool in only a small percentage of voice disorder patients, and is "somewhat useful" in an additional limited number. The author's indications for, and limitations of, stroboscopy are summarized in Table 12-3.

The most important clinical application of stroboscopy are: (1) to differentiate submucosal cysts from mucosal nodules; (2) to determine the tissue consisten-

cy and thickness of mucosal neoplasms, including nodules, leukoplakia, and carcinoma; (3) to assess vocal fold muscle tone; and (4) to assess recovery of normal vocal fold function after surgery (by a return of normal mucosal waves). Among the indications for stroboscopy, it is important to note that few require the magnification provided by TL. In other words, stroboscopy during TFL is sufficient to diagnose most conditions, in this author's opinion, although there are other experienced laryngologists who disagree and believe that TL should be performed in addition to TFL in most new cases, and instead of TFL in many follow-up cases. These colleagues (including RT Sataloff, MD [personal communication, 2001]) argue that the superior optics and magnification of TL can reveal subtle structural abnormalities that may be missed during stroboscopy with

Very Useful

Assessing alteration of the mucosal waves caused by previous trauma or surgery

Assessing vocal fold mobility and/or tone after paralysis

Diagnosing superior laryngeal nerve paresis or paralysis

Differentiating vocal nodules from submucosal cysts

Useful

Identifying early or small vocal fold lesions, such as nodules, papillomas, and carcinomas

Assessing thickness and/or depth of invasion of midmembranous vocal fold carcinomas

Assessing the tissue consistency and thickness of any mucosal lesion

Not Useful

Assessing vocal fold dysfunction when there is primary or compensatory supraglottic contraction

Assessing invasion of vocal fold carcinoma that involves the anterior commissure or arytenoid

Differentiating laryngeal dystonia from muscle tension dysphonia

Differentiating most functional from most organic voice disorders

TABLE 12-3. *Indications for, and Limitations of, Stroboscopy*

TFL alone; but all agree that it is essential to include TFL also to assess laryngeal biomechanics.

In patients who do not have organic vocal fold lesions, the information obtained from TFL is crucial, especially in the diagnosis of functional, inflammatory, and neuromuscular voice disorders. Although high-speed video systems are available for laryngology, currently employed video systems provide useful slow-speed video (30 frames per second). Frame-by-frame review of the TFL examination allows the voice clinician to evaluate laryngeal biomechanics critically. Even when stroboscopy is not possible because marked supraglottic contraction is present (and the vocal folds cannot be visualized directly), usually TFL is still diagnostic.

For many years, TFL has been the author's primary diagnostic examination technique for all voice disorder patients. When considering the relative contributions of the various examination techniques to making an accurate diagnosis, the author estimates that *TFL (with or without stroboscopy) provides the essential diagnostic information 95% of the time, and TL with stroboscopy provides that information 5% of the time.*

LARYNGEAL MUSCLE TENSION PATTERNS (MTPs)

Through fiberoptic examination of normal subjects and patients with voice disorders, consistent observations have been made about laryngeal biomechanics.

The normal biomechanical configuration for effortless phonation (of a sustained vowel) is that the vocal folds approximate along their lengths, "like two hands clapping on a hinge":

Vocal fold closure is achieved without the participation of supraglottic structures, and closure is complete along the entire length of the folds, ie, without a perceptible chink. There is neither front-to-back foreshortening of the folds, nor side-to-side compression by the false vocal cords, and the aryepiglottic folds remain thin and rounded.

Abnormal Patterns of Glottic and Supraglottic Muscle Tension

Abnormal patterns of glottic and supraglottic muscle tension are observed in virtually all patients with voice disorders, regardless of cause. There are four basic patterns that are termed *muscle tension patterns (MTPs)*: type I is glottal, and types II-IV are supraglottal.[1]

Muscle Tension Pattern I (MTP I)

MTP I (Figure 12-1A) was first described by Morrison and colleagues in 1986 as "an open glottic chink," and they associated this finding with what they termed "muscle tension dysphonia."[4] The characteristic finding of MTP I is a gap between the vocal fold free edges during phonation, with a conspicuous posterior gap between the vocal processes. MTP I also has been called a *laryngeal isometric* pattern because it presumably is caused by the simultaneous and inappropriate overcontraction of the posterior cricoarytenoid muscles in opposition to the lateral cricoarytenoid muscles during phonation.

MTP I is seen in most patients with vocal nodules and in about half of patients with conversion aphonia. The voices of patients in the latter group are characteristically a whisper. In patients with vocal nodules, MTP I may be considered both the cause of (and the result of) the nodules; however, patients who undergo successful voice therapy for nodules routinely demonstrate improvement in laryngeal biomechanics well before the actual involution of the lesions.

The assertion that MTP I indicates increased vocal fold tension is substantiated by the observation on stroboscopy that the amplitude of mucosal vibrations at all frequencies is markedly decreased compared to normal. Not surprisingly, the voice associated with MTP I is characteristically harsh, breathy, and strained.

Some voice clinicians believe that an open posterior commissure is a normal variant, particularly in women.

An open posterior commissure may indeed be seen in subjects without any evidence of a voice disorder; however, that "normal variant" pattern looks (and sounds) different from MTP I. With the former, the vocal processes touch and only the portion posterior to the vocal processes is open, producing a small triangular chink. That finding ("posterior-chink in women") may be a function of the examination method—it is commonly seen with per oral TL, but not with TFL—thus, it may be a muscle-tension response to pulling on the tongue, and so forth. With MTP I, the vocal processes are open and the gap between the vocal folds extends the entire length of the folds. MTP I is the TFL finding that correlates with substantially increased vocal fold tension/stiffness.

Muscle Tension Pattern II (MTP II)

MTP II (Figure 12-1B) is characterized by approximation of the false vocal folds. In its mildest form, only the anterior portions of the false vocal folds are compressed—almost approximating or actually just touching. The voice may therefore be only moderately or intermittently abnormal. Complete false vocal fold closure is associated with a severe and pitch-locked dys-

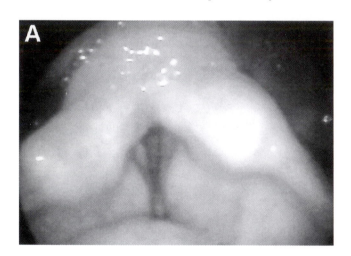
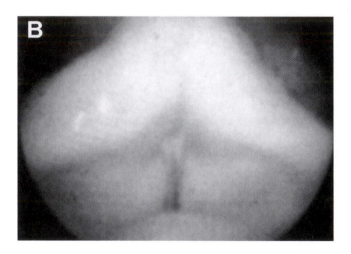

FIGURE 12-1A. *Muscle Tension Pattern I: This sequence of laryngeal photographs (from TFL) shows MTP I, "a laryngeal isometric." This pattern is seen often in patients with muscle tension dysphonias, with or without vocal nodules, and it is sometimes seen in patients with conversion aphonia. Because of the open glottal configuration, MTP I may be confused with hypokinetic voice disorders, or even with abductor-type spasmodic dysphonia. A consistent feature of MTP I is increased tension/stiffness of the vocal folds on stroboscopy. Not surprisingly, when MTP I is present the patient's voice usually sounds breathy and strained.*

FIGURE 12-1B. *Muscle Tension Pattern II: This sequence of laryngeal photographs (from TFL) shows MTP II, so-called plica ventricularis. Although once believed to be a discrete diagnosis, MTP II is now recognized as simply a compensatory laryngeal behavior that is seen in both functional and organic disorders. Of the four muscle tension patterns, MTP II is the one most frequently associated with underlying organic disease. It is common in patients with postoperative dysphonias; it is sometimes seen in patients with vocal fold paresis and paralysis; and it also is common after laryngeal irradiation and/or surgery for carcinoma. Because phonation is achieved by the false vocal folds, the voice in MTP II is pitch-locked and severely dysphonic.*

phonia. In the past, this type of supraglottic contraction was termed dysphonia *plica ventricularis* and was believed to be a discrete diagnosis. However, MTP II is not a diagnosis, but is rather a symptom (and a laryngeal physical finding) associated with a variety of conditions, both primary (functional) and secondary (compensatory).[2]

MTP II is observed most commonly in voice patients with underlying glottal closure problems, eg, paralysis, paresis, presbylaryngis. More than any other MTP, MTP II is usually associated with underlying organic pathology. MTP II tends to be related to attempted compensation for glottal insufficiency. After cordectomy or vertical hemilaryngectomy for cancer, for example, the vocal folds may be incompetent (incapable of closure), so that MTP II results as a compensatory maneuver. Indeed, false-vocal-fold voice may be the only way for such patients to achieve adequate loudness for effective verbal communication.

Muscle Tension Pattern III (MTP III)

MTP III (Figure 12-1C) is characterized by *partial anteroposterior contraction* of the larynx during phona-

tion. Typically, the arytenoids are pulled forward toward the petiole of the epiglottis, obscuring the posterior one-half to two-thirds of the vocal folds. When MTP III is the only finding, the voice may be relatively normal, and MTP III is always seen when one pitches his or her voice at its very lowest pitch. Along with MTP II, MTP III is frequently observed in patients with underlying glottal closure problems.

Muscle Tension Pattern IV (MTP IV)

Extreme anteroposterior contraction, ie, complete sphincter-like closure of the larynx, in which the arytenoids actually contact and squeeze against the petiole, is characteristic of MTP IV (Figure 12-1D). The voice in MTP IV is pitch-locked and severely strained, tense, and dysphonic, as phonation is achieved by vibration of supraglottic structures, usually the arytenoids against the epiglottis.

MTPs and Functional Voice Disorders

Certain MTPs are commonly observed in (but not pathognomonic of) functional, non-organic, voice disorders.[2] Patients with conversion aphonia, for example,

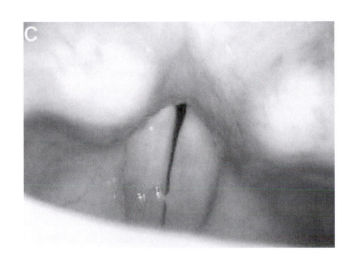
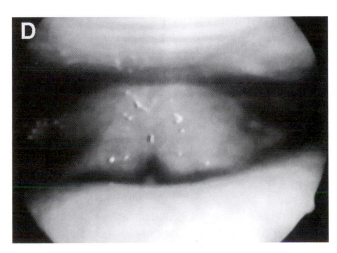

FIGURE 12-1C. *Muscle Tension Pattern III: This sequence of laryngeal photographs (from TFL) shows MTP III, "partial anteroposterior contraction." The pattern is common in patients with muscle tension dysphonias, particularly those with Bogart-Bacall syndrome and those with vocal nodules who are decompensating. Because of the anteroposterior contraction, only the anteriormost portion of the vocal folds can be visualized, and stroboscopy is often suboptimal in patients with MTP III. With MTP III, the voice is variable.*

FIGURE 12-1D. *Muscle Tension Pattern IV: This sequence of laryngeal photographs (from TFL) shows MTP IV, "complete anteroposterior contraction." This pattern resembles the sphincteric larynx: the arytenoids are plastered forward against the petiole; the false vocal folds are foreshortened and approximated; and the aryepiglottic folds are thickened and contracted as well. MTP IV is seen in patients with severe muscle tension dysphonias (including some patients with conversion aphonia), reflux laryngitis, and with severe adductor-type spasmodic dysphonia. MTP IV is the least common MTP. Because of the severity of the A-P contraction, none of the vocal folds can be visualized during phonation, stroboscopy is not possible, and the voice is pitch-locked, harsh, strained, and severely dysphonic.*

usually will demonstrate MTP I or MTP IV. On occasion, because of the open glottic configuration, MTP I may be confused with a hypofunctional condition or with abductor-type spasmodic dysphonia. With MTP IV in particular, visual biofeedback (using TFL) is often effective in restoring the patient's normal voice. MTP II and MTP IV are observed in patients with muscle tension dysphonia, but more commonly such patients have underlying glottal insufficiency.

Bogart-Bacall syndrome is a fairly common cause of vocal fatigue and dysphonia in vocal professionals.[5] The characteristics of this syndrome are a very low-pitched speaking voice, poor breath support for conversational speech, and the finding of MTP III on TFL. This syndrome may occur because the patient consciously (or unconsciously) desires to have a very low-pitched speaking voice. Bogart-Bacall syndrome may be associated with reflux laryngitis. Counseling and voice therapy directed at improving breath support and increasing the pitch of the voice are effective.

Interestingly, MTP III is observed routinely when patients and normal subjects phonate using the lowest pitch of the vocal range. Indeed, the finding of MTP III may be an indicator that the patient is using a habitual speaking pitch that is too low.

Typically, patients with both mature and immature vocal nodules demonstrate MTP I, and some demonstrate MTP III, as well. Those who demonstrate MTP III are usually in the process of vocal decompensation, that is, they are experiencing severe dysphonia and even odynophonia (painful speaking).

The following scenario may be postulated. There is air-wasting caused by traumatic swellings at the juncture of the anterior and middle thirds of the vocal folds—at the point of maximal impact, in the mid-striking zone. In an attempt to maintain normal pitch and volume, vocal fold tension and stiffness are increased. This, in turn, causes a compensatory increase in subglottic pressure to drive the stiffened vocal folds, which then increases the hardness of glottal attack and leading edge friction, so that the swellings (nodules) are further traumatized. Thus, a vicious cycle is created in which swelling and air-wasting lead to increased vocal fold tension and subglottic pressure, which, in turn, further aggravate the swollen nodules.

Over time, vocal fold tension/stiffness progressively increases in a vain attempt to compensate for the air-wasting caused by the lesions. This cycle explains the finding of MTP I (as a manifestation of the increased vocal fold tension/stiffness); when the patient can no longer compensate by increasing the tension of the vocal folds (MTP I), anteroposterior contraction (MTP III) occurs in an attempt to reduce the air-wasting by

covering the open posterior commissure, where the air-wasting is most pronounced. Indeed, both MTP I and III are observed commonly in patients with vocal nodules whose voices have decompensated. Furthermore, during connected speech and singing, these patterns can be seen to worsen with diminishing breath support, especially at the end of phrases when the subglottic pressure is at its lowest.

The Compensatory (Functional Component) of Organic Voice Disorders

Two important general observations have emerged from experience with TFL in patients with voice disorders[2,6-8]:

1. One or more of four MTPs is (are) observed routinely in all patients with bona fide organic voice disorders, and the MTPs appear to be compensatory.

2. For diagnostic purposes, the compensatory MTPs may be removed temporarily (modified) during TFL by softening the vocal tasks, so that the clinician can assess the underlying glottal condition. This is not only desirable, but also necessary, for accurate diagnosis.

The process of temporarily removing compensatory laryngeal behaviors for purposes of diagnostic assessment (during TFL examination or acoustical analysis) is called *unloading*.[6] Unloading is accomplished by literally softening the hardness of the glottal attack. A number of maneuvers may accomplish this, including: (1) use of an aspirate vocal attack, such as saying the phrase, "Harry had a hard head"; (2) use of a breathy glissando; (3) humming (through the nose); and (4) yawning or sighing.

Not surprisingly, compensatory laryngeal behaviors may mask the underlying glottal condition to the point at which the actual diagnosis may be missed. Patients with vocal fold paresis, for example, may exhibit marked supraglottic activity (in an attempt to achieve closure), and if the voice clinician does not unload the patient during examination, he or she may misinterpret the laryngeal findings and inappropriately diagnose a hyperkinetic functional voice disorder. TFL is the only examination method by which the voice clinician can separate the primary laryngeal condition from the compensatory component. Indeed, it is the only examination method that allows unloading.

When compensatory for an organic condition, supraglottic contraction—either front-to-back (MTP III) or from side-to-side (MTP II)—seems to be a consequence of air-wasting at the level of the vocal fold. Virtually all patients with (organic) glottal closure problems demonstrate hyperkinetic laryngeal behaviors, ie, MTP findings. Patients with vocal fold paralysis, for example, demonstrate MTP III. However, the degree of compensatory supraglottic activity is variable. Aerodynamic measurements of patients with unilateral vocal fold paralysis have bimodal distribution, and the aerodynamic variables correlate with the degree of supraglottic contraction. Patients with low resistance and high-flow rates demonstrate relatively little supraglottic activity, while those with high resistance and low-flow rates demonstrate marked supraglottic activity (often MTP II). By comparison, in the unloaded state, all patients with such paralysis have low resistance and high-flow rates.

Other patterns are common. Patients with severe Reinke's edema (polypoid degeneration) often develop MTP II. Presumably, false vocal fold phonation produces a more predictable voice. Patients with spasmodic dysphonia and tremor often demonstrate MTP II, MTP IV, or both. Why patients with spasmodic dysphonia, a hyperkinetic voice disorder, compensate by further overclosing the glottis is still somewhat speculative; however, it is believed that supraglottic phonation, although further degrading the quality of the voice, improves vocal fluency. Notably, patients with reflux laryngitis may develop any of the MTPs.

Finally, it is important to note that some patients with contact ulcers and granulomas, vocal nodules, Reinke's edema, and free-edge leukoplakia have developed the lesions as a result of hyperkinetic laryngeal behaviors, ie, forced glottal closure that is compensatory for a glottal closure problem.[8] In the author's opinion, relatively subtle degrees of vocal fold paresis are common and cannot be diagnosed by per oral examination methods. Table 12-4 summarizes some of the commonly observed MTPs in functional and organic voice disorders.

To summarize, there are four basic patterns of abnormal muscle tension that can be observed in patients with both organic and functional voice disorders; there are the *muscle tension patterns I-IV*:

MTP I   Open posterior glottal chink ("laryngeal isometric")

MTP II   False vocal fold approximation ("plica ventricularis")

MTP III Partial anteroposterior contraction ("foreshortening")

MTP IV   Complete anteroposterior contraction ("sphincter-like closure")

It is important to note that the MTPs are not mutually exclusive, ie, many patients demonstrate two or more MTPs. Furthermore, the MTPs may appear to change from examination to examination, and they should change after initiation of treatment.

Differentiating Hyperfunctional From Hypofunctional Voice Disorders

The emphasis of this chapter has been on the identification and classification of hyperkinetic vocal behaviors and on the associated fiberoptic findings of patients with voice disorders. Theoretically, the differential diag-

A. Common Primary MTP Patterns Seen in Functional Voice Disorders	
1. Conversion aphonia/dysphonia	MTP I or IV
2. Vocal abuse/misuse syndromes	
a. Tension-fatigue syndrome	MTP IV
b. Bogart-Bacall syndrome	MTP III
c. Vocal nodules	MTP I & III
3. Reflux laryngitis	MTP I-IV
4. Postoperative dysphonias	MTP II
B. Commonly Observed Secondary (Compensatory) MTP Patterns	
1. Vocal cord paresis/paralysis	MTP II & III
2. Spasmodic dysphonia	MTP II & IV
3. Polypoid degeneration	MTP II
4. Contact ulcers/granulomas	MTP I-III

TABLE 12-4. *Commonly Observed Muscle Tension Patterns (MTPs) in Functional and Organic Voice Disorders*

nosis for hyperfunctional (hyperkinetic), and for hypo-functional (hypokinetic) voice disorders should be quite different. Unfortunately, in practice, a functional or compensatory component accompanies most voice disorders so that hyperkinetic laryngeal behavior may be seen in truly hypokinetic conditions.

The most important principle in accurate diagnosis is unloading. While unloading usually can be accomplished by simply altering the vocal task during TFL, in some patients it may require a short period of voice therapy. Presented in Table 12-5 are the differential diagnoses of primary and compensatory hyperfunctional and hypofunctional voice disorders, as well as some of the differentiating criteria.

Laryngeal Biomechanics of the Singing Voice

Marked supraglottic contraction has been observed with certain vocal tasks and styles of singing in normal subjects. Yanagisawa et al[7] found that the singing styles of "twang" and "belting" are associated with more supraglottic contraction than other styles, such as opera. In patients with voice disorders, abnormal biomechanical (MTP) findings must be interpreted within the context of vocal dysfunction; however, in healthy vocalists, the significance of MTP findings has not yet been established.

How much muscle tension, based upon the MTP classification, is acceptable, tolerable, or physiologic for a vocalist? When do the MTP findings suggest bad technique, excessive vocal stress, or an imminent vocal problem? Are certain styles of singing intrinsically inefficient or stressful to the vocal apparatus? What is the effect of vocal training on vocal efficiency (on laryngeal biomechanics)? These and other related questions currently are being studied in the hope of establishing normative data so that studies of laryngeal biomechanics can be used to train singers, and what is more important, to prevent vocal dysfunction.

The Center for Voice Disorders of Wake Forest University conducted a study of the laryngeal biomechanics of 100 healthy singers.[3] Half the singers were professionals, half were amateurs, and none had had any vocal difficulty for at least three months before the study.

First, demographic and background data were collected, including information about the training of each subject, his or her medical, social, and vocal histories, as well as practice and performance schedules. Next, a TFL was performed using standardized vocal tasks and the images were recorded on a laser disk for subsequent review. For each of the vocal tasks, 180 frames (30 per second for 6 seconds) were available for review. Each

frame was analyzed subsequently for each of the MTPs, and an MTP score was then computed for each subject for each task. (The MTP score was a percentage of the frames on which one of the MTPs was observed.)

The speaking and singing tasks included:

1. saying the phrase "the cake is great and the rainbow is beautiful"

2. sustaining high and low notes (the highest and lowest notes of the vocal range)

3. singing the last line of the *Star Spangled Banner,* "o'er the land of the free, and the home of the brave," sung 3 times: "on key," then an octave lower, and finally a fourth higher

4. singing a selection from his or her repertoire using his or her style (eg, opera, musical theater, jazz, country & western, etc.). A relatively difficult passage was selected, usually one that demonstrated the passaggio.

While the data have not yet been analyzed statistically, they appear to show several trends:

- Pushing the limits of voice in terms of amplitude (loudness) increases muscle tension scores for similar tasks, regardless of the style of singing.

- Muscle tension is observed routinely when subjects sing the lowest note of their pitch range.

- Singing out of range routinely produces dramatic increases in muscle tension scores.

- Subjects with physical findings consistent with reflux laryngitis generally have increased muscle tension scores.

- Professional singers are generally more efficient (have lower MTP scores) than amateurs.

- Trained singers are generally more efficient (have lower MTP scores) than untrained singers.

An attempt was made to correlate singing style with muscle tension scores. It was not possible to obtain equal representation of professional and amateur singers in each group (for example, there were no professional barbershop singers); and furthermore, it was not possible to get significant numbers of singers in some of the groups (rock singers, for example, hardly ever kept their appointments).

Despite these limitations, interesting data emerged. Successful, professional opera singers, all of whom had training, usually demonstrated remarkably low muscle tension scores. For singing tasks, there were many in this group with muscle tension scores of 0%. On the other hand, gospel singers had little formal vocal train-

I. Hyperfunction
   A. The differential diagnosis of primary hyperadduction
      1. Adductor-type spasmodic dysphonia
      2. Functional voice disorders (muscle tension dysphonias)
         a. Vocal fold nodules
         b. Bogart-Bacall syndrome
         c. Other abuse/misuse/overuse syndromes
   B. The differential diagnosis of secondary (compensatory) hyperadduction
      1. Spasmodic dysphonia (adductor and abductor types)
      2. Vocal fold paresis/paralysis
      3. Vocal fold bowing/atrophy
      4. Reinke's edema
      5. Laryngitis
         a. Gastroesophageal reflux
         b. Viral infection
II. Hypofunction (Hypoadduction)
   A. Differential diagnosis of common glottal closure problems
      1. Parkinsonism
      2. Vocal fold bowing/atrophy
      3. Vocal fold paresis/paralysis
      4. Abductor-type spasmodic dysphonia
      5. Myasthenia gravis
      6. Amyotrophic lateral sclerosis
      7. Other degenerative neuromuscular disorders
   B. The differential diagnosis of compensatory hypoadduction
      1. Adductor-type spasmodic dysphonia
III. Differentiating Hypofunction From Hyperfunction
   A. TFL with unloading
   B. Diagnostic voice therapy (unloading)
   C. Acoustic voice analysis (loaded and unloaded)
      1. Reduced pitch range
      2. Spectrographic analysis
      3. Aerodynamic measurements
      4. Waveform analysis
   D. Laryngeal electromyography (when indicated)

TABLE 12-5. *Differential Diagnosis of Hyperfunction and Hypofunction*

ing; their muscle tension scores were the highest of any group; and in some cases, the MTP scores were 100% for their singing tasks. One bluegrass singer made the following comment about his laryngeal biomechanics (and his muscle tension score), "if it don't hurt, it ain't bluegrass." The relative rank order (of muscle tension scores) for different styles of singing is shown in Table 12-6. They ranged from a low MTP score of 41% for choral singing to a high of 94% for gospel.

SUMMARY

Laryngeal examination by TFL, unlike other methods, does not significantly alter laryngeal biomechanics and is, therefore, an excellent way to evaluate laryngeal function. Four discrete patterns of laryngeal muscle tension, the MTPs, are observed, and these either correspond to specific functional conditions, or may be associated secondarily with laryngeal compensatory behaviors in response to organic conditions.

(Shown in rank order: from lowest muscle tension scores to the highest)
Choral
Art song
Opera
Barbershop
Popular/Jazz
Musical theater
Country & Western
Bluegrass
Gospel
Rock

TABLE 12-6. *Relative Muscle Tension Scores of Different Styles of Singing*

REFERENCES

1. Koufman JA. Approach to the patient with a voice disorder. *Otolaryngol Clin North Am.* 1991;24:989-998.

2. Koufman JA, Blalock PD. Functional voice disorders. *Otolaryngol Clin North Am.* 1991;24:1059-1073.

3. Koufman JA, Radomski T, Joharji GM, Russell GB, Pillsbury DC. Laryngeal biomechanics of the singing voice. *Otolaryngol Head Neck Surg.* 1996;115:527-537.

4. Morrison MD, Nichol H, Rammage LA. Diagnostic criteria in functional dysphonia. *Laryngoscope.* 1986;94:1-8.

5. Koufman JA, Blalock PD. Vocal fatigue and dysphonia in the professional voice user: Bogart-Bacall syndrome. *Laryngoscope.* 1988;98:493-498.

6. Koufman JA, Blalock PD. Diagnosis and subclassification of spasmodic dysphonia: the value of therapeutic "unloading," and of spectral analysis. Presented at the annual meeting of The American Laryngological Association. Los Angeles, CA: May 18, 1993. *Ann Otol Rhinol Laryngol* (submitted for publication).

7. Yanagisawa E, Estill J, Manbrino L, Talkin D. Supraglottic contributions to pitch raising. Videoendoscopic study with spectroanalysis. *Ann Otol Rhinol Laryngol.* 1991;100:19-30.

8. Koufman JA, Postma GN, Cummins MM, Blalock PD. Vocal fold paresis. *Otolaryngol Head Neck Surg.* 2000;122:537-541.

CHAPTER 13

Introduction to the Laboratory Diagnosis of Vocal Disorders

Gwen S. Korovin, MD, FACS

John S. Rubin, MD, FACS, FRCS

As the voice laboratory has evolved over the past thirty years, it has played an ever-increasing role in the diagnosis and treatment of voice disorders. In 1970, only facilities in Syracuse and Chicago, followed by Gainesville and Los Angeles, boasted the presence of laboratories designed solely for the study of voice. We now have nearly 110 voice laboratories throughout the United States and Canada registered with The Voice Foundation (1721 Pine Street, Philadelphia, Pennsylvania 19103).

It is important to remember that voice research did not really begin at that time. We cannot forget the role of the great observations made by many of our predecessors. Interest in the voice dates back as early as the fifth century B.C.[1] The first practical observations of the human vocal folds at work can be credited to Manuel Garcia, who in 1854 first used the dental mirror for observations of the vocal folds.[2] Since that time, many investigators have become interested in voice. Individual studies have been carried out in a multitude of laboratories not designed for voice work alone. These have all contributed greatly to the field as it is today. They laid the foundation upon which modern voice research has been built. Brewer summarized it well when he stated that "historically the voice came first, then the arts of using it more effectively and only lately the science of dealing with its mechanics."[3] We now have the facilities to deal with the science of voice mechanics in a more highly organized and concise manner. A variety of studies can be done in each of these facilities. Greater collaboration between voice laboratories can occur because of awareness of the research being carried out elsewhere. In this way, we hope to make even greater strides in the study of the voice sciences.

THE VOICE LABORATORY

The analysis of phonation depends on the study of three interrelated systems. These include the respiratory, laryngeal, and articulatory systems. The respiratory system serves as the power source. The laryngeal system serves as the oscillator. The articulatory system functions along with the resonators to shape the sound, thus producing voice. Aerodynamic power from the respiratory system must undergo changes from the laryngeal systems. Adjustments and tuning of the vocal tract are then carried out by the articulatory system.[4-6]

These systems are now being studied in the various laboratories, which exist in many varieties and levels of sophistication. An example of an extensive laboratory is the Wilbur James Gould Recording and Research Center at the Denver Center of the Performing Arts, which is producing a great deal of new and exciting data. Many laboratories are affiliated with otolaryngology residency training programs and/or hospitals and as such are used mainly for teaching purposes and clinical evaluations.

These serve to foster interest among residents and students in the field of voice at an early stage in their careers. Many of these also do basic science and/or clinical research, as at the Ames Vocal Dynamics Laboratory at Lenox Hill Hospital in New York City (with which one of the authors [GSK] is connected).

The Role of the Voice Laboratory

The voice laboratory has the capability to provide visual, acoustic, respiratory, aerodynamic, and electrophysiologic information. The laboratory serves as a supplement to the history and physical examination. It should in no way replace this examination, nor should it replace perceptual evaluations of the voice. We should not underestimate the value of the laryngeal mirror examination. It allows us to see the true color and gives an estimate of the true size of the vocal folds. Mirrors that provide three times the magnification of the simple mirror can give even more detail. A majority of lesions can be seen with the mirror. There is minimal anatomic distortion during this examination, although some distortion occurs at the laryngeal entry because of the pulling forward of the tongue.

The laboratory may aid in diagnosis. In most cases, however, vocal disorders are not diagnosed in the voice laboratory. They are diagnosed in the clinical setting, and the diagnosis is supported by the data generated in the laboratory. However, in some cases a lesion that is not readily visible (for example, certain subglottal lesions or glottic scars or partially resolved paralysis of the superior laryngeal nerve) may be uncovered by laboratory assessment. Visual data may provide the diagnosis when the lesion has been missed during the routine examination. In other cases, no lesions or abnormalities are detected on physical examination or during the collection of visual data, but the voice is still disordered. In these cases the laboratory can help in diagnosis by detecting specific respiratory, aerodynamic, neurologic, or other abnormalities. This is especially true of visual analysis techniques, including the fiberoptic and rigid scopes with the addition of the stroboscope. Videokymography or other high-speed visualization techniques may be used in the clinically advanced or research-oriented center.

The voice laboratory provides objective data that not only serve as support for subjective findings of a physical examination, but also can be used for more accurate assessment of treatment outcome. In patients undergoing a surgical procedure, preoperative and postoperative data can be obtained. In patients going through a voice therapy program, pretherapy and post-therapy data can be documented. These findings can then be used as a guide for any necessary further diagnosis and as an evaluation of the success of the therapy. In these ways the voice laboratory helps the patient, the physician, and the therapist.

The voice laboratory allows for the storage of information. Data may be obtained and retrieved for analysis at a later time. This provides a savings of time that was previously wasted for repetitive data collection. Digitization has proven of particular benefit in this regard. New equipment is being developed continually. If a voice recording is stored, it can be evaluated with new, more advanced equipment in the future. In this way, additional information may be obtained. Also, the recording can be used to compare early data with later data on the same patient.

Voice laboratory data can be helpful in providing information for voice teachers and therapists. These data can be an aid in the treatment regimen, in that physicians and therapists can evaluate how the treatment is progressing. A patient and a voice therapist may perceive a subjective improvement. The voice laboratory information can then be used for objective evidence, and further therapy can then be supported.

The voice laboratory can provide essential information for the patient. The patient and the practitioner may be able to view the results of the study simultaneously. Thus, it acts as an instantaneous form of biofeedback, and holds the promise of playing an even greater role in therapy in the future. The patients can gain better insight regarding their problems and in addition gain understanding of the physiology of their vocal instruments. In this way laboratory data are an effective teaching tool and diagnostic aid.

The voice laboratory provides medical and legal documentation. In our increasingly litigious society, it has become of greater importance to keep a permanent record, which may be needed for legal purposes at a later time. Insurance companies may also require the information. In this regard, it is helpful to compare voice data or a voice print to an audiogram. It is rare that any otologic treatment is done without an audiogram, and we are working toward a time in which no vocal treatments will be given without some type of "voicegram."

In discussing the role of the voice laboratory, it becomes of great importance to realize that we are treating the whole patient, not just the laboratory results in isolation. We cannot just look at the numbers. We need to look at the entire picture, which includes all the subjective and objective information. (In some ways, the title of this chapter is misleading. Rather than "the laboratory diagnosis of voice disorders," it should more specifically be "the role of the laboratory as an adjunct to the diagnosis of voice disorders.") As stated by Hirano, the purpose of most tests is basically "not to make a diagnosis of the etiologic disease of the voice disorder but to evaluate one or several aspects of the vocal function."[7]

Others have different views of the role of the voice laboratory, but all have a common thread. Gates and Painter see the voice laboratory as a common meeting ground of the four groups of professionals concerned with people with disordered voices: the laryngologist, the speech-language pathologist, the voice teacher, and the clinical voice scientist.[8]

Gould saw research into voice functions as providing an increasingly valuable means to evaluate problems of voice, and objectively measure speech production in the clinical setting.[4] Martin sees the role of the laboratory to the phonosurgeon as assisting in diagnosing, evaluating operative results, and developing better phonosurgical procedures.[9] von Leden sees the medical application of these scientific measures as offering substantial clinical benefits for both physician and patient, for their sensitivity often permits the discovery of early changes in the larynx before the eyes and ears of the examiner detect the underlying physiologic or pathologic aberrations.[10]

The point is that the role of the voice laboratory differs depending on the orientation of the particular clinician or scientist. However, the voice laboratory plays an important role for all these people. As Gould stated, "The most important scientific study to the laryngologist derived from research in these areas (ie, respiratory, laryngeal, and articulatory) is that which can be applied directly to patient care."[11] This is the ultimate goal.

How to Set Up a Voice Laboratory

In setting up a voice laboratory, it is most important to determine what your needs are. You must decide what it is that you ultimately want to measure. Will you be doing mostly clinical testing? Will it be primarily a research facility? Will you be doing studies in both these areas? This goal must be set early.

It is most helpful when beginning a new venture to visit other working laboratories. The Voice Foundation keeps a list of essentially all the laboratories and could be helpful in this regard. When visiting, it is advisable to try to learn all you can about the equipment. You probably will not want to reproduce an identical laboratory, as your goals may differ. You must also be aware of how much space you have available. This will help determine which equipment you should choose. Attendance at various voice seminars may be very helpful. The Voice Foundation's annual symposium on care of the profes-

sional voice, along with many other voice seminars and workshops throughout the world, can convey valuable, practical information about the working voice laboratory.

It is important to determine the attributes of the planned laboratory personnel—that is, technicians, therapists, physicians, scientists, and so forth—and how much time they will devote to the laboratory. This may play a key role in determining the sophistication of the equipment to be obtained, which will also depend on the patient population available.

Finances are of major importance. Many hospitals and university programs may be able to attract grants and endowments to begin a laboratory. Residency programs may be able to provide funds if the laboratory is to be used for teaching purposes. Although money can be brought in through clinical testing, it may take time to earn back monies that are spent on the laboratory.

TYPES OF ANALYSIS

Visual Analysis

Visual analysis is of great importance in the voice laboratory evaluation. The simple mirror examination done prior to the laboratory studies provides a great deal of information. It is the most widely used method of visualization. The flexible fiberoptic laryngoscope, first introduced by Sawashima and Hirose in 1968, is the next most widely available tool for evaluating the larynx.[12] The fiberoptic scope requires a somewhat powerful light source. A television monitor and recorder can be attached for viewing and videotaping purposes. Advantages of the flexible scope include visualization of the supraglottic laryngeal tract with relatively minor distortion of the anatomy. Disadvantages include some peripheral distortion and the requirement of a strong light source, particularly if stroboscopy is to be used.

The rigid laryngeal telescope (also commonly referred to as a rigid laryngoscope), first introduced by Andrews and Gould in 1971, allows examination of the vocal folds with better light magnification and resolution.[13] By adjusting the angle of visualization, Gould has shown how subcordal and subglottic changes can be seen more easily.[14] The laryngoscope can be attached to a camera, and movements of the folds can be recorded on high-speed film.

The addition of the use of the stroboscope in the clinical setting has been a great technologic advancement. Stroboscopic light allows apparent slow-motion evaluation of vocal fold motion. It gives a clearer, sharper image of the mucosal layer of the vocal fold. The examiner can detect structural or functional changes in the larynx. Minor mucosal changes and early lesions can be diagnosed more easily than with continuous light.

The stroboscope can be used with the flexible fiberoptic scope to give information about vocal fold motion and supraglottic motion during both speech and singing. This provides valuable information to the physician and therapist. When the stroboscope is used with the rigid scope, a closer view of the vocal folds is afforded. Subtle changes of the motion of the glottic and subcordal or subglottic areas can be visualized better.

With any of these methods of visual evaluation, it is important to establish a standardized method of assessment. In one of the author's laboratories (GSK), a form that records the appearance of the vocal folds in full adduction, full abduction, and the paramedian position is used. Symmetry, closure, mobility, amplitude, stiffness, glottal closure, regularity, supraglottal and subglottal movement, and frequency are evaluated. Others use a standardized method proposed by Bless et al that includes an evaluation of fundamental frequency, symmetry of movements, periodicity, glottic closure, amplitude of vibration, mucosal wave, and the presence of nonvibrating portions of the vocal fold.[15] No widespread standard is available at the present time.

Newer methods of high-speed and digital recording have been devised and allow for even more accurate visualization. Some computer equipment can allow frame-by-frame analysis, but this is present in the more research-oriented voice laboratories only. Videokymography, a technique which allows for real-time evaluation of the mucosal wave at a single site on the true vocal fold, is now available commercially. It provides further information on mucosal wave patterns in different pathologic states.[16]

Electroglottography allows further evaluation of the vibratory signal. It traces the opening and closing of the glottis. The traces can be superimposed with the visual images and thus can be correlated. An interesting feature of electroglottography is that not only does it represent an optimal choice for fundamental frequency (F_0) measurement,[6] but it can be used also for measurement of continuous (connected) speech. The technology is still in its infancy, but it is commercially available.[17,18] The technique may be difficult in some subjects because of obesity or other anatomic factors.[6]

Photoglottography, in which the opening and closing of the glottis modulates a beam of light, also provides an electrical signal simple enough for reliable F_0 determination. The technique is somewhat invasive, however.[6]

Acoustic Analysis

The tape recorder remains the most valuable basic tool for the voice laboratory. Analog recordings can be converted to digital, which can then be used for data storage. Digital recording has been replacing the use of the standard analog system. It is arguably more precise and of longer-lasting, higher quality, although some investigators remain concerned about distortion introduced by the digitization and compression process. Data from digital recording are immediately computer-capable, allowing on-line analysis. Alternatively, data can be stored for use at a later date. Digital video computer stroboscopes are now commercially readily available in which both the image and the sound are digitized and stored directly on the hardware or as an individual CD or on Zip disks.

The stopwatch is another useful and simple tool in the voice laboratory. The maximum phonation time and the "S/Z" ratio are both simple measures to obtain, with useful clinical correlations.

The phonetogram is a measure of the maximal phonational frequency range at varying intensities. This is the range of vocal frequencies encompassing the modal and falsetto registers. Its extension is from the lowest tone sustainable in modal register to the highest tone sustainable in falsetto.[19] It is used commonly in European laboratories. One drawback is that it is time consuming.

Sound spectrographic analysis, the dissection of the acoustic wave into its most basic components, is used widely in the research and clinical laboratory. Sound spectrography resolves a periodic waveform into a series of sine waves of different frequencies, amplitudes, and phase relationships. The fundamental frequency and harmonics can be determined. Different ratios have been established to compare the information obtained. These allow comparison and greater standardization of data. Hundreds of scientific papers have been published on applications of sound spectrography. Spectrographic categorizations of hoarse voices were made over thirty years ago.[20]

While most disorders of the larynx do not, in and of themselves, appear to have significant influence on the mean speaking F_0, F_0 variability and range do seem to reflect tissue changes.[6] Such variability has been evaluated in the voice laboratory.

Many kinds of packaged systems have been developed to aid in the acoustic analysis of the voice.[6] These allow the measurement of fundamental frequency, intensity, and pitch. They are interfaced with microcomputers, allowing analysis and quantification of various acoustic characteristics of phonated speech. More technologically sophisticated packages continue to be under development.

The *Visipitch* is a self-contained analog fundamental frequency analyzer. It was designed specifically for ease of clinical use. It provides an oscilloscopic display of F_0 and of relative intensity over time. The *Visipitch* is used regularly in many clinics. It is particularly useful as a feedback tool for the therapist and patient.[6, 21]

In addition, the vocal demodulator that has been developed by Winholtz at the Denver Center has been evaluated for office use and may provide a simple way of measuring fundamental frequency.[22]

Jitter, shimmer, and harmonic-to-noise ratio are other acoustic analyses offered regularly in different commercially available acoustic packages.

Jitter is the name commonly given to frequency (period) perturbation. It is the variability of the F_0. Jitter measurements tend to be concerned with short-term F_0 variation. (In continuous speech, variability is reflected in pitch sigma.) Jitter, then, is a measure of frequency variability not accounted for by voluntary changes in F_0. A considerable body of literature confirms the usefulness of jitter assessment in laryngeal pathology.[6,23]

Measures of amplitude perturbation (shimmer) serve to quantify short-term instability of the vocal signal. Some feel it is as important as jitter in its contribution to perception of hoarseness. Amplitude perturbation is a measure based on the peak amplitude of each phonatory cycle.[24]

Assuming that the pure (average) periodic wave is increasingly contaminated by random noise as hoarseness worsens, this degree of contamination can be expressed as a periodic harmonic-to-noise amplitude ratio. Harmonic-to-noise ratio can be described, relatively simply, as the mean amplitude of the average wave divided by the mean amplitude of the isolated noise components for the train of waves. For convenience, it is expressed in decibels. A characteristic feature of hoarseness is the replacement of harmonics by noise energy (aperiodic sound intensifying at the expense of periodic signal).[6]

Jitter, shimmer, harmonic-to-noise ratio. and mean F_0 are basic tests of acoustic analysis readily available in many commercially available programs. As the algorithms vary between packages, great care must be exercised when comparing results with other packages.

In setting up a laboratory, it is important to evaluate all the different systems available and determine which of these are most appropriate for your individual needs.

Aerodynamic Analysis

The vocal tract is an aerodynamic sound generator and resonator system. The basis for aerodynamic analysis is respiratory analysis. The volume of air that the lungs can hold, the pressures that can be developed, and the characteristics of airflow (the rate of change of the volume) are all critical elements in the production and maintenance of voice. Basic pulmonary function testing, available in most pulmonary laboratories, gives information regarding tidal volume, functional residual capacity, inspiratory capacity, total lung capacity, vital capacity, forced vital capacity, forced expiratory volume, and maximal mid-expiratory volume. Instrumentation is readily commercially available. For example, a flow transducer attached to an anesthetic-type face mask will permit evaluation of airflow.

Studies of airflow efficiency offer valuable information to physicians. Four parameters measured traditionally in the laboratory are subglottal pressure, supraglottal pressure, glottal impedance, and volume velocity of airflow at the glottis. Different calculations can then be done to determine such things as mean flow rate, glottal resistance, and the phonation quotient.

Transglottal airflow can be measured by a newer technique called flow glottography. One method of airflow measurement is the inverse filtering technique. Although inverse filtering was formerly tedious, a simplified method by Rothenberg has made it simpler to use in the clinical research setting.[5] Air volume can be measured with a wet spirometer, a device which has not changed much since its invention over 100 years ago, or a dry spirometer. Two types of portable dry spirometry are in current use: one, a mechanical type, and the other a flow transducer and integrator circuit system. Lung volume changes can be determined by change in the chest wall (rib cage and abdominal size). Articulatory and phonatory volumes can be measured by a pneumotachograph, which can show very small volume changes in time periods involving only a fraction of a second (unlike the spirometer).[6]

Electromyography

Laryngeal electromyography[15] is an objective method available to study the neural function of laryngeal muscle activity. It helps to determine which muscles are in use during different phonatory conditions. Electromyography can be used to follow a patient with laryngeal paralysis. Differentiation between peripheral laryngeal nerve paralysis or paresis, central neurologic disorders, and arytenoid fixation or dislocation may be determined. Its importance has increased, proportionate to the number of centers now utilizing it. Laryngeal electromyography is also a useful adjunct in administration of botulinum toxin for various problems. The equipment can be made available as part of a voice laboratory, or it can be used in conjunction with neurologists or physiatrists in their laboratories. Laryngeal electromyography is discussed in detail in another chapter (Chapter 15).

COST AND EFFECTIVENESS

Voice laboratories vary from the very rudimentary to the very advanced; the level of sophistication is often dependent on the need. When a voice laboratory is being planned, it is important to determine cost versus effectiveness.

The voice committee of the International Association of Logopedics and Phoniatrics (IALP) sent out a questionnaire in an attempt to determine the most frequently used examinations.[7] The laryngeal mirror, a tape recording, perceptual evaluation, and measures of mean phonation time and fundamental frequency were the most commonly used. The information determined in this study is of great value because these four measures can all be done at low cost in an office setting. They may be all that is necessary for the most rudimentary laboratory. Packaged systems are offered by several companies to provide a means to measure a multitude of functions. A voice laboratory in a hospital setting provides a more central facility that can be used by physicians and therapists in a particular region. It may be easier to fund, as grants and endowments may come from the hospital. Staffing is easier as no one individual is responsible for the entire laboratory and equipment as is the case in the office setting.

In evaluating cost versus effectiveness, it is helpful to keep in mind the words of Ingo Titze, who said, "Many instruments are not necessarily a blessing. A few good instruments usually are."[25] To further evaluate costs versus effectiveness, we must remember that in many ways we are still testing the tests. We know the importance of objective data and documentation. Just as audiograms are an integral part of the otologic evaluation, vocal dynamics evaluation is becoming more of an integral part of the voice evaluation. However, it has not been determined which tests will remain as essential parts of the "voicegram." Vocal testing is undergoing continual changes. We are using many tests in attempts at "cross validation." The question of reliability and reproducibility is slowly being answered. The question of which tests to do in which patients is of continuing importance in our changing economic climate.

THE VOICE TEAM

The treatment of vocal disorders is highly dependent on the voice team. The essential team members include the physician (laryngologist), the therapist (speaking or singing), and the voice scientist. Specialists should familiarize themselves with the voice laboratory and its clinical applications. Only through cooperation and collaboration of the specialists can we truly improve the care of our patients.

Others, including various medical specialists (pulmonologists, endocrinologists, gastroenterologists, gynecologists, neurologists, allergists, maxillofacial specialists, or physical therapists) may also be called in for aid at various times.

Interlaboratory cooperation becomes an integral part of the field of voice as a whole. It is only through the cross-fertilization of different voice specialists and laboratory facilities that we have achieved today's level of sophistication. Teamwork is truly an essential part of the laboratory diagnosis of voice disorders. Herein lies the future of voice science.

REFERENCES

1. von Leden H. The cultural history of the layrnx and voice. In: Gould WJ, Sataloff JR, eds. *Voice Surgery*. St. Louis, MO: Mosby Year Book; 1993:3-65.

2. von Leden H. The cultural history of the human voice. In: Lawrence VL, ed. *Transcripts of the 11th Symposium: Care of the Professional Voice*, part 2. New York, NY: The Voice Foundation; 1982:116-123.

3. Brewer DW. Voice research: the next ten years. *J Voice*. 1989;3(1):7-17.

4. Gould WJ. The clinical voice laboratory: clinical application of voice research. *Ann Otol Rhinol Laryngol*. 1984;93(4):346-350.

5. Sundberg J. *The Science of the Singing Voice*. DeKalb, IL: Northern Illinois University Press; 1987.

6. Baken RJ. *Clinical Measurement of Speech and Voice*. San Diego, CA: College-Hill Press; 1987.

7. Hirano M. Objective evaluation of the human voice: clinical aspects, *Folia Phoniatr (Basel)*. 1989;41:89-144.

8. Korovin GS. Introduction to the Laboratory Diagnosis of Voice Disorders. In: Rubin JS, Sataloff RT, Korovin GS, Gould WJ, eds. *Diagnosis and Treatment of Voice Disorders*. New York, NY: Igaku-Shoin; 1995:262-268.

9. Martin GF. The contribution of the speech sciences to the development of phonosurgery. In Gould WJ, Sataloff RT, Spiegel JR, eds. *Voice Surgery*. St. Louis, MO: Mosby Year Book; 1993:97-122.

10. von Leden H, Mooie P, Timcke R. Laryngeal vibrations: measuremented the glottic wave. Part III;

the pathologic laryna. *Arch Otolaryngol.* 1960; 71:16-35.

11. Gould WJ. The clinical voice laboratory: clinical application of voice research. *J Voice.* 1988;1(4):305-309.

12. Sawashima M, Hirose H. New laryngostics technique by use of fibre optics. *J Acoust Soc Am.* 1968;43:168-170.

13. Andrews AN Jr, Gould WJ. Laryngeal and nasal-frigical indirect telescope. *Ann Otol Rhinol Laryngol.* 1977;88:627.

14. Gould WJ. Why is there a need for this conference? In: Cooper JA, ed. *Assessment of Speech and Voice Production: Research and Clinical Applications.* Bethesda, MD: NIDCD Monograph; 1990:1-4.

15. Bless DM, Hirano M, Feder RJ. Videostroboscopic evaluation of the larynx. *Ear Nose Throat J.* 1987;66:289-296.

16. Svec J. On vibration properties of human vocal folds: voice registers bifurcations, resonance characteristics, development and application of videokymography (Ph.D. thesis). Rigksuniversiteit gromingen, the Netherlands; 2000.

17. Fourcin AJ. Voice quality and electrolaryngology. In: Ball M, Kent R, eds. *Handbook of Voice Quality Measurement.* San Diego, CA: Singular Publications; in press.

18. Barry WJ, Goldsmith MJ, Fuller HC, Fourcin AJ. Stability of voice frequency measures in speech. *Twelfth Int. Cong Phon Sci (Univ de Provence).* 1991;2:38-4.

19. Hollien ll, Dew D, Philips P. Phonational frequency ranges of adults. *J Speech Hearing Res.* 1971;14:755-760.

20. Yanagihara N. Significance of harmonic changes and voice components in hoarseness. *J Speech Hearing Res.* 1967;10:531-541.

21. Horii Y. Automatic analysis of voice fundamental frequency and intensity using a *Visipitch. J Speech Hearing Res.* 1983;26:467-471.

22. Winholtz WS, Ramig LO. Vocal tremor analysis with the vocal demodulator. *J Speech Hearing Res.* 1992;35:562-579.

23. Kitajima K, Tanabe M, Isshiki N. Pitch perturbation in normal and pathogical voice. *Studia Phonologica.* 1975;9:25-32.

24. Takahashi H, Koike Y. Some perceptual dimensions and acoustical correlates of pathologic voices. *Acta Otolaryngologica.* 1975;338(suppl):1-24.

25. Titze IR. Measurements for the assessment of voice disorders. In: Cooper JA, ed. *Assessment of Speech and Voice Production: Research and Clinical Applications.* Bethesda, MD: NIDCD Monograph; 1990:42-49.

CHAPTER 14

Measuring Vocal Fold Function

Raymond H. Colton, PhD

Peak Woo, MD

THE PHYSIOLOGY OF PHONATION

What is commonly known as the voice is the product of the vibratory motion of the vocal folds and the resonant effects of the vocal tract. The vocal folds constitute the major (but not only) source of periodic sound for speech. The vocal folds move to and fro to interrupt the egressive air stream and thus produce an acoustic disturbance. Sound is nothing more than alternating regions of higher-than-normal and lower-than-normal regions of air pressure produced at a rate someone can hear. The exact form of the acoustic disturbance produced by the vocal folds is dependent on the exact pattern of vocal fold movement and its interaction with the air stream.

The shape of the acoustic pulse determines the frequencies present in the complex tone produced by the vocal folds. For example, consider the effect of decreasing the closing time of the vocal folds (top panel of Figure 14-1) on the amplitude of the higher frequencies (bottom panel of Figure 14-1). Physiologically, a decreased closed time could be the result of increased vocal fold tension. The acoustic pulse is generated at the instant of closing:[1] the more rapid closing time results in the increased amplitudes at the higher frequencies.

Increased air turbulence through the glottis may also affect the acoustic pulse produced, primarily by increased noise levels. Increased air turbulence may be produced in a variety of ways including incomplete vocal fold closure, the presence of a mass on one or both vocal folds, and irregularities on the surface of the vocal folds. Such pathologic conditions may also affect the frequency and stability of vibration.

It appears clear that the vibratory motion of the vocal folds and their interaction with the air stream determine the acoustic output of the vocal folds. This acoustic output after modification by the resonators determines the listener's perception of the voice. A pathologic lesion, when it affects the vibratory motion of the vocal folds, affects the acoustic pulse produced and therefore affects the listener's perception of the voice. However, the abnormality may affect some vibratory features more than others. In order to understand the effect of pathologic lesions on vibratory motion and the production of the acoustic pulse, the vibratory characteristics of the vocal folds should be studied. Part of that study includes careful observation and, where possible, the measurement of vibratory motion and parameters of the acoustic pulse produced. In this chapter, we review the nature of normal vibratory motion, the various ways we have to measure it, and the measurement of its acoustic product.

Physiologic Properties of Phonation

In order to understand phonatory physiology, one must recognize that there are two major properties

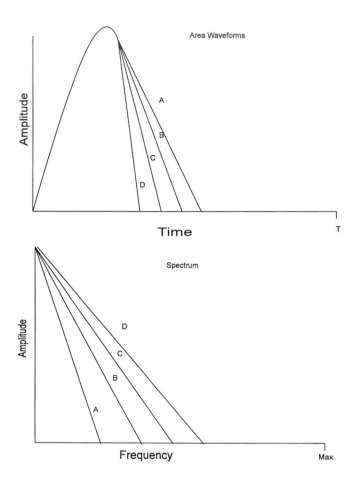

FIGURE 14-1. *The relationship between the shape of the glottal volume velocity waveform and the acoustic properties of the sound. Four glottal pulses, A to D, differing in the abruptness of the change to zero flow at glottal closure, are shown. Shown in the bottom panel are the associated spectra. (Redrawn from Fig. 9-3 Löfqvist.[1])*

important to vocal fold vibration. The first is the *myoelastic* properties of the vocal folds and the second is *aerodynamics* of the air stream. This subject is discussed in greater detail in Chapter 7.

Myoelastic Properties of the Vocal Folds

The myoelastic properties of the vocal folds include the muscles that make up the vocal folds or affect the size, shape, and tension of the vocal folds together with other nonmuscle tissue present in the vocal folds.

The thyroarytenoid (TA) muscle constitutes the bulk of the vocal folds. Its contraction affects the length, mass, and tension of the vocal folds. Together with the cricothyroid (CT), it can affect the relative stiffness of the various layers of the vocal folds and control the fundamental frequency, intensity, and pulse shape of the

vocal fold tone. Additional effects can be produced by the interarytenoid and the lateral cricoarytenoid muscles, which because they are the major adductors of the vocal folds affect the resistance of the vocal folds to opening by the pressures beneath the vocal folds. The posterior cricoarytenpoid (PCA), the only abductor of vocal folds, could affect phonation by influencing the degree of glottal opening during phonation.

Muscle tissue and nonmuscle tissue affect the elasticity and stiffness of the vocal folds.[2-5] Elasticity is a mechanical property that restores the shape of the folds after they have been deformed by an external force. Together they determine the exact pattern of vibration and the relative coupling of the various layers of the vocal folds.[6-9] Both properties affect the frequency of vibration of the vocal folds and the intensity of the voice source. Also affected is the shape of the acoustic disturbance that determines the frequency composition of the tone.

Aerodynamic Properties

Air pressure and airflow are the two aerodynamic properties important in vocal fold vibration. Pressure immediately beneath the vocal folds (subglottal pressure) is responsible for the blowing of the vocal folds open during a cycle of vibration. The magnitude of the subglottal air pressure is dependent on (1) the force of the respiratory system and (2) the magnitude of vocal fold adduction. The latter is reflected in the duration of the closed phase of the vocal folds.

Airflow through the glottis interacts with the vocal folds to produce vibration. The magnitude of the airflow depends on the subglottal air pressure and the magnitude and duration of the glottal opening. Airflow may be laminar or turbulent or both. Turbulent airflows result in the creation of noise or aperiodic vibration.

Vocal Fold Vibration

The vocal folds are a layered structure, with each layer having a differential effect on the movement of the folds depending on the degree of muscle activity, the degree of coupling of the various layers, and the degree of muscle tension. As reported by Hirano,[6,9,10] the vocal fold layers are (1) the epithelium, (2) the lamina propria, and (3) the muscle. The lamina propria consists of the three layers called (1) superficial, (2) intermediate, and (3) deep. Each layer may exhibit different mechanical characteristics. The degree of coupling between the various layers is responsible for the mucosal wave.

The mucosal wave is a wavelike motion along the surface of the vocal folds starting below the folds and progressing to and along the upper surface to the lateral boundaries of the folds. It is similar to the wave created on the surface of a pond when an object is thrown into the water. It probably originates well below the upper surface of the vocal folds,[11] created perhaps by a combination of air pressure increases and the Bernoulli effect. When viewed from above with conventional stroboscopic techniques, it starts at the medial margin of the folds and travels at about a rate of 0.5 to 2 m/s laterally.[12]

Not all phonation produces a mucosal wave, as the wave depends on a loose coupling between the epithelium and the underlying layers of the folds. At higher pitches, the vocal folds are tensed and the coupling between the layers is very high. Thus, usually little or no mucosal wave is visible at higher fundamental frequencies of vocal fold vibration.

Modes of Vibration of the Vocal Folds

There are several modes of vibration of the vocal folds.[13] The most common is that typically heard during speech; its area-versus-time waveform is illustrated in Figure 14-2. Other modes of vibration are described by the terms *creaky voice, falsetto voice, vocal fry, twang,* and *cry.* Each appears to have a different area-versus-time waveform, as illustrated in Figure 14-3. When there is a pathologic lesion on the vocal folds, the mode of vibration may be altered and new modes created. Some of these abnormal modes include breathy voice, hoarse voice, tremor voice, and harsh voice. The specific mode of vibration is determined by many physiologic factors, and it in turn determines the nature of the acoustic pulse created. Although the area-versus-time waveform of the vocal folds is not the acoustic pulse, the two are closely related.[14] Measurements of the area-versus-time

waveform of the vocal folds can be used to obtain estimates of the acoustic pulse, and from the acoustic pulse, an analysis of the frequency components of the tone can be made. A listener's perception of a voice is determined by the combination of the fundamental frequency, intensity, and spectrum of the vocal sound.

There are many parameters of the voice one could observe and measure. Some are physiologic, some acoustic, and some perceptual. Although all can be quantified, instruments are readily available to capture and analyze physiologic and acoustic events. These are the focus of this chapter.

WHAT TO MEASURE ABOUT VOCAL FOLD VIBRATION

Myoelastic Properties

Muscle Activity

The measurement of muscle activity is important for several reasons. It provides evidence of (1) innervation of a muscle, that is, whether the muscle is receiving a

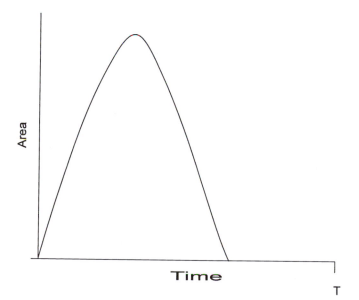

FIGURE 14-2. *Example of an area-versus-time waveform for a normal speaker.*

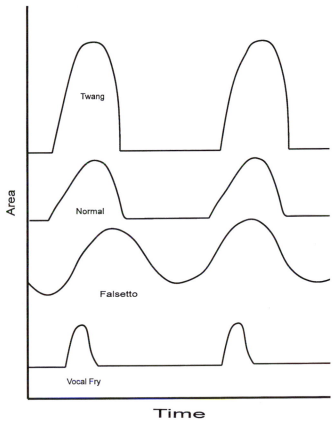

FIGURE 14-3. *Examples of area-versus-time waveforms for various modes of vocal fold vibration.*

nerve impulse, (2) muscle tone, that is, whether the muscle is firing to maintain itself in a state of readiness for contraction, (3) abnormal electrical activity in the muscle, that is, whether there are unusual bursts or levels of activity, especially when unexpected, and (4) muscle timing, that is, when the muscle begins and ends its firing. The magnitude of muscle activity is an indirect reflection of the tension exerted in and on the vocal folds.[15-17] Tension is important in controlling the frequency, intensity, and wave shape during phonation. Therefore, EMG studies are important to determine the roles of the various muscles of the larynx on phonation and their effect on the control of frequency, intensity, and waveform. When a muscle abnormality is suspected as a cause of a voice problem, there is also considerable justification for performing an examination of muscle function, yet EMG is not a routine procedure in most offices or clinics. A more complete discussion of EMG techniques and findings is presented in Chapter 15.

EMG is performed when there is suspected muscle abnormality, for example, when spasmodic dysphonia (SD), essential tremor, spasticity, myasthenia gravis (MG), or muscle dystonias are present. It has found routine use in the treatment of SD when BOTOX is injected into selected muscles of the larynx. EMG is used to verify the muscle to be injected, study the characteristics of muscle activity, and observe the effects of the BOTOX on muscle activity.[18-22]

EMG may be also used for intraoperative monitoring in order to differentiate between a true vocal fold paralysis, a fixed arytenoid, posterior glottal stenosis, abnormal reinnervation, and/or paradoxic vocal fold movement.[23-29] The advantage of intraoperative EMG (IEMG) is that it may make it easier to visualize the muscle of interest and it may be of immediate value to the surgeon for planning. In Figure 14-4 is an example of an IEMG record of a patient with an immobile vocal fold. Note the small amount of activity at rest in the left TA muscle and the absence of activity on the right (denervated) side. Even during the cough and swallow, activities typically showing large EMG activity, there is no activity in the muscle on the right side.[29]

The type of measurements that can be made from electromyograms is shown in Table 14-1. Amplitudes are usually expressed in terms of volts or fraction thereof (milli- or microvolts). Time is usually in seconds or frac-

tions thereof. Analysis of EMG spectrum is sometimes necessary because the EMG trace is usually the sum of many individual muscle fibers,* each of which may have different firing rates. It may be possible from such an analysis to identify specific muscle fiber types that may be involved during contraction.[30]

Contact Area of the Vocal Folds

Electroglottography (EGG) is a technique for recording the contact area of the vocal folds during vibration. It involves the passage of a high-frequency, small-amplitude current through the neck and vocal folds. The amount of current flow depends on the resistance (actually impedance) of the tissues in the current path. The current flow is negligible when air spaces are reached. Thus, when the vocal folds touch, there is a small current flow; when they open, current flow is markedly reduced. Only a small portion of the current flow recorded shows the effects of the vocal folds; the largest component of the signal is caused by slow movements of the larynx and other structures in the neck. However, when amplified and appropriately filtered to remove the very slow components of the signal, a good representation of normal vocal fold contact area as a function of time can be obtained.

Interpretation of the EGG waveform requires a thorough knowledge of normal vocal fold vibration and an awareness of the problems and limitations of the technique. A good model relating EGG waveform characteristics and the actual pattern of vibration of the vocal folds is invaluable.[31-34] One such model is shown in Figure 14-5. The EGG waveform is probably most valid when the vocal folds are touching or close to touching. When the folds are completely open, the EGG waveform may be affected by many random current fluctuations that may have little relationship to vibration.

EGG traces are best interpreted within the context of other techniques that record vocal fold vibration. One such technique involves the recording of transglottal airflow such as shown in Figure 14-5. EGG may also be combined with photoglottography (see later) in order to simultaneously view the glottal area and the vocal fold contact area. Others have combined actual measurements of glottal area as measured from high-speed films with EGG.[32,33,35,36] EGG waveforms also have appeared in synchrony with videostroboscopy.[37-39] Combining the EGG trace with any of these other techniques assists in the proper interpretation of the trace and a more complete understanding of the underlying vibratory pattern.

A number of objective measurements can be obtained from EGG waveforms. First, the EGG may provide a reliable estimate of the fundamental frequency of vibration.[40-42] The amplitude of the EGG trace is arbitrary and subject to electrode placement, the thickness

---

* It is possible to record from a single muscle fiber, in which case the EMG record will contain a single firing frequency. However, this technique involves considerable care and very fine electrodes. A good discussion of single motor unit recordings in the larynx may be found in Lovelace, Blitzer, and Ludlow.[27]

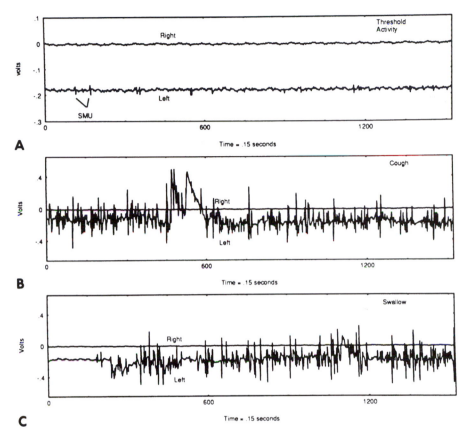

A

B

C

FIGURE 14-4. *(A) Fibrillation potentials on the denervated (right) side of the TA muscle in a patient with immobile vocal folds. There is little or no recruitment compared with the normal (left) side. (B) Activity when the patient coughed. (C) Activity when the patient swallowed. Large recruitment potentials are seen from the left side but none from the right. (Reproduced with permission from Woo P, Arandia H. Interoperative laryngeal electromyographic assessment of patients with immobile vocal fold,* Ann Otol Rhinol Laryngol. *101:799-806, 1992.)*

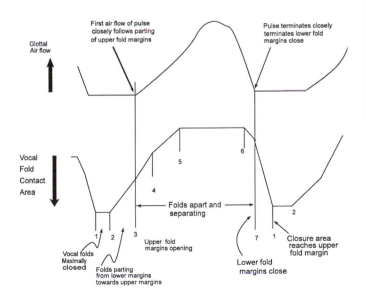

FIGURE 14-5. *A model of the relationship between an EGG waveform and the phases of a normal vocal fold vibratory cycle. (From Rothenberg.[34] Reprinted by permission of the American Speech-Language Hearing Association.)*

Peak or average amplitude of activity
Time of onset or offset of muscle activity
Location and magnitude of any bursts of activity
Spectrum of the EMG

TABLE 14-1. *Measurements That Can Be Made on EMG Records*

of the skin, the thickness of the muscles and other structures in the neck, the amount of fat in the neck, neck size, and so forth. Thus, it is difficult to calibrate easily the amplitude of the trace for the actual vocal fold contact area. What can be stated is that when the trace is maximum (or minimum depending on how the trace is oriented†), the vocal folds are in maximum contact. When the EGG trace is the opposite state, the vocal

---

† Many authors orient the waveform so that an increase in waveform deflection represents increased contact area. Others orient the waveform so that increased vocal fold contact area is shown as a downward deflection, as shown in Figure 14-5.

folds are in minimum contact, presumably open. It is possible to measure timing relationships in the EGG waveform as illustrated in Figure 14-5. From such waveforms, it is possible to measure the *opening* and *closing* time as well as the *closed* time of the vocal folds. It is also possible to measure the *total time* of a cycle of vibration. From the measurements of open time and total time, an *open quotient,* or *abduction quotient,* can be computed. The open quotient (OQ) is the ratio of the open time to the total time. When multiplied by 100, OQ can be expressed as a percentage of the open time. It provides an estimate of the work performed by the vocal folds to produce the acoustic pulse. Another quotient that can be computed is the *closed quotient,* the ratio of the closed time to the total time of vibration. The *speed quotient (SQ)* is the ratio of the opening time to the closing time of the vocal folds. The *speed index (SI)*[43] can be derived from the speed quotient by the following formula:

$$\frac{\text{Opening time} - \text{closing time}}{\text{Opening time} + \text{closing time}} \quad or \quad \frac{SQ - 1}{SQ + 1}$$

According to Hirano et al,[44] the SI is superior to SQ in providing a visual impression of the shape of the glottal waveform. An SI close to -1 implies a very rapid opening phase and a rather slow (or much slower) closing phase. Equal opening and closing times would produce an SI of zero. Slow opening phases and very rapid closing phases produce SIs close to 1. The range of variation of SI is between -1 and +1, whereas SQ ranges between zero and some large positive number. Waveform variations such as these in the acoustic pulse will produce differences in the spectrum of the glottal tone and voice quality.

Glottal Area Variations During the Vocal Fold Cycle

Movement patterns of the vocal folds affect the area of glottal opening. It is possible to record the opening of the glottis using a variety of techniques. These include high-speed photography, videostrobolaryngoscopy, and photoglottography.

High-speed photography captures the motion of the vocal folds by exposing very sensitive film at rates up to 5000 frames per second or more. At these rates, a single cycle of vibration produced at 100 Hz would occupy about 50 frames and the time resolution per frame would be 0.2 ms. This resolution would provide a very good estimate of the details of the vibratory cycle either by measuring the actual movement of the vocal folds or the glottal area changes within the cycle. Considerable information has been collected about the vocal fold vibratory cycle by this technique, in spite of its expense,

the need for expertise, and the time needed for its successful implementation.

Videostrobolaryngoscopy (VSL) is a tool used more and more in the ear, nose, and throat clinic. It is also a good research tool when used appropriately. The patient's voice is analyzed to determine the fundamental frequency, which is used to control the frequency of the light flashes illuminating the vocal folds. Usually there is a slight difference between the two frequencies (about 1 1/2 cycles) in order to produce the illusion of a slow vibratory motion of the vocal folds. Typically, one apparent vibratory cycle occupies about 20 video frames. This rate would produce a time resolution in the apparent vibratory cycle of 50 ms, considerably greater than for high-speed films. On the other hand, stroboscopy is much easier to use, is less expensive, and can be used successfully with a much greater number of patients. Stroboscopy is discussed in further detail in Chapter 11.

In today's cost-conscious health care environment, the single most clinically useful tool in the management of voice problems is undoubtedly the VSL unit. Despite its inherent limitations,[43] it is very simple to use and has become widely accepted in the assessment of vocal vibratory function. Add-on features, such as computer integration and statistics, the fundamental frequency, decibel output, and other waveforms superimposed and displayed on screen (see Figure 14-6), result in conven-

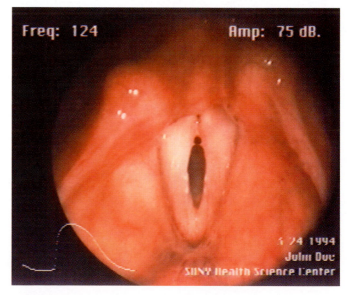

FIGURE 14-6. *Video print of a captured image from a stroboscopic examination. In the upper left corner, the fundamental frequency of the phonation is displayed, whereas the SPL of the phonation is displayed on the upper right corner. In the lower right corner, the data of the examination, the patient's name, and the center performing the examination are displayed.*

ient and practical data collection from patients. Although interpretation of VSL requires some experience, once this experience is gained, a myriad of voice problems and pathologic conditions may be revealed. Objective reporting of VSL observation is not yet standardized. However, automated estimates of glottal areas and amplitudes are being developed using computerized image analysis techniques (Figure 14-7).

Photoglottography is a technique in which a bright light is shown through the vocal folds‡ and recorded using a photocell. The light waveform mirrors the area waveform reasonably well[45-49] and can be used to study the details of the vocal fold vibratory cycle. It has the advantage of being inexpensive, easy to use, and reliable. Of course, it is an indirect measure of actual vocal fold movement and, indeed, an indirect measure of glottal area.

VIDEOKYMOGRAPHY AND HIGH-SPEED DIGITAL IMAGING OF THE LARYNX

Limitations of Videostroboscopy

Videostroboscopy is the most easily applicable technology for assessment of vocal function. However, it has inherent limitations that are based on the principle of stroboscopy. Primarily, stroboscopy is appropriate for examination of pseudo-periodic vibrations. This makes stroboscopy suboptimal for examination of phonations which are not periodic. Rapid changes in periodicity of vocal fold motion makes the frequency detector of the stroboscope unable to keep up. Where the periodicity of vocal vibration may be contaminated by multiple periodic voice sources, the stroboscope may indicate rapidly changing frequencies or frequency doubling which is not in keeping with clinical observations. Because the intrinsic theory and application of stroboscopy is dependent on a periodic voice, many pathologic conditions of voice are not adequately visualized by videostroboscopy. Some specific pathologic conditions where stroboscopic examination fail are in patients with voice characteristics of vocal tremor, voice breaks, and diplophonia. Other pathologic voice conditions that are difficult to resolve with videostroboscopy are short vocal gestures that are not frequency-locked. thus the onset of phonation, offset of phonation, and production of rapid vocal gestures cannot be resolved with conventional means using videostroboscopy. In some pathologic conditions, the voice source is to be examined during the voice production of vocal register transitions. Examination of larynx and vocal fold vibration during the production of voice as it is going from chest voice to head voice, or during voice production as the singer is gliding down from falsetto to modal voice has not been possible with traditional videostroboscopy techniques.

‡ The light usually is directed from above the vocal folds as it is convenient to use the light from the continuous light source often found in routine fiberoptic endoscopy.

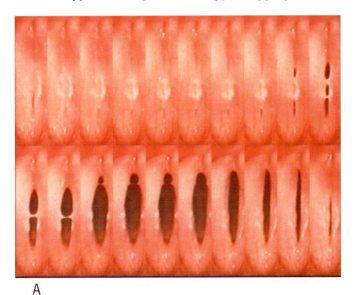

A

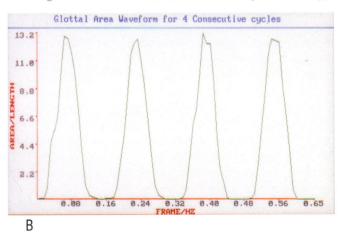

B

Figure 14-7. *(A) Video print of successive captured images of a single "cycle" of vocal fold vibration as captured in a stroboscopic examination. This print was prepared by selecting a small area of interest (eg, the vocal folds), capturing a frame using a video frame grabber, and then advancing the tape one video frame to capture another frame. This process was continued until 20 frames were captured. (B) Plot of glottal area as a function of time for four successive stroboscopic cycles of vocal fold vibration.*

These problems have prompted investigators to find a laryngoscopic method not limited to periodic vibrations. Laryngeal photokymography was first reported by Gall[50] in 1984. With the realization of a line-scanning camera that is practical[51,52] laryngeal videokymography has gained some popularity as a clinical tool for the examination of vocal fold vibration. Ultra-high-speed cinematography, first developed in the Bell Telephone Laboratories in the 1930s, has served as a research tool. This technique is impractical in the clinical arena. This cinematographic technique has been supplanted by digital high-speed imaging systems. With the cost reduction of high-speed digital systems, high-speed digital imaging systems may soon be applicable in the clinical examination of vocal fold vibration. This technique may offer the most powerful method for processing and evaluating vocal fold vibrations. High-speed digital video and videokymography with high-speed line scanning of vocal fold vibration are novel but promising technologies which can be used in basic research and clinical applications.

Videokymography

Videokymography is an imaging system in which a standard CCD camera is used to scan a single line at a defined point of interest at very fast rates and display this line as a rater display on the video monitor. The principle of Videokymography is based on the fact that each video frame is composed of 512 lines at thirty frames per second. By selection of a single line, much greater rates of scanning can be achieved. This single line scanning is achieved at the cost of two-dimensional spatial resolution since only a single line is displayed. The overall scanning rate of a single line scanning camera using conventional camera is on the order if 8,000 frames per second. The successive line from the scanning line camera is displayed on a monitor with the time dimension in the vertical axis. Thus the time scrolls vertically at a rate of 144 consecutive line images per half frame. Each monitor frame represents a time interval of 18.4 milliseconds. The initial development of line scanning CCD camera usable for clinical applications was in Groningen by Schutte and Svec.[51,52] This special CCD video camera can work in two modes. In the first mode, the system functions as a normal black and white commercial video camera. Recordings occur at 50 images per second onto standard videotape. In the second mode, the Videokymography mode, the camera is able to record images of a single cross section of the vibrating portion of the vocal folds at a rate of 7812.5 images per second. Instead of registering the whole image of the vocal folds, the imaging system reads just a single line of the image. The successive line images are presented on a commercial television monitor and show the vibra-

tory pattern of the selected part of the vocal folds. Videokymography uses a standard videolaryngoscopic set-up with a continuous light source. Both the normal and high-speed Videokymography images are recorded and displayed by means of a standard video recorder. Switching between the two modes of the camera is controlled by a foot switch.

Schutte, Svec, and Sram[53] first reported on the clinical use of Videokymography for evaluation of vibratory function. Videokymography is able to display the pattern of vocal fold vibration in one image that summarizes all the vibratory cycles at the line of interest. It is possible to trace the vocal fold vibration in very hoarse and breathy voices where videostroboscopy may fail. By study of different points of interest, differences in phase and amplitude abnormalities between the right and left vocal folds can be detected. By being able to look at every glottal cycle during phonation, quantitative measures may be obtained, which otherwise would be impossible with videostroboscopy. Much as quantification was done in a laborious way with high-speed imaging in the 1950s as a research instrument, Videokymography can be applied in a much simpler method to demonstrate the successive cycle of the glottal vibratory pattern.

In studies of normal and pathologic vocal vibratory function, a considerable amount of information has been documented. In a study of normal vocal folds, one can observe that the normal vocal folds may vibrate irregularly and show asymmetries and irregularities. For example, the production of an abnormal voice by normal vocal apparatus shows abnormal vibratory patterns such as double vocal fold openings in a single glottal cycle, presence of sub harmonic vibratory pattern, and transient phase asymmetries. Videokymography allows for investigation into the normal variability of the vocal mechanism. In a study of subjects with voice disorders, the presence of subtle phase shift abnormalities and cycle-to-cycle asymmetric vibrations could be documented better than with videostroboscopy alone. In a publication using both Videokymography and stroboscopy, the authors concluded that the two techniques are complementary.[53] While the stroboscopy examination gives good spatial resolution of vocal fold vibration and its abnormalities along the length of the vocal fold, Videokymography is especially helpful in irregular vocal fold oscillation where stroboscopy fails. The possibility of line rater display of real time vibratory function of the vocal fold makes this technology desirable in research applications involving dysphonia.

Line scanning using Videokymography may offer many new details on how vocal folds begin and end oscillation and on how the vocal folds behave during rapid laryngeal adjustments. In going from the steady state of vocal fold oscillation to the full cessation of vocal fold oscillation, a number of glottal cycles are necessary to dampen the vibratory amplitude from steady state oscillation to full stop. How pathologic conditions affect the beginning and end of vocal fold oscillation are areas that can be easily observed using Videokymography. The qualitative and quantitative aspects of this is just beginning to be understood.

Despite the clinical availability of Videokymography equipment, there continue to be some disadvantages. One disadvantage of Videokymography is the lack of spatial resolution of the image. The image is displayed as a line tracing with the time axis in the vertical Y-axis. The exact line of scanning must be presumed to be steady during the scanning as one must switch between the regular two-dimensional display modes and the one-dimensional line scanning mode. The interpretation of the line scanning display is not intuitive and requires training, even for those with expertise in videostroboscopy interpretation. Despite the specialized power of line scanning cameras, interpretation of the Videokymography image must still be considered an area most clinicians are not yet ready to apply to day-to-day practice.

High-Speed Video Imaging of Vocal Vibration

Many investigations studying vocal vibratory function have used ultra high-speed photography. The high-speed cinematography results published by Von Leden, Moore, and Timcke showed many examples of variations of normal vibration that could not be resolved easily.[54] These include: dichotic phonation, vocal fry, and asymmetry of cycle-to-cycle vibratory abnormalities. Hirose and coworkers were the first to use a high-speed digital image camera for the observation of vocal fold vibration.[55] Recently, several authors have reported on high-speed video imaging to examine normal and pathologic laryngeal vibrations.[56-58] Improvement in imaging cameras and software has made the digital high-speed imaging camera a clinically available tool in the investigation of vocal fold vibratory abnormalities. One of the systems is available as an add-on camera to the computer digital stroboscopy unit. The camera can record at rates of 2,000 frames per second to 4,000 frames per second in black and white. The resolution is variable. At a frame rate of 2,000 frames per second, the resolution is quite acceptable. The duration of capture is set at two seconds, but this is adjustable depending on how much flash memory is available. Play back of the high-speed video is variable and is usually set at 15 frames per second. Using simple math, a two-second display of high-speed digital requires 4.44 minutes of viewing in slow

motion mode! This makes practical analysis of high-speed video quite cumbersome unless there is a method of data reduction. To reduce the amount of video that must be analyzed, it is possible to define an area of interest from the initial video frame and perform a "digital" Videokymography display of the data. In this way, multiple digital Videokymography displays may be obtained without sacrificing spatial resolution and without laborious viewing of the video display. Furthermore, data reduction of the spatial image using signal and image analysis techniques may be applied. New technologies of signal analysis and image analysis can and certainly will be developed to aid in the clinical assessment of abnormal vocal fold oscillation using this technology.

Two areas where digital high-speed images will offer new insight on vocal fold behavior will be illustrated. The first example is in the initial production of phonation and variation with loudness and frequency changes. The second example is in the clinical investigation of vibratory transient sounds such as voice breaks and diplophonia sounds.

Normal Onset and Offset of Vocal Fold Oscillation

Laryngeal movements and adjustments are seen before and after vocal fold oscillation. First, there is vocal fold adduction with symmetric medial movements. The vocal processes are adducted gently. This is followed by vocal fold oscillation. The event before the vocal fold oscillation and the production of sound is termed the pre-phonatory set. The pre-phonatory set has a variable degree of movement, duration, and approximation. The pre-phonatory set and the actual vibration of the vocal folds may occur in an overlapping manner. Thus while the vocal fold is still being adducted and the vocal process is being placed into position, vocal fold oscillation has already started. Oscillation occurs initially with small oscillations of the medial margin. These then build up to larger oscillations until a set configuration of vocal fold oscillation has been achieved. The steady state of vocal fold vibration can then be defined as having steady state amplitude, phase, and glottal contact. Once the vocal fold oscillations are steady, quasi-periodic vibrations can be seen and one glottal cycle resembles the other. Once steady state oscillation is achieved, the phonatory cycle shows definable open and closed period with defined vibratory amplitude, mucosal wave, and open and closed quotient. The number of glottal cycles necessary before the achievement of full vocal fold oscillation is variable. This appears to be dependent on factors such as frequency, loudness, and glottal attack effort.

At the end of the voice gesture, the vocal folds stop oscillating slowly. The number of glottal cycles for this to occur is variable depending on vocal effort, frequency, and vocal gesture. This slow declination of vocal fold oscillation from the steady state of vibration to the cessation of vibration is termed vocal fold offset. It is believed to be dependent on the stiffness and the mass of the vocal folds. Vocal folds vibrating at loud phonation and low phonation have greater amplitude. The number of cycles for vocal folds to stop vibration is greater in low loud phonation than high soft phonation.

Much new information may be obtained by systematic analysis of the onset and offset phase of vocal fold vibrations in normal and pathologic conditions using high-speed video. One possible application is in the evaluation of the effect of voice therapy. Another is in the evaluation of neurologically based dysphonia such as spasmodic dysphonia.

Clinical Application of High-Speed Imaging in Diplophonia

Vocal pathologies resulting in diplophonia are particularly difficult to resolve with videostroboscopy. This is because the tracking of the frequency of vocal fold vibration by the stroboscope is dependent on a single frequency. When there are two distinct frequencies or when there are multiple sub harmonics of oscillations, the tracking of the stroboscope becomes inaccurate. In a study of patients with diplophonia, multiple etiologies may contribute to the diplophonic sound. Thus, diplophonia may be produced by some normal subjects voluntarily, it may be present in patients with vocal fold paralysis, vocal fold scarring, or in patients with mass lesions. High-speed digital video has been able to define several patterns that are present in patients with diplophonia.

Diplophonia is the consequence of irregular vocal fold vibration. Several interesting patterns were associated with different pathologies. It is useful to analyze these patterns by tension, mass, or stiffness results on vocal fold vibration and further differentiate them by whether there is unilateral or bilateral involvement. There appear to be three major patterns. These are the tension pattern, the stiffness pattern, and the mass pattern.

Tension pattern is best seen in the patient with vocal cord paralysis. The vocal fold that has intrinsic tension will tend to vibrate faster than the vocal fold that is not innervated and therefore flaccid. The intrinsic coupling of the vibration between the vocal folds may result in each vocal fold vibrating in synchrony but this system may fall apart with inadequate breath support or adjustments of the supraglottic articulators. This will then result in two different frequencies of the vocal folds vibrating with the same subglottic pressure. The net effect of two different

vocal folds vibrating at different frequencies is the creation of phase shifts as the vocal folds vibrate in and then out of phase at predictable rates.

Stiffness pattern is seen in patients with scarring laryngitis and other inflammatory effects of the vocal fold cover. In this pattern the patient may be speaking in vocal fry with a predominantly rough voice quality. This is seen as two vibration patterns. A small glottal opening in an alternating manner follows a large glottal opening. The key difference between the stiffness versus the tension pattern is that both vocal folds participate in the alternation of glottal cycle. The sub harmonics that are created may be every other beat, every third beat, or every fourth beat of the fundamental frequency.

Mass pattern is seen when there is another mass that is initiated as an oscillatory structure by the air stream. This may be due to the mass lesion, the arytenoid mucosa, or the false vocal folds. When the mass has periodic vibration it will then contribute to the acoustics. When the mass is on the vocal folds, it may interfere with the affected vocal fold by alteration of the glottal cycle. Because most masses of the vocal folds vibrate at a lower frequency, the resultant periodic sound source will be in one of the sub harmonics of the sound source spectrum.

The role of high-speed digital imaging in clinical care of the patient with dysphonia is just beginning. An ideal role would be as a complementary tool to videostroboscopy. High-speed digital imaging should offer new information on pathology or pathophysiology of phonation that could not otherwise be obtained. The investigation of voices characterized by diplophonia and voice breaks in a variety of voice disorders is an obvious application for high-speed digital imaging.

Glottal Area

The glottal area may be measured using any one of the above techniques and involves sampling the area at successive time points in the vocal fold vibratory cycle. From these area-versus-time waveforms, estimates of the fundamental frequency of vibration can be obtained. If calibration data are available, measurements of the real glottal areas can be made and compared with those of other patients or with those of the same patient at different points during treatment. Measures of peak area and average area are possible. Measurements of OQ, closed quotient, SQ, and SI, as previously defined above, can also be made. In fact, all these measurements were originally defined and made from high-speed films.

Vocal Fold Vibratory Cycle

The vocal fold vibratory cycle, like the glottal area cycle, can be captured using the techniques of high-speed photography, and stroboscopy. In addition, EGG can be used to look at the closing and closed phases of the vocal fold vibratory cycle. The most direct measurements are those made when one is able to visualize the vocal folds, as in high-speed photography and stroboscopy. When visible, measurements of the width and length of the vocal folds are possible as are measurements of the movements of selected points along the length of the vocal folds. The actual speed of movement of the vocal folds can be measured. One potentially important measurement is the speed of the mucosal wave. Such measurements may then be compared with those made on normal speakers.

Aerodynamic Properties

Subglottal Air Pressures

The pressures beneath the vocal folds are important in determining the intensity of the acoustic pulse and the spectrum of the acoustic pulse and indirectly reflect the resistance of the vocal folds to vibration and the fundamental frequency. These pressures may be measured with a variety of techniques, including esophageal balloon, tracheal puncture, and indirect estimates via measurement of intraoral air pressure.

Esophageal balloon movements involve the placement of a latex balloon attached to the end of a catheter into the nose and then into the esophagus. The balloon is positioned in the esophagus immediately behind and below the cricoid cartilage using either direct visualization with x-ray films or, as is most often done, indirect visualization, by measuring the distance from the nares to the balloon tip. Pressures in the subglottal region are reflected in the esophagus through the membrane and muscle sheath connecting the tracheal rings posteriorly. The end of the tube exiting at the nares is connected to a pressure transducer and senses the differential pressures within the esophagus. Care must be taken with this technique as the magnitudes of the pressures are affected by the amount of air in the lungs and the locations on the pressure-volume curve at which the measurements are taken.[59]

Tracheal puncture is a technique in which a needle is inserted between two tracheal rings and perpendicular to the air stream. The needle is connected to a pressure transducer and used to record directly the pressure beneath the vocal folds.[59] An alternative to the puncture technique is to pass a miniature transducer through the vocal folds and allow it to remain in the subglottal area to register pressure variations.[60] This technique has the advantage of recording the rapid fluctuations of pressure that occur during phonation. Both this and the puncture technique are invasive, require care in placement, may require medical attention, and limit the tasks that the patient can perform. Pressure measurements are important in interpreting aerodynamic events and should be performed wherever possible.

Another technique for estimating subglottal pressures involves the measurement of the intraoral pressure produced during the production of stop consonants like /p/ or /b/. The theory[61-63] is that during the production of these consonants, the pressure within the oral cavity is the same as the pressure elsewhere in the respiratory tract if there is no significant closure of the vocal folds. During the production of a voiceless consonant, the vocal folds are not vibrating and therefore should not impose any significant obstruction to the airflow from the lungs. Thus, the pressure behind the oral constriction is the same everywhere and would reflect the pressure available to drive the vocal folds if they were to vibrate.

A patient is asked to produce a series of /pV/ or /bVp/ syllables.§ The intraoral air pressure is recorded as shown in Figure 14-8. Peak pressures during the production of the consonant are measured and used to estimate the subglottal pressure during the initial production of the vowel in the syllable. The technique has found widespread use in estimating subglottal pressure.[64-71]

Pressure is usually reported in pascal units (or subunits called kilopascals, kPa). One Pa is equal to 10^4 dyne/cm^2. Pressure measurements reflect a combination of effects within the larynx and respiratory system. The pressure is affected by the magnitude of the respiratory effort, the intensity of phonation, the fundamental frequency of phonation, and the degree and type of vocal effort used to phonate. Together with airflow and vocal intensity, it can be used to estimate the efficiency of phonation by a patient. Vocal efficiency is defined as the ration of the acoustic power to the aerodynamic power and can be estimated by dividing the acoustic intensity of the utterance by the product of the air pressure and the airflow used to produce the utterance. Although not routinely calculated, vocal efficiency should be a regular

§ Commenting on the Smitheran and Hixon[63] technique for estimating subglottal pressure Rothenberg[62] suggested the use of a /bVp/ syllable in order to reduce the potential effect of aspiration of the /p/ on pressure measurements; he said the additional consonant in the syllable would cause the vocal folds to be adducted again at or just before the articulatory release. This, he claims, would reduce the drop of subglottal pressure caused by the /p/ aspiration. Most investigators have used Smitheran and Hixon's original suggestions on the choice of syllable and have used a simple /pV/ syllable.

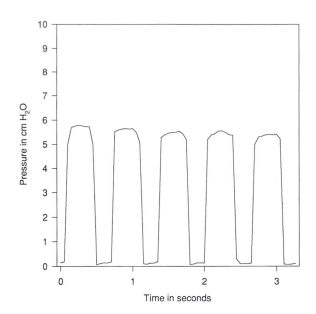

FIGURE 14-8. *Series of intraoral pressure traces recorded during the production of a series of /bVp/ syllables. Measurements of the peak pressure on each syllable are made, and a line is drawn between these peaks. The line is used to estimate the pressure during the production of the vowel in the syllable. Of course, when the vocal folds vibrate, the pressure beneath them decreases. Thus, the estimate is only valid during the initial portion of the vowel.*

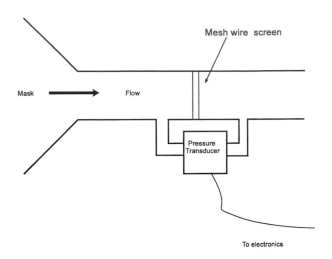

FIGURE 14-9. *Schematic of a pneumotachograph.*

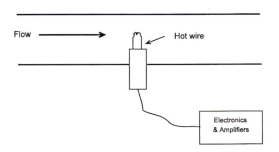

FIGURE 14-10. *Schematic of an HWA.*

measurement of phonatory function for both normal and pathologic speakers.[72-77]

Another measurement that may have great clinical utility is phonation threshold pressure (PTP).[78,79] This is defined as the minimum pressure required to initiate phonation. Titze and his colleagues have shown that peak flow, OQ, and SQ all depend on PTP. Thus, interpretation of these parameters and how they might relate to vocal fold vibration requires knowledge about the magnitude of PTP.

Transglottal Airflow

The airflows through the glottis depend on a number of factors including the subglottal air pressure, the PTP, the resistance of the vocal folds to vibration, and the area of opening of the glottis (for some measurements of airflow). Airflow may be recorded using a pneumotachograph, hot wire anemometer, or the Rothenberg mask.

A pneumotachograph is a tube within which is placed a fine mesh wire screen in order to create a resistance to airflow (see Figure 14-9). The resistance results in a pressure difference across the screen that is measured with a pressure transducer. Greater flows

produce a greater pressure difference; thus, pressure measurements can be used to estimate the airflow rates. The configuration of the mask and tube system determines the frequency response of the system, and standard pneumotachographs, because of their large masks and tubes, typically have a very low frequency response. Airflows measured with a pneumotachograph represent the average flow across several cycles of vibration.

The hot wire anemometer (HWA) may offer a flow-measuring system with a much higher frequency response. It operates on the principle that when air flows, it reduces the temperature of a wire through which a constant amount of current is flowing (see Figure 14-10). This results in a change of resistance of the wire and a change in the voltage across the wire. In this way, changes of airflow are reflected in changes of voltage. The HWA is very sensitive to changes in the ambient temperature and must be operated in a stable temperature environment, or be compensated for any temperature changes. They are also insensitive to

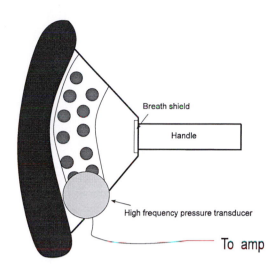

FIGURE 14-11. *Schematic of a circumferentially exhausted face mask.*

changes in the direction of current flow, although modifications have been made to sense flow direction. The HWA measures flows within the immediate vicinity of the wire, flows that may not be representative of the total volume flow of air.[80] However, with care and appropriate electronics, the HWA can be used routinely to measure airflow in the laboratory and clinic.[81-85]

The Rothenberg mask may be thought of a special version of a pneumotachograph. It has the advantage of possessing a much higher frequency response range than a standard pneumotachograph. Consequently, it is capable of recording the rapid airflow variations that occur during a vocal cycle, up to about 2000 Hz.[86,87] The mask is illustrated in Figure 14-11. The airflows recorded with the Rothenberg mask are the product of the flows through the glottis and the effects of the resonators in the vocal tract. In order to obtain estimates of the volume velocity airflow through the glottis, the recorded airflow must be inverse-filtered to remove the resonant effects. Inverse filtering is a technique[70,86,88,89] that reverses the effects of the vocal tract and produces an estimate of the glottal airflow waveform during vibration either from the acoustic signal[89] or from the oral airflow waveform.[86,87] An example waveform derived from inverse filtering of the orally emitted airflow waveform is shown in Figure 14-12. In the same figure, an example of a waveform derived from an HWA is also shown.

Airflow and Airflow Waveforms

The average airflow during a phonation can be measured with any of the techniques discussed. It is an extremely useful measure since it reflects the amount of air used during the phonation and may indirectly reflect the efficiency of phonation (although a better estimate

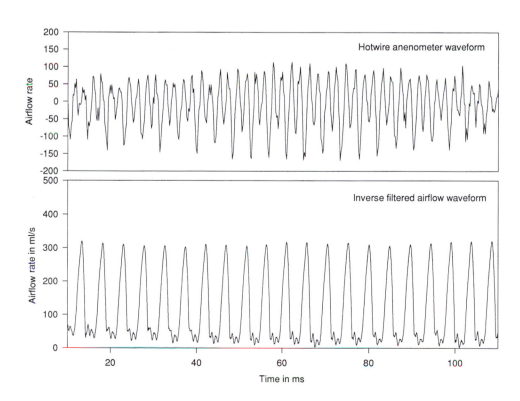

FIGURE 14-12. *Example of waveforms produced by a HWA (top trace) and inverse filtering.*

of vocal efficiency may be obtained by measuring sub-glottal pressure and vocal intensity in addition to air-flow). Patients with phonatory problems show variations of average airflow rate, especially before and after treatment.

The remaining measures must be obtained from a technique that records the airflow rate variations during a cycle of vibration. Peak airflow is the maximum airflow during the cycle, whereas leakage airflow rates‖ reflect the airflows when the vocal folds are presumably closed. Both peak and leakage flows contribute to a high average flow rate, but in average flow, one cannot determine whether its magnitude is primarily determined by large peak flows or by large leakage flows. Open time and OQ can be calculated from recordings obtained with a technique that tracks the airflow variations in a cycle. In addition, opening or closing time or SQ and SI can be calculated from such recordings. These measurements presumably reflect the work done by the vocal folds during a vibratory cycle. Of course, these measurements, because they are made on the airflow pulse, are one step removed from the acoustic pulse that ultimately determines the spectrum and the voice quality of the tone produced.

WHAT TO MEASURE IN THE ACOUSTIC OUTPUT OF THE VOCAL FOLDS

Frequency of Vibration

The frequency of vibration is an important acoustic measurement because it reflects the contributions of muscle activity, passive tissue parameters, subglottal air pressure, and glottal resistance of the vocal folds. The fundamental frequency of the tone produced by the vocal folds reflects their vibrating frequency. It is usually the lowest frequency present in the tone.

Fundamental frequency is determined by the activity of the CT and TA muscles (primarily) and the mass and passive tension of the vocal folds.[90-95] Men, because they have larger larynges than women, typically exhibit lower fundamental frequencies than women[94] or children of either sex. During conversational speech, men typically exhibit average fundamental frequencies between 100 and 150 Hz, whereas women typically have average fun-

damental frequencies between 190 and 250 Hz (see Table 14-2). Fundamental frequency varies as a function of age in both sexes, and its magnitude is higher in the youngest and oldest age groups (see Figure 14-13).

Fundamental frequency also varies during speech production. When fundamental frequency is measured over a reasonably long time period (eg, paragraph, speech, etc.), it is reported as the standard deviation (SD) of frequency, or if fundamental frequency is expressed in semitones FL, pitch sigma.# Fundamental frequency variation may also be measured over a short time duration, usually adjacent cycles of vibration. This variation is referred to as frequency perturbation or jitter. It may be expressed in units of time (usually milliseconds or microseconds) or as a ratio measure of the average period differences divided by the average period of utterance.** Average jitter factors as reported by Casper[96] for three normal speaking adults in three age groups are shown in Table 14-3.

Jitter reflects the stability of vocal fold vibration. It is thought to be the result of irregular neural impulses,[97,98] variations of heart beats,[99-101] and/or variations in the dynamics of tissue response to vibration.[102] Vocal jitter correlates with perceptual judgments of hoarseness and roughness.[103,104] It is known that jitter increases when there is a pathologic lesion on the vocal folds.[105-111]

Vocal Intensity

Vocal intensity refers to the power of the tone produced at the vocal folds. Although it is common to refer to vocal power, rarely is the actual power of the sound measured. Instead, the SPL of the voice sound is measured. This is because it is relatively easy and cheaper to make instruments to measure sound pressure than to measure power. Most microphones are pressure-measuring devices. As there is a known relationship between sound power (intensity) and sound pressure,†† one can

---

‖ Another term for *leakage airflow* is minimum airflow rate. This is simply defined as the minimum flow during the cycle. Practically, both measurements are defined in the same way, but the term *leakage flow* presumes that there is an opening somewhere along the total length of the vocal folds through which air can flow.

In much of the early literature, the results of measurements of fundamental frequency were reported in terms of semitones FL. *FL* refers to the *frequency level* scale that has a base frequency of 16.35 Hz, and the unit of measurement is the semitone. A semitone is a unit with a ratio between two frequencies of 1.059:1 (approximately). Larger units are also defined, such as the octave (2:1 ratio) and tone (1.122:1 ratio). Most western music is based on this scale.

** If the ratio is multiplied by 100, the result is called *jitter factor.* If the ratio is multiplied by 1000, it is referred to as the *jitter ratio.* See Baken[95] for further details.

†† Intensity $\approx$ pressure^2

Speech Condition	Male		Female	
	Mean	SD	Mean	SD
Spontaneous Speech				
In hertz	123.3	19.67		
In semitones	34.98	3.2		
Reading				
In hertz	129.4	19.67	224	20.34
In semitones	35.8	3.2	45.3	3.78

Source: Based on data presented by Hollien et al.[142]

TABLE 14-2. *Mean and Standard Deviation of Fundamental Frequency for Normal Male and Female Young Adults*

easily relate the two measurements. The SPL is actually a ratio measurement of pressure. The reference pressure is about 20 µPa, and the unit of measurement is the decibel (dB).

The average sound pressure level for an utterance can be measured with sound level meters (for example, devices made by B&K Instruments or Radio Shack) or

Fundamental Frequency

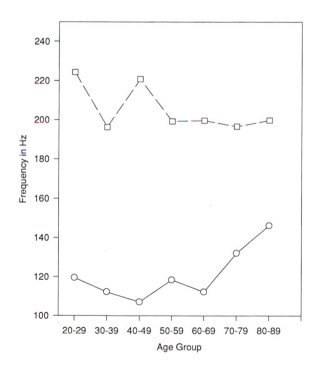

FIGURE 14-13. *Fundamental frequency as a function of age in normal speakers. (Data are based on Hollien et al.[142])* ○ = male. □ = female.

Group	Age Group	Jitter Factor	
		/i/	/u/
Male	20-29	0.80	0.72
	40-49	0.99	0.85
	60-69	0.91	0.84
Female	20-29	0.57	0.58
	40-49	0.65	0.61
	60-69	0.62	0.73

Source: Data based on Casper.[96]

TABLE 14-3. *Mean Jitter Factor Measurements for 20 Normal-Speaking Male and Female Subject Groups in Each of Three Age Decades for the Vowels /i/ and /u/*

with calibrated microphone and amplifier systems. It reflects the approximate energy in the vocal fold tone. However, vocal intensity is also strongly influenced by the vocal tract resonators. Simply spreading or pursing the lips can make a difference of 3 to 5 dB in the measured intensity. Thus, one needs to be cautious about interpreting SPL measurements and must specify the nature of the speech material used.

Sustained vowels probably have the greatest face validity as reflecting the sound power produced by the vocal folds as their major energy is provided by the vocal folds, and if a vowel with little constriction in the vocal tract is used, the intensity is not markedly affected by the vocal tract. The average vocal intensity is also greatly dependent on the speaker. Thus, average vocal intensity is subject to greater variability within an utterance and at different sample times.

The variability of vocal intensity, like fundamental frequency, can vary long and short-term. Long-term variation occurs over sentences, paragraphs, or larger speech utterances. It is usually reported as the standard deviation of the mean. Short-term variation, like frequency perturbation, is the variation of SPL that occurs from one cycle to the next. It is called amplitude perturbation or shimmer and may be reported in average decibels of difference among adjacent cycles or as a ratio of decibel differences divided by the average intensity of the utterance. Some shimmer data for normal-speaking adults are reported in Table 14-4.

Acoustic Spectrum

Spectrum refers to the individual frequency components of a tone and their amplitudes. The vocal folds produce a complex tone consisting of a fundamental frequency and a number of frequencies usually harmonically related to the fundamental frequency. The spectrum of the vocal fold tone may remain reasonably constant over a finite time period or it may change drastically within short periods of time. The instantaneous, or short-term, spectrum reflects the spectral characteristics for a very short period of time, for example, 20 to 30 ms. One method of analyzing and displaying an instantaneous spectrum produces a spectrogram. One could also compute a fast Fourier transform (FFT) to obtain the same results. An example of a vowel segment FFT computed over a time interval of 20 ms is shown in Figure 14-14. It is possible (although not very likely) that another FFT computed 20 ms later than the one shown in Figure 14-14 would show very different results.

If the spectrum is analyzed from recorded speech, it will reflect the characteristics of both the vocal folds and the vocal tract acting as a resonator. If one desires the spectrum of the vocal fold tone, the resonant effects of the vocal tract must be eliminated or neutralized. One method for neutralizing the effects of the vocal tract is by computing the long-term spectrum (LTAS) of an utterance. LTAS is obtained by simply analyzing the spectrum at many points in time of an utterance and averaging the results. Rapid spectral changes associated with consonants are reduced by the averaging technique. The averaged spectrum reflects primarily the long-term spectral characteristics of the utterance, primarily the spectral characteristics of the vocal folds, and the overall resonance characteristics of the vocal tract. An example of

	Shimmer		
Group	/ʌ/	/i/	/u/
Males (*n* = 31)	0.47	0.37	0.33
Females (*n* = 20)	0.33	0.23	0.19

Source: Data for male speakers from Horii;[143] data for female speakers from Sorensen and Horii.[144]

TABLE 14-4. *Mean Shimmer for a Group of Normal Male and Female Speakers Producing the Vowels /ʌ/, /i/, and /u/*

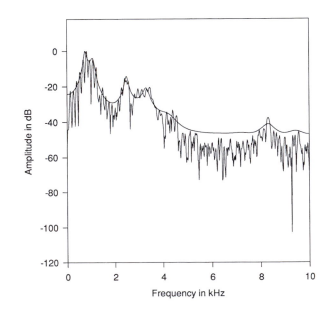

FIGURE 14-14. *FFT of a short segment of a sustained vowel from a normal speaker.*

an LTAS analysis of a simple sentence is shown in Figure 14-15. Note that the strongest part of the spectrum occurs between 500 and 2000 Hz. This spectrum is actually quite different from the spectrum typically associated with the vocal folds (Figure 14-16). However, LTAS may be a measurement of acoustic spectrum as it reflects more closely what a listener might hear from a subject or patient. there have been many reports on the LTAS of normal and pathologic voice production.[112-125] This is a very promising technique and one that can be easily implemented in the ear, nose, and throat or speech pathology clinic.

Phonation Time

There are several measures in which the maximum duration that a subject can produce on a single breath is recorded. These measures presumably reflect the degree of respiratory control or the efficiency of the conversion of airflow and pressures into sound. Maximum phonation time (MPT) is the duration of phonation an individual can produce on one expiratory breath. It is usually recorded on the vowel /ɑ/ and may be considered an index of phonatory control. Some typical MPTs of normal subjects are presented in Table 14-5. There are also data on MPTs of children and the elderly. A summary of the results for normal speakers as a function of age is shown in Figure 14-17. One of the difficulties with MPT is that a patient may not be able to produce a maximum

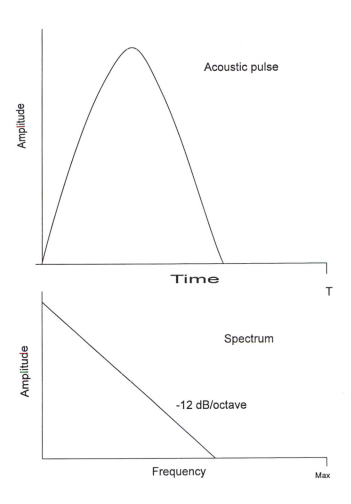

FIGURE 14-16. *Schematic spectrum characteristic of the vocal folds at conversational frequencies.*

time, at least not on the first try. Repeated trials are often needed before a reliable estimate of the true MPT is obtained. Kent et al[126] discussed some of the findings of studies in which the performance of subjects on maximum tests of phonation were investigated. Clear

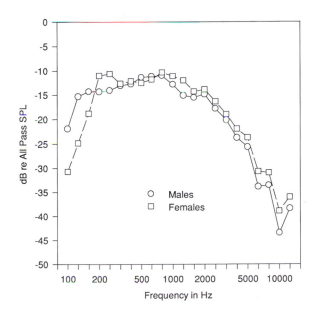

One Third Octave LTAS

FIGURE 14-15. *LTAS of a paragraph produced by male and female speakers.*

Group	Mean	SD	95% Confidence Interval
Male	34.6	11.75	30.2-39.4
Female	25.7	7.5	22.9-28.7

Source: Adapted from Hirano et al.[145]

TABLE 14-5. *Mean Maximum Phonation Times for 25 Normal-Speaking Men and 25 Normal-Speaking Women*

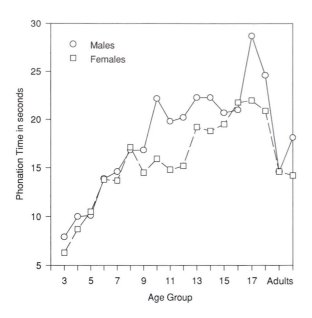

FIGURE 14-17. *Mean MPTs as a function of age. (Data are drawn from references 145 and 146.)*

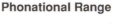
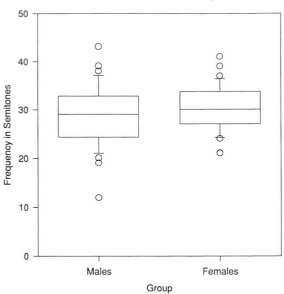

FIGURE 14-18. *Mean phonational ranges, in semitones, of a group of 35 normal-speaking male and 27 normal-speaking female subjects.*

instructions,[127] the number of trials,[128] and effects of modeling[129] were considered, and cautions were provided to those interested in obtaining reliable and valid measurement of MPT. This article also provides an excellent review of the findings relative to MPT and presents considerable data on normal phonation.

The *s/z* ratio is a variant on the concept of maximum phonation time. It is based on the observations by Boone[130] that patients often have a reasonably long production of a voiceless consonant but a much shorter duration of a voice, consonant. Some "normative" data were presented by Eckel and Boone[131] and data in children by Tait, Michel, and Carpenter.[132] The measure has also been used with patients with voice problems.[131,133-135] According to Eckel and Boone, one would expect a normal subject to produce an *s/z* ratio somewhere between 1 and 1.4. Ratios greater than 2.0 are suspect, and such patients should be examined more thoroughly. The *s/z* ratio is meant to be a screening test and does not necessarily have any diagnostic or prognostic value. It may be useful in monitoring the effects of treatment, however.

Phonational and Dynamic Range

Phonational range is the range between the minimum and the maximum frequency an individual can produce, whereas *dynamic range* is the range between the minimum and maximum intensity an individual can produce. Both provide an index of the maximal capabilities of the individual. In Figure 14-18 are some data on

phonational ranges of normal speakers. Most normal speakers can produce a phonational range between 2 and 3 octaves, although trained singers can often produce a much greater range. Some data on dynamic ranges of normal speakers are presented in Figure 14-19. Most normal speakers can produce ranges around 40 dB. Typically, the lowest intensity a normal speaker can produce is about 65 dB SPL, and the largest output is 105 to 110 dB SPL. However, the dynamic range depends on the frequency at which it is obtained. If a speaker is asked to maintain approximately the same frequency for both the minimum and the maximum phonations (a task not easily accomplished), the dynamic range may be much less than 40 dB. For example, the subjects whose data are shown in Figure 14-19 were asked to produce their minimum and maximum intensity levels at the 40th percentage point of their phonational range. The mean intensity ranges were 24.50 dB for the male group and 25.52 dB for the female group.

There are problems with the measurement of both phonational and dynamic ranges, as was noted for MPT. Is the patient producing the minimum and maximal levels? How many trials are needed before stable data are obtained? We have found it useful to start at a comfortable frequency (or intensity) and then ask the patient to produce higher and higher frequencies (or lower and lower frequencies) until no phonation is produced. It is

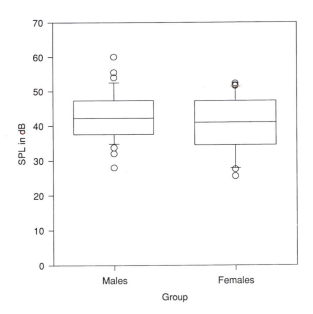

Maximum Dynamic Range

FIGURE 14-19. *Mean dynamic ranges, in decibels, of a group of 35 normal-speaking male and 27 normal-speaking female subjects.*

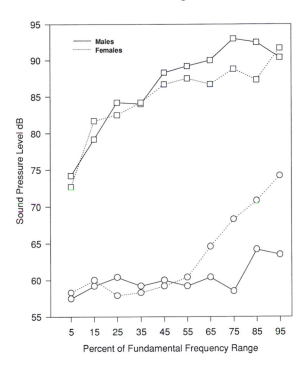

Phonetogram

FIGURE 14-20. *Phonetograms of normal male and female speakers. (Redrawn from data reported by Gramming.[137])*

helpful to present tones from an audio oscillator to the patients so that they can match their production to a target pitch. In some patients, asking them to slowly glide up or down in pitch helps to obtain the end points.

The phonetogram combines the two measurement procedures into a single plot. At selected points along the frequency range of a subject, measurements of the minimum and maximum intensity are obtained. A sample phonetogram of a group of normal subjects is presented in Figure 14-20. The phonetogram has found more extensive use in Europe[136-138] than in the United States. In some cases, the procedure has been automated so that the total time needed for obtaining the data is greatly reduced.[137,139] The phonetogram is not without its problems[140,141] and needs to be carefully interpreted. There is some question if the results obtained and their importance to clinical decisions are worth the time expended.

WHY MEASURE VOCAL FOLD VIBRATION AND ITS ACOUSTIC OUTPUT?

Why should one obtain objective measurements of vocal fold vibration and the acoustic output of phonation? Obviously such information is critical to our understanding of normal voice production, but what value does the expenditure of time, effort, and money

have for the diagnosis and treatment of voice problems? There are several reasons to obtain objective data on vocal function in patients. These are (1) the need for objective documentation of the patient's voice, (2) the need for objective data to assess the results of treatment, (3) the need for data to understand the pathologic vibratory process, (4) the potential need for data to support medical decisions in legal proceedings, and (5) the need to determine the minimal set of clinically relevant measurements.

Objective Documentation of a Patient's Voice

Patients and clinicians do not always remember what the patient sounded like before the start of any treatment. Nor do they remember very precisely. Patients may be concerned with a particular aspect of their voice, whereas the clinician reacts to another aspect. Both the patient's and the clinician's impressions of the patient's voice may be vague or use terms that may have multiple meanings. Impressions of a patient's voice are not always reliable indicators of the nature of the voice problem or its severity. Objective data can provide a reliable "picture" of the patient's voice. Such data can be placed into a patient's record, and the tests can be repeated many times to provide indices of any change that has resulted.

Objective data on different aspects of the voice can be obtained. Laryngoscopic observations describe the physical appearance of the vocal folds. Videorecordings of such examinations provide a permanent record. Stroboscopic data can be obtained to describe the vibratory characteristics of the vocal folds, revealing details about vibration that might be invaluable to a proper diagnosis or to developing the best plan of treatment. Airflow and air pressure data can be used to describe the patient's use of these parameters during vocalization. Acoustic data can be used to present a picture of the frequency, intensity, and stability of phonation. The acoustic spectrum provides a picture of the component frequencies in the voice that eventually listeners perceive when listening to the voice. Acoustic data can also be used to assess the capabilities of the system, capabilities that might be important in rendering a prognosis.

One need not try to obtain all possible data but should be selective and sample the relevant physiologic and acoustic features of a patient's voice. Records in the form of pictures, videotapes, graphs, or numbers obtained after the analysis of selected features of the voice may be included in the patient's record, thus providing an objective picture of the patient's voice.

Objective Data Critical for Properly Assessing Treatment Results

Studies in which data are collected on relevant parameters of the voice before and after a course of treatment are invaluable for evaluating the effects of the treatment. Such data should not be simply used to judge the "success" or "failure" of treatment. Rather they should be used to determine what physiologic (or acoustic) features changed in the voice and what such changes may mean to the functioning of the voice. Such data may help to "fine tune" treatment approaches, especially surgical techniques. Such data are invaluable to assess the techniques used in voice therapy.

Objective data may not always support the patient's (or clinician's) perception of the voice change as a result of treatment. In some cases, the patient may obtain relief of a problem that has little to do with the voice. For example, some patients with voice difficulties complain of difficulty swallowing or liquids aspirating. A surgical procedure may be tried that improves either of these two functions but does little to improve or affect vibratory function. The patient has improved, but the improvement was not with the voice. With voice therapy, a patient may learn to produce voice in a different way that results in a reduction in muscle soreness. Perhaps the muscle sore-

ness was the patient's main concern and the treatment provided the hoped-for relief. However, there may have been little change in the sound of the voice. If there is no change in the voice, one would expect little change in some or all of the measurements obtained before treatment. Patients and clinicians need to be aware of the expected goals of treatment and evaluate objective data on the voice with these goals in mind.

Objective Data Help to Understand the Pathologic Vibratory Process

Proper diagnosis and effective treatment depend on an understanding of the disorder. What is the effect of an observed pathologic condition on vibratory function and how does that affect the production of the pathologic voice? With some abnormalities, the effect may be very subtle. In some patients, there is no observable pathologic lesion, but careful observation and testing may reveal subtle abnormalities in vibratory function. Such abnormalities may be corrected with careful, fine surgery, or with medical management, or may require voice therapy. When the exact nature of the underlying pathophysiology is understood, the likelihood of efficient, effective treatment is greatly increased.

Objective Data for Legal Proceedings

There is a common saying "Ignorance is bliss, but it won't stand up in court." Objective data about a patient's voice, especially before and after treatment, can be critical in justifying treatment decisions in a court of law. Such data provide independent evidence of the exact state of the patient's voice and of the effects of treatment. A simple audiotape recording of a patient's voice, even if unanalyzed, can be an important objective record.

Objective Data to Evaluate Clinically Relevant Measurements

Many potential measurements can be made on the voice. Many have been discussed in this chapter, but the list is by no means complete. Some of these measurements are redundant and may reflect a feature of the voice that has little relationship to the diagnosis or the suggested treatment. Ideally, one would like a small set of measurements that are most relevant to the diagnosis, the prognosis, or both. At the time of the writing of this chapter, there is no such set. Objective data must be collected on many more patients before one could hope to derive the optimum set of measurements one should routinely use in the evaluation of patients with voice problems. Different combinations of measurements may be needed for different needs or patient groups. The set of measurements one requires to obtain a proper diagnosis may not be the same as that one would use to assess the results of treatment. Basic questions about whether such measurements should be solely physiologic or acoustic have not been addressed. Continued research and data collection on normal and pathologic speakers may help to answer these and other questions.

EXAMPLES OF MEASUREMENTS IN PATIENTS WITH PHONATORY DISORDERS

Patients with vocal fold nodules probably constitute the largest number of patients with benign lesions of the vocal folds. In a recent study, systematic ratings of videostroboscopic recordings of 30 patients with nodules were obtained. The patients were all female, and most received voice therapy for treatment of the nodules. The most frequent category for each of eight stroboscopic signs is shown in Figure 14-21. The most frequent glottal configuration (when the vocal folds were most closed) is a posterior chink. The affected fold, that is, the fold or folds with the lesion, had a slightly rough edge, a slightly decreased amplitude, and a slightly decreased lateral extent of the mucosal wave. The other signs were normal. An example of an inverse-filtered airflow and an EGG trace of a nodule patient is shown in Figure 14-22. Relevant acoustic measurements for this patient are reported in Table 14-6.

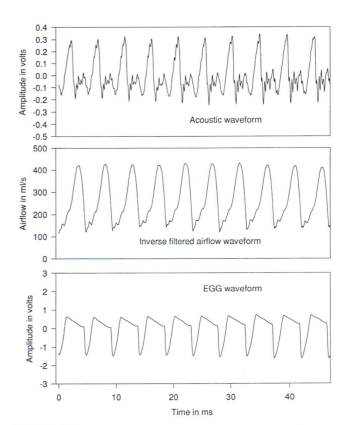

FIGURE 14-22. *Audio trace (top), inverse-filtered airflow trace (middle), and EGG trace (bottom) for a patient with a vocal fold nodule.*

Acoustic, EGG, or airflow measures of vocal fold function usually cannot guide the physician on treatment or diagnosis. For example, even severe vocal nodules may respond to conservative medical and speech therapy management. Vocal function measurements may reveal high flow rates, low signal-to-noise (S/N) ratios, and other findings of pathologic vibratory function. However, vocal function measures serve as only one criterion to assess the results or progress of treatment. Studies are currently in progress to assess voice results using multidimensional methods that include perceptual, videostroboscopic, acoustic, and airflow analysis. It remains to be demonstrated which tests will be most cost-effective and relevant.

Because some vocal fold lesions interfere with the vibratory function of the vocal folds, assessment of mucosal vibratory function by VSL is a cornerstone tool for diagnosis and treatment results. VSL is now routinely used to document the restoration of vocal fold function. To document the restoration of vibratory function, acoustic spectrum analysis and its desired measures in time and frequency domain are useful (ie, S/N ratio, jitter, shimmer, or the ratio of high energy to total energy).

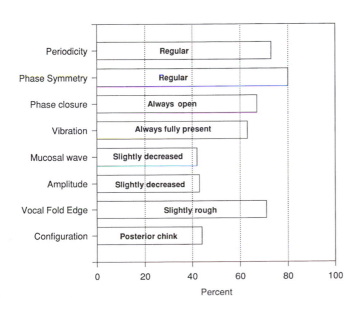

FIGURE 14-21. *Most frequent category for eight strobo-scopic signs in 30 patients with vocal fold nodules. (Data are from Colton et al.[147])*

Measurement	Pretreatment	Post-treatment
Sound pressure level (dB)	77.72	75.3
Fundamental frequency (Hz)	237	248
Phonational range (ST)	23.68	27.75
Dynamic range (DB)	17.25	20.56
Average flow (mL/s)	240.21	317.52
AC flow (mL/s)	204.75	160.25
Leakage flow (mL/s)	157.25	244.46
Open quotient (%)	50.89	63.49
Lung pressure cm H_2O	5.14	5.55
Vocal efficiency	43.66	20.5

TABLE 14-6. *Summary of Pre- and Post-treatment Acoustic and Airflow Measurements for a Patient With a Vocal Fold Nodule Shown in Figure 14-22*

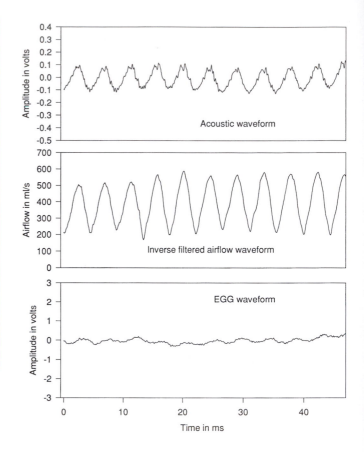

FIGURE 14-23. *Audio trace (top), inverse-filtered airflow trace (middle), and EGG trace (bottom) for a patient with vocal fold paralysis.*

Individuals who undergo treatment often show changes in EGG, VSL, and airflow data, and this gives insight on phonatory physiology. However, because of the wide variety of pathologic conditions and the large variations in function, large cohort studies may be necessary before statistical differences between treatment groups can be demonstrated.

An example of an inverse-filtered airflow and an EGG trace of patient with a left vocal fold paralysis is shown in Figure 14-23. Note the large leakage airflow and the small vibratory airflow component. The level of the EGG is very low, making interpretation of the EGG trace almost impossible. A summary of the aerodynamic and acoustic measurements is presented in Table 14-7.

Patients with vocal fold paralysis who seek treatment have three types of complaints: (1) dyspnea with phonation (short phonation time and high mean flow rates), (2) difficulty being heard in noisy environments (decreased maximum loudness), and (3) a voice lacking in clarity, a decreased S/N ratio, and lowered high-frequency energy (total energy ratio). With successful treatment many of these measures show obvious change. This is used clinically in the operating room during medialization laryngoplasty to monitor the size of the implant as well as to predict the final result.

Although jitter, shimmer, and other acoustic measures of vocal function may be useful, they may not be as important as more direct measures of vocal function. VSL can be used to document the extent of the glottal gap, level differences between the vocal folds, and the site and position of the glottal gap. In patients with vocal fold scarring and vocal fold paralysis, VSL gives some estimate of the rehabilitation potential of the vocal folds.

Phonatory function measures in functional and hyperfunctional voice disorders can be very useful in understanding what is often a clinical challenge. In the highly trained singer and in the patient presenting with subtle yet perplexing dysphagia, advanced measures of phonatory function by EGG and airflow and acoustic methods supplement the information obtained by physical examination and VSL. In many cases, the patients with subtle voice complaints have a paucity of clinical findings by direct laryngoscopy. Yet it is these same complaints that prompt them to seek repeat consultations with otolaryngologists and speech-language

Measurement	Pretreatment	Post-treatment
Sound pressure level (dB)	73.34	75.64
Fundamental frequency (Hz)	233	227
Phonational range (ST)	20.12	20.61
Dynamic range (DB)	13.04	21.09
Average flow (mL/s)	529.56	175.03
AC flow (mL/s)	201.8	185.11
Leakage flow (mL/s)	423.37	95.03
Open quotient (%)	64.45	58.76
Lung pressure cm H_2O	5.26	8.68
Vocal efficiency	7.72	95.69

TABLE 14-7. *Summary of Pre- and Post-treatment Acoustic and Airflow Measurements for a Patient With a Vocal Fold Paralysis Shown in Figure 14-23*

pathologists. They often complain of a lack of timbre to their voice, a veiled voice quality, a loss of singing capability in a specific range, or dysphonia during a transition between chest and head voice manifested as a voice break. Easy vocal fatigue and nonspecific throat pain are other complaints that often defy accurate diagnosis by classic history and physical examination.

In patients with special needs, advanced study of vocal fold vibratory function is often very helpful. In the elderly population with mild vocal fold atrophy, a short closing time on stroboscopy correlates nicely with EGG findings of prolonged opening time. These findings are also consistent with findings of a slight elevation in mean flow rates and an elevation in the expected AC/DC ratio. Analysis using these techniques helps to define the pathophysiology, making patient counseling and treatment planning easier.

Patients who undergo speech therapy for vocal fold nodules or hyperfunctional voice disorders also show internally consistent changes in measures of vocal fold vibratory function. When treatment of vocal fold nodules is successful, the findings on VSL show improved vocal contact, greater amplitude, and normalized glottal contact time. This correlates nicely with an improved AC/DC ratio and acoustic measures such as signal/noise ratio, jitter, and shimmer.

SUMMARY

The voice is the product of many physiologic events that together determine the acoustic output. Measurement of these events takes place in many different domains and illuminates a different, small piece of the puzzle we call voice. Measurement of various aspects of the voice permits an objective quantification of the voice that can be used to assess the status of the voice, the change in the voice that occurs over time, and changes that are the direct result of intervention. No ear, nose, and throat surgeon would think of performing surgery or any treatment on a patient who had a hearing problem without at least an objective audiogram. What is needed for the voice is an objective test such as the audiogram. But as we are dealing with production, we have much less control of the input to the system. There are many possible variations that could result in the observed phenomena, and it takes considerable time, data, model making, and thought to relate the various input considerations to the eventual acoustic output of the voice. Objective data on normal speakers and those with voice problems are needed to advance our understanding about normal voice physiology and what goes wrong.

The clinician who treats a variety of voice disorders must selectively use the myriad of available research and clinical tools to assess phonatory function. Rather than research interests, the clinician's focus is on improving results of the diagnosis and treatment. By selectively using relevant measures, these measures may be used as feedback to improve the treatment techniques.

REFERENCES

1. Löfqvist A. Aerodynamic measurements of vocal function. In: Blitzer A, Brin MF, Sasaki CT, et al, eds. *Neurologic Disorders of the Larynx.* New York, NY: Thieme Medical; 1993:98.

2. Alipour-Haghighi F, Titze I. Viscoelastic modeling of canine vocalis muscle in relaxation. *J Acoust Soc Am.* 1985;78:1939-1943.

3. Colton RH. Physiological mechanisms of vocal frequency control: the role of tension. *J Voice.* 1988;2:208-220.

4. Perlman AL, Titze IR, Cooper DS. Elasticity of canine vocal fold tissue. *J Speech Hear Res.* 1984;27:212-219.

5. Titze I. Comments on the myoelastic-aerodynamic theory of phonation. *J Speech Hear Res.* 1980;23:495-510.

6. Hirano M. Morphological structure of the vocal cord as a vibrator and its variations. *Folia Phoniatr (Basel)*. 1974;26:89-94.

7. Hirano M. Structure of the vocal fold in normal and disease states: anatomical and physical studies. In: Ludlow C, Hart M, eds. *Proceedings of the Conference on the Assessment of Vocal Pathology*. Rockville, MD: American Speech-Language Hearing Association; 1980.

8. Kakita Y, Hirano M, Kawasaki H. Schematical presentation of vibration of the vocal cord as a layer-structured vibrator. *Nippon Jibiinkoka Gakkai Kaiho*. 1976;11:1333-1340.

9. Kakita Y, Hirano M, Kawasaki H, et al. Schematical presentation of vibration of the vocal cords as a layer-structured vibrator: normal larynges. *Jpn J Otol (Tokyo)*. 1976;79:1333-1340.

10. Hirano M, Matsuo K, Kahita Y, et al. Vibratory behavior versus structure of the vocal fold. In: Titze I, Scherer R, eds. *Vocal Fold Physiology*. Denver, CO: Denver Center for the Performing Arts; 1983.

11. Yumoto E, Kurokawa H, Okamura H. Vocal fold vibration of the canine larynx: observation from an infraglottic view. *J Voice*. 1991;5:299-303.

12. Titze IR, Jiang JJ, Hsiao TY. Measurement of mucosal wave propagation and vertical phase difference in vocal fold vibration. *Ann Otol Rhinol Laryngol*. 1993;102:58-63.

13. Stevens KN. Vibration modes in relation to model parameters. In: Stevens KN, Kirano M, eds. *Vocal Fold Physiology*. Tokyo, Japan: University of Tokyo Press; 1981:291.

14. Rothenberg M. Acoustic interaction between the glottal source and the vocal tract. In: Stevens KN, Hirano M, eds. *Vocal Fold Physiology*. Tokyo, Japan: University of Tokyo Press; 1981:305.

15. Hast MH. Physiological mechanisms of phonation: tension of the vocal fold muscle. *Acta Otolaryngol (Stockh)*. 1966;62.

16. Moore DM, Berke GS. The effect of laryngeal nerve stimulation on phonation: a glottographic study using an in vivo canine model. *J Acoust Soc Am*. 1988;83:705-715.

17. Slavit DH, McCaffrey TV, Yanahi E. Effect of superior laryngeal nerve on vocal fold function: an in vivo canine model. *Otolaryngol Head Neck Surg*. 1991;105:857-863.

18. Blitzer A, Brin MF. Treatment of spasmodic dysphonia (laryngeal dystonia) with local injections of botulinum toxin. *J Voice*. 1992;6:365-369.

19. Blitzer A, Brin MF, Fahn S, et al. Localized injections of botulinum toxin for the treatment of focal laryngeal dystonia (spastic dysphonia). *Laryngoscope*. 1988;98:193-197.

20. Blitzer A, Brin MF, Fahn S, et al. Clinical and laboratory characteristics of focal laryngeal dystonia: study of 110 cases. *Laryngoscope*. 1988;98:636-640.

21. Blitzer A, Lovelace RE, Brin MF, et al. Electromyographic findings in focal laryngeal dystonia (spastic dysphonia). *Ann Otol Rhinol Laryngol*. 1985;94:591-594.

22. Brin M, Blitzer A, Fahn S, et al. Adductor laryngeal dystonia (spastic dysphonia): treatment with local injections of botulinum toxin (Botox). *Mov Disord*. 1989;4:287-296.

23. Crumley RL. Laryngeal synkinesis: its significance to the laryngologist. *Ann Otol Rhinol Laryngol*. 1989;98:87-92.

24. Kotby MN, Fadle E, Madkour O, et al. Electromyography and neurography in neurolaryngology. *J Voice*. 1992;6:159-187.

25. Kotby MN, Haugen LK. Critical evaluation of the action of the posterior crico-arytenoid muscles, utilizing direct EMG study. *Acta Otolaryngol (Stockh)*. 1967;70:260-268.

26. Kotby MN, Haugen LK. Clinical application of electromyography in vocal fold mobility disorders. *Acta Otolaryngol (Stockh)*. 1970;70:428-437.

27. Lovelace RE, Blitzer A, Ludlow CL. Clinical laryngeal electromyography. In: Blitzer A, Brin MF, Sasaki CT, et al, eds. *Neurologic Disorders of the Larynx*. New York, NY: Thieme Medical; 1992:66.

28. Thumfart WF. From larynx to vocal ability: new electrophysiological data. *Acta Otolaryngol (Stockh)*. 1988;105:425-431.

29. Woo P, Arandia H. Intraoperative laryngeal electromyographic assessment of patients with immobile vocal fold. *Ann Otol Rhinol Laryngol*. 1992;101:799-806.

30. Burke RE. Motor units: Anatomy, physiology, and functional organization. In: Brooks VB ed. *Handbook of Physiology, section 1, The Nervous System*, vol 2, *Motor Control, part 1*. Bethesda, MD: American Physiological Society; 1981:345.

31. Childers DG, Hicks DM, Moore GP, et al. A model for vocal fold vibratory motion, contact area, and the electroglottogram. *J Acoust Soc Am.* 1986;80:1309-1320.

32. Childers DG, Krishnamurthy AK, Naik JM, et al. Assessment of laryngeal function by simultaneous measurement of speech, electroglottography and ultra-high speed film. *Folia Phoniatr (Basel).* 1983;35:116A.

33. Childers DG, Naik JM, Larar JN, et al. Electroglottography, speech, and ultra-high speed cinematography. In: Titze IR, Scherer RC, eds. *Vocal Fold Physiology: Biomechanics, Acoustics and Phonatory Control.* Denver, CO: Denver Center for the Performing Arts; 1983:202.

34. Rothenberg M. Some relations between glottal air flow and vocal fold contact area. In: Ludlow C, Hart M, eds. *Proceedings of the Conference on the Assessment of Vocal Pathology.* Rockville, MD: American Speech-Language-Hearing Association; 1981.

35. Childers DG, Moore GP, Naik JM, et al. Assessment of laryngeal function by simultaneous synchronized measurement of speech, electroglottography and high-speed film. In: Lawrence V, ed. *Transcripts of the 11th Symposium: Care of the Professional Voice, part 2, Medical/Surgical Sessions: Papers.* New York, NY: Voice Foundation; 1983:234.

36. Hildebrand BH. *Vibratory Patterns of the Human Vocal Cords During Variations in Frequency and Intensity* [dissertation]. Gainesville: University of Florida; 1976.

37. Anastaplo S, Karnell MP. Synchronized videostroboscopic and electroglottographic examination of glottal opening. *J Acoust Soc Am.* 1988;83:1883-1890.

38. Karnell M. Synchronized videostroboscopy and electroglottography. *J Voice.* 1989;3:68-75.

39. Karnell MP, Li L, Panje WR. Glottal opening in patients with vocal fold tissue changes. *J Voice.* 1991;5:239-246.

40. Abberton E, Fourcin AJ. Laryngographic analysis of intonation. *Br J Disord Commun.* 1972;17:24-29.

41. Fourcin AJ. Laryngographic examination of the vocal fold vibration. In: Wyke B, ed. *Ventilatory and Phonatory Control Mechanisms.* London: Oxford University Press; 1974.

42. Fourcin AJ, Abberton E. First applications of a new laryngograph. *Med Biol Illustr.* 1971;21:172-182.

43. Hirano M, Bless DM. *Videostroboscopic Examination of the Larynx.* San Diego, CA: Singular; 1993.

44. Hirano M, Gould WJ, Lambiase A, et al. Movements of selected points on a vocal fold during vibration. *Folia Phoniatr (Basel).* 1980;32:39-50.

45. Coleman RF, Wendahl R. On the validity of laryngeal photosensor monitoring. *J Acoust Soc Am.* 1968;44:1733-1735.

46. Gerratt BR, Hanson DG, Berke GS, et al. Photoglottography: a clinical synopsis. *J Voice.* 1991;5:98-105.

47. Kitzing P. Photo- and electroglottographical recording of the laryngeal vibratory pattern during different registers. *Folio Phoniatr (Basel).* 1982;34:234-241.

48. Kitzing P, Löfqvist A. *Clinical application of combined electro- and photoglottography.* Proceedings of the 17th Congress of Logopedics and Phoniatrics; 1978.

49. Kitzing P, Sonesson B. A photoglottographical study of the female vocal folds during phonation. *Folia Phoniatr (Basel).* 1974;26:138-149.

50. Gall M. Strip Kymography of the glottis. *Arch Otorhinolaryngol.* 1984;240:287-293.

51. Svec JG, Schutte HK. Videokymography: high-speed line scanning of vocal fold vibration. *J Voice.* 1996;10:201-205.

52. Schutte HK, Svec JG, Sram F. Videokymography: research and clinical aspects. *Log Phon Vocol.* 1998;22:152-156.

53. Schutte HK, Svec JG, Sram F. First results of clinical application of videokymography. *Laryngoscope.* 1998;108:1206-1210.

54. Von Leden H, Moore GP, Timcke R. Laryngeal vibrations: measurements of the glottis wave: part 3. The pathologic larynx. W. *Arch Otolaryngol.* 1960;71:16-35.

55. Honda R, Kiritani S, Imagawa H, Hirose H. High-speed digital recording of vocal fold vibration using a solid-state image sensor. In: Baer T, Sasaki C, Harris KS, eds. *Laryngeal Function in Phonation and Respiration.* San Diego, CA: College Hill Press; 1987:485-491.

56. Eysholdt U, Tigges M, Wittenberg T. Proschel U. Direct evaluation of high-speed recordings of vocal fold vibrations. *Folia Phoniatr Logop.* 1996:48: 163-170.

57. Hertegard S, Lindestad PA. *Vocal fold vibrations studied during phonation with high-speed video imaging.* Karolinska Institute, Huddinge University Hospital Phoniatric and Logopedic Progress Report. 1994;9:33-40.

58. Hess MM, Gross M. High-speed, light intensified digital imaging of vocal fold vibrations in high optical resolution via indirect microlaryngoscopy. *Ann Otol Rhinol Laryngol.* 1993;102:502-507.

59. Kunze LH. Evaluation of methods of estimating sub-glottal air pressure. *J Speech Hear Res.* 1964;7:151-164.

60. Perkins WH, Koike Y. Patterns of subglottal pressure variations during phonation. *Folia Phoniatr (Basel).* 1969;21:1-8.

61. Kitajima K, Fjita F. Estimation of subglotta pressure with intraoral pressure. *Acta Otolaryngol (Stockh).* 1990;109:473-478.

62. Rothenberg M. Interpolating subglottal pressure from oral pressure. *J Speech Hear Disord.* 1982;7:218-224.

63. Smitheran JR, Hixon TJ. A clinical method for estimating airway resistance during vowel production. *J Speech Hear Disord.* 1981;46:138-146.

64. Hertegård S, Gauffin J. Insufficient vocal fold closure as studied by inverse filtering. In: Gauffin J, Hammarberg B, eds. *Vocal Fold Physiology: Acoustic, Perceptual, and Physiological Aspects of Voice Mechanisms.* San Diego, CA: Singular; 1991:243.

65. Hillman RE, Holmberg EB, Perkell JS, et al. Objective assessment of vocal hyperfunction: an experimental framework and initial results. *J Speech Hear Res.* 1989;32:373-392.

66. Hillman RE, Holmberg EB, Perkell JS, et al. Phonatory function associated with hyperfunctionally related vocal fold lesions. *J Voice.* 1990;4:52-63.

67. Holmberg EB, Hillman RE, Perkell JS. Glottal airflow and transglottal air pressure measurements for male and female speakers in soft, normal and loud voice. *J Acoust Soc Am.* 1988:84:511-529.

68. Holmberg EB, Hillman RE, Perkell JS, et al. Relationships between SPL and aerodynamic and acoustic measures of voice production: inter- and intra-subject variation. In: *Speech Communication Group Working Papers,* 8th ed. Cambridge, MA: MIT Press; 1992:85.

69. Netsell R, Lotz WK, DuChane AS, et al. Vocal tract aerodynamics during syllable productions: normative data and theoretical implications. *J Voice.* 1991;5:1-9.

70. Perkell JS, Holmberg EB, Hillman RE. A system for signal processing and data extraction from aerodynamic, acoustic, and electroglottographic signals in the study of voice production. *J Acoust Soc Am.* 1991;89:1777-1781.

71. Sundberg J, Titze I, Scherer R. Phonatory control in male singing: a study of the effects of subglottal pressure, fundamental frequency, and mode of phonation on the voice source. *J Voice.* 1993;7:15-29.

72. Isshiki N. Vocal efficiency index. In: Stevens KN, Hirano M, eds. *Vocal Fold Physiology.* Tokyo, Japan: Tokyo University Press; 1981: 93.

73. Isshiki N. Clinical significance of a vocal efficiency index. In: Titze IR, Scherer RC, eds. *Vocal Fold Physiology: Biomechanics, Acoustics and Phonatory Control.* Denver, CO: The Denver Center for the Performing Arts; 1983:230.

74. Schutte H. Integrated aerodynamic measurements. *J Voice.* 1992;6:127-134.

75. Schutte HK. Aerodynamics of phonation. *Acta Otorhinol Belg.* 1986;40:344-357.

76. Tanaka S, Gould W. Vocal efficiency and aerodynamic aspects in voice disorders. *Ann Otol Laryngol.* 1985;94:29-33.

77. Titze IR. Vocal efficiency. *J Voice.* 1992;6:135-138.

78. Titze IR. Phonation threshold pressure—a missing link in glottal aerodynamics. *J Acoust Soc Am.* 1992;91:2926-2935.

79. Titze IR, Sundberg J. Vocal intensity in speakers and singers. *J Acoust Soc Am.* 1992;91:2936-2946.

80. Rothenberg M. Use of a hot-wire anemometer to measure air flow in speech. Unpublished manuscript; 1985.

81. Kitajima K. Airflow study of pathologic larynges using a hot wire flowmeter. *Ann Otol Laryngol.* 1985;94:195-197.

82. Kitajima K, Isshiki N, Tanabe M. Use of a hot wire meter in the study of laryngeal function. *Studia Phonol (Kyoto).* 1978;12:25-30.

83. Teager H. Some observations an oral air flow during phonation. *IEEE Trans Acoust Speech Sig Process.* 1980;28:599-601.

84. Woo P. Phonatory volume velocity recording by use of hot film anemometry and signal analysis. *Otolaryngol Head Neck Surg.* 1986;95:312-318.

85. Yoshiya I, Nakajima T, Nagai I, Jitsukawa S. A bidirectional respiratory flowmeter using the hot wire principle. *J Appl Physiol.* 1975;38:360-365.

86. Rothenberg M. A new inverse filtering technique for deriving the glottal air flow during voicing. *J Acoust Soc Am.* 1973;53:1632-1645.

87. Rothenberg M. Measurement of air flow during speech. *J Speech Heart Res.* 1977;2:155-176.

88. Javkin HR, Antonanzas-Barros H, Maddieson I. Digital inverse filtering for linguistic research. *J Speech Hear Res.* 1987;30:122-129.

89. Miller JR, Mathews MV. Investigation of the glottal waveshape by automatic inverse filtering. *J Acoust Soc Am.* 1963;35:18-76.

90. Titze I, Durham P. Passive mechanisms influencing fundamental frequency control. In: Baer T, Sasaki CH, Harris K, eds. *Laryngeal Function in Phonation and Respiration.* San Diego, CA: College-Hill; 1986:304.

91. Titze IR. On the relation between subglottal pressure and fundamental frequency in phonation. *J Acoust Soc Am.* 1989;85:901-906.

92. Titze IR. Mechanisms underlying the control of fundamental frequency. In: Gauffin J, Hammarberg B, eds. *Vocal Fold Physiology: Acoustic, Perceptual, and Physiological Aspects of Voice Mechanisms.* San Diego, CA: Singular; 1991:129.

93. Titze IR, Luschei ES, Hirano M. Role of the thyroarytenoid muscle in regulation of fundamental frequency. *J Voice.* 1989;3:213-224.

94. Titze I. Physiologic and acoustic differences between male and female voices. *J Acoust Soc Am.* 1989;85:1699-1707.

95. Baken RJ. *Clinical Measurement of Speech and Voice.* Boston, MA: College-Hill; 1987.

96. Casper JK. *Frequency Perturbation in Normal Speakers: A Descriptive and Methodological Study* [dissertation]. Syracuse, NY: Syracuse University; 1983.

97. Baer T. Vocal jitter: a neuromuscular explanation. In: Lawrence V, ed. *Transcripts of the Eighth Symposium: Care of the Professional Voice.* New York, NY: The Voice Foundation; 1979:19.

98. Titze IR. A model for neurologic sources of aperiodicity in vocal fold vibration. *J Speech Hear Res.* 1991;34:460-472.

99. Orlikoff R, Baken R. Consideration of the relationship between the fundamental frequency of phonation and vocal jitter. *Folia Phoniatr (Basel).* 1990;42:31-40.

100. Orlikoff RF, Baken RJ. Fundamental frequency modulation of the human voice by the heartbeat: preliminary results and possible mechanisms. *J Acoust Soc Am.* 1989;85:888-893.

101. Orlikoff RF, Baken RJ. The effect of the heartbeat on vocal fundamental frequency perturbation. *J Speech Hear Res.* 1989;32:576-582.

102. Wong D, Ito MR, Cox NB, et al. Observation of perturbations in a lumped-element model of the vocal folds with application to some pathological cases. *J Acoust Soc Am.* 1991;89:383-394.

103. Coleman RF, Wendahl R. Vocal roughness and stimulus duration. *Speech Monogr.* 1967;34:85-92.

104. Wendahl R. Some parameters of auditory roughness. *Folia Phoniatr (Basel).* 1966;18:26-32.

105. Hartmann E, von-Cramon D. Acoustic measurement of voice quality in central dysphonia. *J Commun Disord.* 1984;17:425-440.

106. Laver J, Hiller S, Beck JM. Acoustic waveform perturbations and voice disorders. *J Voice.* 1992; 6:115-126.

107. Lieberman P. Perturbations in vocal pitch. *J Acoust Soc Am.* 1961; 33:597-603.

108. Lieberman P. Some acoustic measures of the fundamental periodicity of normal and pathologic larynges. *J Acoust Soc Am.* 1963;35:344-353.

109. Nichols A. Jitter and shimmer related to vocal roughness. *J Speech Hear Res.* 1979;22:670-671.

110. Smith W, Lieberman P. Computer diagnosis of laryngeal lesion. *Compt Biomed Res.* 1969; 2:291-303.

111. Sorensen D, Horii Y. Directional perturbation factors for jitter and for shimmer. *J Commun Disord.* 1984;17:143-151.

112. Dejonckere PH. Recognition of hoarseness by means of LTAS. *Int J Rehabil Res.* 1983;6:343-345.

113. Frokjaer-Jensen B, Prytz S. Registration of voice quality. *B & K Tech J.* 1976;3:3-17.

114. Hammarberg B, Fritzell B, Gauffin J, et al. Acoustic and perceptual analysis of vocal dysfunction. *Phoniatr Logoped Prog Rep.* 1980;2:1-17.

115. Hammarberg B, Fritzell B, Schiratzki H. Teflon injection in 16 patients with paralytic dysphonia: perceptual and acoustic evaluations. *J Speech Hear Disord.* 1984;49:72-82.

116. Hollien H, Majewski W. Speaker identification by long-term spectra under normal and distorted speech conditions. *J Acoust Soc Am.* 1977;62:975-980.

117. Hurme P, Sonninen A. Acoustic, perceptual and clinical studies of normal and dysphonia voice. *J Phonet.* 1986;14:489-492.

118. Izdebski K. Overpressure and breathiness in spastic dysphonia. *Acta Otolaryngol (Stockh).* 1984;97:373-378.

119. Kitzing P. LTAS criteria pertinent to the measurement of voice quality. *J Phonet.* 1986;14:477-482.

120. Löfqvist A. The long-time average spectrum as a tool in voice research. *J Phonet.* 1986;14:471-476.

121. Löfqvist A, Mandersson B. Long-term average spectrum of speech and voice analysis. *Folia Phoniatr (Basel).* 1987;39:221-229.

122. Prytz S, Frokjaer-Jensen B. Long-term average spectra analysis of normal and pathological voices. *Folia Phoniatr (Basel).* 1976;78:280.

123. Sonninen A, Hurme P. Clinical and acoustic observations of normal and hoarse voices. In: *Papers in Speech Research.* University of Jyvaskyla; 1982:2.

124. Wendler J, Doherty ET, Hollien H. Voice classification by means of long-term speech spectra. *Folia Phoniatr (Basel).* 1980;32:51-60.

125. Wendler J, Rauhut A, Kruger H. Classification of voice qualities. *J Phonet.* 1986; 14:483-488.

126. Kent RD, Kent J, Rosenbek J. Maximum performance tests of speech production. *J Speech Hear Res.* 1987;52:367-387.

127. Bless D, Hirano M. *Verbal instructions: a critical variable in obtaining optimal performance for maximum phonation time.* Presented at the annual meeting of the American Speech-Language-Hearing Association, Toronto; 1982.

128. Stone RE Jr. Issues in clinical assessment of laryngeal function: contraindications for subscribing to maximum phonation time and optimum fundamental frequency. In: Bless DM, Abbs JH, eds. *Vocal Fold Physiology: Contemporary Research and Clinical Issues.* San Diego, CA: College-Hill; 1983:410.

129. Neiman GS, Edeson B. Procedural aspects of eliciting maximum phonation time. *Folia Phoniatr (Basel).* 1981;33:285-293.

130. Boone DR. *The Voice and Voice Therapy.* 2nd ed. Englewood Cliffs, NJ: Prentice-Hall; 1983.

131. Eckel FC, Boone DR. The *s/z* ratio as an indicator of laryngeal pathology. *J Speech Hear Disord.* 1981;46:147-149.

132. Tait NA, Michel JF, Carpenter MA. Maximum duration of sustained /s/ and /z/ in children. *J Speech Heart Disord.* 1980;45:239-246.

133. Hufnagle J, Hufnagle K. S/Z ratio in dysphonic children with and without vocal cord nodules. *Lang Speech Heart Serv Schools.* 1988;19:418-422.

134. Rastatter MP, Hyman M. Maximum phoneme duration of /s/ and /z/ by children with vocal nodules. *Lang Speech Heart Serv Schools.* 1982; 13:197-199.

135. Shearer W. *s/z* ratio for detection of vocal nodules. *Folia Phoniatr (Basel).* 1983;35:172.

136. Damste PH. The phonetogram. *Pract Otol Rhinol Laryngol.* 1970;32:185-187.

137. Gramming P. *The Phonetogram: An Experimental and Clinical Study* [dissertation]. Lund University, Malmo, Sweden: Malmo General Hospital; 1988.

138. Pabon JP, Plomp R. automatic phonetogram recording supplemented with acoustical voice-quality parameters. *J Speech Hear Res.* 1988;31:710-722.

139. Schutte HK, Seidner W. Recommendation by the Union of European Phoniatricians (UEP): standardizing voice area measurement/phonetography. *Folia Phoniatr (Basel).* 1983;35:286-288.

140. Coleman RF. Sources of variation in phonetograms. *J Voice.* 1993;7:1-14.

141. Titze IR. Acoustic interpretation of the voice profile (phonetogram). *J Speech Hear Res.* 1992;35:21-34.

142. Hollien H, Dew D, Phillips P. Phonational frequency ranges of adults. *J Speech Hear Res.* 1971;14:755-760.

143. Horii Y. Vocal shimmer in sustained phonation. *J Speech Hear Res.* 1980;23:202-209.

144. Sorensen D, Horii Y. Frequency and amplitude perturbation in the voice of female speakers. *J Commun Disord.* 1983;16:57-61.

145. Hirano M, Koike Y, von Leden H. Maximum phonation time and air usage during phonation. *Folia Phoniatr (Basel).* 1968;20:185-201.

146. Finnegan DE. Maximum phonation time for children with normal voices. *J Commun Disord.* 1984; 17:309-317.

147. Colton RH, Woo P, Brewer DW, et al. Stroboscopic signs associated with benign lesions of the vocal folds. *J Voice.* 1995;312-325.

CHAPTER 15

Laryngeal Electromyography

Lucian Sulica, MD

Andrew Blitzer, MD, DDS

Electromyography (EMG) studies electrical activity in muscle. It was first applied to the muscles of the larynx in a systematic way by Faaborg-Andersen and Buchtal in the late 1950s.[1-3] As the only way to investigate neural activity in vivo, laryngeal EMG has greatly expanded its clinical scope in the intervening decades, but no clear consensus exists on its role in laryngology. Despite general acceptance, some misunderstandings persist about its capabilities, and as a result, its potential as well as some of its limitations are underappreciated.

TECHNICAL CONSIDERATIONS

EMG measures electrical activity in muscle by means of electrodes. Although there are several different techniques, all require three components: a ground electrode, which helps to reduce interference, a reference electrode, and a recording electrode.[4] These last two are designated the positive and negative electrodes by convention, which should imply that they carry electrical charge.

Of the various techniques of EMG, the noninvasive method using surface electrodes is the least sensitive and specific, particularly for small muscles close to one another as in the larynx, because of the distance of the electrodes from the motor endplates where electrical activity is normally generated. For the same rea-

son, surface electrodes cannot generally detect spontaneous electrical activity. Thus, surface EMG has been of limited utility in the larynx. However, electrodes placed on the mucosa of the larynx have been used to examine the posterior cricoarytenoid and the cricopharyngeus muscle and to monitor the thyroarytenoid muscles during surgery in the area of the recurrent nerve.[5-7] Surface EMG may also have some utility in biofeedback training.[8,9]

Invasive techniques using either monopolar or concentric needle electrodes offer increased accuracy.[4,10,11] The monopolar needle is solid, insulated except for its tip, and is used to measure potential differences between the tip and a reference electrode on the skin. The concentric electrode is a hollow needle that contains a fine wire in its lumen. It records differences between the outer cannula, functioning as the reference electrode, and the inner wire. The relative advantages and disadvantages of the two types of needle electrodes are extensively debated, but each can be used in most clinical situations. Concentric needles offer significant advantages in the measurement of single motor units and waveforms. It is important to note which type of electrode is used in a given study, as data are not readily comparable between the two.

An advantage of both monopolar and concentric needle electrodes is that they can be easily moved to sample many sites within the same muscle. Yet, in the larynx, the needle may move out of a muscle if the patient swallows or coughs. The problem of needle movement can be overcome with hooked-wire electrodes. In this technique, a 30-gauge wire is bent and placed through the shaft of a needle that is then placed into the muscle. The outside needle is then removed, and recording can commence from the hooked wire (Figure 15-1). Two hooked wires can be used to limit the field being measured, and to give data more like that of a concentric electrode. Hooked-wire electrodes are particularly important for measurements over time, during different activities, or in different positions.[10,12]

At our center, the percutaneous monopolar needle technique is the standard. It is usually performed with the patient in the recumbent position, the neck slightly extended. Local anesthesia is not used, as the procedure is relatively painless and the anesthetic agent may produce artifact in the cricothyroid muscle recording. A

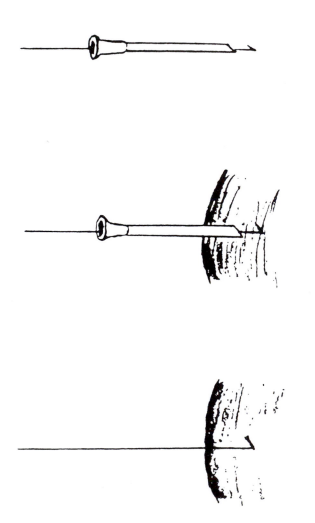

FIGURE 15-1. *A diagram of the insertion of a hooked-wire electrode into muscle.*

ground electrode is placed over the sternum, and a reference lead is placed over the cheek.

In order to investigate the two components of vagal innervation of the larynx, both cricothyroid and both thyroarytenoid muscles are tested and compared, although not necessarily simultaneously. To test the cricothyroid muscle, the needle electrode is passed through the skin overlying the cricothyroid membrane and then along the outside of the cricoid cartilage superiorly and laterally until electrical activity is identified. The patient is asked to turn and raise the head to ensure that the needle is not in the strap muscles. Once the needle is confirmed to be in the right position, spontaneous activity is sought during quiet respiration. Maximum volitional activity is obtained with high-pitched phonation.

The thyroarytenoid-vocalis muscle complex is tested by passing the needle through the skin and the cricothyroid membrane in the midline. It is then advanced superiorly and laterally inside the thyroid cartilage until it pierces the muscle complex and crisp potentials are identified during phonation. Simple manipulation of the needle allows sampling at multiple sites within the muscle.

Occasionally, when there are questions about vocal fold abduction, it is useful to test the posterior cricoarytenoid muscles. The posterior cricoarytenoid muscle is the only abductor of the larynx. Therefore, in patients with respiratory symptoms like stridor or breathy dysphonias, understanding the electrical activity in this muscle is important. In the technique most commonly used by the senior author (AB), the larynx is rotated away from the investigator and the posterior edge of the thyroid lamina is palpated with the thumb.[13] The needle is inserted along the lower half of the posterior edge of the thyroid cartilage, traversing the inferior constrictor. It is advanced until it stops against the cricoid. The needle is then pulled back slightly and the patient is asked to sniff in order to maximally stimulate the posterior cricoarytenoid (Figure 15-2). Another satisfactory technique involves inserting the needle through the cricothyroid membrane at the midline, traversing the lumen of the subglottic space and piercing the posterior lamina of the cricoid cartilage to one side or the other of midline.[14] The electrical signal on the far side of the cartilage represents posterior cricoarytenoid muscle. This can be verified by the patient sniffing. In our experience, this approach is most useful in the young patient whose cartilage has not undergone extensive calcification. A tracheal injection of lidocaine is helpful in avoiding airway irritation.

Thyroarytenoid and posterior cricoarytenoid muscle electrodes may also be placed under endoscopic guidance or under direct vision at operative laryngoscopy.[15,16]

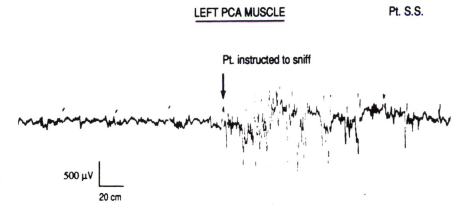

LEFT PCA MUSCLE   Pt. S.S.

Pt. instructed to sniff

500 μV

20 cm

FIGURE 15-2. *A laryngeal EMG record-ing of the PCA muscle showing a burst of activity on sniffing (maximal stimulation).*

PHYSIOLOGY AND PATHOLOGY

An EMG yields a visual signal of electrical activity in muscle, either via oscilloscope, or in all newer systems, a digital trace. In addition, the electrical signal is cou-pled to a speaker and produces audible output. Different types of potentials have specific acoustic signatures that are readily identified by the experienced examiner, and the audible signal is an important part of the EMG exam-ination. There are four characteristics of electrical activity in muscle: morphology or waveform, amplitude, duration, and frequency. Acoustically, the amplitude of an electrical potential generally corresponds to loud-ness, and duration and rise time correspond to pitch.[11]

Electrical activity in muscle is the result of changes in the strong negative resting potential of the muscle cell that in turn result from other electrical or chemical signals. Normally, depolarization is the result of neural stimulation via acetylcholine to the motor endplates of a muscle fiber. All muscle fibers innervated by a given motoneuron form a motor unit. The electrical summa-tion of all their potentials forms a motor unit potential (MUP, also called a motor unit action potential, or a muscle action potential), the basic electrophysiologic component of striated muscle.

A useful classification of EMG findings divides elec-trical activity into three types based on the circum-stance in which it appears: insertional, spontaneous, and volitional.[4,11] Upon insertion, irritation by the nee-dle itself may cause a few individual fibers to depolarize, which yields a burst of spike discharges that extinguish-es quickly. These may take the form of pseudomyotonic "dive bomber" discharges (discussed below) (Figure 15-3). Any such activity persisting beyond 400 milliseconds from needle movement is considered prolonged and a sign of pathologic muscle membrane instability.

Spontaneous activity in normal muscle at complete rest is minimal, usually limited to subthreshold non-propagated depolarizations at the endplate that produce extremely brief, irregular, and low amplitude electrical signals. They make a characteristic hissing or white-noise type sound, and have an initial negative deflection (an upwards deflection of the trace, by convention). This distinguishes them from fibrillation potentials, which have an initial positive deflection and are pathologic. Measurement of spontaneous activity in laryngeal mus-cles is difficult because complete silence is rarely achieved. These muscles are continuously active in res-piration. Spontaneous activity such as fibrillations and positive sharp waves can be more clearly identified in limb muscles, in which complete relaxation can produce electrical silence. In the larynx, electrical silence in and of itself may suggest pathology.

Volitional activity is examined by having the patient contract the muscle with a needle in place. In the larynx, this consists of an action appropriate for the muscle in question: voicing or a Valsalva maneuver for the thy-roarytenoid, sniffing for the posterior cricoarytenoid, or a glissando (slide) for the cricothyroid. Contraction results in the appearance of the MUP. Each MUP has its own characteristics and is thus identifiable throughout an examination, but it is possible to make some gener-alizations.[4,11] The normal MUP is usually bi- or tripha-sic in shape. Phases are counted by noting the number of times the potential crosses the baseline and adding one. Greater than four phases is considered abnormal and termed "polyphasic." This is reflective of a loss of synchrony among the endplates that make up a motor unit.

The duration and amplitude depend on the muscle studied, and are generally proportional to the muscle size.[4] Faaborg-Andersen[1,2] and Buchtal[3] have described laryngeal MUPs of amplitudes ranging from 224 to 358 microvolts. They also found mean durations of 3.5 mil-liseconds in the vocalis and 5.3 milliseconds in the cricothyroid. Their data were obtained with concentric

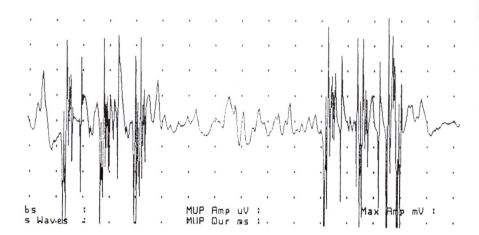

FIGURE 15-3. *A laryngeal EMG recording of the TA muscle showing pseudomyotonic discharges.*

100uV

10ms

needle electrodes. Similar measurements made with monopolar electrodes recorded a mean amplitude of 426 microvolts and duration of 3.5 milliseconds for the vocalis muscle, and 500 microvolts and 4.4 milliseconds for the cricothyroid.[17] MUP duration has been shown to increase with age and with decreasing temperature.[4] Amplitude is also affected by the distance of the needle from the muscle fibers. In order to check this distance, an examiner may measure the rise time of a MUP, the time between the onset of the first negative deflection and its peak. For observations about a given MUP to be valid, its rise time should be less than 200 microseconds.[4,10]

Frequency of MUPs is determined largely by the force of contraction. Besides increasing the frequency of discharge from an individual motor unit, increasing contraction will result in the activation of adjacent motor units. This phenomenon is known as recruitment. At a high level of contraction, multiple motor units will be firing at high frequency, making it impossible to distinguish features of any single MUP either visually or acoustically. This is known as a full interference pattern, and is normally achieved at about 30% of maximum isometric contraction (Figure 15-4).[11] Inability to attain full interference pattern suggests pathology (Figure 15-5).

Like normal findings, abnormalities in EMG may be divided into insertional, spontaneous, and volitional.[4,11] Prolonged insertional activity, defined as depolarizations lasting longer than 400 milliseconds, is suggestive of muscle membrane instability, as in polymyositis and other myopathies. Spontaneous firing of individual muscle fibers at rest indicates denervation or myopathy. This may appear either as spike fibrillations or positive sharp waves (PSW), but their significance is the same (Figures 15-6 and 15-7). Both are marked by an initial positive (downward) deflection and fire with a regular periodicity. Higher frequency runs of spike fibrillations and PSWs, usually prompted by needle movement, that wax and wane in amplitude and frequency are called myotonic discharges. The telltale acoustic signal of myotonic discharge has been likened to the sound of a dive bomber or a motocross bike. Myotonic discharges occur in a variety of intrinsic disorders of muscle such as myositis, myotonic dystrophy, glycogen storage diseases, hyperparathyroidism, and so forth. Fasciculation potentials are the result of spontaneous discharge of all or part of an entire motor unit, which they resemble, except that they occur singly rather than in trains, and at rest, rather than with movement. They are a typical finding in amyotrophic lateral sclerosis, but can appear in any condition of chronic denervation. MUPs that occur in repetitive runs, but generally constant in duration and amplitude, are termed myokymia, and occur in response to a number of factors that alter the biochemical environment of the nerve, such as demyelination, edema, or toxins. Acoustically, myokymia resembles the sound of marching soldiers. Complex repetitive discharges are abrupt onset and offset, multifiber discharges with bizarre morphologies that are thought to signify chronicity of neuromuscular disease.

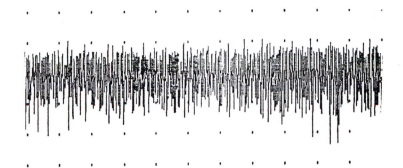

FIGURE 15-4. *A laryngeal EMG recording of the TA muscle during voicing, showing a normal interference pattern.*

1mV

200ms

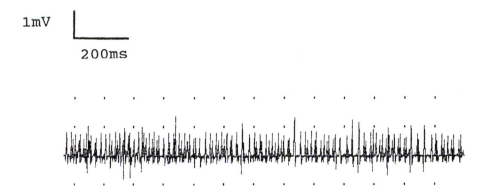

FIGURE 15-5. *A laryngeal EMG recording of the TA muscle during voicing in a patient with vocal fold paresis, showing a decreased interference pattern.*

500μV

200ms

Voluntary contraction may yield abnormal MUPs. In general, large amplitude, long duration MUPs suggest neurogenic disease, whereas small amplitude, short MUPs suggest myopathy.[11] There are several exceptions to this, like early reinnervation potentials and potentials of chronic severe myopathy. Forceful contraction that fails to produce a full interference pattern suggests denervation, as discussed above.

As is evident, the spectrum of abnormal findings in EMG is broad, and reflects the disordered physiology of the disease under investigation. Most findings can occur in a variety of conditions; none is pathognomonic. Whether they carry significance depends on the frequency with which they occur and their clinical context. There are few lists of strict diagnostic criteria for specific diseases in the EMG literature for this reason. The beginning electromyographer may find this frustrating, but with experience, EMG becomes a useful and thought-provoking means of evaluating laryngeal function.

As laryngeal EMG is often applied to conditions of nerve injury, let us examine such a situation as an example of the mutability of electrical findings over time

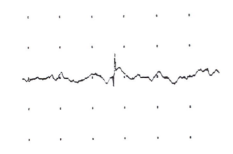

100uV

10ms

FIGURE 15-6. *A laryngeal EMG recording of the TA muscle in a patient with vocal fold paralysis, showing an example of a fibrillation potential suggestive of denervation.*

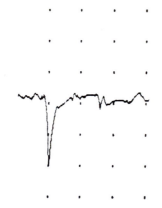

100uV

10ms

FIGURE 15-7. *A laryngeal EMG recording of the TA muscle in a patient with vocal fold paralysis, showing an example of a positive sharp wave, suggestive of a denervating process.*

and the integration of electrical and clinical observations. (The sequence of electrical changes in vocal fold denervation have been well demonstrated in a canine model.[18-20])

Initially, following a nerve injury, no electrical signals can travel to the distal end of any of the compromised axons to prompt release of neurotransmitter. Therefore, no depolarization of the affected motor units occurs. In cases of extreme injury, such as a nerve section, in which all axons are interrupted, there can be electrical silence both at rest and with efforts at movement. Alternately, the injury may be incomplete and some motor units may remain intact. In this case, the examiner asks the patient to activate the muscle—for example, to phonate, in the case of the thyroarytenoid. A nerve injury severe enough to cause symptomatic vocal fold paresis would almost certainly disrupt enough motor units to impair recruitment and cause an incomplete interference pattern at maximal effort. Because of the appearance of the trace of this phenomenon, it is referred to as a "picket-fence" pattern (Figure 15-5).

If the site of nerve injury is unknown, comparison of findings in the cricothyroid and the thyroarytenoid muscle can be helpful. Signs of denervation in both point toward the jugular foramen and the central nervous system, whereas abnormal findings restricted to the thyroarytenoid direct workup along the course of the recurrent laryngeal nerve.

Over time, the resting potential of a muscle cell that receives no neural input falls to near the depolarization threshold.[11] From time to time, it crosses this threshold and the cell fires, repolarizes, and then repeats the cycle. On EMG, this manifests as fibrillation potentials or PSWs—single positive spikes that occur with some regularity (Figures 15-6 and 15-7). There is some variability in how long a muscle must be denervated to produce fibrillations; three weeks is widely quoted in the literature, but it may take up to five weeks.[4,10,11,18] Because of the change in muscle cell resting potential, prolonged insertional activity may also occur, as cells are more likely to depolarize with irritation.[11] In fact, prolonged insertional activity usually precedes the appearance of fibrillations. If no neural ingrowth occurs, fibrillation potentials will persist until the muscle atrophies and is replaced by connective tissue.

If reinnervation occurs, early nerve fibers grow in irregularly to encounter atrophied muscle fibers and disordered neuromuscular junctions.[4,11] The result is motor unit weakness and asynchrony, and thus MUPs of early reinnervation are typically low in amplitude, polyphasic, and prolonged (Figure 15-8). Yet, they provide clear evidence that neural regeneration is occurring. With time, synchronicity improves, although nearly never to preinjury levels. Therefore, the MUP of late reinnervation still tends to be polyphasic and prolonged, although perhaps less so than before. Because the late-reinnervation motor unit generally incorporates many more muscle fibers than a normal, preinjury motor unit, its MUP demonstrates high amplitude—the so-called giant wave.

Because EMG evidence of reinnervation appears before clinical return of function, EMG can have prognostic value. Yet, reinnervation is not synonymous with return of function. The recurrent laryngeal nerve contains fibers for both vocal fold abduction and adduction, and these fibers do not necessarily find their way back to the appropriate motor units. Anomalous regrowth may result in an immobile, albeit reinnervated, vocal fold. EMG findings in this circumstance are not spurious, although they may appear to be. The clinically important phenomenon of synkinesis in the larynx, although appreciated as early as 1963,[20] is often overlooked, although it has implications for voice function and treatment.[21]

In order to make sense of the various electrical findings of denervation, the examiner must first have an idea of the age of the nerve injury. For instance, fibrillation potentials carry different significance at one month following injury than they do one year later. Second, the examiner must combine the EMG examination findings with those of the laryngoscopic examination. Finally, comparison with previous EMGs is often useful to see if reinnervation is ongoing or has reached a plateau.

CLINICAL APPLICATIONS OF LARYNGEAL ELECTROMYOGRAPHY

Laryngeal EMG is useful in separating mechanical from neurogenic causes of vocal fold immobility.[16,20-24] EMG has been found to be more reliable than computed tomography scanning (CT) for this purpose,[23] and offers a safer and less costly alternative to operative endoscopy. Conditions such as cricoarytenoid arthritis and or arytenoid dislocation generally yield near-normal EMGs, although Yin and coauthors have cautioned that patterns of myopathy or neuropathy may occur in long-standing arytenoid dislocation, and have emphasized the importance of testing multiple sites within the muscle.[25] Neurogenic vocal fold immobility, on the other hand, can show a wide variety of abnormal electrical activity, as described above.

In cases of denervation, comparison of findings in muscles innervated by the superior laryngeal nerve (cricothyroid) and the recurrent laryngeal nerve (thyroarytenoid) can indicate the site of lesion.[26] Abnormal findings in both muscles suggest an injury proximal to the branching of the superior nerve form the main trunk of the vagus, whereas abnormalities isolated to the thyroarytenoid direct investigation into lower neck and the mediastinum.

With respect to prognosticating return of vocal fold function, researchers have reported rates of 69% to 90% correct prediction of return of motion.[27-30] These results are difficult to interpret and reconcile with each

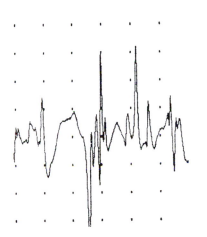

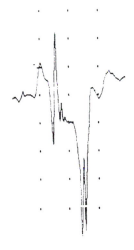

FIGURE 15-8. *A laryngeal EMG recording of the TA muscle showing two examples of polyphasic potentials suggestive of a repair process.*

100uV

10ms

A

B

other because much depends on the criteria used in each study. In general, though, the preservation of normal-morphology MUPs, suggesting incomplete nerve injury, is a positive sign and a good argument for early EMG examination following neural injury.[19,30] Polyphasic MUPs are more problematic, but also generally improve chances of return of function. However, the absence of motor unit potentials, either normal or polyphasic, and the presence of fibrillations and PSWs, are reliable indicators of poor prognosis.[27,30]

Setting strict criteria for reinnervation can create the impression that it is an all-or-none phenomenon, whereas it more likely occurs on a continuum that includes misdirected growth resulting in synkinetic muscular activity.[21,31-34] Some studies have dismissed immobile vocal folds that demonstrate electrical signs of reinnervation as false positives, whereas, these are probably more appropriately considered cases of synkinetic reinnervation. Synkinesis can be confirmed by the presence of muscle activation in tasks that a given muscle would be expected to remain quiet, or by simultaneous activation of abductor and adductor muscles monitored with hook-wire electrodes. Even with persistent vocal fold immobility, voice quality with synkinesis can be near normal because of restoration of muscle tone.[21] In summary, EMG evidence of reinnervation is not syn-

onymous with return of function. In prognosticating return of function to a denervated vocal fold, as in other aspects of clinical EMG, serial examinations and clinical correlation are helpful.

More widespread use of laryngeal EMG has created a new appreciation for the entity of laryngeal nerve paresis and for isolated superior laryngeal nerve palsy.[35-39] Both conditions may cause vocal fold bowing, and EMG can help distinguish between bowing caused by these neurologic factors and from bowing caused by other factors such as atrophy, sulcus vocalis, and postsurgical scarring.

Laryngeal EMG is an essential tool in the investigation of disorders of vocal fold mobility associated with a wide variety of systemic neurologic conditions, including hereditary sensory and motor neuropathy,[40] postpolio syndrome,[41,42] the Parkinson-plus syndromes,[43,44] and in distinguishing upper from lower motor neuron lesions.[45] With multiple muscle samples, the diagnosis of bulbar palsy (anterior horn cell disease), primary lateral sclerosis, Arnold-Chiari malformation, or syringomyelia can be entertained.[10] When there is regular, slow, repetitive firing of MUPs in the larynx, with synchronous firing of muscles in the palate and pharynx, the diagnosis of myoclonus is easily made (Figure 15-9). A regular 4- to 8-Hz repetitive signal can suggest essen-

Larynx

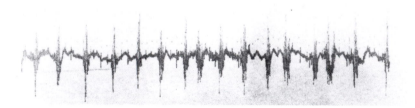

Palate

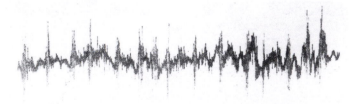

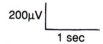

200μV

1 sec

FIGURE 15-9. *A simultaneous recording of the EMG of the TA muscle and plate showing a synchronous myoclonic electrical pattern.*

tial tremor. Once again, evaluation of extralaryngeal muscles may be useful. In some patients, the amplitude and numbers of potentials decrease with repetitive function or repetitive stimulation. This is suggestive of myasthenia gravis (Figure 15-10). If this is found, edrophonium (Tensilon) injection, followed by repeat testing, should show a return to normal activity.[10] The diagnosis can be confirmed in the usual manner with acetylcholine receptor antibody testing, although antibodies have been reported positive in only about 10% of cases of myasthenia gravis involving primarily the larynx.[46]

Patients with spasmodic dysphonia have been studied extensively, and certain EMG characteristics have helped differentiate spasmodic dysphonia from other disorders. An effective method is to synchronize the EMG with the voice-spectrogram and measure the delay from the onset of electrical activity to the onset of sound. It is characteristically delayed in patients with spasmodic dysphonia by 500 milliseconds to 1 second (normal: 0 to 200 milliseconds) (Figure 15-11).[10,47]

EMG can be used for intraoperative monitoring of the recurrent laryngeal nerve during surgeries that place this structure at risk. Hooked-wire electrodes can be placed into the thyroarytenoid-vocalis muscle com-

agents, including paralytics and local agents, can inhibit electrical activity in muscle.

EMG has proved to be the ideal method of guiding therapeutic injection of botulinum toxin. A hollow needle can be used as a monopolar electrode to inject toxin where the electrical signal is crisp, loud, and high-pitched, indicating that motor endplates, and therefore nerve terminals, are nearby.[50] Because botulinum toxin acts at nerve terminals to prevent the release of acetylcholine, this method serves to minimize the dose needed for a therapeutic effect and increases accuracy of placement, thereby reducing diffusion and unintended effects.

Finally, surface EMG is an evolving tool in biofeedback therapy of both speech and swallowing disorders.[8,9]

SUMMARY

In the years since the seminal work of Faaborg-Andersen and Buchtal, electromyography (EMG) has become a useful tool for the laryngologist. It is valuable in making distinctions between mechanical limitation and denervation in the immobile vocal fold. In the case

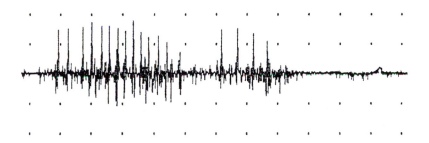

FIGURE 15-10. *A laryngeal EMG recording of the TA muscle showing decreasing amplitude and numbers of potentials with continued function, suggestive of myasthenia gravis.*

500uV

200ms

plex endoscopically, or surface electrodes can be placed on top of the postcricoid area or attached to the endotracheal tube at the level of the vocal folds in order to provide warning when the recurrent nerve is stimulated.[6,48,49] Surgeons should be aware that anesthetic

of denervation, it can point to the site of lesion and provide prognostic information that guides treatment. EMG is an integral part of the investigation of neurologic disorders affecting the larynx. Intraoperatively, it can be used to monitor the recurrent laryngeal nerves during

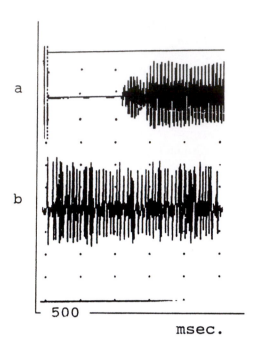

FIGURE 15-11. *(A) Voice spectrogram and (B) electromyogram of patient with spasmodic dysphonia, showing a greater than 1-second delay between the onset of electrical activity and the onset of voice.*

procedures that put these structures at risk. EMG is the standard method of directing therapeutic injection of botulinum toxin, and has been used in biofeedback therapy for speech and swallowing disorders

Although EMG yields measurable data, it is in essence a qualitative test. The comparison with endoscopy and imaging studies made by Woodson is apt.[51] EMG diagnosis of neuromuscular disease is based on patterns of abnormalities and change over time, and, like the other tests, requires clinical correlation.

The most important contribution of EMG to laryngology has been to catalyze interest in mechanisms of neural control of the larynx. The resulting refinement of electrodiagnostic approaches to the larynx, including quantitative and single-fiber EMG and evoked potential testing, should, with time, yield as much insight into these mechanisms as we now have into the structure and function of vocal fold mucosa.

REFERENCES

1. Faaborg-Andersen K. Electromyographic investigation of intrinsic laryngeal muscles in humans. *Acta Physiol.* 1957;41(suppl 140):1-149.

2. Faaborg-Andersen K, Buchtal F. Action potentials from internal laryngeal muscles during phonation. *Nature.* 1956;177:340-341.

3. Buchtal F. Electromyography of intrinsic laryngeal muscles. *J Exp Physiol.* 1959;44:137-148.

4. Aminoff MJ. Clinical Electromyography. In: Aminoff MJ, ed. *Electrodiagnosis in Clinical Neurology.* 4th ed. Philadelphia, PA: Churchill Livingstone; 1999:223-252.

5. Fujita M, Ludlow CL, Woodson GE, et al. A new surface electrode for recording from the posterior cricoarytenoid muscle. *Laryngoscope.* 1989;99:316-320.

6. Khan A, Pearlman RC, Bianchi DA, Hauck KW. Experience with two types of electromyography monitoring electrodes during thyroid surgery. *Am J Otolaryngol.* 1997;18:99-102.

7. Guindi GM, Higenbottam TW, Payne JK. A new method for laryngeal electromyography. *Clin Otolaryngol.* 1981;6:271-278.

8. Andrews S, Warner J, Stewart R. EMG biofeedback in the treatment of hyperfunctional dysphonia. *Br J Disord Commun.* 1986;21:353-369.

9. Hillel AD, Robinson LR, Waugh P. Laryngeal electromyography for the diagnosis and management of swallowing disorders. *Otolaryngol Head Neck Surg.* 1997;116:344-348.

10. Lovelace RE, Blitzer A, Ludlow C. Clinical laryngeal electromyography. In: Blitzer A, Brin MF, Sasaki CT, et al, eds. *Neurologic Disorders of the Larynx.* New York, NY: Thieme Medical Publishers; 1992:66-82.

11. Campbell WW. Needle Electrode Examination. In: Campbell WW, ed. *Essentials of Electrodiagnostic Medicine.* Baltimore, MD: Williams & Wilkins; 1999:93-116.

12. Hirano M, Ohala J. Use of hooked-wire electrodes for electromyography of the intrinsic laryngeal muscles. *J Speech Hearing Res.* 1969;12:362-373.

13. Blitzer A, Brin MF, Stewart C, Fahn S. Abductor laryngeal dystonia: a series treated with botulinum toxin. *Laryngoscope.* 1992;102:163-167.

14. Mu LC, Yang SL. A new method of needle-electrode placement in the posterior cricoarytenoid muscle for electromyography. *Laryngoscope.* 1990;100:1127-1131.

15. Thumfart WF. Electromyography of the larynx and related technics. *Acta Otorhinolaryngol Belg.* 1986;40:358-376.

16. Woo P, Arandia H. Intraoperative laryngeal electromyographic assessment of patients with immobile vocal fold. *Ann Otol Rhinol Laryngol.* 1992;101:799-806.

17. Rodriquez AA, Myers BR, Ford CN. Laryngeal electromyography in the diagnosis of laryngeal nerve injuries. *Arch Phys Med Rehabil.* 1990;71:587-590.

18. Shindo ML, Herzon GD, Hanson DG, Cain DJ, Sahgal V. Effects of denervation on laryngeal muscles: a canine model. *Laryngoscope.* 1992;102:663-669.

19. Mu L, Yang S. An experimental study on the laryngeal electromyography and visual observations in varying types of surgical injuries to the unilateral recurrent laryngeal nerve in the neck. *Laryngoscope.* 1991;101:699-708.

20. Siribodhi C, Sundmaker W, Adkins JP, Bonner FJ. Electromyographic studies of laryngeal paralysis and regeneration of laryngeal motor nerves in dogs. *Laryngoscope.* 1963;73:148-163.

21. Blitzer A, Jahn AF, Keidar A. Semon's law revisited: an electromyographic analysis of laryngeal synkinesis. *Ann Otol Rhinol Laryngol.* 1996;105:764-769.

22. Rontal E, Rontal M, Silverman B, Kileny PR. The clinical differentiation between vocal fold paralysis and vocal cord fixation using electromyography. *Laryngoscope.* 1993;103:133-137.

23. Sataloff RT, Bough ID, Spiegel JR. Arytenoid dislocation: diagnosis and treatment. *Laryngoscope.* 1994;104:1353-1361.

24. Hoffman HT, Brunberg JA, Winter P, Sullivan MJ, Kileny PR. Arytenoid subluxation: diagnosis and treatment. *Ann Otol Rhinol Laryngol.* 1991;100:1-9.

25. Yin SS, Qiu WW, Stucker FJ. Value of electromyography in differential diagnosis of laryngeal joint injuries after intubation. *Ann Otol Rhinol Laryngol.* 1996;105:446-451.

26. Quiney RE. Laryngeal electromyography: a useful technique for the investigation of vocal cord palsy. *Clin Otolaryngol.* 1989;14:305-316.

27. Min YB, Finnegan EM, Hoffman HT, Luschei ES, McCullough TM. A preliminary study of the prognostic role of electromyography in laryngeal paralysis. *Otolaryngol Head Neck Surg.* 1994;111:770-775.

28. Hirano M, Nosoe I, Shin T, Maeyama T. Electromyography for laryngeal paralysis. In: Hirano M, Kirchner J, Bless D, eds. *Neurolaryngology: Recent Advances.* Boston, MA: College Hill; 1987:232-248.

29. Thumfart W. Electromyography of the larynx. In: Samii M, Gannetta PJ, eds. *The Cranial Nerves.* Berlin: Springer Verlag; 1981:597-606.

30. Parnes SM, Satya-Murti S. Predictive value of laryngeal electromyography in patients with vocal cord paralysis of neurogenic origin. *Laryngoscope.* 1985;95:1323-1326.

31. Crumley RL. Laryngeal synkinesis: its significance to the laryngologist. *Ann Otol Rhinol Laryngol.* 1989;98:87-92.

32. Crumley RL. Laryngeal synkinesis revisited. *Ann Otol Rhinol Laryngol.* 2000;109:365-371.

33. Nahm I, Shin T, Watanabe H, et al., Misdirected regeneration of the injured recurrent laryngeal nerve in the cat. *Am J Otolaryngol.* 1993;14:43-48.

34. Hiroto I, Hirano M, Tomita H. Electromyographic investigation of human vocal cord paralysis. *Ann Otol Rhinol Laryngol.* 1968;77:296-304.

35. Simpson DM, Sternman D, Graves-Wright J, Sanders I. Vocal cord paralysis: clinical and electrophysiologic features. *Muscle Nerve.* 1993;16:952-957.

36. Koufman JA, Postma GN, Cummins MM, Blalock PD. Vocal fold paresis. *Otolaryngol Head Neck Surg.* 2000;122:537-541.

37. Dursun G, Sataloff RT, Spiegel JR, Mandel S, Heuer RJ, Rosen DC. Superior laryngeal nerve paresis and paralysis. *J Voice.* 1996;10:206-211.

38. Dray TG, Robinson LR, Hillel AD. Idiopathic bilateral vocal fold weakness. *Laryngoscope.* 1999;109:995-1002.

39. Tanaka S, Hirano M, Chijiwa K. Some aspects of vocal fold bowing. *Ann Otol Rhinol Laryngol.* 1994;103:357-362.

40. Dray TG, Robinson LR, Hillel AD. Laryngeal electromyographic findings in Charcot-Marie-Tooth disease type II. *Arch Neurol.* 1999;56:863-865.

41. Robinson LR, Hillel AD, Waugh PF. New laryngeal muscle weakness in post-polio syndrome. *Laryngoscope.* 1998;108:732-734.

42. Driscoll BP, Gracco C, Coelho C, et al. Laryngeal function in postpolio patients. *Laryngoscope.* 1995;105:35-41.

43. Guindi GM, Bannister R, Gibson WP, Payne JK. Laryngeal electromyography in multiple system

atrophy with autonomic failure. *J Neurol Neuro surg Psychiatry.* 1981;44:49-53.

44. Isozaki E, Osanai R, Horiguchi S, Hayashida T, Hirose K, Tanabe H. Laryngeal electromyography with separated surface electrodes in patients with multiple system atrophy presenting with vocal cord paralysis. *J Neurol.* 1994;241:551-556.

45. Palmer JB, Holloway AM, Tanaka E. Detecting lower motor neuron dysfunction of the pharynx and larynx with electromyography. *Arch Phys Med Rehabil.* 1991;72:214-218.

46. Mao VH, Abaza M, Spiegel JR, et al. Laryngeal myasthenia gravis: report of 40 cases. *J Voice.* 2001;19:122-130.

47. Blitzer A, Lovelace RE, Brin MF, Fahn S, Fink ME. Electromyographic findings in focal laryngeal dystonia (spasmodic dysphonia). *Ann Otol Rhinol Laryngol.* 1985;94:591-594.

48. Lipton RJ, McCaffrey TV, Litchy WJ. Intraoperative electrophysiologic monitoring of laryngeal muscle during thyroid surgery. *Laryngoscope.* 1988;98: 1292-1296.

49. Mermelstein M, Nonweiler R, Rubinstein EH. Intraoperative identification of laryngeal nerves with laryngeal electromyography. *Laryngoscope.* 1996;106:752-756.

50. Brin MF, Blitzer A, Stewart C, Fahn S. Treatment of spasmodic dysphonia (laryngeal dystonia) with local injections of botulinum toxin: review and technical aspects. In: Blitzer A, Brin MF, Sasaki CT, Fahn S, Harris KS, eds. *Neurologic Disorders of the Larynx.* New York, NY: Thieme Medical Publishers; 1992:214-228.

51. Woodson GE. Clinical value of laryngeal EMG is dependent on experience of the clinician. *Arch Otolaryngol Head Neck Surg.* 1998;124:476.

CHAPTER 16

Laryngeal Photography and Videography

Eiji Yanagisawa, MD, FACS

Brian P. Driscoll, MD, FACS

H. Steven Sims, MD

The Spanish-born singing teacher Manuel Garcia is credited with the first successful visualization of the intact larynx. In 1854, using a dental mirror, with a hand-held mirror for reflecting sunlight, he was able to visualize the movements of his own vocal folds.[1] The first successful photographs of the larynx were taken by Thomas French of New York in 1882. Using a box camera with an attached laryngeal mirror and a device to concentrate sunlight (Figure 16-1A), he was able to produce surprisingly good quality black-and-white photographs (Figure 16-1B).[2,3]

Since the early photographs of the larynx by French, many other methods of laryngeal documentation have been described. These include: (1) indirect laryngoscopic photography,[4,5] (2) direct laryngoscopic photography,[4,6-9] (3) fiberscopic photography,[10-28] (4) telescopic photography,[19,21-24,26-48] and (5) microscopic photography.[5,29,49-58] Although many have contributed to the evolution and refinement of laryngeal documentation, several authors merit special mention.

In 1941, P. Holinger, J. D. Brubaker and J. E. Brubaker introduced the Holinger and Brubaker 35 mm camera.[6,8] This camera, although expensive and bulky, set a new standard for laryngeal photography. Most would agree that the clarity, color, and brilliance of these photographs have not been surpassed even by today's standards. This system is no longer used.

In 1954, Yutaka Tsuiki of Tohoku University, Japan, was the first to "televise" the larynx. He used a "tele-endoscope" attached to a large television camera. He predicted the importance of video recording the larynx as a method of documentation and teaching.[59]

In 1963, Oscar Kleinsasser of Cologne adapted the Zeiss otologic microscope for laryngoscopic use by utilizing a 400 mm objective lens.[51-53] Later with the use of a photoadapter, beam splitter, and single lens reflex (SLR) camera, he produced extremely high-quality pictures of the larynx.[52]

In 1968, Sawashima and Hirose of Tokyo introduced the flexible laryngoscope.[14] This instrument is now standard equipment for the practicing otolaryngologist. The quality of photodocumentation through this instrument, although acceptable, is not of high resolution. The advent of modern telescopes such as the Hopkins rod lens (Karl Storz), the Lumina optic system (Wolf), and the full Lumen system (Nagashima) has made superb endoscopic documentation of the larynx easy. These instruments provide brilliant, magnified images of high resolution and significant depth of field. The use of these instruments by Paul Ward, George Berci, and Bruce Benjamin has brought very high standards to laryngeal photography.[19,32-36,44,46,48] The excellent articles by Benjamin describing his methods of laryngeal photography are highly recommended.[33,60] Videotape recording

(VTR), as pioneered by Koichi Yamashita, has become the standard technique of the serious endoscopist who requires high-quality documentation of laryngeal form and function.[18,19,21] Recent advances in video technology produce images of such high quality that Kantor, Berci, Partlow, et al described a technique of *video-microlaryngoscopy* in which the operation is performed while viewing the larynx on a television screen.[39]

There have been essentially three methods of laryngeal documentation: (1) still photography, (2) videography, and (3) cinematography. Cinematography has been totally replaced by videography because of the time and

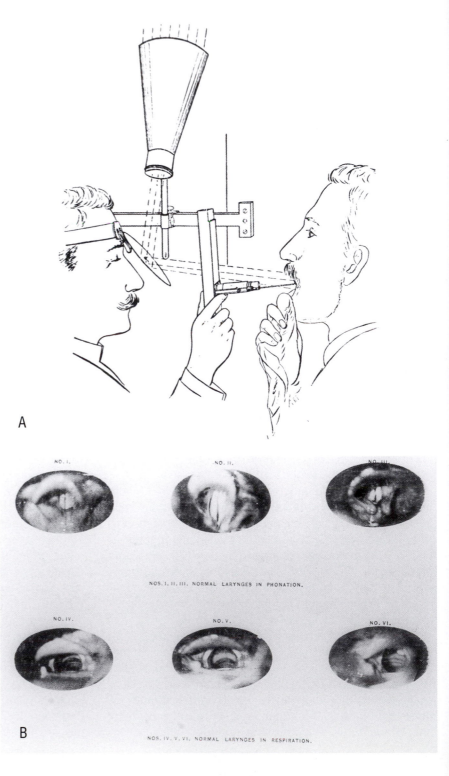

FIGURE 16-1. *(A) Dr. French's method of laryngeal documentation used in 1882. He used a sunlight concentrator as a light source. The light was then reflected off a forehead reflector onto a laryngeal mirror. (B) Sample photographs taken by Dr. French.*

expense required of the former and the ever-increasing quality of the latter. Still photography retains an important role in laryngeal documentation, although it lacks the dynamics required to study laryngeal function. Digital imaging is the newest technology for permanently recording images using a computer. This technique can also be applied to laryngeal documentation.

A discalimer: This chapter describes the techniques of still photography and videography of the larynx employed by the senior author (EY). The authors describe equipment that they regularly use. Other brands or makes not described could also be used successfully. Digital imaging is also discussed.

STILL PHOTOGRAPHY OF THE LARYNX

Still photography is the traditional method of laryngeal photography. There are numerous methods in which one can "take a picture" of the larynx. Many of these methods provide high-quality color slides for publication or presentation. The basic equipment is a 35 mm single lens reflex (SLR) camera (Figure 16-2) combined with a light source and a means of visualizing the larynx, such as the laryngeal mirror, laryngoscope, flexible fiberscope, rigid telescope, or operating microscope. Laryngeal photography has recently been made even easier with the use of the newer 35 mm SLR cameras with built-in autowinders combined with the TTL (Through The Lens) electronic flash system.

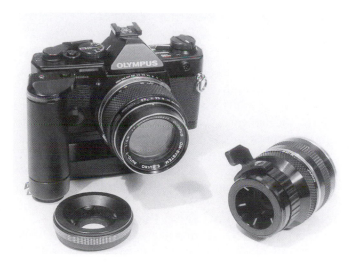

FIGURE 16-2. *The single-lens-reflex (SLR) system for still photography. (Top left) Olympus OM-2 35 mm SLR camera with an autowinder and 100 mm macrolens. (Bottom left) Karl Storz quick-connect adapter. (Bottom right) Olympus SMR coupler to which a 2X extender is attached.*

Still Photography in the Office

Indirect Still Laryngoscopic Photography

This method is difficult, unpredictable, and requires an experienced photographer. During indirect mirror laryngoscopy (ML) using a fiberoptic headlight as the light source, the laryngeal image appearing in the mirror is photographed. This is accomplished with a 35 mm SLR camera on a tripod to which a 100 mm telephoto lens, such as the Nikon Medical close-up lens, and a ring light are attached. ASA 400 or faster Ektachrome film is recommended. In the authors' experience, satisfactory results are obtained only 20% of the time.

Fiberscopic Still Laryngeal Photography

Although this technique produces a grainy image that is inferior in resolution to that of the telescope, there are distinct advantages to its use. Full functional examination of the larynx can be accomplished with one insertion, even in difficult patients in whom other techniques of laryngeal examination would be difficult or impossible, for example, small children, immobilized adults, and those with a hypersensitive gag or unusual supraglottic anatomy that makes visualization of the anterior larynx difficult with the telescope.

This technique can be accomplished with a number of flexible scopes such as the Olympus ENF-P3 (3.4 mm) or L3 (4.2 mm), Machida 4L (4.0 mm) or 3L (3.3 mm), or Pentax FNL-10S (3.5 mm).[15,16,25]

The senior author's recommended equipment for photodocumentation consists of: (1) the Olympus OM-2 35 mm SLR camera with an autowinder, clear-glass focusing screen 1-9, and 2X teleconverter; (2) Olympus ENF-P2 or P3 fiberscope (the authors' choice); (3) Olympus SMR endoscopic coupler (Figure 16-2); (4) Karl Storz xenon cold light source 487C, 610, or 615; and (5) Ektachrome ASA 400 or 800 daylight film. The camera is set on automatic mode with the appropriate ASA setting. The flexible scope is connected to the 2X teleconverter, which is attached to the SLR camera using either the SMR endoscopic coupler or the 100 mm macrolens with the Karl Storz quick-connect adapter (Figure 16-2). The fiberscope is then advanced to the hypopharynx through an anesthetized (4% lidocaine) and vasoconstricted (3% ephedrine) nose. The images are centered and focused in the viewfinder of the camera, and the larynx is photographed during inspiration and phonation (Figure 16-3A). The clearest pictures are taken immediately after phonating /i/ (Figure 16-3B). It should be noted that the laryngeal image occupies a small portion of the photographic field, and much of what the camera sees is blackened out. This situation

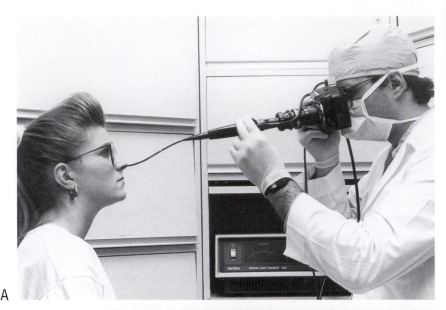

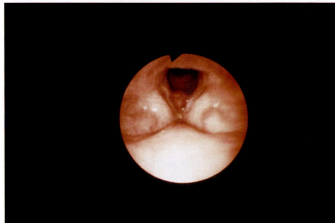

FIGURE 16-3. *(A) Method of fiberscopic laryngeal photography in the office. (B) Photograph taken with the above method showing a laryngeal polyp.*

will cause the metering system in most automatic cameras to overexpose the photograph, thus washing out the laryngeal image. To prevent this, the compensation dial of the camera should be set at -1 or -2 to underexpose the image by 1 or 2 f-stops. A series of photographs should be taken with appropriate bracketing of the shots. When a xenon light source is not available, faster films (ASA 800 or greater) should be used.

More recently the authors have employed the TTL endoscopic flash photography technique as recommended by Karl Storz (Figure 16-4A). This technique uses the Nikon 5005 camera, which is set to manual at a shutter speed of 1/30 of a second, and any aperture setting except *S*. The Karl Storz 610 light source is set at auto TTL and attached to the camera with a 570MN connection cord (Figure 16-4A and B). The fiberscope is connected to the camera by the Karl Storz 593 T2 lens, and the focal length can be set from 30 mm to 140 mm. The

authors routinely use 140 mm as it produces a larger image. Using the TTL system obviates the need to underexpose the image or bracket the photographs. In the authors' hands the success rate of the older method is approximately 50%, which rises to 80% with the TTL system. The readers are advised to consult the Karl Storz company for updated system information.

Telescopic Still Laryngeal Photography

This provides the clearest laryngeal images available in the office. The equipment used by the authors includes: (1) the Olympus 35 mm SLR OM-2 camera system described for fiberscopic laryngoscopy; (2) a telescope, such as the Kay 9105 (70 degree), the Karl Storz rigid telescope 8706 CL (70 degree), the Nagashima SFT-1 (with an "Olympus-type" eyepiece) (70 degree), the Karl Storz right-angled telescope 8702D (90 degree), or the Stuckrad magnifying telescope (Wolf) (90 degree);

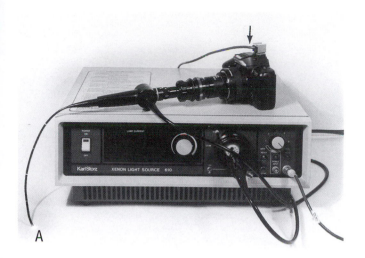

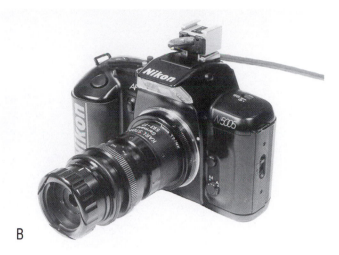

FIGURE 16-4. *(A) Fiberscopic electronic flash still photography system showing Nikon SLR camera, with the Karl Storz 35–140 mm adapter, 570MN TTL light cord (arrow), and the Karl Storz 610 light source. (B) Enlarged view of the Nikon N5005 with Karl Storz 35–140 mm zoom lens adapter.*

(3) a xenon light source (Karl Storz 487C, 610, 615); and (4) ASA 400 or 800 Ektachrome daylight film.

With the soft palate and posterior tongue anesthetized, the patient's tongue is grasped and protruded. The telescope is advanced into the mouth, being careful not to induce gagging by touching the posterior tongue or pharynx (Figure 16-5A). Having the patient vocalize a high-pitched /i/ raises and fully exposes the larynx in most cases. Pictures can be taken during respiration and phonation. The exposures should be bracketed using the automatic compensation dial. Repeated insertions are usually required. The success rate with this method is 70–80% (Figure 16-5B).[26,28,47,61] The Karl Storz TTL system as described for the fiberscope can also be used in this setting.

Microscopic Still Laryngeal Photography

The necessary equipment includes: (1) the Zeiss operating microscope with a straightforward eyepiece and the 250 or 300 mm objective lens, (2) a 35 mm SLR camera, (3) a photoadapter, and (4) Ektachrome ASA 320 Tungsten film.

In this technique, the larynx is exposed with a laryngeal mirror and viewed through the microscope. The wall-mounted scope is easier to manipulate and is recommended if available. The microscope is locked during photography to limit camera-shake aberrations. Although some report good results with this method, in the authors' hands the success rate is less than 20%. The difficulty in exposing the larynx while focusing the operating microscope is the disadvantage.

Still Photography in the Operating Room

Direct Laryngoscopic Photography

There are two methods of photographing the larynx directly through the laryngoscope. The first utilizes a 100 mm or 200 mm telephoto lens attached to a 35 mm SLR camera on a tripod (Figure 16-6A and B). Ektachrome Tungsten ASA 320 is used. If the Dedo or Ossoff photographic laryngoscope with two large fiberoptic cables is used, no additional light sources are needed. The major difficulty with this technique is that it is cumbersome. Interruption of the operation and readjustment of the camera and tripod are necessary with each new photograph of the larynx. The success rate is 70–80%. The image obtained with this method may be small but quite satisfactory.

The second method requires an aperture-preferred automatic 35 mm SLR camera, such as the Nikon FE or the Olympus OM-2 with a 50 mm macrolens attached. If the newer autofocus cameras such as the Nikon 6006 or 8008 are used, they should be focused manually. This prevents the camera from focusing on the edge of the laryngoscope. Ektachrome Tungsten ASA 320 film is used. For this technique the camera is hand-held, and the larynx is focused through the laryngoscope and photographed (Figure 16-7A). The resulting image, although small, is quite recognizable (Figure 16-7B). The photograph may be cropped and enlarged. The authors feel this is the simplest method of laryngeal photography, and it is recommended for the occasional laryngeal photographer.

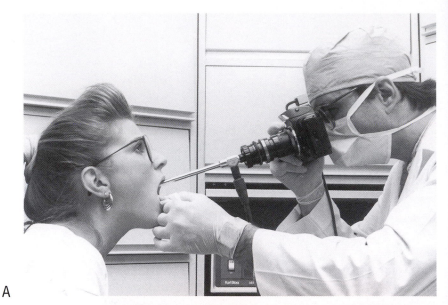

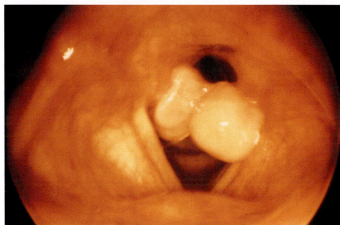

A

B

FIGURE 16-5. *(A) Method of telescopic still photography in the office. (B) Photograph taken with this method showing post-intubation granulomas.*

Telescopic Laryngeal Photography

In the operating room, telescopic laryngeal photography is accomplished by passing a telescope, attached to a 35 mm SLR camera and light source, through the laryngoscope and then photographing the larynx.[32,33]

The setup the authors use includes the Hopkins 0 degree straightforward telescope 8700A with the Karl Storz 487C or 615 xenon light source (Figure 16-8A). The telescope is attached to the Olympus OM-2 camera with a 100 mm macrolens, a Karl Storz quick-connect adapter, a 1-9 focusing screen and an autowinder. ASA 400 Ektachrome daylight film is used.

This method is highly successful (greater than 90%) and produces excellent pictures of the larynx (Figure 16-8B). The major drawbacks are the expense of the special telescope and adapters and the need to interrupt surgery to photograph the larynx. One can also use a Nikon automatic camera with the Karl Storz TTL flash system.

Microscopic Laryngeal Photography

Laryngeal photography through the operating microscope can be accomplished with or without the use of a photoadapter.[26,50-52,54-58] High-quality images of varying magnification are possible with this technique.

Microscopic Photography With the Use of a Photoadapter

Microscopic photography with the use of a photoadapter requires the following equipment: (1) an operating microscope (the authors prefer Zeiss), (2) a beam splitter, (3) a photoadapter, (4) an automatic 35 mm SLR camera, and (5) a ring adapter for the camera. High-speed Ektachrome Tungsten ASA 320 film is used. After the laryngoscope is suspended, the microscope with the attached beam splitter, photoadapter, and 35 mm SLR camera are positioned for microlaryngoscopy (Figure 16-9A). Photographs can now be taken at any time. Two

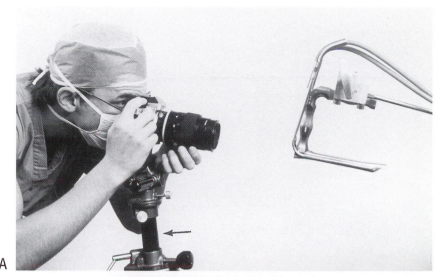

FIGURE 16-6. *(A) Method of direct laryngeal photography in the operating room with a SLR camera and a 100 mm lens mounted on a tripod (arrow). (B) Photograph taken with this method showing a pedunculated vallecular cyst lying on the top of the epiglottis.*

major advantages of this technique are that the surgeon is the photographer and there is minimal disruption of the operation. Other advantages include the following: (1) one can photograph at varying magnifications (6X, 10X, 25X, and 40X) (Figure 16-9B), (2) the full-field image of the larynx at higher magnifications obviates the need for copying and enlarging the slides for presentation, and (3) with the use of a Telestill or dual photoadapter, TV and movie documentation are possible.

The disadvantages are: (1) the expense of the beam splitter and the photoadapter, (2) the shallow depth of field, especially at high magnification, and (3) the need for brilliant illumination, such as that provided by the Dedo or Ossoff (Pilling) photographic laryngoscope. The success rate is approximately 70%.

Microscopic Photography Without the Use of a Photoadapter

This simple, inexpensive means of laryngeal photography known as the *microscopic macrolens technique*[26,58]

requires only: (1) the Zeiss operating microscope, (2) an *aperture-preferred* automatic 35 mm SLR camera, such as the Nikon FE, Pentax ME, or Olympus OM-2, (3) a 50 mm macrolens, and (4) the Dedo or Ossoff photographic laryngoscope. Ektachrome Tungsten ASA 320 film is used.

During microscopic laryngoscopy, the larynx is focused through the microscope with the eyepiece set at 0. The microscope is then locked in place. With the camera focused at infinity and the aperture wide open (usually f3.5), the camera is placed on the microscope eyepiece, and the laryngeal image is centered and brought into sharp focus through the camera (Figure 16-10A). The picture is then taken. Surprisingly good quality photographs, with a success rate of 70–80%, can be taken with this simple technique (Figure 16-10B). Some disadvantages are that occasionally it may be difficult to hold the camera still on the eyepiece, and it requires interruption of surgery. The ultimate success of this technique depends on illumination, critical focusing, and the stability of the patient, microscope, and camera.

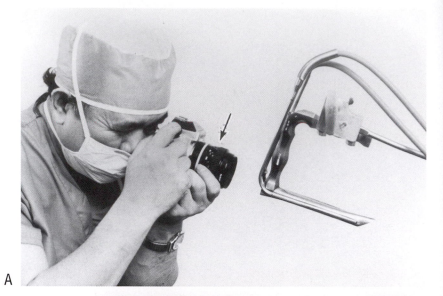

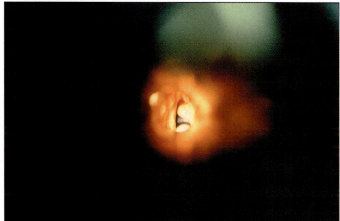

FIGURE 16-7. *(A) Method of laryngeal photography in the operating room using a hand-held SLR camera with a 50 mm macrolens (arrow). (B) Photograph taken with this technique showing a laryngeal polyp.*

VIDEOGRAPHY OF THE LARYNX

Recent technologic advances such as the light-sensitive charge-coupled device (CCD) video cameras, xenon light sources, and improved endoscopic equipment have made videographic documentation of the larynx a highly successful and versatile practice. Video images can be obtained through the use of the flexible fiberscope, the rigid telescope, or the operating microscope. Hard copies of excellent quality can be provided instantly by the color video printers.

Videography of the Larynx in the Office

Fiberscopic Videolaryngoscopy

Fiberscopic videolaryngoscopy[23,25,26,28,62-64] is the most widely used technique for video documentation of the larynx. It is the easiest and best tolerated technique and allows a full endoscopic examination of the upper aerodigestive tract with one pass. It allows evaluation of both the form and the function of the larynx, along with simultaneous voice recording. The following equipment is needed: (1) a flexible fiberscope, (2) a color video camera, (3) a video camera adapter, (4) a light source (xenon is preferred), (5) a video recorder (3/4", 1/2", 8 mm), and (6) a color monitor. The fiberscopes available include the Olympus ENF-P3, P4, or L3, Machida ENT 4L or 3L, and Pentax FNL 10S or 15S. There are many fine-quality miniature single-chip CCD video cameras available for fiberscopic videolaryngoscopy. These include: (1) Karl Storz Supercam 9060B (7 lux) and Telecam (3 lux) (Figure 16-11); (2) Olympus OTV-S3 or SC; (3) Toshiba CCD (10 lux) (distributed by Nagashima) (Figure 16-11); (4) Elmo EC-202 CCD (10 lux) and Elmo MN 401X (5 lux) or CN 401E (distributed by Videomedics and Nagashima) (Figure 16-12); (5) Panasonic GP KS 152 (5 lux); (6) Aztec VID 1 (7 lux); and (7) Wolf Endocam CCD (10 lux). Some of these cam-

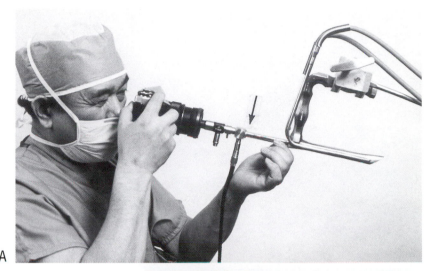

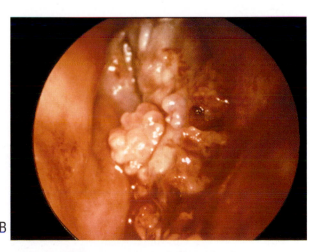

FIGURE 16-8. *(A) Method of telescopic still photography in the operating room with the Hopkins 8700A telescope (arrow). (B) Photograph of transglottic tumor taken with this method.*

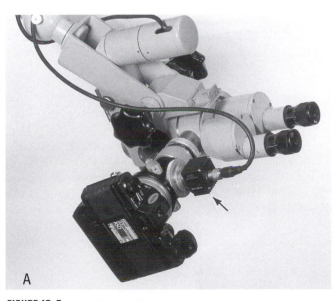

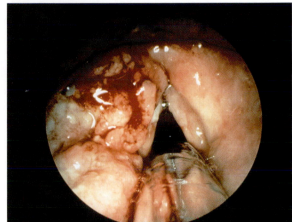

FIGURE 16-9. *(A) Method for microlaryngoscopic still photography using the SLR camera attached to the Zeiss operating microscope via a photoadapter. Also note a miniature CCD camera on the photoadapter (arrow). (B) Photograph of extensive squamous cell carcinoma taken with this technique.*

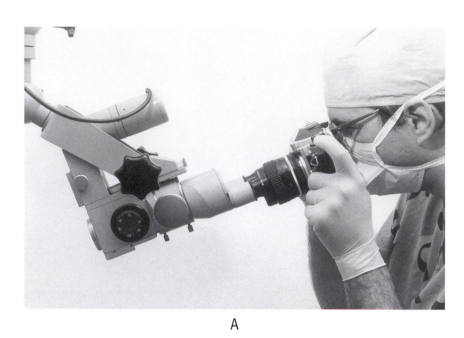

A

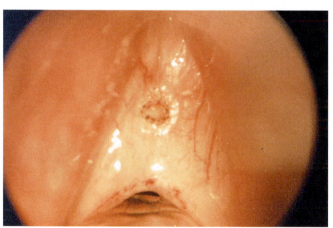
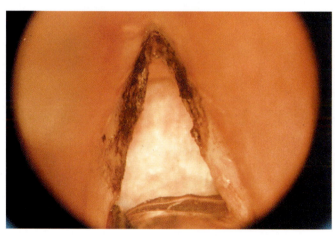

B

FIGURE 16-10. *(A) Method of microscopic still photography without photoadapter ("microscopic macrolens technique"). (B) Photographs of laryngeal web, before and after CO_2 laser excision, taken with this technique.*

eras are equipped with C-mount couplers and require special adapters for the endoscopes while others have built-in nondetachable adapters (Figure 16-11). The cost of these single-chip video cameras ranges in price from $2,000 to $5,000 (1999). More recently, three-chip high-resolution cameras have become available. They include the Karl Storz Tricam 9070N and Stryker 780, which cost about $18,000–$20,000.

Yanagisawa et al advocated the use of home video cameras for videolaryngoscopy in the early 1980s.[22,28,48] They were able to obtain excellent results with reasonably priced ($1,000–$1,500) home video cameras. Some of

these cameras include: (1) Olympus Movie 8 VX801-62 (7 lux), (2) Ricoh R620 CCD (4 lux), and (3) Ricoh R66 (4 lux) (Figure 16-12). With the use of the Karl Storz quick-connect adapter, the fiberscope could be attached to the video camera lens. These home video cameras are not used any more because they are obsolete, and much smaller, reasonably priced CCD cameras are now available. Figure 16-11 demonstrates a comparison of the sizes and shapes of the old home video cameras and the newer compact CCD cameras. The examination is performed in the same manner as that described for fiberscopic still photography (Figure 16-13A).

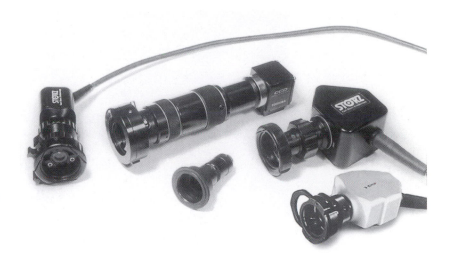

FIGURE 16-11. *Miniature CCD video cameras (left to right): 1) Karl Storz supercam camera with a built-in adapter; 2) Toshiba C-mount CCD camera with Nagashima zoom lens videoadapter; 3) Elmo EC-102 miniature CCD camera with a C-mount adapter; 4) Karl Storz Tricam 3-chip CCD camera; 5) Stryker 782 3-chip camera.*

The most significant advantage of fiberscopic video-laryngoscopy is the ease of examination. Other advantages are that (1) it is rapid, (2) it is comfortable for the patient, (3) children and uncooperative adults may be examined, (4) it allows evaluation of form and function along with simultaneous voice recording, and (5) it allows limited examination of the subglottis and trachea. Its major disadvantage is that the image produced is smaller, more distorted, and of lower resolution when compared to the telescopes. The use of larger endoscopes such as the Olympus ENF-L3 helps to decrease the impact of edge distortion by providing a larger distortion-free area in the center of the image.

Other disadvantages include: (1) it requires greater illumination because of the small diameter of the scope, (2) it requires a light-sensitive camera (low lux), and (3) it tends to produce the moiré effect (multiple abnormal color strips) on the television screen, interfering with detailed interpretation. The overall success rate approaches 95%, even when used in infants and children (Figure 16-13B).

The senior author currently uses the Olympus ENF-P3 (3.4 mm) and ENF-L3 (4.2 mm) fiberscopes attached to a lightweight three-chip CCD camera with a xenon light source for optimal images. The wider nasal cavity is sprayed with topical anesthetic (4% lidocaine) and decongestant (3% ephedrine). With the patient in an upright sitting position, the fiberscope is passed along the floor of the nose, through the velopharyngeal port, and down to the oropharynx. When one obtains the desired image on the monitor, illumination and focus are optimized and recording begins. A panoramic view of the larynx, the pharynx, and the base of the tongue is obtained. The scope is advanced to the vallecula, then over the epiglottis into the laryngeal vestibule (Figure 16-3). Close-up views of the glottis, true and false vocal folds, and vestibule (and sometimes even the subglottis) can be obtained as well as views of any lesions. If the moiré effect (unwanted color strips) is seen on the monitor, the camera is turned relative to the endoscope.

When the image is too dark for diagnostic purposes and/or for documentation, the authors recommend the

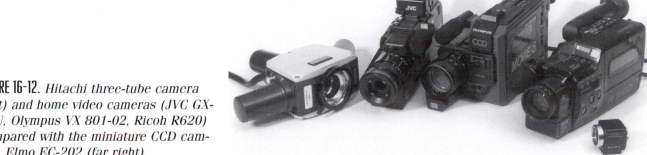

FIGURE 16-12. *Hitachi three-tube camera (left) and home video cameras (JVC GX-N8U, Olympus VX 801-02, Ricoh R620) compared with the miniature CCD camera, Elmo EC-202 (far right).*

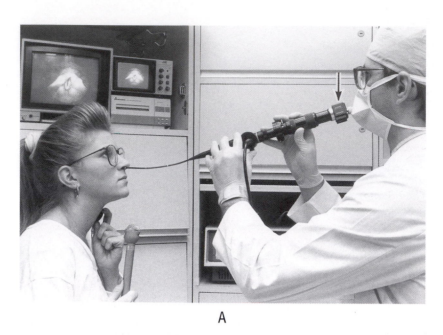

A

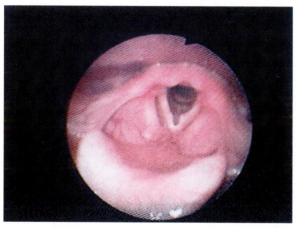 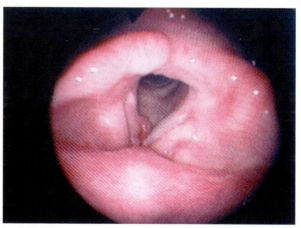

B

FIGURE 16-13. *(A) Method of flexible fiberscopic videolaryngoscopy in the office using the miniature CCD camera, Elmo EC-202 (arrow). (B) Images of laryngeal nodules taken with Olympus ENF-P3 (3.6 mm) (left) and laryngeal polyps taken with Olympus ENF-L (4.4 mm) (right). Note the difference in size of the images created with these different scopes. The images were produced with a Sony UP-5000 video printer.*

following: (1) use an extra-light-sensitive video camera (low lux), (2) increase the video camera sensitivity by using the gain control switch, (3) advance the tip of the fiberscope very close to the vocal folds, (4) change the image size by using a zoom adapter for a micro CCD camera, or (5) use a fiberscope with a large diameter such as the Olympus ENF-L3 (4.2 mm) (Figure 16-13B). The image and color quality can also be improved during printing using adjustment control of the color video printer (Figure 16-13B).

Telescopic Videolaryngoscopy

Telescopic videolaryngoscopy[23,26,28,62-66] is performed using much the same technique as the fiberscopic method, except that the telescope is passed through the mouth and the camera is connected to a telescope instead of a fiberscope. This method gives a brilliant picture and is particularly well-suited for diagnosing subtle changes in laryngeal structure.

The necessary equipment includes a single- or three-chip CCD miniature camera or a video camera, and a rigid telescope such as the (1) Karl Storz 8706CL, (2) Kay Elemetrics 9105, (3) Nagashima SFT-1, (4) Wolf Stuckrad, and (5) Karl Storz 8702D. These telescopes are attached to the CCD camera via a special adapter if the CCD camera does not have a built-in adapter. The 70 degree telescope such as the Nagashima SFT-1, Karl Storz 8706CL and Kay Elemetrics 9105 permit excellent visualization of the anterior commissure and posterior portions of the larynx, and make them especially useful for laryngostroboscopy.

The examination is performed in the following manner: (1) the patient's soft palate and posterior tongue are anesthetized with 4% Xylocaine (lidocaine), (2) the scope is dipped in warm water or sprayed with defogger, (3) the patient's tongue is grasped by the examiner with one hand while the scope is inserted with the other hand, keeping the glossoepiglottic fold in the midline while advancing the scope, ensuring optimal (midline) orientation of the larynx (Figure 16-14A), and (4) video recording is begun when the vocal folds are in clear focus (Figure 16-14B).

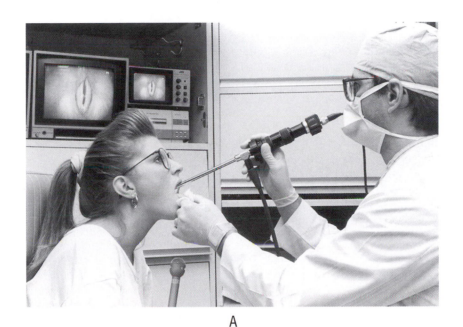

A

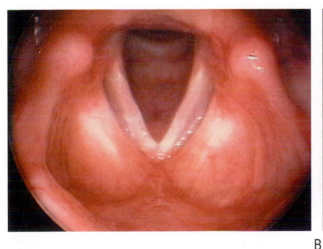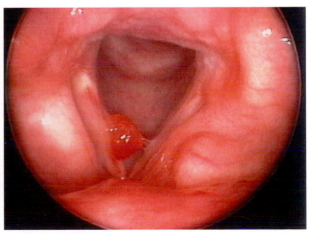

B

FIGURE 16-14. *(A) Method of telescopic videolaryngoscopy in the office using the 70 degree Nagashima SFT-1 telescope attached to the miniature CCD camera, Elmo EC-202 with Nagashima videoadapter. (B) Images of a normal larynx (left) and a laryngeal polyp (right) taken with this method. The images were produced with a Sony UP-5100 video printer.*

The major benefit of this system is the superior optics offered by the telescope. This provides (1) a wide-angle view of the larynx with a large, clear image and (2) a close-up view of the larynx to detect subtle anatomic lesions. The larger diameter of the scope also allows for increased light transmission and a much brighter and clearer stroboscopic image. The disadvantages of this technique include the following: (1) children and some adults with hyperactive gag reflexes may be unable to tolerate the examination, (2) fogging of the scope requires cleaning and reinsertion, and (3) voice and vocal mechanics may be distorted.

The authors prefer the telescopic examination because of the superior image produced (Figure 16-14B): the image is larger, brighter, and sharper than that of the fiberscope. This translates to increased diagnostic capabilities for subtle laryngeal changes. In the authors' hands, this technique has a 90% success rate.

Microscopic Videolaryngoscopy

This technique is similar to that described for microscopic still photography in the office using the Zeiss operating microscope. The only difference is that a video camera hookup is used instead of an SLR camera. This technique (as one might expect) is time-consuming and awkward. The authors have abandoned this technique in favor of the techniques described above.

Videography in the Operating Room

Telescopic Videolaryngoscopy

In the operating room, telescopic videolaryngoscopy[62,64-66] is accomplished with the use of the straight-forward Hopkins rigid telescope 8700A, a miniature CCD camera (Figure 16-15A), and a xenon light source. In this setting, the miniature CCD camera is more useful and convenient than the home video camera. After the laryngoscope is suspended, the telescope is placed through the laryngoscope and the image is centered. The advantage of this system is the splendid image quality (Figure 16-15B). With the use of a color video printer, still images can be obtained easily during or after the procedure. The major disadvantages are that (1) it requires interruption of the surgical procedure, and (2) it is difficult to document surgical technique.

The senior author always passes the 0° telescope for documentation prior to microlaryngoscopic surgery as he believes telescopic videolaryngoscopy provides the best possible laryngeal images. In selected cases, he uses the other angled telescopes (30°, 70°, 90°, 120°). The 30° and 70° telescopes allow excellent visualization of the anterior commissure. The 70° and 90° telescopes are useful for evaluation and documentation of laryngeal ventricles. The inferior border of the true vocal fold lesion can be readily identified with the 70° or 120° telescopes. The involvement of the anterior commissure by an anterior lesion of the vocal fold can be precisely identified with the 30° and 70° telescopes in most cases.

Telescopic video documentation of subglottic lesions in a tracheotomized patient can be performed through a tracheotomy opening using the Hopkins 4 mm 70° telescope.

Microscopic Videolaryngoscopy

Microscopic videolaryngoscopy[26] remains the single most convenient and effective method to teach and doc-

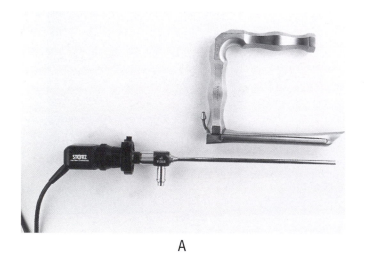

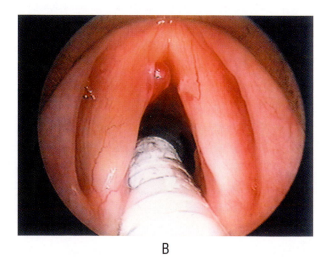

A   B

FIGURE 16-15. *(A) Telescopic videolaryngoscopy in the operating room using the Dedo laryngoscope and the Karl Storz Supercam CCD miniature camera attached to the 8700A 0 degree telescope. (B) Image of a laryngeal polyp taken with this system. The image was produced with a Sony UP-5100 video printer.*

ument microsurgery of the larynx. This is the authors' preferred method of operative documentation.[26]

The equipment used includes: (1) a photographic laryngoscope such as the Dedo or Ossoff (these laryngoscopes have two channels that house large-bore fiberoptic cables); (2) a light source, such as the Pilling 2X; (3) the (Zeiss) operating microscope with a straight eyepiece and 400 mm objective lens (Figure 16-16A); (4) a beam splitter; (5) a photoadapter, such as the Zeiss or Telestill photoadapter; (6) a miniature CCD camera or pickup tube camera (Figure 16-16A); (7) a video recorder; and (8) a color TV monitor. With their small size and weight, the miniature CCD cameras interfere minimally with the operative procedure. However, the more expensive and bulkier three-tube cameras, such as the Hitachi DK5050 or Ikegami ITC-350 M, produce video images of excellent quality (Figure 16-16A and B). For those seeking the highest-quality images, the three-tube cameras have been replaced with the newer three-chip cameras, such as the Sony DXC-750 ($16,000) and Hitachi, Ikegami, or Stryker three-chip camera. Sony introduced a moderately priced three-chip CCD camera, Sony DXC 960 MD (approximately $6,000) in 1993.

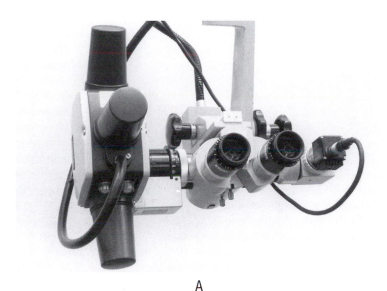

A

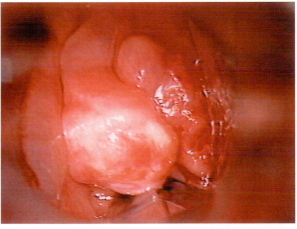 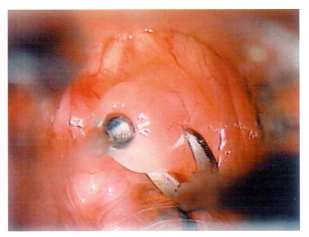

B

FIGURE 16-16. *(A) Techniques for microscopic videography. Coupled to the left of the Zeiss microscope is the Hitachi three-tube camera attached to a beam splitter. By comparison, coupled to the right of the scope is the Elmo EC-202 mini CCD camera attached to the Zeiss photoadapter. (B) Images taken with this technique demonstrating obstructive laryngeal polyps (left) and excision of a polyp with scissors (right). Images were produced with a Sony UP-5100 video printer.*

Some of the multiple advantages of this system are: (1) minimal interference with the operative procedure, (2) live viewing by an unlimited audience, (3) equipment that is readily available in most medical centers, (4) variability of magnification, facilitating precise documentation of small lesions, (5) pediatric and adult use, (6) video documentation for teaching surgical techniques, and (7) the capability of producing instant color prints of publishable quality when a color video printer is used. Among the disadvantages are: (1) the depth of field is shallower, (2) instrumentation is more difficult, as the microscope is between the surgeon and the patient, (3) at times surgery must be carried out through one eyepiece because of the small proximal opening of the laryngoscope, and (4) refocusing at various magnifications may be necessary.

Kantor-Berci Telescopic Video Microlaryngoscope

In 1990, Kantor, Berci, Partlow et al introduced a new approach to microlaryngeal surgery and its documentation.[39] Their method is akin to performing endoscopic sinus surgery. Using a specially designed *microlaryngoscope* that houses a rigid telescope with attached camera, they are able to both video-record and perform the operation while viewing a high-resolution TV screen (Figure 16-17A and B). The required equipment includes: (1) a Kantor-Berci videomicrolaryngoscope (Karl Storz 8590 VJ) (an improved model is now available) and Lewy (or other) laryngoscope holder; (2) a Karl Storz Supercam micro CCD video camera; (3) a xenon light source (Karl Storz 615, or 487C); (4) a large, high-resolution TV monitor and recorder; and (5) a color video printer (Sony UP-5000).

Some of the advantages of the Kantor-Berci system include the following: (1) it gives a clear, sharp image with excellent depth of field, (2) it facilitates instrumentation of the larynx, as the microscope is not between the surgeon and patient, and (3) it provides superior documentation. Some disadvantages are that: (1) the equipment is costly, (2) specialized equipment such as the angled forceps are needed, (3) it requires a dedicated video camera, (4) refocusing may be necessary (Supercam camera) when the zoom lens is used, (5) there is some image distortion, (6) at the time of writing no pediatric laryngoscope is available, and (7) depth perception may be impaired because the system creates a monocular image.

In a series of patients, the senior author (EY) has compared this technique with the standard microscope technique at the same setting. While the Kantor-Berci system is an effective means of documenting laryngeal surgery and offers superior visualization of the anterior larynx with an excellent depth of field, the microscopic system has the advantage of variable magnification with a depth of field that is generally better than expected, and permits true binocular vision.

Video Image Transfer to Print and Slide

Video images can be transferred to either prints or slides, in color or black and white. This can be accomplished in several ways.

Production of Prints

This can be accomplished instantaneously while videotaping, or at a later viewing through the use of the video printers (Figure 16-18A-C).[26,41] The authors initially used the Sony UP-5000 (Figure 16-18A) but currently prefer the Sony UP-5100 or UP-5500 color video printer, which produces a superior high-resolution image. However, this unit is quite expensive ($7,000 to $8,000). The more affordable Sony CVP G700 ($1,500) or Sony DPM 1000 ($400) (Figure 16-18B), which produces very acceptable images, may be used. However, the time required to produce a print is longer with less expensive printers. Black-and-white prints for publication can also be made by photographing the color video printouts using black-and-white film (such as ASA 400 Tri-X or T-Max). Prints can also be made using a computer, as described in the following digital imaging section.

Production of Slides

There are several methods of producing slides from video images. The first is to photograph the video image on the TV screen (TV screen photography) (Figure 16-18 D-F).[26,62-64,67] The equipment necessary is: (1) a 35 mm SLR camera, (2) Ektachrome Daylight ASA 400 color film, (3) a 50 mm macrolens, (4) a tripod, and (5) an orange-colored filter (Kodak CC40R or Tiffen CC40) when using color film. The camera is placed on the tripod (Figure 16-18D), and the laryngeal image on the TV screen is brought into focus. The shutter speed should be one-half per second or slower (thus the need for the tripod) to cut out interference (raster) lines. For best results the room should be dark to avoid glare on the TV screen, and the video player should be in the play mode. In the pause mode, unwanted horizontal lines may be seen either at the top or bottom of the screen. Each photograph is usually bracketed (-1, 0, +1) using the exposure compensation dial on the camera. This is the least expensive method of producing quite satisfactory results.

The second method of slide production is to copy the color video printouts using color slide film (Ektachrome ASA 320 Tungsten film). This is a practical, much less expensive way.

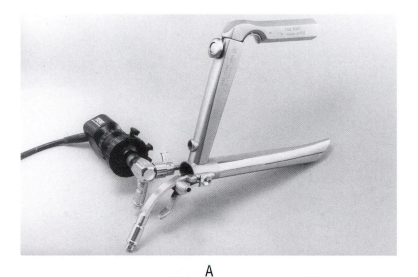

A

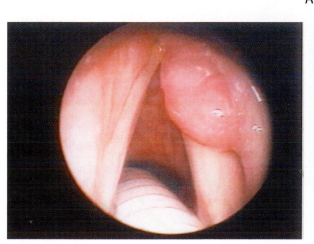 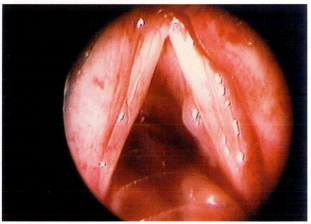

B

FIGURE 16-17. *(A) Kantor-Berci's video microlaryngoscopic technique. Karl Storz Supercam CCD miniature camera is attached to the specially designed telescope (Karl Storz 8575A) and inserted into the built-in channel on the left side of the Kantor-Berci video microlaryngoscope (Karl Storz 8590B). (B) Images taken with this technique showing a false vocal fold polyp (left) and laryngeal polyp (right). Images were produced with a Sony UP-5100 video printer.*

The third method is to use a video/slide making system such as Sony Slidemaker MD, which receives RGB video signals from a color printer (Sony UP 5100/5500) and allows one to photograph the desired image with its attached 35 mm camera (ISO 100 or Polachrome ISO 40 color slide film).

The fourth method is by the use of the Stryker Surgislide Slidemaker (Figure 16-18G). This is a relatively new analog image capture device for the production of 35 mm slides from either a video camera during videography or a prerecorded video image later. The recommended film is ASA 100 Professional Daylight Ektachrome. A 35 mm automatic SLR camera is attached to the front of the image capture device. This system produces excellent color slides. The advantage of the Stryker Slidemaker is the ability to capture images directly onto 35 mm slide film without the need for additional hardware or software. However, the disadvantage is its high cost (approximately $9,000).

Documentation by Digital Imaging

Digital imaging is the newest technology for permanently recording images without film. An image obtained via a video camera can now be converted to an electronic signal that a computer can read, record, and store in a digital fashion.

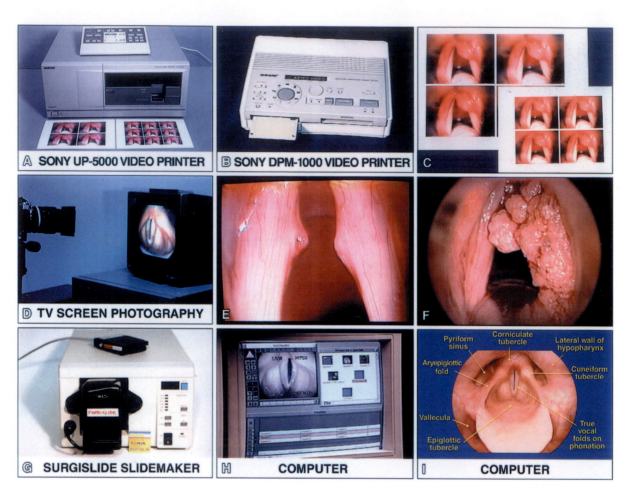

FIGURE 16-18. *Video image transfer to prints and slides. (A) Sony color video printer UP-5000. (B) Sony DPM-1000 color video printer. (C) Color video prints produced by Sony UP-5100 and by Sony CVP-G700. (D) TV screen photography. (E) Image of laryngeal nodules produced by TV screen photography. (F) Image of transglottic laryngeal carcinoma produced by TV screen photography. (G) Stryker Surgislide slide maker. (H) Digitized laryngeal image on the computer screen, which can be annotated. Prints are made using a digital color printer. (I) Annotated image of the normal larynx produced by a digital color printer Sony UP-5500.*

The image can be digitized from a video camera, a digital camera (still or video), a videotape, a slide, a print, or a negative.

There are a number of advantages to digital imaging: (1) the image is produced immediately and thus can be "re-shot" if needed, (2) the image can be transferred via modem to other computers for immediate consultation, (3) the image does not degrade with time, (4) various types of editing of the image are possible, (5) images taken over time can be displayed on one screen, (6) storage and retrieval of images is much simpler, and (7) photographic quality resolution is possible (though expensive). Disadvantages include the initial start-up expense and the time needed to master the system.[68]

Laryngeal documentation can be accomplished by digitizing images from prerecorded videotape (Figure 16-18H and I). Video recording has been the senior author's method for many years. Software is available that can capture video images either as still frames or as full-motion video. These digitized images may be made into composite pictures, labeled, and saved as a computer file. The computer system we use for digital imaging is a Macintosh Quadra 950 with 64 MB of RAM and a 4 GB hard disk with Avid Media Suite Pro and Adobe Photoshop. The image may be printed with a digital printer. The authors use the Sony UP-5500 digital color video printer, which utilizes a dye sublimation printing process. This printer produces high-quality photo-realistic prints suitable for publication (Figure 16-18I), although the printer is quite expensive (approximately $9,000). Less expensive digital color printers are available. Color slides may be obtained by photographing these computer prints. Alternatively, the computer file may be transferred to photo prints or 35 mm slides by a computer service bureau, usually via high-capacity removable storage devices such as Zip disks, optical drives, or compact disks (CDs).

More recently, still digital image capture devices such as the Sony DKR-700 Digital Still Recorder, the Stryker Digital Capture System SDC, and the Stryker Digital Capture System SDC Pro have become available and can be used for laryngeal imaging. The digital recording systems such as the Kay Digital video recording system (DVRS) and the Pentax Electronics video recording system are useful for digital imaging of the larynx.

Sony Digital Still Recorder

The Sony DKR-700 (Figure 16-19A) is a compact digital still recorder. It captures the images and stores them on convenient high capacity 2.5 inch Sony MD data disks. The images can be easily retrieved, sorted, and annotated. It can store 100 noncompressed images on a MD data disk. The advantages of Sony DKR-700 include its compatibility with popular software programs. A disadvantage of the Sony DKR-700 is its long capture time (approximately 28 seconds). This means that during these 28 seconds, the surgeon cannot take another picture. This is unacceptable for laryngeal documentation unless the capture time is shortened in future versions of this product.

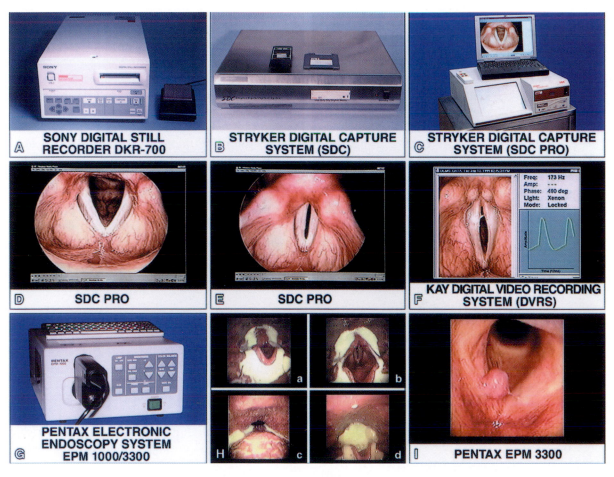

FIGURE 16-19. *Documentation by digital imaging. (A) Sony digital still recorder DKR-700. (B) Stryker Digital Capture System SDC. It captures still images only. (C) Stryker Digital Capture System SDC Pro. It captures both still and motion images. (D) Computer still image of the larynx on inspiration captured by Stryker SDC Pro. (E) Computer still image of the larynx on phonation captured by Stryker SDC Pro. (F) Still computer image of stroboscopic view of the vocal folds on phonation captured by Kay digital video recording system. Note on-screen display of an EGG waveform. (G) Pentax electronic endoscopy system EPM 1000 (a newer smaller version of EPM 3300). This is an excellent device to capture still images in single and multiple image formats. (H) Still images of swallowed milk in various stages taken with Pentax EPM 3300. (I) Computer still image of the laryngeal polyp captured by Pentax EPM 3300.*

Stryker Digital Capture System SDC

The Stryker SDC (Figure 16-19B) is a device which instantly transports surgical images to a high density computer disk. Software is available which allows for annotation and enhancement of the images. This system is simple to operate. No adjustments are necessary. Images can be saved as a standard bit-map file, which means that they are uncompressed. Image capture time is very fast (about one second) and the system is quite acceptable for laryngeal documentation. The cost of this system is approximately $10,000.

Stryker Digital Capture System SDC Pro

The Stryker SDC Pro (Figure 16-19C-E) capture device is a newer version of the Stryker SDC and can be used to record still images or video segments. Housed within the device are a central processing unit (CPU) and hard drive that can capture digital images or streaming video onto a writeable CD (compact disk). The CD system included within the Stryker SDC Pro digital capture device is the CDWriter Plus 9100 series.

The CD has become the standard for data storage, accessible using either a Macintosh or Windows based operating system. A single CD may hold approximately 650 images captured in bit-map (BMP) format, or approximately 12,000 images in compressed Joint Photographic Expert Group (JPEG) format. Alternatively, a single CD may record up to 20 minutes of continuous video, and a CD may contain a mixture of both still images and video. Capture is nearly immediate without hardware delay.

Advantages to the new Stryker SDC Pro system include the ability to capture not only still images but also streaming video. Although the Zip format used for the Stryker SDC is a popular medium for storage, the CD is a more universally accepted medium for data storage and retrieval. The Stryker SDC Pro allows for the import of images and video into popular software applications for digital annotation, such as Microsoft PowerPoint.

The Stryker SDC Pro system is an excellent technique for documentation of still and motion images of the larynx. The main disadvantages of this system is its high cost (approximately $13,000).

Kay Digital Video Recording System (DVRS)

The Kay digital video recording system (DVRS) (Figure 16-19F) is a newer version of its previous 9100 Stroboscopy Recording System based on VHS or S-VHS videotape recorders. Unlike its predecessor, the DVRS records video images directly to computer storage media. It captures both full-motion video and high-resolution still images. Audio and video are captured together. Image retrieval is easy. It allows instantaneous review of the data, and allows on-screen display of important information such as an EGG waveform (Figure 16-19F).

Pentax Electronic Endoscopy System EPM 1000/3300

The Pentax electronic videoendoscopic system (Figure 16-19G-I) is a highly integrated digital imaging system, utilizing the Pentax EPM 3300 (the EPM 1000 is a smaller unit used for laryngoscopic imaging) and a flexible electronic videolaryngoscope. It was primarily developed for the evaluation of gastrointestinal disorders. However, more recently it has been used for evaluation of the larynx and pharynx. It is useful for the study of swallowing disorders (Figure 16-19H). The Pentax flexible electrolaryngoscope, which has a CCD chip at the tip of the endoscope, provides remarkably clear images of the larynx and hypopharynx (Figure 16-19I). Images of various stages of swallowing of milk taken with the Pentax system are shown in Figure 16-19H.

The Pentax electronic videoendoscopy system has an excellent image capture device. It captures instantaneously. Images can be obtained in single, four, or nine-in-one formats and can be videoprinted right after the examination. The main disadvantage is its cost.

So far, all chip-tip camera flexible endoscopes have had their camera systems combined with their light sources. Therefore, despite their excellent image quality, they cannot be connected to a stroboscope. Recently, Olympus has developed a prototype chip-tip laryngoscope that works with any light source (including a stroboscope) and shows great promise for advancing diagnostic laryngeal imaging (Robert T. Sataloff, MD, personal communication, August 2000).

SUMMARY

Laryngeal documentation can be accomplished by videography, still photography, and digital imaging. Various methods of these modalities in the office and in the operating room setting are described.

Still photography remains a valuable method of laryngeal documentation for those who own or are familiar with still photographic equipment. The photographic images obtained through the telescope are clearly superior to those captured through the fiberscope. The main disadvantage of still photography is that one cannot see the results until the films are developed.

At the beginning of this new century (2000), videography is the most versatile and useful means of laryngeal documentation because it permits excellent demonstration of anatomy, pathology, and physiology with simultaneous voice recording. It also serves as an important source for digital imaging. With the use of a color video printer, high-resolution video prints of laryngeal pathology can be obtained instantaneously for medical records and educational purposes. The image can also be replayed immediately after the procedure and shown to the patient.

Videography of the larynx in the office can be accomplished by using a flexible fiberscope or a rigid telescope. Fiberscopic documentation results in images with less resolution but permits examination of laryngeal motion and can be performed in children and adults with hyperactive gag reflexes. Telescopic documentation provides superior structural images with high resolution.

Videography of the larynx in the operating room can be accomplished by means of microscopic, telescopic, and direct laryngoscopic videolaryngoscopy. Microscopic video documentation is currently the preferred method of documenting laryngeal pathology and teaching microlaryngeal surgery. Telescopic videography through the laryngoscope using a (0°, 30°, 70°, 90°, or 120°) telescope produces the clearest images of the larynx.

Digital imaging is the newest technology for permanently recording images without film. Digital imaging of the larynx can be accomplished by transferring video images from a prerecorded videotape into a computer. High-quality color prints can be produced utilizing a dye sublimation digital color printer. Digital imaging of the larynx can now be accomplished without film or videotape by utilizing a newer digital image capture device such as the Stryker Digital Capture System. This device captures laryngeal still images from a video camera and quickly transports them to a computer disk from which slides and prints can be generated. The newer digital capture systems record both still and motion images.

Advantages of digital imaging include: (1) safe, long-term storage without image degradation, (2) easy computer manipulation and retrieval, and (3) production of superior quality images using a digital printer. Disadvantages are the high cost of the system and the constantly evolving technologic improvements, which make the systems obsolete quickly and make upgrades necessary.

As this new technology improves and the cost of digital imaging decreases, the use of digital imaging of the larynx will likely become widespread.

REFERENCES

1. Garcia M. Observations on the human voice. *Proc R Soc Lond.* 1855;7:399-420.

2. French TR. On photographing the larynx. *Trans Am Laryngol.* 1882;4:32-35.

3. French TR. On a perfected method of photographing the larynx. *NY Med J.* 1884;4:655-656.

4. Ferguson GB, Crowder WJ. A simple method of laryngeal and other cavity photography. *Arch Otolaryngol.* 1970;92:201-203.

5. Padovan IF, Christman NT, Hamilton LH, et al. Indirect microlaryngoscopy. *Laryngoscope.* 1973; 83:2035-2041.

6. Holinger PH. Photography of the larynx, trachea, bronchi and esophagus. *Trans Am Acad Ophthalmol Otolaryngol.* 1942;46:153-156.

7. Holinger PH, Tardy ME. Photography in otorhinolaryngology and bronchoesophagology. In: English GM, ed. *Otolaryngology.* Vol 5. Philadelphia, PA: Lippincott; 1986 chap 22.

8. Holinger PH, Brubaker JD, Brubaker JE: Open tube, proximal illumination mirror and direct laryngeal photography. *Can J Otolaryngol.* 1975;4:781-785.

9. Rosnagle R, Smith HW. Hand-held fundus camera for endoscopic photography. *Trans Am Acad Ophthalmol Otolaryngol.* 1972;76:1024-1025.

10. Brewer DW, McCall G. Visible laryngeal changes during voice study. *Ann Otol Rhinol Laryngol.* 1974;83:423-427.

11. Davidson TM, Bone RC, Nahum AM. Flexible fiberoptic laryngo-bronchoscopy. *Laryngoscope.* 1974;84:1876-1882.

12. Hirano M. *Clinical Evaluation of Voice (Disorders of Human Communication, 5).* New York, NY: Springer-Verlag Wien; 1981.

13. Inoue T. Examination of child larynx by flexible fiberoptic laryngoscope. *Int J Pediatr Otorhinolaryngol.* 1983;5:317-323.

14. Sawashima M, Hirose H. New laryngoscopic technique by use of fiberoptics. *J Acoust Soc Am.* 1968;43:168-169.

15. Selkin SG. Flexible fiberoptics for laryngeal photography. *Laryngoscope.* 1983;93:657-658.

16. Selkin SG. The otolaryngologist and flexible fiberoptics—photographic considerations. *J Otolaryngol.* 1983;12:223-227.

17. Silberman HD, Wilf H, Tucker JA. Flexible fiberoptic nasopharyngolaryngoscope. *Ann Otol Rhinol Laryngol.* 1976;85:640-645.

18. Yamashita K. Endonasal flexible fiberoptic endoscopy. *Rhinology.* 1983;21:233-237.

19. Yamashita K. *Diagnostic and Therapeutic ENT Endoscopy.* Tokyo, Japan: Medical View; 1988.

20. Yamashita K, Mertens J, Rudert H. Die flexible Fiberendoskopie in der HNO-Heildunde. *HNO.* 1984;32:378-384.

21. Yamashita K, Oku T, Tanaka H, et al. VTR endoscopy. *J Otolaryngol Jp.* 1977;80:1208-1209.

22. Yanagisawa E. Videolaryngoscopy using a low cost home video system color camera. *J Biol Photogr.* 1984;52:9-14.

23. Yanagisawa E. Videolaryngoscopy. In: Lee KJ, Stewart CH, eds. *Ambulatory Surgery and Office Procedures in Head and Neck Surgery.* Orlando, FL: Grune & Stratton; 1986:chap 6.

24. Yanagisawa E, Carlson RD. Physical diagnosis of the hypopharynx and the larynx with and without imaging. In: Lee KJ, ed. *Textbook of Otolaryngology and Head and Neck Surgery.* New York, NY: Elsevier; 1989:chap 37.

25. Yanagisawa E, Yamashita K. Fiberoptic nasopharyngolaryngoscopy. In: Lee KJ, Stewart CH, eds. *Amburatory Surgery and Office Procedures in Head and Neck Surgery.* Orlando, FL: Grune & Stratton; 1986:31-40.

26. Yanagisawa E, Yanagisawa R. Laryngeal photography. *Otolaryngol Clin North Am.* 1991;24:999-1022.

27. Yanagisawa E, Carlson RD, Strothers G. Videography of the larynx—fiberscope or telescope? In: Clement PAR, ed. *Recent Advances in ENT—Endoscopy.* Brussels, Belgium: Scientific Society for Medical Information; 1985:175-183.

28. Yanagisawa E, Owens TW, Strothers G, et al. Videolaryngoscopy—a comparison of fiberscopic and telescopic documentation. *Ann Otol Rhinol Laryngol.* 1983;92:430-436.

29. Alberti PW. Still photography of the larynx—an overview. *Can J Otolaryngol.* 1975;4:759-765.

30. Albrecht R. Zur Photographie des Kehlkopfes. *HNO.* 1956;5:196-199.

31. Andrew AH. Laryngeal telescope. *Trans Am Acad Ophthalmol Otolaryngol.* 1962;66:268.

32. Benjamin B. Technique of laryngeal photography. *Ann Otol Rhinol Laryngol.* 1984;93:(suppl 109).

33. Benjamin B. *Diagnostic Laryngology—Adults and Children.* Philadelphia, PA: Saunders; 1990.

34. Berci G. *Endoscopy.* New York, NY: Appleton-Century-Crofts; 1976.

35. Berci G, Caldwell FH. A device to facilitate photography during indirect laryngoscopy. *Med Biol Illus.* 1963;13:169-176.

36. Berci G, Calcaterra T, Ward PH. Advances in endoscopic techniques for examination of the larynx and nasopharynx. *Can J Otolaryngol.* 1975;4:786-792.

37. Gould WJ. The Gould laryngoscope. *Trans Am Acad Ophthalmol Otolaryngol.* 1973;77:139-141.

38. Hahn C, Kitzing P. Indirect endoscopic photography of the larynx—a comparison between two newly constructed laryngoscopes. *J Audiov Media Med.* 1978;1:121-130.

39. Kantor E, Berci G, Partlow E, et al. A completely new approach to microlaryngeal surgery. *Laryngoscope.* 1991;101:678-679.

40. Konrad HR, Hopla DM, Bussen J, et al. Use of video tape in diagnosis and treatment of cancer of larynx. *Ann Otol Rhinol Laryngol.* 1981;90:398-400.

41. Mambrino L, Yanagisawa E, Yanagisawa K, et al. Endoscopic ENT photography—a comparison of pictures by standard color films and newer color video printers. *Laryngoscope.* 1991;101:1229-1232.

42. Muller-Hermann F, Pedersen P. Modern endoscopic and microscopic photography in otolaryngology. *Ann Otol Rhinol Laryngol.* 1984;93:399.

43. Oeken FW, Brandt RH. Lupenkontrolle endolaryngealer Operationen Modifikation der Schwenklupenhalterung nach Brunings. *HNO.* 1967;15:210-211.

44. Steiner W, Jaumann MP. Moderne otorhinolaryngologische Endoskopie beim Kind. *Padiat Prax.* 1978;20:429-435.

45. Stuckrad H, Lakatos I. Uber ein neues Lupenlaryngoskop (Epipharyngoskop). *Laryngol Rhinol Otol.* 1975;54:336-340.

46. Ward PH, Berci G, Calcaterra TC. Advances in endoscopic examination of the respiratory system. *Ann Otol Rhinol Laryngol.* 1974;83:754-760.

47. Yanagisawa E. Office telescopic photography of the larynx. *Ann Otol Rhinol Laryngol.* 1982;91:354-358.

48. Yanagisawa E, Casuccio JR, Suzuki M. Video laryngoscopy using a rigid telescope and video home system color camera—a useful office procedure. *Ann Otol Rhinol Laryngol.* 1981;90:346-350.

49. Jako GJ. Laryngoscope for microscopic observations, surgery and photography. *Arch Otolaryngol.* 1970;91:196-199.

50. Jako GJ, Strong S. Laryngeal photography. *Arch Otolaryngol.* 1972;96:268-271.

51. Kleinsasser O. Entwicklung und Methoden der Kehlkopffotografie (Mit Beschreibung eines neuen einfachen Fotolaryngoskopes). *HNO.* 1963;1:171-176.

52. Kleinsasser O. *Microlaryngoscopy and Endolaryngeal Microsurgery.* Philadelphia, PA: Saunders; 1968.

53. Kleinsasser O. *Tumors of the Larynx and Hypopharynx.* New York, NY: Thieme; 1988:124-130.

54. Olofsson J, Ohlsson T. Techniques in microlaryngoscopic photography. *Can J Otolaryngol.* 1975;4:770-780.

55. Scalo AN, Shipman WF, Tabb HG. Microscopic suspension laryngoscopy. *Ann Otol Rhinol Laryngol.* 1960;69:1134-1138.

56. Strong MS. Laryngeal photography. *Can J Otolaryngol.* 1975;4:766-769.

57. Tardy ME, Tenta LT. Laryngeal photography and television. *Otolaryngol Clin North Am.* 1970;3:483-492.

58. Yanagisawa E, Eibling DE, Suzuki M. A simple method of laryngeal photography through the operating microscope—"Macrolens technique." *Ann Otol Rhinol Laryngol.* 1980;89:547-550.

59. Tsuiki Y. *Laryngeal Examination.* Tokyo, Japan. Kanehara Shuppan; 1956.

60. Benjamin B. Art and science of laryngeal photography. (Eighteenth Daniel C. Baker, Jr, Memorial Lecture). *Ann Otol Rhinol Laryngol.* 1993;102:271-282.

61. Yanagisawa E, Carlson RD. Videophotolaryngography using a new low cost video printer. *Ann Otol Rhinol Laryngol.* 1985;94:584-587.

62. Yanagisawa E. Documentation. In: Ferlito A, ed. *Neoplasms of the Larynx.* Edinburgh, Scotland: Churchill Livingstone; 1993:chap 21.

63. Yanagisawa E, Weaver EM. Videolaryngoscopy: equipment and documentation. In: Blitzer A, et al, eds. *Office-Based Surgery in Otolaryngology.* New York, NY: Thieme; 1998:chap 25.

64. Yanagisawa E. Videography and laryngeal photography. In: Ferlito A, ed. *Diseases of the Larynx.* London, England: Arnold, 2000:chap 7.

65. Yanagisawa E, Horowitz JB, Yanagisawa K, et al. Comparison of new telescopic video microlaryngoscopic and standard microlaryngoscopic techniques. *Ann Otol Rhinol Laryngol.* 1992;101:51-60.

66. Yanagisawa K, Yanagisawa E. Current diagnosis and office practice—technique of endoscopic imaging of the larynx. *Curr Op Otolaryngol Head Neck Surg.* 1996;4:147-153.

67. Yanagisawa K, Shi J, Yanagisawa E. Color photography of video images of otolaryngological structures using a 35 mm SLR camera. *Laryngoscope.* 1987;97:992-993.

68. Stone JL, Peterson RL, Wolf JE. Digital imaging techniques in dermatology. *J Am Acad Dermatol.* 1990;23:913-917.

CHAPTER 17

3D Laryngeal CT Scan for Voice Disorders

Virtual endoscopy—Virtual dissection

Jean Abitbol, MD, Albert Castro, MD,
Rodolphe Gombergh, MD, Patrick Abitbol, MD

HISTORY

X-ray

Radiology developed as a result of both the understanding of electricity and the ability to create a vacuum lamp. Sir Wilhelm Croobes, a physician, and a president of the Royal Society of Medicine in London, performed the first experiment to create the cathodic-ray tube in 1856. He found that a few particles of gas remain in the vacuum tube when used as a vehicle of electricity. The molecules of radiation matter in front of the cathode that escape and bombard the surfaces they meet are the cathodic rays.

It was the experiment known as the "Shadow of the Maltese Cross" in which Professor W. Goodspeed, from the University of Pennsylvania in Philadelphia, and the English photographer, William Jennings, performed the first "ray photography" with a Crookes tube.[1-3] This experiment took place in 1890 and is considered the embryology of radiology.[4] William C. Roentgen, considered the "father of radiology" performed the first x-ray for medical purposes in 1895 when he x-rayed his wife's hand. He gave his name to the process of x-ray of the photonic emission. The medical applications of Roentgen rays (x-rays) began in 1896 and WC Roentgen was awarded the Nobel prize in 1901 for his pioneering work.[5-7]

By the end of the 19th century, Otto Glasser reported on the works of 23 pioneers in radiology in the United States alone.[8] For example, in Chicago, in 1896, the surgeon James Burry successfully x-rayed his hands, assisted by an engineer, Charles Ezra Scribner. At the 1896 Medical Society of Philadelphia Meeting, Henry Ware Cattell presented the first communication on radiology. Following this meeting, WW Keen and EP Davies published 'Medical Applications of X-rays or Roentgen Rays' in the *American Journal of Medical Sciences,* in March of 1896. Thus, the principles and applications of x-rays were established.

Kymography

Kymography was first described by Kaestle, Riedor, and Rosenthal in 1909, in Munich. They used a number of plates running at a speed of 5 cm/sec producing an illusion of a movement: it was also called the radio-cinema. Thus, the Roentgen cinema developed, and allowed the study of the movements of organs inside the body with x-rays.[9] HP Mosher, in 1927, studied the movements of the tongue, the epiglottis, and the hyoïd bone during speech and swallowing, which was the first cineradiograph of the vocal tract.[10] In September 1945, G. Henny, and B. Boone, published in the *American Journal of Roentgenology,* "electrokymography for heart." They studied the parallelism between the electrocardiogram

(ECG) and the radiographic movements, while recording their data.[11]

Tomography

The radiograph is a projection of an organ on a film called summation. Tomography is a slice by slice image of the organ. Laryngeal radiotomography, developed by André Bocage in 1921, was the first to image "slice the body" with slice-thickness from 1 mm to 10 mm. The principle was to move synchronously the plate and the tube, with the patient being immobile, so the synchronous motion of these parameters would print a specific and precise area of the organ to study.

In 1935, Georges Massiot and his son, Jean, made the first recorded tomography collecting all their data on film.[12-14] Until the early 1960s, the radiograph was merely a view of one plane. Tomography of the lungs or the larynx was interesting and very useful for diagnosis, but it had shortcomings. The density of the tissue was useful in distinguishing a tumor from normal tissue.

Air is used as a differentiating contrast medium within soft tissues when processing radiographs of the vocal tract.[15] However, the overlapping cervical spine disturbs the anterior-posterior views. To try to avoid this disturbance, high-kilovolt (120 kV) filtered radiographs and tomographs have been used with a copper filter placed in front of the x-ray tube to enhance the air-soft tissue interface by obscuring bone shadows.[16,17] There are series of anterior-posterior views at 5 mm intervals from the cervical spine to the thyroid cartilage. The images may be acquired during respiration or sustained phonation on /i/. The radiation exposure will be very high if multiple slices are taken. The most helpful tomography of the larynx is the anterior-posterior view or frontal view avoiding the cervical spine shadow. The lateral plane yields very little additional information. Tomography shows the laryngeal surface and is useful in examination of any soft tissue, benign or malignant mass, laryngocele, or thickening of the mucosa. However, the anterior commissure, the posterior wall of the glottic space, the cricoarytenoid and cricothyroid joints are poorly visualized. This new technology using multiple and complex movements of the x-ray tube and the receptor improved very satisfactorily the imaging quality.[18]

Conventional and Numerized Radiology

Today, conventional diagnostic x-ray technology utilizes a numerized technique, both direct and indirect.

The direct technique uses an x-ray tube instead of a film as its receptor. This receptor sends the data to a computer, and the result is an image summation. It is then possible to analyze, to magnify, and to distinguish bone from soft tissue, but it is limited to one plane. The indirect technique instead of a receptor uses a support which can be digitalized in a computer and analyzed in the same way as the direct technique.

Computerized Tomography Scanning: CT Scan

In 1967, Hounsfield studied a new concept with the EMI corporation, the analysis of x-ray data with appropriate software.[19] This idea occurred to him when he was asked by EMI to perform research on the shape of blood cells. He studied all angles of these structures, first in two dimensions and later in three dimensions, and found the computer to be crucial in his work. Hounsfield had the idea to take multiple radiographs, with frames being computerized with a specific program. This process was the birth of computerized tomography. Hounsfield published his first manuscript on this subject "Computerized Transverse Axial Scanning" in 1973 in the *British Journal of Radiology* with J. Ambrose, who developed the clinical applications. Cormach and Hounsfield received the Nobel prize in 1979 for this discovery.

Initially, axial transverse tomography was the only possible connection to the computer. Thus, it was named computerized tomography (CT). In 1990, spiral CT was available with one detector, in 1993 it was used with two detectors, and in 1999, it was a technique utilizing multiple detectors. At the same time, important computer advances occurred. In 1995, the first work station with multiplane imaging became available; and in 1999, volume-rendering and transparency techniques became practical.

Magnetic Resonance Imaging: MRI

In 1946, 51 years after Roentgen created the x-ray, Edward Purcell and Felix Bloch developed magnetic resonance imaging (MRI), and in 1952 were awarded the Nobel prize for their work. They analyzed the behavior of the body's own protons on a magnetic field (instead of using x-rays, which bombard the body and the plate), after having been excited by a magnetic system. The protons are oriented with an accurate spin. The first MRI was performed in New York by Demadiour in 1977[20] with the capability of distinguishing tumor mass from normal tissue by analysis of the tissue density. This imaging is often called "protonic imaging" because it uses the variations of the magnetic field or gradient. The x-rays are called "calcic imaging" because they use the photonic transmission of x-rays that are strongly absorbed by the human body because of its high percentage of calcium. MRI is capable of multiplanar, high-resolution imaging and may be superior or more accurate for soft tissue definition compared to the CT scan.[21-23] There is no exposure to irradiation with MRI; however, artifacts are numerous because of the respiratory movements, the pulsatile flow of the carotid and other arteries. These artifacts may be reduced by using fast-spin echo techniques. The sections may be 3 to 5 mm, parallel to the vocal folds and perpendicular to the vocal folds. Fatty tissue yields a high signal and gives a very satisfactory anatomic analysis of the paraglottic space. The ossified cartilage will give a bright signal, the non-ossified cartilage, a low signal. MRI must never be used if a patient has surgical clips (after thyroïd surgery), pacemakers, or cochlear implants.

Other Techniques

Xeroradiography

Xeroradiography is performed with wider latitude of exposure with edge enhancement; thus, images have a higher resolution with a better contrast.[24] It has provided a large amount of information on laryngeal cartilages, on the soft tissues, and a precise analysis of the ventricles. It has proven accurate when looking for foreign bodies and in distinguishing a subglottic mass not always visible on stroboscopy. It is also a technique that the author (JA) has used to analyze vocal tract behavior during sustained vowels "a," "i," "u." Today, xeroradiography is no longer available because of the high exposure to radiation required, which, compared to numerized radiology and CT scan, is 5 times higher.[24,25]

Fluoroscopy—Laryngography

Fluoroscopy is rarely used to study the larynx, partly because of the high radiation exposure. Pharyngolaryngography with barium contrast was commonly used for the visualization of the posterior wall of the tongue, the vallecula, the pyriform sinuses, and the posterior wall of the hypopharynx, in the 1980s.[26]

Positron Emission Tomography: PET Scan

Positron emission tomography or PET scan is a relatively new and interesting imaging technique based on the difference in the uptake and metabolism of glucose, H_2O_3, or fluorine 18-FDG. PET scans should prove very useful in future laryngeal research for voice fatigue and can be compared with the other techniques.[27]

ANATOMY RELATED TO RADIOGRAPHY

Phylogenetically, the larynx is an organ which functions as a constrictor-dilator mechanism in the airway. From amphibians to mammals, the larynx develops as a complex structure of cartilages, muscles, and mucosa primarily from branchial arches in utero. At 6 weeks, the epiglottis is seen at the base of the third and fourth pharyngeal arches. At 8 weeks, the thyroid, the cricoid, and the arytenoid cartilages are formed. Around 10 to 12 weeks, the vocal folds are individualized. At 7 months, the larynx is anatomically and functionally a sketch of an adult larynx. An understanding of the skeletal elements and articulations of the vocal tract is necessary to avoid misdiagnosis when interpreting imaging of the larynx.

Cartilages of the Larynx

The cartilages of the larynx, including the thyroid, cricoid, arytenoid, and corniculates consist of three components: non-ossified hyaline cartilage, a cortical bone marrow cavity containing fatty tissue, and scattered bony trabeculae. Enchondral (such as thyroid cartilage) ossification starts around 30 years of age. The ossification process follows specific patterns in each cartilage.[28,29] The epiglottis and the arytenoids are composed of yellow fibrocartilage that does not usually ossify. However, in our series, on helical CT scan at around 70 years of age, the authors have seen numerous ossified arytenoids.[30,31] On CT scan, ossified cartilage shows a high-alternating, outer and inner cortex, and a central, low-alternating medullary space. Non-ossified hyaline cartilage and non-ossified fibro-elastic cartilages have the same attenuation values of soft tissue.[32-38]

The angle of the two laminae of the thyroid or "shield of the folds" is approximately 110° in children, 120° in females, and 90° in males.[39]

The cricoarytenoid joint depends on the articular surface, as described by Lampert in 1926.[40] The facets of the cricoid are cylindrically curved with an axis sharply inclined horizontally. The angles between the horizontal plane and the cricoarytenoid joint axis are primate specific: 25° for the Mycetes, 55° for the *Macacas*, and 55° to 60° for *Homo sapiens*. These facets do not exist in non-primates.[41,42]

The cricoid cartilage is a complete ring with a height of 2.5 cm at the posterior arch and 0.75 cm at the anterior arch.

The arytenoids measure around 1.2 cm in height and are mobile and symmetric. The corniculate cartilages are at the apices of the arytenoids. The virtual dissection used in helical CT scanning by the authors shows the facet of the arytenoids.

The cricothyroid joint lies between the convex articular facet of the thyroid inferior horn and the flat articular facet of the posterolateral surface of the cricoid cartilage.

The cricoarytenoid joint is a saddle-shaped synovial joint with a strong capsular ligament. The arytenoid joints have complex sliding, rocking, and tilting movements described for decades by the observations gained through indirect and direct laryngoscopy but never by a CT scan "virtual arthroscopy" in vivo. Because of their low mass, they allow abduction-adduction in less than 0.1 second. This joint is critical for understanding not only the function of the laryngeal framework but also the source of most laryngeal pathologies.[43,44]

Soft Tissues of the Larynx

Radiography depends on tissue density in the larynx.

1. The mucosa of the larynx shows no enhancement except with a specific algorithm with the vocal-scan (the technique utilized by the authors to generate the images illustrated in this chapter)

2. Muscular tissue has no relevant enhancement in the conventional CT scan but does with the vocal-scan

3. Connective tissue is usually not seen except with the vocal-scan, which has a cross-sectional imaging capacity that is ideally suited to differentiate the different compartments of the larynx and hypopharynx. The paraglottic space is symmetric between the mucosa and the laryngeal framework, and extends into the aryepiglottic folds. The supraglottic region (ventricles, false vocal folds) is adjacent to the pre-epiglottic space. The aryepiglottic folds separate the endolarynx (anteromedially) from the piriform sinuses (posteromedially). At the glottic level the medial boundary is the conus elasticus of the vocal ligament to the upper edge of the cricoid cartilage and joins the cricothyroid membrane anteriorly. The cricothyroid membrane posterolaterally forms the lateral boundary of the paraglottic space.[45,46] Also, at the glottic level, the thyroarytenoid muscle forms the bulk and shape of the vocal fold, which also occupies most of the volume of the paraglottic space.[47]

Dynamic Aspects of the Larynx

For the first time, laryngeal movements were observed and analyzed radiographically by the authors using three-dimensional (3D) CT, which allows observations of the movements of cartilages and joints. The anatomy of the soft tissues is well known and does not need any further explanation to understand the "virtual

dissection."

The first roentgenologic laryngeal closure study was published in 1940 by Lindsay demonstrating the behavior of a laryngocele during phonation.[48] These tomograms also showed that the laryngeal airway is closed by apposition of both the vocal folds and the vestibular folds. The first observation by the way of laryngeal cineradiography during breathing was published by Ardran, Kemp, and Manen in 1953.[49] They noted that the larynx falls slightly on inspiration and rises on expiration and that the lumen widens on inspiration and narrows during expiration. These findings were confirmed in 1956 by Fink.[50] The first functional tomographies were produced 10 years later in 1966, by Ardran et al. They studied the role of the epiglottis, the cricoid, and the arytenoid cartilages and the ventricles during breathing and phonating.[51,52] R. Fink, in a retrospective on the human larynx, emphasized the role of the cricoarytenoid joint.[53,54] The vocal scan brings us a better understanding of the dynamic and functional aspects of this joint and the cricothyroid joint. It demonstrates the movements of the cricoarytenoid joint laterally, anteriorly and posteriorly.

In the movie *Voice Performers and Voice Fatigue* by the author Jean Abitbol, in 1988, a parallel study between xerography and the flexible laryngoscope gave a satisfactory analysis of the physiology of the larynx during phonation.[55]

CLINICAL AND MULTIMEDIA EVALUATION OF LARYNGEAL DISEASES

Laryngeal diseases usually have a typical clinical history and generally do not require extensive imaging. The laryngologist can assess the laryngeal mass with his or her simple clinical examination, videolaryngoscopy, or videolaryngostroboscopy. The numerous techniques of laryngeal evaluation, developed in the last two decades, have provided an accurate approach of the diagnosis of laryngeal pathologies. The "good morning doctor" from the patient can provide diagnostic guidance by analysis of his or her maximum phonation time and voice characteristics. Listening to the patient's voice is the indispensable first step.

Manuel Garcia developed the first method of indirect laryngoscopy in 1854. This examination is still routinely used, as it provides assessment of the real color of the mucosa and gives information in three dimensions.[56] The stroboscopic light became the second fundamental step in laryngeal examination. To be able to see the vocal folds in slow motion has brought forth a new harvest of unknown diagnoses and misdiagnoses. Video or computerized stroboscopy of the larynx may be stored on tape or DVD and can be compared with other examinations. Photographs of the larynx provide objective data that are helpful when comparing the laryngeal imaging before and after treatment.

Objective acoustic measures such as spectrographic analysis, fundamental F_0 measurements, formants, shimmer, and jitter during speech and singing are also valuable.

Electromyography has become a valuable clinical tool in the evaluation of vocal fold paresis or immobility, and allows for accurate location of the branch of the recurrent nerve or the superior laryngeal nerve that is impaired.[57]

Nowadays, radiology of the larynx is not only used to confirm pathology but also assists in diagnosis as with the 3D CT scan to visualize a "virtual dissection." The data gained from both clinical videolaryngoscopy and imaging provide a better understanding of the disease and lead to a better strategy for therapy.

CT SCAN

How does a CT scan work? What was the basis for development of the vocal scan?

Basics of Helical CT Scan

Principles

As previously discussed, x-rays are photons with a wavelength from 10^{-4} nm to 10^2 nm, are produced by the tube, and require an important power supply.

The x-ray tube moves with a circular movement and x-ray data are gathered by a detector. The table on which the patient lies moves horizontally. This dual movement creates a helical figure in a virtual cylinder.

Projections of data collected are digitized. This revolutionary method was a major radiologic advance in the ability to assess density of the mass. Hounsfield had the ingenious idea to detect x-rays with a crystal, thus producing a visible light spectrum. The CT scan improved resolution dramatically by permitting smaller, more discrete image slices. The detectors are crystals, which increase the sensitivity, and thus, the different densities may be analyzed by the computer. Data analysis was made possible once the computer became available. Algorithms then allowed reconstruction imaging.

Acquisition

- The slice-thickness is defined by the collimation of x-rays (Figures 17-1 through 17-5).

- The flux of photons depends on the power supply of the tube (120 kV usually, at 15 mA). The flux is limited by the heat effect.

- The speed of the table on which the patient lies going in to the gantry is measured in mm/sec. It is related to the collimation.

- Pitch $= \dfrac{\text{Table incrementation during each gantry rotation}}{\text{Collimation}}$

- The time of the spiral is linked to the volume acquisition and the slice-thickness.

Reconstruction

Algorithms that improve resolution are used. Here a 360° rotation technique is used. There are two rotations of the tube (720°). Then, the image parameters are calculated for a 360° reconstruction essentially doubling the amount of information in the computer from which the image is resolved, thereby enhancing detail. Table speed, related to "pitch" is also important. The more rapidly the table is moving, the more the thickness slices increase.

Applications for Acquisition

The gantry angles used in helical CT scanning are almost the same as those used in conventional CT. For the helical CT scan of the larynx, the gantry angles are parallel to the vocal folds during abduction and adduction.

Inaccurate gantry angle may cause a misdiagnosis with an artificial thickening of the anterior commissure, and the interposed laryngeal ventricle may disturb the evaluation of the paraglottic space.[58,59]

However, misdiagnoses decrease with the practical application of the 3D CT scan with sagittal, coronal, and 120° planes that the authors use, the ability to retrospectively study the images, along with the collaboration of a radiologist and a laryngologist, but a zero risk of misdiagnosis never exists.

Contrast

The rapid acquisition of the helical CT has dramatically decreased the use of intravenous contrast. The contrast dose is reduced by at least one-third for better enhancement of the main vessels and of the soft tissues (thyroarytenoid muscle, cricothyroid membrane).[60]

Approximately, 150 ml of intravenous contrast is required if there is an angulation of the gantry and 100 ml if not. Prior to the scan 46 mg of contrast medium at a rate of 1 ml/sec are injected and followed by infusion at a rate of 0.5 ml/sec.

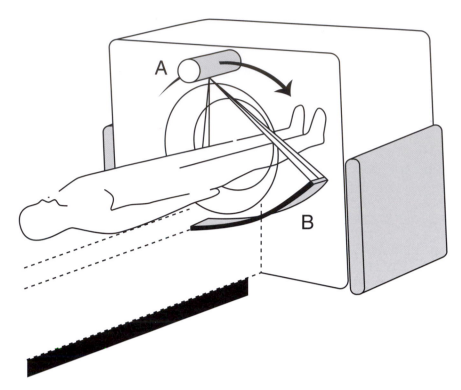

FIGURE 17-1. *X-ray tube with a double detector: A: x-ray tube; B: double detector.*

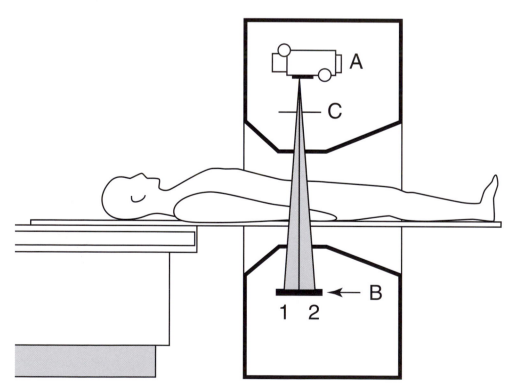

FIGURE 17-2. *A: x-ray tube; B: double detector; C: collimation.*

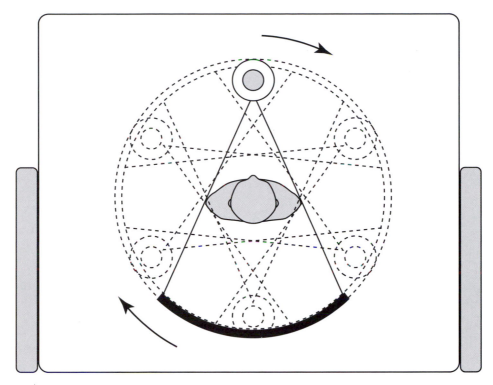

FIGURE 17-3. *Acquisition. X-ray tube and detectors move simultaneously. The patient is inside the gantry.*

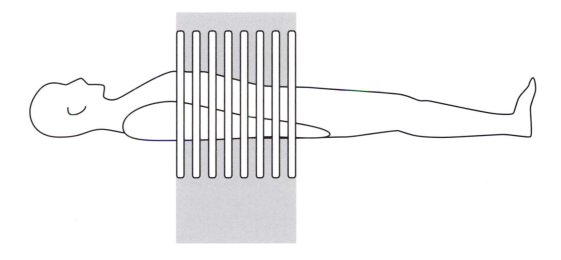

FIGURE 17-4. *Conventional CT scan: slice by slice requiring 30 minutes for acquisition. Each slice needs 6 to 10 seconds with a relapse time of 10 to 20 seconds.*

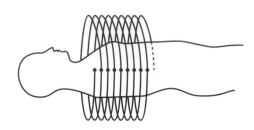

FIGURE 17-5. *Helical CT scan—The spiral technique allows a 20 second acquisition time.*

Slice-Thickness/Collimation

The best image quality, as illustrated in this chapter, is obtained when the interval of reconstruction is equal to the slice-thickness with overlapping slices.[61]

For example, an acquisition set obtained with a 3 mm collimation can be reconstructed into images of 3 mm (same slice-thickness) in 1 mm increments only resulting in 2 mm overlap of adjacent images.

Pitch

It is proportional to collimation. Increasing the pitch will decrease the longitudinal resolution; that is why a pitch of 1 seems to be the optimal level for preserving the Z-axis resolution. It allows multiplane reconstruction for the arytenoids and the laryngeal joints.

Power Supply

The tube current is a critical factor in helical CT: 200-250 amps and 120 kV are used. If the power supply is not adequate, increased noise, poor contrast enhancement, and grainy images will result.

Applications for Reconstruction

Reconstruction

Accurate and adequate algorithms are necessary for high-quality reconstruction, which depends on slice-thickness, slice overlapping, and contrast resolution.

Slice-thickness is used for a volumetric acquisition and, retrospectively, a reconstruction. Because data acquisition is volumetric, the scanning time of the patient is not increased and the slice-thickness used during the scanning does not have to be equal to the slice-thickness used for reconstruction. To improve the images, the reconstruction can also be obtained with slice overlapping. For laryngeal pathology, we use a 0.6 mm reconstruction interval made with 1 mm collimation through the laryngeal framework. This technique has been performed in the temporal bone.[62] The 3D information displayed is used for diagnosis and aids in planning phonosurgery. To ensure better quality of the

images and, thus, more accurate diagnosis, the larynx must be studied with at least two helical acquisitions.[63]

Principles of the CT Scan

Technology with very powerful computers bring us to the third dimension: "virtual endoscopy," and "transparent body."

Evaluation of the tissue density is possible and from this point, the quality of the structures are more precise. To render homage to Hounsfield the units of density in CT were named Hu (Hounsfield unit), the scale is from -1000 to +1000.

Air = -1000 Hu;

Water = 0 Hu; and

Bone = +1000 Hu.

There exist 2000 levels of shades in black and white from -1000 Hu to +1000 Hu. To distinguish the different structures' density and, thus, the different type of tissue, a color is applied on the Hu scale for better definition and imaging.

The color chosen to analyze our frames in 3D CT scan has proven to be indispensable. It should be recalled that the human eye can distinguish only 20 levels of gray but 250,000 colors. It is necessary to adapt the image to the location to be explored. The image is distinguished by two parameters: the width and the density of the window. The more the window is decreased, the more density differentiation is appreciated. Therefore, the threshold of the window must be equal to the average tissue density to be imaged (Figure 17-6). The screen is coupled with a color laser printer to obtain a hard copy and recorded on CD-ROM or a DVD. With this machine, it is possible to do a fly-through, and the CT scan has proven irreplaceable in the diagnosis of deep lesions, which are hard to see. Thus, CT and MR imaging are more useful in these cases.[64-69]

The laryngeal joints are very well observed with the 3D CT scan.

CT is very helpful in cricoarytenoid joint injury when preparing the surgical strategy.

Angiography is helpful in conjunction with 3D CT for providing a better understanding of the laryngeal physiology and pathologies such as angiomas and paragangliomas.[70]

Vocal Scan

Helical computer assisted tomography scanning or helical CT scan has been improved by the advances in computer technology. Planes are stored to create the 3D imaging. The program with an accurate workstation can perform reformations/reconstructions. All the planes may be used. For the vocal scan, the authors have deter-

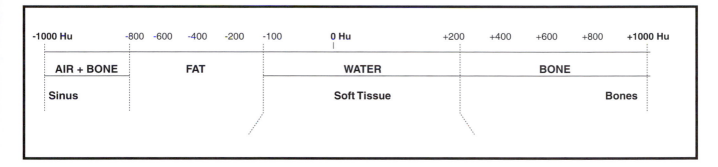

-1000 Hu		-800	-600	-400	-200	-100	0 Hu		+200	+400	+600	+800	+1000 Hu
AIR + BONE			FAT				WATER			BONE			
Sinus							Soft Tissue						Bones

FIGURE 17-6. *Hounsfield units: Density of the tissue in Hu.*

mined specific parameters, including orientation of the plane, measurement of tissue density in Hounsfield units (Hu), the time exposure, and the "shadow" work.

Acquisition

Technical advances have not only improved image quality in the last two decades, but also the way in which such images are obtained.

Conventional CT Scanners

Conventional CT scanners need sophisticated cables to couple the x-ray and detector assembly to the recon-struction process. It also needs high voltage. The proto-col for individual scans was performed with a 2 second scan time separated by a 6 second interscan delay. This delay allows time to re-orient the source-detector assembly within the gantry, time for table movement, and a short breath for the patient.[71]

The patient lies on a sliding table. The table moves into a gantry, a central circular aperture housing the x-ray source and detectors. The slices are parallel to the vocal folds. The imaging procedure is performed from the inferior maxilla to the sixth cervical vertebra. The more detail needed, the thinner the slices must be and the longer the imaging time required. With the conven-tional CT scan, most images are 1 to 2 mm thickness-slices, every 3-5 mm. The patient moves the prescribed distance through the gantry for each slice; the table moves 3 mm, one image shot, 3 mm, another image is shot with a total imaging time of approximately 20 to 30 minutes.

Vocal Scan

The authors use a spiral CT scanner. The procedure is much faster, requiring only 20 seconds exposure time. The spiral CT scanner moves the subject continuously in a circle and creates a volume acquisition imaging. These data are collected and stored. The first step is a multi-planar study (coronal, sagittal, and axial). Then the analysis begins for three-dimensional imaging. The

images are colored regarding the tissue density. We have 2000 levels of gray or 2000 Hu, which are converted to color. The advantages are enormous: rapid acquisition time, few motion artifact, a color and 3D picture, and animation.[72,73]

Intravenous contrast may be required for some pur-pose (laryngeal arteries) or pre-surgical mapping of a hemorrhagic mass (angioma). Data are recorded in the computer with an adequate program capable of analyz-ing every detail, both from the technical point of view (scale of density rendering) and the anatomic point of view (for example, if the focus of analysis is on the joints or on the vocal ligament), which are intimately linked. The laryngologist must work with and interpret the images with the radiologist at the workstation to change some parameters of contrast if the pathology being eval-uated is not visible on the first images. The Hu must be chosen to identify the specific lesion; protocols have been developed accordingly.

One of the successes of the helical CT scan from the very beginning was the ability to analyze the anterior commissure that was previously impossible to see with computed tomography. The anterior commissure was found to have a mean width of 1-1.6 mm in normal sub-jects.[74]

Vocal Scan Reconstruction

The helical CT reconstruction requires multiple angles for the same structures to be analyzed. With the helical CT, there is a 360° view with a complete gantry rotation. During the procedure, the patient moves con-tinuously through the gantry.

Mathematical interpolation with specific parameters allows the reconstruction through the computer. Parameters include collimation, table speed or incre-mentation, and image reconstruction intervals. Although the slice-thickness of collimation is pre-set before the scan, the computer can generate overlapping images. If a 2 mm collimation is used, slices may be reconstructed every 1 mm. For example, in laryngeal imaging a 1 cm collimation with a 20 sec helical exposure, covering 20 cm of tissue along the Z-axis has a pitch of 1.

Advantages of Helical CT Scan

The advantages of helical CT technology are numerous.[75-78]

1. The procedure is fast; in a single 20 second interval an entire vocal tract is helicallly scanned and ready to be reconstructed in 3D.

2. Helical CT is able to eliminate respiratory artifacts and is able to reconstruct overlapping images at arbitrary intervals on the workstation. The 3D CT scan gives a very high quality image with the reconstruction, not only of the image but also of a virtual mobility between two scanning points. For example, aperture and closure of the glottis can be generated from helical acquisitions; this has dramatically improved the scope of analysis for the vocal tract (and also for the entire body).

3. Helical CT has the ability to shift the location of slice reconstruction and create new images, retrospectively, with the image and the laryngologist in front of the screen of the workstation.

4. In some instances, helical CT scan has replaced the conventional CT in laryngeal imaging as numerized radiology did for conventional radiology. Improved vascular identification allows easier separation of mass lesions from vessels. The contrast enhancement is tremendously improved by the choice of the filter with reconstruction having the same advantages observed in thoracic or color imaging.

Limits of Helical CT Scan

The limits of the helical CT are few as described below:

- The chainsaw artifact: a few slices are missing; this problem is solved by overlapping imaging.

- The lego effect is caused by squared edges of each slice at the convexity. This artifact is corrected by using a smoothing algorithm during the 3D reconstruction or by using a thinner slice-thickness during scanning (1 mm).

- The threshold selection is a crucial factor. 3D images depend both on the algorithm and the threshold chosen during reconstruction.

- Artifacts related to metallic objects (dental crowns, bridges, surgical clips, and prostheses and cochlear implants).

- Volume rendering will create an artificially smooth surface of the endolaryngeal structures.

Image quality also depends on the power source. A high power is needed, especially in large patients, in which the images may be excessively grainy. Refinements in detection technology, higher-heat-capacity of x-rays tubes, and improvements in new workstations will advance the possibilities in achieving optimal images.

Although helical CT allows a rapid acquisition and reduces artifact such as respiratory misregistration, the swallowing artifacts may still cause degradation of images in the vocal tract study. A near perfect acquisition technique is needed.[79]

Virtual Endoscopy and Virtual Dissection

The post-processing of helical CT data allows creation of a reconstruction from axial slices into a high-quality picture of variable orientation. The virtual endoscopy was described for the first time in 1994 by Vining et al.[80,81] They used an accurate three-dimensional software, the voxel viewer, and a silicon graphics machine. Computer simulations allow creation of virtual endoscopy. A "virtual dissection" from the lumen of the larynx and trachea to the vessels and muscles is performed via the applications of acquisitions and reconstructions. In other words, 3D imaging is accurately created, recorded, and printed.[82-85]

Previously, diagnosis of airway disease was only possible by invasive endoscopy, considered the gold standard for the evaluation of airway obstruction. Virtual endoscopy may prove to be a non-invasive technique to diagnose the nature and the degree of airway obstruction.[86] The anatomy of interest was separated from the surrounding anatomy by a process called image segmentation. A threshold value was determined for each anatomic object to optimally observe its volume elements or voxels. For vocal folds an upper threshold of -100 Hounsfield unit (Hu) and a lower threshold of -700 Hu was used.

The reconstructed anatomy or the "virtual dissection" can be observed from the lumens as in endoscopy, being considered a virtual endoscopy. It is similar to surgical dissection, isolating each soft tissue, muscle, artery, membrane, and ligament; thus, it is a virtual dissection.

The virtual dissection is registered to the helical data set, thus allowing axial, coronal, and sagittal planes.[87-90] Computed tomography virtual endoscopy is a nominative radiologic technique that produces visualization of intraluminal surfaces in 3D reconstruction of air/tissue or fluid/tissue interfaces rarely seen with MRI imaging. Axial helical CT imaging is performed with the patient in the supine position, holding his/her breath or phonating a sustained vowel /"i"/ for 20 seconds if possible.

The following parameters are used: collimation thickness of 2 mm, pitch factor of 1-1.5, and reconstruction interval of 2 mm. The reconstructed axial CT data images are archived on digital tape and transferred to "a voxel workstation" for review and post- processing.[91] The 3D virtual dissection or virtual endoscopy are reconstructed from the axial CT data using a navigator software package on the workstation. This results in a surface-shaded display of the lumen from inside.[92-94] A satisfactory evaluation of the surface can also be performed. The images travel via a fly-through path of the lumen from the larynx to the trachea or from the trachea to the larynx.[95,96] Imaging the subglottic space, visible from the trachea, or an inferior perspective is possible. A movie loop of the fly-through path is created and archived. Data are also archived on CD-ROM. The total time to create a fly-through path is less than 10 minutes if studying the ventricles, the vocal folds, the subglottic space, and the trachea. Videolaryngoscopy with a flexible and rigid scope has been performed and compared to the helical 3D CT scan or vocal scan. However, with this technique an inferior view of the vocal fold is impossible.[73,97]

CT scan and MRI enable us to evaluate the deep structures of the larynx, from the vocal ligament to the laryngeal articulators. Although CT scan in 3D and MR imaging is excellent, helical 3D CT scan enables much faster image acquisition and muliplanar or three-dimensional image reconstruction. Videolaryngostroboscopy and vocal scan demand a close, regular, interdisciplinary cooperation in order to have a better understanding of the pathology and to facilitate an accurate therapeutic strategy. This cooperation is of particular importance in pre- and post-therapeutic evaluation of laryngeal neoplasm and carcinoma. CT of the vocal tract may be obtained with dynamic incremental scanning or helical scanning being superior.

For the vocal scan: helical acquisition with 1.2 to 1.5 mm collimation and 1 to 1.5 pitch produces images with excellent details.[98] The acquisition technique requires examination of a patient in supine position, with a hyper-extended neck, instructing the patient to resist swallowing or coughing and to hold the breath or to sustain vowel phonation of /"e"/ for 20 seconds. The software is crucial to obtaining three-dimensional volume reconstruction and so-called virtual endoscopy. The surface renderings simulate endoscopic views of the inner surface of the vocal tract by means of computer-generated ray casting.

The practical values of virtual endoscopy are numerous, accomplished by the "virtual dissection," enhancing surgical preparation. Because of the rapid image acquisition, the vocal scan is also performed during phonation on different vowels and different tones in order to analyze the real movements of the vocal tract during singing and speaking. Vocal scans are always reconstructed with a specific standardized soft tissue algorithm.

CASES

Authors' protocols: The examination is accomplished during a period of 20 seconds with a power supply of 120 kV and 150 amps. The machine is a CT gold spiral Elcint-Picker. It works with multiple detectors. Slice-thickness is 1.3 mm every 0.6 mm with a pitch of 2.

First series imaged in this vocal tract protocol: The air is imaged throughout the entire vocal tract. Slice-thickness: 2.7 mm every 1.3 mm with a pitch of 1.5.

The second series is during free breathing (holding one's breath will provide good imaging) and examines soft tissues of the laryngeal muscles and mucosa with the surface-shaded display. Slice-thickness is 1.3 mm every 0.6 mm with a pitch of 2.

The third series is used for evaluating the laryngeal framework, articulations, and cartilages, chiefly the arytenoids. This series has a slice-thickness of 0.6 mm every 0.3 mm with a pitch of 2.

The authors have named this 3D CT scan technique of the vocal tract the "vocal scan," and the protocol is illustrated in Figures 17-7 to 17-30.

SUMMARY

For decades, CT and MR imaging have provided images with satisfactory details of the vocal tract. At the dawn of the third millenium, the dynamic of incremental scanning with helical scanning has already created a new horizon for a better understanding of laryngeal structure and function. Moreover, the vocal scan with volume acquisition, and virtual endoscopy by fly-through (virtual dissection) gives an indispensable adjunct to the new generation of otolaryngologists performing simulation surgery and dynamic anatomic study.

ACKNOWLEDGMENT

With special thanks to Jean-Bernard Lenczner, MD, Radiologist; Director du Centre Jean Mermoz (Drancy – France) for his contribution.

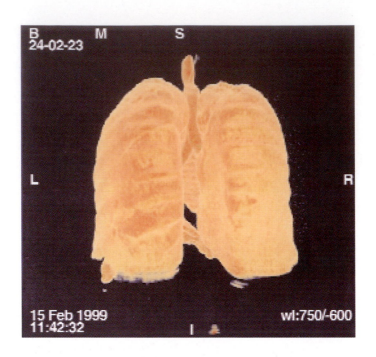

FIGURE 17-7. *The lungs.*

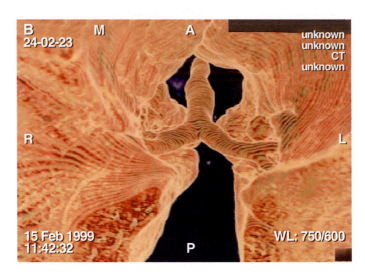

FIGURE 17-8. *Magnified helical CT scan of the carina.*

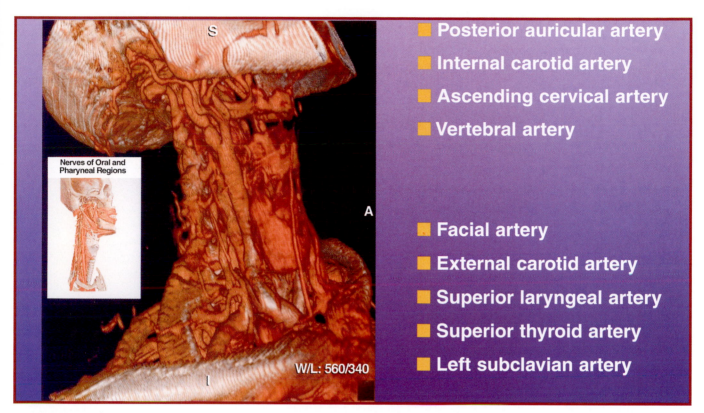

FIGURE 17-9. *Virtual dissection of the neck.*

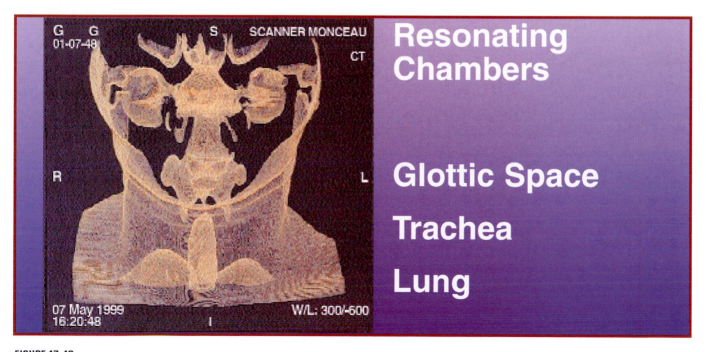

FIGURE 17-10. *Vocal tract transparency: voice production.*

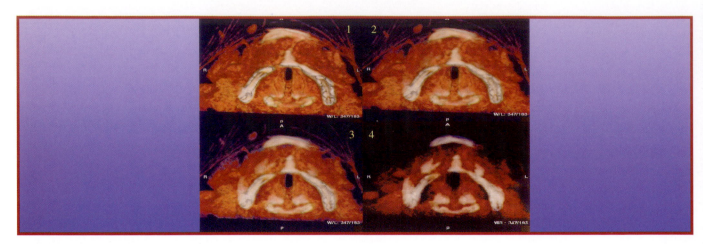

FIGURE 17-11. *Visualization of the glottic area: 4 different transparencies to visualize from the superficial to the deep layer of the cricoarytenoid joint.*

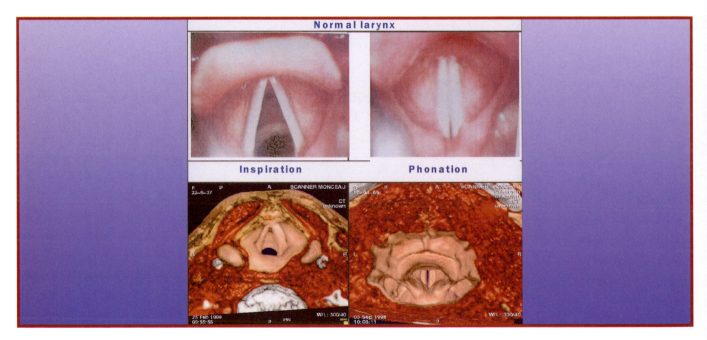

FIGURE 17-12. *Virtual endoscopy provides a superior view in many ways when compared with indirect laryngoscopy in a normal larynx.*

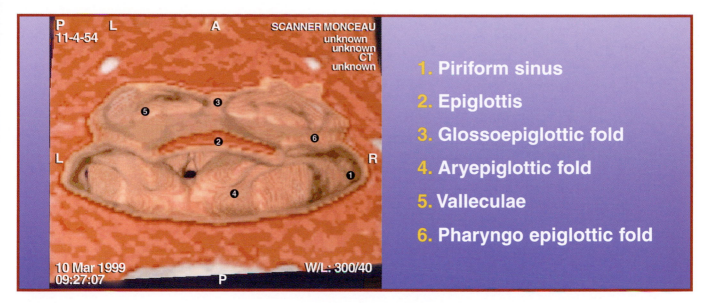

1. **Piriform sinus**
2. **Epiglottis**
3. **Glossoepiglottic fold**
4. **Aryepiglottic fold**
5. **Valleculae**
6. **Pharyngo epiglottic fold**

FIGURE 17-13. *Virtual endoscopy of the larynx from a superior view with a Valsalva maneuver.*

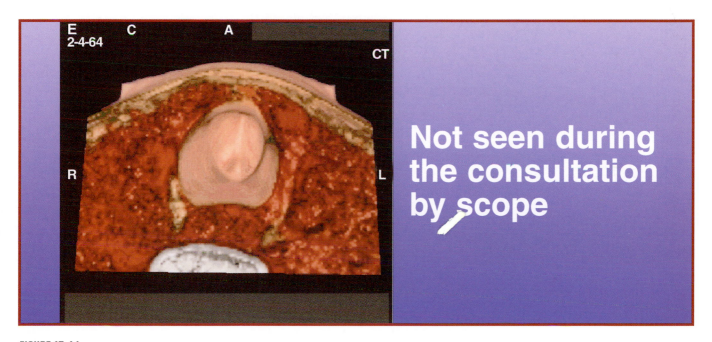

Not seen during the consultation by scope

FIGURE 17-14. *Inferior view of the vocal folds: virtual endoscopy.*

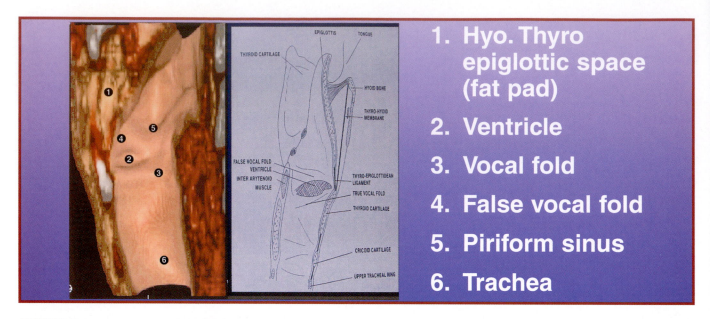

FIGURE 17-15. *Lateral and internal views of the larynx: virtual endoscopy.*

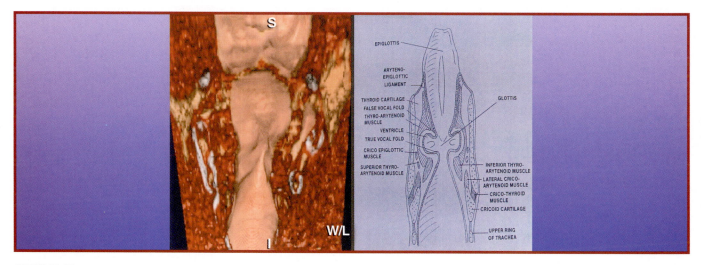

FIGURE 17-16. *Lateral and internal views of the larynx: virtual endoscopy.*

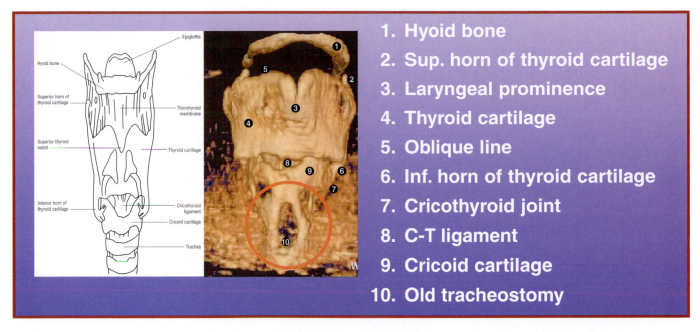

1. **Hyoid bone**
2. **Sup. horn of thyroid cartilage**
3. **Laryngeal prominence**
4. **Thyroid cartilage**
5. **Oblique line**
6. **Inf. horn of thyroid cartilage**
7. **Cricothyroid joint**
8. **C-T ligament**
9. **Cricoid cartilage**
10. **Old tracheostomy**

FIGURE 17-17. *Framework of the larynx (can be used to observe a tracheostomy scar): anterior view (post tracheo).*

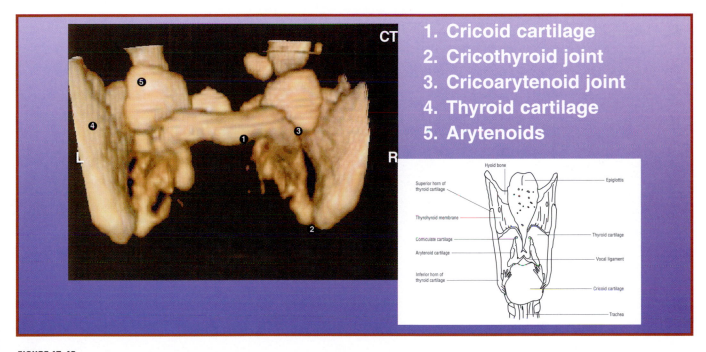

1. **Cricoid cartilage**
2. **Cricothyroid joint**
3. **Cricoarytenoid joint**
4. **Thyroid cartilage**
5. **Arytenoids**

FIGURE 17-18. *Cricoarytenoid joint during slow inspiration: posterior view.*

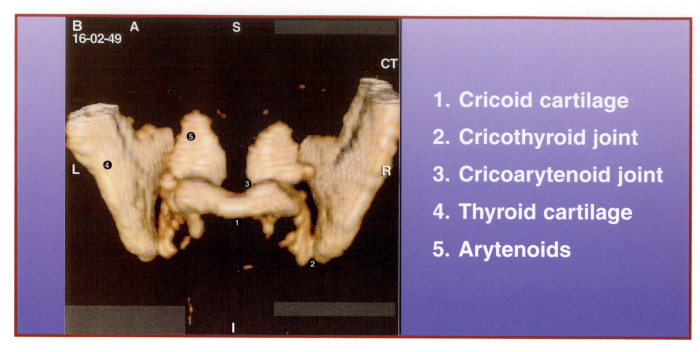

FIGURE 17-19. *Cricoarytenoid joint during phonation with a sustained vowel /i/: posterior view.*

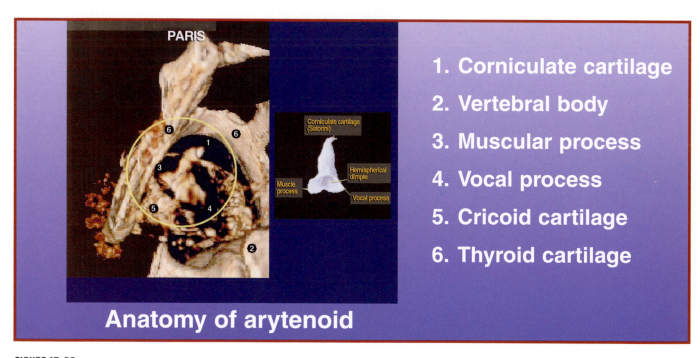

FIGURE 17-20. *Accurate view of the arytenoids: anterosuperior view.*

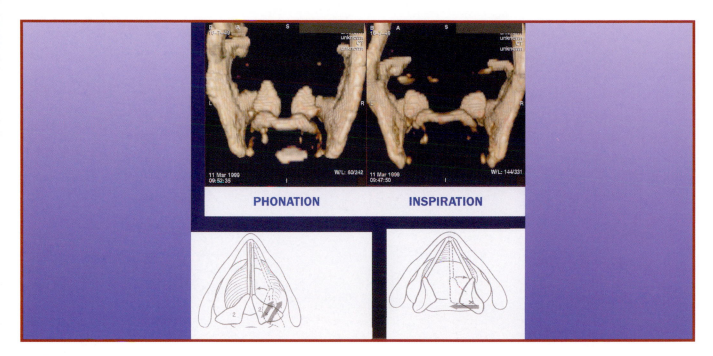

FIGURE 17-21. *Mobility of the arytenoids (1): comparison between phonation and inspiration.*

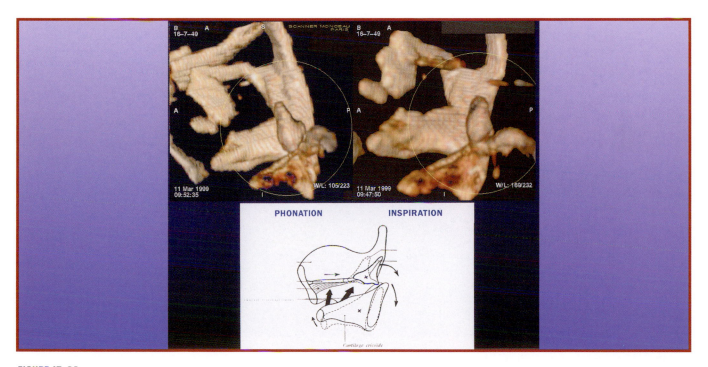

FIGURE 17-22. *Mobility of the arytenoids and the cricothyroid joint (2): comparison between phonation and inspiration.*

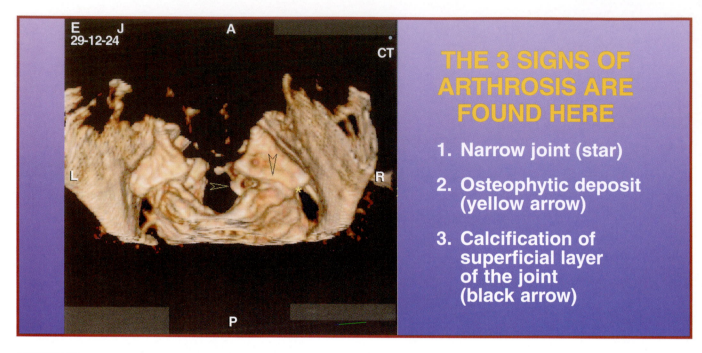

FIGURE 17-23. *Cricoarytenoid arthrosis.*

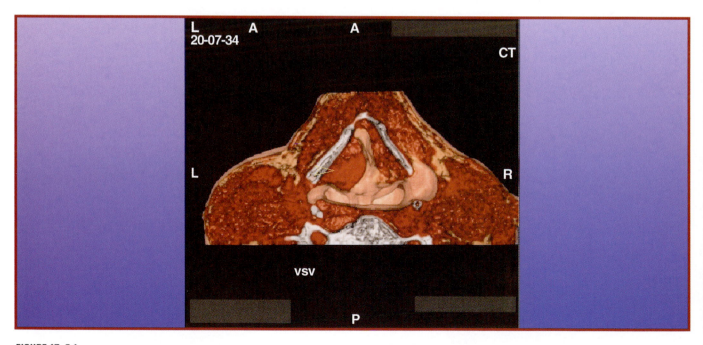

FIGURE 17-24. *Cancer of the left vocal fold.*

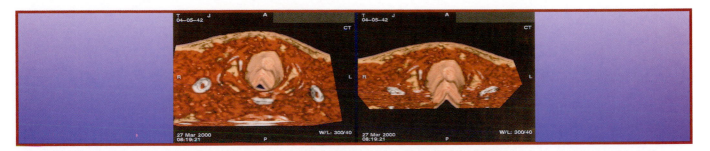

FIGURE 17-25. *Subglottic cancer below the anterior commissure, not visible by fiberoptic laryngoscopy (endotracheal, inferior view).*

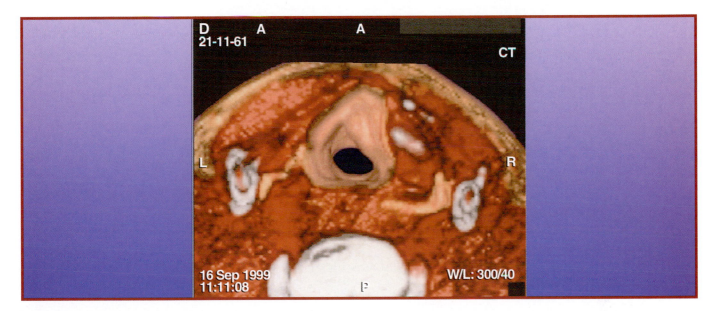

FIGURE 17-26. *Teflon injection (1) in the wrong layer of the right vocal fold (too superficial).*

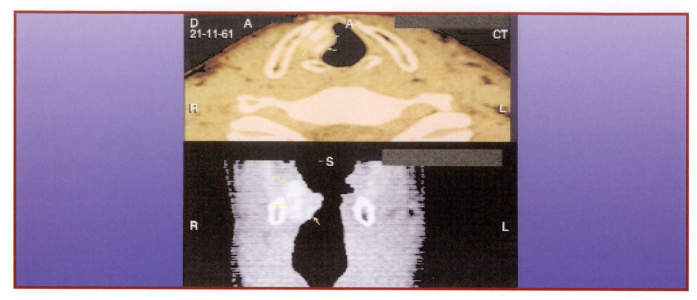

FIGURE 17-27. *Teflon injection (2) in the wrong layer of the right vocal fold (too superficial).*

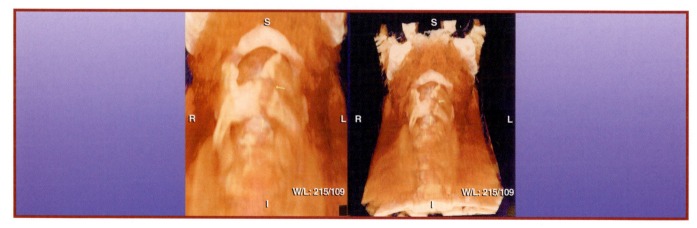

FIGURE 17-28. *Imaging of postsurgical trauma after laryngeal shave (Adam's apple resection) in a transsexual.*

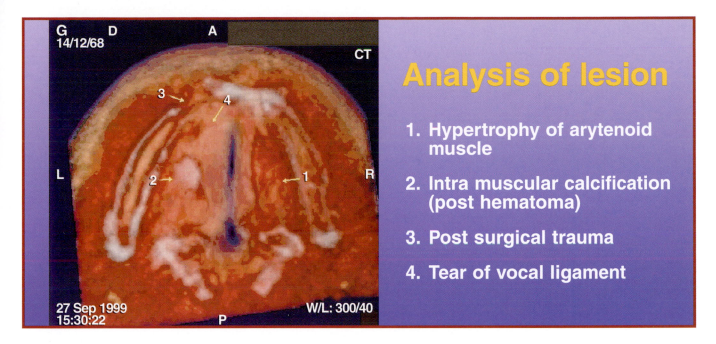

FIGURE 17-29. *Imaging of postsurgical trauma after laryngeal shave (Adam's apple resection) in a transsexual.*

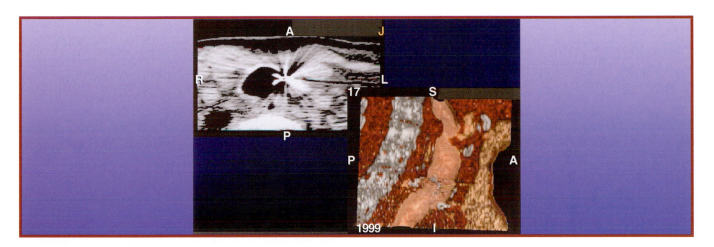

FIGURE 17-30. *Imaging of a postoperative clip and scar in the trachea.*

REFERENCES

1. Albers-Schonberg H. *Die Röntgentechnick.* Hambourg: Lucas Gräfe & Sillem; 1903.

2. Beclere A. La radiographie et la radioscopie dans les hôpitaux. *La Presse Médicale.* 21 Octobre 1899; No. 84.

3. Santini EN. *La Photographie à Travers les Corps Opaques par les Rayons Electriques, Cathodiques et de Roentgen.* Paris: Ch. Mendel;1896.

4. Pfahler GE. The early history of roentgenology in Philadelphia 1899-1920. *Am J of Roentgenol.* 1956;75(1):14-22.

5. Glasser O. The genealogy of the Roentgen rays. *Am J Roentgenol.* 1933;30(2):180-200.

6. Roentgen WC. *Und die Geschichte der Röntgenstrahlen.* Berlin: Springer-Verlag; 1959.

7. Londe A. *Traité Pratique de Radiographie et de Radioscopie.* Paris: Gauthier-Villars; 1898.

8. Glasser O. The genealogy of the Roentgen rays. *Am J Roentgenol.* 1933;30(3):348-367.

9. Lomon, Comandon. La radiocinématographie par la radiographie des écrans renforçateurs. *Bulletins et Mémoires de la Société de Radiologie Médicale de Paris.* 1911:127-135.

10. Mosher HP. X-rays study of movements of the tongue, epiglottis and hyoid bone in swallowing. *Laryngoscope.* 1927;37:235-262.

11. Reynolds RJ. Sixty years of radiology. *Br J Radiol.* 1956;29(341):238-245.

12. Jaubert de Beaujeu. Les écrans renforçateurs. *Annales d'Electrologie et Radiologie.* 1913:155-168.

13. Morgan RH. Screen intensification. *Am J Roentgenol.* 1956;75(1):14-31

14. Schinz HR. *60 Jahre Medizinische Radiologie.* Stuttgart: G. Thieme; 1959.

15. Momose KJ, MacMillian AS Jr. Roentgenologic investigation of the larynx and trachea. *Radiol Clin North Am.* 1978;16:321-341.

16. Maguire GH. The larynx: simplified radiological examination using heavy filtration and high voltage radiography. *Radiology.* 1966;87:102-110.

17. Maguire GH, Beigue RA. Selective filtration: a practical approach to high kilovoltage radiography. *Radiology.* 1965;85:345-351.

18. Ardran GM, Ebrys RE. Tomography of the larynx. *Clin Radiol.* 1965;16:369.

19. Hounsfield GN. Computed medical imaging. *Journal de Radiologie.* 1980;61(6-7):459-468.

20. Laugier A. "De Roentgen à Becquerel. La radiologie a 75 ans. *Concours Médical.* 1971;93(17): 3174-3202.

21. Castelijns JA, Gerritsen GJ, Kaiser MC, et al. Invasion of laryngeal cartilage by cancer: comparison of CT and MR imaging. *Radiology.* 1988;16:199-206.

22. Lufkin RB, Hanafee WN. Application of surface coil to MR anatomy of the larynx. *Am J Roentgenol.* 1985;145:483-489.

23. Lufkin RB, Hanafee WN, Wortham D, Hoover L. Larynx and hypopharynx: MR imaging with surface coils. *Radiology.* 1986;158:747-754.

24. Doust BD, Ting YM: Xeroradiography of the larynx. *Radiology.* 1975;110:727-731.

25. Abitbol J. *Atlas of Laser Surgery.* San Diego, CA: Singular Publishing Group; 1995:101-104.

26. Powers WE, McGee HH, Seaman WB. The contrast examination of larynx and pharynx. *Radiology.* 1957;68:169-172.

27. Kostakoglu L, Wong JC, Barrington SF, Cronin BF, Dynes AM, Maisey MN. Speech-related visualization of laryngeal muscles with fluorine-18-FDG. *J Nucl Med.* 1996;37:1771-1773.

28. Keem JA, Wainwright J. Ossification of the thyroid, cricoid and arytenoid cartilages. *S Afr J Lab Clin Med.* 1958;4:83-118.

29. Yeager VL, Lawson C, Archer CR. Ossification of laryngeal cartilages as it relates to computed tomography. *Invest Radiol.* 1985;17:11-19.

30. Kahane JC. Connective tissue changes in the larynx and their effects on voice. *J Voice.* 1987;1:27-30.

31. Kahane JC. Histologic structure and properties of the human vocal folds. *Ear, Nose Throat J.* 1988;67:322-330.

32. Archer C, Yeager VL: Evaluation of laryngeal cartilages by computed tomography. *J Comput Assist Tomogr.* 1979;3:604-611.

33. Becker M, Hasso AN. Imaging of malignant neoplasms of the pharynx and larynx. In: Taveras JM, Ferrucci JT, eds. *Radiology: Diagnosis-Imaging-Intervention.* Philadelphia, PA. JB Lippincott; 1996:1-16.

34. Becker M, Zbaren P, Delavelle J, et al. Neoplastic invasion of the laryngeal cartilage: reassessment

of criteria for diagnois at CT. *Radiology.* 1997;203:521-532.

35. Becker M, Zbaren P, Laeng H, et al: Neoplastic invasion of the laryngeal cartilage: Comparison of MR imaging and CT with histopathologic correlation. *Radiology.* 1995;194:661-669.

36. Curtin HD. Imaging of the larynx: current concepts. *Radiology.* 1989;173:1-11.

37. Mafee MF, Schild JA, Michael AS, et al. Cartilage involvement in laryngeal carcinoma: correlation of CT and pathologic macrosection studies. *J Comput Assist Tomogr.* 1984;8:969-973.

38. Mancuso AA, Calcaterra TC, Hanafee WN. Computed tomography of the larynx. *Radiol Clin North Am.* 1978;16:195-208.

39. Fink BR. *The Human Larynx: A Functional Study.* New York, NY: Raven Press; 1975:31-48.

40. Lampert H. Zur Kenntnis des Platyrrhinenkehlkopfes. *Morphol Jb.* 1926;55: 607-654.

41. Napier J. *The Roots of Mankind.* New York, NY: Harper and Row; 1970:29.

42. Napier JR, Walker AC. Vertical clinging and leaping—a newly recognized category of locomotor behavior of primates. *Folia Primatol.* 1967;6:204-219.

43. Von Leden H, Moore P. The larynx and voice: the function of the normal larynx (Motion Picture). *Arch Otolaryngol.* 1957;66:735.

44. Yanagihara N, Von Leden H. The cricothyroid muscle during phonation. Electromyographic, aerodynamic, and acoustic studies. *Ann Otol Rhinol Laryngol.* 1996;75:987-1006.

45. Curtin HD. The larynx. In: Som PM, Curtin HD, eds. *Head and Neck Imaging.* 3rd ed. St Louis, MO: Mosby; 1996:612-707.

46. Mancuso AA. Evaluation and staging of laryngeal and hypopharyngeal cancer by computed tomography and magnetic resonance imaging. In: Silver CE, ed. *Laryngeal Cancer.* New York, NY: Thieme; 1991:46-94.

47. Mafe MF, Schild JA, Valvassori GE, Capek V. Computed tomography of the larynx: correlation with anatomic and pathologic studies in cases of laryngeal carcinoma. *Radiology.* 1983;147:123-128.

48. Lindsay JR. Laryngocele ventricularis. *Ann Otol Rhinol Laryngol.* 1940;49:661-673.

49. Ardran GM, Kemp FH, Manen L. Closure of the larynx. *Br J Radiol.* 1953;26:497-509.

50. Fink BR. The mechanism of closure of the human larynx. *Trans Am Acad Ophthalmol Otolaryngol.* 1956;60:117-127.

51. Ardran GM, Kemp FH, Manen L. The mechanism of the larynx. Part 1 : the movement of the arytenoid and cricoid cartilages. *Br J Radiol.* 1966;39:641-654.

52. Ardran GM, Kemp FH, Manen L. The mechanism of the larynx. Part 2: the epiglottis and closure of the larynx. *Br J Radiol.* 1967;40:372-389.

53. Fink BR. *The Human Larynx: A Functional Study.* New York, NY: Raven; 1975:48-52.

54. Maue WM. *Cartilages, Ligaments and Articulations of the Adult Human Larynx* [dissertation] University of Michigan, Ann Arbor, MI: University Microfilms; 1970.

55. Abitbol J. *Voice Performers and Voice Fatigue.* San Diego, CA: Singular Publishing Group; 1987.

56. Garcia M. *Observations on the human voice. Proc Roy Soc (London).* 1855;7:399-420.

57. Sataloff RT, Abaza M, Mandel S, Manon-Espillat R. Laryngeal electromyography. *Curr Opin Otolaryngol Head Neck Surg.* 2000;8:524-529.

58. Metes A, Hoffstein V, Direnfeld V, Chapnick JS. Three-dimensional CT reconstruction and volume measurements of the pharyngeal airway before and after maxillofacial surgery in obstructive sleep apnea. *J Otolaryngol.* 1993;22:20-24.

59. Bushberg JT, Seibert JA, Leidholdt EM, Boone JM. X-ray computed tomography. In: Passano III, WM, ed. *The Essential Physics of Medical Imaging.* Baltimore, MD: Williams & Wilkins; 1994:239-290.

60. Spreer J, Krahe T, Jung G, et al. Spiral versus conventional CT in routine examinations of the neck. *J Comput Assist Tomogr.* 1995;19(6):905-910.

61. Craven CM, Nak KS, Blanshard KS, et al. Multispiral three-dimensional computed tomography in the investigations of craniosynostosis: technique optimization. *Br J Radiol.* 1995;68:724-730.

62. Hermans R, Marchal G, Feenstra L, et al. Spiral CT of the temporal bone: value of image reconstruction at submillimetric table increments. *Neuroradiology.* 1995;37:150-154.

63. Schmalfuss IM, Mancuso AA. Protocols for helical CT of the head and neck. In: *Helical (Spiral) Computed Tomography.* Philadelphia, PA: Lippincott-Raven; 1998:11-23.

64. Mancuso AA, Hanafee WN. *Computed Tomography and Magnetic Resonance of the Head and Neck.*

2nd ed. Baltimore, MD: Williams & Wilkins; 1985:241-357.

65. Robert Y, Rocourt N, Chevalier D, Duhamel A, Carcasset S, Lemaitre L. Helical CT of the larynx: a comparative study with conventional CT scan. *Clin Radiol.* 1996;521:882-885.

66. Rodenwaldt J, Niehaus HH, Kopka L, Grabbe E. Spiral CT in arytenoid cartilage dislocation: the optimization of the study parameters with a cadaver phantom and its clinical evaluation. *Rofo Fortschr Geb Rontgenstr Neuen Bildgeb Verfahr.* 1998;168:180-184.

67. Barnes GT, Lakshminarayanan AV. Conventional and spiral computed tomography: physical principles and image quality considerations. In: Lee JKT, Stanley RL, Sagel SS, Heiken JP, eds. *Computed Body Tomography With MRI Correlation.* Philadelphia, PA: Lippincott-Raven; 1998:1-20.

68. Sataloff RT, Rao VM, Hawkshaw M, Lyons K, Spiegel JR. Cricothyroid joint injury. *J Voice.* 1998;12:112-116.

69. Schaefer SD. Use of CT scanning in the management of the acutely injured larynx. *Otolaryngol Clin North Am.* 1991;24:31-36.

70. Konowitz PM, Lawson W, Som PM, Urchen ML, Breakstone BA, Biller HF. Laryngeal paraganglioma: update on diagnosis and treatment. *Laryngoscope.* 1988;98:40-49.

71. Brink JA. Technical aspects of helical (spiral) CT. *Radiol Clin North Am.* 1995;33:825-841.

72. Silverman PM, Zeiberg AS, Sessions RB, Troost TR, Davros WJ, Zeman RK. Helical CT of the upper airway: normal and abnormal findings on three-dimensional reconstructed images. *Am J Roentgenol.* 1995;165:541-546.

73. Yumoto E, Sanuki T, Hyodo M, Yasuhara Y. Three-dimensional endoscopic mode for observating laryngeal structures by helical computed tomography. *Laryngoscope.* 1997;107:1530-1537.

74. Kallmes DF, Phillips CD. The normal anterior commissure of the glottis. *Am J Roentgenol.* 1997;168:1317-1319.

75. McEnery KW, Wilson AJ, Murphy WA Jr, Marushack MM. Spiral CT imaging of the musculoskeletal system: a phantom study. *Radiology.* 1992;185:118.

76. Ney DR, Fishman EK, Kawashima A, Robertson DD Jr, Scott WW. Comparison of helical and serial CT with regard to three-dimensional imaging of musculoskeletal anatomy. *Radiology.* 1992;185:865-869.

77. Silverman PM, Korobkin M. High resolution computed tomography of the normal larynx. *Am J Roentgenol.* 1983;140:875-880.

78. Silverman PM, Zeiberg AS, Sessions RB, Troost TR, Zeman RK. Three-dimensional (3-D) imaging of the hypopharynx and larynx using helical CT: comparison of radiological and otolaryngological evaluation. *Ann Otol Rhinol Otolaryngol.* 1995;104(6): 425-431.

79. Suojanen JN, Mukherji SK, Wippold FJ. Spiral CT of the larynx. *Am J Neuroradiol.* 1994;15:1579-1582.

80. Vining DJ, Shifrin RY, Haponik EF, et al. Virtual bronchoscopy. *Radiology.* 1994;193-261.

81. Frankenthaler R, Moharir VM, Kikinis R, et al. Virtual otoscopy. *Otolaryngol Clin North Am.* 1998;31:183-192.

82. Vining DJ, Liu K, Choplin RH, et al. Virtual bronchoscopy: relationship of virtual reality endobronchial simulations to actual bronchoscopic findings. *Chest.* 1996;109:549-553.

83. Brink JA, Heiken JP, Wang G, et al. Helical CT: principles and technical considerations. *Radiographics.* 1994;14:887-893.

84. Zeiberg AS, Silverman PM, Sessions RB, et al. Helical (spiral) CT of the upper airway with three dimensional imaging: technique and clinical assessment. *Am J Roentgenol.* 1996;166:293-299.

85. Lacrosse M, Trigauz JP, Vanbeers BE, et al. 3D spiral CT of the tracheobronchial tree. *J Comput Assist Tomogr.* 1995;19:341-347.

86. Burke AJ, et al. Evaluation of airway obstruction using virtual endoscopy. *Laryngoscope.* 2000; 110:23-29.

87. Jolesz FA, Lorensen WE, Shinmoto H, et al. Interactive virtual endoscopy. *Am J Roentgenol.* 1997;169:1229-1235.

88. Rodenwaldt J; Kopka L. Roedel R, et al. 3D virtual endoscopy of the upper airway: optimization of the scan parameters in a cadaver phantom and clinical assessment. *J Comput Assist Tomogr.* 1997;21(3):405-411.

89. Fried MV, et al. Virtual laryngoscopy. *Ann Otol Rhinol Laryngol.* 1999;108(3):221-226.

90. Moharir, et al. Computer-assisted three-dimensional reconstruction of head and neck tumors. *Laryngoscope.* 1998;108:1592-1598.

91. Wiegand DA, Channin DS. The surgical workstation: surgical planning using generic software. *Otolaryngol Head Neck Surg.* 1993;109:434-440.

92. Eisele DW, Richtsmeier WJ, Graybeal JC, Koch WM, Zinreich SJ. Three-dimensional models for head and neck tumor treatment planning. *Laryngoscope.* 1994;104:433-439.

93. Pototschnig C, Veolklein C, Dessl A, Giacomuzzi S, Jaschke W, Thumfart WF. Virtual endoscopy in otorhinolaryngology by postprocessing of helical computed tomography. *Otolaryngol Head Neck Surg.* 1998;119:536-539.

94. Gallivan RP, et al. Head and neck computed tomography virtual endoscopy: evaluation of a new imaging technique. *Laryngoscope.* 1999;109:1570-1579.

95. Vining DJ, Liu K. Choplin RH, Haponik EF. Virtual bronchoscopy: relationships of virtual reality endobronchial simulations to actual bronchoscopic findings. *Chest.* 1996;109:549-553.

96. Vining DJ, Shifrin RY, Grishaw EK. Virtual colonoscopy [abstract]. *Radiology.* 1994;193:446.

97. Gilani S, Norbash AM, Ringl H, Rubin GD, Napel S, Terris DJ. Virtual endoscopy of the paranasal sinuses using perspective volume rendered helical sinus computed tomography. *Laryngoscope.* 1997;107:25-29.

98. Suojanen JN, Mukherji SK, Wippold FJ: Spiral CT of the larynx. *Am J Neuroradiol.* 1993;15:1579-1582.

CHAPTER 18

The Evaluation of Voice Outcomes and Quality of Life

Michael S. Benninger, MD
Glendon M. Gardner, MD

The ability to objectively evaluate both the normal and the disordered human voice has improved dramatically in the last two decades, driven by better understanding of the anatomy and physiology, and development of new technologies. With this information, the voice clinician can now make reproducible assessments, recommend treatment, and measure the effects of interventions. Despite the exponential growth in assessment capabilities, there is no agreed-upon gold standard for evaluating voice.

Over the past decade, there has also been a movement in the medical community to assess the impact of disease, treatment or nontreatment, on the patient's perception of quality of life. In simplest terms, this quality of life evaluation has been called an assessment of "outcome," and efforts to objectively measure changes in outcome have led to creation of validated outcomes measurement tools or instruments. Although outcomes assessment in relationship to voice is in its infancy, there has been great progress. This chapter describes the outcomes and quality of life movement and reviews contemporary outcomes assessment as it relates to the abnormal human voice.

QUALITY OF LIFE AND OUTCOMES

Health is a multidimensional concept that, according to the World Health Organization, incorporates physical, mental, and social states.[1] Handicap is defined as "… a social, economic, or environmental disadvantage resulting from an impairment or disability," and disability is defined as "… restriction or lack of ability manifested in the performance of daily tasks."[2] The degree of change in the parameters of physical, mental, or social status is considered to represent an outcome. These outcomes, however, depend on a number of factors including the baseline level of function, other concomitant medical conditions, a person's perception of quality of life, and cultural or societal influences. In general, medical care strives to prevent and eliminate disease and thereby improve the quality of a patient's life. Traditionally, assessment of only one's physical function was used to determine the impact of health or disease. Such practice limits the ability to assess the emotional or social impact of disease or its treatment. An acknowledgment of these limitations led to the development of a whole new way of looking at health and disease, and has been coined the "outcomes" movement.

Traditional assessment of outcomes in medicine has been largely through the perspective of the treating physician or other clinician (such as nurses or speech-language pathologists). Therefore, an outcome was identified via changes in the physical examination, an improvement or change in symptoms and functions, or changes in laboratory tests or x-ray examinations. Classically, the simplest two measurements of an outcome of treatment are the presence or absence of disease, or the patient living or dying. Despite their simplicity, these gross measures are very important in relationship to medical care. However, although these distinctions are significant, they are often inadequate for assessing the general impact on quality of life. For example, surgical treatment may be successful for the management of a vocal fold polyp yielding complete return of normal voice function. However, if the treatment of the polyp resulted in a missed important business appointment, missed audition or performance, or even the ability to cheer at a sports event, the impact on quality of life might be significantly different from the unequivocal success as perceived by the surgeon.

The medical profession's early attempts to assess quality of life have revolved around questionnaires which served to identify key issues that patients may have in relationship to their disease.[3] These questionnaires usually focused on questions that the physician or other person administrating the questionnaire felt were important, often not including factors that the person completing the questionnaire was most concerned about. Over time, following multiple revisions and adaptations, these questionnaires have tended to address, to some degree, both of these perspectives. Furthermore, questionnaires were not statistically validated, and, therefore, one could not be sure that they truly measured what was intended to be measured, or that responses by individuals with disease, were different from those without disease. It was also not clear whether or not the questionnaire maintained its validity over time so that a person who had no change in status would answer questions similarly at different times.

The realization that there are many critical issues related both to the presence of a disease or the treatment of the disease, and efforts to measure the entire impact of health on individuals and society, are what have driven the outcomes movement. Outcomes research attempts to observe patients in their typical clinical environment, and uses patient-centered measures.

MEASURING QUALITY OF LIFE

Quality of life measurement instruments have been developed to attempt to measure the multidimensional nature of health. The questions and items within these tests usually cluster around broad health-related areas that can be measured in direct relationship to disease or response to treatment. Probably the best recognized and utilized quality of life measurement tool is the *Medical Outcomes Study 36 Item Short Form General-Health Survey,* or "SF-36."[4-6] This instrument is self-administered by individuals and assesses eight domains of

health that are commonly affected by disease or its treatment: physical functioning, role functioning, social functioning, mental health, bodily pain, general health, vitality, and health transition.[4-6] Each of these subscales provides a score that is reliable and a valid measure of health for that particular dimension. The SF-36 has been used to evaluate a wide range of health issues and to compare quality of life as it relates to different disease processes.[7]

One of the disadvantages of general health measurement tools to evaluate specific disorders is that they may not assess well the specific impact of the disease on an individual and how it may be affected by other medical conditions. This has led to an effort to develop disease-specific outcomes measurements tools.[8] The creation of these outcomes measurement tools requires a comprehensive, statistically validated assessment of reliability, predictability, reproducibility, responsiveness, and interpretability. In general, they should be easy to use (low burden) and should assist in the evaluation of the specific problems they were designed to assess.

The human voice is unique in all of the animal kingdom, and is the fundamental method of human communication. The range of frequency and flexibility of sound production allows the voice to express emotions of the human soul. The voice laughs and cries, yells and whispers, sings and hums, recognizes danger or placidity. For a "professional vocalist," both singers and speakers, the voice serves as the primary source of livelihood and income. It allows most others a means to carry out the activities of their occupation or avocation. In general, people take the voice for granted. It is there when you need it, and it usually performs at the level of expectation of the individual. Even for the professional vocalist who may have spent years refining the quality and attributes of his/her voice, it is usually dependable and predictable. When the voice fails any person, the impact on general communication for social and occupational needs gains importance. When the voice fails the professional vocalist, the impact is often even more substantial, if not devastating, and potentially career ending.

It has been difficult to develop measures to assess voice quality and health impact. Most of the present measurements deal with objective specifics of voice production; the mechanics of voice production, such as posture, support, and resonance; or specific physiologic actions such as vocal fold vibration. Although these measures have great value and are critical for improved understanding and training of the voice, they fail to measure either the importance of voice production and the impact of voice disorders on the overall quality of life of the voice user or the effects from an intervention or treatment. Even with objective tests, there are no generally agreed-upon gold standards of measurement. Furthermore, different objective tests have been designed for different measures of function, such as fundamental frequency, frequency range, airflow parameters, perturbation, or vocal fold vibration. Variation occurs between clinicians in the performance and interpretation of these tests. Such limitations have prevented valid comparisons of the impact of an intervention in different environments or comparisons of two different interventions.

Although it would be expected that improvements in objective tests would correlate with improvements in outcome, severity of disease as measured by these tests does not necessarily measure the impact to an individual. Minimal variations in pitch would likely have a much greater impact for a performing vocalist than in a person who has minimal voice demands. A cured small laryngeal cancer may prevent a singer or other speaker from performing. The impact on their quality of life would be expected to be greater and likely to be represented poorly by objective tests.

With the development of general quality of life surveys such as the SF-36, the clinician can assess the impact of disease or treatment on quality of life. Furthermore, comparisons can be made between patients and others without the disorder or between patients with two or more different disorders. Our recent study showed that there are significant differences in perception of quality of life between dysphonic (disordered voice) patients and unaffected average people in the United States.[7] When evaluating the specific domains of the SF-36, we found that the domains of "role function emotion" and "role function physical" were both significantly different between dysphonic and non-dysphonic people. These two domains deal with the ability to perform work and other daily tasks as a result of the physical or emotional impact of their disorder. As voice problems might be expected to have an impact on work and other daily activities, this finding is not unexpected. The "social functioning" score was also worse in dysphonic patients. Because "physical functioning," "vitality," and "mental health" scores were also worse for dysphonic patients than for normals, it can be seen that these voice disorders affect a broader sense of well-being than the specific symptoms. Objective tests of voice function or standard questionnaires would not be expected to measure these quality of life impacts.

THE VOICE HANDICAP INDEX

Traditionally, outcomes for patients with voice disorders have been measured with a clinical or biomedical frame of reference. The variables that are used to indi-

cate a favorable or unfavorable treatment outcome do not rely on attitudinal input from the patients. In an effort to shift the focus from the clinicians' judgments to patients' self-perceptions of their voice disorders, we developed the *Voice Handicap Index* (VHI).[8] (See Figure 18-1.) The VHI consists of 30 statements that reflect the variety of experiences that a patient with a voice disorder may encounter. Patients note a frequency of each experience on a 5-point equally appearing scale (never—0, almost never—1, sometimes—2, almost always—3, always—4), with a maximal total score of 120. The VHI is able not only to measure the physical effects of their voice problem but also the functional and emotional aspects, or subscales. The VHI is scored for each of these three individual subscales and a total score. Therefore, it can serve as an independent, objective measure of the impact on quality of life of voice dysfunction.

Our studies show that the quality of life impact of a disordered voice is substantial even when compared to other chronic diseases such as angina, sciatica, chronic sinusitis, or back pain, particularly in the areas of social functioning and role playing.[7] Overall, however, other chronic diseases tend to produce worse scores than dysphonia.

Because the SF-36 is scaled only relating to the individual domains and not for a total score, direct overall total comparisons to the VHI cannot be made. Nonetheless, by evaluating the individual domains, a comparison of quality of life impact of various disorders can be made between the SF-36 and VHI. For example, when attempting to correlate the VHI with the SF-36, strong correlations were found between the total VHI scores and the individual subscales to the SF-36 domains of social functioning, role functioning, emotional and physical, and mental health. The greatest disability of voice patients is in the functional areas, as was validated by our study in assessing the relationship of the VHI to the SF-36.[7] Because patients with voice disorders generally do not have significant changes in bodily pain, general health, vitality, and general physical functioning, the VHI would not be expected to be very sensitive to changes in these domains of the SF-36.

Patients with vocal fold paralysis had worse scores in many of the domains of the SF-36 than other dysphonic patients, particularly in the domains of role playing, emotional and physical functioning.[7] This is likely caused by the impact of vocal fold paralysis on lifting and straining and other daily activities. In general, patients with paralysis appear to be more disabled and have poorer overall quality of life than the other categories of patients with dysphonia, as measured by both the SF-36 and VHI. When evaluated with the VHI, the

Voice Handicap Index (VHI)

Instructions: These are statements that many people have used to describe their voices and the effects of their voices on their lives. Check the response that indicates how frequently you have the same experience.
(Never = 0 points: Almost Never = 1 point; Sometimes = 2 points; Almost Always = 3 points; Always = 4 points)

		Never	Almost Never	Sometimes	Almost Always	Always
F1.	My voice makes it difficult for people to hear me.					
P2.	I run out of air when I walk.					
F3.	People have difficulty understanding me in a noisy room.					
P4.	The sound of my voice varies throughout the day.					
F5.	My family has difficulty hearing me when I call them throughout the house.					
F6.	I use the phone less often than I would like.					
E7.	I'm tense when talking with others because of my voice.					
F8.	I tend to avoid groups of people because of my voice.					
E9.	People seem irritated with my voice.					
P10.	People ask, "What's wrong with your voice?"					
F11.	I speak with friends, neighbors, or relatives less often because of my voice.					
F12.	People ask me to repeat myself when speaking face-to-face.					
P13.	My voice sounds creaky and dry.					
P14.	I feel as though I have to strain to produce voice.					
E15.	I find other people don't understand my voice problem.					
F16.	My voice difficulties restrict my personal and social life.					
P17.	The clarity of my voice is unpredictable.					
P18.	I try to change my voice to sound different.					

FIGURE 18-1. *The Voice Handicap Index (VHI). The figure shows the 30 items included in the Voice Handicap Index with instructions as to how to complete the form. The questions are itemized by letter and number. The letters (P, F, E) are representative of the three subscales (Physical, Functional, Emotional). The scores for each of the items with the same letter can be added to give the subscale score. The three subscale scores are added to give a total score. A change in 8 points for an individual subscale or 18 points for the total score is considered a significant change.[8] Copyright American Speech-Language-Hearing Association. Reprinted with permission. Adapted from Jacobson, Johnson, Grywalski, et al. Journal of Speech Pahtology. 1997;6:66-70. (Continues)*

		Never	Almost Never	Sometimes	Almost Always	Always
F19.	I feel left out of conversations because of my voice.					
P20.	I use a great deal of effort to speak.					
P21.	My voice is worse in the evening.					
F22.	My voice problem causes me to lose income.					
E23.	My voice problem upsets me.					
E24.	I am less outgoing because of my voice problem.					
E25.	My voice makes me feel handicapped.					
P26.	My voice "gives out" on me in the middle of speaking.					
E27.	I feel annoyed when people ask me to repeat.					
E28.	I feel embarrassed when people ask me to repeat.					
E29.	My voice makes me feel incompetent.					
E30.	I'm ashamed of my voice problem.					

P Scale   _____
F Scale   _____
E Scale   _____
Total Scale   _____

Please circle the word that matches how you feel your voice is today.

Normal   Mild   Moderate   Severe

FIGURE 18-1. *The Voice Handicap Index (VHI). (Continued)*

vocal fold edema group had better scores for the total, functional, and physical scores than the patients with vocal fold masses (such as nodules or polyps). Individuals with vocal fold paralysis in general had worse scores than other individuals with voice disorders as measured by the VHI.[7]

In a subsequent study, we attempted to compare the VHI and its three subscales to various objective tests. We were able to show that the functional subscale of the VHI correlated well with both signal to noise ratio (SNR) and maximum phonatory time (MPT). Other measures, such as jitter, shimmer, fundamental frequency, semitones, and airflow volume had little correlation with the patients' perception of the quality of life impact of their voice disorder as measured by the VHI.[9] Although these specific measures did not correlate with the VHI, as the voices of patients worsened, as measured by the objective laboratory parameters, a corresponding change in the VHI scores occurred.[9] The relationship between objective laboratory measures and the VHI cannot be seen as interchangeable. There are corresponding appropriate changes in both with worsening voice, but only strong correlations in SNR and MPT. This may suggest that the tests may likely measure different parameters of voice. It also may suggest that the objective laboratory tests now used may measure specific parameters of voice, but not the global impact of a voice disorder on the patient's emotional, functional, and physical perception of health.

The VHI, therefore, is a statistically validated, objective test that can be used to measure the emotional, physical, functional, and total quality of life impact of a voice disorder. It can be used to measure the response to treatment or nontreatment, to perform research related to voice, or to evaluate patients in different clinical environments. In the absence of definitive, established gold standards for measuring voice, the VHI may serve as the template for assessing voice outcome. Finally, the VHI can be used along with other objective tools or tests to assess the characteristics of an individual's voice and the impact of those characteristics on quality of voice and quality of life.

SUMMARY

The future challenges related to outcomes research in voice will revolve around the application of these types of instruments to allow identification of factors important to the patient. The first challenge is to determine the severity of a patient's handicap or disability from a particular disorder. This will have an impact on the aggressiveness of treatment, or, in some cases, the decision whether or not to treat. The second challenge is to utilize outcomes research to identify the best treatment. This may also be used to develop new treatments that take into consideration the vocalist's response to treatment. Finally, voice outcomes research should focus on how improvement of a specific disorder will influence the global quality of life for the voice user and for his/her family.

The future for outcomes research in voice is bright. There is much effort directed at improvement of quality of life and measurement. These efforts in combination with traditional voice evaluations, basic voice research science, and prospective, randomized clinical trials should have a dramatic impact on voice care in the future. The application of objective outcomes tools such as the VHI and the SF-36 to performing vocalists will ensure that the global impact on quality of life is measured.

REFERENCES

1. World Health Organization. The economics of health and disease. *WHO Chronicle.* 1971;25:20-24.

2. World Health Organization. *International Classification of Impairments, Disabilities and Handicaps: A Manual of Classification Relating to the Consequences of Disease.* Geneva, Switzerland: World Health Organization; 1980.

3. Benninger MS, Gardner GM, Jacobson BH, Grywalski C. New dimensions in measuring voice treatment outcomes. In: Sataloff R. *Professional Voice.* Clifton Park, NY: Delmar; 1996.

4. Ware JE, Sherbourne CD. The MOS 36-item Short Form Health Survey (SF-36). I. Conceptual framework and item selection. *Med Care.* 1992;30:473-483.

5. McHorney CA, Ware JE, Raczek AE. The MOS 36-item Short Form Health Survey (SF-36). II. Psychometric and clinical tests of validity in measuring physical and mental health constructs. *Med Care.* 1993;31:247-263.

6. McHorney CA, Ware JE, Lu JF, Sherbourne CD. The MOS 36-item Short Form Health Survey (SF-36). III. Tests of data quality, scaling, assumptions and reliability across diverse patient groups. *Med Care.* 1994;32:40-66.

7. Benninger MS, Ahuja AS, Gardner G, Grywalski C. Assessing outcomes for dysphonic patients. *J Voice.* 1998;12:540-550.

8. Jacobson BH, Johnson A, Grywalski C, et al. The Voice Handicap Index (VHI): development and validation. *J Speech Lang Pathol.* 1997;6:66-70.

9. Ahuja A, Benninger MS, Grywalski C, Gardner G. Correlation between the Voice Handicap Index with objective acoustic and aerodynamic measurements. *J Voice.*

CHAPTER 19

Voice Impairment, Disability, Handicap, and Medical/Legal Evaluation

Robert T. Sataloff, MD, DMA, FACS

Medical care of singers and actors inspired the development of voice as a subspecialty of laryngology. Although the interest was originally aesthetic and scientific, the broader practical importance of voice dysfunction soon became apparent. It is intuitively obvious that dysphonia in a great singer is not only an artistic and cultural tragedy, but also a disability that may result in the loss of millions of dollars annually for some performers. However, as our discipline has evolved, it became clear that singers are not the only professional voice users. Voice professionals include also actors, clergy, politicians, teachers, sales personnel, secretaries, and anyone else whose ability to make a living is diminished or interrupted by voice disturbance.

As awareness of the importance of the human voice has grown, so too have legal issues surrounding voice dysfunction. Some voice disorders arise out of an individual's employment and may be covered under Workers' Compensation laws in some jurisdictions. Such cases might include vocal nodules developing in a school-teacher, or dysphonia in a shop foreman who suffers a laryngeal fracture while working and can no longer be heard over the noise at his/her job site. However, Workers' Compensation statutes are usually quite specific and vary greatly from one jurisdiction to another. The fact that a health problem is causally related to employment does not guarantee that it will be compensable under Workers' Compensation statutes in any

given case. Other legal avenues may be pursued in some cases, such as civil suits under Tort law; physicians should be familiar with their roles in different types of legal proceedings and the financial implications for the patient of the applicable law. Hearing loss illustrates this issue particularly well. A given hearing loss may be compensated at the rate of $18,000 in Rhode Island, $108,940 in Pennsylvania, or at an unlimited level (depending upon jury verdict) for a railroad worker subject to the Federal Employer's Liability Act. If a given injury (dysphonia, hearing loss, etc) is covered under Workers' Compensation law in a given jurisdiction, then compensation is determined by that statute, and the worker is generally prohibited from suing the employer outside the Workers' Compensation system. If the injury is not covered specifically in the applicable Workers' Compensation statute, then the employee may be able to file a civil suit and recover a potentially unlimited amount of compensation. Other cases are not causally related to work, such as a patient who develops dysphonia following endotracheal intubation, thoracic surgery, or laryngeal surgery. Yet, such vocal injuries may have profound effects on the patient's earning potential, and redress may be sought under Tort law.

It is helpful for physicians to understand the accepted definitions of impairment, disability, and handicap. These terms are defined well by the World Health Organization.[1] An impairment is "any loss or abnormality of psychological, physiological, or anatomical structure or function."[1, p47] The abnormalities of losses that constitute an impairment may be temporary or permanent, and they involve the existence of a defect of a bodily structure, including mental defects. A disability resulting from an impairment is "any restriction or lack...of ability to perform an activity in the manner or within the range considered normal for a human being."[1, p143] Disabilities are characterized by abnormalities of customarily expected performance of activities. They may be temporary or permanent, and there may be direct consequences of impairment, or individual responses to an impairment (such as psychologic reactions). A handicap is "a disadvantage for a given individual, resulting from an impairment or a disability, that limits or prevents the fulfillment of a role that is normal (depending on age, sex, and social and cultural factors) for that individual."[1, p183] Handicaps reflect the consequences for the individual resulting from an impairment and/or disability in terms of social, cultural, environmental, and economic impact.[2]

VOICE IMPAIRMENT, DISABILITY, AND HANDICAP

In order to help guide fair and reasonable determination of impairment and disability for voice, guidelines developed for other body systems and functions have been helpful. The World Health Organization's *International Classification of Impairments, Disabilities and Handicaps* provides a classification scheme that is quite useful for many conditions, but it does not furnish specific compensation guidelines for most conditions. In the United States (and in some other countries) the American Medical Association's *Guides to The Evaluation of Permanent Impairment* (referred to as *The Guides*) have become the standard.[2] *The Guides* rate many impairments and disabilities throughout the body in terms of their percentage impairment of the whole person. At present, even *The Guides* does not provide a sufficient and sophisticated approach to the evaluation of voice impairment and disability. Various other publications of international repute also cover voice impairment disability in inadequate depth.[2,3] This chapter contains suggestions to modify and improve existing guidelines.[2] Additional information about assessing voice handicap may be found in the chapter on Outcomes Measures (Chapter 18).

For many years, *voice* and *speech* were treated by the medical profession (and the first four editions of the AMA *Guides*) as one subject under the heading *speech*. In the last 20 years, voice and voice science have evolved as independent subspecialties in otolaryngology and speech-language pathology. Therefore, technology and standards of practice now permit appropriate consideration of both aspects of verbal communication. The upcoming fifth edition of the AMA *Guides* will contain preliminary changes that acknowledge and begin to rectify this problem. *Voice* refers to production of sound of a given quality, ordinarily using the true vocal folds. *Speech* refers to the shaping of sounds into intelligible words. The disability and handicap associated with severe impairment of *speech* are obvious: if a person cannot speak intelligibly, verbal communication in social environments and the workplace is extremely difficult or impossible. However, *voice* disorders have been underappreciated for so long that their significance may not be as immediately apparent. Nevertheless, if a voice disorder results in hoarseness, breathiness, voice fatigue, decreased vocal volume, or other similar voice disturbances, the worker may be unable to be heard in the presence of even moderate background noise, to carry on telephone conversations for prolonged periods, or to perform other work-related (and social) functions. Communication with hard-of-hearing family members and friends may also be particularly difficult and frustrating.

Numerous conditions, both physical and environmental, can result in voice or speech disturbances. An extensive review of their etiologies, diagnoses, and treatments is beyond the scope of this discussion. Information on this subject is contained elsewhere in this book and in other literature.[4-7] Briefly, voice and speech dysfunction may be caused by trauma (brain, face, neck, chest), exposure to toxins and pollution, cerebrovascular accident, voice abuse, cancer, psychogenic disorders, and other causes. This chapter concentrates on the consequences of voice and speech dysfunction and also synthesizes information introduced in previous writings.[2,8,9]

EVALUATION

Evaluation of a person with speech or voice complaints begins with a thorough history. Inquiry should include questions regarding the patient's professional and avocational vocal needs and habits, voice use patterns, problems prior to the onset of the current complaint, the time and apparent cause of the onset of voice and speech dysfunction, and any evaluations and interventions that have been tried to improve voice function. It is also essential to obtain information about environmental irritants and pollution, which may influence the voice greatly.[6] The voice may be impaired not only by mucosal irritants and inhalant toxicity, but also by any substances that decrease lung function or neurologic function (including neurotoxins such as heavy metals).

However, a thorough history must include information about virtually all body systems, as maladies almost anywhere in the body may be causally related to voice complaints. The details of a comprehensive voice and speech history, and physical examination are beyond the scope of this brief chapter and may be found in other literature and elsewhere in this book.[7] The physical examination should include thorough evaluation of the structures in the head and neck, and evaluation of other parts of the body, as appropriate, based on history and physical assessment of the patient. A thorough evaluation of voice and speech is also mandatory.

For the purposes of this chapter, it should be assumed that the evaluation of voice and speech involves an assessment of a person's ability to produce phonation and articulate speech, and does not involve assessment of content, language, or linguistic structure. At the present time, there is no single, universally accepted measure to quantify voice or speech function. Therefore, the standard of practice requires the use of a battery of tests.

Various tests and objective measures of voice have been clinically available since the late 1970s. Tests such as strobovideolaryngoscopy, acoustic analysis, phonatory function assessment, and laryngeal electromyography (EMG) are recognized as appropriate and useful in the evaluation of speech and voice disorders.[10-14] Some or all of these tests may be necessary in selected cases in order to determine the severity of a voice disorder and establish the presence of organic versus nonorganic voice/speech impairment and disability.

Evaluation of voice requires visualization of the larynx by a physician trained in laryngoscopy (usually an otolaryngologist) and determination of a specific medical cause for the voice dysfunction. Assessment of voice quality, frequency range, intensity range and endurance, pulmonary function, and function of the larynx as a valve (airflow regulator) can be performed easily and inexpensively. Normative values for these assessments have been established in the literature and are discussed elsewhere in this book.[7,11,14] More sophisticated techniques to quantify voice function (spectrography, inverse filtering, etc) may be helpful in selected cases. Slow-motion assessment of vocal fold vibration using strobovideolaryngoscopy (an established procedure that was first described more than 100 years ago) is often medically necessary to establish an accurate diagnosis.

In keeping with standard practice to establish the presence and amount of impairment and disability, a battery of tests is required to determine *audibility, intelligibility,* and *functional efficiency* of voice and speech. Audibility permits the patient to be heard over background noise. Intelligibility is the ability to link recognizable phonetic units of speech in a manner that can be understood. Functional efficiency is the ability to sustain voice and speech at a rate and for a period of time sufficient to permit useful communication.

Many approaches are available for speech assessment, most of which are described in standard speech-language pathology textbooks.[4] However, for the purposes of determining impairment and disability, the method recommended in the AMA *Guides* is employed most commonly.[2] This assessment protocol uses "The Smith House" reading paragraph, which reads as follows:

> Larry and Ruth Smith have been married nearly fourteen years. They have a small place near Long Lake. Both of them think there's nothing like the country for health. Their two boys would rather live here than any other place. Larry likes to keep some saddle horses close to the house. These make it easy to keep his sons amused. If they wish, the boys can go fishing along the shore. When it rains, they usually want to watch television. Ruth has a cherry tree on each side of the kitchen door. In June they enjoy the juice and jelly.

The patient is placed approximately eight feet from the examiner in a quiet room. The patient is then instructed to read the paragraph so that the examiner can hear him or her plainly, and so that the patient can be understood. Patients who cannot read are asked to count to 100 (and should be able to do so in under 75 seconds). Patients are expected to be able to complete at least a 10-word sentence in one breath, sustain phonation for at least 10 seconds on one breath, speak loudly enough to be heard across the room, and maintain a speech rate of at least 75 to 100 words per minute. The advantages of the system described in *The Guides* are simplicity, and wide application for disability determination. However, this approach does not take advantage of many standardized speech evaluation tests, of technology for better quantification, or of techniques available to help identify psychogenic and intentional voice and speech dysfunction. These advanced methods should be used at least when the results of simple confrontation testing are unconvincing or equivocal; ideally, they should be used in all cases. In addition, it does not address the issue of workers whose native language is something other than English. No specific passages have been assigned for various languages. However, appropriate passages may be drawn from the phoniatric or speech-language pathology literature of appropriate countries and used by a medical examiner whose command of the specific language is sufficient to permit valid and reliable interpretation of the patient's responses.

In most respects, the medical evaluation of a person sent for medical/legal purposes or independent medical evaluation (IME) is the same thorough examination that should be performed for all patients with voice and speech disorders. However, for medical/legal purposes, it is important for physicians to be certain that they thoroughly understand the occupational needs and demands of the patient. One schoolteacher's professional vocal needs may be very different from those of another schoolteacher, even in the same school district. Similar differences occur among all voice professionals, including singers, telephone operators, and many others whose occupations depend upon voice and speech. Understanding the individual circumstances is essential in formulating an accurate, rational, and defensible opinion regarding causation and consequences of a voice/speech problem. All such information must be thoroughly documented, and the rationale for the physician's conclusions must be apparent.

There is a substantial difference in physician responsibilities for the "patient" at the conclusion of a medical/legal encounter compared with patients evaluated medically only. Ordinarily, we are accustomed to providing our patients with information, diagnoses, treatment recommendations, and to ordering appropriate studies. Such communication is not appropriate in many medical/legal settings, and the physician, patient, and referring professional (often an attorney) may be better served by having the physician's conclusion communicated in writing in a formal medical/legal report. The physician should be careful not to express opinions until they have been formed to a reasonable degree of medical certainty. This often requires gathering of additional information (such as work records), which may not be available at the time of the initial examination.

Great care should be taken to avoid expressing opinions prematurely, as retracting them later can be confusing, awkward, and can impugn the physician's medical and legal credibility. Formulating accurate conclusions that can be supported is important to help establish what happened and its consequences, and to support recommendations for patient assistance, in some cases. For example, people in vocally intensive occupations (schoolteachers, stockbrokers) who require voice surgery and/or extensive voice therapy may be well served by a leave of absence, acquisition of assistive devices (such as microphones), and by other modifications in performance routine that may have an unexpectedly great impact on their work environment and job security.

Judgments regarding short-term and long-term disability issues may have profound effects upon an individual's life and a business' economy; in some cases, they may require an employer to pay a disabled worker the equivalent of many years' salary, on top of the cost associated with replacement of the employee. Such recommendations should be made firmly when appropriate

and should never be made when they are not truly medically necessary (particularly prolonged leaves of absence). Formulating accurate and fair opinions in these matters requires thorough understanding of all relevant facts, and often reflection and review on the part of the physician.

SUGGESTED CRITERIA FOR DETERMINING VOICE AND/OR SPEECH IMPAIRMENT

An appropriate determination of voice-related disability requires a comprehensive understanding of voice science and medicine, legal definitions and issues, and consideration of the vocal needs of each individual with a voice/speech impairment.

For the purposes of classifying voice and/or speech impairment and disability, audibility, intelligibility, and functional efficiency must be taken into account. Audibility permits the patient to be heard over background noise. It generally reflects the condition of the voice. Disability determination should be based on subjective and objective assessments of voice and speech, on reports pertaining to the patient's performance in everyday living and occupational situations and on instruments such as the *Vocal Handicap Index*.[15] The reports or evidence should be supplied by reliable observers. For the nonprofessional voice user, the standard of evaluation should be the normal speaker's performance in average situations for everyday living. For the professional voice user, the standard of evaluation is the expected performance in professional and everyday situations of comparable voice professionals. Table 19-1 summarizes suggested voice and speech impairment criteria, modified in part from those set forth in the AMA *Guides*. In evaluating functional efficiency, *everyday speech communication* should be interpreted as including activities of daily living, and also routine voice and speech requirements of the patient's profession. A judgment is made regarding the patient's speech and voice capacity with regard to each of the three columns of the classification chart (Table 19-1). The degree of impairment of voice/speech is equivalent to the greatest percentage of impairment recorded in any one of the three columns of the classification chart.

For example, a particular patient's voice/speech impairment is judged to be the following: Audibility, 10% (Class 1); Intelligibility, 50% (Class 3), and Functional Efficiency, 30% (Class 2). This patient's voice/speech impairment is judged to be equivalent to the greatest impairment, 50%.

Converting an impairment of voice and speech into impairment of the whole person requires knowledge of

Classification	Audibility	Intelligibility	Functional Efficiency
Class 1 0%–14% speech impairment	Can produce voice of intensity sufficient for *most* of the needs of everyday speech communication, although this sometimes may require effort and occasionally may be beyond patient's capacity.	Can perform *most* of the articulatory acts necessary for everyday speech communication, although listeners occasionally may ask the patient to repeat, and the patient may find it difficult or impossible to produce a few phonetic units.	Can meet *most* of the demands of articulation and phonation for everyday speech communication with adequate speed and ease, although occasionally the patient may hesitate or speak slowly.
Class 2 15%–34% speech impairment	Can produce voice of intensity sufficient for *many* of the needs of everyday speech communication; is usually heard under average conditions; however, may have difficulty in automobiles, buses, trains, stations, restaurants, and so forth.	Can perform *many* of the necessary articulatory acts for everyday speech communication. Can speak name, address, and so forth and be understood by a stranger, but may have numerous inaccuracies; sometimes appears to have difficulty articulating.	Can meet *many* of the demands of articulation and phonation for everyday speech communication with adequate speed and ease, but sometimes gives impression of difficulty, and speech may sometimes be discontinuous, interrupted, hesitant, or slow.
Class 3 35%–59% speech impairment	Can produce voice of intensity sufficient for *some* of the needs of everyday speech communication, such as close conversation; however, has considerable difficulty in such noisy places as listed above; the voice tires rapidly and tends to become inaudible after a few seconds.	Can perform *some* of the necessary articulatory acts for everyday speech communication; can usually converse with family and friends; however, strangers may find it difficulty to understand the patient, who often may be asked to repeat.	Can meet *some* of the demands of articulation and phonation for everyday speech communication with adequate speed and ease, but often can sustain consecutive speech only for brief periods; may give the impression of being rapidly fatigued.
Class 4 60%–84% speech impairment	Can produce voice of intensity sufficient for a *few* of the needs of everyday speech communication; can barely be heard by a close listener or over the telephone, perhaps may be able to whisper audibly but has no louder voice.	Can perform a *few* of the necessary articulatory acts for everyday speech communication; can produce some phonetic units; may have approximations for a few words such as names of own family members; however, unintelligible out of context.	Can meet a *few* of the demands of articulation and phonation for everyday speech communication with adequate speed and ease, such as using single words or short phrases, but cannot maintain uninterrupted speech flow; speech is labored, rate is impractically slow.
Class 5 85%–100% speech impairment	Can produce voice of intensity sufficient for *none* of the needs of everyday speech communication.	Can perform *none* of the articulatory acts necessary for everyday speech communication.	Can meet *none* of the demands of articulation and phonation for everyday speech communication with adequate speed and ease.

TABLE 19-1. *Voice and Speech Impairment Guide*

the individual's occupational voice and speech require-ments. These may be divided into three classes, as fol-lows (note that these criteria are this author's (RTS) rec-ommendations, and are not yet accepted AMA guide-lines):

Class 1:   Voice/speech impairment should not result in significant change in ability to perform necessary occupational func-tions. Little or no voice/speech required for most daily occupational require-ments. Examples: manuscript typist, data-entry clerk, copy editor.

Class 2:   Voice/speech is a necessary component of daily occupational responsibilities, but not the principal focus of the indi-vidual's occupation. Impairment of voice or speech may make it difficult or impossible for the individual to perform his or her occupation at his or her pre-impairment level. Examples: stockbro-ker, non-trial attorney, supervisor in a noisy shop.

Class 3:   Voice/speech are the primary occupa-tional asset. Impairment seriously diminishes the individual's ability to perform his or her job, or makes it impossible to do so. Examples: class-room teacher, trial attorney, opera singer, broadcast announcer.

Table 19-2 is intended as a guideline for converting the percentage of voice/speech impairment to percent-age impairment of the whole person.

THE "WORTH" OF A VOICE

While improved, standardized guidelines for the esti-mation of vocal impairment and disability such as those proposed above may be helpful, no such guidelines are universally applicable to each individual case. If such guidelines are accepted by the AMA *Guides*, they may come to govern voice impairment and disability determi-nation in Workers' Compensation cases and jurisdictions that include speech and voice within their Workers' Compensation statutes. In other jurisdictions, and in sit-uations in which the vocal impairment is not causally related to employment, legal redress for voice impair-ment is generally determined under Tort law. In such cases, a judge or jury determines the degree of impair-ment and disability and the value of compensation, gen-erally based on expert testimony. Reference to docu-

ments such as the AMA *Guides* may be included, but many other factors are introduced into testimony to help the judge or jury establish whether a loss is compensable (someone was at fault), and, if so, the amount of com-pensation that is appropriate. Malpractice actions are generally handled in this fashion; and malpractice suits for dysphonia occur frequently. In some cases, they are (arguably) justified. As recently as 1999, this author (RTS) has reviewed actions in which "vocal cord strip-ping" was used in young professional singers as the first treatment for vocal nodules, and the surgery resulted in profound, bilateral vocal fold scar. In such instances, arguments frequently center on that singer's true artistic skill and potential for life earnings (determination of damages). Other cases involve famous, established singers for whom enormous earning ability is well-docu-mented and financial losses in the millions are relatively easy to estimate. In such cases, arguments focus on issues of informed consent, accuracy of diagnosis, appro-priateness of surgery, and whether the dysphonia was caused by a deviation from the standard of care or simply to a recognized complication such as unfavorable scar.

In all such instances, otolaryngologists have an obli-gation to their profession and the public. As distasteful as medical legal aspects of voice disorders may be, we must be prepared to evaluate them honestly and dispas-sionately. Our evaluation should draw on all the scien-tific, clinical, and technologic advances that have enhanced the practice of laryngology/voice, and should be influenced by an awareness of the standard of prac-tice in impairment and disability determination as set forth in publications such as the AMA *Guides*.

We must be prepared to recognize that dysphonia may result in substantial disability and loss of earnings for many of our patients. When such problems occur as an unavoidable consequence of surgery, we must be prepared to help juries and judges understand the unpredictabilities of surgery. However, when they occur because of deviations or violations of the standard of care, we must also be willing to recognize that the patient may be entitled to compensation in accordance with our country's legal system. We must also recognize that, to some extent, the pressures exerted by the med-ical-legal climate have worked to improve the standar of care and still exert pressure on our profession to remain current with the latest advances and changes in the state-of-the-art care. Maintaining currency is particular-ly important in a rapidly evolving discipline such as laryngology/voice.

Case Reports

Case one is a 42-year-old female, former teacher, now an elementary school guidance counselor, who returned

% Speech Impairment	% Impairment of the Whole Person Occupational Class 1	% Impairment of the Whole Person Occupational Class 2	% Impairment of the Whole Person Occupational Class 3
0	0	0	0
5	2	4	5
10	4	8	10
15	5	10	15
20	7	14	20
25	9	18	25
30	10	20	30
35	12	24	35
40	14	28	40
45	16	32	45
50	18	36	50
55	19	38	55
60	21	42	60
65	23	46	65
70	24	48	70
75	26	52	75
80	28	56	80
85	30	60	85
90	32	64	90
95	33	66	95
100	35	70	97

TABLE 19-2. *Speech Impairment Related to Impairment of the Whole Person*

to work seven years ago following a ten-year hiatus. Within the first month, she experienced a sudden onset of hoarseness. She continued to work for several months before seeking medical attention. Initial evaluation by an otolaryngologist revealed vocal folds nodules, and relative voice rest for four days was recommended. She had no improvement in her voice. She then saw a speech therapist weekly for two years with no improvement. She then underwent excision of bilateral vocal fold masses. Her voice improved for six months, after which her hoarseness returned. She was again diagnosed with recurrent vocal fold nodules and gastroesophageal reflux disease.

She was referred to this author (RTS) two years following surgery, with complaints of constant hoarseness and voice fatigue. She was unable to project her voice well and unable to sing although she would have liked to. She had been treated for gastroesophageal reflux disease for the past year. She had year-round allergy symptoms but stated they were "now better controlled since she started receiving injections."

Physical examination revealed a moderately hoarse and breathy voice. Strobovideolaryngoscopy revealed a broad-based, solid, white mass of her right vocal fold with a fibrotic mass of the left vocal fold; arytenoid erythema and edema consistent with gastroesophageal reflux disease; bilateral superior surface varicosities and scarring apparent upon stroboscopic visualization. Laryngeal EMG revealed mild bilateral superior laryngeal nerve paresis. No neuromuscular junction abnormalities were noted. Objective voice evaluations were completed and revealed decreased intensity, phonation time, harmonic-to-noise ratio, acoustic measures and (s/z) ratio.

There was no improvement in the appearance of her vocal fold lesions following six weeks of aggressive medical treatment for the reflux laryngitis disease. Voice therapy was unsuccessful over the six-week period despite excellent compliance by the patient. The patient was taken to the operating room for excision of the bilateral lesions. Biopsy revealed adult-onset laryngeal papillomatosis, not "nodules" as had been diagnosed by her previous physician.

The patient required two subsequent laryngeal operations within one year in an attempt to eradicate disease and improve her phonatory function. She will continue to require ongoing surveillance by a laryngologist for recurrence of papillomata, and surveillance for the development of laryngeal carcinoma. She will require ongoing voice therapy and treatment for her reflux disease. When she is able to return to work, she will require a personal amplification system to help with vocal projection. Her vocal prognosis is guarded. Her impairment would be noted as 60%-84% (Class 4).

Case two is a 38-year-old male factory worker who has worked at the same chemical plant for twenty years. He started in the rubber division and ten years later switched to the plastics and chemical division. He was working in a management position stating he was responsible for "everything that blows up." He suffered an inhalation injury two years ago resulting from heavy exposure to vinyl chloride fumes when three reactors malfunctioned. He underwent microlaryngoscopy and excision of bilateral "vocal fold polyps" one year after this injury. His voice improved after surgery and he remained out of work for approximately six weeks following surgery. One month after returning to work, he was exposed to anhydrous ammonia fumes and experienced immediate dyspnea and sudden and severe hoarseness. He underwent a second microlaryngoscopy and vocal fold polypectomy. He attempted to return to work but became aphonic after three days.

He reported voice deterioration after voice use and any exposure to fumes, perfumes, smoke, or gasoline and that his hoarseness was now associated with shortness of breath. He also experienced chronic globus sensation. He was undergoing psychologic counseling for stress-related problems secondary to his voice problems and he also had to quit smoking.

His voice was harsh, hoarse, slightly breathy, and pressed. Strobovideolaryngoscopy revealed bilateral vocal fold scarring, decreased mucosal wave, hypervascularity, and mucosal irregularities. Objective voice measures revealed marked abnormalities in harmonic-to-noise ratio, shimmer, and maximum flow rate.

This individual had a mucosal vocal fold injury secondary to inhalation of noxious fumes, initially vinyl chloride, and airway hyperactivity causing dysphonia and dyspnea. Additional surgery was recommended. The vocal fold mucosa never returned to normal nor did his voice quality. Five years later he developed progressive hysplastic vocal fold changes (leukoplakia).

This case illustrates the scope of the shortcomings of *The Guides'* current rating system. It does not take into account significant, medically proven symptom fluctuation, or specific occupational vocal requirements. When this patient was at home, protected from fumes, or pollution, he would be rated Class 3 on the basis of audibility. Once he enters the work environment, or many other everyday settings, his impairment becomes a Class 5. Considering the impact on his life and employability, it is reasonable to assign him a Class 5 rating.

Case three is a 28-year-old male singer and songwriter. He developed vocal difficulties one year ago while recording an album. He had been singing and performing rock and roll for ten years with no prior vocal difficulties. While recording his album, he experienced loss of midrange, decreased volume, breathiness, and hoarseness. He was not ill at the time. Three months later he was diagnosed with a left vocal fold polyp and surgical excision of the lesion was performed the following month. The patient had additional complaints of his voice being worse is the morning, frequent throat clearing, and a globus sensation. He was given advice concerning control of his reflux laryngitis symptoms and placed on a reflux protocol. He remains unhappy with his vocal progress to date.

Strobovideolaryngoscopy revealed a right vocal fold mass, left vocal fold scar, reflux laryngitis, and superior laryngeal nerve paresis. The mass and scar were typical sequelae of hemorrhage, as suggested by his history of sudden voice change while recording. Examination of his singing voice revealed excess tension in the jaw and tongue, hoarseness, and decreased range. Laryngeal EMG was advised and revealed a 20% decrease in function of the left superior laryngeal nerve. Additionally, he had abnormalities in electroglottography (EGG) quasi open quotient, AC flow, minimal flow, maximum flow rate, s/z ratio, maximum phonation time, and acoustic measurements.

This case illustrates an important shortcoming of the current rating system. According to the current method, he would be rated Class 2 on the basis of audibility. Yet, as a professional singer, he is totally disabled from this work-related injury. A classification scheme that considered the individual's professional voice needs would classify him as Class 5.

SUMMARY

As the field of laryngology/voice evolved over time, considerations of voice impairment and disability are evolving. All laryngologists should be familiar with these developments, as well as substantive developments in medical, surgical, and postsurgical voice management. Physicians must be extremely diligent about obtaining all the facts before arriving at a diagnosis and rendering an opinion. Misdiagnoses of voice and speech disorders are common, and somewhat understandably so, because of the dramatic recent advances in the standard of voice/speech care. Nevertheless, misdiagnosis is serious for both medical and medical/legal reasons and can generally be avoided. Information on the latest techniques in voice evaluation is available through The Voice Foundation*, the literature cited in this article, and through numerous other sources. In medical/legal settings, it is advisable for physicians to consider not only the standard of care, but moreover the state of the art. They should also complement their medical expertise with a reasonable understanding of legal issues, including not only definitions of impairment and disability, but also the legal theories and jurisdiction under which a case is being managed. Such knowledge will enhance our abilities to help not only our patients' voices, but also each patient as a person.

REFERENCES

1. *International Classification of Impairments, Disabilities and Handicaps*. Geneva, Switzerland: World Health Organization; 1980.

2. *Guides to the Evaluation of Permanent Impairment*. 4th ed. Chicago, IL: American Medical Association;1993.

3. Glorig A, Sataloff RT. Audiological system. In: Demeter SL, Andersson GBJ, Smith GM, eds. *AMA Disability Evaluation*. St. Louis, MO: Mosby-Yearbook, Inc; 1996:482-498.

4. Aronson A. *Clinical Voice Disorders*. 3rd ed. New York, NY: Thieme Medical Publishers; 1990.

5. Rubin J, Sataloff RT, Korovin G, Gould WJ. *The Diagnosis and Treatment of Voice Disorders*. New York, NY: Igaku-Shoin Medical Publishers, Inc; 1995.

6. Sataloff RT. The impact of pollution on the Voice. *Otolaryngol Head Neck Surg*. 1992;106(6):701-705.

7. Sataloff RT. *Professional Voice: Science and Art of Clinical Care*. 2nd ed. San Diego, CA: Singular Publishing Group; 1997.

8. Sataloff RT. Voice and speech impairment and disability. In: Sataloff RT, ed. *Professional Voice: Science and Art of Clinical Care*. 2nd ed. San Diego, CA: Singular Publishing Group; 1997:795-801.

9. Sataloff RT, Abaza MM. Impairment, disability and other medical/legal aspects of dysphonia. *Otolaryngol Clin North Am*. In press.

10. Baken RJ. *Clinical Measurement of Speech and Voice*. Boston/Toronto/San Diego: College-Hill Press, Little Brown and Co; 1987.

11. Hirano M. *Clinical Examination of the Voice*. New York, NY: Springer-Verlag; 1981.

12. Sataloff RT, Spiegel JR, Carroll LM, Schiebel BR, Darby KS, Rulnick RK. Strobovideolaryngoscopy in professional voice users: results and clinical value. *J Voice*. 1988;1(4):359-364.

13. Sataloff RT, Spiegel JR, Hawkshaw M. Strobovideolaryngoscopy: results and clinical value. *Ann Otol Rhinol Laryngol*. 1991;100(9):725-727.

14. Sataloff RT. The human voice. *Sci Am*. 1992;267(6):108-115.

15. Benninger MS, Gardener GM, Jacobson BH, Grywalski C. New dimensions in measuring voice treatment outcomes. In Sataloff RT, ed. *Professional Voice: The Science and Art of Clinical Care*. 2nd ed. San Diego, CA: Singular Publishing Group; 1997:789-794.

UNIT 3

Management

CHAPTER 20

Common Medical Diagnoses and Treatments in Patients with Voice Disorders

Robert T. Sataloff, MD, DMA, FACS

Mary J. Hawkshaw, RN, BSN, CORLN

Joseph R. Spiegel, MD, FACS

Laryngologists specializing in voice devote the majority of their practices to the medical management of benign voice disorders. Indeed, although most of us are active surgeons, the good voice specialist takes pride in avoiding the need for laryngeal surgery through expert medical management. Success depends not only upon a good laryngologist, but also on the availability of a voice team, including a speech-language pathologist, voice scientist, singing voice specialist, and medical consultants who have acquired special knowledge about voice disorders (neurologists, pulmonologists, endocrinologists, internists, allergists, and others). This chapter provides an overview of many of the benign voice problems encountered by otolaryngologists, and current nonsurgical management concepts.

There are numerous medical conditions that adversely affect the voice. Many have their origins primarily outside the head and neck. This chapter is not intended to be all-inclusive, but rather to highlight some of the more common and important conditions found in professional voice users seeking medical care.

In the 2,286 cases of all forms of voice disorders reported by Brodnitz in 1971,[1] 80% of the disorders were attributed to voice abuse or to psychogenic factors resulting in vocal dysfunction. Of these patients, 20% had organic voice disorders. Of women with organic problems, about 15% had identifiable endocrine causes. A much higher incidence of organic disorders, particu-larly reflux laryngitis, acute infectious laryngitis, and benign vocal fold masses, is found in one of the author's (RTS) practice.

VOICE ABUSE

When voice abuse is suspected or observed in a patient with vocal complaints, he or she should be referred to a laryngologist who specializes in voice, preferably a physician affiliated with a voice care team.

Common patterns of voice abuse and misuse will not be discussed in detail in this chapter. They are covered elsewhere in the literature,[2] and elsewhere in this book. Voice abuse and/or misuse should be suspected particularly in patients who complain of voice fatigue associated with voice use, whose voices are worse at the end of a working day or week, and in any patient who is chronically hoarse. Technical errors in voice use may be the primary etiology of a voice complaint, or may develop secondarily as a result of a patient's efforts to compensate for voice disturbance from another cause.

Speaking in noisy environments, such as cars and airplanes, is particularly abusive to the voice, as are back-stage greetings, postperformance parties, choral conducting, voice teaching, and cheerleading, to name a few. With proper training, all these vocal activities can be done safely. However, most patients, surprisingly even singers, have little or no training for their speaking voice.

If voice abuse is caused by speaking, treatment should be provided by a licensed, certified speech-language pathologist in the United States, or by a phoniatrist in many other countries. Training the speaking voice in many cases will benefit singers greatly not only by improving speech, but also by indirectly helping singing technique. Physicians should not hesitate to recommend such training, but it should be performed by an expert speech-language pathologist who specializes in voice. Many speech-language pathologists who are well trained in swallowing rehabilitation, articulation therapy, and other techniques are not trained in voice therapy for the speaking voice, and virtually none are trained through their speech and language programs to work with singing.

Specialized singing training also may be helpful to some voice patients who are not singers, and it is invaluable for patients who are singers. Initial singing training teaches relaxation techniques, develops muscle strength, and is symbiotic with standard speech therapy. Abuse of the voice during singing is an even more complex problem, as discussed elsewhere in this book.

INFECTION AND INFLAMMATION

Upper Respiratory Tract Infection Without Laryngitis

Although mucosal irritation usually is diffuse, patients sometimes have marked nasal obstruction with little or no sore throat and a "normal" voice. If the laryngeal examination shows no abnormality, a singer or professional speaker with a "head cold" should be permitted to use his/her voice and be advised not to try to duplicate his or her usual sound, but rather to accept the insurmountable alterations in self-perception caused by the change in the supraglottic vocal tract and auditory system. The decision as to whether performing under those circumstances is advisable professionally rests with the voice professional and his or her musical associates. The patient should be cautioned against throat clearing, as this is traumatic and may produce laryngitis. If a cough is present, non-narcotic medications should be used to suppress it.

Laryngitis With Serious Vocal Fold Injury

Hemorrhage in the vocal folds and mucosal disruption associated with acute laryngitis are contraindications to speaking and singing. When these are observed, treatment includes strict voice rest in addition to correction of any underlying disease. Vocal fold hemorrhage in voice professionals is most common in premenstrual women who are using aspirin products or nonsteroidal

anti-inflammatory drugs (NSAIDs) for dysmenorrhea. Severe hemorrhage or mucosal scarring may result in permanent alterations in vocal fold vibratory function. In rare instances, surgical intervention may be necessary. The potential gravity of these conditions must be stressed, for singers are generally reluctant to cancel an appearance. As von Leden observed, it is a pleasure to work with "people who are determined that the show must go on when everyone else is determined to goof off."[3] However, patient compliance is essential when serious damage has occurred. At present, acute treatment of vocal fold hemorrhage is controversial. Most laryngologists allow the hematoma to resolve spontaneously. Because this sometimes results in an organized hematoma and scar formation requiring surgery, some physicians advocate incision along the superior edge of the vocal fold and drainage of the hematoma in selected cases. Further study is needed to determine optimal therapy guidelines.

Laryngitis Without Serious Damage

Mild to moderate edema and erythema of the vocal folds may result from infection or from noninfectious causes. In the absence of mucosal disruption or hemorrhage, they are not absolute contraindications to voice use. Noninfectious laryngitis commonly is associated with excessive voice use in preperformance rehearsals. It may also be caused by other forms of voice abuse and by mucosal irritation produced by allergy, smoke inhalation, and other causes. Mucous stranding between the anterior and middle thirds of the vocal folds is seen commonly in inflammatory laryngitis. Laryngitis sicca is associated with dehydration, dry atmosphere, mouth breathing, and antihistamine therapy. Deficiency of mucosal lubrication causes irritation and coughing and results in mild inflammation. If no pressing professional need for performance exists, inflammatory conditions of the larynx are best treated with relative voice rest in addition to other modalities. However, in some instances, speaking and singing may be permitted. The patient should be instructed to avoid all forms of irritation and to rest the voice at all times except during warm-up and performance. Corticosteroids and other medications discussed later may be helpful. If mucosal secretions are copious, low-dose antihistamine therapy may be beneficial, but it must be prescribed with caution and should generally be avoided. Copious, thin secretions are better than scant, thick secretions or excessive dryness. The patient with laryngitis must be kept well hydrated to maintain the desired character of mucosal lubrication. The patient should be instructed to "pee pale," consuming enough water to keep urine diluted. Psychologic support is crucial. For example, it is often helpful for the physician to intercede on a singer's behalf and to convey "doctor's orders" directly to agents or theater management. Such mitigation of exogenous stress can be highly therapeutic.

Infectious laryngitis may be caused by bacteria or viruses. Subglottic involvement frequently indicates a more severe infection, which may be difficult to control in a short period of time. Indiscriminate use of antibiotics must be avoided; however, when the physician is in doubt as to the cause and when a major voice commitment is imminent, vigorous antibiotic treatment is warranted. In this circumstance, the damage caused by allowing progression of a curable condition is greater than the damage that might result from a course of therapy for an unproven microorganism while culture results are pending. When a major concert or speech is not imminent, indications for therapy are the same as for the nonsinger or nonprofessional speaker.

Voice rest (absolute or relative) is an important therapeutic consideration in any case of laryngitis. When no professional commitments are pending, a short course of absolute voice rest may be considered, as it is the safest and most conservative therapeutic intervention. This means absolute silence and communication with a writing pad. The patient must be instructed not to whisper, as this may be an even more traumatic vocal activity than speaking softly. Whistling through the lips also involves vocal fold activity and should not be permitted. So does the playing of many musical wind instruments. Absolute voice rest is *necessary* only for serious vocal fold injury such as hemorrhage or mucosal disruption. Even then, it is virtually never indicated for more than seven to ten days. Three days are often sufficient. Some excellent laryngologists do not believe voice rest should be used at all. However, absolute voice rest for a few days may be helpful in patients with laryngitis, especially those gregarious, verbal singers who find it difficult to moderate their voice use to comply with relative voice rest instructions. In many instances, considerations of finances and reputation mitigate against a recommendation of voice rest. In advising performers to minimize vocal use, Punt counseled, "Don't say a single word for which you are not being paid."[4] This admonition frequently guides the ailing singer or speaker away from preperformance conversations and backstage greetings and allows a successful series of performances. Patients should also be instructed to speak softly and as infrequently as possible, often at a slightly higher pitch than usual; to avoid excessive telephone use; and to speak with abdominal support as they would in singing. This is relative voice rest, and it is helpful in most cases.

An urgent session with a speech-language pathologist is extremely helpful for discussing vocal hygiene and in providing guidelines to prevent voice abuse. Nevertheless, the patient must be aware that some risk is associated with performing with laryngitis even when performance is possible. Inflammation of the vocal folds is associated with increased capillary fragility and increased risk of vocal fold injury or hemorrhage. Many factors must be considered in determining whether a given speech or concert is important enough to justify the potential consequences.

Steam inhalations deliver moisture and heat to the vocal folds and tracheobronchial tree and may be useful. Some people use nasal irrigations although these have little proven value. Gargling has no proven efficacy, but it is probably harmful only if it involves loud, abusive vocalization as part of the gargling process. Some physicians and patients believe it to be helpful "moistening the throat," and it may have some relaxing or placebo effect. Ultrasonic treatments, local massage, psychotherapy, and biofeedback directed at relieving anxiety and decreasing muscle tension may be helpful adjuncts to a broader therapeutic program. However, psychotherapy and biofeedback, in particular, must be expertly supervised if used at all.

Voice lessons given by an expert teacher are invaluable. When technical dysfunction is suggested, the singer or actor should be referred to his/her teacher. Even when an obvious organic abnormality is present, referral to a voice teacher is appropriate, especially for younger actors and singers. Numerous "tricks of the trade" permit a voice professional to overcome some of the impairments of mild illness safely. If a singer plans to proceed with a performance during an illness, he or she should not cancel voice lessons as part of the relative voice rest regimen; rather, a short lesson to ensure optimal technique is extremely useful.

Sinusitis

Chronic inflammation of the mucosa lining the sinus cavities commonly produces thick secretions known as postnasal drip. Postnasal drip can be particularly problematic because it causes excessive phlegm, which interferes with phonation, and because it leads to frequent throat clearing, which may inflame the vocal folds. Sometimes chronic sinusitis is caused by allergies and can be treated with medications. However, many medications used for this condition cause side effects that are unacceptable in professional voice users, particularly mucosal drying. When medication management is not satisfactory, functional endoscopic sinus surgery may be appropriate.[5] Acute purulent sinusitis is a different matter. It requires aggressive treatment with antibiotics, sometimes surgical drainage, treatment of underlying conditions (such as dental abscess), and occasionally surgery.[5]

Lower Respiratory Tract Infection

Lower respiratory tract infection may be almost as disruptive to a voice as upper respiratory tract infection. Bronchitis, pneumonitis, pneumonia, and especially reactive airway disease impair the power source of the voice and lead to vocal strain, and sometimes injury. Lower respiratory tract infections should be treated aggressively, pulmonary function tests should be considered, and bronchodilators (preferably oral) should be used as necessary. Coughing is also a very traumatic vocal activity, and careful attention should be paid to cough suppression. If extensive voice use is anticipated, nonnarcotic antitussive agents are preferable because narcotics may dull the sensorium and lead to potentially damaging voice technique.

Tonsillitis

Tonsillitis also impairs the voice through alterations of the resonator system and through technical changes secondary to pain. Although there is a tendency to avoid tonsillectomy, especially in professional voice users, the operation should not be withheld when clear indications for tonsillectomy are present. These include, for example, documented severe bacterial tonsillitis six times per year. However, patients must be warned that tonsillectomy may alter the sound of the voice, even through there is no change at the vocal fold (oscillator) level.

Other Infections

Autoimmune deficiency syndrome (AIDS) is becoming more and more common. This lethal disease may present as hoarseness and xerostomia. Unexplained oral candidiasis, *Candida* infections of the tracheobronchial tree, and respiratory infections with other unusual pathogens should raise a physician's suspicions. However, it should also be remembered that infections with *Haemophilus influenzae, Streptococcus pneumoniae*, and common viruses are the most frequent pathogens in AIDS patients, just as they are in patients without AIDS. This disease should be considered in patients with frequent infections.

The laryngologist must also be alert for numerous other acute and chronic conditions that may cause laryngeal abnormalities, or even vocal fold masses that may be mistaken for malignancy and biopsied unnecessarily. Tuberculosis is being seen more often in modern practice. Although laryngeal lesions used to be associated with extensive pulmonary infection, they are now usually associated with much less virulent disease, often only a mild cough. Laryngeal lesions are usually localized.[6,7]

Sarcoidosis, a granulomatous disease, demonstrates laryngeal symptoms in 3% to 5% of cases.[8] Noncaseating granulomas are found in the larynx, and the false vocal folds are involved frequently, producing airway obstruction rather than dysphonia. Less common diseases, including leprosy,[9,10] syphilis,[11] scleroderma,[12] typhoid,[13] typhus,[13] and other conditions, may produce laryngeal lesions that may mimic neoplasms and lead the laryngologist to obtain unnecessary biopsy of lesions that can be cured medically.

Confusing lesions may also be caused by a variety of mycotic infections, including histoplasmosis,[14-16] coccidiomycosis,[17] cryptococcosis,[18] blastomycosis,[19,20] actinomycosis,[21,22] candidiasis,[23] aspergillosis,[24-26] mucormycosis,[27] rhinosporidiosis,[28] and sporotrichosis.[29] Parasitic diseases may also produce laryngeal masses. The most prominent example is leishmaniasis.[30] More detailed information about most of the conditions discussed above is available in an excellent text by Michaels.[31] Some viral conditions may also cause laryngeal structural abnormalies, most notably papillomas. However, herpes virus, variola, and other organisms have also been implicated in laryngeal infection.

SYSTEMIC CONDITIONS

Aging

This subject is so important that it has been covered extensively in other literature.[32] Many characteristics associated with vocal aging are actually deficits in conditioning, rather than irreversible aging changes. For example, in singers, such problems as a "wobble," pitch inaccuracies (singing flat), and inability to sing softly are rarely caused by irreversible aging changes, and these problems can usually be managed easily through voice therapy and training.

Hearing Loss

Hearing loss is often overlooked as a source of vocal problems. Auditory feedback is fundamental to speaking and singing. Interference with this control mechanism may result in altered vocal production, particularly if the person is unaware of the hearing loss. Distortion, particularly pitch distortion (diplacusis) may also pose serious problems for the singer. This appears to cause not only aesthetic difficulties in matching pitch, but also vocal strain, which accompanies pitch shifts.[33] In-depth discussion is not presented here as this subject is discussed in other literature.[2]

Respiratory Dysfunction

The importance of "the breath" has been well recognized in the field of voice pedagogy. Respiratory disorders are discussed at length in other literature.[34] Even a mild degree of obstructive pulmonary disease can result in substantial voice problems. Unrecognized exercise-induced asthma is especially problematic in singers and actors, because bronchospasm may be precipitated by the exercise and airway drying that occurs during voice performance. In such cases, the bronchospastic obstruction on exhalation impairs support. This commonly results in compensatory hyperfunction.

Treatment requires skilled management and collaboration with a pulmonologist and a voice team.[35] Whenever possible, patients should be managed primarily with oral medications; the use of inhalers should be minimized. Steroid inhalers should be avoided altogether whenever possible. It is particularly important to recognize that asthma can be induced by the exercise of phonation itself,[36] and in many cases a high index of suspicion and methacholine challenge test are needed to avoid missing this important diagnosis.

Allergy

Even mild allergies are more incapacitating to professional voice users than to others. This subject can be reviewed elsewhere.[37] Briefly, patients with mild intermittent allergies can usually be managed with antihistamines although they should never be tried for the first time immediately prior to a voice performance. Because antihistamines commonly produce unacceptable side effects, trial and error may be needed in order to find a medication with an acceptable balance between effect and side effect for any individual patient, especially a voice professional. Patients with allergy-related voice disturbances may find hyposensitization a more effective approach than antihistamine use, if they are candidates for such treatment. For voice patients with unexpected allergic symptoms immediately prior to an important voice commitment, corticosteroids should be used rather than antihistamines, in order to minimize the risks of side effects (such as drying and thickening of secretions) that might make voice performance difficult or impossible. Allergies commonly cause voice problems by altering the mucosa and secretions and causing nasal obstruction. Management will not be covered in depth in this brief chapter. However, it should be recognized that many of the medicines commonly used to treat allergies have side effects deleterious to voice function, particularly dryness and thickening of secretions. Consequently, when voice disturbance is causally related to these conditions, more definitive treatment through allergic immunotherapy should be considered. This is especially important to professional voice users.

Gastroesophageal Reflux Laryngitis

Gastroesophageal reflux laryngitis is extremely common among voice patients, especially singers.[38] This is a condition in which the sphincter between the stomach and esophagus is inefficient, and acidic stomach secretions reflux (reach the laryngeal tissues), causing inflammation. The most typical symptoms are hoarseness in the morning, prolonged vocal warm-up time, halitosis and a bitter taste in the morning, a feeling of a "lump in the throat," frequent throat clearing, chronic irritative cough, and frequent tracheitis or tracheobronchitis. Any or all of these symptoms may be present. Heartburn is not common in these patients, so the diagnosis is often missed. Prolonged reflux also is associated with the development of Barrett's esophagus, esophageal carcinoma, and laryngeal carcinoma.[32,38]

Physical examination usually reveals erythema (redness) of the arytenoid mucosa. A barium swallow radiographic study with water siphonage may provide additional information but is not needed routinely. However, if a patient complies strictly with treatment recommendations and does not show marked improvement within a month, or if there is a reason to suspect more serious pathology, complete evaluation by a gastroenterologist should be carried out. This is often advisable in patients who are over 40 years of age or who have had reflux symptoms for more than five years. Twenty-four hour pH monitoring of the esophagus is often effective in establishing a diagnosis. The results are correlated with a diary of the patient's activities and symptoms. Bulimia should also be considered in the differential diagnosis when symptoms are refractory to treatment and other physical and psychologic signs are suggestive.

The mainstays of treatment for reflux laryngitis are elevation of the head of the bed (not just sleeping on pillows), antacids, H_2 blockers or proton pump inhibitors, and avoidance of eating for three to four hours before going to sleep. This is often difficult for singers and actors because of their performance schedule, but if they are counseled about minor changes in eating habits (such as eating larger meals at breakfast and lunch), they usually can comply. Avoidance of alcohol, caffeine, and specific foods is beneficial. Medications that decrease or block acid production may be necessary. It must be recognized that control of acidity is not the same as control of reflux. In many cases, reflux is provoked during singing because of the increased abdominal pressure associated with support. In these instances, it often causes excessive phlegm and throat clearing during the first ten or fifteen minutes of a performance or lesson, as well as other common reflux laryngitis symptoms even when acidity has been neutralized effectively. Laparoscopic Nissen fundoplication has proven extremely effective and should be considered a reasonable alternative to lifelong medication in this relatively young patient population.[38]

Endocrine Dysfunction

Endocrine (hormonal) problems warrant special attention. The human voice is extremely sensitive to endocrinologic changes. Many of these are reflected in alterations of fluid content of the lamina propria just beneath the laryngeal mucosa. This causes alterations in the bulk and shape of the vocal folds and results in voice change. Hypothyroidism is a well-recognized cause of such voice disorders, although the mechanism is not fully understood.[39-42] Hoarseness, vocal fatigue, muffling of the voice, loss of range, and a sensation of a lump in the throat may be present even with mild hypothyroidism. Even when thyroid function tests results are within the low-normal range, this diagnosis should be entertained, especially if thyroid-stimulating hormone levels are in the high-normal range or are elevated. Thyrotoxicosis may result in similar voice disturbances.[43]

Voice changes associated with sex hormones are encountered commonly in clinical practice and have been investigated more thoroughly than have other hormonal changes. Although a correlation appears to exist between sex hormone levels and depth of male voices (higher testosterone and lower estradiol levels in basses than in tenors),[44] the most important hormonal considerations in males occur during the maturation process.

When castrato singers were in vogue, castration at about age 7 or 8 resulted in failure of laryngeal growth during puberty, and voices that stayed in the soprano or alto range and boasted a unique quality of sound.[45] Failure of a male voice to change at puberty is uncommon today and is often psychogenic in etiology.[1] However, hormonal deficiencies such as those seen in cryptorchidism, delayed sexual development, Klinefelter's syndrome, or Fröhlich's syndrome may be responsible. In these cases, the persistently high voice may be the complaint that causes the patient to seek medical attention.

Voice problems related to sex hormones are most common in female singers.[46] Although vocal changes associated with the normal menstrual cycle may be difficult to quantify with current experimental techniques, unquestionably they occur.[2,46-50] Most of the ill effects are seen in the immediate premenstrual period and are known as laryngopathia premenstrualis. This common condition is caused by physiologic, anatomic, and psychologic alterations secondary to endocrine changes. The vocal dysfunction is characterized by decreased vocal efficiency, loss of the highest notes in the voice, vocal fatigue, slight hoarseness, and some muffling of the voice. It is often more apparent to the singer than to the listener. Submucosal hemorrhages in the larynx are more common in the premenstrual period.[48] In many European opera houses, singers used to be excused from singing during the premenstrual and early menstrual days ("grace days"). This practice is not followed in the United States and is no longer in vogue in most European countries. Premenstrual changes cause significant vocal symptoms in approximately one-third of singers. Although ovulation inhibitors have been shown to mitigate some of these symptoms,[49] in some women (about 5%),[51] birth control pills may deleteriously alter voice range and character even after only a few months of therapy.[52-55] When oral contraceptives are used, the voice should be monitored closely. Under crucial performance circumstances, oral contraceptives may be used to alter the time of menstruation, but this practice is justified only in unusual situations. Symptoms very similar to laryngopathia premenstrualis occur in some women at the time of ovulation.

Pregnancy results frequently in voice alterations known as laryngopathia gravidarum. The changes may be similar to premenstrual symptoms or may be perceived as desirable changes. In some cases, alterations produced by pregnancy are permanent.[56,57] Although hormonally induced changes in the larynx and respiratory mucosa secondary to menstruation and pregnancy are discussed widely in the literature, the author has found no reference to the important alterations in abdominal support. Uterine muscle cramping associated with menstruation causes pain and compromises abdominal support. Abdominal distension during pregnancy also interferes with abdominal muscle function. Any singer whose abdominal support is compromised substantially should be discouraged from singing until the abdominal impairment is resolved.

Estrogens are helpful in postmenopausal singers but generally should not be given alone. Sequential replacement therapy is the most physiologic regimen and should be used under the supervision of a gynecologist. Under no circumstances should androgens be given to female singers even in small amounts if any reasonable therapeutic alternative exists. Clinically, these drugs are most commonly used to treat endometriosis, or post-menopausal loss of libido. Androgens cause unsteadiness of the voice, rapid changes of timbre, and lowering of the fundamental frequency (masculinization).[58-62] These changes are usually permanent.

Recently, we have seen increasing abuse of anabolic steroids among body builders and other athletes. In addition to their many other hazards, these medications may alter the voice. They are (or are closely related to) male hormones; consequently, they are capable of producing masculinization of the voice. Lowering of the fundamental frequency and coarsening of the voice produced in this fashion are generally irreversible.

Other hormonal disturbances may also produce vocal dysfunction. In addition to the thyroid gland and the gonads, the parathyroid, adrenal, pineal, and pituitary glands are included in this system. Other endocrine disturbances may alter voice as well. For example, pancreatic dysfunction may cause xerophonia (dry voice), as in diabetes mellitus. Thymic abnormalities can lead to feminization of the voice.[63]

Neurologic Disorders

There are numerous neurologic conditions that may adversely affect the voice. They are discussed in other literature[64,65] and elsewhere in this book. Some of them, such as myasthenia gravis, are amenable to medical therapy with drugs such as pyridostigmine (Mestinon). Such therapy frequently restores the voice to normal. An exhaustive neurolaryngologic discussion is beyond the scope of this chapter. Nevertheless, when evaluating voice dysfunction, laryngologists must consider numerous neurologic problems, including Parkinson's disease, various other disorders that produce tremor, drug-induced tremor, multiple sclerosis, dystonias, and many other conditions. Spasmodic dysphonia (SD), a laryngeal dystonia, presents particularly challenging problems. This subject is covered in detail in another chapter. Stuttering also provides unique challenges. Although still poorly understood, this condition is noted for its tendency to affect speech while sparing singing.

Vocal fold hypomobility may be caused by paralysis (no movement), paresis (partial movement), arytenoid dislocation, cricoarytenoid joint dysfunction, and laryngeal fracture. Differentiating among these conditions is often more complicated than it appears at first glance. A comprehensive discussion is beyond the scope of this chapter, and the reader is referred to other literature.[65] However, in addition to a comprehensive history and physical examination, evaluation commonly includes strobovideolaryngoscopy, objective voice assessment, laryngeal electromyography, and high-resolution computed tomography (CT) of the larynx. Most vocal fold motion disorders are amenable to treatment. Voice therapy should be used first in virtually all cases. Even in many patients with recurrent laryngeal nerve paralysis, voice therapy alone is often sufficient. When therapy fails to produce adequate voice improvement in the patient's opinion, surgical intervention is appropriate.

General Health

As with any other athletic activity, optimal voice use requires reasonably good general health and physical conditioning. Abdominal and respiratory strength and endurance are particularly important. If a person becomes short of breath from climbing two flights of stairs, he or she certainly does not have the physical stamina necessary for proper respiratory support for a speech, let alone a strenuous musical production. This deficiency usually results in abusive vocal habits used in vain attempts to compensate for the deficiencies.

Systemic illnesses, such as anemia, Lyme disease, mononucleosis, AIDS, chronic fatigue syndrome, or other diseases associated with malaise and weakness may impair the ability of vocal musculature to recover rapidly from heavy use and may also be associated with alterations of mucosal secretions. Other systemic illnesses may be responsible for voice complaints, particularly if they impair the abdominal muscles necessary for breath support. For example, diarrhea and constipation that prohibit sustained abdominal contraction may be reasons for the physician to prohibit a strenuous singing or acting engagement.

Any extremity injury, such as a sprained ankle, may alter posture and therefore interfere with customary abdominothoracic support. Voice patients are often unaware of this problem and develop abusive, hyperfunctional compensatory maneuvers in the neck and tongue musculature as a result. These technical flaws may produce voice complaints, such as vocal fatigue and neck pain, that bring the performer to the physician's office for assessment and care.

Anxiety

Voice professionals, especially singers and actors, are frequently sensitive and communicative people. When the principal cause of vocal dysfunction is anxiety, the physician can often accomplish much by assuring the patient that no organic problem is present and by stating the diagnosis of anxiety reaction. The patient should be counseled that anxiety is normal and that recognition of it as the principal problem frequently allows the performer to overcome it. Tranquilizers and sedatives are rarely necessary and are undesirable because they may interfere with fine motor control. For example, beta-adrenergic blocking agents such as propranolol hydrochloride have became popular among performers for the treatment of preperformance anxiety. Beta-blockers are not recommended for regular use; they have significant effects on the cardiovascular system and many potential complications, including hypotension, thrombocytopenic purpura, mental depression, agranulocytosis, laryngospasm with respiratory distress, and bronchospasm. In addition, their efficacy is controversial. Although they may have a favorable effect in relieving performance anxiety, beta-blockers may produce a noticeable adverse effect on singing performance.[66] Although these drugs have a place under occasional, extraordinary circumstances, their routine use for this purpose not only is potentially hazardous but also violates an important therapeutic principle. Performers have chosen a career that exposes them to the public. If such persons are so incapacitated by anxiety that they are unable to perform the routine functions of their chosen profession without chemical help, this should be considered symptomatic of an important underlying psychologic problem. (See chapter 29 by Rosen et al for further details.) For a performer to depend on drugs to perform is neither routine nor healthy, whether the drug is a benzodiazepine, a barbiturate, a beta-blocker, or alcohol. If such dependence exists, psychologic evaluation should be considered by an experienced arts-medicine psychologist or psychiatrist. Obscuring the symptoms by fostering the dependence is insufficient. However, if the patient is on tour and will only be under a particular otolaryngologist's care for a week or two, the physician should not try to make major changes in his or her customary regimen. Rather, the physician should communicate with the performer's primary otolaryngologist or family physician to coordinate appropriate long-term care.

As professional voice users constitute a subset of society as a whole, all the psychiatric disorders encountered among the general public are seen from time to time in voice professionals. In some cases, professional voice users require modification of the usual psychologic treatment, particularly with regard to psychotropic medications. Detailed discussion of this subject can be found elsewhere in the literature.[67]

When voice professionals, especially singers and actors, suffer a significant vocal impairment that results in voice loss (or the prospect of voice loss), they often go through a psychologic process very similar to grieving.[67] In some cases, fear of discovering that the voice is lost forever may unconsciously prevent patients from trying to use their voices optimally following injury or treatment. This can dramatically impede or prevent recovery of function following a perfect surgical result, for example. It is essential that otolaryngologists, performers, and their teachers be familiar with this fairly common scenario, and it is ideal to include an arts-medicine psychologist and/or psychiatrist as part of the voice team.

Other Psychologic Problems

Psychogenic voice disorders, incapacitating psychologic reactions to organic voice disorders, and other psychologic problems are encountered commonly in young voice patients. They are discussed in other literature.[67]

Substance Abuse

The list of substances ingested, smoked, or "snorted" by many people is disturbingly long. Whenever possible, patients who care about vocal quality and longevity should be educated about the deleterious effects of such habits upon their voices and upon the longevity of their careers by their physicians and teachers. A few specific substances have already been discussed earlier.

STRUCTURAL ABNORMALITIES

Nodules

Nodules are callous-like masses of the vocal folds that are caused by vocally abusive behaviors and are a dreaded malady of singers or actors. Occasionally, laryngoscopy reveals asymptomatic vocal nodules that do not appear to interfere with voice production; in such cases, the nodules should not be treated. Some famous and successful singers have had untreated vocal nodules throughout their careers. However, in most cases nodules result in hoarseness, breathiness, loss of range, and vocal fatigue. They may be caused by abusive speaking rather than improper singing technique. Voice therapy always should be tried as the initial therapeutic modality and will cure the vast majority of patients even if the nodules look firm and have been present for many months or years. Even apparently large, fibrotic nodules often shrink, disappear, or become asymptomatic with six to twelve weeks of voice therapy with good patient compliance. Even in those who eventually need surgical excision of the nodules, preoperative voice therapy is essential to prevent recurrence. Care must be taken in diagnosing nodules. It is almost impossible to make the diagnosis accurately and consistently without strobovideolaryngoscopy and good optical magnification. Vocal fold cysts are commonly misdiagnosed as nodules, and treatment strategies are different for the two lesions. Vocal nodules are confined to the superficial layer of the lamina propria and are composed primarily of edematous tissue or collagenous fibers. Basement membrane reduplication is common. They are usually bilateral and fairly symmetric.

Caution must be exercised in diagnosing small nodules in patients who have been singing or speaking actively. In many singers, for example, bilateral, symmetric soft swellings at the junction of the anterior and middle thirds of the vocal folds develop after heavy voice use. No evidence suggests that patients with such "physiologic swelling" are predisposed to the development of vocal nodules. At present, the condition is generally considered to be within normal limits. The physiologic swelling usually disappears with 24 to 48 hours of rest from heavy voice use. The physician must be careful not to frighten the patient by misdiagnosing physiologic swellings as vocal nodules. Nodules carry a great stigma among voice professionals, and the psychologic impact of the diagnosis should not be underestimated. When nodules are present, these patients should be informed with the same gentle caution used in telling a patient that he or she has a life-threatening illness.

Submucosal Cysts

Submucosal cysts of the vocal folds are probably also traumatic lesions that are the result of a blocked mucous gland duct in many cases. However, they may also be congenital or occur from other causes. They often cause contact swelling on the contralateral side and can be initially misdiagnosed as nodules. They can usually be differentiated from nodules by strobovideolaryngoscopy when the mass is observed to be obviously fluid-filled. They may also be suspected when the nodule (contact swelling) on one vocal fold resolves with voice therapy while the mass on the other vocal fold does not resolve. Cysts may also be discovered on one side (occasionally both sides) when surgery is performed for apparent nodules that have not resolved with voice therapy. The surgery should be performed superficially and with minimal trauma, as discussed in a separate chapter, and elsewhere.[32] Cysts are ordinarily lined with thin squamous epithelium. Retention cysts contain mucus. Epidermoid cysts contain caseous material. Generally, cysts are located in the superficial layer of the lamina propria. In some cases, they may be attached to the vocal ligament.

Polyps

Vocal *polyps*, another type of vocal fold mass, usually occur on only one vocal fold. They often have a promi-

nent feeding blood vessel coursing along the superior surface of the vocal fold and entering the base of the polyp. The pathogenesis of polyps cannot be proven in many cases, but the lesion is thought to be traumatic and sometimes starts as a hemorrhage. Polyps may be sessile or pedunculated. They are typically located in the superficial layer of the lamina propria and do not involve the vocal ligament. In those arising from an area of hemorrhage, the vocal ligament may be involved with post-hemorrhagic fibrosis that is contiguous with the polyp. Histologic evaluation most commonly reveals collagenous fibers, hyaline degeneration, edema, thrombosis, and often bleeding within the polypoid tissue. Cellular infiltration may also be present. In some cases, even sizable polyps resolve with relative voice rest and a few weeks of low-dose steroid therapy (eg, Methylprednisone 4 mg twice a day). However, most require surgical removal. If polyps are not treated, they may produce contact injury on the contralateral vocal fold. Voice therapy should be used to ensure good relative voice rest and prevention of abusive vocal behavior before and after surgery. When surgery is performed, care must be taken not to damage the leading edge of the vocal fold, especially if a laser is used, as discussed later. In all laryngeal surgery, delicate microscopic dissection is now the standard of care. Vocal fold "stripping" is an out-of-date surgical approach formerly used for benign lesions that often resulted in scar and/or poor unserviceable voice function. It is no longer an acceptable surgical technique in most situations.

Granulomas

Granulomas usually occur in the cartilaginous portion of the vocal fold near the vocal process, or on the medial surface of the arytenoid. They are composed of collagenous fibers, fibroblasts, proliferated capillaries, and leukocytes. They are usually covered with epithelium. Granulomas are associated with gastroesophageal reflux laryngitis and trauma (including trauma from voice abuse and from intubation). Therapy should include reflux control, voice therapy, and surgery if the granuloma continues to enlarge or does not resolve after adequate time and treatment.

Reinke's Edema

Reinke's edema is characterized by an "elephant ear," floppy vocal fold appearance. It is often observed during examination in many nonprofessional and professional voice users and is accompanied by a low, coarse, gruff voice. Reinke's edema is a condition in which the superficial layer of lamina propria (Reinke's space) becomes edematous. The lesion does not usually include hypertrophy, inflammation, or degeneration, although other terms for the condition include polypoid degeneration, chronic polypoid corditis, and chronic edematous hypertrophy. Reinke's edema is often associated with smoking, voice abuse, reflux, and hypothyroidism. Underlying conditions should be treated. However, the condition may require surgery if voice improvement is desired. The surgery should only be performed if there is a justified high suspicion of serious pathology such as cancer, if there is airway obstruction, or if the patient is unhappy with his or her vocal quality. For some voice professionals, abnormal Reinke's edema is an important component of the vocal signature. Although the condition is usually bilateral, surgery should generally be performed on one side at a time.

Sulcus Vocalis

Sulcus vocalis is a groove along the edge of the membranous vocal fold. The majority are congenital, bilateral, and symmetric, although post-traumatic acquired lesions occur. When symptomatic (they often are not), sulcus vocalis can be treated surgically if sufficient voice improvement is not obtained through voice therapy.

Scar

Vocal fold scar is a sequela of trauma and results in fibrosis and obliteration of the layered structure of the vocal fold. It may markedly impede vibration, and consequently cause profound dysphonia. Recent surgical advances have made this condition much more treatable than it used to be, but it is still rarely possible to restore voices to normal in the presence of scar.[32, 68]

Hemorrhage

Vocal fold hemorrhage is a potential disaster in singers. Hemorrhages resolve spontaneously in most cases, with restoration of normal voice. However, in some instances, the hematoma organizes and fibroses, resulting in scar. This alters the vibratory pattern of the vocal fold and can result in permanent hoarseness. In specially selected cases, it may be best to avoid this problem through surgical incision and drainage of the hematoma.[69] In all cases, vocal fold hemorrhage should be managed with absolute voice rest until the hemorrhage has resolved (usually about one week) and relative voice rest until normal vascular and mucosal integrity have been restored. This often takes six weeks, and sometimes longer. Recurrent vocal fold hemorrhages are usually caused by weakness in a specific blood vessel, which may require surgical cauterization of the blood vessel using a laser, or microscopic resection of the vessel.[32,70,71]

Papilloma

Laryngeal papillomas are epithelial lesions caused by human papilloma virus. Histology reveals neoplastic epithelial cell proliferation in a papillary pattern, and viral particles. At the present time, symptomatic papillomas are treated surgically, although alternatives have been recommended to the usual laser vaporization approach.[32,71,72] Recently, cidofovir injected into the lesion has shown considerable promise.[73]

Cancer

A detailed discussion of *cancer of the larynx* is beyond the scope of this chapter. The prognosis for small vocal fold cancers is good, whether they are treated by radiation or surgery. Although it may seem intuitively obvious that radiation therapy provides a better chance of voice conservation than even limited vocal fold surgery, later radiation changes in the vocal fold may produce substantial hoarseness, xerophonia (dry voice), and voice dysfunction. Consequently, from the standpoint of voice preservation, optimal treatments remain uncertain.[74] Prospective studies using objective voice measures and strobovideolaryngoscopy should answer the relevant questions in the near future. Strobovideolaryngoscopy is also valuable for follow-up of patients who have had laryngeal cancers. It permits detection of vibratory changes associated with infiltration by the cancer long before they can be seen with continuous light. Stroboscopy has been used in Europe and Japan for this purpose for many years. In the United States, the popularity of strobovideolaryngoscopy for follow-up of cancer patients has increased greatly in recent years.[2]

The psychologic consequences of vocal fold cancer can be devastating, especially in a professional voice user.[67] They may be overwhelming for nonvoice professionals as well. These reactions are understandable and expected. In many patients, however, psychologic reactions may be as severe following medically "less significant" vocal fold problems such as hemorrhages, nodules, and other conditions that do not command the public respect and sympathy afforded to a cancer. In many ways, the management of related psychologic problems can be even more difficult in patients with these "lesser" vocal disturbances.

Unusual Vocal Fold Masses

When vocal fold masses are mentioned, laryngologists usually think of nodules, cysts, polyps, and cancer. While these are certainly the most common problems in clinical practice, many other conditions must be kept in mind. Collagen vascular diseases and other unusual problems may also produce laryngeal masses. Rheumatoid arthritis may produce not only disease of the cricoarytenoid and cricothyroid joints, but also consequent neuropathic muscle atrophy,[75] and rheumatoid nodules of the larynx.[76] Rheumatoid arthritis with or without nodules may produce respiratory obstruction. Gout may also cause laryngeal arthritis. In addition, gouty tophi may appear as white submucosal masses of the true vocal fold. They consist of sodium urate crystals in fibrous tissue and have been well documented.[77,78]

Amyloidosis of the larynx is rare but well recognized.[79,80] Amyloidosis is most common in the false vocal folds. Urbach-Wiethe disease (lipoid proteinosis)[81] often involves the mucous membrane of the larynx, usually the vocal folds, aryepiglottic fold, and epiglottis. Other conditions such as Wegener's granulomatosis and relapsing polychondritis may also involve the larynx. They are less likely to produce discrete nodules, but the diffuse edema associated with chondritis, and necrotizing granulomas, may produce significant laryngeal and voice abnormalities leading to surgical intervention. Granular cell tumors may involve the larynx and can be misdiagnosed easily as laryngeal granulomas.[82] Unusual laryngeal masses may also be caused by trauma.

A few rare skin lesions may also involve the larynx, producing significant lesions and sometimes airway obstruction. These include pemphigus vulgaris, seen in adults between 40 and 60 years of age. Pemphigus lesions may involve the mucosa, including the epiglottis.[83] Epidermolysis bullosa describes a group of congenital vesicular disorders usually seen at birth or shortly thereafter. This condition may cause laryngeal stenosis.[75]

Other Conditions

Numerous other conditions could be included in this chapter. For a more comprehensive discussion of the subjects covered above the reader is referred to other literature.[2]

MEDICAL MANAGEMENT FOR VOICE DYSFUNCTION

Medical management of many problems affecting the voice involves not only care prescribed by the otolaryngologist, but also voice therapy, which is provided by an interdisciplinary team. The roles and training of the principal members of the team are covered in detail elsewhere in this book and in other literature.[84-86] This chapter provides a brief introduction to their roles in the medical milieu.

Speech-Language Pathologist

An excellent speech-language pathologist is an invaluable asset in caring for professional voice users and other voice patients. However, otolaryngologists and singing teachers should recognize that, like physicians, speech-language pathologists have varied backgrounds and experience in treatment of voice disorders. In fact, most speech-language pathology programs teach relatively little about caring for professional speakers and nothing about professional singers. Moreover, few speech-language pathologists have vast experience in this specialized area, and no fellowships in this specialty exist. Speech-language pathologists often subspecialize. A speech-language pathologist who expertly treats patients who have had strokes, stutter, have undergone laryngectomy, or have swallowing disorders will not necessarily know how to manage professional voice users optimally or even other less demanding voice patients. The otolaryngologist must learn the strengths and weaknesses of the speech-language pathologist with whom he or she works. After identifying a speech-language pathologist who is interested in treating professional voice users, the otolaryngologist should work closely with the speech-language pathologist in developing the necessary expertise. Assistance may be found through otolaryngologists who treat large numbers of singers or through educational programs such as the Voice Foundation's Symposium on Care of the Professional Voice. In general, therapy should be directed toward vocal hygiene, relaxation techniques, breath management, and abdominal support.[84]

Speech (voice) therapy may be helpful even when a singer has no obvious problem in the speaking voice but significant technical problems singing. Once a person has been singing for several years, a singing teacher may have difficulty convincing him or her to correct certain technical errors. Singers are much less protective of their speaking voices, however. A speech-language pathologist may be able to teach proper support, relaxation, and voice placement in speaking. Once mastered, these techniques can be carried over fairly easily into singing through cooperation between the speech-language pathologist and singing teacher. This "back door" approach has been extremely useful. For the actor, coordinating speech-language pathology sessions with acting voice lessons, and especially with training of the speaking voice provided by the actor's voice teacher or coach, is often helpful. In fact, we have found this combination so helpful that we have added an acting voice trainer to our medical staff. Information from the speech-language pathologist, acting voice trainer, and singing teacher should be symbiotic and should not conflict. If major discrepancies exist, bad training from one of the team members should be suspected and changes should be made.

Singing Voice Specialist

Singing voice specialists are singing teachers who have acquired extra training to prepare them for work with injured voices, in collaboration with a medical voice team.[85] They are indispensable for singers.

In selected cases, singing lessons may also be extremely helpful to nonsingers with voice problems. The techniques used to develop abdominal and thoracic muscle strength, breath control, laryngeal and neck muscle strength, and relaxation are very similar to those used in speech therapy. Singing lessons often expedite therapy and appear to improve the outcome in some patients.

Otolaryngologists who frequently care for singers are often asked to recommend a voice teacher. This may put them in an uncomfortable position, particularly if the singer is already studying with someone in the community. Most physicians do not have sufficient expertise to criticize a voice teacher, and we must be extremely cautious about recommending that a singer change teachers. However, no certifying agency standardizes or ensures the quality of a singing teacher. Although one may be slightly more confident of a teacher associated with a major conservatory or music school or one who is a member of the National Association of Teachers of Singing (NATS), neither of these credentials ensures excellence, and many expert teachers have neither affiliation. However, with experience, an otolaryngologist can ordinarily develop valid impressions. The physician should record the name of the voice teacher of every patient and observe whether the same kinds of voice abuse problems occur with disproportionate frequency in the pupils of any given teacher. Technical problems can cause organic abnormalities such as nodules; therefore, any teacher who has a high incidence of nodules among his or her students should be viewed with cautious concern. The physician should be particularly wary of teachers who are reluctant to allow their students to consult a doctor. The best voice teachers usually are quick to refer their students to an otolaryngologist if they hear anything disturbing in a student's voice. Similarly, voice teachers and voice professionals should compare information on the nature and quality of medical care received and its success. No physician cures every voice problem in every patient, just as no singing teacher produces premiere stars from every student who walks through the studio. Nevertheless, voice professionals must be critical, informed consumers and accept nothing less than the best medical care.

After seeing a voice patient, the otolaryngologist should speak with and/or write a letter to the voice teacher (with the patient's permission) describing the findings and recommendations as he or she would to a physician, speech-language pathologist, or any other referring professional. An otolaryngologist seriously interested in caring for singers should take the trouble to talk with and meet local singing teachers. Taking a lesson or two with each teacher provides enormous insight as well. Taking voice lessons regularly is even more helpful. In practice, the otolaryngologist will usually identify a few teachers in whom he or she has particular confidence, especially for patients with voice disorders, and should not hesitate to refer singers to these colleagues, especially singers who are not already in training.

Pop singers may be particularly resistant to the suggestion of voice lessons, yet they are in great need of training. The physician should point out that a good voice teacher can teach a pop singer how to protect and expand the voice without changing its quality or making it sound "trained" or "operatic." It is helpful to point out that singing, like other athletic activities, requires exercise, warm-up, and coaching for anyone planning to enter the "big league" and stay there. Just as no major league baseball pitcher would play without a pitching coach and warm-up time in the bullpen, no singer should try to build a career without a singing teacher and appropriate strength and agility exercises. This approach has proved palatable and effective. Physicians should also be aware of the difference between a voice teacher and a voice coach. A voice teacher trains a singer in singing technique and is essential. A voice coach is responsible for teaching songs, language, diction, style, operatic roles, and so on, but is not responsible for exercise and basic technical development of the voice.[85]

Acting-Voice Trainer

The use of acting-voice trainers (drama voice coaches) as members of the medical team is new.[86] This addition to the team has been extremely valuable to patients and other team members. Like singing voice specialists, professionals with education in theater arts utilize numerous vocal and body movement techniques that not only enhance physical function, but also release tension and break down emotional barriers that may impede optimal voice function. Tearful revelations to the acting-voice trainer are not uncommon, and, like the singing teacher, this individual may identify psychologic and emotional problems interfering with professional success that have been skillfully hidden from other professionals on the voice team and in the patient's life.

Others

A psychologist, psychiatrist, neurologist, pulmonologist, and others with special interest and expertise in arts-medicine are also invaluable to the voice team. Every comprehensive center should seek out such people and collaborate with them, even if they are not full-time members of the voice team.

SURGERY

A detailed discussion of laryngeal surgery is beyond the scope of this chapter and may be found elsewhere in this book and in other literature.[2] However, a few points are worthy of special emphasis. Surgery for vocal nodules should be avoided whenever possible and should almost never be performed without an adequate trial of expert voice therapy, including patient compliance with therapeutic suggestions. A minimum of six to twelve weeks of observation should be allowed while the patient is using therapeutically modified voice techniques under the supervision of a speech-language pathologist and ideally a singing voice specialist. Proper voice use rather than voice rest (silence) is correct therapy. The surgeon should not perform surgery prematurely for vocal nodules under pressure from the patient for a "quick cure" and early return to performance. Permanent destruction of voice quality is a very real complication.

Even after expert surgery, voice quality may be diminished by submucosal scarring, resulting in an adynamic segment along the vibratory margin of the vocal fold. This situation produces a hoarse voice with vocal folds that appear normal on indirect examination under routine light, although under stroboscopic light the adynamic segment is obvious. No reliable cure exists for this complication. Even large, apparently fibrotic nodules of long standing should be given a chance to resolve without surgery. In some cases the nodules remain but become asymptomatic and voice quality is normal. Stroboscopy in such patients usually reveals that the nodules are on the superior surface rather than the leading edge of the vocal folds during proper, relaxed phonation (although they may be on the contact surface and symptomatic when hyperfunctional voice technique is used and the larynx is forced down).

When surgery is indicated for vocal fold lesions, it should be limited as strictly as possible to the area of abnormality. Virtually no place exists for "vocal fold stripping" in patients with benign disease. Submucosal resection through a laryngeal microflap used to be advocated. In fact, the technique was introduced and first published by one of the authors (RTS). Microflap technique involved an incision on the superior surface of the vocal fold, submucosal resection, and preservation of the mucosa along the leading edge of the vocal fold. The concept that led to this innovation was based on the idea that the intermediate layer of the lamina propria should be protected to prevent fibroblast proliferation. Consequently, it seemed reasonable to preserve the mucosa as a biologic dressing. This technique certainly produced better results than vocal fold stripping. However, close scrutiny of outcomes revealed a small number of cases with poor results and stiffness beyond the limits of the original pathology. Consequently, the technique was abandoned in favor of a mini-microflap, or of local resection strictly limited to the region of pathology.[87] Lesions such as vocal nodules should be removed to a level even with the vibratory margin rather than deeply into the submucosa. This minimizes scarring and optimizes return to good vocal function. Naturally, if concern about a serious neoplasm exists, proper treatment takes precedence over voice preservation. Surgery should be performed under microscopic control. Preoperative and postoperative objective voice measures are essential to allow outcome assessment and self-critique. Only through such study can we improve surgical technique. Outcome studies are especially important in voice surgery as all our technical pronouncements are anecdotal because there is no experimental model for vocal fold surgery. The human adult is the only species with a layered lamina propria.

Lasers are an invaluable adjunct in the laryngologists' armamentarium, but they must be used knowledgeably and with care. Considerable evidence suggests that healing time is prolonged and the incidence of adynamic segment formation is higher with the laser on the vibratory margin than with traditional instruments. Two early studies raised serious concerns about dysphonia after laser surgery.[88,89] Such complications may result from using too low a wattage, causing dissipation of heat deeply into the vocal fold; thus, high power density for short duration has been recommended. Small spot size is also helpful. Nevertheless, many laryngologists caring for voice professionals avoid laser surgery in most cases pending further study. When biopsy specimens are needed, they should be taken before destroying the lesion with a laser. If a lesion is to be removed from the leading edge, the laser beam should be centered in the lesion, rather than on the vibratory margin, so that the beam does not create a divot in the vocal fold. The CO_2 laser may be particularly valuable for cauterizing isolated blood vessels responsible for recurrent hemorrhage. Such vessels are often found at the base of a hemorrhagic polyp. However, a nonlaser technique has proven even better for managing these vessels.[70] At the suggestion of Jean Abitbol, MD, the author has been placing a small piece of ice on the vocal fold immediately before laser use to help dissipate heat and help prevent edema (personal communication, 1983). No studies on the efficacy of this maneuver exist, but the technique appears helpful.

Voice rest after vocal fold surgery is controversial. Although some laryngologists do not recognize its necessity at all, many physicians recommend voice rest for approximately one week, or until the mucosal surface has healed. Even after surgery, silence for more than seven to ten days is nearly never necessary and represents a real hardship for many patients.

Too often, the laryngologist is confronted with a desperate patient whose voice has been "ruined" by vocal fold surgery, recurrent or superior laryngeal nerve paralysis, trauma, or some other tragedy. Occasionally, the cause is as straightforward as a dislocated arytenoid that can be reduced.[90,91] However, if the problem is an adynamic segment, decreased bulk of one vocal fold after "stripping," bowing caused by superior laryngeal nerve paralysis, or some other complication in a mobile vocal fold, great conservatism should be exercised. None of the available surgical procedures for these conditions is consistently effective. If surgery is considered at all, the procedure and prognosis should be explained to the patient realistically and pessimistically. The patient must understand that the chances of returning the voice to professional quality are very slim and that it may be made worse. Zyderm collagen (Xomed) injection has been studied and is helpful in some of these difficult cases.[92] Zyderm collagen, presently, is not approved by the FDA for use in the vocal fold. If used at all, the material should be used under protocol with Institutional Review Board approval. However, human collagen can be used and does not have the same shortcomings. Collagen may be particularly helpful for small adynamic segments. In one of the author's (RTS) opinion, the best technique for extensive vocal fold scarring is the recently introduced method of autologous fat implantation into the vibratory margin.[93]

Occasionally, voice professionals inquire about surgery for pitch alteration. Such procedures have been successful in specially selected patients (such as those undergoing sex-change surgery), but they do not consistently provide good enough voice quality and range to be performed on a professional voice user.

DISCRETION

The excitement and glamour associated with caring for voice patients, particularly a famous performer, naturally tempt the physician to talk about a distinguished patient. However, this tendency must be tempered. Having it known that he or she has consulted a laryn-

gologist, particularly for treatment of a significant vocal problem, is not always in a voice professional's best interest. Famous singers, actors, politicians, and other professional voice users are ethically and legally entitled to the same confidentiality we ensure for our other patients.

VOICE MAINTENANCE

Prevention of vocal dysfunction should be the goal of all professionals involved in the care of professional voice users. Good vocal health habits should be encouraged in childhood. Screaming, particularly outdoors at athletic events, should be discouraged. Promising young singers who join choirs should be educated to compensate for the Lombard effect. The youngster interested in singing, acting, debating, or other vocal activities should receive enough training to prevent voice abuse and should receive enthusiastic support for performing works and activities suitable for his or her age and voice. Training should be continued during or after puberty, and the voice should be allowed to develop naturally without pressure to perform operatic roles prematurely.

Excellent regular training and practice are essential, and avoidance of irritants, particularly smoke, should be stressed early. Educating voice professionals about hormonal and anatomic alterations that may influence the voice allows him or her to recognize and analyze vocal dysfunction, compensating for it intelligently when it occurs. The body is dynamic, changing over a lifetime, and the voice is no exception. Continued vocal education, training, and monitoring are necessary throughout a lifetime, even in the most successful and well-established voice professionals. Vocal problems even in premiere singers are commonly caused by cessation of lessons, excessive schedule demands, and other correctable problems, rather than by irreversible alterations of aging. Anatomic, physiologic, and serious medical problems may affect the voices of patients of any age. Cooperation among the laryngologist, speech-language pathologist, acting teacher, and singing teacher provides an optimal environment for cultivation and protection of the vocal artist.

REFERENCES

1. Brodnitz F. Hormones and the human voice. *Bull NY Acad Med.* 1971;47:183-191.

2. Sataloff RT. *Professional Voice: Science and Art of Clinical Care.* 2nd ed. San Diego, CA: Singular Publishing Group; 1997:1-1069.

3. von Leden H. *Presentation at the Seventh Symposium on Care of the Professional Voice.* The Juilliard School, New York; June 16, 1978.

4. Punt NA. Applied laryngology—singers and actors. *Proc R Soc Med.* 1968;61:1152-1156.

5. Spiegel JR, Sataloff RT, Hawkshaw M, Hoover CA. Sinusitis. In: Sataloff RT, ed. *Professional Voice: Science and Art of Clinical Care.* 2nd ed. San Diego, CA: Singular Publishing Group; 1997:437-440.

6. Bull TR. Tuberculosis of the larynx. *Br Med J.* 1996;2:991-992.

7. Hunter AM, Millar JW, Wightman AJ, et al. The changing pattern of laryngeal tuberculosis. *J Laryngol Otol.* 1981;95:393-398.

8. Divine KD. Sarcoidosis and sarcoidosis of the larynx. *Laryngoscope.* 1965;75:533-569.

9. Munor MacCormick CE. The larynx in leprosy. *Arch Otolaryngol.* 1957;66:138-149.

10. Binford CH, Meyers WM. Leprosy. In: Binford CH, Connor DH, eds. *Pathology of Tropical and Extraordinary Disease.* Vol 1. Washington, DC: Armed Forces Institute of Pathology; 1976:205-225.

11. MacKenzie M. *A Manual of Diseases of the Throat and Nose.* Vol 1. *Diseases of the Pharynx, Larynx and Trachea.* London, England: J. & A. Churchill; 1884.

12. Astacio JN, Goday GA, Espinosa FJ. Excleroma. Experiences en El Salvador. *Seconda Mongrafia de Dermatologia Iberolatino-Americana.* (Suplemento AO 1). Lisboa, Portugal; 1971.

13. Hajek M. *Pathologie und Therapie der Erkrankungen des Kehlkopfes, der Luftrohre und der Bronchien.* Leipzig: Curt Kabitzsch; 1932.

14. Withers BT, Pappas JJ, Erickson EE. Histoplasmosis primary in the larynx. Report of a case. *Arch Otolaryngol.* 1977;77:25-28.

15. Calcaterra TC. Otolaryngeal histoplasmosis. *Laryngoscope.* 1970;81:111-120.

16. Gould WJ, Sataloff RT, Spiegel JR. *Voice Surgery.* St. Louis, MO: Mosby Year Book; 1993:1-359.

17. Friedmann I. Diseases of the larynx. Disorders of laryngeal function. In: Paparella MM, Shumrick DA, eds. *Otolaryngology.* 2nd ed. Philadelphia, PA: Saunders Publishing; 1980:2449-2469.

18. Reese MC, Conclasure JB. Cryptococcosis of the larynx. *Arch Otolaryngol.* 1975;101:698-701.

19. Bennett M. Laryngeal blastomycosis. *Laryngoscope.* 1964;74:498-512.

20. Hoffarth GA, Joseph DL, Shumrick DA. Deep mycoses. *Arch Otolaryngol.* 1975;97:475-479.

21. Brandenburg JH, Finch WW, Kirkham WR. Actinomycosis of the larynx and pharynx. *Otolaryngology.* 1978;86:739-742.

22. Shaheen SO, Ellis FG. Actinomycosis of the larynx. *J R Soc Med.* 1983;76:226-228.

23. Tedeschi LG, Cheren RV. Laryngeal hyperkeratosis due to primary monilial infection. *Arch Otolaryngol.* 1968;82:82-84.

24. Rao PB. Aspergillosis of the larynx. *J Laryngol Otol.* 1968;83:377-379.

25. Ferlito A. Clinical records: primary aspergillosis of the larynx. *J Laryngol Otol.* 1974;88:1257-1263.

26. Keir SM, Flint A, Moss JA. Primary aspergillosis of the larynx simulating carcinoma. *Human Pathol.* 1983;14:184-186.

27. Anand CS, Gupta MC, Kothari MG, et al. Laryngeal mucormycosis. *Indian J Otolaryngol.* 1978;30:90-92.

28. Pillai OS. Rhinosporidiosis of the larynx. *J Laryngol Otol.* 1974;88:277-280.

29. Lyons GD. Mycotic disease of the larynx. *Ann Otol.* 1966;75:162-175.

30. Zinneman HH, Hall WH, Wallace FG. Leishmaniasis of the larynx. Report of a case and its confusion with histoplasmosis. *Am J Med.* 1961;31:654-658.

31. Michaels L. *Pathology of the Larynx.* Berlin: Springer-Verlag; 1984.

32. Sataloff RT, Spiegel JR, Rosen DC. The effects of age on the voice. In: Sataloff RT, ed. *Professional Voice: Science and Art of Clinical Care.* 2nd ed. San Diego, CA: Singular Publishing Group; 1997:259-267.

33. Sundberg J, Prame E, Iwarsson J. Replicability and accuracy of pitch patterns in professional singers. In: *Vocal Fold Physiology: Controlling Chaos and Complexity.* Sydney, Australia: Singular Publishing Group; 1996:291-306.

34. Spiegel JR, Sataloff RT, Cohn JR, Hawkshaw M. Respiratory dysfunction. In: Sataloff RT, ed. *Professional Voice: Science and Art of Clinical Care.* 2nd ed. San Diego, CA: Singular Publishing Group; 1997:375-386.

35. Spiegel JR, Sataloff RT, Cohn JR, et al. Respiratory function in singers. Medical assessment, diagnoses and treatments. *J Voice.* 1988;2(1):40-50.

36. Cohn JR, Sataloff RT, Spiegel JR, et al. Airway reactivity-induced asthma in singers (ARIAS). *J Voice.* 1991;5(4):332-337.

37. Cohn JR, Spiegel JR, Hawkshaw M, Sataloff RT. Allergy. In: Sataloff RT, ed. *Professional Voice: Science and Art of Clinical Care.* 2nd ed. San Diego, CA: Singular Publishing Group; 1997:369-374.

38. Sataloff RT, Castell DO, Katz PO, Sataloff DM. *Reflux Laryngitis and Related Disorders.* San Diego, CA: Singular Publishing Group; 1999:1-112.

39. Ritter FN. The effect of hypothyroidism on the larynx of the rat. *Ann Otol Rhinol Laryngol,* 1964. 67:404-416.

40. Ritter FN. Endocrinology. In: Paparella M, Shumrick D, eds. *Otolaryngology.* Vol 1. Philadelphia, PA: W.B. Saunders; 1973;727-734.

41. Michelsson K, Sirvio P. Cry analysis in congenital hypothyroidism. *Folia Phoniat.* 1976;28:40-47.

42. Gupta OP, Bhatia PL, Agarwal MK, Mehrotra ML, Mishr SK. Nasal pharyngeal and laryngeal manifestations of hypothyroidism. *Ear Nose Throat J.* 1977;56(9):10-21.

43. Malinsky M, Chevrrie-Muller C, Cerceau N. Etude clinique et electrophysiologique des alterations de la voix au cours des thyrotoxioses. *Ann Endocrinol.* (Paris). 1977;38:171-172.

44. Meuser W, Nieschlag E. Sexual hormone und Stimmlage des Mannes. *Deutsch Med Wochenschr.* 1977;102:261-264.

45. Brodnitz F. The age of the castrato voice. *J Speech Hearing Disord.* 1975;40:291-295.

46. Sataloff RT, Emerich KA, Hoover CA. Endocrine dysfunction. In: Sataloff RT, ed. *Professional Voice: Science and Art of Clinical Care.* 2nd ed. San Diego, CA: Singular Publishing Group; 1997:291-298.

47. Schiff M. The influence of estrogens on connective tissue. In: Asboe-Hansen G, ed. *Hormones and Connective Tissue.* Copenhagen, Denmark: Munksgaard Press; 1967:282-341.

48. Lacina V. Der Einfluss der Menstruation auf die Stimme der Sangerinnen. *Folia Phoniat.* 1968:20:13-24.

49. Wendler J. Cyclicly dependent variations in efficiency of the voice and its influencing by ovulation inhibitors. Zyklusabhangige Leistungsschwankungen der Stimme und ihre Beeinflussung durch Ovulationshemmer. *Folia Phoniatr* (Basel). 1972; 24(4):259-277.

50. von Gelder L. Psychosomatic aspects of endocrine disorders of the voice. *J Comm Disord.* 1974;7:257-262.

51. Christine Carroll, MD Arizona State University at Tempe: Personal communication with Dr. Hans von Leden. September, 1992.

52. Dordain M. Etude Statistique de l'influence des contraceptifs hormonaux sur la voix. *Folia Phoniat.* 1972;24:86-96.

53. Pahn V, Goretzlehner G. Stimmstorungen durch hormonale Kontrazeptiva. *Zentralb Gynakol.* 1978;100:341-346.

54. Schiff M. "The pill" in otolaryngology. *Trans Am Acad Ophthalmol Otolaryngol.* (J-F) 1968;72:76-84.

55. Brodnitz F. Medical care preventive therapy (panel). In: Lawrence V, ed. *Transcripts of the Seventh Annual Symposium, Care of the Professional Voice.* New York, NY: The Voice Foundation; 1978;3:86.

56. Flach M, Schwickardi H, Simen R. Welchen Einfluss haben Menstruation and Schwangerschaft auf die augsgebildete Gesangsstimme? *Folia Phonat.* 1968;21:199-210.

57. Deuster CV. Irreversible Stimmstorung in der Schwangerscheft. *HNO.* 1977;25:430-432.

58. Damste PH. Virilization of the voice due to anabolic steroids. Folia Phoniat. 1964;16:10-18.

59. Damste PH. Voice changes in adult women caused by virilizing agents. *J Speech Hear Disord.* 1967; 32:126-132.

60. Saez S, Francoise S. Recepteurs d'androgenes: mise en evidence dans la fraction cytosolique de muqueuse normale et d'epitheliomas pharyngolarynges humains. *C R Acad Sci (Paris).* 1975; 280:935-938.

61. Vuorenkoski V, Lenko HL, Tjernlund P, Vuorenkoski L, Perheentupa J. Fundamental voice frequency during normal and abnormal growth, and after androgen treatment. *Arch Dis Child.* 1978;53:201-209.

62. Bourdial J. Les troubles de la voix provoques par la therapeutique hormonale androgene. *Ann Otolaryngol (Paris).* 1970;87:725-734.

63. Imre V. Hormonell bedingte Stimmstorungen. *Folia Phoniat.* 1968;20:394-404.

64. Deems DA, Sataloff RT. Spasmodic dysphonia. In: Sataloff RT, ed. *Professional Voice: Science and Art of Clinical Care.* 2nd ed. San Diego, CA: Singular Publishing Group; 1997:499-506.

65. Sataloff RT, Mandel S, Rosen DC. Neurologic disorders affecting the voice in performance. In: Sataloff RT, ed. *Professional Voice: Science and Art of Clinical Care.* 2nd ed. San Diego, CA: Singular Publishing Group; 1997:479-498.

66. Gates GA, Saegert J, Wilson N, Johnson L, Sheperd A, Hearnd EM. Effects of beta-blockade on singing performance. *Ann Otol Rhinol Laryngol.* 1985; 94:570-574.

67. Rosen DC, Sataloff RT. *Psychology of Voice Disorders.* San Diego, CA: Singular Publishing Group; 1997:1-261.

68. Sataloff RT. Vocal fold scar. In: Sataloff RT, ed. *Professional Voice: Science and Art of Clinical Care.* 2nd ed. San Diego, CA: Singular Publishing Group; 1997:555-561.

69. Sataloff RT, Spiegel JR, Hawkshaw M, Rosen DC. Vocal fold hemorrhage. In: Sataloff RT, ed. *Professional Voice: Science and Art of Clinical Care.* 2nd ed. San Diego, CA: Singular Publishing Group; 1997:541-554.

70. Hochman I, Sataloff RT, Hillman R, Zeitels S. Ectasias and varicies of the vocal fold: clearing the striking zone. *Ann Otol Rhinol Laryngol.* 1999; 108(1):10-16.

71. Zeitels SM. Phonomicrosurgical techniques. In: Sataloff RT, ed. *Professional Voice: Science and Art of Clinical Care.* 2nd ed. San Diego, CA: Singular Publishing Group; 1997:647-658.

72. Zeitels SM, Sataloff RT. Phonomicrosurgical resection of glottal papillomatosis. *J Voice.* 1999; 13(1):123-127.

73. Wellens W, Snoeck R, Desloovere C, et al. Treatment of severe laryngeal papillomatosis with intralesional injections of Cidofovir [(S)-1-(3-Hydroxy-Phosphonylmethoxypropyl) Cytosine, HPMPC, Vistide®]. In: McCafferty G, Coman W, Carroll R, eds. Sydney; 1997. Bologna, Italy: Monduzzi Editor; 1997:455-549.

74. Spiegel JR, Sataloff RT. Laryngeal cancer. In: Sataloff RT, ed. *Professional Voice: The Science and Art of Clinical Care.* 2nd ed. San Diego, CA: Singular Publishing Group; 1997:673-688.

75. Wolman L, Drake CS, Young A. The larynx in rheumatoid arthritis. *J Laryngol.* 1965;79:403-404.

76. Bridger MWM, Jahn AF, van Nostrand AWP. Laryngeal rheumatoid arthritis. *Laryngoscope.* 1980;90:296-303.

77. Virchow R. Seltene Gichtablagerungen. *Virchows Arch Pathol.* 1868;44:137-138.

78. Marion RB, Alperin JE, Maloney WH. Gouty tophus of the true vocal cord. *Arch Otolaryngol.* 1972;96:161-162.

79. Stark DB, New GB. Amyloid tumors of the larynx, trachea or bronchi; report of 15 cases. *Ann Otol Rhinol Laryngol.* 1949;58:117-134.

80. Michaels L, Hyams VJ. Amyloid in localized deposits and plasmacytomas of the respiratory tract. *J Pathol.* 1979;128:29-38.

81. Urbach E, Wiethe C. Lipoidosis cutis et mucosae. *Virchows Arch Pathol Anat.* 1929;273:285-319.

82. Sataloff RT, Hawkshaw M, Ressue J. Granular cell tumor of the larynx. *Ear Nose Throat J.* 1998;77(8):582-584.

83. Charow A, Pass F, Ruben R. Pemphigus of the upper respiratory tract. *Arch Otolaryngol.* 1971; 93:209-210.

84. Rulnick RK, Heuer RJ, Perez KS, Emerich KA, Sataloff RT. Voice therapy. In: Sataloff RT, ed. *Professional Voice: Science and Art of Clinical Care.* 2nd ed. San Diego, CA: Singular Publishing Group; 1997:699-720.

85. Emerich KA, Baroody MM, Carroll LM, Sataloff RT. Singing voice specialist. In: Sataloff RT, ed. *Professional Voice: Science and Art of Clinical Care.* 2nd ed. San Diego, CA: Singular Publishing Group; 1997:735-745.

86. Freed SL, Raphael BN, Sataloff RT. The role of the acting voice trainer in medical care of professional voice users. In: Sataloff RT, ed. *Professional Voice: Science and Art of Clinical Care.* 2nd ed. San Diego, CA: Singular Publishing Group; 1997:765-774.

87. Sataloff RT, Spiegel JR, Heuer RJ, et al. Laryngeal mini-microflap: a new technique and reassessment of the microflap saga. *J Voice.* 1995;9(2):198-204.

88. Abitbol, J. Limitations of the laser in microsurgery of the larynx. In: Lawrence VL, ed. *Transactions of the Twelfth Symposium: Care of the Professional Voice.* New York, NY: The Voice Foundation; 1984.

89. Tapia RG, Pardo J, Marigil M, Pacio A. Effects of the laser upon Reinke's space and the neural system of the vocalis muscle. In: Lawrence VL, ed. *Transactions of the Twelfth Symposium: Care of*

the Professional Voice. New York, NY: The Voice Foundation; 1984:289-291.

90. Sataloff RT, Feldman M, Darby KS, Carroll LM, Spiegel JR. Arytenoid dislocation. *J Voice.* 1988;1(4):368-377.

91. Sataloff RT, Bough ID, Spiegel JR. Arytenoid dislocation: diagnosis and treatment. *Laryngoscope.* 1994;104(10):1353-1361.

92. Ford CN. Bless DM. Collagen injected in the scarred vocal fold. *J Voice.* 1988;1(1):116-118.

93. Sataloff RT, Spiegel JR, Hawkshaw M, Rosen DC, Heuer RJ. Autologous fat implantation for vocal fold scar. *J Voice.* 1997;11(2):238-246.

CHAPTER 21

Congenital Anomalies of the Larynx

Ted L. Tewfik, MD, FRCSC

Steven E. Sobol, MD

Congenital anomalies of the larynx are a common reason for consultation in pediatric otolaryngology. Symptoms of congenital laryngeal anomalies frequently present at birth but may be delayed. The clinical findings range from subtle changes in feeding or speech, to life-threatening respiratory obstruction.

Stridor is a sign of upper respiratory obstruction. Generally, inspiratory stridor suggests obstruction above the glottis while expiratory stridor indicates a lesion lower in the subglottis or trachea. Biphasic stridor suggests a glottic or subglottic obstruction.

Anomalies of the larynx are the major cause of neonatal stridor, accounting for 60% of such cases,[1] and must be differentiated from tracheal anomalies, bronchial or other acquired lesions.[2]

In this chapter, we review the common congenital anomalies of the larynx in terms of their epidemiology, etiology, clinical presentation, diagnosis, and management.

LARYNGOMALACIA

Epidemiology

Laryngomalacia is the most common congenital anomaly of the larynx, accounting for 60% of all cases.[3] Male infants are affected twice as commonly as females.[4]

Etiology and Pathogenesis

The exact cause of laryngomalacia is not known. Theories include abnormal development of the cartilaginous structures and immaturity of neuromuscular control.[5]

The epiglottis derives from the third and fourth branchial arches. Overgrowth of the third arch portion of the epiglottis results in elongation and lateral extension of the mature structure, which may be seen in patients with laryngomalacia.[3] There is some evidence that the laryngeal cartilages are intrinsically weaker in patients with laryngomalacia.[6] Other histologic studies, however, have shown no difference between normal and affected children.[7]

Immature neuromuscular control may be responsible for the arytenoid prolapse seen in laryngomalacia.[8] This theory is supported by the finding that children with laryngomalacia have an increased incidence of hypotonia, associated with gastrointestinal reflux (GER), obstructive sleep apnea, and failure to thrive.[9] However, there is no increase in the incidence of laryngomalacia in premature infants who are classically hypotonic.[10]

In a recent prospective study, Gianonni et al,[11] observed GER in 64% of patients with laryngomalacia. They concluded also that GER was significantly associated with severe symptoms and a complicated clinical course.

Clinical Presentation

The most common symptoms of laryngomalacia include noisy respiration and inspiratory stridor, accentuated by supine positioning, feeding, and agitation, and relieved by neck extension and prone positioning. Symptoms are usually absent at birth, begin within the first few weeks of life, increase over several months, and resolve by eighteen months to two years of age. Less commonly, the child may experience feeding difficulties but rarely failure to thrive. Respiratory distress and cyanosis are also rare.

On examination, the child with laryngomalacia is usually within the normal range of growth, appears healthy, and does not exhibit signs of respiratory distress (nasal flaring, supraclavicular or intercostal indrawing, and/or cyanosis). The cry is normal and strong. Head and neck examination is usually normal.

Flexible endoscopy may reveal several characteristic abnormalities such as[12]:

1. Elongation and lateral extension of the epiglottis (omega shaped), which falls posteroinferiorly on inspiration,

2. Redundant, bulky arytenoids, which prolapse anteromedially on inspiration,

3. Shortening of the aryepiglottic folds, resulting in tethering the arytenoids to the epiglottis,

4. Inward collapse of the aryepiglottic folds (with the cuneiform cartilages) on inspiration.

Expiration results in the expulsion of these supraglottic structures with unimpeded flow of air. The vocal folds can usually be visualized and have normal structure and function in patients with laryngomalacia (Figure 21-1).[10]

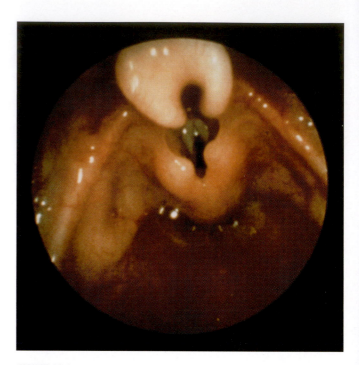

FIGURE 21-1. *Laryngomalacia: Omega-shaped epiglottis and short epiglottic folds. (Courtesy of Dr. J. Paul Willging of Cincinnati)*

Shah and Wetmore[13] proposed a classification for laryngomalacia based on the clinical presentation and anatomic site of collapse. The severity of the *s*tridor, *w*eight gain, *a*ge of presentation, and the *n*eurologic status (SWAN) represent the clinical factors. The adoption of similar classifications should facilitate documentation and statistical analyses of management and outcome in future reports (Table 21-1).

Type I	Inward collapse of A/E folds, corniculate and cuneiform cartilages. Obstruction occurs as these cartilages are drawn inward during inspiration.
Type II	A long tubular epiglottis (exaggerated omega-shaped) curls on itself and contributes to the obstruction.
Type III	Anterior, medial collapse of the corniculate and cuneiform cartilages to occlude the laryngeal inlet during inspiration.
Type IV	Posterior inspiratory displacement of the epiglottis against the posterior pharyngeal wall, or inferior collapse of the vocal folds.
Type V	Short A/E folds.

TABLE 21-1. *Types of Laryngomalacia[13]*

Diagnosis

The classic history and endoscopic examination are usually sufficient to establish a diagnosis of laryngomalacia in cases of mild to moderate stridor.

Radiographic studies may suggest a diagnosis of laryngomalacia and should be performed to rule out coexisting anomalies of the airway (tracheomalacia, innominate artery compression, or vascular rings of the trachea).[4,14] Inspiratory plain films of the neck may show inferior and medial displacement of the epiglottis and arytenoids. Fluoroscopy may reveal supraglottic collapse and hypopharyngeal dilatation.

Microlaryngoscopy and rigid bronchoscopy under general anesthesia should be performed when the child is experiencing respiratory distress or there is suggestion of coexisting anomalies on radiologic imaging.[15]

Multiple authors have reported on the effects of acid and pepsin on the larynx and tracheobronchial tree. Persistent edema in patients with GER is a common finding in infants with laryngomalacia.[16] A band of inflammation beneath the epithelium associated with the presence of intra-epithelial eosinophils appear to be a histologic indication for concurrent reflux in laryngomalacia.[17]

Management

The majority of patients with laryngomalacia can be managed by observation given that the condition is generally self-resolving by 12-18 months of age.

Medical management of documented esophageal reflux disease should be employed as this is known to contribute to laryngomalacia.[18] The therapy includes positioning measures and medications (Table 21-2).

Surgical management is indicated for respiratory complications of laryngomalacia:

1. Tracheotomy is indicated for acute respiratory distress and should be left in place until the supraglottic pathology resolves with age.[4]

Drug (Generic) (Trade name)	**Dosage**	**Class**
Cimetidine (Tagamet)	Neonate: 5-10 mg/kg/day po in div. doses q8-12h	H-2 receptor antagonist
	Infant: 10-20 mg/kg/day po in div. doses q6-12h	
	Child: 20-40 mg/kg/day po in div. doses q6h	
Ranitidine (Zantac)	Child & infant > 1 month old: 5-10 mg/kg/day po in 2-3 div. doses	
Famotidine (Pepcid)	1-2 mg/kg/day po in 2 div. doses	H-2 receptor antagonist
Omeprazole (Prilosec)	Infant: 0.5 mg/kg po q24h	H+/K+ ATPase inhibitor
	Child: 0.7-3.3 mg/kg po q24h	
Cisapride (Propulsid)	Neonate & Infant : 0.1 mg/kg/dose po 8h	Prokinetic agent
	Child: 0.1-0.2 mg/kg/dose po q6-8h	
Metoclopramide (Reglan)	Neonates, infants, & children: 0.4-0.8 mg/kg/day in 4 div. doses	Prokinetic agent

TABLE 21-2. *Commonly Used Medications for the Treatment of GER*[18]

2. Supraglottoplasty avoids the need for tracheotomy. In this procedure, the laryngeal inlet is widened by removing a wedge of the aryepiglottic folds bilaterally, trimming the epiglottis, removing the corniculate and cuneiform cartilages and redundant arytenoid mucosa. The procedure is usually performed using laser surgery. Patients are extubated the day after surgery.[10] Relief of respiratory symptoms has been shown to occur in excess of 80% of cases.[19] Complications of the bilateral procedure include the development of posterior supraglottic stenosis, which may be prevented by unilateral endoscopic supraglottoplasty (Figures 21-2 and 21-3).[20] In our opinion, it is always advisable to avoid excessive excision, and reassess the patient if symptoms persist.

Complications

Although some studies have quoted a high percentage of respiratory distress in patients with laryngomalacia,[21,22] the vast majority of patients resolve without complications.[15] Complications in rare cases include chest deformities, attacks of cyanosis, obstructive apnea, pulmonary hypertension, right heart failure, and failure to thrive.

VOCAL FOLD PARALYSIS

Epidemiology

According to Cotton and Prescott[23] vocal fold paralysis is the second most common congenital anomaly of the larynx. It represents 15% of all congenital laryngeal anomalies; however, other authors list its incidence around 10%.[24] There is no gender difference in the prevalence of this anomaly. The paralysis may be either bilateral or unilateral. Approximately half of all cases of bilateral vocal fold paralysis are congenital.[25,26]

Etiology and Pathogenesis

Overall, the most common cause of bilateral vocal fold paralysis is Arnold-Chiari malformation, followed by birth trauma causing excessive strain on the cervical spine; one-third of cases are idiopathic.[26-30] Birth trauma induced vocal fold paralysis may be bilateral or unilateral and is responsible for approximately 20% of cases, usually following high-forceps or abnormally presenting deliveries. Fifty percent of patients with bilateral vocal fold paralysis have associated anomalies. Other acquired cases of bilateral vocal fold paralysis may be secondary to central neuromuscular immaturity cerebral palsy, hydrocephalus, myelomeningocele, spina bifida, hypoxia, hemorrhage, or infection.[29]

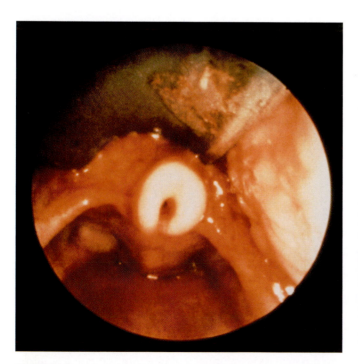

FIGURE 21-2. *Laryngomalacia associated with obstructive sleep apnea. (Courtesy of Dr. J. Paul Willging of Cincinnati)*

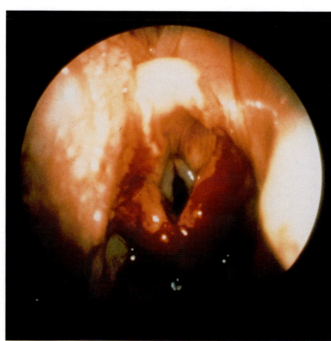

FIGURE 21-3. *Same patient in Figure 21-2, after supraglottoplasty. (Courtesy of Dr. J. Paul Willging of Cincinnati)*

Whereas a central nervous system defect is usually responsible for bilateral vocal fold paralysis, unilateral disease is usually secondary to peripheral nerve pathology.[27] The most common cause of unilateral vocal fold paralysis is iatrogenic following cardiac surgery.[27,28] Blunt trauma causing traction injuries to the recurrent laryngeal nerve may be responsible for a number of cases.[28] Lesions in the mediastinum such as tumors or vascular malformations may be the cause of certain cases of unilateral vocal fold paralysis.

Clinical Presentation

Bilateral vocal fold paralysis presents in children with near-normal phonation and progressive airway obstruction, manifesting as biphasic or inspiratory stridor at rest, exacerbated by agitation. Respiratory compromise becomes more pronounced with age as the oxygen requirements increase.[31] Obstruction can progress to a state of respiratory distress requiring airway intervention. Aspiration is common with bilateral vocal fold paralysis, often resulting in recurrent chest infections.

Unilateral vocal fold paralysis may present during the first few weeks of life or may go unnoticed because of the paucity of respiratory symptoms. The most common symptoms are a hoarse, breathy cry, which may be aggravated by agitation. Feeding difficulties and signs of aspiration may also be present in children with unilateral vocal fold paralysis.

Head and neck examination may reveal the presence of other cranial nerve deficits. A full examination should be performed in patients with vocal fold paralysis to rule out associated anomalies.

Diagnosis

Bilateral vocal fold paralysis is suggested by a history of early inspiratory stridor associated with signs of respiratory distress and abnormal voice or cry.[32] If the child is stable, flexible endoscopy may be performed allowing for dynamic visualization of vocal fold movement. The limitations of this diagnostic modality, however, are the inability to palpate the cricoarytenoid joint and visualize the rest of the upper airway. Rigid laryngobronchoscopy should be done to confirm the diagnosis and to assess the airway for other anomalies. If the diagnosis is uncertain, the procedure should be repeated one week later to confirm the diagnosis.

Flexible endoscopic examination is usually sufficient to establish a diagnosis of unilateral vocal fold paralysis. In the presence of respiratory distress, rigid bronchoscopy should also be done to rule out the presence of concurrent airway anomalies.

Radiographic imaging for patients with vocal fold paralysis can be performed both for diagnosis and to rule out concurrent pathology. Ultrasound of the larynx can be used to assess vocal fold function in patients unable to tolerate endoscopy or as a non-invasive follow-up study in patients with known paralysis.[33] Patients with bilateral vocal fold paralysis should have imaging of the central nervous system to rule out abnormalities or injuries. Patients with unilateral vocal fold paralysis should have radiographic studies (CT mediastinum and neck) to rule out other lesions compromising the function of the recurrent laryngeal nerve.

Experimental studies using laryngeal electromyography (EMG) are currently under way to help in the diagnosis of idiopathic cases;[34] however, several centers have been using EMG routinely for clinical purposes since the early 1990s (R. T. Sataloff—personal communication, 2002).

Management

Patients with bilateral vocal fold paralysis may need urgent airway intervention, usually achievable by endotracheal intubation. Tracheotomy is necessary to relieve the obstruction and should remain in place for at least two years to allow for spontaneous recovery, which occurs completely in more than half of patients.[26] Supportive measures are also necessary for the patient with bilateral vocal fold paralysis to ensure that adequate nutrition is received while preventing aspiration.

If recovery does not occur, consideration should be given to vocal fold lateralization procedures in an effort to decannulate the patient. Arytenoidectomy produces reliable results in maintaining a patent airway and achieving decannulation. Transverse laser cordotomy has had early success in allowing decannulation in older children and adults. Some authors advocate early lateralization procedures in patients with bilateral vocal fold paralysis in order to prevent complications of long-term tracheotomy.[35-37]

The majority of cases of unilateral vocal fold paralysis can be managed by observation, ensuring that respiratory and feeding difficulties do not develop. Upright positioning is usually sufficient to alleviate aspiration difficulties. Rarely, intubation may be necessary to acquire a stable airway in distressed patients.

CONGENITAL SUBGLOTTIC STENOSIS

Epidemiology

Congenital subglottic stenosis is defined as subglottic narrowing in the absence of endotracheal intubation or any other apparent cause.[31] It is the third most common congenital anomaly of the larynx,[4,23] and is the most common laryngeal anomaly to require tracheotomy in infants.[38] Males are affected twice as commonly as females.

Etiology and Pathogenesis

Incomplete recanalization of the laryngotracheal tube during the third month of gestation will lead to different degrees of congenital subglottic stenosis. At the extreme spectrum of this condition is complete laryngeal atresia (see below), which results from complete failure to recanalize the lumen in the tenth week of gestation.[39]

Classification

Congenital subglottic stenosis can be classified according to the gross and histologic characteristics of the obstruction.[4] Membranous congenital subglottic stenosis is the result of circumferential submucosal hypertrophy with excess fibrous connective tissue and mucous glands.[40] On examination, it usually appears as circumferential, soft-tissue thickening, which is compressible. It is the most common and mild form of congenital subglottic stenosis.

Cartilaginous subglottic stenosis is the result of abnormal development of the cricoid cartilage and usually appears as an elliptically shaped narrow lumen of the subglottis,[40,41] The defect is usually lateral thickening of the cricoid cartilage, but may also be caused by anteroposterior narrowing, in some cases.

Holinger[42] described different types of cricoid cartilage abnormalities associated with congenital subglottic stenosis. They include elliptical-shaped cricoid, subglottic laryngeal cleft, flattened cricoid, large anterior lamina, generalyzed thickening, as well as a rare anterior submucous cleft.

Clinical Presentation

The manifestations of congenital subglottic stenosis usually appear in the first few months of life. The stenosis is not evident until the child develops an acute inflammatory process, which further compromises the subglottic space.[43] The clinical presentation during this period does not differ from that of infectious laryngotracheobronchitis (croup). Biphasic stridor with or without respiratory distress is the most common presenting symptom. The child may have a barking cough, but the cry is usually normal.

Suspicion of congenital subglottic stenosis should be aroused when these symptoms are recurrent or if they are prolonged beyond the normal duration of infectious croup despite adequate medical therapy.[15,44] Another clinical scenario that should arouse suspicion of congenital stenosis is in asymptomatic children who are dif-

ficult to intubate, or decannulate. Children with Down's syndrome are at increased risk of having congenital subglottic stenosis and may present in this fashion.

On examination, the child with congenital subglottic stenosis may or may not be in significant respiratory distress (nasal flaring, supraclavicular or intercostal indrawing, cyanosis). Head and neck examination is usually normal.

Flexible endoscopy does not adequately assess the subglottis but is important to rule out vocal fold paralysis and other glottic abnormalities.

Diagnosis

Congenital subglottic stenosis is usually suggested by a history of recurrent episodes of croup. Rigid bronchoscopy under general anesthesia should be done to confirm the diagnosis, plan future management, and assess the airway for other anomalies. The stenosis should be evaluated in terms of its length and diameter, which may be adequately assessed by passing a scope or endotracheal tube of known outer diameter through the stenosis. The largest tube or scope to pass through the airway is a good measure of the lumen diameter.[45] A diagnosis of congenital subglottic stenosis is made when the lumen diameter is less than 4 mm in a term infant or 3 mm in a preterm infant.[43] The findings at endoscopy are characteristically less severe than in children with acquired subglottic stenosis.

Radiographic evaluation may help to assess the subglottic airway prior to bronchoscopy or when the diagnosis is unclear. Plain lateral or AP x-rays will show a characteristic narrowing at the level of the subglottis.[46]

Management

Most cases of congenital subglottic stenosis will resolve spontaneously with growth of the child and can be managed conservatively. During episodes of acute laryngotracheobronchitis, patients with congenital subglottic stenosis should be managed aggressively in order to avoid intubation, as this increases trauma to the airway.[43] Less than half of all children with congenital subglottic stenosis will require surgical airway intervention.[47]

Endotracheal intubation and tracheotomy may be required in patients who have significant airway compromise. Most children who require tracheotomy can be decannulated by 3-4 years of age when the subglottic space matures to a sufficient diameter.

Laryngotracheoplasty is usually unnecessary but may be required to reconstruct the airway in patients who cannot be decannulated. In neonates who fail extubation, anterior cricoid split should be considered when the pathology is anterior glottic or subglottic. The patient weight should be more than 1,500 grams.[45,48,49] A vertical split is carried through the lower thyroid cartilage, the cricoid cartilage, and the first two tracheal rings.[31] An endotracheal tube is used as a stent for approximately seven days before extubation.[50] In properly selected patients, the anterior cricoid split results in less hospitalization, morbidity, and mortality when compared to tracheotomy.[49] Medical treatment of gastroesophageal reflux, and use of antibiotics and steroids during the intubation period, should be routine in patients undergoing open procedures.

Laser ablation has a limited role in the management of congenital subglottic stenosis and is usually reserved for soft lesions less than 5 mm in thickness.

SUBGLOTTIC HEMANGIOMA

Epidemiology

Subglottic hemangiomas account for 1.5% of all congenital anomalies of the larynx.[3,4] Females are affected twice as commonly as males.[51]

Etiology and Pathogenesis

Subglottic hemangiomas result from vascular malformations derived from mesenchymal rests of vasoactive tissue in the subglottis.[1] Histologically, the majority of these lesions are composed of capillary-like vessels as opposed to the cavernous hamangiomas, which present often in older patients.[52]

Clinical Presentation

The child with a subglottic hemangioma is usually asymptomatic at birth. As the lesion rapidly increases in size from 2-12 months of age, the baby develops progressive respiratory distress, which is at first intermittent and then continuous. The symptoms are similar to that of infectious croup, presenting with biphasic stridor, barking cough, normal or hoarse cry, and failure to thrive. Some patients may develop airway obstruction significant enough to necessitate intervention. After the first year of life, most patients will have a progressive resolution of their symptoms as the lesion regresses spontaneously by 5 years of age.[51,53,54]

On examination, the child with a subglottic hemangioma may or may not be in significant respiratory distress (nasal flaring, supraclavicular or intercostal indrawing, and/or cyanosis). Head and neck examination is usually normal. Cutaneous hemangiomas are present in half of these patients.[4]

Flexible endoscopy does not demonstrate the lesion but is necessary to rule out other laryngeal anomalies (Figure 21-4).

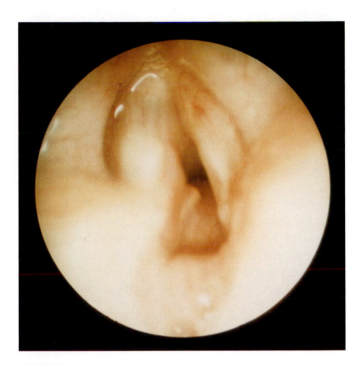

FIGURE 21-4. *Posterior subglottic hemangioma. (Courtesy of Dr. J. Paul Willging of Cincinnati)*

Diagnosis

Rigid bronchoscopy under general anesthesia is necessary to establish diagnosis of subglottic hemangiomas. The lesion usually presents as a smooth, compressible submucosal mass, located posterolaterally in the subglottis.[55] It may be unilateral or bilateral and may extend to the upper trachea. It is usually sessile, pink-blue in color, and easily compressible. When the diagnosis is unclear, biopsy of the lesion should be undertaken with caution because of the risk of significant hemorrhage.[51]

Plain x-rays of the neck may aid in making the diagnosis prior to endoscopy. Anteroposterior views will show an asymmetric narrowing of the subglottis, and lateral views will demonstrate posterior subglottic soft-tissue density.

Management

Observation is usually sufficient for subglottic hemangiomas that do not cause significant airway obstruction. A substantial number of patients, however, will require surgical intervention at some point during the acute growth phase to relieve airway obstruction.

Surgical approaches in patients with subglottic hemangiomas can be classified as open or endoscopic. The goal is to establish an adequate airway. It should be emphasized that all surgical interventions in cases of subglottic hemangiomas should be as conservative as possible, to avoid iatrogenic subglottic stenosis.[56]

Open surgical procedures may be necessary in the acute setting to establish an airway or can rarely be employed to resect lesions not amenable to endoscopic approaches.[57] Tracheotomy is usually necessary to secure the airway, and should be left in place until the lesion regresses spontaneously, usually by 5 years of age.

Steroid injection into small or moderate-sized hemangiomas may precipitate involution secondary to suppression of estradiol stimulation of the lesion and increased responsiveness to vasoconstrictors.[58] Steroids have been found to decrease the size and increase the rate of involution of hemangiomas, and may be considered as adjuvant therapy in certain cases.[59,60] However, the use of systemic steroid therapy is insufficient as a sole treatment option for the majority of subglottic hemangiomas.

Other endoscopic surgical techniques that have been described include carbon dioxide laser ablation,[4] electrocautery,[61] intralesional interferon,[62] or sclerosing agent injection. Of these, endoscopic laser ablation is most frequently successful for the treatment of small, unilateral lesions.[55,63] Recurrence of the hemangioma can occur in certain cases where the lesion extends beyond the submucosa and go undetected at the time of surgery.

External beam irradiation and radioactive gold implants have a 93% success rate at curing subglottic hemangiomas[52] but are not used because of the increased risk of thyroid cancer.[64] Finally, selective embolization of large laryngeal hemangiomas may be used in cases refractory to other therapies.[65]

Hughes et al[66] studied the safety and efficacy of individualized management to determine the various strategies in avoiding tracheostomy. They concluded the morbidity and the need for tracheostomy in congenital subglottic hemangioma cases can be minimized using a combination of therapeutic modalities. The treatment should be individualized according to the severity of the symptoms and the morphology of the lesion.

LARYNGEAL WEBS

Epidemiology

Laryngeal webs are rare congenital anomalies of the larynx.

Etiology and Pathogenesis

Incomplete recanalization of the laryngotracheal tube during the third month of gestation will lead to different degrees of laryngeal webs. The extreme of this situation is complete laryngeal atresia (see below). The most common site of development of laryngeal webs is at the anterior part of the vocal folds, although they may be present as posterior interarytenoid, subglottic, or supraglottic webs.[67,68]

Clinical Presentation

Laryngeal webs may present with symptoms ranging from mild dysphonia to significant airway obstruction depending on the size and location of the web. Stridor is rare except in cases of posterior interarytenoid webs. These cases typically present with airway obstruction in the presence of a normal voice or cry.[69] One third of children with laryngeal webs have associated anomalies of the respiratory tract, most commonly subglottic stenosis.[70] When respiratory distress is out of proportion to that caused by the web itself, other anomalies should be ruled out.

On examination, the child with a laryngeal web may or may not be in significant respiratory distress (nasal flaring, supraclavicular or intercostal indrawing, and/or cyanosis). Head and neck examination is usually normal.

Flexible endoscopy may reveal the presence of a laryngeal web but is insufficient in evaluating the extent of the anomaly (Figures 21-5 and 21-6).

Diagnosis

Rigid laryngoscopy and bronchoscopy under general anesthesia are necessary to assess the site, thickness, horizontal, and vertical extent of the web. The web may appear as a thin, translucent defect involving the anterior part of the vocal folds or as a thick fibrous structure, which extends inferiorly into the subglottis. The posterior glottis is usually not involved but may be

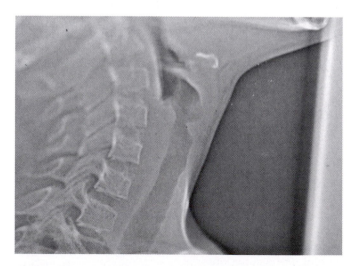

FIGURE 21-5. *Laryngeal web with subglottic extension as seen on lateral neck x-ray. (Courtesy of Dr. J. Paul Willging of Cincinnati)*

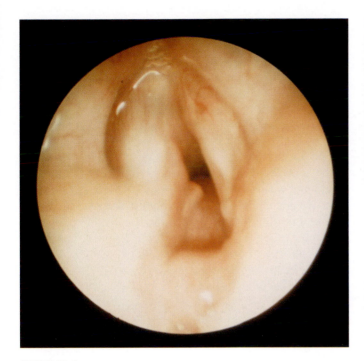

FIGURE 21-6. *Congenital web of the glottis. (Courtesy of Dr. J. Paul Willging of Cincinnati)*

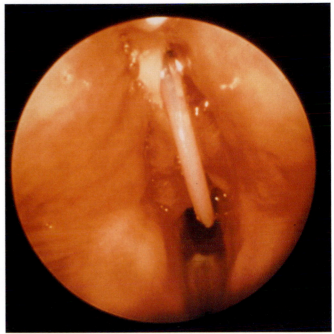

FIGURE 21-7. *Same patient in Figure 21-6, after keel placement. (Courtesy of Dr. J. Paul Willging of Cincinnati)*

closed by the presence of an interarytenoid web, which prevents vocal fold abduction. These posterior webs are best visualized when the examination is done without an endotracheal tube in place.

Radiographic evaluation may help to assess the site and extent of the laryngeal web prior to bronchoscopy and the presence of concurrent congenital subglottic stenosis. Lateral plain x-rays will show a characteristic sail sign representing persistent tissue between the vocal folds and subglottis.

Management

Management of laryngeal webs ranges from observation to emergent tracheotomy depending on the thickness of the lesion. Thin anterior webs may be lysed endoscopically using the cold knife or laser.[71] Endoscopic placement of a keel may be needed to prevent recurrence (Figure 21-7).

Thicker anterior webs may require a tracheotomy and a laryngofissure approach to remove redundant soft tissue, with postoperative stenting.[71] Revision procedures may be required in certain cases, especially those with complicated webs.

Posterior laryngeal webs are not managed adequately by either endoscopic or open techniques and are often best treated with tracheotomy and watchful waiting.[69]

LARYNGOTRACHEOESOPHAGEAL CLEFT (LTEC)

Laryngotracheoesophageal clefts (LTECs) are rare anomalies with a midline defect between the posterior larynx and trachea and the anterior wall of the esophagus of varying length. Severe forms of the defect are lethal.

Classification

LTEC has been classified into 3 categories by Evans[72]:

> Type I (31%)—Cleft is limited to the interarytenoid region above the vocal folds. This type does not involve the cricoid cartilage.
>
> Type II (47%)—This type includes the cricoid and extends into the cervical trachea.
>
> Type III (22%)—This type involves the thoracic trachea.

A modification of this classification was proposed by Benjamin and Inglis.[73] In this classification, type I cleft is limited to the supraglottic lumen above the vocal folds. Type II is a partial cleft of the cricoid extending below the level of the vocal folds, and type III involves the whole cricoid cartilage and may extend to the cervical tracheoesophageal septum. Type IV involves a major part of the tracheoesophageal wall in the thorax.

Associated Anomalies

Moungthong and Holinger[74] reported on their experience with LTEC in 1997. Cardiovascular anomalies were the most frequently seen. Examples include pulmonary valvular stenosis, aberrant innominate artery, patent ductus arteriosus, aortic valvular stenosis, and ventricular septal defect. Pulmonary agenesis, bronchoesophageal fistula, tracheoesophageal fistula, rudimentary uterus, and congenital blindness were also documented.

Diagnosis and Clinical Findings

Type I or the supraglottic type (Benjamin and Inglis classification)[73] is the most difficult to diagnose. The clinician may be alerted by feeding difficulties, husky cry, or aspiration pneumonia. Stridor, coughing, and cyanotic episodes precipitated by feeding are all symptoms that may vary in severity depending on the extent of the cleft.

The differential diagnosis should include tracheoesophageal fistula, esophageal atresia, and choanal atresia.

Chest x-ray may demonstrate pneumonia and the lateral view may show the anterior displacement of the nasogastric tube.

The definite diagnosis is made endoscopically. Suspension microlaryngoscopy is necessary to avoid missing the subtle defect (Figure 21-8).

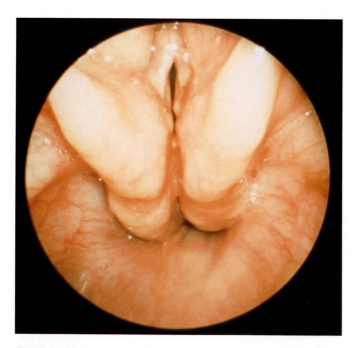

FIGURE 21-8. *Laryngeal cleft (type III). (Courtesy of Dr. J. Paul Willging of Cincinnati)*

Management

Prevention of the gastroesophageal reflux is important in all types of clefts (see Table 21-2).

Type I (Benjamin and Inglis classification)[73] is usually corrected with growth and requires nursing in the upright position and thickening of the formula. Endoscopic repair may be needed to correct the cases that do not respond to the conservative measures. Types II and III can be corrected through a cervical incision, while type IV may require lateral thoracotomy incision combined with a cervical approach. Others use an anterior, transtracheal repair. The pleura is used for interposition in the thoracic defect and the sternocleidomastoid muscle for the cervical portion. Primary closure of small defects (those with redundant mucosa), and the use of costal cartilage graft interposition (for type III) have also been described.[74]

LARYNGEAL ATRESIA

Epidemiology

Laryngeal atresia is an uncommon congenital anomaly of the larynx.[75] There are only a few reports of documented survivors of such lesions.[76]

Etiology and Pathogenesis

Failure of recanalization of the laryngotracheal tube during the third month of gestation will lead to laryngeal atresia.

Clinical Presentation

Laryngeal atresia presents as acute airway obstruction in the newborn immediately after clamping of the umbilical cord. Examination reveals a neonate with severe respiratory distress, marked by the presence of strong respiratory efforts and the inability to inhale air or cry. Complete laryngeal obstruction is known to cause secondary changes, including enlarged hypoechogenic lungs, dilated trachea, and fetal hydrops.[77]

Without an immediate tracheotomy (intubation is unsuccessful), death is imminent. The exception to this is in a child who has a concurrent tracheoesophageal fistula of sufficient size to permit the passage of air distal to the obstruction.

Diagnosis

Diagnosis of laryngeal atresia should be done endoscopically after securing the airway with a tracheotomy tube.

The presence of polyhydramnios may alert the physician to the prenatal diagnosis of laryngeal atresia, allowing for management preparation prior to birth.[78] However, if a concomitant tracheoesophageal fistula is present, the absence of polyhydramnios will make the prenatal diagnosis more difficult.[79]

Management

Laryngeal atresia requires immediate tracheotomy at birth. If the diagnosis is anticipated, clamping of the umbilical cord should be avoided until the tracheotomy is secured in order to maximize oxygenation.[76,79] In cases where a fistula is present, mask ventilation and esophageal intubation can be performed as a temporary measure until a tracheotomy is done.[79]

LARYNGEAL CYSTS AND LARYNGOCELES

Epidemiology

Laryngeal cysts are uncommon congenital anomalies of the larynx. Congenital saccular cysts represent 25% of all laryngeal cysts.

Etiology and Pathogenesis

Laryngeal cysts are caused by obstruction of the laryngeal saccule orifice in the ventricle, leading to retention of mucus.[80] Ductal cysts arise from blockage of submucosal mucous glands and can occur in the vallecula, subglottis, or the vocal folds. Ductal cysts are common in the subglottis after prolonged intubation caused by irritation and blockage of submucosal glands.

Laryngoceles are air-filled dilatations of the saccule arising from increased endolaryngeal pressure in the presence of congenital tissue weakness at the level of the saccular orifice.[81]

Clinical Presentation

Laryngeal cysts may present with mild symptoms to varying degrees of airway obstruction, inaudible or muffled cry or dysphagia. Children typically present with stridor soon after birth, in some cases necessitating tracheotomy.[81,82] In a small number of cases, the saccular swelling may be seen as an external neck mass.

Laryngoceles are usually symptomatic intermittently when inflamed or infected, and may present as a mass in the neck.[83]

Diagnosis

Endoscopy reveals the presence of a bluish-pink cystic lesion behind the aryepiglottic fold (lateral cyst) or emanating from the ventricle and protruding into the laryngeal lumen (anterior cyst) (Figure 21-9).

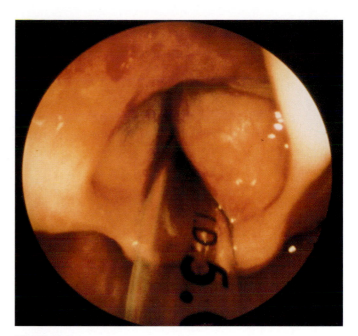

FIGURE 21-9. *Fullness of the right aryepiglottic fold caused by a saccular cyst. (Courtesy of Dr. J. Paul Willging of Cincinnati)*

Management

If emergent management of a saccular cyst is necessary, endotracheal intubation is usually possible. Needle aspiration or incision of the lesion may be done as a temporizing measure but definitive management requires endoscopic or open complete cyst excision to prevent recurrence. Ductal cysts can be removed using forceps or laser excision if they are symptomatic.

Laryngoceles can be treated using endoscopic approach or through open surgical technique, and need only be addressed if they are symptomatic.[81]

LARYNGEAL LYMPHANGIOMAS

Epidemiology

Laryngeal lymphangiomas are rare congenital anomalies of the larynx. There are only several reports of cases confined to the larynx, and most cases of laryngeal obstruction are secondary to the effects of external compression from adjacent lymphangiomas.[71,84] Half of all cases are diagnosed in the neonatal period, and 75% by 1 year of age.[4]

Etiology and Pathogenesis

Lymphangiomas originate from lymphatic vessel malformations. Lymphangiomas are classically subclassified as simple (capillary), cavernous (dilated lymphatic channels), and cystic hygromas (discrete cystic spaces).

Clinical Presentation

Lymphangiomas may be asymptomatic or present with dysphonia and significant airway obstruction when they attain a large size. Upper respiratory tract infections may precipitate symptoms by causing a rapid increase in the size of these lesions.[4]

Diagnosis

Diagnosis of a lymphangioma should be done endoscopically only after securing an airway.

Management

Tracheotomy is often necessary to establish an airway in patients with laryngeal lymphangiomas. Their large size and locally invasive nature often complicate excision of these lesions. Moreover, because these lesions tend to grow over time and involve vital structures, complete excision is often difficult. Laser ablation of these lesions is the mainstay of current therapy and staged procedures are often needed to attain control of the airway. Sclerosing agents are currently under investigation as a possible modality of treatment for laryngeal lymphangiomas.[85] Radiation therapy is not effective in the treatment of these lesions and is associated with secondary malignancies.

GENETIC AND CENTRAL NEUROMUSCULAR ANOMALIES

Cri-du-chat syndrome is caused by a terminal deletion on the short arm of chromosome 5 (5p13.3, 5p14.1, 5p14.2, or 5p14.3) or rarely by interstitial deletion. An attempt to localize the developmental field affected in cri-du-chat syndrome was made by Kjaer and Niebuhr from Denmark.[86] They found that specific malformations occurred in the bony contours of the sella tursica and the clivus in cri-du-chat patients with terminal deletions. These specific regions develop around the notochord where the neurons to the larynx have migrated ventrally.

The frequency of the syndrome is 1 in 50,000 births. Approximately 1% of profoundly retarded patients are diagnosed with cri-du-chat syndrome. Affected individuals exhibit microcephaly, hypotonia, and cardiovascular defects. The characteristic mewy cry (cat cry) is present only during infancy. The high-pitched stridor is the result of interarytenoid muscle paralysis in an elongated larynx with a floppy epiglottis. Faces of these patients are round with hypertelorism and broad nasal root.[87,88]

Arthrogryposis multiplex congenita is associated with multiple joint disorders and central nervous system abnormalities. Laryngeal manifestations include bilateral vocal fold paralysis, hypertrophy of the cricopharyngeus, and supraglottic redundancy similar to laryngomalacia. These children almost always require tracheotomy, and prognosis is poor.[89]

Plott's syndrome, an X-linked disorder, is associated with laryngeal adductor paralysis.[90]

Table 21-3 includes other syndromes and conditions associated with laryngeal and/or tracheal anomalies.

SUMMARY

In this chapter we present an overview of the different congenital anomalies of the larynx. The most common anomaly is laryngomalacia. It accounts for approximately 60% of all cases. The symptoms include inspiratory stridor that is accentuated by supine position, feeding, and agitation. The child with laryngomalacia is usually healthy and has a normal cry. Flexible laryngoscopy is essential to make the diagnosis. Omega-shaped epiglottis, redundant bulky arytenoids, and short aryepiglottic folds are characteristic signs. The majority of patients can be managed conservatively, and the condition usually resolves by 12-18 months.

Vocal fold paralysis accounts for 15% of congenital anomalies of the larynx. The most common cause of bilateral vocal fold paralysis is Arnold-Chiari malformation. Birth trauma accounts for 20% of all cases. Aspiration is common in bilateral paralysis. CT scan is essential to rule out lesions compromising the recurrent laryngeal nerve. The majority of unilateral vocal fold paralysis are managed by observation; however, tracheotomy is necessary in bilateral cases.

Congenital subglottic stenosis is the most common laryngeal anomaly to require tracheotomy in infants. Biphasic stridor is the most common symptom. A diagnosis of the condition is made when the luminal diameter is less than 4 mm in the full-term infant. Most cases resolve spontaneously, and laryngotracheoplasty is required in patients who cannot be decannulated.

Subglottic hemangioma constitutes 1.5% of all congenital anomalies of the larynx. The symptoms include biphasic stridor and barking cough with or without failure to thrive. Most cases resolute gradually in 4-5 years. Rigid endocopy is essential to make the diagnosis. If the airway obstruction is significant, a surgical procedure may be needed. The treatment has to be individualized, depending on the clinical picture.

Laryngeal webs are rare laryngeal anomalies. The symptoms vary according to the size and location of the web. The treatment options also depend upon the airway status and the morphology of the lesion.

Syndrome or condition	MIM No. POSSUM No. [A]	Inheritance[B]	Ear, nose, and throat manifestations	Other manifestations
Adducted thumb syndrome, Christian syndrome or craniosynostosis, arthrogryposis, cleft palate	*201550 3591	AR	Myopathic face, micrognathia, cleft palate, low-set ears, abnormal shape of ears, torticollis, laryngomalacia, dysphagia	Craniosynostosis, microcephaly, downward slanting palpebral fissures, telecanthus, ophthalmoplegia, pectus excavatum, adducted thumbs, contractures, mental retardation, seizures, hypotonia, early death
Agnathia, synotia, microstoma or otocephaly syndrome	202650 3478	sporadic	Absence of mandible, micrognathia, small nostrils, choanal atresia, microstomia, aglossia, blind mouth, cleft palate, low-set ears, ears fused in the midline, middle ear anomalies, bilobed epiglottis, rudimentary vocal folds, webbed neck	Epicanthal folds, epibulbar dermoids, abnormal rib number, vertebral anomalies, dextrocardia, situs inversus, hypoplastic lungs, renal agenesis, cardiac defects, holoprosencephaly, lethal
Atelosteogenesis, type 3	4761		Midface hypoplasia, microstomia, micrognathia, cleft palate, flat nasal bridge, anteverted nostrils, low-set ears, helix hypoplastia, stenosis of the external auditory canal, laryngomalacia	Prominent forehead, hypertelorism, long clavicles, atlantoaxial instability, scoliosis, cleft of vertebral bodies, multiple joint dislocations, rhizomelic short/bowed limbs
Bilateral ptosis, vocal fold paralysis	4792	AD	Vocal fold paralysis, abnormal cry	Failure to thrive, normal intelligence, ptosis

TABLE 21-3. *Syndromes and Conditions Associated With Congenital Anomalies of the Larynx 91 (Continues)*

Syndrome or condition	MIM No.[A] POSSUM No.[A]	Inheritance[B]	Ear, nose, and throat manifestations	Other manifestations
Chondrodysplasia punctata, X-linked recessive	*302950 3737	XLR	Small nose, broad nasal bridge, anteverted nostrils, deafness, short neck, laryngeal abnormality	Cicatricial alopecia, ichthyosis, coarse hair, frontal bossing, short stature, MR (del Xp22)
Chromosome 5, partial del 5p or Cri-du-chat syndrome	3073		High, shrill mewing cry, broad cheeks, cleft lip/palate, micrognathia, broad nasal bridge, small posteriorly angulated ears, preauricular tags, laryngeal abnormality	Microcephaly, round face, hypertelorism, hypotonia, heart defects, cryptorchidism, epicanthic folds, moderate to severe MR
Chromosome 7, partial dup 7q	3076		Micrognathia, beaked nose, everted lips, cleft palate, macroglossia, anteverted or bat ears, short neck, hearing abnormality, laryngeal abnormality	Short stature, macrocephaly or hydrocephalus, frontal bossing, hypertelorism, cryptorchidism, single palmar crease, MR
Craniofacial digital genital anomalies	4163		Narrow face, pointed chin, microstomia, micrognathia, anteverted ears, abnormal cry, laryngeal abnormality	Hypotelorism, cryptophthalmos (not obligatory), ambiguous genitalia, hypospadias, cryptorchidism, anal stenosis or atresia, thymic aplasia, hypotonia, MR
Cryptophthalmos, multiple congenital anomalies (MCA) syndrome, or Fraser syndrome	*219000 3179	AR	Asymmetric face, coloboma of nostrils, choanal atresia, cleft lip/palate, low-set ears, atresia of the external auditory canal	Hypertelorism, cryptophthalmos (not obligatory), ambiguous genitalia, hypospadias, cryptorchidism, anal stenosis or atresia, thymic aplasia, hypotonia, MR

TABLE 21-3. *Syndromes and Conditions Associated With Congenital Anomalies of the Larynx* [91] *(Continues)*

Syndrome or condition	MIM No. POSSUM No.[A]	Inheritance[B]	Ear, nose, and throat manifestations	Other manifestations
De la Chapelle dysplasia or atelosteogenesis type 2, or neonatal osseous dysplasia	*256050 3847	AR	Cleft palate, folded-down ears, abnormal neck, laryngeal stenosis, bronchomalacia	Short ribs, scoliosis, severely hypoplastic ulna and fibula, bowed limbs, bifid humeral metaphysis, lethal
Diastrophic dysplasia	*222600 3185	AR	Cauliflower ears, calcified ear cartilage, cleft palate, micrognathia, conductive deafness, tracheal and laryngeal abnormality, abnormal cry	Short stature, short/bowed limbs, hitch-hiker thumbs, contractures, cryptorchidism, epiphyseal or metaphyseal abnormality, brachydactyly, dislocated hips, kyphoscoliosis, respiratory obstruction
Distal muscular atrophy, deafness	158580 4621	AD	Sensorineural deafness, vocal fold paralysis, abnormal cry	Scoliosis, distal muscular atrophy, muscle weakness, abnormal gait
Facio-auriculo-vertebral dysplasia, oculo-auriculo-vertebral dysphasia, or Goldenhar syndrome	164210 3339	AD AR	Facial asymmetry, triangular face, macrostoma, micrognathia, cleft palate, deafness, epibulbar dermoids, preauricular pits or tags, microtia or anotia, tracheoesophageal fistula, laryngeal abnormality	Intrauterine growth retardation (IUGR) microcephaly, microphthalmos, coloboma of eyelid, iris, and retina, oligodontia, hypoplastic lungs, dysplastic kidney, vertebral defects, agenesis of corpus callosum, hydrocephalus, MR
Farber lipogranulomatosis, generalized lipogranulomatosis, or acid ceramidase deficiency	*228000 3436	AR	Hoarseness of voice caused by vocal fold thickening, macroglossia, thickened gingiva, hamartoma of mouth	Painful/swollen joints and subcutaneous nodules, cloudy cornea, lymphadenopathy, hepatosplenomegaly, diffuse osteoporosis, nephropathy, seizures MR

TABLE 21-3. *Syndromes and Conditions Associated With Congenital Anomalies of the Larynx* [91] *(Continues)*

Syndrome or condition	MIM No. POSSUM No.[A]	Inheritance[B]	Ear, nose, and throat manifestations	Other manifestations
Fraser-Jéquier-Chen syndrome	4306		Laryngeal cleft, beaked nose, high narrow palate, low-set ears, preauricular tags	Pancreatic and renal dysplasia, short limbs, genital anomalies, imperforate anus, brachydactyly, polydactyly
Hydrolethalus syndrome	*236680 3567	AR	Micrognathia, flattened or cleft nose, glossoptosis, low-set ears, tracheal/laryngeal abnormality	Hydrocephalus, micropolygyria, polydactyly, segmental lung defect, heart defect
Hypothalamic-hamartoblastoma syndrome, or ano-cerebro-digital syndrome, or Pallister-Hall syndrome	*146510 3471	AR	Flat face, glossoptosis, cleft palate, anteverted nostrils, micrognathia, prominent and low-set ears, ear cartilage deficiency, laryngeal cleft, tracheal abnormality	IUGR, macrocephaly, prominent occiput, abnormal sella turcica, hypothalamic hamartomas, agenesis of corpus collosum, hypopituitarism, scoliosis, genital anomalies, heart defects, imperforate anus, postaxial polydactyly or syndactyly, lethal
Hypothyroidism, spiky hair, deafness	241850 4622	XLR	Choanal atresia, cleft palate, micrognathia, bifid epiglottis	Spiky hair, scalp alopecia, borderline mental retardation, spasticity, hypothyroidism
Infantile type sialuria	*269920 4308	AR	Coarse facies, speech deficit, laryngeal abnormality	Neonatal ascites, short stature, hepatic fibrosis, hepatomegaly, ataxia/athetosis, moderate to severe MR (storage disorder)
Keutel syndrome or pulmonary stenosis, brachydactyly, deafness, cartilage defect	*245150 3675	AR	Sensorineural deafness, midface hypoplasia, short philtrum, calcified ears, laryngeal/tracheal abnormality	Brachydactyly, soft tissue calcification, abnormal ossification, syndactyly, carpal fusion, peripheral pulmonary stenosis, heart defects, immunologic or hematologic abnormalities, MR

TABLE 21-3. *Syndromes and Conditions Associated With Congenital Anomalies of the Larynx* [91] *(Continues)*

Syndrome or condition	MIM No. POSSUM No.[A]	Inheritance[B]	Ear, nose, and throat manifestations	Other manifestations
Killian–Teschler-Nicola syndrome, or Pallister mosaic syndrome, or chromosome 12, mosaic tetrasomy 12P	3800	Sporadic	Coarse facies, broad nasal bridge, anteverted nostrils, long philtrum, large and low-set ears, thickened helix, cleft palate, short neck, laryngeal abnormality	Sparse hair, irregular skin pigmentation, accessory nipples, puffy eyelids, cataracts, optic nerve abnormality, inguinal/umbilical hernia, diaphragmatic hernia, genital anomalies, imperforate anus, caudal appendage, seizures, hypotonia, moderate to severe MR
Laryngeal abductor paralysis, MR, or Plott syndrome	308850 4008	XLR	Bilateral vocal fold paralysis, myopathic face, abnormal cry, dysphagia	Failure to thrive, MR, optic nerve abnormality, hypotonia
Laryngeal hypoplasia, encephalocele	4672		Laryngeal atresia, low-set and abnormal ears	Stillbirth, abnormal placenta, hydrops fetalis, contractures of large joints, other elbow and wrist deformities, horseshoe kidney, hydrocephalus, encephalocele
Laryngeal web, congenital heart disease	4156	AD	Laryngeal web, subglottic stenosis, abnormal cry	Short stature, heart defect
Laryngotracheoesophageal cleft, unilateral pulmonary hypoplasia	4341		Laryngotracheoesophageal cleft, tracheoesophageal fistula, partial tracheal agenesis, micrognathia, microstomia, low-set ears	Abnormal rib structures, vertebral anomalies, heart defect, hypoplastic lung, pancreas/spleen abnormality
MR, hypopituitarism, distal arthrogryposis	208080 4799	AR	Square face, midface hypoplasia, short nose, depressed bridge, anteverted nostrils, micrognathia, prominent ears, laryngeal abnormality	Failure to thrive, frontal bossing, ridged metopic sutures, delayed skeletal maturation, ulnar deviation of fingers, contractures, hypopituitarism, hydrocephalus, severe MR

TABLE 21-3. *Syndromes and Conditions Associated With Congenital Anomalies of the Larynx* [91] *(Continues)*

Syndrome or condition	MIM No. POSSUM No.[A]	Inheritance[B]	Ear, nose, and throat manifestations	Other manifestations
Metaphyseal chondrodysplasia, Kaitila type	250230 4064	AR	Tracheobronchomalacia, thickened gingivae, broad alveolar ridge	Thoracolumbar kyphosis, sciolosis, hypermobile joints, cone-shaped apiphyses, brachydactyly, pectus deformity (progressive)
Metaphyseal chondrodystrophy, Sussman type	4197	AR	Midface hypoplasia, laryngeal/tracheal abnormality	Short stature, short limbs, blue sclerae, cardiomyopathy, vertebral segmentation defects, spindle-shaped fingers
Multiple congenital anomalies, Hood-Hartwell type	4797		Laryngeal atresia, micrognathia, beaked nose, short philtrum, abnormal helix	Hypertelorism, delayed skeletal maturation, hypoplastic lungs, hypoplastic kidneys, ureteric reflux
Omphalocele, larynx/pharynx hypoplasia	182210 4022	AR	Broad nasal bridge, abnormal columella, down-turned mouth angles, thin lips, abnormal cry, pharyngeal and laryngeal hypoplasia	High-arched eyebrows, hypertelorism, scoliosis, omphalocele, hypotonia, MR
Opitz-Frias syndrome, G syndrome, or Opitz oculo-genital-laryngeal syndrome, type 2	*145410 3239	AD XLD	Broad nasal bridge, anteverted nostrils, cleft palate, posteriorly angulated ears, micrognathia, dysphagia, laryngeal abnormality	Hypertelorism, hypospadias, scrotal/anal anomalies (in the spectrum of BBBG syndrome)
Pachyonychia congenita or Jadassohn-Lewandowsky syndrome	*167200 4181	AD AR	Dysphonia secondary to thickening of the posterior commissure of the larynx, deafness (conductive), oral leukoplakia, natal teeth	Onycholysis, thickened nails, palmoplantar hyperkeratosis, cutaneous cysts, corneal leukokeratosis

TABLE 21-3. *Syndromes and Conditions Associated With Congenital Anomalies of the Larynx* [91] *(Continues)*

Syndrome or condition	MIM No. POSSUM No.[A]	Inheritance[B]	Ear, nose, and throat manifestations	Other manifestations
Shy-Drager syndrome	146500 4664	AR	Vocal fold paralysis, speech defect	Decreased sweating, irregular respiration, hypotension, bowel and bladder incontinence, psychosis, tremor with no intellectual deterioration
Smith-Lemli-Opitz syndrome, type 2	*268670 3645		Micrognathia, tented upper lip, short philtrum, cleft or high-arched palate, glossoptosis, low-set ears, short webbed neck, dysphagia, laryngeal abnormality	Short limbs, polydactyly, syndactyly, overlapping fingers, dislocated hip, heart defects, ambiguous genitalia, dysplastic kidneys, unilobular lungs, abnormal pancreas, agenesis of corpus callosum, MR
Thoraco-laryngo-pelvic dysplasia or thoracopelvic dysostosis	187770 3606	AD	Laryngeal hypoplasia	Respiratory distress, short stature, pectus deformity, short ribs, short round ilium, shallow sciatic notch, hypoplastic lungs
Toriello-Carey syndrome or Pallister syndrome	217980 4568	AR	Short nose, anteverted nostrils, cleft palate, glossoptosis, low-set ears, posteriorly angulated ears, sensorineural deafness, short neck, laryngeal abnormality	Microcephaly, agenesis of corpus callosum, short palpebral fissures, telecanthus, inguinal hernia, hypospadias, cryptorchidism, small hands, clinodactyly of 5th finger, heart defect, hypotonia (early death)
Tracheal agenesis association	2849		Laryngeal atresia, abnormal esophagus, tracheal agenesis	Limb deficiencies, wide carrying angle of elbow, abnormal palmar dermatoglyphics, hypoplastic thumbs, lung segmental defects, duodenal atresia, imperforate anus

TABLE 21-3. *Syndromes and Conditions Associated With Congenital Anomalies of the Larynx* [91] *(Continues)*

Syndrome or condition	MIM No. POSSUM No.[A]	Inheritance[B]	Ear, nose, and throat manifestations	Other manifestations
Ulnar-mammary syndrome of Pallister	*181450 *3420*	AD	Facial asymmetry, jaw abnormality, cleft soft palate, laryngeal abnormality	Asymmetric hypoplasia of ulnar rays, breast hypoplasia, scoliosis, small penis, cryptorchidism, apparent absence of sweat glands, imperforate hymen, pyloric stenosis
Urbach-Weithe syndrome, lipoid proteinosis, or hyalinosis cutis et mucosae	*247100 *4830*	AR	Macroglossia, yellow infiltration of larynx, hoarseness of voice, tracheal abnormality	Subcutaneous yellow nodules, increased skin pigmentation, intracranial calcification, seizures, hyperlipidemia
Velo-cardio-facial syndrome or Shprintzen syndrome	#192430 *3132*	AD	High nasal bridge, cleft palate (often submucous), micrognathia, microtia, conductive deafness, nasal speech, laryngeal abnormality	Short stature, microcephaly, heart defects, ocular abnormalities, thymic aplasia, MR

[A]MIM: **M**endelian **I**nheritance in **M**an. A Catalog of Human Genes and Genetic Disorders, by Victor A. McKusik, 11th ed, The Johns Hopkins University Press, Baltimore, MD, 1994. **POSSUM**: **P**icture **o**f **S**tandard **S**yndromes and **U**ndiagnosed **M**alformations, by Agnes Bankier et al., Murdoch Institute, Royal Children's Hospital, Victoria, Australia.

[B]AD: autosomal dominant; AR: autosomal recessive, XLD: X-linked dominant, XLR: X-linked recessive

* Confirmed gene and inheritance

Phenotype that can be caused by mutation in any of 2 or more genes.

MR: Mental retardation

TABLE 21-3. *Syndromes and Conditions Associated With Congenital Anomalies of the Larynx 91*

The chapter also incudes other less common congenital laryngeal anomalies such as laryngotracheoesophageal clefts (LTEC), laryngeal atresia, cysts, and lymphangiomas, as well as a comprehensive table (Table 21-3) of congenital syndromes and conditions associated with laryngeal anomalies.

ACKNOWLEDGMENT

The authors would like to thank Dr. J. Paul Willging of Cincinnati for contributing the photographs to this chapter.

REFERENCES

1. Batsakis JG. *Tumors of the Head and Neck—Clinical and Pathological Considerations.* 2nd ed. Baltimore, MD: Williams & Wilkins; 1979:220-221.

2. Leung AK, Cho H. Diagnosis of stridor in children. *Am Fam Physician.* 1999;60:2289-2296.

3. Holinger PH, Brown WT. Congenital webs, cysts, laryngoceles and other anomalies of the larynx. *Ann Otol Rhinol Laryngol.* 1967;76:744-752.

4. Willging JP, Cotton RT. Congenital anomalies of the larynx. In: Tewfik TL, Der Kaloustian VM, eds. *Congenital Anomalies of the Ear, Nose, and Throat.* New York, NY: Oxford University Press; 1997:383.

5. Belmont JR, Grundfast K. Congenital laryngeal stridor (laryngomalacia): etiologic factors and associated disorders. *Ann Otol Rhinol Laryngol.* 1984;93:430-437.

6. Shulman JB, Hollister DW, Thibeault DW, Krugman ME. Familial laryngomalacia—a case report. *Laryngoscope.* 1976;86:84-91.

7. Keleman G. Congenital laryngeal stridor. *Arch Otolaryngol.* 1953;58:245-248.

8. Martin JA. Congenital laryngeal stridor. *J Laryngol Otol.* 1963;77:290-294.

9. Grundfast KM, Harley E. Vocal cord paralysis. *Otolaryngol Clin North Am.* 1989;2:569-597.

10. Zalzal GH, Anon JB, Cotton RT. Epiglottoplasty for the treatment of laryngomalacia. *Ann Otol Rhinol Laryngol.* 1987;96:72-76.

11. Gianonni C, Sulek M, Friedman EM, Duncan NO 3rd Gastroesophageal reflux association with laryngomalacia: a prospective study. *Int J Pediatr Otorhinolaryngol.* 1998;43:11-20.

12. Chen JC, Holinger LD. Congenital laryngeal lesions: pathology study using several microsections and review of the literature. *Pediatr Pathol.* 1994;14:301-325.

13. Shah UK, Wetmore RF. Laryngomalacia: a proposed classification form. *Int J Pediatr Otorhinolaryngol.* 1998;46:21-26.

14. Friedman EM, Williams M, Healy GB, McGill TG. Pediatric endoscopy: a review of 616 cases. *Ann Otol Rhinol Laryngol.* 1984;93:517-519.

15. Holinger PH. Clinical aspects of congenital anomalies of the larynx, trachea, bronchi and esophagus. *J Laryngol Otol.* 1961;75:1-18.

16. Matthews BL, Little JP, McGuirt WF Jr, Koufman JA. Reflux in infants with laryngomalacia: results of 24-hour double-probe pH monitoring. *Otolaryngol Head Neck Surg.* 1999;120:860-864.

17. Iyer VK, Pearman K, Raafat F. Laryngeal mucosal histology in laryngomalacia: the evidence for gastro-oesophageal reflux laryngitis. *Int J Pediatr Otorhinolaryngol.* 1999;49:225-230.

18. Clinical Pharmacology. In: Gold Standard Multimedia. Available at: http://www.gsm.com. Accessed July 31, 2000.

19. Sichel JY, Dangoor E, Eliashar R, Halperin D. Management of congenital laryngeal malformations. *Am J Otolaryngol.* 2000;21:22-30.

20. Kelly SM, Gray SD. Unilateral supraglottic epiglottoplasty for severe laryngomalacia. *Arch Otolaryngol Head Neck Surg.* 1995;121:1351-1354.

21. Fearon B, Ellis D. The management of long term airway problems in infants and children. *Ann Otol Rhinol Laryngol.* 1971;80:669-677.

22. Friedman EM, Vastola P, McGill TJ. Chronic pediatric stridor: etiology and outcome. *Laryngoscope.* 1990;100:277-280.

23. Cotton RT, Prescott AJ. Congenital anomalies of the larynx. In: Cotton RT, Myers CM III, eds. *Practical Pediatric Otolaryngology.* Philadelphia, PA: Lippincott-Raven; 1998:497-513.

24. Hughes CA, Dunham ME. Congenital anomalies of the larynx and trachea. In: Westmore RF, Muntz HR, McGill TJ, eds. *Pediatric Otolaryngology.* New York, NY: Thieme Publications; 2000:778.

25. Holinger LD. Etiology of stridor in the neonate, infant and child. *Ann Otol Rhinol Laryngol.* 1980;89:397-400.

26. Cohen SR, Geller KA, Burns JW, Thompson JW. Laryngeal paralysis in children: long-term retrospective study. *Ann Otol Rhinol Laryngol.* 1982;9:417-424.

27. Gentile RD, Miller RH, Woodson GE. Vocal cord paralysis in children 1 year of age or younger. *Ann Otol Rhinol Laryngol.* 1986;95:622-625.

28. Rosin DF, Handler SD, Potsic WP, et al. Vocal cord paralysis in children. *Laryngoscope.* 1990;100: 1174-1179.

29. Holinger LD, Holinger PC, Holinger PH. Etiology of bilateral abductor vocal cord paralysis. *Ann Otol Rhinol Laryngol.* 1976;85:428-436.

30. Ferguson CF. Congenital abnormalities of the infant larynx. *Otolaryngol Clin North Am.* 1970;3:185-200,

31. McGill TJ, Healy GB. Congenital and acquired lesions of the infant larynx. A refresher survey. *Clin Pediatr.* 1978;17:584-589.

32. Takamatsu I. Bilateral vocal cord paralysis in children. *Nippon Jibiinkoka Gakkai Kacho* [Journal of the Oto-rhino-laryngological Society of Japan]. 1996;99:91-102.

33. Friedman EM. Role of ultrasound in the assessment of vocal cord functions in infants and children. *Ann Otol Rhinol Laryngol.* 1997;106:199-209.

34. Berkowitz RG. Laryngeal electromyography findings in idiopathic congenital bilateral vocal cord paralysis. *Ann Otol Rhinol Laryngol.* 1996;105: 207-212.

35. Bower CM, Choi SS, Cotton RT. Arytenoidectomy in children. *Ann Otol Rhinol Laryngol.* 1994;103:271-278.

36. Kirchner FR. Endoscopic lateralization of the vocal cord in abductor paralysis of the larynx. *Laryngoscope.* 1979;89:1779-1783.

37. Narcy P, Contencin P, Viala P. Surgical treatment of laryngeal paralysis in infants and children. *Ann Otol Rhinol Laryngol.* 1990;99:124-128.

38. Tucker GF, Osoff RH, Newman AN, Holinger LD. Histopathology of congenital subglottic stenosis. *Laryngoscope.* 1979;89:866-877.

39. Tucker JA, O'Rahilly R. Observations on the embryology of the human larynx. *Ann Otol Rhinol Laryngol.* 1986;95:336-347.

40. Smith RJ, Catlin FI. Congenital anomalies of the larynx. *Am J Dis Child.* 1984;138:35-39.

41. Holinger LD, Oppenheimer RW. Congenital subglottic stenosis: the elliptical cricoid cartilage. *Ann Otol Rhinol Laryngol.* 1989;98:702-706.

42. Holinger LD. Histopathology of subglottic stenosis. *Ann Otol Rhinol Laryngol.* 1999;108:101-111.

43. Healy GB. Subglottic stenosis. *Otolaryngol Clin North Am.* 1989;22:599-606.

44. Fearon B, Crysdale WS, Bird R. Subglottic stenosis in the infant and child: methods and management. *Ann Otol Rhinol Laryngol.* 1978;87:645-648.

45. Myer CM III, O'Connor DM, Cotton RT. Proposed grading system for subglottic stenosis based on endotracheal tube sizes. *Ann Otol Rhinol Laryngol.* 1994;103:319-323.

46. Dunbar JS. Upper respiratory tract obstruction in infants and children. *Am J Roentgen.* 1970;109:227-246.

47. Holinger PH, Kutnick SL, Schild JA, Holinger LD. Subglottic stenosis in infants and children. *Ann Otol Rhinol Laryngol.* 1976;85:591-599.

48. Holinger LD, Stankiewicz JA, Livingstone GL. Anterior cricoid split: the Chicago experience with an alternative to tracheotomy. *Laryngoscope.* 1987;97:19-24.

49. Rosenfeld RM, Bluestone CD. Does early expansion surgery have a role in the management of congenital subglottic stenosis? *Laryngoscope.* 1993;103:286-290.

50. Cotton RT: Prevention and management of laryngeal stenosis in infants and children. *J Pediatr Surg.* 1985;20:845-851.

51. Benjamin B, Carter P. Congenital laryngeal hemangioma. *Ann Otol Rhinol Laryngol.* 1983;92:448-455.

52. Brodsky L, Yoshpe N, Ruben RJ. Clinico-pathological correlates of congenital subglottic hemangiomas. *Ann Otol Rhinol Laryngol.* 1983;105 (suppl):4-18.

53. Pitanguy I, Caldeira AM, Calixto CA, Alexandrino A. Clinical evaluation and surgical treatment of hemangiomata. *Head Neck Surg.* 1984;7:47-59.

54. Riding K. Subglottic hemangioma. a practical approach. *J Otolaryngol.* 1992;21:419-421.

55. Healy GB, Fearon B, French R, McGill T. Treatment of subglottic hemangioma with carbon dioxide laser. *Laryngoscope.* 1980;90:809-813.

56. Cotton RT, Tewfik TL. Laryngeal stenosis following carbon dioxide laser in subglottic hemangioma. Report of three cases. *Ann Otol Rhinol Laryngol.* 1985;94:494-497.

57. Seid AB, Pransky SM, Kearnes DB. The open surgical approach to subglottic hemangioma. *Int J Pediatr Otorhinolaryngol.* 1993;26:95-96.

58. Hawkins DB, Crockett DM, Kahlstrom EJ, MacLaughlin EF. Corticosteroid mangement of airway hemangiomas: long-term follow-up. *Laryngoscope*. 1984;94:633-637.

59. Cohen SR, Wang CI. Steroid treatment of hemangioma of the head and neck in children. *Ann Otol Rhinol Laryngol*. 1972;81:584-590.

60. Hoeve LJ, Kuppers GL, Verwoerd CD. Management of infantile subglottic hemangioma: laser vaporization, submucus resection, intubation, or intralesional steroids? *Int J Pediatr Otorhinolaryngol*. 1997;42:179-186.

61. Davidoff AM, Filston HC. Treatment of infantile subglottic hemangioma with electrocautery. *J Pediatr Surg*. 1992;27:436-439.

62. Ohlms LA, Jones DT, McGill TJ, Healy GB. Interferon alpha-2a therapy for airway hemangiomas. *Ann Otol Rhinol Laryngol*. 1994;103:1-8.

63. Healy G: Treatment of subglottic hemangioma with the carbon dioxide laser. *Laryngoscope*. 1980;90:809-813.

64. Fisher JM. Cancer in the irradiated thyroid. *N Engl J Med*. 1975;292:975-977.

65. Konior RJ, Holinger L, Russell EJ. Superselective embolization of laryngeal hemangioma. *Laryngoscope*. 1988;98:830-834.

66. Hughes CA, Rezaee A, Ludemann JP, Holinger LD. Management of congenital subglottic hemangioma. *J Otolaryngol*. 1999;28:223-228.

67. Cohen SR. Congenital glottic webs in children. A retrospective review of 51 patients. *Ann Otol Rhinol Laryngol (suppl)*. 1985;121:2-16.

68. McHugh H, Loch J. Congenital webs of the larynx. *Laryngoscope*. 1942;52:43.

69. Benjamin B, Mair EA. Congenital interarytenoid web. *Arch Otolaryngol Head Neck Surg*. 1991;117:1118-1121.

70. Benjamin B. Congenital laryngeal webs. *Ann Otol Rhinol Laryngol*. 1983;92:317-326.

71. McGill T. Congenital diseases of the larynx. *Otolaryngol Clin North Am*. 1984;17:57-62.

72. Evans JNG. Management of the cleft larynx and tracheoesophageal clefts. *Ann Otol Rhinol Laryngol*. 1985;94:627-630.

73. Benjamin B, Inglis A. Minor congenital laryngeal clefts: diagnosis and classification. *Ann Otol Rhinol Laryngol*. 1989;98:417-420.

74. Moungthong G, Holinger LD. Laryngotracheoesophageal clefts. *Ann Otol Rhinol Laryngol*. 1997;106:1002-1011.

75. Gatti W, MacDonald E, Orfei E. Congenital laryngeal atresia. *Laryngoscope*. 1987;97:966-969.

76. Okada T, Ohnuma N, Tanabe M, et al. Long-term survival in a patient with congenital laryngeal atresia and multiple malformations. *Pediatr Surg Int*. 1998;13:521-523.

77. Kalache KD, Franz M, Chaoui R, Bollman R. Ultrasound measurements of the diameter of the fetal trachea, larynx and pharynx throughout gestation: applicability to prenatal diagnosis of obstructive anomalies of the upper respiratory digestive tract. *Prenat Diagn*. 1999;19:211-218.

78. Watson WJ, Thorp JM Jr, Miller RC, et al. Prenatal diagnosis of laryngeal atresia. *Ann J Obstet Gynecol*. 1990;163:1456-1457.

79. Cohen MS, Rothschild MA, Moscoso J, et al. Perinatal management of unanticipated congenital laryngeal atresia. *Arch Otolaryngol Head Neck Surg*. 1998;124:1368-1371.

80. DeSanto LW. Laryngocele, laryngeal mucocele, large saccules and laryngeal cassular cysts: a developmental spectrum. *Laryngoscope*. 1974;84:1291-1296.

81. Civantos FJ, Holinger LD. Laryngocele and saccular cysts in infants and children. *Arch Otolaryngol Head Neck Surg*. 1992;118:296-300.

82. Mitchell DB, Irwin BC, Bailey CM, Evans JN. Cysts of the infant larynx. *J Laryngol Otol*. 1987;101:833-837.

83. Canalis RF, Maxwell DS, Hemenway WG. Laryngocele—an updated review. *J Otolaryngol*. 1977;6:191-199.

84. Cohen SR, Thompson JW. Lymphangiomas of the larynx in infants and children: a survey of pediatric lymphangiomas. *Ann Otol Rhinol Laryngol (suppl)*. 1986;127:1-20.

85. Mikhail M, Kennedy R, Cramer B, Smith T. Sclerosing of recurrent lymphangioma using OK-432. *J Pediatr Surg*. 1995;30:1159-1160.

86. Kjaer I, Niebuhr E. Studies of the cranial base in 23 patients with cri-du-chat syndrome suggest a cranial developmental field involved in the condition. *Am J Med Genet*. 1999;82:6-14.

87. Benjamin B. Congenital disorders of the larynx. In: *Otolaryngology—Head and Neck Surgery*. 3rd ed. St. Louis, MO: Mosby; 1999:262-284.

88. Tewfik TL, Teebi AS, Der Kaloustian VM. Selected syndromes and conditions. In: Tewfik TL, Der Kaloustian VM, eds. *Congenital Anomalies of the Ear, Nose, and Throat.* New York, NY: Oxford University Press; 1997:460.

89. Cohen SR, Isaacs H. Otolaryngological manifestations of arthrogyposis multiplex congenita. *Ann Otol Rhinol Laryngol.* 1976;85:484-490.

90. Plott D. Congenital laryngeal abductor paralysis due to nucleus ambiguus dysgenesis in three brothers. *N Engl J Med.* 1964;271:593.

91. Tewfik TL, Teebi AS, Der Kaloustian VM. Syndromes and conditions associated with anomalies of the larynx and trachea. In: Tewfik TL, Der Kaloustian VM, eds. *Congenital Anomalies of the Ear, Nose, and Throat.* New York, NY: Oxford University Press; 1997:393-398.

CHAPTER 22

Voice Disorders in the Pediatric Population

Reza Rahbar, DMD, MD, FACS

Gerald B. Healy, MD

It is estimated that alteration of voice is present in up to 25% of the general pediatric population, and 6-40% of school-aged children.[1-3] Voice disorders can cause emotional and social handicaps because of unintelligible voice quality. Etiology is multifactorial; therefore, proper evaluation and understanding of vocal physiology, neurologic, systemic, inflammatory, and psychologic factors are required. Today, a multidisciplinary approach to the diagnosis and treatment of voice disorders is essential.

The purpose of this chapter is to present an overview of the developmental anatomy of the larynx, as well as selected voice disorders and their medical and surgical management in the pediatric population.

VOICE AND LARYNGEAL DEVELOPMENT

At birth the larynx is approximately one-third the size of that of an adult. The newborn larynx sits at the level of the third or fourth cervical vertebra and rises even higher with swallowing. The superior location of the larynx places the epiglottis at the level of the palate, which explains obligate nasal breathing during the first several months of life. The larynx gradually descends to the level of C6-C7 by the age of 15.[4] The hyoid bone and thyroid cartilage are not separated at birth but separate as the larynx descends in the neck. The epiglottis is furled, and the aryepiglottic folds are shorter than in the adult. The laryngeal introitus of newborns and children is T-shaped with a bulkier epiglottis and proportionately larger arytenoid cartilages. The adult vocal fold is formed by five distinct layers: mucosal epithelium; three layers of the lamina propria (superficial, intermediate, deep); and the thyroarytenoid or vocalis muscle.[5] However, the newborn lamina propria is formed in one layer, and there is no vocal ligament.[6] An immature vocal ligament is observed after 4 years of age. The length of the vocal fold at birth ranges from 6-8 mm and increases to 8-16 mm by adolescence.[4] The infant vocal fold is half membranous and half cartilaginous, whereas the adult vocal fold is three-fifths membranous and two-fifths cartilaginous. The fundamental frequency of the infant voice at birth is 400 to 500 Hz, and it is on average 286.5 Hz by age 7 years for both sexes.[7] At puberty, the male thyroid cartilage develops a 90-degree angle anteriorly, while the female cartilage remains at a 120-degree angle. As these changes take place, the fundamental frequency of male voice lowers more than that of the female. The average voice fundamental frequency for an adult female is about 210 Hz, and that of the adult male is 120 to 130 Hz.[8]

TERMINOLOGY AND CLASSIFICATION

Voice disorders can be divided into different categories. However, there is no consensus as to the terminology and classification systems. *Voice* refers to sounds produced by the vocal folds. *Speech* is the final outcome of sound from the larynx as it is modified by pharyngeal and oral cavity resonance. *Aphonia* is described as no recognizable laryngeal tone. *Dysphonia* is any abnormality in the quality of the voice (frequency, amplitude, phonation time, and resonance). *Congenital* airway lesions are present at birth and are manifest by an altered cry or respiratory distress. *Acquired* airway lesions are more likely to affect older children and are frequently recognized by alterations in the voice. *Psychogenic* voice disorders refer to any voice disorder without organic pathology, which presents as laryngeal muscle misuse with a psychoemotional etiology. *Functional* voice disorders refer to conditions primarily caused by incorrect vocal technique (resonatory, articulatory, phonatory).[4]

VOICE EVALUATION

Evaluation of the larynx is an essential part of the assessment of a child with a voice disorder. Flexible nasoendoscopy (available in size 3 mm or smaller) should be a routine part of the examination. It allows for the evaluation of laryngeal anatomy and vocal fold function, thus possibly determining the nature of dysphonia. The use of rigid endoscopes and stroboscopy (with flexible or rigid endoscopes) has been popularized in the past decade. This allows for obtaining quantitative and qualitative data on vocal fold function. Further evaluation may be undertaken by utilizing microlaryngoscopy under general anesthesia, imaging including PA and lateral neck x-rays, ultrasound, computerized tomography (CT) or magnetic resonance imaging (MRI) of the larynx, and objective analysis in a voice laboratory.

CONGENITAL VOICE DISORDERS

Congenital laryngeal disorders are covered in greater detail in Chapter 21. Some of the more common disorders are reviewed briefly in this chapter to emphasize their clinical management.

Vocal Fold Paralysis

Vocal fold paralysis (VFP) may present at birth or in the first few months of life. It is the second most common laryngeal disorder in neonates.[2] The absence or decrease in vocal fold mobility can be unilateral or bilateral. It may present as dysphonia, feeding difficulty, and/or stridor.

Unilateral vocal fold paralysis is four times more common than bilateral, and is more likely to have a peripheral rather than a central cause. Impairment of the vagus nerve can occur anywhere along its course

from the brain through the neck, chest, and larynx. Left VFP is more common than right because of the longer course of the left recurrent laryngeal nerve (RLN). Unilateral paralysis usually presents with a weak cry, but an adequate airway. Causes of congenital unilateral vocal fold paralysis include birth trauma with stretch injury to the RLN (forceps, difficult or breech delivery), chest lesions (cardiac and great vessel abnormalities, mediastinal tumors or cysts), tracheal or bronchial malformations, infections, CNS malformations, congenital muscular disorders or idiopathic.[9]

Bilateral VFP generally presents with the vocal folds in the paramedian position. The airway is compromised because of inability to abduct the cords. The infant's voice and cry are generally normal, but stridor, retractions, and cyanosis frequently are present. Bilateral vocal fold paralysis usually has a central cause such as hydrocephalus, Arnold-Chiari malformation, or meningomyelocele.

Flexible laryngoscopy is currently the most commonly used method for the diagnosis of vocal fold paralysis. Ultrasonic evaluation of vocal fold mobility has also been described and is quite useful.[10] Several studies have reported that the natural history of vocal fold paralysis is toward spontaneous recovery.[11,12] The prognosis is better for unilateral, acquired, or right-sided paralysis. The overall recovery rate for congenital VFP is about 50%.[2]

Management of vocal fold paresis in children is controversial. Factors that should be considered include: etiology, unilateral or bilateral involvement, severity of the symptoms, and prognosis for recovery. Many surgical modalities have been proposed, and no single procedure is applicable to all cases. Surgical options include Gelfoam injection, fat injection, collagen injection, thyroplasty (vocal fold medialization or lateralization), arytenoidectomy, partial cordotomy, and reinnervation techniques (ansa hypoglossi, ansa-strap-nerve muscle pedicle implantation).

Laryngocele

A laryngocele is an abnormal dilatation of the saccule filled with air. It is rarely seen in the pediatric population. Anatomically it is divided into three groups depending on the extension of the cyst: 1) *Internal laryngocele:* located in the anterior ventricle and with extension superiorly and posteriorly to the false vocal fold, but remaining within the laryngeal framework; 2) *External laryngocele:* dilated cyst piercing through the thyrohyoid membrane with cephalad extension; 3) *Combined laryngocele:* has both internal and external components. Diagnosis is confirmed with endoscopy, and computerized tomography can be helpful. The most common surgical treatment includes endoscopic marsupialization or an external approach through a laryngofissure for complete removal.

Laryngeal Web

A laryngeal web is a membrane of variable thickness that is formed during the embryogenesis of laryngotracheal groove (Figure 22-1). A majority of laryngeal webs (75%) are located anteriorly at the level of the true vocal folds with a posterior glottic opening.[4] Webs are associated with hoarseness and a weak or absent cry. Cohen and colleagues (1982) reported the largest series of congenital glottic web, 51 patients over a 30-year period.[11] In this series, hoarseness was the most common presentation, and tracheotomy was required in 38% of cases with thick webs.

Treatment depends on the degree of the airway compromise, consistency, and thickness. A thin glottic web can be lysed endoscopically (scissors, or surgical laser) without the need for stenting. The authors have employed topical application of Mitomycin-C successfully to decrease the degree of scar formation and restenosis postoperatively. The management of thick glottic web is more challenging. The surgical method utilized (endoscopic, laryngofissure with stenting, temporary tracheotomy) and time of surgery should be individualized.

Ductal Cysts

Ductal cysts or retention cysts may occur anywhere in the larynx (Figure 22-2). Patients often present with hoarseness and weak cry. The etiology is unknown, but is thought to be caused by local irritation causing obstruction of the submucosal glands and their dilated collecting ducts. They may also present in the subglottic

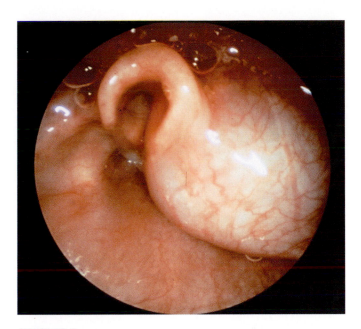

FIGURE 22-2. *Supraglottic congenital laryngeal cyst.*

area secondary to intubation trauma. Surgical treatment includes endoscopic removal with forceps or laser.

Saccular Cysts

Saccular cysts arise as a result of obstruction of the saccular orifice. They are fluid-filled and lack communication with the airway. Airway obstruction may occur intermittently as the cyst impedes upon the airway lumen, or may be continuous with ongoing inspiratory stridor. Saccular cysts are divided into two groups: 1) *Anterior saccular cysts:* located between the false and true vocal folds; 2) *Lateral saccular cysts:* extending into the false vocal fold and aryepiglottic fold. Diagnosis is made by flexible fiberoptic laryngoscopy or direct laryngoscopy. Initial treatment is usually by surgical laser vaporization of the cyst and its contents or by resection with "cold" instruments. Endoscopic or external excision may be required in recurrent cases.

Laryngeal Hemangioma

Laryngeal hemangioma most commonly presents in the subglottic area. Cutaneous hemangiomas are found in 50% of patients with airway hemangiomas.[13] The most common presenting symptoms include progressive biphasic stridor, barking cough, and hoarseness. The natural history is one of growth over the first 6 to 18 months of life, followed by gradual regression. Diagnosis is confirmed by endoscopy, and biopsy is generally not indicated because of the risk of bleeding. Treatment is based on the symptoms and includes observation, steroids (systemic or injection), surgical laser excision,

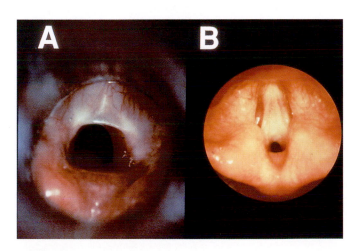

FIGURE 22-1. *(A) Thin glottic web. (B) Thick glottic web.*

open surgical excision, systemic interferon, and in some cases, tracheotomy.[13-15]

Laryngeal Cleft

A laryngeal cleft is caused by the failure of closure of the tracheoesophageal septum at approximately 35 days' gestation. Laryngeal clefts are divided into four types depending on their extent: *Type I* is confined to the interarytenoid space above the level of the vocal folds; *Type II* represents a partial cricoid cleft; *Types III and IV* transverse the cricoid completely and extend through various levels of the trachea down to the carina (Figure 22-3). Alternative classifications are also used (see Chapter 21).

It is a rare anomaly, most commonly presenting with stridor and/or aspiration. Respiratory distress and cyanosis are usually precipitated by feeding. Diagnosis is confirmed with endoscopy, but barium swallow is also an important diagnostic tool. The first line of management for a small laryngeal cleft is thickening of the feeding. Small clefts with persistent aspiration can be repaired endoscopically or through a laryngofissure. Laryngeal clefts with extension to the trachea usually require a combination of transcervical and thoracotomy approach, and large clefts may require emergency management.

ACQUIRE VOICE DISORDERS

Vocal Fold Nodules

The most common cause of voice disorders in children is vocal fold nodules. It is estimated that more than one million children in the United States have vocal fold nodules, with the lesion being more common in boys than girls.[2] Nodules are often associated with behavioral problems, family conflict, or aggressive behavior. Vocal fold nodules occur from overuse and/or misuse of the larynx causing mechanical trauma of the vocal fold mucosa at the point of maximum impact. Patients present with hoarseness, throat clearing, or cough. There is no dependable correlation between the size of the nodule and the degree of dysphonia.[16] They are often bilateral and located at the junction of the anterior one-third and the posterior two-thirds of the vocal fold. Nodules may appear rounded or fusiform. A fusiform or spindle-shaped thickening is more commonly seen in children, whereas discrete nodules are more common in adults (Figure 22-4).

The diagnosis of vocal fold nodules is made by flexible or rigid laryngoscopy, and videostroboscopy should be performed to help differentiate nodules from cysts and other lesions. Treatment modalities depend on the age of the patient, symptoms, level of cooperation to undergo voice therapy, and the size and firmness of the nodules. It is difficult to assess the success rate of the different treatment modalities because of questions regarding accuracy of diagnosis and the lack of controlled studies and adequate follow-up. However, treatment in a young cooperative child is primarily conservative, focusing on behavior modification, relaxation techniques, and speech therapy. Surgical removal may be necessary if the nodules have become very hyalinized and fibrotic. The surgical method of choice is microlaryngeal dissection. Long-term results are generally good, and postoperative voice therapy is recommended.

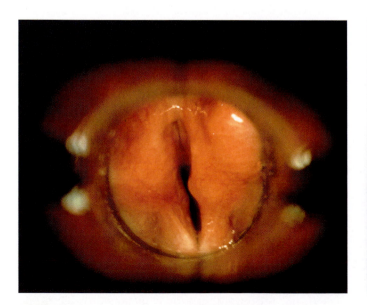

FIGURE 22-3. *Interarytenoid laryngeal cleft.*

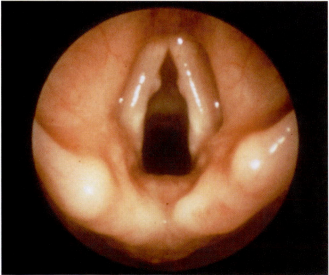

FIGURE 22-4. *Vocal fold nodules.*

Recurrent Respiratory Papillomatosis

Recurrent respiratory papillomatosis (RRP) is the most common benign neoplasm of the larynx. RRP is a therapeutic challenge because of the tendency to reoccur and spread to different areas of the airway. It is thought that the etiology is secondary to exposure to HPV during the birth process.[17,18] RRP most commonly presents in the upper and lower aspect of the ventricles, laryngeal surface of the epiglottis, and vocal folds. The trachea is the next most common site of involvement. The voice is characteristically low, harsh, breathy, or aphonic (Figure 22-5).

The diagnosis is usually made in infancy or early childhood with direct laryngoscopy and biopsy. Papillomas appear as an exophytic, pedunculated mass that may be single or multiple. The treatment of choice is microsuspension laryngoscopy with surgical laser or microforceps removal of the papillomas. The goal of surgery is to establish a stable airway and acceptable voice. Caution should be exercised so as not to cause web/scar in the anterior or posterior glottis.

A variety of medical therapeutic trials have been attempted to lower the high rate of recurrence in these patients. Several studies using interferon in association with CO_2 laser have shown a marked reduction of the disease or a decrease in the number of surgical procedures needed to control the airway.[19-21] Although there are no long-term results, adjunctive treatment with antiviral agents such as acyclovir, ribavirin, cidofovir, and photodynamic therapy have also been advocated.

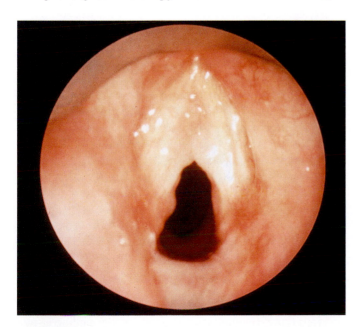

FIGURE 22-5. *Laryngeal papillomas, symmetrically involving both true vocal cords.*

Laryngeal Polyps

Unlike vocal fold nodules, polyps in children are usually unilateral and may be sessile or pedunculated. In many cases, they are thought to be caused by vocal abuse and straining leading to vocal fold edema, hemorrhage, and polypoid changes. They can present with hoarseness, intermittent voice changes, inability to sustain a tone, and breathiness. Voice therapy is always recommended, and laser or microdissection have both been advocated for their removal.

Laryngeal Granuloma

Laryngeal granuloma usually presents secondary to traumatic intubation, prolonged intubation, and/or reflux esophagitis. These children present with hoarseness and habitual throat clearing. Biopsy will show nonspecific granulation tissue covered with hyperplastic squamous epithelium.[22] The primary treatment is management of the underlying gastroesophageal reflux disease. Adjunctive voice therapy is recommended. Surgical management with the laser or microlaryngeal dissection is reserved for lesions not responding to medical treatment or those causing airway obstruction.

ABNORMAL RESONANCE AND VOICE DISORDERS

The cause of abnormal voice quality can be lack of proper resonance after production of a normal voice at the glottic level. These disorders are common in children and can be divided into two broad categories of *hyponasality* and *hypernasality*. Proper diagnosis can be difficult by listening alone and might require further evaluation by an experienced speech-language pathologist. In general, closing the child's nose during speech may help to distinguish between these two categories. If speech improves, the underlying defect is *hypernasality*, and if no change is noted, the problem is *hyponasality*.

Hyponasality is caused by obstruction of the nasal cavity, most commonly from adenoid hypertrophy. This results from a lack of nasal sounds *n, m, ng*. Other causes resulting in anterior or posterior nasal obstruction are turbinate hypertrophy, allergies, sinusitis, septal deviation, choanal stenosis, and tumors of the nose and nasopharynx. The goal of treatment is the resolution of nasal obstruction medically or surgically.

Hypernasality is associated with audible escape of air from the nose during speech production caused by velopharyngeal insufficiency (VPI). Multiple factors such as the velopharyngeal sphincter, adenoid size, and status of the soft palate musculature affect the quality of the speech. Nasal sounds such as *m, n, ng* are produced with the VP sphincter open. However, nonnasal sounds require a varying degree of VP closure. It is estimated that a sphincter gap of more than 0.2 cm^2 can result in VPI. This results in excessive air escape through the nose and the reduction of intraoral air pressure necessary for the production of consonants.[8]

The most common cause of hypernasality is cleft palate. The incidence of VPI even after cleft palate repair has been reported as high as 75%.[8] Velopharyngeal insufficiency can also present after adenoidectomy, and is estimated to occur in 1 in 1,500 cases.[8] Critical preoperative evaluation for conditions such as submucous cleft, occult submucous cleft palate, and a history of nasal regurgitation and hypernasality is of utmost importance to avoid postadenoidectomy VPI.

Speech therapy is the first line of treatment for hypernasality. Use of a prosthetic device and obturator is recommended to improve VP closure, provide some biofeedback, and improve the results of speech therapy. Surgical options for VPI include procedures such as pharyngeal flap and pharyngoplasty.[7,8]

IATROGENIC VOICE DISORDERS

Intubation Injury

The incidence of voice disorders in children following prolonged intubation is unknown. Traumatic and prolonged intubation can lead to a variety of glottic and subglottic injuries such as: cricoarytenoid fixation, arytenoid dislocation, vocal fold paralysis, glottic web formation, and subglottic stenosis (Figure 22-6). Internal trauma to the larynx by traumatic or prolonged intubation can cause pressure injury to the RLN as it enters the larynx at the cricothyroid joint, causing vocal fold paralysis. This must be differentiated from cricoarytenoid fixation and dislocation by direct palpation of the arytenoids during laryngoscopy.

At the glottic level, posterior glottic stenosis is the most common presentation of intubation injury. It has been classified into four different types: *Type I:* vocal process adhesion; *Type II:* interarytenoid scar; *Type III:* unilateral cricoarytenoid fixation with or without interarytenoid fixation; *Type IV:* bilateral cricoarytenoid fixation with or without interarytenoid fixation.[23]

Voice changes in these children range from hoarseness, breathiness, and lower fundamental frequency to aphonia. Evaluation includes flexible fiberoptic or rigid laryngoscopy, direct microlaryngoscopy and bronchoscopy, palpation of the arytenoids for mobility, and videostroboscopy in a cooperative child. Treatment includes endoscopic or external approaches to lyse the adhesions, vocal fold lateralization, or cartilage grafting to address the posterior glottic scarring leading to vocal

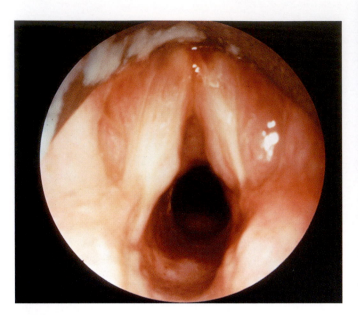

FIGURE 22-6. *Healed erosion at posterior commissure in former premature infant. Also note subglottic stenosis.*

fold fixation. Early institution of voice therapy is essential to maximize vocal function and to prevent acquisition of abusive compensatory speech habits.

Caustic Ingestion

Any history of caustic ingestion in a child requires a complete evaluation of the upper airway to rule out injuries to the areas of the oral cavity, hypopharynx, esophagus, and larynx. The site and severity of the injury varies based on the type and quantity of the caustic material. For example, crystal *Drano* most commonly affects the anterior oral cavity (lip, tongue), while *Liquid-Plummer* and *Plunge* mainly cause injury to the esophagus and stomach.[24] Laryngeal injuries are common with more severe caustic agents such as lye and acid ingestion. The method of injury in these agents involves mucosal coagulation necrosis presenting as burns in the area of the supraglottis and epiglottis.

These patients present with hoarseness or aphonia and respiratory distress. Initial management is stabilization of airway, most commonly requiring tracheotomy. Endoscopic laser excision or laryngofissure with or without stenting are the recommended procedures for the treatment of the glottic stenosis in these patients. The role of newer modalities such as Mitomycin-C remains unknown.

Laryngeal Trauma

Laryngeal trauma is uncommon in the pediatric age group because of the high position of the larynx in the neck (C3, C4). Also, the pediatric larynx is protected anteriorly by the inferior projection of the mandible, and posteriorly by the rigid cervical spine.[25] However, external trauma, either blunt or sharp, can cause laryngeal framework trauma and injury to the recurrent laryngeal nerve. This is most often seen in the pediatric population with motor vehicle accidents, clothes-line-type bicycle injuries, sports injuries, or gunshot wounds.

The management of the pediatric airway with a laryngeal trauma requires complete cooperation and coordination between the otolaryngologist, anesthesiologist, and other services involved. The risk and benefits of endotracheal intubation with regard to the stability of the airway and the possibility of further mucosal injury should be addressed. The option of awake, local tracheotomy in an uncooperative child with an unstable airway is not recommended. Establishment of a secure airway in these patients should be done under direct visualization with a rigid bronchoscope, and tracheotomy should be performed over the bronchoscope.

Surgical Trauma

Iatrogenic vocal fold paralysis (VFP) caused by surgical trauma is less common in the pediatric age group compared to adults. In general, any procedure in the thorax or neck (thyroid surgery; repair of tracheo-esophageal fistula; excision of neck mass: cervical teratoma, schwannoma, lymphatic malformation) may cause damage to the vagus or recurrent laryngeal nerve. In the pediatric population, cardiac and thoracic procedures are the most common cause of VFP. Zhar and Smith reported temporary or permanent vocal fold paralysis of 8.8% in children following ligation of patent ductus arteriosus.[26] Although unilateral VFP is the most common presentation, bilateral VFP often presents following surgical treatment of cerebellopontine angle or posterior fossa masses (meningioma, arachnoid cyst, astrocytoma, medulloblastoma).

The cry or voice characteristics of a traumatic vocal fold paralysis are the same as the congenital presentation. Unilateral vocal fold paralysis is manifested by a weak and breathy voice, whereas bilateral vocal fold paralysis may produce a breathy voice or more commonly a normal voice, but with respiratory compromise and stridor.

HORMONE INDUCED VOICE CHANGES

Androgen Deficiency

Normal pubertal voice changes in male and female adolescents are dependent on hormonal changes. For example, medical castration because of chemotherapy, radiation therapy, surgery, trauma, or hypophyseal hypogonadism prevents normal development and the secondary voice changes affected in a male adolescent. Hormone replacement and phonosurgery may be needed for improvement of the voice quality in these patients.

Hypothyroidism

Hypothyroidism occurs with increasing frequency throughout life. The prevalence of hypothyroidism is about one in 3,500 to 4,000 infants born in North America or Europe. It is six times more common in girls than boys. Hypothyroidism affects virtually every organ system. Children with congenital hypothyroidism (cretinism) present with severe mental and growth retardation. Voice disorders in these patients are common because of flaccidity and myxedematous infiltration of the laryngeal musculature.[27]

GENETIC DISORDERS AND SYNDROMES

Ehlers-Danlos Syndrome

The characteristic voice of infants with Ehlers-Danlos syndrome is low and monotonous.[28] This is thought to occur as a result of the overelasticity of the vocal ligament in these infants.

Plotts's Syndrome

It is a hereditary neuromuscular dysfunction of the larynx described by Plott in 1964.[29] Plotts's syndrome is X-linked and associated with mental retardation. It presents as a weak cry and breathy voice. Fiberoptic laryngoscopy confirms paralysis of the laryngeal abductors.

Cri du Chat Syndrome

This is a rare syndrome first reported by Lejeune in 1963.[7] It is caused by partial deletion of the short arm of chromosome 5. The affected infants have a characteristic high-pitched cry with long duration that resembles the mewing of a cat. The endolarynx is said to be elongated and curved with a floppy epiglottis. The fundamental frequency of these infants is an average of 860 Hz, whereas the average infant cry is 500 to 530 Hz.[7] Other associated anomalies in these infants include microcephaly, hypertelorism, micrognathia, low-set ears, oral clefts, and mental retardation.[30] In general, prognosis is poor.

Hurler's and Hunter's Syndromes

Hurler's and Hunter's syndromes are transmitted as an autosomal recessive trait, causing lipid storage disease (mucopolysaccharidosis). These patients present with hoarseness and vocal fatigue because of the deposition of metabolites in the larynx.

Von Recklinghausen Neurofibromatosis

Von Recklinghausen disease is an autosomal dominant with high penetrance. The most common site of presentation of neurofibromatosis in the airway is at the supraglottic and glottic levels. The most common presentation is hoarseness and dyspnea. Direct laryngoscopy and biopsy is needed to confirm the diagnosis. These lesions have a benign course, and treatment is based on the severity of symptoms, as well as the size and location of the lesion. Endoscopic excision is the treatment of choice for smaller lesions. An external approach (laryngofissure, or lateral pharyngotomy with lateral thyrotomy) may be needed for excision of larger lesions.

Craniofacial Abnormalities

Craniofacial dysmorphic features in patients with cleft lip and palate, Down's syndrome, Crouzon's syndrome, and others, may result in an alteration in voice quality interfering with intelligibility of speech. As the result of compensatory mechanisms, there is hyperadduction of the false vocal folds during the speech. These patients present with a rough and tense voice. Treatment must be individualized based on craniofacial dysmorphic features contributing to the problem, followed by speech therapy.

VOICE DISORDERS IN HEARING IMPAIRED CHILDREN

Development of normal speech and voice is dependent on normal auditory function and stimulation. Children with a hearing deficit may manifest voice disorders as early as 12 months of age. The type and severity of the voice disorder depends on the degree of hearing loss and lack of auditory stimulation. The voice of these children typically has a monotonous tone and higher mean fundamental frequency. Amplification (hearing aids, cochlear implant) and speech therapy are essential for improvement and the development of normal speech and voice quality.

PSYCHOGENIC VOICE DISORDERS

Stress-related voice disorders can present in children. The underlying psychologic problems are related to tensional symptoms, adjustment, personality, or anxiety disorders. The typical presentation is called *conversion aphonia,* in which the child presents with a whispered voice and loss of normal voice quality. Older children and adolescents can present with a more severe form of the voice abnormality called *functional vocal fold spasm;* only isolated case reports can be found in the literature.[31] These patients present with episodes of hoarseness associated with dyspnea resem-

bling laryngospasm or an asthma attack. They are often misdiagnosed as having spasmodic dysphonia, a condition that is extremely uncommon in children. Optimal management requires psychotherapy or psychologic counseling in conjunction with speech therapy.[32]

INFLAMMATORY LESIONS AND VOICE DISORDERS

Any inflammatory or infectious process can cause edema and erythema of the laryngeal mucosa. Depending on the etiology, systemic manifestation may be mild and voice changes with dysphonia may present as the only sign. Bacterial and viral infections are the most common form of inflammatory processes affecting the larynx. Fungal laryngitis can be seen in immunocompromised children or those on long-term inhaled steroids. The spectrum of disease and management are similar in children and adults and are covered elsewhere throughout this book.

LARYNGEAL NEOPLASM AND VOICE DISORDERS

Malignant tumors of the pediatric larynx are rare. The most common neoplasm in the pediatric age group is rhabdomyosarcoma. Other malignancies involving the larynx have also been reported, including squamous carcinoma, neuroectodermal tumor of infancy, lymphoma, and mucoepidermoid carcinoma.[33-35] Benign neoplasms include neurofibromas, hamartomas, adenomas, and chondromas. Hoarseness is the most common initial presentation of any laryngeal neoplasm. Respiratory distress and stridor are later manifestations as the tumor grows. Because of low suspicion, there is usually a delay in the diagnosis. Because of the aggressive nature of laryngeal malignancy in children, management often includes the combination of surgery, radiation, and chemotherapy, depending on the tumor histology and the stage of the disease.[34,35]

REFERENCES

1. Wilson DK. *Voice Problems of Children.* 3rd ed. Baltimore, MD: Williams & Wilkins; 1987.

2. Choi SS, Cotton RT. Surgical management of voice disorders. *Pediatr Clin North Am.* 1989;36:1535-1549.

3. Zajac DJ, Farkas Z. Dindzans LJ, et al. Aerodynamic and laryngographic assessment of pediatric vocal function. *Pediatr Pulmonol.* 1993;15:44-51.

4. Morrison M, Rammage L. *The Management of Voice Disorders.* London, England: Chapman and Hall Medical; 1994.

5. Hirano M, Bless DM. Videostroboscopic examination of the larynx. San Diego, CA: Whurr; 1993.

6. Pengilly AJ. Pediatric voice disorders. In: Cotton RT, Myer CM, III eds. In: *Practical Pediatric Otolaryngology.* Philadelphia, PA: Lippincott-Raven; 1999:75-95.

7. Aronson AE. *Clinical Voice Disorders, an Interdisciplinary Approach.* New York, NY: Thieme-Stratton; 1980:57-61.

8. Maddern BR, Campbell TF, Stool S. Pediatric voice disorders. *Otolaryngol Clin North Am.* 1991;24:1125-1140.

9. Scott-Brown WG. *Scott-Brown's Otolaryngology,* 5th ed. Evans JNG, ed. Vol 6. *Paediatric Otolaryngology.* London, England: Butterworth; 1987:412-419.

10. Friedman EM, Vastola AP, McGill TJ, et al. Chronic pediatric stridor: etiology and outcome. *Laryngoscope.* 1990;100:277-280.

11. Cohen SR, Geller KA, Birns JW, et al. Laryngeal paralysis in children: a long-term retrospective study. *Ann Otol Rhinol Laryngol.* 1982;91:417-424.

12. Emery PJ, Fearon B. Vocal cord palsy in pediatric practice: a review of 71 cases. *Int J Pediatr Otorhinolaryngol.* 1984;8:147-154.

13. Froehlich P, Stamm D, Floret D, et al. Management of subglottic hemangioma. *Clin Otolaryngol.* 1995;4:336-339.

14. Seid AB, Ransky SM, Kearns DB. The open surgical approach to subglottic hemangioma. *Int J Pediatr Otorhinolaryngol.* 1993;22:85-90.

15. MacArthur CJ, Senders CW, Katz J. The use of interferon Alpha-2A for life-threatening hemangioma. *Arch Otolaryngol Head Neck Surg.* 1995;121:690-693.

16. von Leden H. Vocal nodules in children. *Ear Nose Throat J.* 1985;64:29-41.

17. Quick CA, Krzyzed RA, Watts SL, et al. Relationship between condylomata and laryngeal papillomata: clinical and molecular virological evidence. *Ann Otol.* 1980;89:467-471.

18. Kashima HK, Kessis T, Mounts P, et al: Polymerase chain reaction identification of human papillomavirus DNA in CO_2 laser plume from recurrent respiratory papillomatosis. *Otolaryngol Head Neck Surg.* 1991;104:191-195.

19. Leventhal B, Kashima HK, Mounts P, et al. Long-term response of recurrent respiratory papillomatosis to treatment of lymphoblastoid interferon alpha-n1. *N Engl J Med.* 1991;325:613-617.

20. Healy GB, Gelber RD, Trowbridge AL, Grundfast KM, Ruben RJ, Price KN. Treatment of recurrent respiratory papillomatosis with human leukocyte interferon—results of a multicenter randomized clinical trial. *N Engl J Med.* 1988;319:401-407.

21. Lundquist PG, Haglund S, Carlson B, et al. Interferon therapy in juvenile laryngeal papillomatosis. *Otolaryngol Head Neck Surg.* 1984;92:386-391.

22. Benjamin B, Croxson G. Vocal nodules in children. *Ann Otol Rhinol Laryngol.* 1987;96:530-531.

23. Irving RM, Baily CM, Evans JNG. Posterior glottic stenosis in children. *Int J Pediatr Otorhinolaryngol.* 1993;28:11-23.

24. Holinger LD, Tucker GF. Jr Trauma. In: *Otolaryngology—Head and Neck Surgery.* 2nd ed. St. Louis, MO: Mosby-Year Book; 1993:2331-2338.

25. Brown PM, Schaefer SD. Laryngeal and esophageal trauma. In: *Otolaryngology—Head and Neck Surgery.* 2nd ed. St. Louis, MO: Mosby-Year Book; 1993:1864-1874.

26. Zhar RIS, Smith RJH. Vocal fold paralysis in infants twelve months of age and younger. *Otolaryngol Head Neck Surg.* 1996;114:18-21.

27. Cohen SR, Thompson JW, Geller KA, et al. Voice change in the pediatric patient. *Ann Otol Rhinol Laryngol.* 1983;92:437-443.

28. Scott-Brown WG. Scott-Brown's Otolaryngology. 5th ed. Stell PM, ed. Vol 5. *Laryngology.* London, England: Butterworth; 1987:119-144.

29. Plott D. Congenital laryngeal abductor paralysis due to nucleus ambiguus dysgenesis in three brothers. *N Engl J Med.* 1964;271:593-596.

30. Jones KI. *Smith's Recognizable Patterns of Human Malformation.* 4th ed. Philadephia, PA: Saunders Publishing; 1988:40-114.

31. Froese AP, Sims P. Functional dysphonia in adolescence: two case reports, *Can J Psychiatry.* 1987;32:389-391.

32. Morrison MD, Nichol H, Rammage LA. Diagnostic criteria in functional dysphonia. *Laryngoscope.* 1986;94:1-5.

33. Ohlms LA, McGill T, Healy GB. Malignant laryngeal tumors in children: a 15-year experience with four patients. *Ann Otol Rhinol Laryngol.* 1994;103:686-688.

34. Gindhart TD, Johnston WH, Chism SE, et
    al.Carcinoma of the larynx in childhood. *Cancer.*
    1980;46:1683-1687.

35. Mitchell DB, Humphreys S, Kearns DB.
    Mucoepidermoid carcinoma of the larynx in a
    child. *Int J Pediatr Otorhinolaryngol.* 1988;
    15:211-215.

CHAPTER 23

The Larynx: A Hormonal Target

Jean Abitbol, MD

Patrick Abitbol, MD

Endocrinology is a science, which started with voice. In 400 BC, Aristotle described the effect of castration on the songbird. Galen was the first to describe and to name the thyroid gland. It was another 1,500 years before Leonardo da Vinci began the study of the numerous endocrine organs. *De Humanis Corporis Fabrica*,[1] published in 1543, provided the first text on human anatomy and endocrine glands. The word "hormone" comes from the Greek *hormao*, which means to arouse.

Endocrinology is the study of the relationship between two cells via a molecule: the hormone. This molecule stimulates, via the bloodstream, a response in a distant organ. The methods of communication by messenger molecules from one cell to another are called:

- Autocrine: the molecule that has an impact on the cell where it has been synthesized

- Paracrine: the molecule that has an impact on the cells adjacent to the cell that has synthesized the molecule

- Endocrine: the molecule enters the bloodstream without any excretory channel

All hormonal activity needs a target organ or target cells with specific receptors. If their actions are limited in time, they may have an irreversible impact.

The mediators between the central nervous system and the glands are the supra-chiasmic nuclei and the hypothalamus with its indispensable partner, the pituitary gland. Hence, any information processed will have a wide range of responses adapted to physical and psychologic stimuli.[2] The principles of hormonal action are based on the understanding of the genome, and the concept of receptors, which can be located on the cell membrane or its nucleus.

GENOME

The primary function of the gene is to produce a specific protein. The hormones act as commander. The genome for a haploid eukaryotic cell consists of approximately 100,000 genes. The action of a hormone is mediated by specific receptors: either on the membrane of the cell, and/or on the nucleus. The expression of the gene depends on the receptors or more precisely, on the number of activated receptors.[3]

TWO KINDS OF RECEPTORS

Membrane receptors are not liposoluble. Leutinizing hormone (LH), follicle stimulating hormone (FSH), thyroid stimulating hormone (TSH), growth factors, and insulin activate them. These hormones stimulate a specific receptor, which follows a complex biomechanical chain of events leading to the formation of the mRNA via the transcription factor.[4]

Nuclear receptors. In order to act directly on the nucleus, hormones must be liposoluble to cross the cell membrane. They include steroid hormones, sex hormones, thyroid hormones, and active vitamin metabolites such as retinoids, vitamin A metabolites, and vitamin D. These hormones go through the cell membrane and activate directly the intracellular receptors in the nucleus. From then on, the hormone–gene journey is the same as for membrane receptors. It leads to the formation of the mRNA via the transcription factor.

ENDOCRINE ORGAN

There are 8 endocrine glands:

1. The *pituitary gland* is located in the sella turcica inside the sphenoid bone. It is divided in two parts: the anterior part or adenohypophysis that secretes FSH, LH, adrenocorticotrophic hormone (ACTH), growth hormone (GH), and the posterior part, which is a transmitter and a reserve for neurohormones.

2. The *pineal gland,* located at the junction of the cerebrum, the brain stem and the cerebellum, is fixed on the roof of the third ventricle. It is an appendage of the brain and secretes melatonin. It is an evolutionary relic of fish.

3. The *thyroid gland* is located in front of the trachea between the second and the fifth cartilage rings. It secretes the thyroxin hormones: T_3 and T_4.

4. The *parathyroid glands,* located at the posterior aspect of the thyroid gland, are 4 in number. They secrete parathormone.

5. The *adrenal gland* with the adrenal cortex and the adrenal medulla is located above the kidney. The adrenal cortex secretes mineralocorticoids, glucocorticoids, and androgens. The adrenal medulla, like the paraganglia, secretes catecholamines (adrenaline and noradrenaline) and dopamines.

6. The *thymus* is located in the upper part of the thorax, posterior to the sternum. It secretes the hormone thymosin.

7. The *pancreas* secretes glucagon and insulin.

8a. The *testicles* secrete androgens and 25% of the total daily production of 17β-estradiol (the remainder being derived by conversion of both testicular and adrenal androgens in peripheral tissues).

8b. The *ovaries* secrete estrogen (E), progesterone (P), and the androgen dehydro-epiandrosterone (DHEA).

The endocrine organs without glands are:

- The cerebrum for endorphins. The suprachiasmic nucleus (SCN), the gyrus, the hypothalamus, the posterior part of the hypophysis for endorphins, catecholamines, dopamines, and cytokines

- The epithelium of the digestive tract: the gastric epithelium for gastrin, secretin

- The kidney, the placenta, and heart: for renin–angiotensin

THE LARYNX IS A HORMONAL TARGET

The voice is at the crux of the psyche and the hormonal world. Voice mutation is controlled by sex hormones. The voice is changed by the hypothalamic–pituitary axis through its endocrine impact and, during everyday life, because of the hormones of the cerebrum. Emotional stress and the psyche may also provide the hormonal trigger to induce a change in voice production.

The common denominators of endocrine effects on laryngeal structures are numerous: The actions of estrogens and progesterone produce changes in the extravascular spaces and modification of glandular secretions; by the action of progesterone, there is modification of nerve transmission speed; by the action of androgen, hypertrophy or atrophy of striated muscles occurs as well as calcification of cartilages. The thyroid hormones also affect dynamic function of the vocal folds.

Sex Hormones and the Larynx

Does voice have a chromosomal sex? The voice changes with advancing years, with the scars of life, with its physical and emotional conditions, but the essential element that remains constant is that voice has a sex chromosome: XY for males, XX for females. However, this issue is not as clear-cut as it may appear. Consider the principal effects caused by the three main sex hormones, estrogen, progesterone and androgens.

Estrogen

Estrogens are present in women and at very low levels in men. They have a hypertrophic and proliferative effect on mucosa. They reduce the desquamating effect of the superficial layers and cause differentiation and complete maturation of fat cells. The degree of cytoplasmic acidophilia and of nuclear pyknosis, as noted in gynecologic cervical smears and in smears from the vocal folds, is a measure of this maturational effect. Estrogens have no effect on striated muscles. Their effects on cerebral tissue are well known. Among other things, they are theorized to reduce the risk of contracting Alzheimer's disease.[5]

Progesterone

As its name implies, this hormone promotes gestation and, thus, is only present in adult women with ovulatory cycles. The central action of estrogen is the modification of steroid hormone activity by affecting receptor concentration. Estrogen increases target tissue responsiveness to itself, to progesterone, and to androgens by increasing the concentration of its own receptors and that of the intracellular progesterone and androgen receptors. The effects of progesterone can be felt only if there has previously been estrogenic influence of the tissues.[6,7] The progesterone receptor is induced both by estrogen and progestin. Estrogen exerts its influence on the progesterone receptor gene.[8] Apparently, this is the only known case of hormonal harmony in the human organism, wherein the influence of estrogens is a prerequisite to allow the action of progesterone to take place, as only estrogens will trigger the possibility of action and of growth in the receptor sites of progesterone. Progesterone has an antiproliferative effect on mucosa and accelerates desquamation. Hence, there is no satisfactory cellular differentiation. In the authors' study on uterine cervical and vocal fold smears, the pathologist is not able to distinguish between the two samples. Basophil cells have been observed on both slides. Therefore, there is a menstrual-like cycle on the vocal fold epithelium. Furthermore, one can observe a drying-out of the mucosa with a reduction in secretions of the glandular epithelium. Progesterone has a diuretic effect by its action on sodium metabolism, which is opposed to that of aldosterone. Estrogen increases capillary permeability and allows the passage of intracapillary fluids to the interstitial space. Progesterone decreases capillary permeability, thus trapping the extracellular fluid out of the capillaries and causing tissue congestion. This congestion is quite apparent in the breasts, in the lower abdominal and pelvic tissues, as well as in the vocal folds, where it causes premenstrual dysphonia.

Some synthetic progestins, such as the derivatives of nortestosterone, have an androgenic effect caused by active metabolites. They have a masculinizing effect on the female voice. They should never be prescribed in voice professionals if there is any therapeutic alternative, as discussed below.

Androgens

Testosterone is the essential male hormone, secreted by the testis.[9] In women, androgens are secreted principally by the adrenal cortex and formed as derivatives of aldosterone, but they are also secreted by the *theca interna* of the ovaries. Studies have shown that androgens cause an increase in the female libido.[10-11] Furthermore, there is a masculinizing action when the concentration of testosterone is greater than 150 micrograms/dl.[12] Androgens are essential for male sexuality, but they cause in women an often-irreversible masculinizing effect at doses greater than 200 micrograms/dl. Man is the only primate with adrenal glands that secrete an important amount of dehydroepiandrosterone (DHEA), that is converted to androstenedione. In skin, these androgens cause acne, seborrhea, and hirsutism. In mucosa, they cause a loss of hydration with a reduction in glandular secretions. In muscles, they cause a hypertrophy of striated muscles with a reduction in the fat cells in skeletal muscles. There is also a reduction in the whole body fatty mass.[13] Anabolic steroids increase the volume and the power of the muscular mass, and may lead to definitive male voice, which may be an irreversible effect.

Puberty

The influence of sex hormones at puberty is modulated through the hypothalamus–pituitary axis. Puberty usually lasts from 2 to 5 years, and occurs between the ages of 12 to 17.

The passage from childhood to adulthood is marked by appearance of secondary sexual characteristics, as well as the physical and physiologic changes that are peculiar to each sex. The hypothalamo–hypophyseal pituitary axis and its testicular or ovarian response determine and influence the physical, psychic, and emotional sexuality of the person. In the Western world, the average age at which puberty begins is around 12 years for girls and 13 years for boys. In the girl, estrogen and progesterone secretion will lead to a woman's voice. In the boy, testosterone will yield a man's voice: a fundamental frequency one-third lower than a child's voice for the woman and an octave lower for the man; the pulmonary capacity, the cardiovascular apparatus, the level of hemoglobin, and the striated muscle mass all increase in man. Androgens are the most important hormones responsible for the passage of the boy-child voice to the man's voice, and their impact is irreversible. The thyroid prominence or Adam's apple appears, the vocal folds lengthen and become rounded, and the epithelium thickens with the formation of three distinct layers. The laryngeal mucus becomes more viscous. The arytenoids become bigger. The thyroarytenoid ligaments become thicker and more powerful. The anterior portion of the cricothyroid muscle broadens, becomes more resistant, and its contraction will permit a head voice. Closure of the cricothyroid space induces a forward tilt of the thyroid cartilage. The anterior commissure is thus brought downwards and backwards, thereby shifting the glottic plane from the horizontal. The horizontal projection of the vocal fold is therefore shortened, which may contribute to the ability to produce high notes.

The Castrato: A Pure Example of the Impact of Sex Hormone on Voice

In the fifteenth century the Roman Catholic Church wanted to have high pitched, feminine voices in the chapel choirs, but without any women. The ecclesiastic world followed scrupulously the maxim of St Paul, *"mulieres in ecclesiae taceant"* or *"women should not be heard in the Church."*[14] Castration, to keep the beauty of the feminine voice, was an eccentricity of the Church at that time, for which voice was more important than virility. To allow the castrato to have a feminine voice, the castration had to be performed before any sign of puberty, before any secretion of testosterone. Even at that time, the importance of the definitive and indelible hormonal influence of testosterone had been recognized. The castrato has a powerful crystalline voice with an exceptional register. It is an ambiguous voice. The voice comes from a body born XY, but one that has never been clothed by testosterone, and, hence, this voice does not have a male print.

Castrati had the external skeletal envelope of a male with a lung capacity of 5 liters. They also possessed the muscular abdominal and pelvic girdle necessary to sustain a male voice. This is caused by growth hormones, adrenal hormones, and thyroid hormones. Their resonating chambers were defined by a male-type bony architecture. However, the vocalis muscle is highly sensitive to the impact of male hormones, and in particular to the lack of androgens. They, therefore, keep their child-like characteristics. Vocal folds having kept a child-like configuration and being made to vibrate in a female register by the power of a man in a male skeletal environment define the quality of the voice. However, this is not the whole story. As in any musical instrument, there must exist a harmony between the two vocal folds vibrating one against the other, the power of the pulmonary bellows producing the sound energy, and the resonating chambers that allow the amplification and the coloring of the voice. This harmony is especially tenuous in the creation of an operatic castrato voice. This is why during the Renaissance many were called, but few chosen. According to written reports and to the one wax cylinder recording made in 1904, the castrato had a voice, with a range of 3 to 4 octaves. He could hold a note for some 120 seconds and could work his voice for up to 8 hours per day.[14]

THE FEMALE VOICE

In females, voice breaks are much less apparent. The female voice is not a child-like voice: it is 3 tones lower and has 5 to 12 formants, as opposed to the pediatric voice, which only has 3 to 6 formants. In females, there is little development of the thyroid cartilage or of the cricothyroid membrane. The vocal muscle thickens slightly, but remains very supple and quite narrow. The squamous mucosa also differentiates into three distinct layers on the free edge of the vocal folds. The sub- and supraglottic glandular mucosa becomes hormone-dependent to estrogens and progesterone. The ovaries start to work. The first menstrual cycles appear, at first rather irregularly and then regularly. The hormonal rhythm is also modulated through the hypothalamo–hypophyseal axis by the action of FSH and LH on the ovary. Menstrual cycles will continue for the next forty years. For each cycle, the follicular and the luteal phases are distinguishable and linked together by ovulation.[15] During the follicular phase, the secretion of estrogens increases progressively, activated by FSH between day 4 and day 8, and reaching a peak on day 13 of the cycle. LH reaches its peak on day 14, leading to ovulation. The egg is snapped up by the fallopian tube. The luteal phase allows the creation of a new endocrine gland: the corpus luteum, that secretes progesterone and estrogen.

The exocervical squamous mucosa has three layers: the lamina propria, and the chorion, with a basal and a parabasal membrane. The junction between the different cells is relatively large in the first part of the cycle and less so in the second phase. This intercellular space is therefore hormone-dependent (Figure 23-1). Its important effect on the human voice is discussed in the section on premenstrual voice syndrome. The endocervix has a glandular ciliated epithelium with serous and mucous glands which is also extremely hormone-dependent. Estrogens produce fluid mucus and progesterone produces thick mucus. At menopause, there is atrophy of the mucosa of the uterine cervix with relative conservation of the glandular secretions as long as there is continued secretion of estrogens. The presence of androgens causes a thickening of the cervical mucosa, a loss of its suppleness and sheen, as well as a drying-out of the sero-mucous glands. We observe the same effects in the larynx. The glandular cells are above and under the free edge of the vocal folds (Figure 23-2). In the ovary, the cells of the granulosa and of the theca interna secrete estrogens. Progesterone is secreted only by the corpus luteum, which disappears at menopause. Testosterone and its derivatives are produced by the cells of the theca interna and transported to the cells of

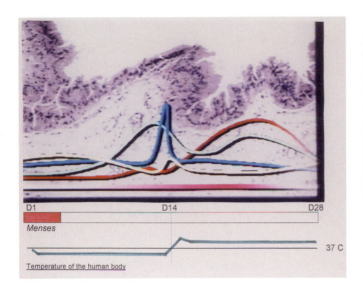

FIGURE 23-1. *Menstrual cycle displayed of FSH–LH–β–estradiol–progesterone.*

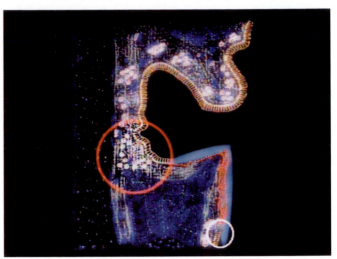

FIGURE 23-2. *Sagittal slide of the laryngeal structure: glandular cells above and under the vocal free edge.*

the granulosa, where they are changed to estradiol.[16] At menopause, and this is even more apparent as the ovaries have practically stopped producing estrogens, the androgen derivatives are changed to estrones in the fat cells by cytochrome P450.[17] Thus, the development of a masculine voice at menopause varies with each individual case and depends on each woman's hormonal profile.

The difference between the male and the female voice involves not only the hormonal effect on the muscle and the mucosa, but also the framework. The gender-related dimorphism of the thyroid cartilage results in significant differences of laryngeal framework dimensions. The post-pubertal thyroid cartilage angle in the male is 90°, and in the female 120°.[18]

The Premenstrual Syndrome (PMS)

Before discussing the premenstrual *"voice"* syndrome (PMVS), a review of the premenstrual syndrome is presented. Review of the extensive literature concerning this syndrome discloses many controversies.[19-23] Although more than 150 symptoms have been ascribed to PMS,[24] it is now agreed that the symptom constellation is rather specific and well defined. Between puberty and menopause, women experience a menstrual cycle averaging 28 days. Each menstrual cycle is determined by the hypothalamus–pituitary axis. Many factors may disturb this cycle: From emotion to hyperexercise, from diet to any illness, the perfect rotation of ovulation may be broken.[25-33]

The fetus at 5 months has 5 to 7 million follicles in the ovaries. At birth there are 2 million follicles, at puberty, 300,000 follicles, near menopause (around 48 years old), 15,000 follicles, and fewer than 1,000 follicles after menopause, at approximately age 55.[34] These follicles produce progesterone after ovulation takes place; it is secreted for 14 days during the second half of the cycle. The clinical aspects of premenstrual syndrome exhibit two environmental sets: the estrogen environment and the progesterone environment. Characteristic symptoms of the estrogen environment are breast tenderness, irritability, and reflux. Characteristic symptoms of the progesterone environment are depression and a decrease of menses. There may be mixed influences. Both of these environments could be associated with the premenstrual voice syndrome, but estrogens are usually involved. To be able to diagnose a premenstrual syndrome, the symptoms must appear 6 to 8 days prior to the onset of menstruation and disappear during or near the end of the menses. Symptoms can appear at menarche, with the first menstrual period, after a first pregnancy, or at other times. We have observed more cases after cessation of the use of an oral contraceptive pill. The key factor in explaining this syndrome is the change in the estrogen/progesterone (E/P) ratio. Vitamin and mineral deficiencies appear to be contributing factors, which may increase the hormonal imbalance, particularly magnesium, vitamin B6, vitamin A, and iron.[35-37] Generally speaking, clinical findings may include nervous tension, mood swings, irritability, and anxiety, associated with generalized edema. Dysphonia, weight gain, swelling of the legs, breast tenderness, and bloating also may occur. PMS can be associated with insulin impairment, headache, increased appetite, fatigue, and sometimes dizziness. These symptoms can be mixed in any individual. The estrogen/progesterone ratio is usually elevated, because of a very mild temporary estrogen excess and mild progesterone deficiency. It may be associated with a slight hypothyroidism, an adrenal dysfunction, and an endorphin impairment.[38] The physiologic basis of these symptoms is the impact of the estrogen and progesterone on the membrane of the cells and on the wall of the capillaries.

The estrogens increase the cellular permeability in one way; "it is a one-way street" from the intracellular to the extracellular space, and from the intracapillary to the extracapillary space.

Progesterone increases the cellular permeability both ways; "It is a two-way street." The flow goes from the intracellular to the extracellular space, from the intracapillary to the extracapillary space, and also from the extracellular to the intracellular space and from the extracapillary to the intracapillary space (Figure 23-3).

Flow from the intracellular space to the extracellular space and inside the lumen of the capillaries produces an optimal E/P ratio. There is almost no edema during this period of the cycle. However, if progesterone is lacking the E/P ratio is not optimal and flow will go only in one direction, by estrogen effect. The permeability of the same membrane is blocked in the way back. The liquid is trapped outside of the cell, in the extracellular space, creating edema. This may explain why more than 90% of Reinke's space edema is found in adult women, although tobacco is a major etiologic factor.[38]

The Premenstrual Voice Syndrome (PMVS)

The premenstrual voice syndrome has been recognized for centuries (Figure 23-4). It has been reported by female singers at La Scala de Milano, at the Opera Houses of Vienna and of Salzburg, in the *diaries kept by these opera houses*. This suggests some explanation for the custom that used to be followed at European opera

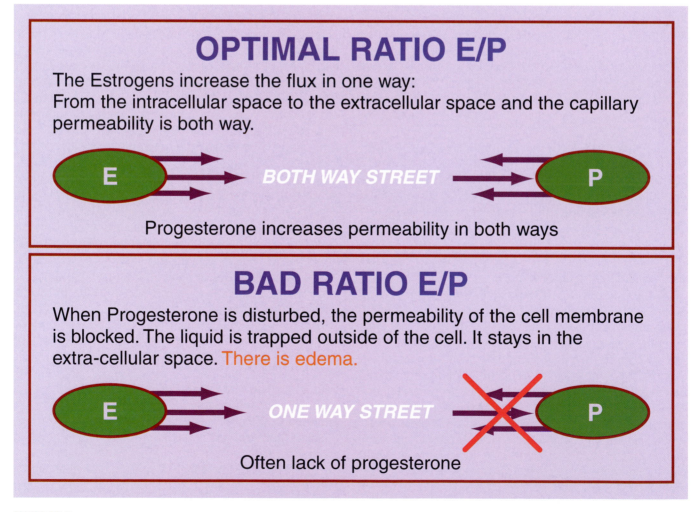

FIGURE 23-3. *Ratio estrogens/progesterone during PMVS.*

houses. For example, the female singers at the Opera of La Scala de Milano used to have "Grace Days." They were not asked to sing during the premenstrual period and while menstruating, but were still paid. Perhaps this abandoned practice should be reconsidered.

Prior to menses, vascular modifications occur and increase the vocal fold mass. The vocal fold edema will decrease the fundamental frequencies during these periods.[39] Ovarian hormones have numerous effects on voice production.[40-42] They may aggravate abnormal movement in some neuromotor disorders[43,44]; moreover, they influence the sensory thresholds,[45] disturb muscle stretch, and impair the flexibility of the cricoarytenoid joint. Changing hormonal levels will influence these parameters. Therefore, it is reasonable to find in some cases, not only an alteration of the voice during the premenstrual phase, but also during ovulation. Information about midcycle voice condition, and during the ovulation phase, should be asked of every woman who suffers premenstrual voice syndrome to yield a complete analysis of the hormonal effects on phonation.

In 1986,[46] Meiri reported that when the nerve terminals of a frog were exposed to progesterone, the acetylcholine released at the neuromuscular junction increased tremendously. It has also been found that the level of norepinephrine in a woman's blood increases with the LH spike at ovulation.[47] These experiments stress the influence of the threshold levels of neurotransmitters.[42-48] These data reflect the importance of the hypothalamic–pituitary axis. It was noted by Wyke[49] that ovarian hormone levels might affect the threshold of laryngeal sensitivity through the baroreceptors: the sensitivity of these receptors is reduced by increasing the severity of pitch disturbance. Since 1983 it has been shown that there are estrogen receptors in the human larynx[50] that play a role in the premenstrual voice syndrome. Besides the direct impact on the mucosal fold, there is also an indirect impact through the laryngeal

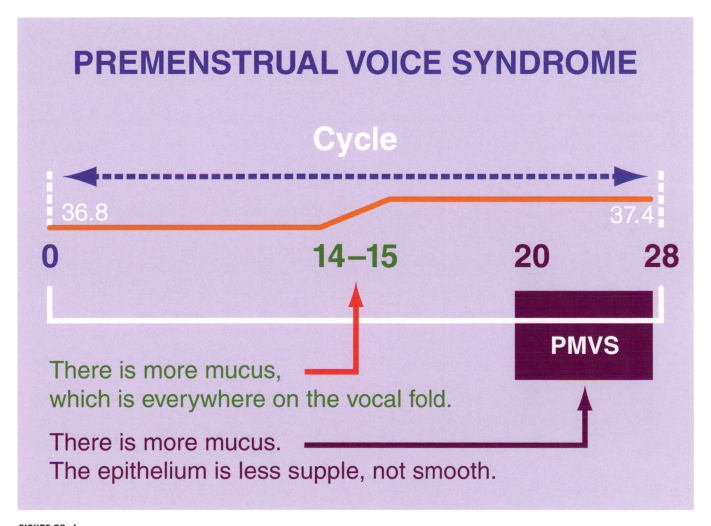

FIGURE 23-4. *Premenstrual voice syndrome.*

nerves. The increased temperature before and after ovulation will increase the velocity of the conduction of the nerve signal. At menses, there is a drop of body temperature, which will decrease nerve conduction velocity. Laryngeal feedback is thereby altered.[51]

Estrogens cause substantial thickening of the endometrial mucosa and an increase in the secretions of the endocervical glandular cells. A similar hormonal effect is noted within the laryngeal mucosa, with an increased secretion from the glandular cells above and below the vocal folds.[52] Similarly, in some patients, the estrogen/progesterone influence also modifies the structure of the laryngeal mucosa just before ovulation, and the tonal quality of the voice can be slightly altered by the presence of mucus on the vocal folds. This increase in production of mucus does not usually affect the speaking or the singing voice. Before menses, vocal symptoms are much more pronounced. Morphologically and functionally, the cervix, the distal part of the uterus, is independent of the endometrium. Just before ovulation, there is slight edema. In fact, the cervix acts like a true hormonal trigger in response to estrogens and progesterone in the epithelium, its chorion, and its squamous and glandular cells.

Progesterone increases the viscosity of the secretions of the glandular cells and the level of acidity, but it decreases their volume, causing a relative dryness. A surprising correlation between cervical and vocal fold smears has been demonstrated as shown by the slide on Figure 23-5.[52]

During the premenstrual period, high gastric acid levels often aggravate esophageal reflux, which is commonly noted during this period. The dryness of the vocal folds, reduced tone of the vocal muscle, edema of the vocal folds, and venous dilation of the microvarices, together, cause the premenstrual voice syndrome.

The clinical signs of the premenstrual voice syndrome from the authors' experience[53] *are* (Figure 23-6)

- Vocal fatigue, decreased pitch, colorless timbre; loss of vocal power;
- Endoscopic laryngoscopy shows microvarices, slight edema of the middle third of the folds, posterior chink, and often inflammation of the posterior wall;
- Stroboscopy reveals diminished laryngeal motion, agility, coordination, and mucosal vibrations: a "chrono-kinetic" impairment;
- Spectrography demonstrates the loss of certain harmonics with a more metallic and husky voice. Narrowed range, a loss of high notes and disturbed pianissimo are found in singers, but low tones are rarely affected.

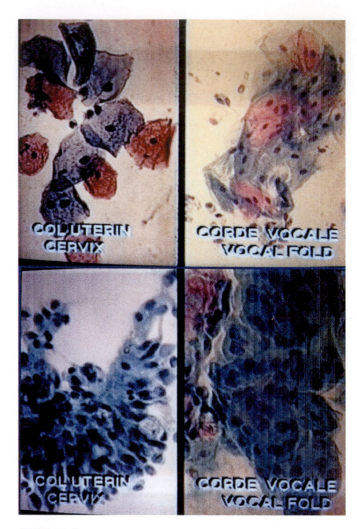

FIGURE 23-5. *Smear test: the parallelism is amazing.*

The above signs are frequently associated with other well-known signs such as increased nervousness, irritability, pelvic pains, a bloated sensation, and asthenia.[54-56]

Physiologically and anatomically:

The *vascular signs:* of patients with a premenstrual voice syndrome:

- 70% demonstrated premenstrual dilation of microvarices, with reactive edema: microvarices (Figure 23-7), microhemorrhage (Figure 23-8), or multiple vascular lesions (Figure 23-9);
- 10% demonstrated a submucosal vocal fold hematoma (Figure 23-10). These hematomas often result in a normal, but easily fatigued, speaking voice. Singing may be impossible.[53]

The *mucosal signs* have been noted in all patients who complain of premenstrual dysphonia. These include:

ACOUSTIC ANALYSIS

- Narrow register
- Lack of high harmonics
- Loss of intensity
- Loss of high pitch
- Maximum Phonation Time (MPT)
- Jitter and Shimmer

STROBOSCOPY

- Microvarices, dilatation of capillaries, varicoses
- Asymmetrical vibration: lack of amplitude
- Ephemeral nodules: hour-glass shape
- Thickness of mucus: "sticky"
- Edema of arytenoids and posterior wall: reflux
- Posterior linkage
- Slight edema on the middle third of the vocal fold

FIGURE 23-6. *Voice parameters during PMVS.*

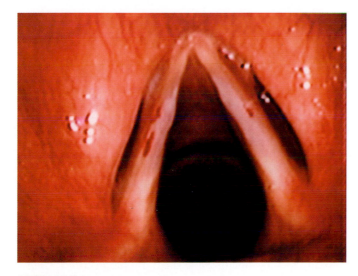

FIGURE 23-7. *Microvarices.*

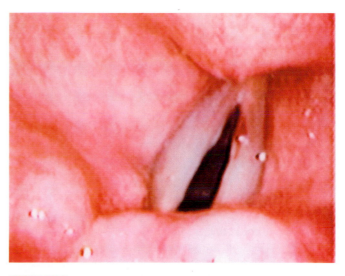

FIGURE 23-8. *Microvarices + microhemorrhage.*

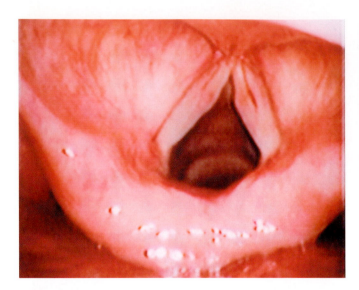

FIGURE 23-9. *Microvarices, + edema + hemorrhage.*

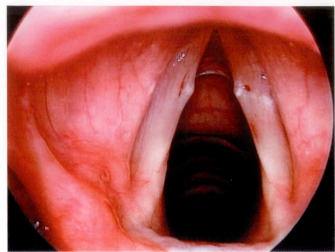

FIGURE 23-11. *Microvarices and nodules.*

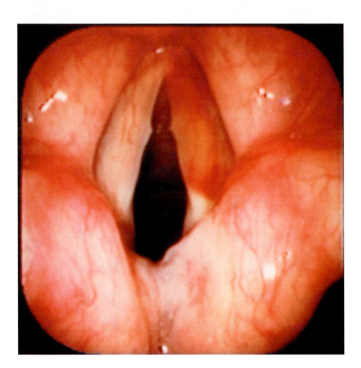

FIGURE 23-10. *Hemorrhage.*

- Edema of the vocal mucosa
- Thickened and diminished glandular secretions, which lead to dryness of the larynx
- Abnormal videostroboscopic findings, including impaired mucosal amplitude and asymmetric vocal fold vibrations, as well as vocal fold nodules without or with microvarices (Figure 23-11). These nodules are bilateral and symmetric and are usually almost asymptomatic. They are

located on the middle third of the vocal folds and lead to a lowering of the register by about 2 to 3 tones, giving a "blues" voice.

Muscular signs were noted in 60% of PMVS patients, including:

- Decreased muscular tone;
- Diminished power of contraction of the vocal muscle after a 10 second sustained phonation of the vowel /i/;
- Vocal fold closure achieved with the participation of the false folds in high pitch;
- Gap between the free edges during phonation and a posterior chink.

Inflammatory signs:

- 3% had a very inflamed nasopharyngeal mucosa;
- 2% had an allergic-type tracheitis with bronchospasm.[53]

In the author's experience (JA), in a study of female patients of childbearing age not taking oral contraceptives, it was noted that about 33% of women suffered from a vocal premenstrual syndrome.

Multifactorial elements explain the PMVS: the effects of estrogen and progesterone on the vocal fold mucosa, on the vocal ligament, on the blood vessels, on the lubrication, and on the psychologic state may explain the premenstrual voice syndrome. The involvement of aldosterone has often been raised, but is controversial.[57-58] Progesterone and estrogens have a synergistic effect.[59] Attempted explanations of the rheologic effects on tissues have included the progesterone/aldosterone ratio and the progesterone/estrogen ratio,[60,61] but there is currently no definitive conclusion. Objectively, one can note:

- A loss of tone in all striated muscles (the vocal muscles, the abdominal musculature, and the intercostal muscles, resulting in reduced pulmonary effort);

- Relaxation of the cardia muscles constituting the angle of Hiss, leading to episodes of gastro-esophageal reflux. Acid reflux may cause posterior laryngitis with edema of the posterior third of the vocal folds and a reduced mobility of the edematous cricoarytenoid joints;

- Edema in the interstitial tissues and in Reinke's space. This edema is normally reversible, but less so in smokers, who, after some years, develop Reinke's edema or pseudomyxedema that leads to a masculine voice caused by vocal fold thickening (Figure 23-12). It may occur in women from the age of 35 on, but never after menopause. A woman who has not suffered from pseudomyxedema before her menopause will rarely suffer from it during the menopause;

- Dilation of the microvarices that may be complicated by small ruptures leading to a hematoma. This explains why vocal professionals should abstain from taking aspirin or NSAIDs at this time. Overuse of these drugs increases the risk of such complications, especially in the "emotionally stressed" performer, who is over-rehearsing or overperforming.

The respiratory, and nasopharyngeal mucosa are also subject to allergic inflammatory effects. During the

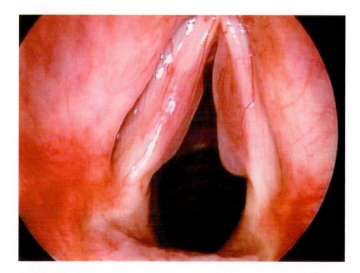

FIGURE 23-12. *Reinke's edema + microvarices, increase during PMVS.*

premenstrual period, a tenfold increase in allergic response is noted in 2% of patients. Hence, the estrogen-progesterone effect leads to a thickening of laryngeal mucus, frequent throat clearing and a reduction of hydration of the free edges of the vocal folds. Vocal lubrication is reduced and vocal fatigue becomes apparent after about 25-30 minutes of phonation.

Treatment of the Premenstrual Voice Syndrome

Generally, hormonal treatment is not necessary for premenstrual voice syndrome; natural remedies are usually satisfactory (Figure 23-13). In light of what we now understand about edema, insulin impairment, neurotransmitter disturbance, low levels of serotonin, and endorphin deficiency, it is clear that multifactorial treatment is appropriate. This therapy is individualized for each woman. In our practice, we have noted good results with natural remedies, including multivitamins and minerals such as: vitamins A, B6, B5, C, and E, and minerals including Mg, Cu, P, Fe, Ca, and Zn. These remedies are combined with vascular therapy and anti-edema drugs, such as bromelaines from pineapples; prostaglandin inhibitors, such as mefenamic acid; and with anti-reflux treatment. This treatment is prescribed for 10 days per month: 8 days before the menses and 2 days during the menses. Also, during this period, we suggest the following diet: low protein, vegetables (carrots), fibers, olive oil, and no alcohol. Great care must be taken never to prescribe progesterone with potential androgenic metabolites, as this may lead to a permanently masculine voice.

Complications of premenstrual voice syndrome may occur. The most significant is recurrent vocal fold hemorrhage, which leads to hemorrhagic masses. Surgery may be necessary in such cases. (Figures 23-14 to 23-18: on the same patient, we see in Figures 23-14 and 23-15, laryngoscopic examination; Figures 23-16 and 23-17, laser phonosurgery; and Figure 23-18, results two months after laser surgery.)

Timing of Phonosurgery in Women

Finally, one must also consider the risk of trauma by endotracheal intubation for any surgery performed during the premenstrual period. Procedures on voice professionals, requiring general anesthesia, must be performed with great care to avoid any direct trauma by the endotracheal tube during intubation and/or trauma caused by rotating the head during surgery. Such care will minimize the risks of post-intubation granulomas and submucosal hematomas of the vocal folds. Blood vessels are very fragile during this period of the cycle. Without question, if surgery is emergent, it must be

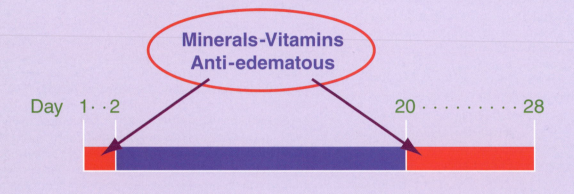

TIMING OF MEDICAL TREATMENT
Premenstrual Voice Syndrome

1. **Iron + Mg: 10 days per month**
2. **Minerals-Vitamins: "*à la carte*"**
3. **Anti-edematous**

FIGURE 23-13. *Timing of medical treatment: premenstrual voice syndrome.*

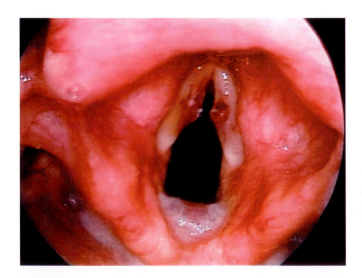

FIGURE 23-14. *Complications of PMVS (1): hemorrhagic nodules during breathing.*

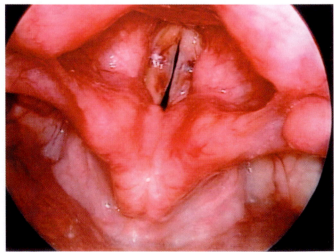

FIGURE 23-15. *Complications of PMVS (2): during phonation.*

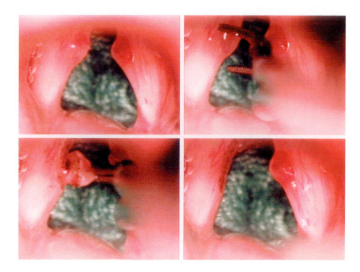

FIGURE 23-16. *Complications of PMVS (3): laser surgery, left side.*

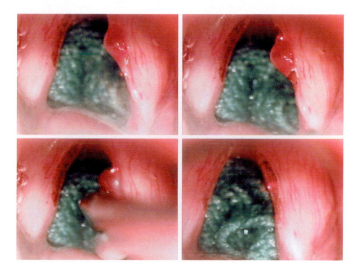

FIGURE 23-17. *Complications of PMVS (4): laser surgery, right side.*

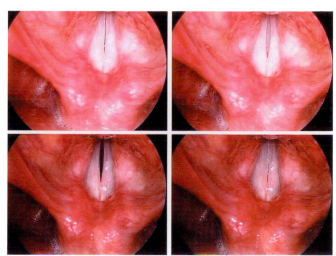

FIGURE 23-18. *Complications of PMVS (5): two months after surgery.*

Phonosurgery should be performed ideally between day 5 and day 20 after menses.

The Perimenopausal Female

Perimenopausal symptoms are well recognized. Hot flashes are the most common symptom. Irregular cycles, anxiety, irritability, fatigue, inappropriate emotional response, insomnia, drying of the throat, drying and thinning of the gastrointestinal tract, vaginal dryness, dizziness, muscle weakness, and weight changes are some of the perimenopausal symptoms. Osteoporosis and cardiopulmonary changes, such as palpitations, high blood pressure, and shortness of breath occur and must be treated. The impact on the voice is very unpredictable and may take more than 15 years following the onset of the perimenopausal symptoms just described.

The Menopausal Voice Syndrome

During menopause, the hormonal climate is greatly altered and may result in changes in the voice. The menses become irregular and vary in quantity as progesterone's influence is reduced premenopause. The disappearance of ovarian follicles leads to the end of menstruation and of progesterone secretion.[62,63] The hypothalamic–hypophyseal axis is greatly altered and there is an increase in FSH and LH secretions that stimulate the ovaries. The ovaries become a unique endocrine organ, as their secretions change, consisting not only of estrogens but also of male hormones. Henceforth, androgens are free to act and their effects are numerous.[64-68] Androgens act on the cerebral cortex, especially the left hemisphere; on the genital organs (uterus, ovaries, breasts); on sebaceous glands; on stri-

done; however, if there is no emergency, when the patient has premenstrual voice syndrome, surgery should be postponed. The author (JA) prescribes pre-phonosurgery medical treatment for 2 months with minerals, vitamins, anti-edema, and anti-reflux medications. In voice professionals, even if they do not have clinical signs of PMVS, the authors prescribe the same treatment. Other surgeons may reschedule the surgery for a different point in the menstrual cycle. In addition to the risks noted above, premenstrual changes may lead to excessive removal of the lesion because of edema of the vocal fold, which distorts the limits of the lesion. The healing process may be impaired or prolonged.

ated muscles, and on the vocal muscles and the vocal mucosa. This has been demonstrated by comparing smears of the vocal folds and cervical smears (Figure 23-19), which exhibit a striking parallelism, in that there is relative mucosal atrophy with basophils, but there also appears to be muscular atrophy that worsens with age and with diminished use of the voice (Figure 23-20). Glandular cells usually located only above and under the vocal folds become more sparse. Hence, there is reduced hydration of the free edges of the vocal folds,[69] resulting in dryness during phonation, leading rapidly to vocal fatigue and to dysphonia. This vocal syndrome is progressive and is especially noticeable in voice professionals: including but not limited to popular singers, opera singers, comedians, barristers, hostesses, and schoolteachers. This gradual deterioration is noticed in high notes and in soft singing. Many women consult physicians more often because they are worried about general menopausal symptoms than because of actual vocal symptoms.

The menopausal voice syndrome presents the following clinical signs:

- During dynamic vocal assessment, acoustically, there is a slight loss in speed of staccato tones at the extremes of range, a loss of intensity, a narrowed range, and a loss of formants in the high tones (hardly noticeable in the day-to-day spoken voice). Anatomically, the vocal folds show a thinner mucosa and a reduced vibratory amplitude;

- Vocal fold cytology is consistent with cervical cytology revealing an atrophic mucosa with

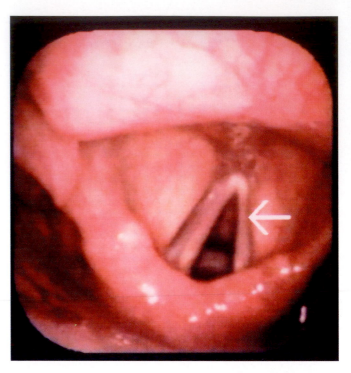

FIGURE 23-20. *Atrophic changes of the right vocal fold.*

basophils present and a reduction in glandular cells in the mucosa of the ventricular band;

- Unilateral or bilateral vocalis muscle atrophy (Figure 23-21);

- Thinning of the vocal fold mucosa with a reduction in amplitude during phonation and asymmetry of the vocal folds noted during stroboscopy;

- The mucosa loses its pearly-white appearance and becomes dull, sometimes with microvarices becoming visible during the premenopausal phase;

- The cricoarytenoid joints move normally, but this diminishes after the age of 65 years, with a loss of the suppleness of the ligaments and with arthrosis;

- The electroglottograph signal is less strong and irregular, bearing witness to the reduced resistance of the vocal fold vibrations;

- The spectral acoustic analysis of the voice shows a 20% to 30% power reduction in the speaking voice, the projected voice, and the singing voice and a narrowed range with the loss of some frequencies.

This seems to vary with individual cases. The vocal "athletes" such as singers and actors may find that two or three tones are altered, but for them, this may be of

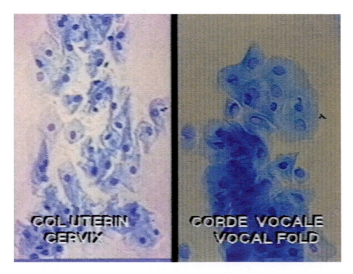

FIGURE 23-19. *Smear test at menopause: the parallelism is amazing.*

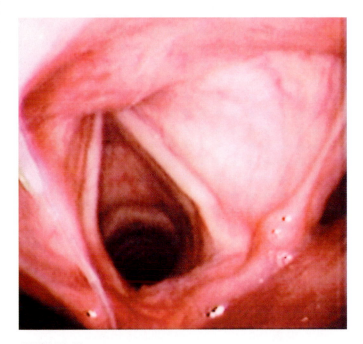

FIGURE 23-21. *Atrophic changes of both vocal folds.*

dramatic importance. The timbre appears to be flat and colorless, as some harmonics have been lost. A loss of melody may be noted in the spoken and the speaking voice.

The authors consider menopausal patients to fit into two broad types: the "Modigliani" types, rather thin and slender, with little adipose tissue, and the "Rubens" types, with a rounded figure.

Since 1978, MacDonald et al[70] demonstrated that estrogen synthesis can take place in fat cells in men and in women. The relationship between obesity and the increase in estrone secretion with reference to the subject's age has also been proven. Cytochrome P450 is responsible for this biosynthesis of estrone from androgens in the fat cells,[16,71-73] and the gene involved is Cyp19. Transcription of P450 aromatase in fat cells increases with age (Figure 23-22).

Androstenedione and other androgen derivatives are transformed to estrogens in lipocytes. More recently, it has been shown that this transformation not only takes place in the lipocytes, but also in the cells of the stroma, in contact with and surrounding the fat cells. These cells

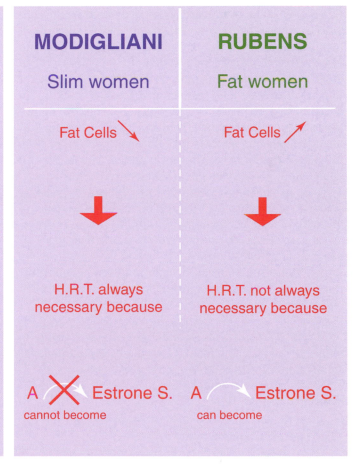

FIGURE 23-22. *Physiopathology of the impact of fat cells in menopausal women.*

can therefore be considered to be "pre-lipocytes." This action is increased by the influence of glucocorticoids.[74-76] Hence, the major site for estrogen synthesis in the menopausal woman is the lipocyte, and the same applies for the obese man.[77-81] It seems to be why an obese tenor has a low testosterone level, as the testosterone is trapped by the adipose tissues and undergoes transformation. In contrast, the deep bass with a slim body has a higher testosterone level, as there is no mass of adipose tissue to lead to estrone metabolism. As we grow older, the lean muscle mass diminishes and the fat mass increases, with a new body cell distribution. Glucocorticoids contribute to the increase in the fat mass, thus showing that great care must be taken when prescribing steroids to a menopausal patient.[82]

Estrone is an estrogen with a weaker action on the target organs than estradiol. Its synthesis in the fat cells is multifactorial. It is stimulated by glucocorticoids, by cAMP (cyclic adenosine monophosphate) and its derivatives but is inhibited by many growth factors.[82] The lipocytes also possess a cellular membrane with insulin specific receptors that allow glucose entry into the cells, thus allowing oxidation and lipogenesis. Maintenance of this property allows the absorption of glucose by the specific receptors of these cells. In the middle of the cell membranes of striated muscle, there is a loss of insulin response with a reduction of insulin receptors. These muscle cells become insulin resistant and insulin secretion increases by the feedback mechanism, resulting in hyper-insulinism. This secondary hyper-insulinism allows fat cells to increase their glucose uptake, as they still have their insulin-specific receptors with an increase in the number of fat cells. The obese patient becomes more obese, and the muscle cells become even leaner.

Glucocorticoids accelerate this process by causing atrophy of the muscle cells and increasing the mass of fat cells, thus contributing to the secondary hyper-insulinism. Fat cells are specific target organs for glucocorticoids.[68,83,84]

An obese menopausal woman possesses significant risks for the transformation of androgens to estrones and estrone sulfate.[85]

More precisely,[86] the adrenal glands will produce 95% and the ovary, 5% of androstenedione. Estrone is indirectly and predominantly secreted by the adrenals at an average of 3,000 µg per day. Conversion occurs in peripheral tissues; adipose tissue is active in aromatization:

- if obese, 3,000 µg, 7% become estrone (200 µg per day) and
- if slender, 3,000 µg, only 1.5% is active in aromatization

The "Rubens" type is certainly much less dependent on hormone replacement therapy than the "Modigliani" type, but needs close attention.

The "Modigliani" patient has little adipose mass, and hence androgens are only slightly transformed to estrones or estrone sulfate, if at all.[87-89] The androgenic action is strong and is often triggered rapidly. In these cases, the authors feel that hormonal replacement therapy for voice professionals is essential[90-92] unless it is contraindicated medically.

Hormone replacement therapy therefore needs careful control, because of the risk of a secondary hyper-estrogenemia.[85] As the fat cell mass increases, the level of endogenous estrogens also increases. If the hormone replacement dose remains high, it may result in a classical hyper-estrogenemia syndrome (tense feeling in the breasts, flatulence, edema, and irritability). Each case must be given individual attention.

Treatment of the Menopausal Voice Syndrome

At menopause, alternative medicine and diet control appear to help reduce symptoms. Multivitamins, minerals, and good hydration are advised: vitamins A, B6, B5, C, E, and vitamin D, as well as minerals Mg, Cu, Zn, P, Fe, and Ca are prescribed by the senior author (JA).

Anti-reflux treatment is usually advisable in an obese woman. The drugs prescribed are taken continuously for 3 months. Hormone replacement therapy is individualized. A gynecologist with special interest in endocrinology, or an endocrinologist, is the best clinician to judge the correct hormone replacement treatment according to the indications and contraindications of each individual, including in the assessment not only vocal symptoms, but also the more common manifestations such as hot flashes, osteoporosis, and cardiovascular and metabolic impairment.[93] Speech therapy is also helpful for many patients with voice disturbance.[94] The therapeutic synergy between hormone replacement therapy, alternative medicine and diet therapy, and voice therapy in selected cases yields a very satisfactory voice result.[95-96] Hormone replacement therapy also improves the quality of life with the prevention or delay of osteoporosis, of cardiovascular risks, of certain central nervous system (CNS) diseases, of dermatologic aging changes, and with the maintenance of an active libido.

Sex Hormone Medication and Voice Disorders

Anabolic steroids may result in a masculine voice. In some athletes, anabolic steroids have been used to enhance athletic performance and appearance. The tragedy in women was that these drugs were often given around the immediate post-pubertal period. Their voices became deeper and never returned to normal. Although the peri-pubescent voice *may* be particularly sensitive, permanent androgenic voice virilization can occur in women of any age.[97] Altered vocal parameters are observed after 2 to 4 months on androgen containing drugs, and sometimes sooner. The pitch drops by as much as 3 to 6 tones; the register narrows from 2 octaves to 1 octave and attaining high notes becomes very difficult.[98,99]

Treatment is first to stop all androgenic hormones. Unfortunately, most of the vocal changes are usually irreversible. Surgery of the laryngeal framework or endoscopic laser surgery may be indicated in certain instances to return the voice to a feminine range. Other surgical techniques to give a higher pitch have also been described by the senior author (JA).[100-102]

Most current contraceptive pills do not affect the voice permanently. Some of the "older birth control pills," prescribed 20 years ago, contained synthetic progesterone components with androgenic side effects and these may still be encountered occasionally in some countries.

As previously stated, the castrato has a feminine voice, and was never exposed to testosterone. The child has a feminine voice, range, and also was never exposed to testosterone. During the childbearing years, a female voice professional must never take male hormones or hormones with androgenic metabolites such as certain progesterones, if she wants to maintain her feminine voice. The menopausal woman will keep her feminine voice if physiologic androgens are not allowed a "free reign" when estrogens and progesterones disappear. Androgens are the only hormones capable of producing a male voice. Hence, early treatment at the first sign of menopause or, in certain cases, perimenopause, is critically important.

In Summary

The voice of a woman changes with the cycle of life and with the aging process. It is constantly under hormonal influence. Before puberty, there is no progesterone. The voice is childlike, supple, and with no vocal fold edema. During the childbearing years, progesterone is produced. About one-third of women suffer from a vocal premenstrual syndrome associated with vocal fatigue and decreased range. At menopause, there is no production of progesterone, there are few estrogens, and androgens appear. In a "Rubens" type female, the fat cells will metabolize the androgens to estrones. In a "Modigliani" type of physiognomy, the androgen impact will predominate. Hormone replacement therapy is often indispensable in voice professionals in order to avoid the development of a male voice and presbyphonia.[103,104]

LARYNGOPATHIA GRAVIDARUM

In the author's experience, 15% of women exhibit a vocal change during the last 5 months of pregnancy, almost always associated with rhinitis. In a 1942 study, Schemer reported approximately 20% of women exhibit voice changes during the last trimester of pregnancy.[96] The symptoms are the same as in the PMVS because of a progesterone environment.

INTERSEXUALITY, HYPOPHYSEAL DISORDERS

Chromosomal Abnormalities

Turner's syndrome[105,106] and Klinefelter's syndrome[107] are typical examples of inter-sexuality and voice disorders. Some groups of hermaphrodites have both ovaries and testicles, but this is rare. The voice is then under the sole control of the testosterone level, above 200 μg/dl, and because of its concentration, the voice has masculine characteristics. In this population with ovaries and testicles, or in transsexuals, the speaking voice may be transformed artificially by phonosurgery in male to female and by androgen therapy and/or surgery in female to male individuals.

Gonadotrophic Disorders

Gonadotrophic Adenoma

In Men

A lack of LH secretion (because of a physical compression of the cells by the adenoma so that the hormones are not able to be released into the bloodstream), will result in a lack of testosterone. This leads to decreased libido with asthenia. Intensity of the voice is weak, the range becomes narrow, the pitch does not change, the voice has fewer harmonics, and the timbre is thin.

In Women

The voice does not change, but there is an indirect consequence on the voice, a reduced muscular tone in the vocal folds, resulting from the impact of other hormones such as ACTH or TSH.

Hypergonadotrophic Disorders

In Men

High FSH levels are almost always associated with testicular deficiency. Hypoandrogenous symptoms appear such as gynecomastia, defects of spermatogenesis, and a higher or falsetto voice.

The testicle is smaller than normal by approximately 40%.[107] Klinefelter's syndrome XXY is the most common etiology. This genetic disease is associated with structural abnormalities of the long bones, excessive growth, and very high levels of FSH and LH.

The testosterone/estradiol ratio is elevated, because the testicle is an important secretor of estradiol.

• The larynx is lengthened, with long, thin vocal folds. The arytenoids are less mobile.

• The voice has a narrow range with loss of timbre as well as power.

Similar symptoms are observed in mosaic patients 46 XY/XXY and also in 46 XX males of the morphotype.[108]

Noonan's syndrome[109] is very rare. Here, LH and FSH levels are high and the testicular secretion is low. There is mental retardation and cryptorchidism. It is an autosomal dominant syndrome 46 XY. As there is a similarity in physical profile with Turner's syndrome with webbed neck, short stature, it is also known as the male Turner's syndrome. Voice is affected because of a depressed nasal bridge, a high arched palate, dental malocclusion, pectus excavatum, and hypotonia. The voice has female characteristics, with vocal atonia, a narrow register, and a shift of the register in the high tones.

Infection with the mumps virus may lead to testicular failure. Usually, it is a failure of spermatogenesis, but sometimes the testosterone producing Leydig cells may also be damaged.[110] There is lack of testosterone and the voice is like a pseudo "castrato."

These symptoms may also appear in males with diminished blood flow to the testicles, with bilateral testicular torsion, following chemotherapy or irradiation, and before puberty.

If similar problems occur after puberty, the voice lacks strength, but the timbre remains masculine.

The most severe testicular deficiency is caused by pathology of both testicles. Occasionally, it may be caused by a problem with gonadotrophins, receptors, or antibodies.

In Women

The FSH level is greater than twice normal during the follicular phase. There is a hypo-estrogenic syndrome with amenorrhea. When these symptoms appear before 40 years of age, they indicate an early menopause or a premature ovarian deficiency.[111]

LH is also high. There is no progesterone, and a very low level of estrogens.

The pathognomonic signs are hot flashes with insomnia, and vaginal dryness. In these women, menopause appears before menarche!

The vocal symptoms are similar to those of menopause, but more dramatic. Similar problems may be observed after irradiation or chemotherapy.

Autoimmune diseases may also be involved. Antibodies to both the FSH receptors and the LH receptors have been found in patients suffering from lupus erythematosus.[112]

Hypogonadotrophic Disorders

In Men

Lack of testosterone with low or normal levels of FSH and LH indicate abnormal hypothalamic function resulting in alterations in quantity and rhythm of the gonadotropin-releasing-hormone (GnRH) production. The voice is less powerful, higher pitched, and weak, similar to a senile voice. This is caused by a decrease in bulk of the vocal muscle, yielding a high voice, and a thinning of the epithelium causing a loss of vibratory amplitude and, hence, of vocal power.

In Women

These patients frequently suffer from insomnia, chronic illness or excess emotional stress, indulge in excessive physical exercise like athletes, and have difficulty maintaining their ideal weight. Basically, they have suffered from a major physical or psychologic upheaval.

Maintaining a balance of hypothalamic secretions with the environment is fundamental. It may be destabilized by external or internal factors. For example, stage fright may induce in a voice professional many responses, some positive and some negative. She may lose her vocal timbre because of an adrenalin-induced vasoconstriction; she may become amenorrheic through inhibition of FSH and LH secretion; she may also give a "once-in-a-lifetime" great performance because of the effect of endorphins from the hypothalamus.

In the polycystic ovarian syndrome (PCOS), androgen excess is typical, with amenorrhea or oligomenorrhea usually starting at adolescence. This leads to an irreversible masculinization of the voice.[113,114]

Growth Hormone

Growth Hormone Insufficiency

The body appearance is abnormal in this condition. The bones are small; there is a protuberant forehead, with very small hands and feet, and a small skull. The skin is thin. Some males may have a microphallus. The striated muscles are small and slim. However, the fat/muscle-mass ratio and the weight-to-height ratio tend to be normal during prepuberty.

The voice in childhood and in male adults is rather peculiar; the resonance cavities are abnormal. The sinus cavities and the nasal fossae are small. Dental eruption is delayed and permanent teeth are irregularly positioned. Bone aging is also very delayed. The lungs are also small.

The thyroid cartilage stays immature for a long time. The vocal fold epithelium is thin, and the amplitude of vibrations during phonation is diminished. The vocal fold muscle is thin and short. The voice is high pitched, but intensity is satisfactory. The register is appropriate. In males, a child-like vocal characteristic occurs, while in women, there is an almost-normal female voice. However, both show a lack of harmonics with a pediatric formants structure.[115,116]

Growth Hormone Excess

Hypersomatotropism and acromegaly are the common conditions resulting from excess of GH. There is an increase in connective tissue throughout the entire body as a result of this excess of secretion. There are transformations of the skin and the connective tissue, as well as facial tissue swelling and acromegaly[117,118] The patient may be recognized by a weak feeling of the handshake or an increase in heel pad thickness, with hypertrophy of distal bones (hands and feet). Gigantism throughout the skeleton (costal bones, inferior and superior maxillary, frontal bone protuberance, vertebral bones, and joints) is observed.

Women grow excess hair and have excessive perspiration because of sebaceous gland hypertrophy.

There is substantial androgen-like effect *except* on striated muscles and gonadal development at puberty. Cartilage growth is prolonged. Body proportions are eunuch-like. The liver, kidneys, thyroid gland, and other internal organs are all increased in size. There is often thickening of the heart's ventricular walls and the cardiac septum, which results in hypertension.

Other abnormalities include:

1. the resonance cavity abnormalities
   - the skin of the face and the lips are thickened
   - the sinus cavities enlarge
   - there is often prognathism
   - the soft palate and uvula are enlarged and thickened
   - the nasal and oropharyngeal tissues are very thick and less flexible
   - respiratory function is decreased (weak)[118]

2. laryngeal anomalies (observations based on personal [JA] experience):

- the epiglottis is enlarged
- the thyroid cartilage is increased in size
- the mobility of the cricoarytenoid joint is impaired
- the laryngeal mucosa is thickened: the vocal folds have a very thick epithelium with essentially normal vibration, and elongated thyroarytenoid muscle
- the voice is deep, of low intensity, and often a narrowed range, but the harmonics and formants are within normal limits

THYROID DISORDERS

Mechanisms of Thyroid Hormone Action

Thyroid gland function has many physiologic effects on fetal growth, maintainance of body weight, the basal metabolic rate, and particularly on cellular differentiation and development. The syndrome of cretinism illustrates the impact of thyroid hormone during development, and suggests that there is a multifactorial effect during the production of other hormones. The thyroid gland plays a crucial role during puberty. It influences the range of the voice and influences the growth parameters. In adulthood, it will affect the metabolic parameters. Basal metabolic rate is increased in hyperthyroidism and decreased in hypothyroidism.

Innervation of the thyroid gland is provided by the sympathetic and parasympathetic nervous systems. The adrenergic nerve fibers and the sympathetic nerve fibers originate from the superior cervical ganglia. The acetylcholinesterase-positive fibers, the parasympathetic fibers, come from the jugular ganglia. Both the cholinergic and the adrenergic fibers are localized around the blood vessels, between the thyroid follicles.

This close association between the thyroid follicles, the thyroid vessels (with their laryngeal branches), and the sympathetic and parasympathetic systems probably partially explains the direct impact on psycho-emotional status and on T_3 and T_4 production.[119,120] The author (JA) has noted that thyroid inflammation comes and goes at times of stress, and in some premenstrual syndromes.

Hyperthyroidism

Hyperthyroidism, of which Graves' disease is the most common kind, is caused by overproduction of thyroid hormone. It is considered to be of an autoimmune etiology and its main symptoms are goiter, weight loss, tremor, agitation, diarrhea, sweating, and an ophthalmopathy. The ophthalmic manifestations such as exophthalmus, extra-ocular muscle hypertrophy, orbital edema, and an exposed cornea may be serious; this infiltrative ophthalmopathy is still not very well understood because it is independent of the thyroid hormone level in the plasma.

Voice disorders are poorly defined and are especially caused by muscular hyperstimulation by the elevated levels of thyroxin. Anxiety increases and the voice becomes hoarse and tremulous. The vocal folds appear hypervascularized and hyperkinetic.[121] Laryngo-pharyngeal-esophageal reflux associated with gastric hypermotility causes posterior edema of the larynx, often with a chronic cough and dysphonia. An increase in the respiratory rate, and a reduction in vital capacity have been seen.

Hyperthyroidism is very frequently associated with a hypervascular thyroid. In such cases, it has been the author's (JA) observation that the vocal folds look hypoxic. A "laryngeal artery steal syndrome" could explain this aspect: the blood being diverted by the goiter; however, this is only a clinical hypothesis, and an empiric deduction. The vocal fold muscles are weak and vocal fatigue occurs. Examination of the vocal folds also often shows a glottic chink during phonation with a loss of amplitude in the vibrations of the epithelium resulting in a hoarse and breathy voice. High pitches are very hard to maintain; low pitches are weak but possible. Similar observations have been made after total thyroidectomies where the laryngeal arteries have been ligated (personal observations).

Hypothyroidism

Hypothyroidism is caused by a lack of thyroxin production. If congenital and untreated, it will lead to cretinism and a small larynx.[122,123] Hearing is decreased. Speech is slow, hesitant, and movements are clumsy. Examination of the larynx shows muscle stiffness. The vocal folds are rarely hypertrophied, but the epithelium is dry and has a narrow amplitude during vibration. There is mucosal edema. The cricoarytenoid joint may be stiff and pain may occur during speaking. The vocal folds are pale; and in some patients, there may be Reinke's edema. There is voice fatigue, hoarseness, and weak intensity. The range is narrow and confined to low tones. The Maximum Phonation Time (MPT) is reduced.

Respiration is altered, with characteristics of dyspnea and shortness of breath, nasal congestion, and a low oxygen saturation, which is often associated with sleep apnea. Sleep apnea is common because of enlargement of the tongue, hypertrophy of oropharyngeal muscles with interstitial edema and muscle fiber

enlargement, respiratory muscle weakness, and depression of the respiratory center.[124]

PINEAL GLAND

The pineal gland is an endocrine gland in mammals, while in fish, it is photoreceptive. It is a small, unpaired central structure, an appendage of the brain. The pineal weight is around 130 mg. Its role in reptiles and birds is mixed: photoreceptor and secretory function. The principal cellular component is the pinealocyte. In human, both photoreceptive function and pinealocyte secretion exist. The gland, richly vascularized, is chiefly innervated by sympathetic nerve fibers from the superior cervical ganglion. Pineal denervation abolishes the rhythmic synthesis of melatonin and the light-dark control of its production.[125] The main role of this gland is to organize the body rhythms and the light-dark cycles by inducing the secretion of the pineal hormone melatonin. The retina and the gut also secrete melatonin. Melatonin is secreted by the influences of the SCN (suprachiasmicnucleus), the body clock synchronized with the retina. It is synthesized during the dark phase of the day. It affects the central nervous system. Melatonin influences the GnRH secretion. It has an effect, as in all other striated muscles, on the quality of the voice through its influence on the CNS at different times of the day and night, as is well known by voice professionals traveling with jet lag.

PARATHYROID DISORDERS

Hypoparathyroidism

Hypoparathyroidism causes hypocalcemia. It stops or slows down the calcification of the larynx and may cause osteomalacia. Hypocalcemia may cause muscle cramps, hyper-excitability and spasmodic contractions. It may also lead to lethal complications such as laryngospasm or a heart attack. Stridor, arrhythmia, and muscle fatigue with spastic muscle contraction are typical of hypocalcemia. It may also lead to paresthesias, circumoral tingling, and, ultimately, tetany. Chvostek's sign will help in the diagnosis, as will Trousseau's sign (a compression of the vessels of the upper arm gives a tetanic state). Voice fatigue, hoarseness, and, rarely, aphonia are observed. Videolaryngoscopy shows the development of vocal fold tetany when the subject is asked to phonate the vowel \a\. During times of emotional stress, these symptoms are aggravated because the patient "consumes" more and more calcium when stressed, and also because of decreased blood supply caused by the vasoconstriction.

In actors and other voice professionals, these signs must be looked for to avoid and prevent serious consequences before going onstage and treated by giving calcium replacement therapy and vitamin D.

Hyperparathyroidism

Hyperparathyroidism causes hypercalcemia, with gastrointestinal, renal, musculoskeletal, and central nervous systems symptoms.

Muscle weakness and hyporeflexia are observed as are dysphonia and aphonia.

ADRENAL DISORDERS

Adrenal Insufficiency

Adrenal insufficiency was the first endocrine disorder described as an endocrine disease by Addison, and was named Addison's syndrome by Trousseau in 1856.[126-128] Addison's disease is a deficiency of the adrenal cortex with hypoproduction of cortisol and aldosterone. Weakness, muscular hypofunction, a weak larynx, and dysphonia are observed.[129] The adrenal cortex controls the tone of striated muscles by controlling the supply of energy to the muscle cells.

In adrenal insufficiency, the subject appears weak, always tired, and the muscular toxins cannot be eliminated. The voice is normal for about 10 minutes and then, suddenly, it breaks, with a husky voice leading to aphonia. The vocal folds vibrate normally for a few minutes and then stop, almost like an intermittent claudication. The vocal fold muscles soon become pathologic. Shouting and singing become almost impossible and the range becomes very narrow. It is easier for the patient to speak in a reclined position than in a standing position.

Congenital Adrenal Hyperplasia

Excess adrenal androgen produces abnormalities. In females, there is an androgenic effect, and in males, a hyperandrogenic effect.[130] The voice is stronger, the male voice is powerful with a wide range, and the female voice is more often a contralto with powerful musculature. The child with signs of virilization, also called "Hercules child," may be caused by hyperproduction of hormones of the adrenal cortex.

The hypersecretion of adrenalin acts as an antidote to muscle fatigue.

DIABETES MELLITUS

Diabetes mellitus is an endocrine disease of the pancreas. More than 10 million people in the United States and 14 million in Europe are diabetic. This pathology is a defect in the metabolic pathways of glucose.

Coronary artery disease and eye problems such as diabetic retinopathy with microaneurysms, conjunctival and irideal hemorrhages resulting from glycogen deposits, depigmentation, and neovascularization are the most dramatic complications. Neural pathology may present as an acute or chronic peripheral neuropathy, involving the limbs as well as the cranial nerves in the head and neck. The autonomic nervous system may also be affected.

As far as voice disturbance is concerned, involvement of the spinal cervical nerves is the most commonly observed mononeuropathy. It causes vocal fatigue because of pain, sensory loss, and weakness of the cervical muscles by an alteration of sympathetic and parasympathetic function. Occasionally, involvement of the third, fifth, sixth, seventh, eighth, and twelfth cranial nerves has been described.[131,132]

The dysphonia can be associated with dysphagia and aspiration. Vocal fold paralysis may rarely be seen with a peripheral lesion of the vagus nerve or a nuclear or supranuclear lesion.[129] Thus, in cases of vocal fold paralysis or paresis, a test of carbohydrate metabolism (glucose) should be done to rule out diabetes. Diabetes may also cause capillary pathology, and poor oxygenation of the vocal fold muscles, with vocal fatigue.

Voice disorders may also occur because of hearing loss caused by diabetes. Thus, in these patients, when there is dysphonia, an audiogram should be performed. In infectious laryngitis with reflux, the management of diabetes is critically important.

CUSHING'S SYNDROME

Harvey Cushing was the first to incorporate the following symptoms into one specific disease: obesity, diabetes, hirsutism, and adrenal hyperplasia.[133] Cushing's syndrome is a symptom complex that reflects excessive tissue exposure to cortisol. The etiologies are usually characterized by excessive ACTH production from a corticotrophic adenoma. Pseudo-Cushing's syndrome can result from long-term steroid therapy.

The typical patient presents with symptoms of virilization, hypokalemia, and high cortisol excretion.

The physical examination reveals hypertension, obesity, abnormal fat distribution (moon face), decreased proximal muscle strength, and menstrual irregularity in women.[134,135]

In our experience, the male voice is not affected. The singing voice is usually normal. In women, it will depend on the influence of the secretion of the dehydro-epiandrosterone from the adrenal gland. Nevertheless, the disease increases weakness of the voice and a loss of high notes.

SUMMARY

This chapter would not be complete without mention of an article in *Nature* by Bennett et al in 1995. They reported that in man, the cerebral projection of speech was not only on the left hemisphere but also on the right side, the side of emotions.[136]

The vocal imprint is characteristic to each individual. It reveals personality and translates emotions. The voice evolves with age and is hormone dependent. The human voice is fluid, both charming and sensual. It bears the scars of life, as well as its joys and pleasures. Nevertheless, the human voice remains intangible, and a fertile field for future research in the cycle of life.

REFERENCES

1. Vesalius A. *De Humanis Corporis Fabrica.* Base; 1543.

2. Harris GW. Neural control of the pituitary gland. *Physiol Rev.* 1948;28:139-179.

3. Darnell J, Lodish H, Baltimore D. *Molecular Cell Biology.* New York, NY: Scientific American Books; 1990.

4. Gammelhoft S, Kahn CR. Hormone signaling via membrane receptors. In: De Groot LJ, ed. *Endocrinology.* Philadelphia, PA: WB Saunders; 1995:49.

5. Asthana S, Craft S, Baker LD, et al. Cognitive and neuroendocrine response to transdermal estrogen in postmenopausal women with Alzheimer's disease: results of a placebo-controlled, double-blind, pilot study. *Psychoneuroendocrinology.* 1999;24(6):657-677.

6. Kerr JB, Sharpe RM. Follicle stimulating hormone induction of Leydig cell maturation. *Endocrinology.* 1985;116:2592-2604.

7. Grossmann A, Kruxeman A, Perry L, et al. A new hypothalamic hormone, CRF, specifically stimulates the release of adrenocorticotrophin and cortisol in man. *Lancet.* 1982;1:921-922.

8. Chauchereau A, Savouret J-F, Milgrom E. Control of biosynthesis and post-transcriptional modification of the progesterone receptor. *Biol Reprod.* 1992;46:174.

9. De Kretser DM, Kerr JB. The cytology of the testis. In: Knobil E. Neill J, eds. *The Physiology of Reproduction.* New York, NY: Raven; 1988;837-932.

10. Sherwin BB, Gelfand MM, Brender W. Androgen enhances sexual motivation in females: a prospective, cross-over study of sex steroid administration in the surgical menopause. *Psychosom Med.* 1985;17:339-351.

11. Persky H, Driesbach L, Miller WR. The relation of plasma androgen levels to sexual behaviors and attitudes of women. *Psychosom Med.* 1982;44:305-319.

12. Longcope C. Adrenal and gonadal androgen secretion in normal female. *Clin Endocrinol Metab.* 1986;15:213-228.

13. Moltz L, Schwartz U. Gonadal and adrenal androgen secretion in hirsute females. *Clin Endocrinol Metab.* 1986;15:229-245.

14. Bouvier RF. *Le Chanteur des Rois.* Paris: Albin Michel; 1943;12-31.

15. Gougeon A. Dynamics of follicular growth in the human: a model from preliminary results. *Human Reproduction I.* 1986;81-87.

16. MacDonald PC, Dombroski RA, Casey ML. Recurrent secretion of progesterone in large amounts: an endocrine/metabolic disorder unique to young women? *Endocr Rev.* 1991;12:372-401.

17. Harada N. A unique aromatas (P450arom) MRNA formed by alternative use of tissue specific exons I in human skin fibroblasts. *Biochem Biophys Res Commun.* 1992;189:1001-1007.

18. Friedrich G, Lichtenegger R. Surgical anatomy of the larynx. *J Voice.* 1997;11(3):345-355.

19. Barnhart KT, Freeman EW, Sondheimer SJ. A clinician's guide to the premenstrual syndrome. *Med Clin North Am.* 1995;79:1457-1472.

20. Richardson JT. The premenstrual syndrome: a brief history. *Soc Sci Med.* 1995;41:761-767.

21. Smith S. The premenstrual syndrome; diagnosis and management. *Fertil Steril.* 1989;53:527-543.

22. Facchinetti F, et al. Oestradiol/progesterone imbalance and the premenstrual syndrome. *Lancet.* 1983;2:1302.

23. Munday MR, Brush MG, Taylor RW. Correlations between progesterone, oestradiol and aldosterone levels in the premenstrual syndrome. *Clin Endocrinol.* 1981;14:1-9.

24. Rubinow DR, Roy-Byrne P. Premenstrual syndrome: overfire from a methodological perspective. *Am J Psychiatr.* 1984;141:163-172.

25. Brayshaw ND, Brayshaw DD. Thyroid hypofunction in premenstrual syndrome. *New Engl J Med.* 1986;315:1486-1487.

26. Aganoff JA, Boyle GJ. Aerobic exercise, mood states and menstrual cycle symptoms. *J Psychosom Res.* 1994;38:183-192.

27. Choi PY, Salmon P. Symptom changes across the menstrual cycle in competitive sportswomen, exercisers and sedentary women. *Br J Clin Psychol.* 1995;34:447-460.

28. Steege JF, Blumenthal J. The effects of aerobic exercise on premenstrual symptoms in middle-aged women: a preliminary study. *J Psychosom Res.* 1993;37(2):127-133.

29. Weyerer S, Kupfer B. Physical exercise and psychological health. *Sports Med.* 1994;17:108-116.

30. Byrne A, Byrne DG. The effects of exercise on depression, anxiety and other mood states: a review. *J Psychosom Res.* 1993;37:565-574.

31. Dua J, Hargreaves L. Effect of aerobic exercise on negative affect, positive affect, stress, and depression. *Percept Mot Skill.* 1992;75:355-361.

32. Lafontaine TP, et al. Aerobic exercise and mood: a brief review, 1985-1990. *Sports Med.* 1992;13:160-170.

33. Longcope C, et al. The effect of a low fat diet on oestrogen metabolism. *J Clin Endocrinol Metab.* 1987;64:1246-1250.

34. Hodgen GD. The dominant ovarian follicle. *Fertil Steril.* 1982;38:281-300.

35. Chihal HJ. *Premenstrual Syndrome: A Clinic Manual.* 2nd ed. Dallas, TX: Essential Medical Information Systems; 1990:18-47.

36. Jones MM. The premenstrual syndrome; part 1. *Br J Scx Med.* 1983;10:9-11.

37. Abraham GE. Nutritional factors in the etiology of the premenstrual tension syndromes. *J Reprod Med.* 1983;28:446-464.

38. Mortola. The premenstrual syndrome. *Reprod Endocrinol Surg Tech.* 1995;2:1635-1647.

39. Frable M. Hoarseness, a symptom of premenstrual tension. *Arch Otolaryngol.* 1962;75:80-82.

40. Lewis PD, Harrison MJG. Involuntary movement in patients taking oral contraceptives. *Br Med J.* 1969;4:404-405.

41. Riddoch D. Jefferson M. Bickerstaff ER. Chorea and the oral contraceptives. *Br Med J.* 1971;4:217-218.

42. Cogen PH, Zimmerman EA. Ovarian steroid hormones and cerebral function. *Adv Neurol.* 1979;26:123-133.

43. Gordon JH, Borison RL, Diamond BI. Modulation of dopamine receptor sensitivity by estrogen. *Biol Psychiatry.* 1980;15:389-396.

44. Miller NH, Gould WJ. Fluctuating sensorineural hearing impairment associated with the menstrual cycle. *J Aud Res.* 1967;7:373-385.

45. Procacci P, Zoppi M, Maresca M, Romano S. Studies on the pain threshold in man. In: Bonica JJ, ed. *Advances in Neurology. International Symposium on Pain.* Vol. 4. New York, NY: Raven Press; 1974:107-113.

46. Meiri H. Is synaptic transmission modulated by progesterone? *Brain Res.* 1986;385:193-196.

47. Rosner JM, Nagle CA, de Laborde NP, et al. Plasma levels of norepinephrine during the periovulatory period and after LH-RH stimulation in women. *Am J Obstet Gynecol.* 1976;124:567-572.

48. Coffey CE, Ross DR, Ferren EL, Bragdon AC, Hurwitz BJ, Olanow CW. The effect of lithium on the on-off phenomenon in Parkinsonism. *Adv Neurol.* 1983;37:61-73.

49. Wyke BD. Laryngeal myotatic reflexes and phonation. *Folia Phoniatr.* 1974;26:249-264.

50. Newman SR, Butler J, Hammond EH, Gray SD. Preliminary report on hormone receptors in the human fold. *J Voice.* 2000;14:72-81.

51. Higgins MB, Saxman JH. Variation in vocal frequency perturbation across the menstrual cycle. *J Voice.* 1989;3:233-243.

52. Abitbol J, de Brux J, Millot G, et al. Does a hormonal vocal cord cycle exist in women? Study of vocal premenstrual syndrome in voice performers by videostroboscopy-glottography and cytology on 38 women. *J Voice.* 1989;3:157-162.

53. Abitbol J. *The Female Voice* [movie 22 min]. San Diego, CA: Singular Publishing Group; 1997.

54. Silverman EM, Zimmer CH. Effect of the menstrual cycle on voice quality. *Arch Otolaryngol.* 1978;104:7-10.

55. Montagnani CF, Arena B, Maffulli N. Estradiol and progesterone during exercise in healthy untrained women. *Med Sci Sports Exerc.* 1992;24:764-768.

56. Edman CD, MacDonald PC. The role of extraglandular estrogens in women in health and disease. In: James VHT, Serio M, Giusti G, eds. *The*

Endocrine Function of the Human Ovary. New York, NY: Academic Press; 1976:135-140.

57. Meisfelt RL. The structure and function of steroid receptor proteins. *Crit Rev Biochem Mol Biol.* 1989;24:101-117.

58. Munday MR, Brush MG, Taylor RW. Progesterone, aldosterone levels in premenstrual syndrome. *J Endocrinol.* 1977;73:21-22.

59. Mortola JF, Girton L. Fischer U. Successful treatment of severe premenstrual syndrome by use of gonadotrophin-releasing hormone agonist and estrogen/progestin. *J Clin Endocrinol Metab.* 1991;71:252-260.

60. Taylor AE, Schneyer A, Sluss P, Crawley WF Jr. Ovarian failure, resistance and activation. In: Adashi EY, Leung CK, eds. *The Ovary.* New York, NY: Raven Press; 1993.

61. O'Brien PM, Selby C, Symonds EM. Progesterone, fluids and electrolytes in premenstrual syndrome. *Br Med J.* 1981;280:1161-1163.

62. Adashi EY. The climateric ovary: an androgen-producing gland. *Reprod Endocrinol Surg Tech.* 1995;2:1745-1757.

63. Applegarth LD. Emotional implications. *Reprod Endocrinol Surg Tech.* 1995;2:1953-1968.

64. Chang RJ, Judd HL. The ovary after menopause. *Clin Obstet Gynecol.* 1981;24:181.

65. Chodzko-Zajko WJ, Ringer RL. Physiological aspects of aging. *J Voice.* 1987;1:18-26.

66. Fedor-Feyberg P. The influence of estrogens on the well-being and mental performances in climateric and post-menopausal women. *Acta Obstet Gynecol Scand.* 1979;64:1-6.

67. Grodin JM, Siiteri PK, MacDonald PC. Source of estrogen production in postmenopausal women. *J Clin Endocrinol Metab.* 1973;36:207-214.

68. Hemsell DL, Grodin JM, Brenner PF, Siiteri PKK, MacDonald PC. Plasma precursors of estrogens II. Correlations of the extent of conversion of plasma androstenedione to estrone with age. *J Clin Endocrinol Metab.* 1974;38:476-479.

69. Buchsbaum HJ. *The Menopause.* New York, NY: Springer-Verlag; 1987.

70. MacDonald PC, Edman CD, Hernsell DI, Porter JC, Citeri PK. Effect of obesity on conversion of plasma androstenedione to estrone in post-menopausal women with and without endometrial cancer. *Am J Obstet Gynecol.* 1978;130:448-452.

71. Inkster SE, Brodie AMH. Expression of aromatase cytochrome P-450 in premenopausal and post-menopausal human ovaries and immunocytochemical study. *J Clin Endocrinol Metab.* 1991;73:717.

72. Sasano H, Okamoto M, Mason JL, et al. Immunolocalization of aromataze, 17α-hydroxylase and side-chain-cleavage P-450 in the human ovary. *J Reprod Fertil.* 1989;85:163-169.

73. Zhao Y, Nichols JE, Buln SE, Mendelson CR, Simpson ER. Aromatase P450 gene expression in human adipose tissue. *J Biol Chem.* 1995;270:16449-16457.

74. Edman CD, MacDonald PC. The role of extraglandular estrogens in women in health and disease. In: James VHT, Serio M, Giusti G, eds. *The Endocrine Function of the Human Ovary.* New York, NY: Academic Press; 1976:135-140.

75. Evans DJ, Hoffmann RG, Kalkhoff RK, Kissebah AH. Relationship of androgenic activity to body fat topography, fat cell morphology, and metabolic aberrations in premenopausal women. *J Clin Endocrinol Metab.* 1983;57:304-310.

76. Hauner H, Schmid P, Pfeiffer EF. Glucocorticoids and insulin promote the differentiation of human adipocyte precursor cells into fat cells. *J Clin Endocrinol Metab.* 1987;64:832-835.

77. Nagamani M, Hannigan EV, Dinh VT, Stuart CA. Hyperinsulinemia and stromal luteinization of the ovaries in postmenopausal women with endometrial cancer. *J Clin Endocrinol Metab.* 1988;67:144.

78. Perel E, Killinger DW. The interconversion and aromatization of androgens by human adipose tissue. *J Steroid Biochem.* 1979;10:623-627.

79. Roncari DAK. Hormonal influences on the replication and maturation of adipocyte precursors. *Int J Obesity.* 1981;5:547-552.

80. Schneider J, Bradlow HL, Strain G, Levin J, Anderson K, Fishman J. Effects of obesity on estradiol metabolism: decreased formation of non-uterotropic metabolites. *J Clin Endocrinol Metab.* 1983;56:973-978.

81. Bulun SE, Mahendroo MS, Simpson ER. Aromatase gene expression in adipose tissue: relationship to breast cancer. *J Steroid Biochem Molec Biol.* 1994;49:319-326.

82. Struhle U, Boshart M, Klock G. Stewart F, Schultz G. Glucocorticoid and progesterone specific effects are determined by differential expression of

the respective hormone receptors. *Nature (London)*. 1989;339:6329-6332.

83. Mattingly RF, Huang WY. Steroidogenesis of the menopausal and post-menopausal ovary. *Am J Obstet Gynecol*. 1969;103:679-693.

84. Exton JH. Regulation of gluconeogenesis by glucocorticoids. In: Baxter JD, Rousseau GG, eds. *Glucocorticoid Hormone Action*. Berlin: Springer Verlag; 1979:535-546.

85. Odell WD. The menopause and hormonal replacement: In: DeGroot L, ed. *Endocrinology*. Philadelphia, PA: WB Saunders; 1995;2129-2137.

86. Emperaire JC. Gynécologie *Endocrinienne du Praticien*. Paris: Editions Frison-Roche; 1995.

87. Tsai-Morris CH, Aquilana DR, Dufau ML. Cellular localization of rat testicular aromatase activity during development. *Endocrinology*. 1985;116:38-46.

88. Vermeulen A. The hormonal activity of the post-menopausal ovary. *J Clin Endocrinol Metab*. 1976;42:247.

89. Waterman MR, Simpson ER. Regulation of adrenal cytochrome P-450 activity and gene expression. *Rev Toxicol*. 1987;98:259-287.

90. Wotiz HH, Davis JW, Lemon HM, Gut M. Studies in steroid metabolism. V. The conversion of testosterone-4-C^{14}-to estrogens by human ovarian tissue. *J Biol Chem*. 1956;222:487.

91. Gambrell RD Jr. The menopause: benefits and risks of estrogen-progestogen replacement therapy. *Fertil Steril*. 1982;37(4):457-474.

92. Rabinovici J, Rothman P, Monroe SE, Nerenberg C, Jaffe RB. Endocrine effects and pharmacokinetic characteristics of a potent new gonadotropin-releasing hormone antagonist (Ganirelix) with minimal histamine-releasing properties: studies in postmenopausal women. *J Clin Endocrinol Metab*. 1992;75:1220.

93. Schiff M. The influence of estrogens on connective tissue. In: Asboe-Hansen G, ed. *Hormones and Connective Tissue*. Copenhagen: Munksgaard Press; 1967:282-341.

94. Applegarth LD. Emotional implications. *Reprod Endocrinol Surg Tech*. 1995;2:1953-1968.

95. Brodnitz F. Hormones and the human voice. *Bull NY Acad Med*. 1971;47:183-191.

96. Gramming P, Sundbert J, Ternstrom S, Leanderson R, Perkins W. Relationship between changes in voice pitch and loudness. *J Voice*. 1988;2:118-126.

97. Hammarback S, Damber JE, Backstrom T. Relationship between symptom severity and hormone changes in women with premenstrual syndrome. *J Clin Endocrinol Metab*. 1989;68:125.

98. Sunderberg J. *The Science of the Singing Voice*. Dekalb: Northern Illinois University Press; 1987.

99. Tarneaud J. *Traité Pratique de Phonologie et de Phoniatrie; La Voix, la Parole, le Chant*. Paris, France: Librairie Maloine; 1941.

100. Abitbol J. *Atlas of Laser Surgery*. San Diego, CA: Singular Publishing Group; 1995.

101. Abitbol J, Abitbol P. *Laser Voice Surgery* [movie 31 min]—21 Cases of Laser Voice Surgery. San Diego, CA: Singular Publishing Group; 1996.

102. Isshiki N. Mechanical and dynamic aspects of voice production as related to voice therapy and phonosurgery. *Otolaryngol Head Neck Surg*. 2000;122:782-793.

103. Abitbol J, Abitbol P. *The Feminine Voice and the Cycle of Life* [movie 22 min]. Bayacedez-Abitbol; 1998.

104. Abitbol J, Abitbol P. Sex hormones and the female voice. *J Voice*. 1999;13:444-446.

105. Lippe B. Turner's syndrome. *Endocrinol Metab Clin North Am*. 1991;20:121-152.

106. Ranke MB, Pfugler H, Rosendahl W, et al. Turner's syndrome: spontaneous growth in 150 cases and review of the literature. *Eur J Pediatr*. 1983;141:80-88.

107. Klinefelter HF. Klinefelter's syndrome: historical background and development. *South Med J*. 1986;79:1089-1094.

108. Bandmann HJ, Breite R, eds. *Klinefelter's Syndrome*. Berlin: Springer Verlag; 1984.

109. Sharland M, Burch M, McKenna WM, Paton MA. A clinical study of Noonan's syndrome. *Arch Dis Child*. 1992;67:178-183.

110. Del Castillo EB, Trabucco A, De la Balze FA. Syndrome produced by absence of the germinal epithelium without impairment of the Sertoli or Leydig cells. *J Clin Endocrinol Metab*. 1947;7:493-502.

111. Rebar RW, Erickson GF, Yen SSC. Idiopathic premature ovarian failure: clinical and endocrine characteristic, *Fertil Steril*. 1982;37:35-41.

112. Taylor AE, Schneyer A, Sluss P, Crowley WF Jr. Ovarian failure, resistance and activation. In: Adashi EY, Lung CK, eds. *The Ovary*. New York, NY: Raven Press; 1993.

113. Stein IF, Leventhal ML. Amenorrhea associated with bilateral polycystic ovaries. *Am J Obstet Gynecol.* 1935;29:181-191.

114. Yen SSC. The polycystic ovary syndrome. *Clin Endocrinol.* 1980;12:177-208.

115. Tanner JM, Whitehouse RH. A note on the bone age at which patients with "isolated" growth hormone deficiency enter puberty. *J Clin Endocrinol Metab.* 1975;41:788-790.

116. August GP, Lippe BM, Blethen SL, et al. Growth hormone treatment in the United States: demographic and diagnostic features of 2331 children. *J Pediatr.* 1990;116:899-903.

117. Grunstein RR, Ho KY, Sullivan CE. Sleep apnea in acromegaly. *Ann Intern Med.* 1991;115:527-531.

118. Daughaday WH. Pituitary gigantism. *Endocrinol Metab Clin North Am.* 1992;21:633-637.

119. Pakarinen A, Hakkinen K, Alen M. Serum thyroid hormones, thyrotropin and thyroxine binding globulin in elite athletes during very intense strength training at one week. *J Sports Phys Fitness.* 1991;31:142-146.

120. Ziegler MG, Morrissey EC, Marshall LL. Catecholamine and thyroid hormones in traumatic injury. *Crit Care Med.* 1990;18:253-258.

121. Malinsky M, et al. Etude clinique et electrophysi-ologique des altérations de la voix au cours des thyrotoxicoses. *Ann Endocrinol (Paris).* 1977;38:171-172.

122. Watnakunakorn C, Hodges RH, Evans TC. Myxedema: a study of 400 cases. *Arch Intern Med.* 1965;116:183-190.

123. Khaleeli AA, Griffith DG, Edwards RHT. The clinical presentation of hypothyroid myopathy and its relationship to abnormalities in structure and function of skeletal of muscle. *Clin Endocrinol.* 1983;19:365-376.

124. Siafakas NL, Salesiotou V, Filaditaki V, et al. Respiratory muscle strength in hypothyroidism. *Chest.* 1992;102:189-194.

125. Klein DC. Photoneural regulation of the mammalian pineal gland. In: Evered D, Clark S, eds. *Photoperiodism, Melatonin and the Pineal. Ciba Foundation Symposium.* Vol. 117. London: Pitman; 1985:38-56.

126. Addison T. *On the Constitutional and Local Effect of Disease of the Supra Renal Capsules.* London: Highly; 1855.

127. Trousseau A. Bronze Addison's disease. *Arch Gen Med.* 1856;8:478-492.

128. Vita JA, Silverberg SJ, Goland RS, et al. Clinical clues to the cause of Addison's disease. *Am J Med.* 1985;78:461-466.

129. Clements RS Jr. Diabetic neuropathy: New concepts of its etiology. *Diabetes.* 1979;28:608-611.

130. New MI, Gertner JM, Speiser PW, Del Balzo P. Growth and final height in classical and nonclassical 21-hydroxylase deficiency. *Acta Pediatr JPN.* 1988;30(suppl):79-88.

131. Ellenberg M. Diabetic neuropathy: clinical aspects. *Metabolism.* 1976;25:1627-1655.

132. Rontal M, Rontal E. Lesions of the vagus nerve: diagnosis, treatment and rehabilitation. *Laryngoscope.* 1977;87:72-86.

133. Cushing H. *The Pituitary Body and Its Disorders: Clinical States Produced by Disorders of the Hypophysis Cerebri.* Philadelphia, PA: JD Lippincott; 1912.

134. Ross J, Linch DC. Cushing's syndrome killing diseases: discriminatory value of signs and symptoms aiding early diagnosis. *Lancet.* 1982:646-649.

135. Urbanic RC, Georges JM. Cushing's disease: 18 years' experience. *Medicine.* 1981;60:14-24.

136. Abitbol J. *Les Coulisses de la Voix—Norma.* Bruxelles: Labor; 1994;42-65.

CHAPTER 24

Laryngopharyngeal Reflux and Voice Disorders

James A. Koufman, MD

Milan Amin, MD

It has been estimated that half of otolaryngology (ORL) patients with laryngeal and voice disorders have laryngopharyngeal reflux (LPR) as the primary cause or as a significant etiologic cofactor.[1] This appears to be true for patients with diverse clinical manifestations.[1,2] Although still controversial, many voice clinicians (including the authors) recommend that LPR be routinely assessed in patients with laryngeal and voice disorders. This point of view is still not accepted (or recognized) by all otolaryngologists. Even among otolaryngologists who have a relatively high index of suspicion for LPR, it appears that this disorder is still often underdiagnosed and undertreated. There appears to be a four-part explanation:

1. *Patients with LPR usually deny symptoms of heartburn and/or regurgitation.* Fewer than half of ORL patients with LPR documented by pH monitoring complain of heartburn or regurgitation, symptoms that clinicians have traditionally felt must be present in order to diagnose reflux disease.[2-4]

2. *The findings of LPR on laryngeal examination vary considerably, and laryngeal edema, a hallmark of LPR, is often unappreciated as a positive finding.* Most otolaryngologists rely solely on the findings of erythema or of *posterior laryngitis* (red arytenoids and piled-up, hypertrophic, posterior commissure mucosa) as the

diagnostic sine qua non of LPR. Unfortunately, these findings are not present in many LPR patients. In the authors' experience, edema (and not erythema) is the principal, and most common, finding of LPR. The edema may be diffuse, or it may create the illusion of sulcus vocalis, an appearance that is the result of subglottic edema in Reinke's space.

3. *Traditional diagnostic tests for gastroesophageal reflux disease (GERD) lack both sensitivity and specificity for LPR.* Barium esophagography, radionuclide scanning, the Bernstein acid-perfusion test, and esophagoscopy with biopsy are all often negative in LPR patients. This is probably because most LPR patients do not develop esophagitis, which is typically observed in gastroenterology patients with GERD.[2,3,5] In addition, LPR is frequently intermittent, and exacerbations depend to some extent upon ever-changing dietary and lifestyle factors.[2]

4. *Therapeutic trials using traditional antireflux therapy often fail in LPR patients, so that clinicians may falsely conclude that LPR is not present.* The traditional treatment for GERD, particularly in the patient with esophagitis, includes dietary and lifestyle modifications and use of antacids, H2-blockers, and/or proton pump inhibitors (PPIs). Such treatment fails to control

LPR in up to 50% of patients.[2] In many cases, the treatment dose is inadequate, and the duration of the therapeutic trial too short.[6] Many clinicians believe that a therapeutic trial of antireflux therapy of several weeks' duration is adequate, but that is not the case. Patients with long-standing LPR often require months of optimal treatment with nearly complete acid suppression with PPIs to resolve their symptoms.[6]

Only within the last two decades, with the availability of new diagnostic methods and treatments, have researchers begun to elucidate the clinical patterns and mechanisms of LPR.[2-5] It now appears that patients with LPR are quite different from typical gastroenterology (GI) patients with heartburn and esophagitis (ie, GERD). How are ORL patients different? Why do ORL patients usually deny heartburn? What are the differences in the mechanisms of LPR and GERD?

The old paradigm of LPR is erroneously based upon the esophagitis model of GERD. Although we still lack ideal diagnostic methods to define the mechanisms and patterns of LPR, a new paradigm is emerging. Two advances are providing some of the answers to the above questions. First, ambulatory 24-hour double-probe (simultaneous esophageal and pharyngeal) pH monitoring (pH-metry) is now generally available as a diagnostic test, and pH-metry effectively documents LPR with a high degree of specificity and sensitivity. Second, compared to previous treatments, PPIs more effectively turn off gastric acid. These drugs are quite effective when compared with H2-blockers.[7,8] As a result of these diagnostic and therapeutic tools, data are beginning to confirm some of the previously controversial clinical observations.

HOW AND WHY ARE ORL PATIENTS WITH LPR DIFFERENT FROM GI PATIENTS WITH GERD?

Ossakow et al[3] compared the symptoms and findings of reflux disease in two discrete groups: ORL patients (n = 63) and GI patients (n = 36). They reported that hoarseness was present in 100% of the ORL patients and 0% of the GI patients, and that heartburn was present in 89% of the GI patients, but in only 6% of the ORL patients. Other authors also have reported a low incidence of heartburn as a symptom in ORL patients with LPR.[2,4] Heartburn is a symptom of esophagitis, and most ORL patients do not have esophagitis. Wiener et al[5] studied 32 ORL patients with hoarseness and found that although pH-metry was abnormal in 78%, esophageal manometry was normal in 100% and esophagoscopy with biopsy was normal in 72%.

Koufman[2] found that only 18% (23/128) of ORL patients with LPR had any findings of esophagitis on barium esophagography. By comparison, esophagitis is found in most GI patients.

It may seem counterintuitive that LPR patients do not also have GERD, and thus, some clinicians remain skeptical about the new paradigm of LPR. However, if the available data are examined from a pathophysiologic perspective, the mechanisms of LPR and GERD are found to differ significantly. Both LPR and GERD are caused by mucosal injury from acid and pepsin exposure.[2] The esophagus has certain protective mechanisms that prevent mucosal injury (bicarbonate production, mucosal barrier, and peristalsis), whereas the pharynx and larynx do not.[2] It takes much less acid/pepsin exposure to cause tissue damage in the pharynx and larynx than in the esophagus. Thus, even if a patient does not have enough reflux to develop esophagitis (and its principal symptom heartburn), he/she still may develop symptomatic LPR.

The clinical manifestations and findings of reflux disease are different in GI and ORL patients, because the mechanisms of GERD and LPR are different. Usually, GI patients have esophageal dysmotility and lower esophageal sphincter (LES) dysfunction, whereas ORL patients generally have good esophageal motor function, but faulty upper esophageal sphincter (UES) function.

GI patients with GERD experience abnormal supine nocturnal esophageal reflux, but only uncommonly experience upright reflux; in contrast, LPR patients experience abnormal daytime upright reflux, but not supine nocturnal reflux.[1-3,5] Not surprisingly, esophageal motility is much more frequently abnormal in GI patients than in ORL patients.[5] In addition, it has been shown experimentally that instilling acid in the distal esophagus of normal subjects and of patients with esophagitis usually results in a prompt increase in tone of the UES.[9] This response does not appear to be intact in ORL patients with LPR.

In summary, it appears that significant differences in esophageal (dys)function may explain many of the clinical differences between LPR and GERD; Table 24-1 summarizes those differences.

CLINICAL MANIFESTATIONS OF LPR

In a large series of LPR patients, dysphonia (hoarseness) was found to be the most common symptom (92%).[2] The pattern of dysphonia was either chronic or intermittent. Patients with intermittent dysphonia often complained that they suffered from "laryngitis" that lasted for days or weeks, several times a year.[2] Additional symptoms were experienced by the majority of the patients: chronic throat clearing (50%), chronic cough

	GERD	LPR
Symptoms		
Heartburn and/or regurgitation	Yes	No
Hoarseness, cough, dysphagia, globus	No	Yes
Findings		
Esophagitis	Yes	No
Laryngeal inflammation	No	Yes
Test results		
Esophageal biopsy (inflammation)	Yes	No
Abnormal esophageal radiography	Yes	Sometimes
Abnormal esophageal pH monitoring	Yes	Often
Abnormal pharyngeal pH monitoring	No	Yes
Pattern of reflux		
Supine (nocturnal)	Yes	Sometimes
Upright (awake)	Sometimes	Yes
Response to treatment		
Dietary and lifestyle modifications	Yes	Sometimes
Rate of success with H2-blockers*	50%	50%
Rate of success with proton pump inhibitors*	90%	90%

*Assuming adequate dosage and duration of therapy.

Table data derived from Koufman.[2]

TABLE 24-1. *Differences Between LPR and GERD*

(44%), globus (33%), and dysphagia (27%). More than half of the patients denied having any heartburn whatsoever; 13% had two or fewer episodes per week, and only 10% complained of more frequent or daily heartburn.[2]

Although most patients with LPR present with mild to moderate dysphonia as the primary symptom, some suffer from more serious, even life-threatening, conditions (Table 24-2). Less common laryngeal manifestations of LPR include laryngospasm, arytenoid fixation, laryngeal stenosis, and carcinoma.[1,2] LPR is also asso-

ciated with the development of polypoid degeneration (Reinke's edema),[1,10] vocal nodules,[1,11] and functional voice disorders.[1,12-14]

Patients with airway obstruction and malignant neoplasia are considered to have life-threatening LPR. Those with other, less severe symptoms and findings are subgrouped into the mild or moderate groups, not only based upon the severity of the clinical situation, but also taking into account the vocal needs and occupation of the patient.

Symptoms

Chronic dysphonia

Intermittent dysphonia

Vocal fatigue

Vocal breaks

Chronic throat clearing

Excessive throat mucus

"Postnasal drip"

Chronic cough

Dysphagia

Globus

Conditions in Which LPR is the Cause or a Causative Cofactor

Reflux laryngitis

Subglottic stenosis

Carcinoma of the larynx

Contact ulcers and granulomas

Posterior glottic stenosis

Arytenoid fixation

Paroxysmal laryngospasm

Vocal nodules

Polypoid degeneration

Laryngomalacia

Sudden infant death syndrome

Pachydermia laryngis

Recurrent leukoplakia

TABLE 24-2. *LPR Symptoms and Associated Laryngeal Conditions*

Reflux and Functional ("Non-Organic") Voice Disorders

The term *functional voice disorder* (FVD) applies to a variety of vocal abuse, misuse, or overuse syndromes. These conditions are also called *muscle tension dysphonias* (MTDs), because transnasal fiberoptic laryngoscopy (TFL) shows abnormal patterns of laryngeal biomechanics. The most commonly observed pattern is supraglottic contraction, either anteroposterior contraction (foreshortening of the vocal folds) and/or false vocal fold approximation/compression.[13,14]

The FVD group of conditions is often associated with the secondary development of histopathologic changes of vocal folds, which include hematomas, nodules, ulcers, granulomas, and Reinke's edema. With the availability of pH-metry, data suggest that 70% of patients with these functional lesions have LPR in addition to abnormal laryngeal biomechanics.[1,13]

As part of the evaluation of each patient with an FVD, the clinician should elicit a *reflux history*. In addition, patients who have laryngeal erythema, edema, or thick mucus in the endolarynx should be suspected of having LPR. This is not to say that treatment of LPR alone will resolve most FVDs. However, this is the case in some patients. On the other hand, failure to treat LPR, when it is present, may delay or prevent resolution of the FVD.

It is important to note that the laryngeal findings of LPR may be subtle in the face of significant supraglottic contraction. The appearance of a (subglottic) groove giving each of the vocal folds the appearance of a sulcus *(pseudosulcus)* should alert the clinician to the possibility of LPR. Likewise, the presence of thick endolaryngeal mucus is often a sign of LPR. This finding is probably the result of a local tissue inflammatory response to chronic irritation.

Granulomas

The etiology of granulomas of the vocal process are multifactorial, but LPR should always be suspected. Granulomas usually result from the combination of acute mucosal ulceration of the vocal process, LPR, and chronic vocal trauma caused by throat clearing and/or a hard glottal attack.[15,16] By itself, chronic vocal trauma can lead to vocal fold ulcers and granulomas; however, in the majority of cases LPR is a cofactor. The clinician should, in each case, consider each of the possible contributing etiologic factors and correct each if therapy is to be effective. In the case of granulomas, effective antireflux therapy is sufficient to allow healing in the majority of patients within eight months, as long as vocally abusive behaviors also are corrected.[15,16]

Paroxysmal Laryngospasm

Laryngospasm is an uncommon complaint, but patients who experience this frightening symptom are usually able to describe events in vivid detail.[17] If the clinician mimics severe inspiratory stridor, the patient will confirm that his or her breathing during an attack does indeed sound similar. Laryngospasm is often paroxysmal, and it usually occurs without warning. The attack awakens some patients. In others, the attacks occur during the day. In some cases, the attacks may have a predictable pattern, for example, during exercise. Some patients are aware of a relationship between LPR and the laryngospasm attacks, others are not.[17]

In a canine model, Loughlin et al[18] showed that chemoreceptors ("taste buds") on the epiglottis responded to acid stimulation at pH of 2.5 (or lower) by triggering reflex laryngospasm. The afferent limb of this reflex is supplied by the superior laryngeal nerve, and nerve interruption abolished the laryngospasm reflex.[18]

In the authors' experience, the majority of patients with paroxysmal laryngospasm respond well to PPI therapy. Antireflux surgery (fundoplication) may be necessary in patients who fail medical treatment.[17,19]

Polypoid Degeneration (Reinke's Edema)

Polypoid degeneration results from chronic laryngeal irritation over a period of many years. It is almost always bilateral and occurs most frequently in elderly female smokers. Nevertheless, it is seen in nonsmoking patients with LPR or hypothyroidism.

Polypoid degeneration may improve with antireflux therapy and cessation of smoking, but most patients with these lesions require surgical treatment as well. It is interesting to note that this group of patients has been reported to have a very high incidence (41%) of prolonged postoperative dysphonia (defined as more than four weeks).[20] This, in part, may have to do with continued (or inadequately treated) LPR after surgery.

Most patients with polypoid degeneration have abnormal pH-metry.[1] Consequently, LPR should be considered in the differential diagnosis, and, at the very least, patients undergoing vocal fold surgery for this condition should receive intense antireflux treatment prior to surgery and during the perioperative period.

Laryngeal Stenosis

Excluding trauma, LPR is the primary cause of subglottic and posterior laryngeal stenosis.[2,21,22] Chronic, intermittent, or chronic-intermittent LPR can cause, or indefinitely perpetuate, a laryngeal disorder. Using a canine model, it has been shown that intermittent (three times per week only) applications of acid and pepsin to the subglottic region following mucosal injury results in nonhealing ulceration of the cricoid, and even subglottic stenosis.[22] LPR documented by pH-metry has been found in 92% of stenosis cases.[2] In the authors' experience, intensive antireflux treatment (with PPIs or fundoplication) is highly successful in leading to decannulation in the majority of patients with stenosis.

The traditional dichotomy between *mature* and *immature* stenoses probably represents an oversimplification. *Immature* implies that massive edema and granulation tissue are present and that the inflammatory process is ongoing. *Mature* implies that acute inflammation has resolved, and that the stenosis is composed of mature fibrous tissue with thin (normal) overlying epithelium. Surgical attempts to correct immature stenosis usually fail unless the underlying inflammatory process is controlled. Conversely, mature stenoses usually can be corrected. In reality, many cases are neither mature nor immature, but somewhere in between. The same also may be true of many acquired laryngeal webs. In the authors' opinion, pH-metry and intense antireflux therapy are indicated in all stenosis cases.

Carcinoma of the Larynx

The most important risk factors for the development of laryngeal carcinoma are tobacco and alcohol; however, LPR also appears to be an important cofactor, especially in nonsmokers.[23,24] The senior author reported 31 consecutive cases of laryngeal carcinoma in which LPR was documented in 84%, but only 58% were active smokers.[2] The exact relationship between LPR and malignant degeneration remains to be proved, but the available pH-metry data suggest that most patients who develop laryngeal malignancy both smoke and have LPR.[24] In addition, leukoplakia and other premalignant appearing lesions may resolve with antireflux therapy.[2]

Tobacco and alcohol adversely influence almost all the body's antireflux mechanisms—they delay gastric emptying, decrease lower esophageal sphincter pressure and esophageal motility, decrease mucosal resistance, and increase gastric acid secretion[2]—and thus, strongly predispose one to reflux. pH-metry, followed by rigorous antireflux treatment, is recommended for all patients with laryngeal neoplasia, with or without other risk factors.

DIAGNOSIS

When a patient presents with dysphonia, globus, dysphagia, chronic throat clearing and cough, and/or "too much throat mucus," symptoms that suggest LPR, the clinician should perform a complete otolaryngologic examination, fiberoptic laryngoscopy, and consider pH-metry as well as a screening examination of the esophagus, ie, barium esophagography or esophagoscopy. Double-probe pH-metry has tremendous advantages over any other diagnostic method, because it is both highly sensitive and specific.[25-27] Furthermore, pH-metry reveals the pattern of reflux, so that subsequent treatment can be custom-tailored for each patient.[26] For example, if the patient does not have supine nocturnal reflux, then elevation of the head of the bed need not be recommended.

pH metry has been available for many years, and standards (normal values) have been established in many laboratories.[1,2,5,25,26] For the esophageal probe, the most important parameter is considered to be the percentage of time that the pH is less than 4, and this measurement is usually recorded for time in the upright position, time in the supine position, and the total time of the study.[2,25,26] For the upright period, the upper limit of normal is approximately 8.0% and for the supine, approximately 2.5%.[2,25,26] However, in many patients (especially professional voice users), lesser exposures may be associated with clinical symptoms.

Why the Pharyngeal Probe is Essential in Diagnosing LPR

Pharyngeal (double-probe) pH monitoring, with the second (proximal) probe being placed behind the larynx, just above the cricopharyngeus, when positive, is by definition diagnostic of LPR.[2,26] At our institutions, and at most places doing such testing, *any* pharyngeal acid exposure is considered to be abnormal.[2] Figure 24-1 shows an example of a portion of a double-probe pH study in which reflux is seen in both the esophageal and the pharyngeal probes.

Double-probe pH-metry is particularly important in LPR patients because otherwise the diagnosis might be missed. Recently, it was shown that the sensitivity of single-probe esophageal pH monitoring for LPR was only 62%, and its positive predictive value was only 49%.[27] In other words, were it not for the pharyngeal probe findings, many patients would falsely be presumed not to have LPR. Pharyngeal pH monitoring is necessary in ORL/LPR patients because it dramatically increases the diagnostic yield.[27]

Screening Examinations of the Esophagus

It is advisable to obtain a barium swallow/esophagogram or perform esophagoscopy in LPR patients because this allows the otolaryngologist to assess the integrity of the esophagus. Although a barium esophagram is not a sensitive test for diagnosing LPR, it may demonstrate significant abnormalities that might otherwise be missed.[28] In a series of 128 patients, the results of barium study revealed that 18% had esophagitis, 14% had a lower esophageal ring, and 3% had a peptic stricture.[2] Barium swallow, then, is used as a screening test. Patients with abnormal findings on barium swallow should have esophagoscopy.

Figure 24-2A shows the appearance of a peptic stricture that was an incidental finding. The patient presented with dysphonia, chronic throat clearing, cough, and dysphagia. He had grossly abnormal pH-metry (upright and supine). A biopsy of the esophagus was recommended, but the patient refused. He was treated with omeprazole 20 mg b.i.d. and after three months was asymptomatic. A repeat barium examination, performed five months after the initial study, showed that the stricture had almost resolved (Figure 24-2B).

Recently, transnasal fiberoptic esophagoscopy was introduced. This examination method requires only topical nasal anesthesia; no sedation is necessary; and the procedure is well tolerated by patients. In the future, this examination may replace radiographic imaging of the esophagus in LPR patients.

TREATMENT

The treatment of acid-related disorders has evolved over time, and has often followed the development of new medications. Initial treatment regimens relied upon dietary and lifestyle changes and the administration of antacids. Such regimens were only minimally effective in treating LPR.

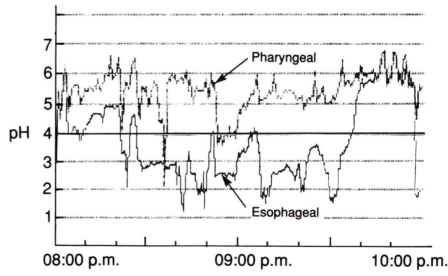

FIGURE 24-1. *Example of double-probe pH study. Pharyngeal reflux is shown. For a pharyngeal reflux event to be considered positive, a precipitous pH drop (below 4.0) in the pharyngeal probe must be immediately preceded by a similar pH drop in the esophageal probe.*

With the introduction of H2-receptor antagonists, the results of treatment of these disorders improved. Studies demonstrate that about 50% of reflux patients improve on H2-blockers, leaving a significant proportion of patients without benefit.[29,30] This is largely caused by the inability of this class of medication to inhibit meal-stimulated acid secretion. Furthermore, some patients eventually develop a tolerance to H2-blockers, limiting the long-term effectiveness of these medications.[31,32]

In the 1980s, a new class of drugs was introduced in the United States, proton pump inhibitors (PPIs). These drugs directly target H^+-K^+ ATPase, the key enzyme in the final acid production pathway within the parietal cell. The elimination or marked suppression of acid production accomplished two things: it reduced exposure of damaged tissues to an acidic environment, and more importantly, it reduced the activity of pepsin, which requires an acidic pH for activation.

Clinical trials have confirmed the superiority of PPIs to H2-blockers both in symptom relief and in mucosal healing.[33,34] Theoretically, this is because PPIs act at the final pathway of acid production, as opposed to H2-blockers, which modulate acid output through blocking stimulation of the parietal cell. Because of this, PPIs have the ability to more completely suppress acid production (basal and meal-stimulated).

PPIs have been particularly effective in improving the healing rate in patients with LPR. While H2-blockers are often effective in treating GERD patients, merely "turning the acid down" is not sufficient treatment for most LPR patients. The acid must be virtually "turned off," because the larynx is far more susceptible to injury from refluxate than the esophagus.[2,22] The larynx lacks the protective mechanisms and barriers that the esophagus has to prevent damage from acid and pepsin exposure. These include a lack of acid buffering capability, the absence of normal peristalsis to clear the refluxate, and the presence of a thinner, more susceptible mucosal lining. Optimal treatment of LPR therefore requires essentially complete cessation of acid-pepsin injury if healing is to occur.

However, PPIs are not effective in all reflux patients, especially with once-daily dosing. Studies done on once-a-day dosing have demonstrated significant failure rates.[35,36] Other studies have demonstrated that the average morning dose of PPI lasts an average of only

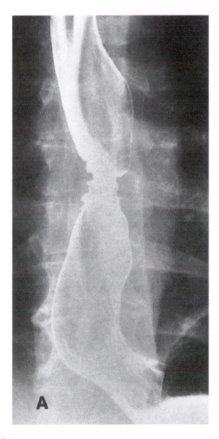
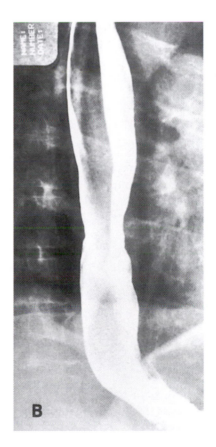

FIGURE 24-2. *Example of peptic stricture seen on barium swallow before (A) and after (B) treatment with proton pump inhibitor therapy.*

13.8 hours,[37] and that the evening dose lasts just 7.5 hours.[38] There have been reports of LPR treatment failures, even on high-dose PPI therapy[36-39]; we found a medical treatment failure rate of 10% in LPR patients receiving PPIs (up to four times per day).[36]

In contrast to GERD, the symptoms of patients with LPR do not resolve in days or weeks; often it takes several months for resolution to occur.[2,6] One follow-up study revealed that fewer than half of patients treated with PPIs are completely well (all symptoms and findings resolved) by four months of treatment.[40] Despite the fact that they are not completely effective in all patients, PPIs are still considered the standard therapy for patients with moderate to severe findings or complications of LPR.[6]

For reasons mentioned above, a minimum of twice-daily dosing is recommended for LPR. The medication should be taken when the patient arises in the morning and late in the afternoon, prior to the evening meal. Finally, the recommended duration of initial therapy with PPIs should be six months.[2,6]

Therapeutic Algorithms

When treating patients with LPR, the severity of the symptoms and findings, the presence of neoplastic lesions, the potential for development of life-threatening complications, the response to previous therapy, the results of pH-metry, the age and occupation of patient, the presence of comorbidities, and compliance issues all influence management. In addition, consideration must be given not only to initial treatment but also to long-range management.

Treatment of Mild to Moderate LPR

For many otolaryngologists, this group comprises the majority of patients with LPR. Such patients typically present with symptoms of intermittent dysphonia, chronic throat clearing, globus pharyngeus, and dysphagia, and findings such as laryngeal edema and posterior laryngitis. It is appropriate for the otolaryngologist to adopt a less aggressive approach to the management of patients in this group. It is not essential to obtain pH-metry routinely in such patients prior to treatment. Initial treatment may be with H2-blockers, antacids, dietary and lifestyle modifications. The latter include: smoking cessation (if the patient smokes), weight reduction (if the patient is overweight), avoidance of overeating and night eating, a low-fat diet, and avoidance of known refluxogenic foods, such as coffee, chocolate, mints, and soda.

Antireflux therapy has two simultaneous goals: to arrest the inflammatory process in the larynx by abolishing gastric acid and, if possible, to reconstitute the body's normal antireflux defenses. The initial six-month period of medical therapy should be used to optimize reversible risk factors that are within the patient's control. Some patients report, for example, that LPR seems to decrease significantly when their weight is close to ideal or with smoking cessation.

If it works, the combination of dietary and lifestyle modifications, antacids, and H2-blockers is a cost-effective therapy. If this regimen fails, the dose of the H2-blocker may be escalated, and if the patient still fails, he/she should be placed on a PPI, starting at a twice-daily dose. The dose of the PPI may also be escalated to achieve a therapeutic response, and adequate time must be given for healing to occur.

The patient who appears to be failing high-dose PPI therapy may be a nonresponder. Such patients should undergo pH-metry while on medication to evaluate drug efficacy. If the patient fails this study, the dose or type of PPI may be adjusted, or a referral made for fundoplication.[41] Serious consideration must also be given to obtaining a referral to a gastroenterologist, as severe reflux may have a serious underlying pathology.

Regardless of the level of medical treatment, it should be continued for a minimum of six months. If the patient becomes asymptomatic after this interval, medication may be decreased or discontinued. However, it is important to counsel patients prior to decreasing or terminating treatment that LPR may relapse. Many patients have disease-free intervals of months or years, but eventually suffer recurrences. Some LPR patients need continual treatment for a lifetime.

The chronic-intermittent pattern of LPR requires the clinician to individualize treatment. Some relatively asymptomatic LPR patients, especially professional vocalists, may need close, long-term follow-up to prevent the development of significant recurrent symptoms, especially because early intervention for recurrences is desirable for such patients.

After six months of therapy, assuming that the patient's symptoms have resolved, if the patient has been started on a PPI, the PPI dose should be tapered and an H2-blocker prescribed. Patients should be warned that he/she might experience a rebound or worsening of reflux symptoms for a few days following cessation of the PPI. After the patient has been on H2-blockers for 6-8 weeks, the patient should be re-examined. If the patient has recurrent symptoms or findings, medication should again be escalated in a stepwise fashion over a period of weeks or months. If medical treatment appears to be failing at a significant dose of H2-blocker, the patient may need to be restarted on a PPI.

Treatment of Moderate to Severe LPR

Ideally, all patients with laryngeal carcinoma, acquired webs and stenoses, and laryngospasm should undergo pH-metry before treatment is initiated; however, this is not always possible, particularly if the patient requires emergency surgical treatment such as tracheotomy. Nevertheless, every effort should be made to obtain pH-metry prior to treatment in this group of patients because: 1) it establishes the diagnosis of LPR; 2) it determines the severity of the LPR (and establishes a baseline); 3) it allows treatment to be individualized; and 4) it may justify unconventional treatment, eg, early fundoplication. For similar reasons, an examination of the esophagus should be performed.

The minimum initial treatment in these patients should be with a PPI at a twice-daily dose, as well as with dietary and lifestyle modifications. A t.i.d. starting dose may be advisable for patients weighing over 200 pounds. Optimal dosing can be adjusted using pH-metry in individuals who do not appear to be responding to treatment. In the event that the patient is unable to take orally administered medicine, an intravenous ranitidine drip should be employed, and the gastric contents should be neutralized using antacids if the patient's stomach is intubated.

In selected cases, those with the most severe form of LPR, particularly young patients (under 40 years of age), fundoplication should be considered as an early alternative.[41] If, for example, a young person presents with subglottic stenosis and laryngeal airway obstruction, with no prior history of trauma or intubation, and pH evidence of severe LPR with a very low LES pressure (less than 6 mm Hg) on manometry, fundoplication may be an advisable alternative to medical treatment.

For most patients, PPIs are the treatment of choice for the first six months, or until such time as the clinical situation that prompted the intervention has resolved. For example, it is injudicious to stop the PPI in the laryngeal stenosis patients still being treated for the stenosis. As some of these patients present with airway obstruction severe enough to require tracheotomy, PPI treatment should be continued until the patient has been successfully decannulated, and it is clear that the LPR is under control, the latter being confirmed by repeat pH-metry. In practice, most patients with stenosis will require either chronic PPI therapy or fundoplication. The same is true for many patients with carcinoma of the larynx, especially nonsmokers who develop carcinoma. In this group, the risk of the patient developing new neoplastic lesions exceeds the risks of definitive long-term antireflux treatment.

When omeprazole (the first PPI) was introduced in the United States in 1989, the Food and Drug Adminis-

tration recommended that it be used in a dose of 20 mg per day for only 6-8 weeks. This overly conservative recommendation was made because omeprazole in large doses for a prolonged period had been shown to produce carcinoid tumors in laboratory animals. It was soon clear that this regimen was woefully inadequate to treat many LPR patients. Fortunately, long-term PPI therapy has been studied extensively in Europe. It is now clear that these drugs are safe, and that they must be employed in larger doses and for prolonged periods.

In patients with life-threatening LPR over the age of 60 years, chronic, long-term, twice-daily PPI treatment is recommended. On the other hand, if the patient has only supine or upright reflux disease, and not both, a single daily dose may suffice for maintenance after the acute phase of the illness has resolved. However, considerable variability is seen, and treatment must be individualized.

For patients under 40 years of age requiring long-term antireflux therapy, fundoplication is usually recommended. For patients between the ages of 40 and 60 years, treatment is selected on an individual basis. In this group, the severity of LPR and the underlying condition are considered, as well as the preferences and overall medical condition of the patient.

Fundoplication as a surgical antireflux treatment is highly effective; however, it does appear to require special technical expertise. Surgical antireflux procedures are a real therapeutic option for some patients, particularly young patients with severe reflux disease. Fundoplication is often recommended for patients with subglottic and tracheal stenosis, as this group appears to have a very high failure rate with medical treatment, and a high likelihood of developing recurrent airway problems later on if medical treatment subsequently fails. Laparoscopic fundoplication has proved highly successful and eliminates much of the morbidity associated with the traditional approach.[41]

SPECIAL CONSIDERATIONS

LPR in Pediatric Patients

Pediatric patients also suffer from LPR. Dysphonia, laryngospasm, laryngomalacia, and pulmonary disorders, such as asthma, have been shown to be related to reflux in infants and children.[2,42-45] Experimental data also suggest that SIDS may be reflux-related.[43,44] Diagnostic pH-metry is especially useful in pediatric patients, because they seldom complain of reflux symptoms, and because so little is known about LPR in the pediatric population.[43]

The treatment algorithm presented above applies to infants and children, but PPIs are cautiously prescribed for patients less than 16 years of age. Therefore, H2-blockers are the mainstays of medical treatment for most children.[42] For pediatric patients with severe of life-threatening complications of LPR, we do recommend the use of PPIs. If there is evidence of medical treatment failure, the patient should be retested while on treatment. If the repeat pH-metry is abnormal, then fundoplication may be indicated.

Xerostomia and LPR/GERD

Xerostomia is often encountered in otolaryngologic practice. In addition to being common after irradiation, xerostomia is also seen with Sjogren's syndrome, scleroderma, most other collagen vascular diseases, cystic fibrosis, and with the use of many medications (eg, anticholinergics, antihypertensives, antihistamines). Xerostomia is a major contributing factor in the development of complications of reflux disease, both LPR and GERD. This is because salivary bicarbonate is needed to restore the intraluminal esophageal pH after a reflux episode.[46] Without normal saliva, the esophageal pH remains very low for an extended period of time. In normal people, the process of pH neutralization takes several swallows (3-5 minutes) following the initial reflux event. In patients with xerostomia, each reflux episode (physiologic or otherwise) is associated with a prolonged period of esophageal acid exposure.

Korsten et al[47] studied sixteen patients with xerostomia caused by head and neck irradiation or medication. All had normal esophageal motility; however, pH-metry and esophageal acid clearance were markedly abnormal in these patients. In addition, the findings of esophagitis were significantly more common in the xerostomia group compared with controls, suggesting that salivary bicarbonate is critical to preventing mucosal damage.

Surgery for Vocal Process Granulomas

Surgical removal of vocal process granulomas is often an exercise in futility, as these lesions usually recur.[16] As mentioned above, most are the result of both LPR and chronic vocal process trauma. The majority of these lesions resolve within eight months with antireflux (PPI) therapy and with good vocal hygiene (correction of vocally abusive behaviors). Surgical removal of granulomas is, however, indicated in four situations[16]:

1. *When granulomas cause airway obstruction.* Airway obstruction from granulomas is uncommon but sometimes occurs. This is a rather obvious indication for surgical removal.

2. *When carcinoma is suspected (for biopsy).* The majority of vocal process granulomas appear as smooth, shiny, bilobed, gray-white masses on the arytenoids. When a granuloma appears to spread anterior to the vocal process or takes on a ragged, keratotic appearance, the possibility of carcinoma must be entertained, and excisional biopsy is indicated.

3. *When granulomas mature and become fibroepithelial polyps.* On occasion, after an extensive period of treatment, a granuloma may take on the appearance of a mature, pedunculated, fibroepithelial polyp. When this occurs, additional medical treatment often fails to eradicate the lesion, and it should be excised.

4. *To restore the voice in selected cases.* Uncommonly, granulomas may produce severe dysphonia. Removal may be indicated in selected cases in which the patient needs to use his or her voice for professional purposes.

Timing of Surgery for Reinke's Edema, Vocal Nodules and Cysts, and Papillomas

Few patients with benign vocal fold lesions require emergency surgery, and many patients with vocal fold lesions also have LPR.[1] It behooves the otolaryngologist to aggressively treat LPR prior to surgery. The authors recommend that antireflux therapy (double-dose PPI) should be instituted a minimum of 2-6 months prior to elective vocal fold surgery, and treatment should be continued postoperatively until healing is complete and normal stroboscopy has returned. The routine use of perioperative antireflux therapy, in our experience, appears to decrease postoperative complications of laryngeal surgery (eg, web information in papilloma patients).

SUMMARY

LPR is an elusive, ubiquitous, and pernicious cause of laryngeal inflammatory and neoplastic disorders; it appears to be clinically distinct from classic GERD. Frequently underdiagnosed and undertreated, LPR is believed to be an etiologic factor in approximately half of patients with laryngeal and voice disorders. The pervasive and serious nature of LPR in such patients demands that clinicians caring for patients with voice disorders consider this diagnosis in almost every case.

REFERENCES

1. Koufman JA, Amin MR, Panetti M. Prevalence of reflux in 113 consecutive patients with laryngeal

and voice disorders. *Otolaryngol Head Neck Surg.* 2000;123:385-388.

2. Koufman JA. The otolaryngologic manifestations of gastroesophageal reflux disease (GERD): a clinical investigation of 225 patients using ambulatory 24-hour pH monitoring and an experimental investigation of the role of acid and pepsin in the development of laryngeal injury. *Laryngoscope.* 1991;101:1-78.

3. Ossakow SJ, Elta G, Colturi T, Bogdasarian R, Nostrant TT. Esophageal reflux and dysmotility as the basis for persistent cervical symptoms. *Ann Otol Rhinol Laryngol.* 1987;96:387-392.

4. Al Sabbagh G, Wo JM. Supraesophageal manifestations of gastroesophageal reflux disease. *Semin Gastrointest Dis.* 1999;10:113-119.

5. Wiener GJ, Koufman JA, Wu WC, Cooper JB, Richter, JE, Castell DO. Chronic hoarseness secondary to gastroesophageal reflux disease: documentation with 24-h ambulatory pH monitoring. *Am J Gastroenterol.* 1989;84:1503-1508.

6. Koufman J, Sataloff RT, Toohill R. Laryngopharyngeal reflux: consensus report. *J Voice.* 1996;10: 215-216.

7. Jansen JB, Van Oene JC. Standard-dose lansoprazole is more effective than high-dose ranitidine in achieving endoscopic healing and symptom relief in patients with moderately severe reflux oesophagitis. The Dutch Lansoprazole Study Group. *Aliment Pharmacol Ther.* 1999;13:1611-1620.

8. Maton PN, Orlando R, Joelsson B. Efficacy of omeprazole versus ranitidine for symptomatic treatment of poorly responsive acid reflux disease—a prospective, controlled trial. *Aliment Pharmacol Ther.* 1999;13:819-826.

9. Gerhardt DC, Shuck TJ, Bordeaux RA, Winship DH. Human upper esophageal sphincter. Response to volume, osmotic and acid stimuli. *Gastroenterology.* 1978;75:268-274.

10. Rothstein SG. Reflux and vocal disorders in singers with bulimia. *J Voice.* 1998;12:89-90.

11. Kuhn J, Toohill RJ, Ulualp SO et al. Pharyngeal acid reflux events in patients with vocal cord nodules. *Laryngoscope.* 1998;108:1146-1149.

12. Ross JA, Noordzji JP, Woo P. Voice disorders in patients with suspected laryngopharyngeal reflux disease. *J Voice.* 1998;12:84-88.

13. Koufman JA, Blalock PD. Functional voice disorders. *Otolaryngol Clin North Am.* 1991;24:1059-1073.

14. Koufman JA. Medicine in the vocal arts. *NC Med J.* 1993;54:79-85.

15. Havas TE, Priestley J, Lowinger DS. A management strategy for vocal process granulomas. *Laryngoscope.* 1999;109:301-306.

16. Koufman JA. Contact ulcer and granuloma of the larynx. In: Gates G, ed. *Current Therapy in Otolaryngology—Head and Neck Surgery.* 5th ed. St. Louis, MO: Mosby Publishers; 1993:456-459.

17. Loughlin CJ, Koufman JA. Paroxysmal laryngospasm secondary to gastroesophageal reflux. *Laryngoscope.* 1996; 106:1502-1505.

18. Loughlin CJ, Koufman JA, Averill DB, et al. Acid-induced laryngospasm in a canine model. *Laryngoscope.* 1996;106:1506-1509.

19. Toohill RJ, Kuhn JC. Role of refluxed acid in pathogenesis of laryngeal disorders. *Am J Med.* 1997;103:100S-106S.

20. Koufman JA, Blalock PD. Is voice rest never indicated? *J Voice.* 1989;3:87-91.

21. Bain WM, Harrington JW, Thomas LE, Schaefer SD. Head and neck manifestations of gastroesophageal reflux. *Laryngoscope.* 1983;93:175-179.

22. Little FB, Koufman JA, Kohut RI, Marshall RB. Effect of gastric acid on the pathogenesis of subglottic stenosis. *Ann Otol Rhinol Laryngol.* 1985;94:516-519.

23. Ward PH, Hanson DG. Reflux as an etiological factor of carcinoma of the laryngopharynx. *Laryngoscope.* 1988;98:1195-1199.

24. Koufman JA, Burke AJ. The etiology and pathogenesis of laryngeal carcinoma. *Otolaryngol Clin North Am.* 1997;30:1-19.

25. Richter JE, ed. *Ambulatory Esophageal pH Monitoring: Practical Approach and Clinical Applications.* New York, NY: Igaku-Shoin; 1991.

26. Postma GN. Ambulatory pH monitoring methodology. *Ann Otol Rhinol Laryngol.* 2000;184(suppl): 10-14.

27. Johnson PE, Amin MA, Postma GN, Belafsky PC, Koufman JA. *pH Monitoring in Patients with Laryngopharyngeal Reflux (LPR): Why the Pharyngeal Probe is Essential?* Presented at the Annual Meeting of the American Academy of Otolaryngology—Head and Neck Surgery, Washington, DC, September 26, 2000. In press.

28. Ott DJ. Gastroesophageal reflux disease. *Radiol Clin North Am.* 1994;32:1147-1166.

29. Scott M, Gelhot AR. Gastroesophageal reflux disease: diagnosis and management. *Am Fam Physician.* 1999;59:1161-1199.

30. Klinkenberg-Knol EC, Meuwissen SG. Treatment of reflux oesophagitis resistant to H2-receptor antagonists. *Digestion.* 1989;44(suppl 1):47-53.

31. Smith JT, Gavey C, Nwokolo CU, Pounder RE. Tolerance during 8 days of high-dose H2-blockade: placebo-controlled studies of 24-hour acidity and gastrin. *Aliment Pharmacol Ther.* 1990;4(suppl 1):47-63.

32. Wilder-Smith CH, Ernst T, Gennoni M, Zeyen B, Halter F, Merki HS. Tolerance to oral H2-receptor antagonists. *Dig Dis Sci.* 1990;35:976-983.

33. Vigneri S, Termini R, Leandro G et al. A comparison of five maintenance therapies for reflux esophagitis. *N Engl J Med.* 1995;333:1106-1110.

34. Skoutakis VA, Joe RH, Hara DS. Comparative role of omeprazole in the treatment of gastroesophageal reflux disease. *Ann Pharmacother.* 1995;29:1252-1262.

35. Leite LP, Johnston BT, Just RJ, Castell DO. Persistent acid secretion during omeprazole therapy: a study of gastric acid profiles in patients demonstrating failure of omeprazole therapy. *Am J Gastroenterol.* 1996;91:1527-1531.

36. Amin MR, Postma GN, Johnson P, Digges N, Koufman JA. Proton pump inhibitor resistance in the treatment of laryngopharyngeal reflux. 2000 (unpublished work).

37. Chiverton SG, Howden CW, Burget DW, Hunt RH. Omeprazole (20 mg) daily given in the morning or evening: a comparison of effects on gastric acidity, and plasma gastrin and omeprazole concentration. *Aliment Pharmacol Ther.* 1992;6:103-111.

38. Peghini PL, Katz PO, Bracy NA, Castell DO. Nocturnal recovery of gastric acid secretion with twice-daily dosing of proton pump inhibitors. *Am J Gastroenterol.* 1998;93:763-767.

39. Bough ID Jr, Sataloff RT, Castell DO, Hills JR, Gideon RM, Spiegel JR. Gastroesophageal reflux laryngitis resistant to omeprazole therapy. *J Voice.* 1995;9:205-211.

40. Grontved AM, West F. pH monitoring in patients with benign voice disorders. *Acta Otolaryngol Suppl.* 2000;543:229-231.

41. Dallemagne B, Weerts JM, Jeahes C, Markiewicz S. Results of laparoscopic Nissen fundoplication. *Hepatogastroenterology.* 1998;45:1338-1343.

42. Halstead LA. Role of gastroesophageal reflux in pediatric upper airway disorders. *Otolaryngol Head Neck Surg.* 1999;120:208-214.

43. Little PJ, Matthews BL, Glock MS, et al. Extraesophageal pediatric reflux: 24-hour double-probe pH monitoring of 222 children. *Ann Otol Rhinol Laryngol Suppl.* 1997;169:1-16.

44. Wetmore RF. Effects of acid on the larynx of the maturing rabbit and their possible significance to the sudden infant death syndrome. *Laryngoscope.* 1993;103:1242-1254.

45. Faubion WA Jr, Zein NN. Gastroesophageal reflux in infants and children. *Mayo Clin Proc.* 1998;73:166-173.

46. Helm JF, Dodds WJ, Riedel DR, Teeter BC, Hogan WJ, Arndorfer RC. Determinants of esophageal acid clearance in normal subjects. *Gastroenterology.* 1983;85:607-612.

47. Korsten MA, Rosman AS, Fishbein S, Shlein RD, Goldberg HE, Biener A. Chronic xerostomia increases esophageal acid exposure and is associated with esophageal injury. *Am J Med.* 1991;90:701-706.

CHAPTER 25

Infectious and Inflammatory Disorders of the Larynx

Robert S. Lebovics, MD, FACS

H. Bryan Neel III, MD, PhD

LARYNGEAL PHYSIOLOGY AND IMMUNOLOGICAL RESPONSES

The larynx is a complex organ situated in the mid-neck that is involved in the functions of phonation and respiration as well as protection of the airway and aiding in deglutition. This organ consists of a network of cartilages and glandular elements, lined by either squamous or respiratory epithelium. The cricoarytenoid joint is a synovial joint, subject to systemic disorders that also affect joints elsewhere in the body. The larynx is innervated by an extensive neural network, subjecting it to disorders of impaired neural function. The lymphatic drainage and anatomic boundaries also have major therapeutic implications when dealing with malignancy. This chapter focuses on those disorders that alter normal laryngeal physiology by either an infectious organism or secondary to a systemic immune disorder mediated by a common inflammatory pathway.

Humans possess an efficient system of physical, cellular, and molecular host defenses. Usually the first level of protection is provided by a specialized epithelium and additional epidermal barriers. Local secretions from the sinonasal tract can contain such antimicrobial substances as lysozyme, or certain types of immunoglobulin G and A (IgG and IgA) antibodies that block microbial adherence and proliferation. The regular flow of fluids through the hollow tube of the pharynx and larynx, in addition to normal mucociliary flow, further prevents the internal spread of infectious organisms that might be colonizing the airway. Environmental trauma, systemic disorders, and large bacterial or viral burdens may, however, overwhelm the physical integrity of these natural barriers.

When external tissue surfaces are penetrated, additional immune mechanisms are recruited, and thus an inflammatory response is elicited. Inflammation can be regarded as the body's natural response to injury. Teleologically it serves to contain and/or eliminate the offending stimulus, and thereby allow for eventual tissue healing.

While inflammation is a necessary protective response, it is clearly a double-edged sword. Severe, prolonged, or inappropriate inflammatory responses can occur in the larynx as in any organ system, and can result in the loss of normal function with consequent morbidity. Often, the challenge for the physician or surgeon is to provide supportive care for the patient until the inflammatory process subsides, or to modulate the inflammatory response through pharmacologic intervention.

Inflammation is a complex cascade of events, involving elements of both cellular and humoral immunity. Either antigen-specific or nonspecific responses may occur. However, the less specific ones have the advantage of being rapidly available during periods of acute infection and may permit the survival of the host until specific focused responses arrive via the immune system. The early or acute phase is characterized by vasodilation, increased vascular permeability, localized release of chemical mediators, and activation of reflex neuronal mechanisms. These lead to Virchow's classic signs of inflammation: pain, redness, heat, and swelling.

Polymorphonuclear leukocytes, lymphocytes, and macrophages are the host's primary acute-phase defense cells. They are highly mobile and short lived in blood cells, and yet they rapidly enter sites of infection to ingest and destroy bacteria. Chemotactic factors produced at the site of inflammation often direct the mobilized pool of polymorphonuclear cells to the site of injury. Several hours later, monocytes are recruited and transform into tissue macrophages. These cells are responsible for the presentation of antigen to T cells, and the production of interleukin-1 (IL-1), tumor necrosis factor (TNF), and interleukin-6 (IL-6) (Table 25-1).

The various stimulating factors, singly or in combination, may promote fever, stimulate hepatic acute-phase responses, and trigger catabolic responses. Lymphocytes and macrophages may respond with an elaborate array of colony-stimulating factors, which will further promote the production of leukocytes in the bone marrow. Depending on the nature of the infection or tissue insult, either a predominantly neutrophilic or a monocytic-lymphocytic infiltrate will predominate. This complex interplay of cascading and amplification continues either until the offending stimulus is eradicated and the tissue returns to normal, or until it is effectively walled off by a granulomatous inclusion. This allows a state of chronic inflammation to persist without a formal and complete resolution of the initial insult.

The larynx, because of its numerous structures and complex architecture, in addition to its critical life-sustaining functions, can frequently present symptoms in a rapid and forceful manner. Because it is the conduit of the body's airflow to and from the lungs, decreased ventilation or complete obstruction can result in either morbidity or mortality.[1] It is, therefore, of critical importance to all clinicians to recognize and diagnose inflammatory and infectious alterations of the larynx promptly, so that normal physiology can be restored and, in more extreme cases, life can be preserved.

COMMON INFECTIOUS DISORDERS OF THE LARYNX

Signs and Symptoms of Laryngeal Disease

A focused history includes information about changes in voice, breathing patterns, and swallowing, in addition to allergic, infectious, and systemic disorders. Persistent unexplained changes in the voice are pathognomonic of a laryngeal disorder. Other symptoms include cough, which can be dry or productive. Pain may be present or referred through branches of the vagus nerve to other regions of the head and neck, for example, the ears. Dysphagia and odynophagia may be associated with neoplastic lesions of the larynx. Besides examination of the neck and throat, physical examination should include, when safe, an indirect mirror examination, flexible fiberoptic endoscopy, and/or rigid endoscopy preferably with a stroboscope. Vocal fold dys-

	Time	Products	Function
Mast cells	Immediate	Histamine, arachidonic acid metabolites	Central to initiation of allergic response
Neutrophils	0 to 6 hours	Proteolytic enzymes, oxygen radicals	Early phagocytosis control of extracellular pathogens
Monocytes	>6 hours	Pro-inflammatory cytokines: IL-1, IL-6, TNF-α Anti-inflammatory cytokines: IL-10	Initiation and modulation of cellular immunity antigen processing
Lymphocytes T cells B cells	Hours to days	T cells: lymphokines, IL-2, γ-interferon B cells: antibody	Antigen-specific responses to pathogens

TABLE 25-1. *Cells of the Inflammatory Response*

function, mucosal alterations, purulent infections of the larynx, mass lesions, structural abnormalities, and occasionally subglottic lesions will be evident on these examinations. Listening to the voice and to the sounds of breathing can also shed light on a pathologic process.

Acute Epiglottitis

Rapidly progressive cellulitis of the epiglottis and its surrounding tissues in the supraglottic airway can cause acute airway obstruction. In infants and children, the causative agent is almost always *Haemophilus influenzae* type B, and bacteremia is present invariably. In adolescents and adults with acute bacterial epiglottitis, the clinical presentation may be less fulminant, and other organisms may be causative. Frequently, the patient complains of dysphagia, odynophagia, and fever that progress over 1 to 2 days. Depending on the degree of respiratory obstruction, stridor may or may not be present. Like a child, an adult with epiglottitis prefers to lean forward, occasionally drooling secretions. Because the caliber of the airway is larger in the adult, intubation or tracheotomy may not be necessary, but the *possibility of imminent complete airway obstruction* mandates prompt management.[2] An edematous, cherry-red epiglottis and surrounding pharyngeal mucosa are the characteristic findings on examination, which *in adults* is best done with fiberoptic instrumentation to confirm the diagnosis. *In infants and children, fiberoptic examination is contraindicated.* A lateral x-ray of the neck may reveal an enlarged epiglottis or the so-called thumb sign. Most hospitals in the United States have protocols established in conjunction with departments of otolaryngology, pediatrics, and anesthesiology to both diagnose and manage the pediatric patient with epiglottitis. In children, an airway must always be secured.

Older patients can be managed by admission to an intensive care unit where adequate clinical monitoring is available until the possibility of airway obstruction has passed. Although fiberoptic examinations are recommended in adults, these procedures should be performed only after preparation has been made to secure an airway by either endotracheal intubation or tracheotomy. After blood cultures are obtained, appropriate antibiotic treatment should be initiated. This is usually a combination of ampicillin and chloramphenicol, although in many centers today a cephalosporin such as cefuroxime has been substituted. Oxygen is administered as dictated by oxygen saturation measurement, using pulse oximetry or arterial blood gas determination. Humidified air by face tent is advisable. If respiratory obstruction worsens, airway protection is required, preferably with endotracheal intubation. Glucocorticoids have been administered as part of the

treatment, but are of unproven benefit. With an appropriate antibiotic, resolution of acute symptoms usually occurs within 48 hours. A child should not be extubated, nor an adult patient removed from an intensive care setting, unless the acute cellulitis of the epiglottis has resolved, as confirmed endoscopically.

Croup (Laryngotracheal Bronchitis)

Croup is a syndrome produced by acute infection of the lower air passages. It is seen most commonly in children below the age of 3 years. The most common pathogen is the parainfluenza virus, although a variety of respiratory viruses can also be found. *Mycoplasma pneumoniae* can produce laryngotracheal bronchitis and/or a croup-like syndrome. The pathophysiology is primarily one of circumferential mucosal inflammation in the subglottic larynx and trachea, and there are variable involvement and spasms of the vocal folds. The epiglottis is usually not involved. The clinical hallmarks include a barking cough with or without stridor and hoarseness. Croup can be distinguished clinically from epiglottitis by lateral x-rays of the neck. Management of severe croup requires hospitalization with close observation and possible intensive care observation. Humidification and oxygen supplementation are given, but rarely is endotracheal intubation required. Nebulized racemic epinephrine can be used and usually helps temporarily. The use of intravenous steroids still remains controversial.

OTHER BACTERIAL INFECTIONS OF THE LARYNX

Laryngeal Diphtheria

Diphtheria still occurs in certain areas of the United States and in other countries, and can infect children who are either immune-compromised or who have not received appropriate immunizations. Laryngeal diphtheria may be insidious because it can occur in a clinical setting in which the pharynx appears normal, that is, there is no silver-gray membrane on the pharynx. Usually, diphtheric laryngitis develops over several days with hoarseness that progresses to complete airway obstruction. Diagnosis is confirmed by a smear of the membranous exudate from either the pharynx or larynx, or if antimicrobial smears and cultures are positive for *Corynebacteria diphtheriae* organisms. In this clinical setting, antimicrobial treatment (frequently a penicillin) in addition to an antitoxin should be administered parenterally, concurrent to or after emergent securing of the airway. Paralysis of the palatal pharyngeal swallowing sequence may occur, and nasogastric tube feeding may be required to help minimize aspiration.[3] The incidence and severity of complications are usually related to the stage of disease at the time that diagnosis and treatment are initiated. Treatment with both antimicrobial agents and antitoxin should not be delayed until positive laboratory cultures are obtained, if there is reasonable clinical suspicion of the diagnosis. Laryngeal diphtheria now occurs almost exclusively in unimmunized individuals. In some patients, cardiomyopathy can occur secondary to the toxin.[3]

Perichondritis of the Larynx

Infection and/or inflammation, followed by necrosis of the laryngeal cartilage, can be associated with different types of acute and chronic diseases. The mucoperichondrium over the laryngeal cartilage is generally a tough resilient barrier to infectious organisms. However, once it is penetrated, its limited vascular supply predisposes to the formation of granulation tissue and/or necrosis and suppuration of the underlying larynx. Etiologic mechanisms are varied; they include iatrogenic causes such as trauma, including trauma from laryngeal surgery or tracheotomy. Inappropriately large endotracheal tubes and feeding tubes are also among the iatrogenic causes of cartilage destruction.[4-6] More commonly today in the United States, external beam irradiation to the larynx can predispose to perichondritis, particularly because of a diminished vascular supply to the tissues. In addition, the normal flora of the oropharynx, hypopharynx, and larynx can be altered by treatment with external beam irradiation. As such, gram-negative rods become part of the normal colonizing bacteria within this portion of the aerodigestive tract, and they may become causative pathogens in laryngeal perichondritis.

Signs and symptoms may vary, depending upon the extent of the problem and stage of inflammation. A patient may present with localized tenderness, dysphagia, odynophagia, fetor, or soft tissue swelling over the region of the larynx. Some early features of infection are severe pain, particularly radiating to the ear, in addition to hoarseness and odynophagia. Inflammation and edema of the arytenoid may result in impaired vocal fold mobility, in addition to audible voice changes. If inflammation extends into the cricoarytenoid joint, this may present clinically with fixation of one or both vocal folds. Inflammation of the cricoid cartilage may cause painful swelling, as well as edema over the posterior lamina of cricoid cartilage. This will result in absence of the normal laryngeal crepitus on physical examination. Major necrosis of the cricoid cartilage heralds complete collapse of the upper airway, necessitating emergent tracheotomy.

Initial treatment consists of identifying the cause of inflammation or infection. Any pockets of pus should be drained in the context of securing a stable airway. It must be emphasized, however, that at this stage, surgery is primarily for diagnosis, with only the airway requiring emergent intervention. A complete pathologic and microbiologic diagnosis is necessary to successful long-term management. In most circumstances, treating the underlying infectious or immune disorder will antedate definitive management of the laryngotracheal complex. Additional treatment during the diagnostic phase may include strict voice rest and analgesics. Because it is frequently easier to prevent severe perichondritis of the larynx than to treat the condition, the otolaryngologist should be involved promptly in the management of patients following both blunt and penetrating laryngeal trauma. Apparently adequate respirations and a seemingly normal voice in these cases may be misleading, and major complications can possibly be avoided with early diagnosis.

Tuberculous Laryngitis

The incidence of tuberculosis in the United States has been found to be increasing during the past several years. The majority of tuberculous infections of the larynx are secondary to pulmonary tuberculosis.[7-9] However, atypical forms of acid-fast bacteria can infect the larynx, particularly in patients with altered cellular immunities. Anatomically, the interarytenoid fold in the posterior portion of the larynx is the most common site of active acid-fast disease. The granulomatous, destructive process of the larynx is slow and insidious. Symptoms such as hoarseness, pain, and dysphagia may occur late in the disease process. It is highly advisable that all patients being treated for pulmonary tuberculosis have the larynx and the remainder of the upper aerodigestive tract examined by the otolaryngologist (Figure 25-1).

There are isolated cases of primary laryngeal tuberculosis, but these are uncommon. While the diagnosis of disease is generally established based on characteristic skin testing, chest radiographs, sputum examination, and early morning gastric lavage, the diagnosis of acid-fast involvement of the larynx requires histologic confirmation. In the operating room setting, direct laryngoscopy can reveal ulcerated mucosa, particularly posteriorly in the region of the arytenoid cartilages and in the interarytenoid fold. It is important, however, to obtain a culture via a swab technique. Better chances of culturing infectious acid-fast organisms occur if deep submucosal tissue biopsies are taken and then cut down for biopsy cultures. The microbiology laboratory should be alerted in advance to facilitate cultures, because of

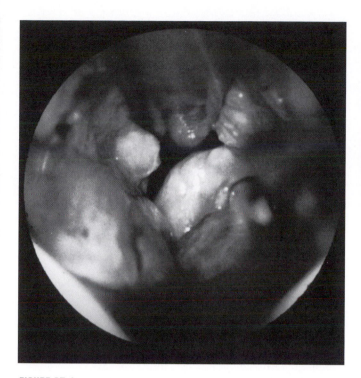

FIGURE 25-1. *Laryngeal tuberculosis—three mass lesions containing* M. tuberculosis. *(Courtesy of Dr. Barry Wenig.)*

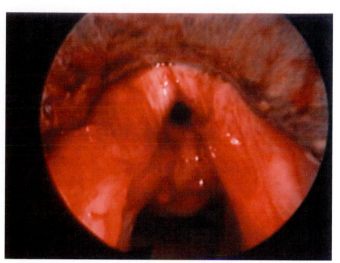

FIGURE 25-2. *Supraglottic stenosis—restenosis of the larynx in a 21-year-old man with common variable hypogammaglobulinemia, who was treated for biopsy-proven nontuberculous mycobacterial infection. He underwent supraglottic laryngectomy to facilitate decannulation 6 months prior to restenosing.*

the difficulties in growing acid-fast organisms. Multiple drug resistances for various mycobacteria are increasing. Therefore, culture and sensitivity testing is crucial in determining long-term chemotherapeutics. In addition to positive biopsy cultures, laryngeal tissues demonstrating histologically invasive acid-fast organisms are critical to substantiating the diagnosis of laryngeal tuberculosis. While treatment is primarily with antimicrobials, airway obstruction and increased aspiration become real clinical issues. A tracheotomy is the safest way to secure an endangered airway. Surgery for secondary stenosis can be performed in the future as clinical circumstances warrant (Figure 25-2).

Leprosy (Hansen's Disease)

Leprosy is a disease caused by infection with *Mycobacterium leprae*. Skin testing in endemic areas suggests that leprosy is in fact highly contagious, as seroconversion is common.[10] Aerosolized droplets from infected nasal secretions are rich in bacteria and constitute one of the primary sources of human-to-human transmission.[11] Skin infection is believed to be transmitted through breaks in the epidermis.[12] Despite widespread exposure in endemic areas, the relative infrequency of clinical leprosy has led to the widely accepted doctrine that prolonged contact with infected

individuals is necessary to contract the disease. More recently, it has been speculated that clinical leprosy may represent reactivation of latent disease, following an immune perturbation in a previously exposed individual.[13] It is similarly believed that host factors such as genetic susceptibility, immunologic status, and nutrition may in part determine susceptibility to infection. It is believed that up to 75% of patients who are exposed to *M. leprae* will clear the disease spontaneously without ever developing clinical signs or symptoms.[12] It is widely accepted that the host immunologic status has a decisive role in the presentation of clinical leprosy.

It is estimated that 12 to 15 million cases of leprosy exist worldwide; approximately one-third of these cases is in India.[14] Approximately 3,000 cases have been registered in the United States, the majority resulting from exposure outside the country.

Virtually all individuals who develop laryngeal leprosy are afflicted with lepromatous cutaneous disease.[11,15] In some studies 30 to 55% of all patients with lepromatous leprosy will develop concomitant laryngeal involvement.[14,16] In concordance with *M. leprae's* predilection for cooler body areas, the epiglottic tip is the area of the larynx most frequently involved with leprosy, where the projection of the epiglottis into the inspired air stream causes air temperature to be approximately 2°C cooler than other areas of the larynx.[14] Although some authors believe that true vocal fold lepromatous nodules are rare, other studies have cited the true vocal folds as the second most frequent location for leprous laryngeal disease; the aryepiglottic fold is involved less frequently. No involvement of the false vocal folds, pyriform apertures, or vallecula has been reported.[14,15] The location of the disease determines the presenting symptoms. Specifically, large lesions of the supraglottic larynx may lead to voice muffling or a "leprous huskiness," a peculiar vocal quality characteristic of laryngeal leprosy.[14] A patient with vocal fold involvement most frequently presents with hoarseness followed by dyspnea and/or dry cough. The patient may also complain of a foreign body sensation, throat pain, or hemoptysis.[10,14] In contradistinction to laryngeal tuberculosis, odynophagia and odynophonia are typically absent.[10]

The appearance of laryngeal leprosy varies considerably. This may consist of simple edema or "congestion," diffuse thickening, subtle discrete pale yellow to pink nodules, or "punched-out" ulcers surrounded by inflammation. Severe fibrosis following a prolonged inflammatory response may lead to a slowly progressive decrease in vocal fold mobility.[12,14,15] The classic pattern of laryngeal disease begins first with the appearance at the epiglottic tip of discrete nodules which, as they continue to develop, enlarge and coalesce into a diffuse irregular thickening, giving the epiglottis a "mulberry appearance."[12,14,15] In later stages the disease may spread to involve the "entire larynx;"[14,15] this may account for the common presentation of laryngeal lesions as "diffuse swelling or thickening."[15] Other less common presentations include punched-out ulcers over the arytenoid cartilages and unilateral or bilateral vocal fold thickening with decreased mobility.[14,15]

The diagnosis of laryngeal leprosy is secured by the identification of the organism in tissue biopsies. The histology of active lepromatous lesions is characterized by marked edema and infiltration by large numbers of epithelioid cells, lymphocytes, and nests of "foamy" histiocytes containing the nonstaining lepra bacilli. Compact, globular masses of free bacilli may also be found scattered throughout the infected tissue. Atrophic stratified squamous epithelium typically overlies the affected areas,[10] and inspection of small nerve bundles and blood vessels and the vocal musculature may reveal bacillus invasion.[16] In unchecked disease, fibrosis with nerve destruction develops, while the overlying epithelium may become hypertrophied and dysplastic. In a large autopsy series of patients with leprosy, 9% were found with cervical vagal nerve involvement; this suggests a possible neuropathic rather than direct infiltrative route of vocal fold paralysis.[16] Following the initiation of treatment, affected tissue is characterized by dense infiltrates of chronic inflammatory cells (largely mononuclear cells and plasmacytes) and occasional fibroblastic infiltrates in the absence of granuloma formation.[15]

The treatment of leprosy as outlined in 1982 by the World Health Organization stratifies patients according to type of presentation. Specifically, for paucibacillary or tuberculoid forms, treatment consists of dapsone 100 mg by mouth every day for 6 months and rifampicin 600 mg by mouth once per month for 6 months. In a patient with multibacillary or lepromatous leprosy, the suggested treatment consists of 2 weeks of dapsone 100 mg/day, rifampicin 600 mg/day, and clofazimine 100 mg/day. Following this 2-week course, the patient is maintained on a regimen of dapsone 100 mg/day, clofazimine 50 mg/day, and rifampicin 600 mg once per month for a minimum of two years.[14] Other authors have recommended that chemotherapy continue until all disease has ceased for at least 3 years, or at least 2 years for tuberculoid and 5 years for lepromatous forms of leprosy.[12] During the commencement of chemotherapy, the clinicians must be vigilant for the onset of erythema nodosum leprosum, an antigen-antibody mediated reaction which can trigger rapid generalized airway edema. It is speculated that this reaction occurs secondary to immune complex deposition in affected areas, and often presents with disseminated painful nodular subcutaneous lesions. Treatment consists of glucocorticoids, thalidomide, clofazimine, and occasionally tracheotomy for erythema nodosum leprosum.[12,13] Relapses are common, particularly in patients with lepromatous forms of leprosy, and the patient may require lifelong antibiotic therapy.[12] Typically early lesions will respond to treatment within a few weeks.[12] Healing occurs with variable amounts of fibrosis, and subsequent airway impairment may require a tracheotomy.[12] Unless there is significant scarring, surgical intervention is usually not necessary in the treatment of laryngeal leprosy.

Laryngeal Syphilis

The spirochete *Treponema pallidum* is the infectious cause of syphilis. Syphilis of the larynx presents clinically during the primary or secondary stage of disease. A gumma usually appears as a characteristically filmy, red, edematous mass that is probably the result of a hypersensitivity reaction to the spirochete. Left untreated, these lesions result in mucosal breakdown, with ulcerations ultimately leading to both perichondritis and fibrosis. There is no particular location that is pathognomonic for syphilis. As the inflammatory process continues, an obstructive cicatricial fibrosis may limit breathing. The epiglottis may be notched or inflamed, and be almost cauliflower-like in its appearance.[17-19]

Hoarseness is usually the presenting symptom. As opposed to acid-fast disease of the larynx, there frequently is no pain associated with the syphilitic inflammatory process. Ulcerative lesions may lead to varying degrees of fibrosis, and respiratory compromise may occur as the gumma progresses. The diagnosis of syphilitic laryngitis is confirmed by both serologic and histopathologic examination.

The prognosis in early lesions that are treated promptly is quite good. In more advanced cases, cartilage destruction may occur, leading to a progressive perichondritis in which vocal fold mobility may be impaired and respiration may be compromised. Occasionally, the airway needs to be secured with a tracheotomy. Patients with laryngeal syphilis also need to be evaluated for systemic manifestations of infection, particularly in the central nervous system.

Penicillins are usually adequate for treating syphilis. While tracheotomy is rarely needed for obstructive lesions, reconstructive surgery might be considered in cases of severe laryngeal stenosis after treatment is completed.

Rhinoscleroma of the Larynx

Klebsiella rhinoscleromatis, also known as the von Frisch bacillus, is the causative bacterium of rhinoscleroma. As in most laryngeal infections, hoarseness, coughing, and occasionally, respiratory compromise may indicate laryngeal involvement. This disease is frequently associated with lesions of the nose, pharynx, tongue, and lower airways. Histologically, the bacteria are found in vacuoles of the characteristic Mikulicz cells. The disease is endemic in both Central America and Eastern Europe. The scleroid lesions usually appear as progressive enlargements of mucosa.[20-22]

The subglottic larynx is the most common location for scleroma of the larynx.[23] Biopsy and culture are the easiest method to establish a diagnosis. On endoscopic evaluation of the larynx, pale areas of swelling may be seen below the vocal folds and in the proximal trachea. If the obstruction is large enough, a tracheotomy is needed. Medical treatment has included antimicrobials, in addition to steroids, theoretically to help minimize fibrosis and scarring. The patient must be evaluated carefully for evidence of rhinoscleroma elsewhere in the upper aerodigestive tract.[24]

Actinomycosis

Actinomycosis is an anaerobic saprophyte that frequently is part of the normal oral flora. The organism becomes pathogenic under special circumstances. As in most infectious processes of the larynx, symptoms include hoarseness, coughing, and occasionally, dysphagia. Endoscopic evaluation followed by histopathologic

analysis of abnormal tissue is required to substantiate the diagnosis. Actinomycosis is difficult to grow in the laboratory; however, its microscopic appearance is self-evident. Histologically, tissues are characterized by numerous granulomata that contain multinucleated giant cells, necrosis, and significant fibrosis. The classic sulfur granule helps to confirm the diagnosis.[25]

Laryngeal tissues that are infected with actinomycosis are generally swollen with a somewhat hard, ligneous feel and light grayish-red hue. Frequently during microscopic laryngoscopy, small sinuses and pits can be seen originating deep in the infected tissues. In addition to characteristic histopathologic findings, actinomycosis should be identified by culture. Necrotic and infected tissue should be debrided. As in all chronic laryngeal infections, if the inflammatory process is allowed to proceed, scarring and fibrosis may occur and result in laryngeal stenosis. Tracheotomy and stenting may be required as part of the airway management. Antimicrobial therapy is usually successful, although prolonged courses of antibiotics (with up to 6 months of oral penicillins) are often utilized to fully eradicate infection.[26-29]

MYCOTIC INFECTIONS OF THE LARYNX

Fungal infections in immunocompetent hosts are rare. Laryngeal mycoses that might be encountered in the United States include blastomycosis, histoplasmosis, and candidiasis. In patients with altered cellular immunities, mycotic infections of the larynx are more common. These particularly involve histoplasmosis and candidiasis, but not blastomycosis. In cases of severe immunocompromise, more uncommon species of fungus may occur.

North American Blastomycosis

Blastomyces dermatitidis is a thick-walled, round, yeast-like fungus. It is endemic in the southeastern portion of the United States as well as the Mississippi River valley. This fungus has been known to cause granulomatous lesions throughout the body, particularly in the lungs, skin, and bone. In the larynx, pyogranuloma formation and fibrosis are seen frequently, and the pathologic picture is completed by a granulomatous reaction with numerous microabscesses.[30] There is hyperplasia of the overlying epithelium with a lymphocytic infiltrate in the submucosa.

Silver-methenamine stains usually demonstrate the presence of the fungal organism, and histologic confirmation with positive culture is usually required for definitive diagnosis. Skin testing has no clinical value in the diagnosis of invasive blastomycosis.

While the presentation of laryngeal blastomycosis is nonspecific, tiny miliary nodules may be seen grossly in more advanced cases. In these cases, a severe inflammatory reaction with mucosal ulceration and bright red granulation tissue is often present.[31,32] Lesions on the true vocal folds may resemble cancer during physical examination. Long-term complications for untreated infection include laryngeal stenosis, particularly fixation of the arytenoids. Amphotericin B, ketoconazole, or itraconazole may be used for treatment.[33,34]

Coccidioidomycosis

The fungus *Coccidioides immitis* is endemic to the southwestern United States and parts of Central and South America. The organism is the causative agent for coccidioidomycosis, also known as valley fever. The fungus *C. immitis* is a spherical, thick-walled, endospore-filled organism in tissue, and exists as a mold in nature. The usual route of infection is by inhalation of the saprophyte. For reasons that are unclear, a more progressive form of infection occurs in black people. Skin tests convert to positive within several weeks of infection, and because the fungus is an inhaled pathogen, it affects primarily the lungs. Histologically, the fungus causes lesions that are tubercle-like granulomata in which an endosporulating spherule is seen on silver-methenamine staining.

Symptoms begin about 2 weeks after exposure, with cough, chest ache, fever, arthralgias, and malaise.[35] As the disease progresses, white females risk developing erythema multiforme. In cases of pulmonary infection, patchy infiltration and mediastinal adenopathy are present, while cavitary lung lesions may be present in more severe cases.

Serologic testing is useful in determining the diagnosis of coccidioidomycosis. Skin testing has value only in epidemiologic studies in endemic areas. Complement-fixation tests are helpful but are not diagnostic if positive. Histologic confirmation of spherules in affected tissue will confirm the presence of invasive fungus. If the lesion is left untreated, voice changes may progress to respiratory insufficiency and subsequent laryngeal stenosis.[36] Treatment is with antifungal medications, using parenteral amphotericin B, oral ketoconazole, or itraconazole.

Histoplasmosis

Disseminated histoplasmosis can present anywhere in the upper airway, including the pharynx or larynx. Histologically, caseating granulomata are frequently seen, and the diagnosis rests on detecting the fungus on special stains or culture. Histologically, granulomas with or without caseation are seen. On routine hematoxylin and eosin stains, pseudoepitheliomatous hyperplasia that mimics the appearance of carcinoma may be seen. The inexperienced pathologist may call this cancer, resulting in wrong treatment. Fungal stains such as Gomori methenamine silver should easily avoid misdiagnosis (Figure 25-3). While most common in the lung, extrapulmonary histoplasmosis has been seen in both the oral cavity and the larynx. Treatment is with ketoconazole, itraconazole, or amphotericin B.[37-40]

Candidiasis

Candida albicans is an oval, budding, yeast-like fungus. It is frequently a normal inhabitant of the oral cavity, gastrointestinal tract, and vagina. Infection of the mouth, also known as thrush, is more frequent in children and in immunosuppressed adults. Microscopic evaluations of mucosal scrapings show the characteristic budding yeast cells and their filaments. Especially in the immunocompetent host, *C. albicans* is uncommon, although laryngeal thrush may be a sign of HIV infection. Oral fluconazole is the drug of choice for laryngeal infection.

IMMUNE DISEASES

Sarcoid of the Larynx

Sarcoid is a systemic granulomatous disease whose etiology is unclear. It primarily affects the lungs and mediastinal lymph nodes. However, multisystem involvement is common. Approximately 5% of patients with pulmonary sarcoid have laryngeal manifestations of their disease.[41] While the presentation of most laryngeal

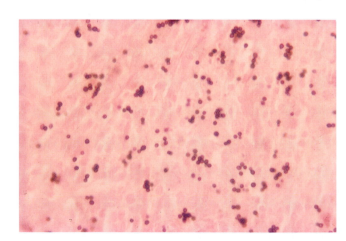

FIGURE 25-3. *Silver-methenamine stain demonstrating invasive hyphal elements in the laryngeal submucosa. This patient had invasive* Histoplasma capsulatum.

infections is similar, that is, progressive hoarseness and occasional pain, sarcoid needs to be distinguished both pathologically and immunologically from other diseases, particularly those involving *Mycobacterium tuberculosis.*

Pulmonary function tests may demonstrate characteristic tracings of extrathoracic pulmonary obstruction. There is a characteristic "honking" voice of sarcoid.[42] On examination, pink, edematous, and turban-like enlargement of supraglottic structures may be considered pathognomonic for laryngeal sarcoid.[43] The incidence of malignancies for patients with sarcoid is greater than the expected incidences for thyroid cancer, laryngeal cancer, and leukemia. The increased cancer risk may be secondary to immunologic factors associated with sarcoid.

Histologically, sarcoid is characterized by noncaseating granulomas, as opposed to infectious organisms of the larynx. On presentation, laryngeal sarcoid usually involves the epiglottis, and contiguous structures such as the aryepiglottic folds and arytenoids often show diffuse, boggy, pale enlargements. Occasionally, the subglottic larynx becomes involved, producing significant airway symptoms. Pain is not a major complaint in most patients.

The diagnosis of sarcoid requires histologic confirmation. In addition, certain laboratory and radiographic findings support the diagnosis of sarcoid. Hypercalcemia and adenopathy of the chest or neck, in the presence of noncaseating granulomata of the lung or epiglottis, help to confirm the diagnosis. Although rarely used today, the Kveim skin test supports the diagnosis. As laryngeal swelling can cause airway obstruction, tracheotomy is required occasionally to support the airway.

Microscopic examination of the involved tissue reveals multiple hard tubercles that are often similar in size to those of acid-fast disease. The tubercle consists of a collection of epithelial cells surrounded by giant cells. In contrast to the findings in other granulomas, the surrounding zone of lymphocytes may be narrow or even absent.[44,45] This might explain why the sarcoid lesions do not undergo caseation necrosis.

Once a diagnosis of laryngeal sarcoid is made, the patient should be referred to an immunologist for systemic evaluation. While no definitive therapy exists, systemic steroids are frequently used in order to minimize symptoms. In cases of less severe obstruction, intralesional injections of steroids have been shown to be helpful, in addition to oral prednisone.[43,46]

AMYLOIDOSIS

Amyloidosis is a group of disorders characterized by deposition of acellular proteinaceous material in tissues.[47] Amyloid aggregates are composed of homogeneous subunits of different proteins which share several common features. All demonstrate a similar tertiary protein structure, the twisted β-pleated sheet. All amyloid deposits contain amyloid P protein, which is identical to serum amyloid P, and all of the primary protein structures are rich in aspartic acid and glutamic acid residues. The resulting structure has a highly polyanionic surface, which may predispose the formation of a β-pleated structure, and presumably contributes to the great stability of the protein aggregates. This characteristic, in turn, allows amyloid to accumulate as a nonreactive proteinaceous deposit that causes structural damage simply by pressure effects on adjacent tissues.[48]

Several subtypes of amyloidosis have been defined, based on the protein makeup of the amyloid deposits and the clinical characteristics of the patient. Primary amyloid (AL) is a product of an immunocyte (plasmacyte) dyscrasia. The proteins in AL amyloid are derived exclusively from immunoglobulin λ and κ chains. This type of amyloidosis occurs in patients with primary systemic amyloidosis, myeloma-associated amyloid, and in most cases of localized amyloidosis such as those involving the larynx.[47,49] There is significant evidence that suggests that the λ chains in AL are more amylogenic than the κ chains.[50] Whereas primary amyloidosis is characterized by the deposition of amyloid in mesenchymal tissues such as the tongue, heart, and gastrointestinal tract, secondary (AA) amyloidosis is associated with deposits mainly in reticuloendothelial organs such as the liver and spleen.[50] AA amyloidosis is associated with chronic destructive inflammatory and infectious diseases such as long-standing tuberculosis and rheumatoid arthritis, and inherited disorders such as familial Mediterranean fever. A third type of amyloid, AF, is a familial variant in which the amyloid subunits are derived from a genetic variant of prealbumin.[51] The protein deposits in AS, "senile" or age-related amyloidosis, are derived from the plasma protein transthyretin. Finally, other variants of amyloidosis include one associated with chronic dialysis in which β$_2$-microglobulin is the protein which forms the protein aggregates.[49]

Laryngeal involvement in amyloidosis is rare, accounting for <1% of all benign laryngeal tumors.[50] Only about 200 cases have been reported in the literature. Those laryngeal lesions that are reported typically are of primary amyloidosis, although a few cases exist of laryngeal involvement as a result of generalized secondary amyloidosis.[50] Prognostic significance has been attached to the appearance of laryngeal amyloidosis as a presenting symptom versus its appearance later in the course of systemic amyloidosis.

The typical patient who presents with laryngeal amyloidosis is in the 40 to 60 age range, and there is a male-to-female predominance of approximately 2:1.[50,52] Amyloidosis is a chronic, slowly progressive disease of insidious onset, characterized by hoarseness, dyspnea, cough, stridor, or odynophagia,[51] and rarely, hemoptysis.[48] The typical lesion of laryngeal amyloidosis is a firm, non-ulcerated, orange-yellow to gray submucosal nodule. Less commonly it may present as one or multiple discrete pedunculated polypoid lesions which may involve any part of the larynx. Several series have noted that the location of amyloid deposits tends to be highest on the ventricles and false vocal folds, somewhat less common in the subglottis and on the aryepiglottic folds, and least common on the true vocal folds.[49,52] The most common clinical presentation is, however, for multiple sites of the larynx to be involved.[49] It is extremely rare for vocal fold fixation or cicatricial stenosis to occur in the context of laryngeal amyloidosis unless other predisposing factors are also present.[10] Various clinical descriptions of amyloidosis include that of a cystic lesion on the true vocal fold[53]; an infiltrating tumor of the true vocal folds and subglottis[51]; multinodular deposits in the subglottis, trachea, and mainstem bronchus[51]; a diffuse infiltrative subglottic narrowing[50]; and an ulcerative process of the anterior commissure with submucosal posterior commissure fullness extending into the subglottis.[50]

Four histologic patterns of amyloidosis have been described. These include amorphous random masses, deposits around blood vessel walls, deposits in continuity with the basement membrane of seromucinous glands, and deposits within adipose tissue.[50,54] Finally, in one series where the laryngeal deposits were carefully subtyped, the amyloidosis was found to be exclusively of the AL type, with more than 60% of the laryngeal deposits displaying a λ light chain staining pattern and 25% with a κ pattern.[49]

In the rare instances of laryngeal amyloidosis secondary to a chronic disease, management focuses upon control of the primary disease. In the much more common isolated laryngeal amyloidosis, the primary treatment is endoscopic surgical removal of nodules that interfere with laryngeal or airway function. In many series it has been demonstrated that if the lesion can be completely excised, there is little or no tendency for recurrence. Because the likelihood of recurrent or residual disease is significant, special care must be taken to avoid traumatization of adjacent normal laryngeal tissues.[53] Removal of amyloid lesions may be complicated by bleeding, because of the propensity of amyloid to infiltrate blood vessels. Advocates of CO_2 laser excision cite improved control of hemorrhage as one advantage of the laser. However, it is cautioned that laser use should be avoided in more extensive lesions because of the significant likelihood of extensive scarring postoperatively.[51,53] In large lesions it often becomes necessary to use external approaches. Although an early study indicated that "coring out" a subglottic lesion was a lasting and effective treatment,[52] more recent series employ laryngofissure for treatment of diffuse subglottic and tracheal amyloidosis. In such studies, excision and curettage of gross lesions has been used, and some have found that repeated curettage as necessary ultimately allows stabilization of the lesions and subsequent decannulation of tracheotomy-dependent patients.[50] Local or systemic steroids are ineffective in controlling or reversing the lesions of amyloidosis.[48,50,55]

In patients with significant subglottic amyloid deposits, bronchoscopy may be merited to determine the extent of the lesions. In addition, pulmonary function tests including flow-volume loops provide a helpful baseline of the patient's airway obstruction as well as differentiating between upper and lower airway obstruction.[48]

Overall, the prognosis for laryngeal amyloidosis is quite good. The need for a tracheotomy is rare,[10] although extensive subglottic lesions may require such measures until they can be controlled or resected.[50] Rarely, death has been reported secondary to amyloidosis; this occurs typically from diffuse tracheobronchial disease and pulmonary failure.[49]

WEGENER'S GRANULOMATOSIS

Wegener's granulomatosis is a multisystem inflammatory disease characterized by vasculitis, granuloma formation, and necrosis. It is of unknown etiology, and it classically affects the upper airway, lungs, and kidneys. The diagnosis requires the exclusion of fungal, mycobacterial, or other infectious agents that may cause similar histologic findings. While the cause of Wegener's granulomatosis is unknown, it is believed to be mediated immunologically.[56,57] The inflammatory events of Wegener's have an unusual affinity for ciliated respiratory epithelium, specifically the nasal cavity, paranasal sinuses, and the upper and lower tracheobronchial tree (Figure 25-4).

In recent years, various serologic markers have been proposed as a sign of disease activity in various autoimmune disorders. In the case of Wegener's granulomatosis, an anti-proteinase 3 antibody has been postulated as a marker of disease activity. This antibody, often interchanged with C-ANCA, is an IgG autoantibody against the neural serinase 3 protein, which is found in the secondary granules of polymorphonuclear cells. To date, a cause-and-effect relationship has not been established

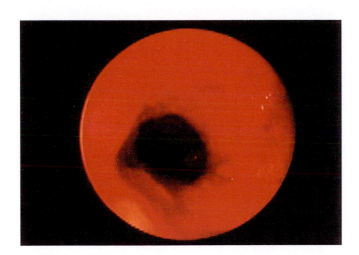

FIGURE 25-4. *Subglottic inflammation—inflamed subglottic larynx that histologically demonstrated necrotizing granulomatous inflammation, multinucleated giant cells, and vasculitis.*

clearly between the proteinase 3 antibodies and an active systemic Wegener's granulomatosis type of vasculitis. The other antineutrophil cytoplasmic antibody, the so-called P-ANCA, refers to a perinuclear staining pattern on immunofluorescence, as opposed to the C-ANCA, which is a cytoplasmic staining pattern on immunofluorescence. An antibody associated with the P-ANCA is more clearly associated with an anti-myeloperoxidase (IgG antibody) that is not felt to be pathognomonic or clearly related to the disease activity in Wegener's granulomatosis. This staining pattern is interpreted by laboratory technicians, and requires expertise and experience in defining the two patterns. The technical differences between the C-ANCA and anti-proteinase 3 antibodies are beyond the scope of this chapter. It is not known whether the anti-proteinase 3 antibodies are causative of the pathologic process or secondary to that process. The possibility of an epiphenomenon needs further elucidation. It is safe to say, however, that patients can have anti-proteinase 3 antibodies and not have Wegener's granulomatosis, and that other patients may clearly have clinicopathologic evidence of Wegener's granulomatosis and have no serologic activity against the proteinase 3 antigen. With that said, however, most rheumatologists and immunologists believe that there is an active correlation between C-ANCA titers and the presence of Wegener's granulomatosis.

Because Wegener's granulomatosis is a clinicopathologic diagnosis at the present time, a physician must identify clearly both the histologic features of the disease as well as its clinical features. This is in order to establish the diagnosis rigorously prior to instituting potentially very toxic treatments. Within the upper airways, one usually sees necrotizing granulomatous vasculitis with multinucleated giant cells and small vessel vasculitis. In the case of renal involvement, the pathologic picture includes necrotizing crescentic glomerulonephritis. In addition to the required tissue from the nose, sinuses, larynx, trachea, and lungs, other organs within the upper airways may contribute to the pathologic diagnosis. Any place where ciliated respiratory epithelium is present is a target organ for this type of vasculitis. Other less common sites of attack include the middle ear and mastoid, the lacrimal system, and ocular system, specifically the sclera. Other clinical evidence of disease would include blood markers that reflect systemic signs of inflammation, for example, acute-phase-reaction markers such as C-reactive protein. In patients who are acutely ill with Wegener's granulomatosis, nearly 100% of patients will demonstrate an elevated erythrocyte sedimentation rate as a marker of systemic inflammation. While these markers are highly sensitive for Wegener's, they are not very specific, as many other inflammatory and autoimmune diseases will cause elevation in acute-phase-reactant titers. Proteinase 3 antibodies are the most promising serologic marker of inflammation to be associated with Wegener's granulomatosis. However, it has to be emphasized that the diagnosis is not made by C-ANCA alone, but that confirmation of disease is still required both clinically and pathologically in order to rigorously and completely establish the diagnosis of Wegener's granulomatosis.

Because the glottic and selected supraglottic structures of the larynx contain squamous epithelium, primary laryngeal involvement in these regions is almost never seen. However, the subglottic larynx contains ciliated respiratory epithelium and is a site for both primary and secondary involvement of inflammation. Approximately 16% of patients with Wegener's granulomatosis develop varying degrees of subglottic stenosis. The spectrum of involvement varies from mild, non-circumferential narrowing or scarring to nearly complete obstruction (Figure 25-5). These changes are characterized by angry red granulomatous inflammation, with infected granulation tissue leading to imminent, complete airway obstruction.

The airway needs to be secured, based on standard clinical criteria. This can be done either by tracheotomy from below or debulking from above. Mechanical debulking may require jet ventilation because airway narrowing may preclude safe intubation, and intubation may obstruct the surgical field. Both the surgeon and the anesthesiologist should be familiar and comfortable with working in a compromised airway with the jet; otherwise, tracheotomy is the safest approach.

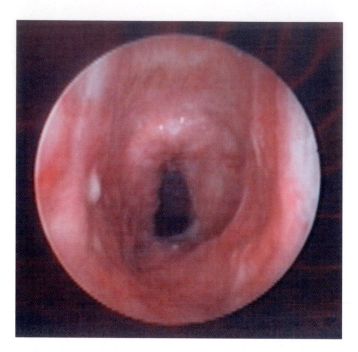

FIGURE 25-5. *Subglottic stenosis—circumferential narrowing of the subglottic larynx in a patient with Wegener's granulomatosis. Histologically the tissue demonstrated acute and chronic inflammation.*

Stenotic lesions of the subglottic larynx in patients with Wegener's granulomatosis may be caused primarily by scar tissue. They are predominantly non-proliferating fibroblasts in a stroma devoid of active inflammatory cells. In patients with primary vasculitis of the subglottic larynx, however, characteristic histopathologic findings might be present. This includes features of acute and chronic inflammation within both mononuclear and polymorphonuclear cell infiltrate. Necrotizing granulomas are present along with multinucleated giant cells and histiocytes. A zone of lymphocytic infiltration classically surrounds the granuloma. Also present is the hallmark of Wegener's granulomatosis involving small vessel vasculitis.[58] The vessel walls are invaded with polymorphonuclear cells that often lead to necrosis of the small vessel and the distal tissues dependent on that blood supply.

The management of subglottic stenosis in Wegener's granulomatosis is complex. It frequently requires individualized and multimodality interventions to achieve satisfactory results.[59] These interventions generally include tracheotomy for airway support prior to long-term management. Long-term airway management may include laser resections of stenotic sites. Mechanical dilatations as well as intralesional injections of long-acting steroid suspensions have been successful. In patients with refractory subglottic stenosis, external approaches including laryngotracheoplasty with anterior and posterior cricoid splits have been used both with and without long-term laryngeal stents. In some cases of laryngotracheoplasty, microvascular free flaps taken from distant sites have aided reconstruction of the subglottic larynx.[59] The theoretical basis for bringing in healthy and independently vascularized tissue is that the hallmark of the disease is a small vessel vasculitis. Once patients are in remission, a new vascular supply to a reconstructed organ may help in long-term healing and decreased scarring.

IDIOPATHIC MIDLINE DESTRUCTIVE DISEASE

Idiopathic midline destructive disease, also known as lethal midline granuloma, is a clinical diagnosis of an inflammatory destructive disease of the midfacial structures. The disease frequently starts in the region of the nose and paranasal sinuses. Lesions come through the midline and often include the laryngotracheal complex. While its etiology has not been elucidated, the present evidence suggests that many cases of idiopathic midline destructive disease are variants of a histiocytic lymphoma. While the underlying pathologic process may be malignancy, there are clearly inflammatory components to this disease that help foment the local destructive process.[60,61]

Patients may present with symptoms anywhere from the nose down to the tracheal carina, and the initiating symptoms may be local to the larynx. Hoarseness, hemoptysis, and dyspnea may be present. Symptomatic airway obstruction may occur early as the disease progresses, and the airway may need to be secured from below with a tracheotomy.

On physical examination the laryngeal mucosa is inflamed and ulcerated, having an almost infected-looking appearance. As in most diseases of unknown etiology in the larynx, a careful history as well as deep mucosal and submucosal biopsies are necessary for diagnosis. Once pathologic confirmation of idiopathic midline destructive disease is obtained, treatment is primarily low-dose external beam irradiation. Because margins in the oncologic sense do not exist in this particular disorder, one should consult a radiation oncologist with knowledge and experience in its treatment. In most cases the radiation fields include normal-looking tissue and possibly asymptomatic distant sites. If progressive laryngeal stenosis causes collapse of the upper respiratory tract, long-term laryngeal rehabilitation is best accomplished with open repair, including microvascular reconstruction to the anterior wall of the cricoid cartilage.

PEMPHIGUS

Pemphigus vulgaris is a bullous disease that predominantly involves the mucous membranes. Both the larynx and the oropharynx may be involved. The disease is generally seen in older patients, with a predilection for people of either Mediterranean or Jewish ancestry. Hoarseness may be the presenting symptom. On fiberoptic examination one may see characteristic bullae that rupture fairly easily. Underneath is denuded epithelium that is frequently covered by a fibrinous, white exudate. On pathologic examination, one finds acantholysis and bullae formation in the epidermis. This ultimately leads to a discontinuity between the basal layers attached to the dermis and the bullae themselves that are attached to the epidermis.

Immunologically, there are deposits of IgG and complement, specifically C3, between the cells within the malpighian layer of the epidermis, and they are pathognomonic for pemphigus vulgaris. In addition, tissue-fixed antibodies of the intracellular substance with the patient's epithelial tissue may be demonstrated by immunofluorescent staining.[62-64]

As in most laryngeal disorders, a history followed by physical examination and mucosal biopsies is critical for establishing the diagnosis. Treatment for this disorder is primarily systemic corticosteroids. Whether additional immune system modulators are required is subject to debate; systemic cytotoxic medication has been promulgated by some as concomitant treatment for the severe form of pemphigus vulgaris. Occasionally, antibiotic treatment is necessary to treat the secondary infection seen over the denuded epithelium on previously ruptured bullae.[64]

RHEUMATOID ARTHRITIS

Rheumatoid arthritis is a systemic immune disorder that affects synovial joints throughout the body. The cricoarytenoid joint is, therefore, subject to degenerative changes as are joints elsewhere in the body. Hoarseness and odynophagia are classic symptoms associated with cricoarytenoid arthritis in addition to a sense of throat fullness that is felt by some. Additionally, referred otalgia, dyspnea, and occasionally, tenderness, are present. In severe cases of bilateral joint disease, stridor may be present.

During physical examination, bright red swelling over the arytenoid may be seen during the acute inflammatory process. The true vocal folds may be edematous, and occasionally, there may be stridor present during inspiration. Occasionally, severe arthritis of the joint may lead to impaired mobility culminating in a fixed vocal fold in the adducted position. As affected patients are treated with anti-inflammatory agents, a more chronic stage may develop that will show roughness and thickening of the mucosa over the arytenoids and a decreased glottic chink. It should be remembered by all physicians that hoarseness may be the presenting symptom of rheumatoid arthritis. In addition to a laryngeal examination, the history should probe for complaints of systemic arthralgias that may or may not have been relieved with anti-inflammatories. Serologic testing, particularly an erythrocyte sedimentation rate and antibodies to the rheumatoid factor, should be considered as part of the immune workup. In severe cases of bilateral joint involvement, tracheotomy may be necessary.

Other collagen vascular diseases may mimic rheumatoid arthritis and present similarly. Reiter's disease and gout are two such diseases that can also affect the larynx. Crohn's disease as well as ankylosing spondylitis have been associated with arthritis of the cricoarytenoid joint. Gastroesophageal reflux disease contributes to the development of many otolaryngologic symptoms, including laryngeal granulomata, cervical dysphagia, subglottic stenosis, and arthritis of the cricoarytenoid joint. In severe cases where an airway needs to be supplemented via tracheotomy, rehabilitation of the airway is difficult. In addition to medical management that might include nonsteroidal anti-inflammatories and corticosteroids, the surgeon might consider vocal fold lateralization techniques to help those desiring decannulation.

RELAPSING POLYCHONDRITIS

Relapsing polychondritis is a rare autoimmune disorder: approximately 30 cases are presently known to exist in the United States. Patients present typically with very painful swellings of the pinna and nose, and progressive loss of the dorsal nasal cartilage support. Loss of this support manifests itself clinically as a saddle-nose deformity. Immunologically, it is thought that there is antibody to cartilage, resulting in a soft, non-springy texture in cartilaginous tissues (Figure 25-6). This loss to the tracheobronchial skeleton manifests itself in impaired breathing.[65] As a consequence of Bernoulli's principle, airway collapse tends to increase as the velocity of air through the tracheobronchial tree is increased. In cases of laryngeal involvement, tracheotomy is frequently necessary to decrease the amount of ventilatory dead space as well as bypass a larynx that functions clinically as with severe laryngomalacia.

A clinical history usually beginning with otalgia and fullness, physical findings of redness, and serologic

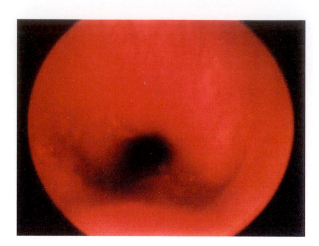

FIGURE 25-6. *Laryngeal collapse—severe chondromalacia demonstrating collapse of the subglottic larynx during respiration in a patient with relapsing polychondritis.*

markers is usually sufficient to confirm the diagnosis.[66] Treatment includes systemic corticosteroids and in many cases cyclophosphamide. Nebulized racemic ephedrine has been advocated for treatment of life-threatening airway edema, which may characterize acute exacerbations of this disease.[67]

Occasionally, management of the laryngotracheal complex as well as the larger airways of the lung, including the secondary and tertiary bronchi, may be managed by submucosal injections of corticosteroids into stenotic segments that appear to have poor function. The long-term prognosis remains poor, but the disease is no longer invariably fatal.

SUMMARY

Many infectious and immunologic disorders may afflict the larynx. Otolaryngologists should be familiar with these challenging disorders, and should remain informed about new developments in diagnosis and treatment.

REFERENCES

1. Lerner DM, Deeb Z. Acute upper airway obstruction resulting from systemic diseases. *South Med J.* 1993;86:623-627.

2. Wolf M, Strauss B, Kronenberg J, et al. Conservative management of adult epiglottitis. *Laryngoscope.* 1990;100:183-185.

3. Parrillo JE, Bone RC. *Critical Care Medicine: Principles of Diagnosis and Management.* St. Louis, MO: Mosby; 1995:1016-1017.

4. McFerran DJ, Abdullah V, Gallimore AP, et al. Vocal process granulomata. *J Laryngol Otol.* 1994;108:216-220.

5. Gould SJ, Howard S. The histopathology of the larynx in the neonate following endotracheal intubation. *J Pathol.* 1985;146:301-311.

6. Mintz DR, Gullane PJ, Thomson DH, et al. Perichondritis of the larynx following radiation. *Otolaryngol Head Neck Surg.* 1981;89:550-554.

7. Soda A, Rubio H, Salazar M, et al. Tuberculosis of the larynx: clinical aspects in 19 patients. *Laryngoscope.* 1989;99:1147-1150.

8. Galietti F, Giorgis GE, Oliaro A, et al. Tuberculosis of the larynx. *Panminerva Med.* 1989;31:134-136.

9. DuPlessis A, Hussey G. Laryngeal tuberculosis in childhood. *Pediatr Infect Dis J.* 1987;6:678-681.

10. Caldarelli DD, Freidberg SA, Harris AA. Medical and surgical aspects of the granulomatous diseases of the larynx. *Otolaryngol Clin North Am.* 1979;12:767-781.

11. Younus M. Leprosy in ENT. *J Laryngol Otol.* 1986;100:1437-1442.

12. Sandberg P, Shum TK. Lepromatous leprosy of the larynx. *Otolaryngol Head Neck Surg.* 1983;91:216-220.

13. Wathen PI. Hansen's disease. *South Med J.* 1996;89:647-652.

14. Soni NK. Leprosy of the larynx. *J Laryngol Otol.* 1992;106:518-520.

15. Gupta OP, Jain RK, Tripathi PP, et al. Leprosy of the larynx: a clinicopathological study. *Int J Lepr Other Mycobact Dis.* 1984;52:171-175.

16. Liu TC, Qiu JS. Pathological findings on peripheral nerves, lymph nodes, and visceral organs of leprosy. *Int J Lepr Other Mycobact Dis.* 1984;52:377-383.

17. Pillsbury HC, Sasaki CT. Granulomatous diseases of the larynx. *Otolaryngol Clin North Am.* 1982;15:539-551.

18. McNulty JS, Fassett RL. Syphilis: an otolaryngologic perspective. *Laryngoscope.* 1981;91:889-905.

19. Lacy PD, Alderson DJ, Parker AJ. Late congenital syphilis of the larynx and pharynx presenting at endotracheal intubation. *J Laryngol Otol.* 1994;108:688-689.

20. Andraca R, Edson RS, Kern EB. Rhinoscleroma: a growing concern in the United States? Mayo Clinic experience. *Mayo Clin Proc.* 1993;68:1151-1157.

21. Soni NK. Scleroma of the larynx. *J Laryngol Otol.* 1997;111:438-440.

22. Fajardo-Dolci G, Chavolla R, Lamadrid-Bautista E, et al. Laryngeal scleroma. *J Otolaryngol.* 1999;28:229-231.

23. Postma GN, Wawrose S, Tami TA. Isolated subglottic scleroma. *Ear Nose Throat J.* 1996;75:306-308.

24. Amoils CP, Shindo ML. Laryngotracheal manifestations of rhinoscleroma. *Ann Otol Rhinol Laryngol.* 1996;105:336-340.

25. Zitsch RP III, Bothwell M. Actinomycosis: a potential complication of head and neck surgery. *Am J Otolaryngol.* 1999;20:260-262.

26. Nelson EG, Tybor AG. Actinomycosis of the larynx. *Ear Nose Throat J.* 1992;71:356-358.

27. Tsuji DH, Fukuda H, Kawasaki Y, et al. Actinomycosis of the larynx. *Auris Nasus Larynx.* 1991;18:79-85.

28. Hughes RA, Paonessa DF, Conway WF. Actinomycosis of the larynx. *Ann Otol Rhinol Laryngol.* 1984;93:520-524.

29. Shaheen SO, Ellis FG. Actinomycosis of the larynx. *J R Soc Med.* 1983;76:226-228.

30. Dumich PS, Neel HB. Blastomycosis of the larynx. *Laryngoscope.* 1983;93:1266-1270.

31. Reder PA, Neel HB. Blastomycosis in otolaryngology: review of a large series. *Laryngoscope.* 1993;103:53-58.

32. Mikaelian AJ, Varkey B, Grossman TW, et al. Blastomycosis of the head and neck. *Otolaryngol Head Neck Surg.* 1989;101:489-495.

33. Suen JY, Wetmore SJ, Wetzel WJ, et al. Blastomycosis of the larynx. *Ann Otol Rhinol Laryngol.* 1980;89:563-566.

34. McCune MA, Rogers RS, Roberts GD. Laryngeal presentation of blastomycosis. *Int J Dermatol.* 1980;19:263-269.

35. Hajare S, Rakusan TA, Kalia A, et al. Laryngeal coccidioidomycosis causing airway obstruction. *Pediatr Infect Dis J.* 1989;8:54-56.

36. Boyle JO, Coulthard SW, Mandel RM. Laryngeal involvement in disseminated coccidioidomycosis. *Arch Otolaryngol Head Surg.* 1991;117:433-438.

37. Sataloff RT, Wilborn A, Prestipino A, et al. Histoplasmosis of the larynx. *Am J Otolaryngol.* 1993;14:199-205.

38. Gerber ME, Rosdeutscher JD, Seiden AM, et al. Histoplasmosis: the otolaryngologist's perspective. *Laryngoscope.* 1995;105:919-923.

39. Reibel JF, Jahrsdoerfer RA, Johns MM, et al. Histoplasmosis of the larynx. *Otolaryngol Head Neck Surg.* 1982;90:740-743.

40. Negroni R, Palmieri O, Koren F, et al. Oral treatment of paracoccidioidomycosis and histoplasmosis with itraconazole in humans. *Rev Infect Dis.* 1987;9(suppl 1):S47-S50.

41. Ellison DE, Canalis RF. Sarcoidosis of the head and neck. *Clin Dermatol.* 1986;4:136-142.

42. Gallivan GJ, Landis JN. Sarcoidosis of the larynx: preserving and restoring airway and professional voice. *J Voice.* 1993;7:81-94.

43. Neel HB III, McDonald TJ. Laryngeal sarcoidosis: report of 13 patients. *Ann Otol Rhinol Laryngol.* 1982;91:359-362.

44. Sakamoto M, Ishizawa M, Kitahara N. Polypoid type of laryngeal sarcoidosis—case report and review of the literature. *Eur Arch Otorhinolaryngol.* 2000;257:436-438.

45. Benjamin B, Dalton C, Croxson G. Laryngoscopic diagnosis of laryngeal sarcoid. *Ann Otol Rhinol Laryngol.* 1995;104:529-531.

46. Bower JS, Belen JE, Weg JG, et al. Manifestations and treatment of laryngeal sarcoidosis. *Am Rev Respir Dis.* 1980;122:325-332.

47. Raymond AK, Sneige N, Batsakis JG. Amyloidosis in the upper aerodigestive tracts. *Ann Otol Rhinol Laryngol.* 1992;101:794-796.

48. Finn DG, Farmer JC. Management of amyloidosis of the larynx and trachea. *Arch Otolaryngol.* 1982;108:54-56.

49. Lewis JE, Olsen KD, Kurtin PJ, et al. Laryngeal amyloidosis: a clinicopathologic and immunohistochemical review. *Otolaryngol Head Neck Surg.* 1992;106:372-377.

50. Fernandes CM, Pirle D, Pudifin DJ. Laryngeal amyloidosis. *J Laryngol Otol.* 1982;96:1165-1175.

51. Simpson GT II, Strong MS, Skinner M, et al. Localized amyloidosis of the head and neck and upper aerodigestive and lower respiratory tracts. *Ann Otol Rhinol Laryngol.* 1984;93:374-379.

52. Djalilian M, McDonald TI, Devine KD, et al. Nontraumatic, nonneoplastic subglottic stenosis. *Ann Otol.* 1975;84:757-763.

53. Talbot AR. Laryngeal amyloidosis. *J Laryngol Otol.* 1990;104:147-149.

54. Barnes EL, Zofar T. Laryngeal amyloidosis: clinicopathological study of seven years. *Ann Otol.* 1977;86:856-862.

55. Mitrani M, Biller HF. Laryngeal amyloidosis. *Laryngoscope.* 1985;95:1346-1347.

56. Hoare TJ, Jayne D, RhysEvans P, et al. Wegener's granulomatosis, subglottic stenosis, and antineutrophil cytoplasm antibodies. *J Laryngol Otol.* 1989;103:1187-1197.

57. Rasmussen N, Petersen J. Cellular immune responses and pathogenesis in C-ANCA positive vasculitides. *J Autoimmun.* 1993;6:227-236.

58. Case records of the Massachusetts General Hospital. Weekly clinicopathological exercises. Case 31-1986. A 39-year-old woman with stenosis of the subglottic area and pulmonary artery. *N Engl J Med.* 1986;7:378-387.

59. Lebovics RS, Hoffman GS, Leavitt RY, et al. The management of subglottic stenosis in patients with Wegener's granulomatosis. *Laryngoscope.* 1992;102:1341-1345.

60. Lu SY, Chen WJ, Eng HL. Lethal midline granuloma: report of three cases. *Changgeng Yi Xue Za Zhi.* 2000;23:99-106.

61. Barker TH, Hosni AA. Idiopathic midline destructive disease—does it exist? *J Laryngol Otol.* 1998;112:307-309.

62. Case records of the Massachusetts General Hospital. Weekly clinicopathological exercises. Case 19-1992. A 56-year-old man with Waldenstrom's macroglobulinemia and cutaneous and oral vesicles. *N Engl J Med.* 1992;326:1276-1284.

63. Nousari HC, Anhalt GJ. Pemphigus and bullous pemphigoid. *Lancet.* 1999;354:667-672.

64. Saunders MS, Gentile RD, Lobritz RW. Primary laryngeal and nasal septal lesions in pemphigus vulgaris. *J Am Osteopath Assoc.* 1992;92:933-937.

65. Estes SA. Relapsing polychondritis. A case report and literature review. *Cutis.* 1983;32:471-476.

66. Batsakis JG, Manning JT. Relapsing polychondritis. *Ann Otol Rhinol Laryngol.* 1989;98:83-84.

67. Gaffney RJ, Harrison M, Blayney AW. Nebulized racemic ephedrine in the treatment of acute exacerbations of laryngeal relapsing polychondritis. *J Laryngol Otol.* 1992;106:63-64.

CHAPTER 26

Neurologic Disorders and the Voice

Marshall E. Smith, MD

Lorraine Olson Ramig, PhD

The laryngeal mechanism is subject to highly complex, extensive neural control; therefore, it is not surprising that disorders of the nervous system have effects on the voice. The phonatory function of the larynx, as well as its roles in respiration and swallowing, can be affected by a wide range of neurologic disorders. These span the entire spectrum of central to peripheral *etiologies* and include trauma, cerebral vascular accidents, tumors, and diseases of the nervous system. Except for the more common problem of laryngeal nerve paralysis and the unusual, but disabling, entity of spasmodic dysphonia, neurologically based voice disorders until recently have been a neglected topic for both basic and clinical research in the fields of otolaryngology, speech pathology, and neurology. It is now more apparent that laryngeal dysfunction is a component of many neurologic disorders and should be a critical consideration in patient assessment and management.[1]

While there have been advances in knowledge of neurologic control of vocalization,[2-5] it is readily apparent that there is little information on laryngeal pathophysiology of many neurologic disorders. The integration between the basic science and clinical realm in neurolaryngology is far from complete. Advances in clinical and research laryngology have begun to bridge this gap. Laryngeal imaging has greatly assisted our ability to visually examine and record laryngeal function.[6-8] In this way, the laryngeal examination has become more accessible as part of a neurologic assessment. Other voice examination techniques include acoustic analysis, glottography, and aerodynamic and electromyographic measures.[9-12] These also have emerging roles in documentation, diagnosis, and assessment of treatment efficacy for neurologic voice disorders.[13-17]

The causes of neurologic disorders of the voice range from common to obscure, depending on the disorder. The "immobile vocal fold" is a frequently encountered clinical problem in otolaryngology. Though speech problems are often associated with the common neurologic conditions of stroke and head injury, the association of *voice* disorders with these conditions has not been systematically described. Eighty-nine percent of the 1.5 million patients with Parkinson's disease in the United States have voice disorders.[18] Essential tremor is the most common movement disorder; it affects the voice in 4 to 20% of cases.[19] Less often encountered are the voice disorders associated with neurologic diseases such as Huntington's disease and cerebellar ataxia. Koufman reviewed a series of 100 consecutive patients seen in a practice with voice complaints.[20] Sixteen had neurologic disorders of the voice, 8 with vocal fold paralysis, and 8 with a variety of other neurologic diseases, including Parkinson's disease, vocal tremor, and myasthenia gravis.

One *framework* for studying neurologic diseases and the voice has come from studies of speech disorders.

Research by Darley et al[21,22] identified different clinically distinguishable types of dysarthrias that could be correlated with pathology in specific areas of the central and peripheral nervous systems. Because many of these neurologic disorders also involve dysphonias, a similar "site-of-lesion" approach was adopted as a tool for classification of neurologic voice disorders.[7,23,24] A general outline of this classic approach is given in Table 26-1.

Aronson has categorized neurologic voice disorders according to the nature of the voice production, whether constant or variable.[25] Five types were described: 1) Relatively constant neurologic voice disorders, including flaccid, spastic (pseudobulbar), mixed flaccid-spastic, and hypokinetic (parkinsonian) dysphonias; 2) Arrhythmically fluctuating neurologic voice disorders, including ataxic, choreic, and dystonic dysphonias; 3) Rhythmically fluctuating dysphonias, including dysphonias of essential voice tremor and palatopharyngolaryngeal myoclonus; 4) Paroxysmal neurologic voice disorder, the sudden abberant phonatory bursts of Gilles de la Tourette syndrome; 5) Neurologic voice disorders associated with loss of volitional phonation, such as apraxia of speech and phonation associated with cerebrovascular accidents. A strength of this classification scheme is its focus on the resulting voice production. However, it does not give direction to the clinician regarding phonatory function to guide treatment interventions.

Recently, Ramig and Scherer[26] proposed a system for considering neurologic voice disorders with specific application to *treatment*. Rather than relating the neurologic disorder to the site of neural damage, this classification system focuses on the existing phonatory dysfunction and resulting voice characteristics. The following categories of neural-based phonatory dysfunction were proposed: *adduction* problems (hypoadduction and hyperadduction), *stability* problems (long-term, eg, tremor and short-term, eg, hoarseness), and *coordination* problems (phonatory incoordination, eg, dysprosody). These categories were used to organize approaches to treatment of neurologic voice disorders,

Classification	Examples
I. Flaccid paresis or paralysis (lower motor neuron)	
A. Muscle	Myopathies, muscular dystrophies
B. Neuromuscular junction	Myasthenia gravis
C. Peripheral nerve	
1. RLN	Trauma, tumor, idiopathic, iatrogenic
2. SLN	(surgery, drugs, radiation), collagen –
3. Upper vagus nerve	vascular, Guillain-Barré
D. Brain stem nucleus	Stroke (Wallenberg's syndrome), Arnold-Chiari malformation, syringobulbia, tumor, trauma
II. Spastic paresis (upper motor neuron)	Pseudobulbar palsy
III. Dyskinetic movement disorders (extrapyramidal system)	Parkinson's disease, essential tremor, dyskinesias, myoclonus, choreas, laryngeal dystonias
IV. Ataxias (cerebellar)	Degeneration, hemorrhage, infarction
V. Apraxias (cortical and subcortical)	Trauma, stroke, tumor, cerebral palsy
VI. Mixed disorders	Amyotrophic lateral sclerosis, multiple sclerosis, Shy-Drager syndrome

TABLE 26-1. *Traditional Classification of Neurologic Voice Disorders Based on Cause*

which focused on modification of laryngeal physical pathology with corresponding changes in perceptual characteristics of voice and *improved functional speech production*. This classification system, in a modified form (Table 26-2) is used to organize the description of neurologic voice disorders in this chapter on the dimensions of *adduction/abduction* and *stability*. It includes mixed disorders that combine features of these two dimensions. Miscellaneous disorders comprise the fourth and fifth types listed by Aronson.[25] Phonatory coordination problems (eg, dysprosody, voice-voiceless contrasts) have been reviewed elsewhere[26] and will not be repeated here as neurologic disorders affecting this dimension frequently overlap with the first two dimen-

Classification	Examples
I. Adduction or abduction problems	
A. Hypoadduction	All lower motor neuron laryngeal paresis or paralysis
	Myasthenia Gravis
	Parkinson's disease
	Parkinsonism
	Shy-Drager syndrome
	Progressive supranuclear palsy
	Traumatic brain injury
B. Hyperadduction	Pseudobulbar palsy
	Huntington's disease
	Adductor laryngeal dystonia (spasmodic dysphonia)
C. Malabduction	Abductor laryngeal dystonia (spasmodic dysphonia)
II. Phonatory instability	
A. Short-term (cycle-to-cycle perturbation, aperiodicity, subharmonics)	Nearly all neurologically based voice disorders
B. Long-term (tremor)	Essential vocal tremor
	Parkinson's disease
	Dystonic tremor
	Cerebellar tremor
	Amyotrophic lateral sclerosis vocal "flutter"
	Palatopharyngolaryngeal myoclonus
	Other respiratory or vocal tract sources
III. Mixed disorders (adduction, abduction, instability)	Amyotrophic lateral sclerosis
	Multiple sclerosis
	Ataxic (cerebellar) dysphonia
	Mixed (abductor-adductor-tremor) spasmodic dysphonia
	Progressive supranuclear palsy
	Shy-Drager syndrome
IV. Miscellaneous disorders	Apraxic dysphonia of cortical dysfunction
	Involuntary phonation of Tourette syndrome

TABLE 26-2. *Classification of Neurologic Voice Disorders Based on Phonatory Dysfunction*

sions. It should be recognized that phonatory function in neurologic disorders can vary and show features of hypoadduction, hyperadduction, malabduction, instability, and/or incoordination at the same time, or that these features may vary during the course of an individual's disease. Nonetheless, the classification provides an outline for observing and interpreting the effects of neurologic disorders on voice that can then guide treatment interventions, be they behavioral, medical, and/or surgical. Treatment of neurologic voice disorders will be reviewed briefly in this chapter but covered extensively elsewhere in this book.

DISORDERS OF ADDUCTION

Disorders of vocal fold adduction accompanying neurologic disorders can range from inadequate adduction (hypoadduction) to excessive adduction (hyperadduction) to inappropriately timed abduction (malabduction).

Hypoadduction

Hypoadduction is observed in many forms and degrees in many neurologic disorders. Damage to any component of the motor unit (muscle, neuromuscular junction, nerve, or nucleus) may result in vocal fold hypoadduction. The most common example of this is vocal fold paralysis. It is also recognized that hypoadduction is found in neurologic diseases of central origin, including Parkinson's disease[27,28] and closed head injury.[29] A primary consequence of hypoadduction is reduced vocal loudness and breathiness.

Hypoadduction Associated With Disorders of the Muscle

Inflammatory myopathies, including polymyositis and dermatomyositis, are unusual conditions that may affect laryngeal function, particularly swallowing.[30] Muscular dystrophies are inherited diseases that yield progressive weakness that is variable in age of onset, distribution, and disability.[30,31] The main laryngeal symptomatology concerns swallowing, yielding oropharyngolaryngeal weakness. Ramig[32] reported increased acoustic aperiodicity and weak, hoarse, and nasal voices in patients with myotonic muscular dystrophy. Myotonic dystrophy is associated mainly with velopharyngeal incompetence.[33,34]

Hypoadduction Associated With Disorders of the Neuromuscular Junction

Interruption of transmission of nerve impulses at the neuromuscular junction may lead to flaccid paresis or paralysis of the vocal folds. Myasthenia gravis (MG) is a neuromuscular disease manifested by weakness and fatigability of voluntary muscles. The incidence of MG has been reported between 2-10 per 100,000.[35,36] Overall, it is seen twice as frequently in women as men, with an even higher ratio in the third and fourth decades. Men usually develop MG in their 50s or 60s.[80] Although neonatal and juvenile forms exist, voice and speech symptoms as initial or secondary symptoms occur primarily in the adult form. An association has been made with thymomas.

MG frequently presents with otolaryngologic symptoms. The most common presenting symptoms are ocular (ptosis and diplopia). It is important to recognize that other head and neck symptoms may be present as an initial manifestation of MG. Carpenter et al reviewed 175 patients with MG.[37] 30 percent had primary symptoms of dysphagia, dysarthria, or dysphonia. Dhillon and Brookes reviewed 48 patients with MG.[38] Nine of their patients had only head and neck symptoms initially, 6 of these complained of dysphonia, usually in conjunction with dysphagia. Calcaterra et al had an even higher percentage of patients in their series present with voice complaints.[39] Of fifty patients with MG, 26 had initial speech complaint: 13 with dysarthria, 5 with hypernasality, 4 with stridor, and 4 with vocal weakness. Vocal fatigue is the major voice complaint in individuals with MG. It may be misdiagnosed as a superior laryngeal nerve paralysis, or bilateral vocal fold paresis/paralysis.[40] These and other reports[41] make the neurolaryngologist and speech pathologist aware that voice and laryngeal involvement may occur as an initial or secondary symptom in MG.

Examination of the larynx in patients suspected of MG should involve observation of the velopharynx for inadequate closure, as well as glottal insufficiency—incomplete adduction or bowing of the vocal folds. The patient should be "stressed" with repetitive vocalizing tasks (reading or counting out loud for 5 minutes) to induce fatigability of involved structures. Phonating or singing a sustained high note for several minutes may induce fatigue with a noticeable drop in pitch of the voice.[42] Fatigability may also be assessed by testing for stapedial reflex decay.[43] Laryngoscopy may raise the suspicion of the examiner to suspect sluggish vocal fold mobility or asymmetry, suggestive of superior laryngeal nerve (SNL) paralysis. Laryngeal EMG of the cricothyroid muscles is helpful to differentiate SLN paralysis from MG.[40] A fluctuation in vocal fold mobility during repeated examinations is suggestive of MG.[80] The diagnosis is made by a *Tensilon* (edrophonium) test. Edrophonium, a short-acting anticholinesterase drug, administered intravenously results in prompt reversal of symptoms.

Improvement in voice and resonance characteristics on spectrograms following edrophonium injection has been documented.[44] Because of the concern for progression to respiratory involvement that may occur in MG, prompt neurologic referral is warranted if MG is suspected.[45] Treatment of MG involves anticholinesterase drugs (eg, pyridostigmine). Steroids are used for severe cases. The effect of thymectomy in treatment of MG is controversial, but is generally recommended in younger patients.[46]

Hypoadduction Associated With Disorders of the Peripheral Nerve (Recurrent Laryngeal Nerve)

Vocal fold paralysis is a common problem resulting in vocal fold hypoadduction, probably the most common neurologic voice disorder seen by the otolaryngologist.[20] This section will generally concern *unilateral vocal fold paralysis* (UVP), as this commonly affects the voice and is much more frequently seen than bilateral vocal fold paralysis. It should be mentioned, however, that bilateral vocal fold weakness may also present with dysphonia and requires an extensive evaluation.[47] Many surveys have reported on the etiologies of vocal fold paralysis. The results of nine surveys involving 1,019 patients were compiled by Terris et al.[48] 36 percent of cases were from neoplasm with 55 percent of these caused by lung cancer. 25 percent were postsurgical, mainly from thyroidectomy. Other causes included idiopathic (14%), inflammatory or medical (13%), and central neurologic (6%). Medical etiologies should be sought in obscure cases, such as vincristine (a chemotherapeutic drug) induced laryngeal neuropathy,[49] or post-polio syndrome associated laryngeal paresis or paralysis.[50-53] The distinction between "idiopathic" and "inflammatory" causes of laryngeal paralysis may be blurred; in many cases "idiopathic" UVP is felt to be an isolated neuropathy caused by virus.[54-56]

The patient symptoms in UVP vary widely. Complaints of hoarse voice and breathy voice are frequent, although it is important to recognize that the voice may be fairly normal.[57] Problems with swallowing, choking, coughing, and aspiration can be found and may be of more immediate concern in considering intervention. The voice in a patient with UVP is usually perceived as reduced in loudness, hoarse, and breathy. Diplophonia may be present. Acoustic findings that often accompany UVP include increased aperiodicity, reduced pitch range and variation, reduced vocal intensity, and decreased harmonics to noise ratio.[57] Variations in glottographic patterns may be seen.[58-60] Glottal aerodynamics often demonstrate high mean airflow rates, and an offset of airflow from baseline ("DC leak"), reflecting glottal insufficiency.[57,61]

There are several factors that influence glottal dynamics and resulting voice in UVP. These include: 1) individual variations in laryngeal framework anatomy[62] and peripheral innervation[63]; 2) the degree and extent of reinnervation[64]; 3) the degree of laryngeal muscle atrophy[65,66]; 4) the time variation of the second and third factors; and, very importantly, 5) individual vocalizing behaviors and laryngeal biomechanics that attempt to compensate for the glottal insufficiency.[67] The particular voice symptoms are created by the complex interaction of the above factors that influence laryngeal biomechanics, particularly in UVP relating to the geometry of the glottic (anterior and posterior) aperture, the three-dimensional position and orientation of the arytenoids, the vertical position of the folds relative to each other, muscle stiffness asymmetries and resulting body-cover relationships, and the interaction of these with glottal airflow and pressures.[7,68]

Laryngoscopy (flexible and rigid telescope) is of critical importance in the evaluation of UVP, as in other voice disorders. Laryngostroboscopy is also very helpful for viewing the effects of UVP on vocal fold position and movement, and glottal closure, mucosal wave asymmetries, and vocal process vertical position.[69] Tomography has also been used in UVP to demonstrate vocal folds on different vertical levels.[70]

The relationship between the location of peripheral laryngeal nerve lesion and the position of the affected vocal fold in UVP seen on laryngoscopy has been a source of controversy. A common notion, promulgated as the "Wagner-Grossman theory," related the position of the vocal fold in vocal fold paralyses to the activity of the cricothyroid muscle.[71] Clinical relevance has been ascribed to this theory by relating glottal configuration to the topognostic localization of site of laryngeal nerve injury.[55,72] In vivo studies have yielded conflicting results.[71,72] Several recent clinical studies have questioned this dogma, pointing to the wide variability in glottal position at various locations of injury.[73-75] A factor complicating this issue is that, in many cases, the exact site and degree of nerve injury are unknown.[7] Neuroanatomic studies have shed light on this controversy. Sanders et al described multiple and variable ipsilateral and crossed interconnections in the peripheral innervation of the human larynx between the superior and recurrent laryngeal nerves.[63] These variations may help explain the spectrum of glottal configurations seen in UVP.

The management of dysphonia secondary to UVP includes behavioral therapy[76] and a variety of surgical techniques. These are covered extensively in other chapters of this book.

Hypoadduction Associated With Disorders of the Peripheral Nerve (Superior Laryngeal Nerve)

Superior laryngeal nerve (SLN) paralysis is less common than recurrent laryngeal paralysis.[77] Causes include surgical trauma (eg, thyroidectomy, carotid endarterectomy), blunt neck trauma, and idiopathic cases. Its presentation may be subtle. Voice complaints may be only of a mild hoarseness, vocal fatigue, or difficulty with projection or singing despite normal speaking voice.[40,78] The laryngeal examination findings in unilateral SLN paralysis have been described as a rotation of the anterior commissure away from and posterior glottis toward the affected (paralyzed) side.[7,77] This maneuver may only be evident by having the patient attempt to phonate at high pitch.[79] Shortening of the vocal fold, unilateral bowing, or scissoring of the vocal folds may be observed.[80] The asymmetry of laryngeal vibration in SLN paralysis may be seen on laryngostroboscopy.[81] This asymmetry has been demonstrated in mathematical simulations[68,82] and animal phonation models of SLN paralysis.[83]

Hypoadduction Associated With Disorders of the Nucleus

Injury to the lower motor neurons of the tenth nerve nucleus results in flaccid laryngeal paralysis and hypoadduction.[23,24] The injury can occur via vascular brain stem infarction of the posterior inferior cerebellar artery. This vascular accident when associated with symptoms of dysphagia and dysarthria, ipsilateral Horner's syndrome, ipsilateral face, and contralateral body pain-temperature impairment, is known as Wallenberg's (lateral pontomedullary) syndrome. Other causes include Arnold-Chiari malformation, syringobulbia, tumor, and trauma.

Hypoadduction Associated With Parkinson's Disease

Hypoadduction is *commonly* associated with the extrapyramidal disorder of idiopathic Parkinson's disease (IPD), a nigrostriatal disorder characterized by dopamine deficiency.[84] Rigidity, tremor, and reduced range of motion are the primary physical pathologies associated with IPD. One in every 100 individuals over 60 and 1 in every 1,000 individuals under age 60 have IPD. While IPD is frequently considered a disease of the elderly, patients have been diagnosed as early as the third decade of life. Patients can live 10-20 years after diagnosis. At least 89% of the 1.5 million individuals with IPD in the United States have a voice disorder.[18]

The voice disorder in IPD is generally characterized by reduced loudness, monotone, hoarseness, and tremor. Reduced volume may be the first *or an early sign of IPD*.[25,85] These voice characteristics are frequently observed in the context of a generalized dysarthria which includes imprecise articulation. The patient with IPD may be unaware that his voice is soft; the reason for this self-perceptual impairment is unclear.[86] The perception of reduced loudness is supported by an acoustic study reporting statistically significantly (2-4 dB at 30 cm) reduced sound pressure level (SPL) in individuals (n = 29) with IPD across a variety of speech tasks when compared to an age-matched control group (n = 14).[87] Reduced SPL has been associated with glottal incompetence and/or bowed vocal folds,[27,28] and with reduced subglottal air pressure.[88] Two recent electromyographic studies of laryngeal muscles in PD report evidence of reduced activation of the TA when compared to a healthy aging group.[11] Decreases in the rate and increases in the variability of motor unit firing in the TA of both aged and PD males were reported by Luschei et al.[12] These findings were interpreted to reflect reduced central drive to the laryngeal motoneuron pools. In contrast, one study[89] reported thyroarytenoid recordings of a single subject with PD. Loss of reciprocal suppression of the TA during inspiration was found, indicative of parkinsonian rigidity. No neurogenic changes were seen to indicate a peripheral neuropathology. Although recordings of reciprocal muscles (posterior cricoarytenoid) were not made, it was thought that the hypokinetic laryngeal movement in PD was related to deterioration in the reciprocal adjustment of the antagonistic muscles.

While dopaminergic (levadopa) treatment has positive effects on the general function of PD, voice and speech symptoms are not consistently alleviated by these pharmacologic treatments.[27,90] Neurosurgical interventions (eg, pallidotomy, adrenal and fetal cell transplants) have been conducted.[91] Findings following these procedures support improved limb function and reduction of medication, but changes in laryngeal and speech mechanism function are not clear.[92,93]

Speech therapy has historically been ineffective for PD.[94,95] However, a recent approach by Ramig and associates,[96-98] the Lee Silverman Voice Treatment (LSVT), which focuses on *improved phonation and sensory awareness*, has generated short and long-term efficacy data.[15-17,99] Significant functional changes in vocal loudness with co-occurring changes in sound pressure level, subglottal air pressure,[88] and vocal fold adduction[28] have been reported following intensive voice treatment (16 sessions in one month). In addition, data support generalized effects of this treatment to articulation,[97] swallowing,[100] and facial expression (J. Spielman and L. Ramig, unpublished data). Recent PET scan findings support evidence of neural changes following treatment.[101] Details of this treatment are summarized elsewhere.[102]

Hypophonia Accompanying Closed Head Injury

Traumatic brain injury yields complex neurologic insults. They usually affect the cortical and subcortical structures as well as others. These injuries may result in voice and speech problems. Voice problems in these patients are described as having decreased loudness. One study found decreases in laryngeal airway resistance and increased glottal airflow in traumatic brain injury patients with voice and speech problems.[29] The same author recently reported a prospective study on acoustic voice analysis of 100 consecutive patients with traumatic brain injury referred for speech problems.[103] Using normative data from CSL (Kay Elemetrics) a high percentage of subjects had elevated scores on amplitude perturbation index, voice turbulence index, and noise-harmonics ratio. These are indicative of hypofunctional phonation and breathiness. Half of subjects had a measurable vocal tremor. Laryngeal biomechanics have not been formally studied via endoscopy in these patients, but information suggests that laryngeal hypoadduction and glottal insufficiency are likely to be found.

Hyperadduction

Hyperadduction is observed in many forms and degrees in various neurologic disorders. It may be constant (such as in the strain-strangle phonation of pseudobulbar palsy), or variable (such as the alternating spastic voice in Huntington's disease and *adductor* spasmodic dysphonia). Laryngeal involvement may be found in all varieties of hyperkinetic movement disorders (chorea, essential tremor, myoclonus, tics, and tardive dyskinesias).[104] It may also be observed as a compensation for hypoadduction. Hyperadduction may involve the true vocal folds and, in many cases, the false folds and supraglottal regions as well.

Hyperadduction Accompanying Upper Motor Neuron Lesions

Pseudobulbar palsy comprises a clinical picture of dysarthria with accompanying dysphonia, dysphagia, and signs of increased jaw jerk and snout reflexes.[105] The primary voice symptoms are harshness, hoarseness, strain-strangle quality, and reduced loudness.[57,106] Duffy and Folger have described disordered voice in 57% of individuals with unilateral upper motor neuron dysarthria.[107] Another clinically distinguishing feature is emotional lability, a reduced threshold for laughing or crying.[25] The term *pseudobulbar palsy* is felt to be inaccurate, as the sites of pathology are supranu-

clear to cranial nuclei, involving bilateral interruption of corticobulbar pathways, most frequently in the internal capsules.[105] The most frequent cause is stroke; other possible etiologies include encephalitis, trauma, and neoplasm.[108]

Voice problems in pseudobulbar palsy occur in the context of dysarthria of speech. The major findings have been summarized by Darley et al as prosodic excess, prosodic insufficiency, articulatory-resonatory incompetence, and phonatory stenosis (harsh, strain/struggle, pitch breaks).[21,22] In a perceptual evaluation of 30 patients, the voices of patients with pseudobulbar palsy were rated generally as monopitch, harsh, and low pitched. Many exhibited a strained voice quality and some had pitch breaks or tremor. The resonance quality may be hypernasal. No studies have reported on laryngoscopy or other measures of phonatory function in these patients. The variability in voice findings in pseudobulbar palsy likely reflects involvement of various structures in the supranuclear neural pathways controlling phonation. No documented studies on behavioral treatment of the dysphonia and dysarthria of pseudobulbar palsy are available.[25]

Hyperadduction Accompanying Quick Hyperkinesia of Huntington's Disease

Choreic movements accompany Huntington's disease, an autosomal dominant disease associated with loss of neurons in the caudate nucleus. The incidence of Huntington's disease is 4 to 8 per 100,000, with the average age of onset 38 years.[104,109] Abnormal, involuntary, abrupt, jerky movements may affect any part of the body. When choreiform movements affect the laryngeal mechanism, voice characteristics include irregular pitch fluctuations and voice arrests. Forced inspirations and expirations, harsh voice quality, excess loudness variations, strain-strangle phonation are classically observed.[21,22] Acoustic analysis reported octave drops (low frequency segments) in sustained phonation of patients diagnosed with Huntington's disease as well as individuals "at risk" for HD[32,110]; voice arrests (both adductor and abductor) and reduced vowel duration were also observed. Clinical endoscopic assessment in one patient revealed rapid adductory and supraglottal jerking movements at rest and during speech production (L. Ramig, clinical observation).

The medical treatment of Huntington's disease involves pharmacologic attempts to control the choreic movements with anti-dopaminergic agents, phenothiazines, benzodiazepines, or anti-seizure medications.[104] The effects of these on voice in HD has not been documented. We have successfully treated an HD patient who demonstrated hyperadductory voice arrests with laryngeal thyroarytenoid botulinum toxin injections (M. Smith, clinical observation).

Hyperadduction Accompanying Dystonia (Including "Adductor Spasmodic Dysphonia")

Spasmodic dysphonia (SD) is a rare but challenging voice disorder generally characterized by effortful, strain/strangle voice quality with frequent voice breaks. It is not a disease, but instead a constellation of voice symptoms and signs.[111] The actual incidence of SD is unknown.[112] SD is now considered more of a descriptive term for several types of voice disorders, including adductor SD and abductor SD. In this disorder, a variety of types of laryngeal dysfunction may be seen, including hyperadduction, malabduction, and phonatory instability.[113-117] These may vary between patients or be found in combination in an individual. The individual's voice symptoms may vary depending on the type and degree of these factors. This section describes the neural bases involving SD and features seen in its most common form, adductor SD.

Research to date indicates that "spasmodic dysphonia" may be considered in most cases as a focal, primary, function-specific, action-induced, laryngeal dystonia.[25,104,118-120] Evidence for the association of spasmodic dysphonia and dystonia comes from several sources, including clinical observations, neurophysiologic studies, and absence of response to voice and behavioral therapy. Important clinical observations have made the association of spasmodic dysphonia with other neurologic diseases, including movement disorders such as Meige's disease.[115,121]

Neurophysiologic studies of SD have been conducted in attempts to establish a neural basis for SD and to localize the neurologic source of abnormalities.[117] Various findings include abnormal electroencephalograms,[122] altered or delayed latencies of evoked auditory brain stem responses,[123] blink reflex response abnormalities,[124,125] altered cerebral regional blood flow,[126] and brain magnetic resonance imaging subcortical[127] or putaminal lesions.[128] Evidence for disordered motor control based on disrupted interconnections between cortex, subcortex, and basal ganglia have been postulated.[117,129] Laryngeal sensory and reflex functions may also play a role. It has been recognized that laryngeal reflex suppression is required for vocalization.[130] Laryngeal adductor reflex response to SLN stimulation has been reliably elicited from awake humans.[131] Abnormalities in inhibitory modulation of this reflex have been measured in patients with spasmodic dysphonia.[132] SD patients who undergo unilateral thyroarytenoid botulinum toxin injection show post-injection reduction in muscle activity of all laryngeal muscles, not just the injected one. This suggests a central modulation of effect through sensory feedback mechanisms.[133] It has been hypothesized that abnormalities in laryngeal reflex suppression during vocalization may be related to the mechanism of phonatory disruption in laryngeal motor control disorders, including spasmodic dysphonia, vocal tremor, Parkinson's disease, and multiple systems atrophy.[5]

The perceptual voice signs and symptoms of adductor spasmodic dysphonia are characterized by a strain and struggle to talk, with accompanying voice breaks or stoppages.[25] Patients may present with a variety of voice qualities, including hoarseness, harshness, or tremor. Voice and pitch breaks may be present. A creaking, fry-type phonation pattern may be seen. Voice symptoms may vary in the individual, based on activity, stress level, and other factors. There is often seen "task specificity" in this voice disorder, as in other dystonias.[119,120,134] Emotional vocalizations such as laughing, crying, or singing are not associated with the symptoms seen in voluntary speech tasks. The difficulty in verbal expression experienced by these patients creates a great deal of stress, anxiety, and depression.[135,136] However, these are not causes of the voice disorder. SD patients do not differ from normal controls in personality trait analysis, unlike individuals with functional voice disorders such as muscle tension dysphonia and vocal nodules.[137]

A comprehensive discussion of adductor laryngeal dystonia and SD is found elsewhere in this book.

Malabduction

Malabduction or "wrong abduction" refers to the inappropriate or mistimed abduction of the vocal folds during phonation. The paired abductor muscles of the intrinsic laryngeal musculature are the posterior cricoarytenoid (PCA) muscles. While the PCA has primarily been considered for its function in respiration, it has also been shown to have an important role in speech and voice. Many speech sounds (eg, stop consonants, fricatives) require the absence of vocal fold vibration. Ludlow et al[138] reported that PCA is active during two specific phonatory tasks during the onset and offset of speech, abduction in the transition from closed glottis to phonation, and abduction in the transition from phonation to open glottis. Malabduction occurs when the vocal folds open inappropriately and allow excess escape of air through the glottis. This results in prolongation of voiceless consonants during speech.

Abductor Spasmodic Dysphonia

Malabduction has generally been associated with the disorder of abductor spasmodic dysphonia. Abductor spasmodic dysphonia is characterized by interruptions of breathy or whispered (unphonated) segments upon a normal or hoarse voice.[25] This type of voice disorder does not necessarily occur in isolation but its characteristic breathy voice breaks may also be a feature associated with other neurologic-based voice disorders such as adductor spasmodic dysphonia, severe vocal tremor, or myoclonus.[7,113] It may be seen as a compensatory behavior to alleviate adductory laryngeal spasms in adductor spasmodic dysphonia.[7,104,139,140] The incidence of abductor spasmodic dysphonia is much less than the adductor variety. In a series of 100 consecutive SD patients, 4 had "pure" abductor SD, and 11 others had malabduction in combination with adductor SD or tremor.[141]

Several studies have reported on objective voice measures in patients with abductor SD. Fiberoptic laryngoscopy demonstrated synchronous and untimely abduction of both true vocal folds, exposing a wide glottic chink,[25,142] and bowing of the vocal folds.[143] Acoustic recordings documented sudden drops in fundamental frequency.[144] Aerodynamic measures found much higher than normal mean airflow rates.[144] Spectrograms demonstrated prolongation of the interval from initial stop consonant (voiced or unvoiced) to vowel, and less energy in higher formants,[145,146] or more high frequency spectral energy during voice breaks.[147] Surprisingly, electromyographic studies of both adductor and abductor SD have failed to demonstrate differentiation of subjects by symptom type, instead showing normal levels and patterns of intrinsic laryngeal muscle activation,[148] with bursts of activity superimposed on these.[149] Another unsuspected finding has been the measurement of abnormal bursts of cricothyroid muscle activity in some abductor SD subjects.[150] Abnormal adductor responses to SLN stimulation have been measured in abductor SD patients.[151] The pattern of reflex response differs from those reported in adductor SD, suggesting differences in laryngeal sensorimotor responses in these disorders.

Advances in the clinical treatment of abductor SD have involved botulinum toxin injection therapy.[150,152,153] Direct electrical stimulation of adductor laryngeal muscles has effectively improved voice production (reduction in voiceless consonant syllable duration) in abductor SD patients.[154] These are discussed elsewhere in this book.

PHONATORY INSTABILITY

Vocal fold vibration is generally not perfectly periodic. A number of factors combine to introduce perturbations (small changes in system behavior) and/or fluctuations (more severe deviations from the norm) into the phonatory mechanism.[155,156] This yields aperiodicity, or minor deviations from periodicity sometimes termed quasi-periodic.[26] Sources of aperiodicity include biomechanical asymmetries,[82,157] variations in neuromuscular control and motor unit firing,[158,159] airflow instabilities,[160] mucus on the vocal folds,[157] glottal source-vocal tract interactions,[161] pulsatile blood flow,[162,163] and chaotic motion resulting from non-linearities in the laryngeal mechanism.[164] These factors, all present in the normal phonatory mechanism, may be exaggerated or amplified in the patient with a neurologic voice disorder. This creates phonatory instability. For purposes of classifying the phonatory effects of instability in neurologic voice disorders it is convenient to separate them into two categories; short-term and long-term.[26,165]

Short-term Phonatory Instability

Short-term instabilities are usually described as the cycle-to-cycle variations in frequency (jitter) and amplitude (shimmer). The effect of short-term instability on speech intelligibility may be associated with the perception of "hoarse-rough" voice quality.[166] Measurements of these variables are affected by physiologic condition,[167] sex,[168] and vowel.[169,170] Short-term phonatory instabilities have been identified in many neurologic voice disorders.[171] Unfortunately, studies have yielded mixed results in distinguishing normal from abnormal voice-disordered populations or differentiating between neurologic voice disorders of various causes.[172,173] Stability measures may have utility in tracking the disease progression of neurologic disorders[171] or documenting efficacy of voice treatment.

Another class of short-term instabilities have also been described.[164] Waveforms seen in both normal and pathologic voice populations (including neurologic voice disorders such as vocal fold paralysis and spasmodic dysphonia) have been found to contain subharmonics, period doubling-tripling-quadrupling and so forth, or alternating aperiodic/periodic segments,[164,174,175] consistent with phenomena seen in low dimensional chaotic dynamical systems.[176] The theory of non-linear dynamics and chaos is being applied to investigate disordered voices in these terms.[164,177,178] As many neurologically impaired voices are not amenable to analysis by traditional perturbation measures,[165] non-linear dynamics may have increasing application in the analysis of neurologic voice disorders.[179,180]

Long-term Phonatory Instability Accompanying Vocal Tremor

Long-term phonatory instability affects vocal fold vibration over a longer time interval than individual glottal cycles. These effects are seen as superimposed on vocal fold vibration throughout the duration of phonatory effort, often lasting seconds. Long-term instabilities are created by *modulation* of the primary signal.[155] The periodic glottal airflow signal is superimposed on by a much slower modulation in frequency (FM) and/or amplitude (AM). This long-term phonatory instability may be normal (physiologic) or abnormal. Vibrato is an excellent example of physiologic vocal modulation.[155,181,182] In neurologic diseases, long-term instability is seen associated with vocal tremor.

Tremor is defined as "any involuntary, approximately rhythmic, and roughly sinusoidal movement."[19] These fluctuations in movement may be observed in various parts of the body. When these movements affect any or several portions of the speech system (respiratory, phonatory, articulatory) they may create vocal tremor. Tremors have been classified by etiology, clinical appearance, and described by frequency, amplitude, body distribution, and exacerbating and relieving factors.[183] Although all individuals have physiologic tremor[14] that occurs with a frequency of 8-12 Hz, abnormal (pathologic) tremor has been reported in the range of 3 to 7 Hz. The tremor frequency is influenced by many factors, including body location and disease type. Tremors are divided into resting tremor and action tremor. Action tremors may be postural (holding a position against gravity), contraction (produced by isometric voluntary contraction), or kinetic/intention (during activity or goal directed movement).[183]

The voice characteristics in vocal tremor have generally been studied from acoustic recordings of sustained vowel phonation. Observation of oscillographic recordings gave information on the amplitude changes of the output.[184-187] With more sophisticated analysis techniques the acoustic signal can be demodulated in amplitude and frequency components.[181,188] These data suggest that in patients with vocal tremor, complex oscillations involving both frequency and amplitude, and variations in these, exist.[181,188-190] Vocal tremor artificially induced by external vibration of the chest, throat, and cheek measured differences in magnitude and synchrony of demodulated acoustic and airflow contours.[191] This suggests differences in vocal output depend on the site of tremor. These patterns may differ in tremors of various neurologic diseases.[111,192] Vocal tremor is a feature of several neurologic diseases, including essential tremor, Parkinson's disease, ataxic dysphonia of cerebellar lesions, amyotrophic lateral sclerosis, and others.

Essential Tremor

Essential tremor (ET) is the most common movement disorder, with a reported prevalence of 4 to 60 per 1,000 people.[19] It is found in all age groups, but generally increases with advancing age. The voice is affected in 4 to 20% of cases,[19] but more frequently the hands or head are involved. A hereditary-familial history of tremor is found in about 50% of cases, and reflects autosomal dominant transmission.[193] A wide variation in reported incidence and inheritance of ET reflects differences in definitions of ET, methodologies of investigation, and symptom overlap with other disorders of movement.[194] Despite much research the pathophysiology of ET is not fully understood.[195] Neurophysiologic research using positron emission tomography suggests that olivocerebellar tracts are abnormal in this condition.[196] A central neurologic oscillator is the cause of ET, but its source or sources are not fully elucidated. Current views describe a disturbance of olivocerebellar rhythmicity, influenced by peripheral somatosensory feedback loops.[195]

Voice problems may be the first symptom for which medical help is sought, as was the case in 13 of 31 patients with ET and vocal tremor reported by Brown and Simonson.[184] Tremor symptoms at various body sites frequently co-exist, and isolated vocal tremor is rarely seen in ET.[197] If isolated vocal tremor alone is found, this is felt to likely be a focal dystonic tremor. As such, vocal tremor of ET may be confused with "spasmodic dysphonia" of laryngeal dystonia.[25,198] Vocal tremor has been described perceptually as quavering or tremulous speech.[25,57,184] The symptoms are most noticeable on vowel prolongation. This is caused by pitch breaks and voice arrests from large amplitude tremor of laryngeal structures that interrupt airflow[25] or allow excess air escape.[199] On laryngeal examination the larynx is usually reported to move both at rest (quiet breathing) with increased movement during phonation.[25] Vertical oscillations in the neck may be visible. Electromyographic study of 8 patients with essential vocal tremor found predominant involvement of the thyroarytenoid muscles as well as other extrinsic laryngeal muscles.[200]

The treatment of essential vocal tremor has involved pharmacotherapy (eg, propranolol, primidone, acetazolamide, alprazolam, phenobarbital) with mixed results.[104] An extensive recent review of pharmacologic treatment of ET concluded that only propranol and primidone have proven efficacy.[201] With each drug about 40-50% of patients experience symptomatic improvement. Unfortunately, the drugs work better for ET of the limbs than axially based (head or voice) tremors. An open label study of primidone in essential voice tremor found it ineffective,[202] but clinical experience suggests it provides benefits to some patients. The two drugs may be used in combination to control ET.[201]

Laryngeal botulinum toxin injections have been shown to be effective in improving voice tremor in ET. In an open trial of 13 vocal tremor patients, 100% of them returned for subsequent injections and had an average of 81 days of best effect.[203] Another study of bilateral injections in 15 patients used perceptual and acoustic assessment of speech and sustained vowel production, and patient self-ratings.[204] Depending on the parameter, 50-65% of patients had improvement in voice. A study of ten patients with ET and vocal tremor did a crossover of unilateral versus bilateral laryngeal injections.[205] By acoustic measures of tremor, a minority showed improvement, but aerodynamic measure of laryngeal airflow and estimated laryngeal airway resistance improved. This was felt to correlate with high patient satisfaction with injections, reflecting perceived reduced vocal effort. The increased laryngeal airflow and improved airflow stability is also an effect of botulinum toxin injections in patients with SD and vocal tremor.[206] Patients with ET and voice tremor tend to be older than SD patients, and may be more prone to laryngeal injection side-effects of dysphagia, choking, and breathiness.[205]

Functional neurosurgical procedures are also available for patients with severe ET and symptoms not controlled with medication. These include stereotactic thalamotomy[207] and deep brain stimulation (DBS) of the ventralis intermedius nucleus of the thalamus.[208-212] DBS is effective in reducing voice tremor in some but not all patients.[208,209] Bilateral DBS appears more effective in reducing vocal and head tremor (which are bilaterally controlled in the CNS) than unilateral DBS.[209,210] However, bilateral DBS has an increased risk of dysarthria as a complication. This can usually be managed with stimulator adjustments.[209,210] Measured improvement in acoustic parameters of vocal tremor after DBS has been documented.[211,212]

Vocal Tremor in Parkinson's Disease

In addition to the other voice abnormalities seen in Parkinson's disease involving hypoadduction, Logemann et al[18] reported that 13.5% of a group of patients with Parkinson's disease had tremulousness of speech. In a similar recent study, perceptual ratings of 45 patients with idiopathic PD found that 20% were rated to have tremor on passage reading (Ramig LO, unpublished data). Vocal tremor is seen mainly in later or more advanced stages of PD.[213] The frequency of vocal tremor in Parkinson's disease has been reported in the range of 5 to 7 Hz, including both frequency and amplitude modulations.[32] Perez and colleagues[214] reported laryngoscopic evidence of tremor in 55% of individuals with PD; vertical laryngeal movement was not uncommon.

Vocal Tremor in Spasmodic Dysphonia

Several studies have documented the presence of vocal tremor in patients with spasmodic dysphonia. This vocal tremor is differentiated from essential tremor in that it is present during phonation but not at rest, other body structures are not generally involved, and there is no family history of tremor.[19,141] Blitzer et al reported that 25% of patients with SD were found to have an irregular tremor.[114] Koufman and Blalock observed tremor in 45% of 100 consecutive SD patients of all varieties (adductor, abductor, mixed, etc).[141] They described "dystonic tremor" as task-specific with crescendo onset just prior to and during phonation, then decrescendo with offset of voicing.

Vocal Tremor of Palatopharyngolaryngeal Myoclonus

An unusual form of myoclonus affects the soft palate, termed palatal myoclonus. It is distinguished from the irregular jerks of limb myoclonus by its periodicity, but is felt not to be a tremor because of nonsinusoidal kinematics.[19] Aronson feels this is a slow form of tremor (usually 1 to 4 Hz) and technically may be a misnomer.[25] Deuschl et al[215,216] distinguish between two forms of palatal tremor. One form, termed essential palate tremor, appears isolated, does not involve other structures, abates during sleep, and is seen in younger patients. The other type, termed symptomatic palatal tremor, is associated with other signs of neurologic involvement that may affect eyes, face, palate, larynx, diaphragm, neck, shoulder, and arm. It may develop after brain stem stroke or hemorrhage and does not diminish during sleep. The neurologic lesions associated with this disorder interrupt the central tegmental tract, the olivo-dentate pathways or contralateral dentate nucleus, and connections via the red nucleus, leading to secondary vacuolar degeneration and hypertrophy of the inferior olive.[217] It may also be termed palatopharyngolaryngeal myoclonus.[25] In this situation it affects speech similarly to essential vocal tremor, causing a quavering voice. When the amplitude of movement is large, voice arrests may appear, resembling spasmodic dysphonia.[25,218] The patient also complains of a clicking or popping sound in the ear, from movement of the palate and pharyngeal muscles that open and close the eustachian tube.[215] Laryngeal dysfunction affecting airway[219] or swallowing[220] may occur. On examination, the rhythmic movement of the palate, pharynx, and larynx (usually bilateral but sometimes unilateral) is seen both at rest and during phonation. Although usually resistant to treatment,[217] symptoms of palatal myoclonus have responded, with varying degrees of success, to treatment with serotonin precursors, carbamazepine, clonazepam, and various surgical approaches.[104] The ear click symptoms have been treated with palate injections of botulinum toxin.[216]

Tremor in Multiple Sclerosis (MS) and Amyotrophic Lateral Sclerosis (ALS)

Long-term phonatory instability has been described in individuals with MS.[221] Evidence of instabilities across the frequency domains of wow (1-2 Hz), tremor (around 8 Hz), and flutter (17-18 Hz) were reported in the sustained phonation of 20 individuals with MS. Aronson identified a distinctive rapid tremor or "flutter" in the voice of individuals with amyotrophic lateral sclerosis (ALS).[25] Acoustic analysis of this tremor identified multiple combinations of levels of amplitude and frequency modulations in the range of 9-13 Hz when compared to control subjects.[192]

MIXED NEUROLOGIC VOICE DISORDERS

Various combinations of ataxic (cerebellar), upper (spastic), and lower (flaccid) motor neuron findings may be found in the "mixed" dysphonias seen in several neurologic diseases. These include cerebellar lesions, ALS, MS, and Parkinson plus syndromes.

Ataxic Dysphonia: Cerebellar Lesions

The function of the cerebellum involves coordination and regulation of skilled movements. The effects of speech and voice from cerebellar lesions are thought to be a breakdown in integration and alterations in motor programming (ataxia).[222] Causes of cerebellar lesions include cerebellar degeneration, infarcts, hemorrhage, or neoplasm. The characteristics of speech and voice in ataxic dysarthria surveyed by Aronson et al (n = 30) included harsh voice (21 patients), monopitch (20 patients), monoloudness (18 patients), poor pitch control or loudness control (bursts of loudness) (24 patients), and vocal tremor (5 patients).[223] The tremor observed in cerebellar disorders is irregular and slow, approximately 3 to 8 Hz.[14] Kent et al[222] reported on the acoustic characteristics of speech in 5 cerebellar patients and found abnormally long vowel and segment durations; they suggested problems with control of fundamental frequency. In another study, long-term phonatory instability (tremor) reflected in pitch fluctuations was found via acoustic analysis of sustained vowels in 6 of 11 subjects with cerebellar atrophy, and 5 of 9 subjects with olivopontocerebellar atrophy.[224] Although the pathophysiology of this disorder suggests reduced laryngeal coordination in abduction/adduction movements,[57] there have been no studies of laryngoscopy or laryngostroboscopy in verification of this.

Amyotrophic Lateral Sclerosis

ALS is a progressive degenerative neurologic disease that affects both upper and lower motor neurons. Its cause is unknown, but findings suggest several etiologies, including autoimmune disorder (antibodies to GMI gangliosides), multifocal conduction block gammopathy, malignancy (eg, lymphoma), and familial/genetic forms.[25,57] The incidence is 0.4 to 1.8 per 100,000. The male to female ratio is about 1.5:1.0. The average age of diagnosis is 58 years, and the disease is uncommon under 40 years of age. The median survival is about 17 months, and 20% of patients with ALS are alive at 5 years. The initial manifestations usually involve muscle weakness, cramps, and fasciculation.[225] One series (n = 123) found that 28% of patients with ALS presented with symptoms in the head, neck, larynx, or voice. 68 percent exhibited slurred speech, 14% hoarseness, and 13% dysphagia as a presenting symptom.[225]

Aronson described the dysphonia of mixed flaccid-spastic dysarthria associated with ALS as a harsh, strain-strangle sound with degrees of breathiness, reduced loudness, audible inhalation, and "wet hoarseness."[25] The wet, gurgling sound is caused by pooling of secretions in the pyriform sinuses and around the glottis. Carrow et al conducted a subjective perceptual voice assessment of 87 patients with motor neuron disease, including ALS.[226] 80 percent had harsh voice quality, 75% hypernasality, 65% breathy voice quality, 63% voice tremor, 60% strain-strangle voice, 38% high pitch, 8% low pitch.

The acoustic characteristics of ALS speech have been the object of recent study. In two studies, Ramig et al documented the progressive neurologic degeneration of voice in ALS with increasing acoustic perturbation measures and decreasing harmonics-to-noise ratio.[13,32] Another study by Strand et al found wide individual variation in acoustic measures of voice in four women with ALS, pointing to the variability in site of and degree of neural involvement in these patients.[227] A "flutter" type of vocal tremor may be present, as described previously.[192] Even ALS patients with perceptually normal voice quality can have acoustically abnormal measures of frequency range and phonatory stability.[228]

Multiple Sclerosis (MS)

MS is a disease of demyelinization of the white matter of the brain, brain stem, and spinal cord. It can disrupt neural function at any level. Symptoms vary in severity and frequently wax and wane, but generally progress. MS can often have otolaryngologic manifestations.[229] Impairment in speech ("scanning speech") has been considered a hallmark symptom of MS (part of

"Charcot's triad"). However, Beukelman et al[230] found that only 23% of 656 MS patients surveyed reported speech or other communication problems. In the series reported by Darley et al[231] most MS patients had normal speech (59%) or minimal speech impairment (29%). When the voice was affected, the main perceptual findings were harshness and impaired loudness control, described as a "spastic-ataxic dysarthria."[231] Less frequently observed were impaired pitch control, inappropriate pitch level, breathiness, and hypernasality. This variety of vocal symptoms suggests that MS patients with voice abnormalities may have problems in both laryngeal adduction (hyperadduction or hypoadduction) and phonatory stability. Speech therapy is thought to benefit patients with MS.[232]

Parkinson Plus Syndromes (Shy-Drager Syndrome, Progressive Supranuclear Palsy)

There are a number of forms of Parkinsonism. The most common is idiopathic PD (80%). The second largest group (12.2%) comprises Parkinsonism plus syndromes.[233] Patients in this group have symptoms of Parkinson's disease and additional neurologic disorders. Two of these include Shy-Drager syndrome and progressive supranuclear palsy (PSP). Shy-Drager is a rare, progressive disorder of the autonomic nervous system.[234] Its syndrome is described by orthostatic hypotension, urinary and rectal incontinence, impotence, loss of sweating, and other autonomic failure. Since the original report, several studies have described respiratory, swallowing, and voice problems in conjunction with bilateral vocal fold paresis/paralysis in these patients.[234-236] The voice is described as monopitch, monoloud, with both strain/strangle and breathy qualities,[57,235] with functional evidence of laryngeal hypo- and/or hyperfunction as well as short and/or long-term phonatory instability.[237] EMG of laryngeal muscles in Shy-Drager syndrome have found denervation of posterior cricoarytenoid and interarytenoid muscles in these patients.[238]

Progressive supranuclear palsy (PSP) is a brain stem neurologic disease of progressive Parkinsonism and ocular motility disturbance.[239] Progressive gait and balance impairment is an early and disabling symptom. Speech difficulties in PSP are reported as a spastic, hypernasal, monotonous, low-pitched dysarthria.[240,241] Imprecise articulation may be the most prominent disordered speech feature of PSP.[241] We have treated a PSP patient with voice problems. Laryngoscopy revealed bowing of the vocal folds, and false fold hyperadduction. Acoustic measures showed decreased vocal intensity. Application of the Lee Silverman Voice Treatment (LSVT) to this patient, and two additional selected patients with Parkinsonism plus syndromes, demonstrated significant improvement pre- to post-treatment as well as maintenance of these changes up to six months.[237]

MISCELLANEOUS NEUROLARYNGEAL DISORDERS

Apraxic Dysphonia

Lesions of the cortex and subcortical regions, such as those caused by stroke, head injury, or tumor, can produce apraxia of phonation, in conjunction with apraxia of respiration and articulation.[25] Phonatory characteristics can vary from mutism to trial-and-error nonspeech to whispered speech, with or without airflow.[106]

Involuntary Vocalization

Verbal and non-verbal vocalizations may be encountered in a variety of neurologic disorders. The most well known of these is Gilles de la Tourette syndrome (TS). TS is a rare, chronic disorder of involuntary motor tics that begins in childhood and persists in adulthood.[242] It is seen predominantly in men, often runs in families, and may have an autosomal dominant mode of inheritance. The involuntary vocalizations in TS range from unintelligible nonverbal noises to verbal tics including coprolalia (repetition of obscene words), echolalia (repetition of the last syllable, word, or sentence spoken by others), or palilalia (repeating by the patient of the last word or sentence in a phrase). The cause of TS is unknown. The symptoms of TS variably respond to dopamine antagonist drugs. This suggests a possible role of dopaminergic hyperactivity in TS.[242] Laryngeal botulinum toxin injection has been used to reduce vocal volume and the social embarrassment of vocal tics.[243-245]

NEUROLARYNGOLOGIC AND VOICE EVALUATION

It has been suggested that the laryngeal system can be regarded as a microcosm of the entire speech mechanism[2] and therefore the larynx may reflect neurologic impairments before other speech components. Neurologic voice disorders can be isolated problems or occur in the context of extensive systemic disease. Because voice disorders have been reported as initial symptoms of various neurologic disorders, such as PD[13] and myasthenia gravis,[30-33] phonatory evaluation should be considered for its contribution to neurologic assessment.[21] The laryngologist, speech pathologist, and neurologist caring for these patients recognize several *key points*. They are aware of 1) disorders for which voice problems and complaints may initially present to the laryngologist or voice clinician, and 2) disorders for which medical, surgical, and/or behavioral intervention may improve laryngeal function, in the context of the individual's general physical condition. These key considerations should not be minimized as voice characteristics may contribute to neurologic differential diagnosis and various intervention procedures may significantly improve quality of life, even in a patient otherwise suffering from a terminal illness. An example that applies particularly to these issues is the patient with early symptoms of bulbar ALS, presented in detail in an excellent review by Hillel et al.[246]

The neurolaryngologic examination involves several components. These include medical history, phonation assessment, general otolaryngology/head and neck examination, laryngeal imaging examination, directed neurologic examination, and, when appropriate, special diagnostic testing.

A careful history of both medical and neurologic symptoms provides the basis for evaluation of the patient with a neurologic voice disorder. The *voice history* includes the nature of the vocal complaint. In general, voice complaint symptoms may be described as hoarseness, vocal fatigue, breathiness, reduced phonational range, aphonia, pitch breaks or inappropriately high pitch, strain/strangle voice, and tremor.[57] One or (frequently) several of these complaints may be given by a patient with a neurologic voice disorder. Voice problems in conjunction with other speech production difficulties such as unclear speech, slurring, or unintelligible speech suggest underlying neurologic disease. The same applies to the presence of concomitant symptoms of dysphagia. The onset and progression of symptoms are elicited, as well as what improves and worsens the voice. Voice and speech problems that are intermittent do not suggest a neurologic disease. When underlying organic neuromotor disease is present, although symptoms may vary to some degree, speech and/or voice is usually not totally normal.[247] Stress worsens most neurologic voice disorders, so this should not be taken as an indication of purely functional etiology of symptoms.[247] Other symptoms of laryngeal dysfunction, ie, swallowing or respiratory complaints, are reviewed; if these also occur, a neurologic disease may be suspected. The patient's complete medication history is discussed. A review of systems pays particular attention to respiratory, gastrointestinal, endocrine, as well as neurologic areas. Questions about fatigue, balance, gait disturbance, tremor, changes in handwriting, sensation, and weakness all pertain to the neurologic system review.

The next portion of the examination comprises the phonation assessment. Ideally, it should be conducted

jointly by the voice/speech pathologist and laryngologist. Separately or together, they assess the quality of the patient's voice, speech, resonance, articulation, and breath support. Such examination begins while listening to the patient relate his/her medical history. In addition, sustained vowel phonation allows evaluation of phonatory stability, tremor, and movement of laryngeal supporting structures. If the patient is a singer and has complaints related to singing, then observation of the patient while singing is mandatory so that the problem may be demonstrated. Professional vocalists may develop neurologic voice disorders; problems during the vocally demanding tasks of singing may be an initial symptom.[248] Testing of the articulators (tongue, lip, jaw) can be done by having the patient rapidly repeat /pa/,/ta/,/ga/. Lack of precision or crispness suggests lower motor neuron or muscular compromise. Sustained phonation of the vowels "ah" and "ee" while alternately pinching and releasing the nares together with reading sentences with high pressure and nasal sounds such as "Suzy stayed all summer" or counting aloud from 60 to 70 can be screening procedures for velopharyngeal incompetence. Increased nasal resonance or nasal air emission during these tasks suggests lack of adequate velopharyngeal closure. Comprehensive assessment of the laryngeal mechanism in the context of motor speech control is summarized by Yorkston et al.[249]

The general otolaryngologic/head and neck examination should be conducted, including assessment of ears, nasal passages, facial structures, oral cavity and oropharynx, nasopharynx, and neck inspection and palpation.

Laryngeal imaging examination is a crucial component of the laryngologist's evaluation. The instrument of choice for examination is the flexible fiberoptic laryngoscope.[81] When no lesion is visible in the larynx in a patient with dysphonia, functional, neurogenic, or psychogenic causes should be investigated. These require visualization of the structures of the speech mechanism dynamically. The flexible fiberoptic laryngoscope allows examination of the larynx, pharynx, palate, and velopharyngeal sphincter at rest and during a variety of tasks, including connected speech, sustained phonation, coughing, singing, and swallowing. This capability is extremely helpful in the assessment of neurologic voice disorders. The rigid laryngeal telescope is also helpful, but not useful in every case. It provides superior image quality for view of the larynx at rest and during sustained vowel phonation, and for viewing the vocal fold mucosal waves under stroboscopic lighting.[10] Video documentation for review and patient education is also an important aspect of the laryngeal imaging examination.

The patient with a neurologic voice disorder may have other neurologic examination findings that aid the physician in diagnosis. These have been reviewed in an excellent summary by Rosenfield.[247] While this neurologic assessment may not replace a complete evaluation by a neurologist, it helps the laryngologist to understand the nature of the illness of which the voice may only be a part. It also facilitates communication with the neurologist about the patient's problem. Components include a cranial nerve examination, assessment of muscle strength and tone (motor and extrapyramidal), and coordination (cerebellar). Although cranial nerve testing is familiar to the otolaryngologist, other aspects of neurologic examination are not. However, these should be routinely performed in cases of suspected neurologic voice disorders. In the elderly patient, a screening examination for tone (resistance to passive movement) may be more revealing than an assessment of muscle strength.[105] Increased tone on passive movement of the limbs may be an upper motor neuron sign, and rigidity of wrist or elbow movement may be an early sign of Parkinson's disease. Coordination and cerebellar function are assessed by observation of gait and Romberg's sign. Following the Romberg test the coordination of the upper extremities is evaluated by finger-nose testing. Observation of the outstretched limbs allows evaluation of postural (cerebellar) tremor. Resting tremor that improves with movement is seen in Parkinson's disease. During the examination the patient is observed for adventitious (unintended or involuntary) movements (eg, tremor of head or limbs, circumoral twitches, blepharospasm, dyskinesias, or dystonias). Observation of the patient's handwriting may be helpful in identifying ataxia or tremor.

Special diagnostic tests are indicated in selected cases. Laryngeal electromyography has been found to be helpful in the diagnostic assessment of vocal fold paralysis, differentiating paralysis from fixation, and in determining prognosis for recovery.[74,250-253] It can provide helpful information in determining etiology and treatment of a variety of neurolaryngologic disorders.[254] The workup of vocal fold paralysis, in the absence of identifiable etiology, involves imaging studies along the entire course of the nerve on the affected side.[48] Regarding spasmodic dysphonia, in the absence of secondary causes for dystonia,[104,255] Rosenfield et al[111] recommended additional medical evaluation with a thyroid-stimulating hormone level (TSH) to identify concomitant hypothyroidism, and Swenson et al[255] suggested a complete blood count and sedimentation rate to rule out systemic vasculitis. In the patient with suspected myasthenia gravis a *Tensilon* test should be performed. Those with presumed underlying central neurologic lesions are evaluated with MRI.

TREATMENT ISSUES RELATED TO NEUROLOGIC DISORDERS OF THE LARYNX

This chapter has organized neurologic disorders of the larynx according to the phonatory dysfunctional dimensions of hypoadduction, hyperadduction, malabduction, and short- and long-term instabilities, and mixed abnormalities. This classification system lends itself to treatment planning that spans the various etiologic factors.

When planning treatment for neurologic disorders of the larynx it is important to consider that patients often have disorders of multiple speech subsystems. Enhancing laryngeal function must be considered in relation to the impact of each subsystem on functional speech production. Recent findings support the key role of phonation in enhancing oral communication in neurologic disorders.[97] Treatment goals must also consider the role of language or cognitive disorders (aphasia, dementia) and the progressive nature of many neurologic diseases when planning treatment to maximize functional communication.

There are various forms of treatment that may affect neurologic disorders of the larynx. Some treatments (neuropharmacologic or neurosurgical) are designed to treat the neurologic disorder and may have co-occurring effects on laryngeal or speech function. Other treatments (behavioral, laryngeal-surgical) are designed to directly treat the phonatory dysfunction and improve the voice. These are ideally conducted by an interdisciplinary, collaborative group such as that formed by the speech pathologist, neurologist, and otolaryngologist to provide the patient who has a neurologic disorder of the larynx with optimal speech intelligibility.[26]

ACKNOWLEDGEMENTS

This work was supported by NIH Grants K08-DC00132 and R01-DC01150 from the National Institute of Deafness and Communication Disorders.

REFERENCES

1. Blitzer A, Brin MF, Sasaki CT, et al, eds. *Neurologic Disorders of the Larynx.* New York, NY: Thieme Medical Publishers; 1992.

2. Barlow SM, Netsell R, Hunker CJ. Phonatory disorders associated with CNS lesions. In: Cummings CW, et al, eds. *Otolaryngology—Head and Neck Surgery.* 1st ed. St Louis, MO: CV Mosby; 1986;2087-2093.

3. Larson CR. Brain mechanisms involved in the control of vocalization. *J Voice.* 1998;2:301-311.

4. Gacek RR, Malmgren LT. Laryngeal motor innervation—central. In: Blitzer A, et al, eds. *Neurologic Disorders of the Larynx.* New York, NY: Thieme Medical Publishers; 1992;29-35.

5. Larson CR, Yoshida Y, Sessile BJ, Ludlow CR. Higher level motor and sensory integration. In: Titze IR, ed. *Vocal Fold Physiology: Frontiers in Basic Science.* San Diego, CA: Singular Publishing Group; 1993;227-275.

6. Ward PH, Berci G, Calcaterra TC. Advances in endoscopic examination of the respiratory system. *Ann Otol Rhinol Laryngol.* 1974;83:754-760.

7. Hanson DG. Neuromuscular disorders of the larynx. *Otolaryngol Clin North Am.* 1991;24:1035-1051.

8. Yanagisawa E. Physical examination of the larynx and videolaryngoscopy. In: Blitzer A, et al, eds. *Neurologic Disorders of the Larynx.* New York, NY: Thieme Medical Publishers; 1992;82-97.

9. Baken R, Orkikoff RF. *Clinical Measurement of Speech and Voice.* 2nd ed. San Diego, CA: Singular Publishing Group; 2000.

10. Bless DM. Measurement of vocal function. *Otolaryngol Clin North Am.* 1991;24:1023-1033.

11. Baker K, Ramig L, Luschei E, Smith M. Thyroarytenoid muscle activity associated with hypophonia in Parkinson disease and aging. *Neurology.* 1998;51(6):1592-1598.

12. Luschei E, Ramig L, Baker K, Smith M. Discharge characteristics of laryngeal single motor units during phonation in young and older adults and in persons with Parkinson disease. *J Neurophysiol.* 1999;81:2131-2139.

13. Ramig LO, Scherer RC, Klasner ER, et al. Acoustic analysis of voice in amyotrophic lateral sclerosis: a longitudinal case study. *J Speech Hear Disord.* 1990;55:2-14.

14. Countryman S, Ramig LA. Effects of intensive voice therapy on voice deficits associated with bilateral thalamotomy in Parkinson's disease: a case study. *J Med Speech-Lang Pathology.* 1993;1:233-249.

15. Ramig L, Sapir S, Fox C, Countryman S. Changes in vocal loudness following intensive voice treatment (LSVT) in individuals with Parkinson disease: a comparison with untreated patients and normal age-matched controls. *Mov Disord.* In press.

16. Ramig L, Countryman S, Thompson L, et al. Comparison of two forms of intensive speech treatment for Parkinson disease. *J Speech Lang Hear Res.* 1995;38:1232-1251.

17. Ramig L, Countryman S, O'Brien C, et al. Intensive speech treatment for patients with Parkinson disease: short and long-term comparison of two techniques. *Neurology.* 1996;47:1496-1504.

18. Logemann JA, Fisher HB, Boshes B, et al. Frequency and occurrence of vocal tract dysfunctions in the speech of a large sample of Parkinson's patients. *J Speech Hear Disord.* 1978;42:47-57.

19. Elble RJ, Koller WC. *Tremor.* Baltimore, MD: Johns Hopkins University Press; 1990.

20. Koufman JA, Isaacson G. The spectrum of vocal dysfunction. *Otolaryngol Clin North Am.* 1991;24:985-988.

21. Darley F, Aronson A, Brown J. Differential diagnostic patterns of dysarthria. *J Speech Hear Res.* 1969;12:246-269.

22. Darley F, Aronson A, Brown J. Clusters of deviant speech dimensions in the dysarthrias. *J Speech Hear Res.* 1969;12:462-496.

23. Ward PH, Hanson DG, Berci G. Photographic studies of the larynx in central laryngeal paresis and paralysis. *Acta Otolaryngol (Stockh).* 1981;91:353-367.

24. Ward PH, Hanson DG, Berci G. Observations on central neurologic etiology for laryngeal dysfunction. *Ann Otol Rhinol Laryngol.* 1981;90:430-441.

25. Aronson AE. *Clinical Voice Disorders.* 3rd ed. New York, NY: Thieme; 1990.

26. Ramig LO, Scherer RC. Speech therapy for neurological disorders of the larynx. In: Blitzer A, et al, eds. *Neurologic Disorders of the Larynx.* New York, NY: Thieme Medical Publishers; 1992:163-181.

27. Hanson DG, Gerratt BR, Ward PH. Cinegraphic observations of vocal pathology in Parkinson's disease. *Laryngoscope.* 1984;92:348-353.

28. Smith ME, Ramig LO, Dromey C, et al. Intensive voice treatment in Parkinson's disease: laryngostroboscopic findings. *J Voice.* 1995;10:354-361.

29. McHenry MA, Wilson RL, Minton JT. Management of multiple physiologic system deficits following traumatic brain injury. *J Med Speech-Lang Path.* 1994;2:59-74.

30. Younger DS, Lange DJ, Lovelace RE, et al. Neuromuscular disorders of the larynx. In: Blitzer A, et al, eds. *Neurologic Disorders of the Larynx.* New York, NY: Thieme Medical Publishers; 1992;246.

31. Mastaglia FL. Genetic myopathies. In: Swash M, Oxbury J, eds. *Clinical Neurology*. New York, NY: Churchill Livingstone; 1991;1286.

32. Ramig LA, Scherer RC, Titze IR, et al. Acoustic analysis of voices of patients with neurological disease: rationale and preliminary data. *Ann Otol Rhinol Laryngol*. 1988;97:164-172.

33. Salomonson J, Kawamoto H, Wilson L. Velopharyngeal incompetence as the presenting symptom of myotonic dystrophy. *Cleft Palate J*. 1988;25:296-300.

34. Hillarp B, Ekberg O, Jacobsson S, Nylander G, Aberg M. Myotonic dystrophy revealed at videoradiography of deglutition and speech in adult patients with velopharyngeal insufficiency: presentation of four cases. *Cleft Palate Craniofac J*. 1994;31:125-133.

35. Fenchiel GM. Clinical syndromes of myasthenia in infancy and childhood. *Arch Neurol*. 1978;35:97-103.

36. Scadding GK, Harvard CWH. Pathogenesis and treatment of myasthenia gravis. *Br Med J*. 1981;283:1008-1019.

37. Carpenter RJ, McDonald TJ, Howard FM. The otolaryngologic presentation of myasthenia gravis. *Laryngoscope*. 1979;89:922-928.

38. Dhillon RS, Brookes GB. Myasthenia gravis in otolaryngological practice. *Clin Otolaryngol*. 1984; 9:27-34.

39. Calcaterra TC, Stern F, Herrmann C, et al. The otolaryngologist's role in myasthenia gravis. *Trans Am Acad Ophthalmol Otolaryngol*. 1972;76:308-312.

40. Dursun G, Sataloff RT, Spiegel JR, Mandel S, Heuer RJ, Rosen DC. Superior laryngeal nerve paresis and paralysis. *J Voice*. 1996;10:206-211.

41. Neiman RF, Mountjoy JR, Allen EL. Myasthenia gravis focal to the larynx: report of a case. *Arch Otolaryngol*. 1975;101:569-570.

42. Walker FO. Voice fatigue in myasthenia gravis: the sinking pitch sign. *Neurology*. 1997;48:1135-1136.

43. Warren WR, Gutmann L, Cody RC, et al. Stapedius reflex decay in myasthenia gravis. *Arch Neurol*. 1977;34:496-497.

44. Rontal M, Rontal E, Leuchter W, et al. Voice spectrography in the evaluation of myasthenia gravis of the larynx. *Ann Otol Rhinol Laryngol*. 1978;87: 722-728.

45. Tyler HR. Neurology of the larynx. *Otolaryngol Clin North Am*. 1984;17:75-79.

46. Oosterhuis JHGH. Myasthenia gravis and other myasthenic syndromes. In: Swash M, Oxbury J, eds. *Clinical Neurology*. New York, NY: Churchill Livingstone; 1991;1368.

47. Dray TG, Robinson LR, Hillel AD. Idiopathic bilateral vocal fold weakness. *Laryngoscope*. 1999; 109:995-1002.

48. Terris DJ, Arnstein DP, Nguyen HH. Contemporary evaluation of unilateral vocal cord paralysis. *Otolaryngol Head Neck Surg*. 1992;107:84-90.

49. Annino DJ, MacArthur CJ, Friedman EM. Vincristine-induced recurrent laryngeal nerve paralysis. *Laryngoscope*. 1992;102:1260-1262.

50. Cannon S, Ritter FN. Vocal cord paralysis in postpoliomyelitis syndrome. *Laryngoscope*. 1987;97: 981-983.

51. Nugent KM. Vocal cord paresis and glottic stenosis: a late complication of poliomyelitis. *South Med J*. 1987;80:1594-1595.

52. Driscoll BP, Gracco C, Coelho C, et al. Laryngeal function in postpolio patients. *Laryngoscope*. 1995;105:35-41.

53. Robinson LR, Hillel AD, Waugh PF. New laryngeal muscle weakness in post-polio syndrome. *Laryngoscope*. 1998;108:732-734.

54. Blau JN, Kapadia R. Idiopathic palsy of the recurrent laryngeal nerve: a transient cranial mononeuropathy. *Br Med J*. 1972;4:259-261.

55. Ward PH, Berci G. Observations on so-called idiopathic vocal cord paralysis. *Ann Otol Rhinol Laryngol*. 1982;91:558-563.

56. Bachor E, Bonkowsky V, Hacki T. Herpes simplex virus type I reactivation as a cause of a unilateral temporary paralysis of the vagus nerve. *Eur Arch Otorhinolaryngol*. 1996;253(4-5):297-300.

57. Colton RH, Casper JK. *Understanding Voice Problems: A Physiological Perspective for Diagnosis and Treatment*. 2nd ed. Baltimore, MD: Williams & Wilkins; 1996.

58. Gerratt BR, Hanson DG, Berke GS. Glottographic measures of laryngeal function in individuals with abnormal motor control. In: Baer T, Sasaki C, Harris K, eds. *Laryngeal Function in Phonation and Respiration*. Boston, MA: Little, Brown, and Co; 1987;521-534.

59. Hanson DG, Gerratt BR, Karin R, et al. Glottographic measures of vocal fold vibration: laryngeal paralysis. *Laryngoscope*. 1988;98:348-353.

60. Jiang J, Lin E, Hanson DG. Glottographic phase difference in recurrent nerve paralysis. *Ann Otol Rhinol Laryngol.* 2000;109:287-293.

61. Woo P, Colton R, Shangold L. Phonatory airflow analysis in patients with laryngeal disease. *Ann Otol Rhinol Laryngol.* 1987;96:549-555.

62. Hirano M, Kurita S, Yukizane K, et al. Asymmetry of the laryngeal framework: a morphological study of cadaver larynges. *Ann Otol Rhinol Laryngol.* 1989;98:135-140.

63. Sanders I, Wu BL, Mu L, et al. The innervation of the human larynx. *Arch Otolaryngol Head Neck Surg.* 1993;119:934-939.

64. Crumley R, McCabe B. Regeneration of the recurrent laryngeal nerve. *Otolaryngol Head Neck Surg.* 1982;92:442-447.

65. Kirchner JA. Atrophy of laryngeal muscles in vagal paralysis. *Laryngoscope.* 1966;76:1753-1765.

66. Quiney RE, Michaels L. Histopathology of vocal cord palsy from recurrent laryngeal nerve damage. *J Otolaryngol.* 1990;19:237-241.

67. Pinho SM, Pontes PA, Gadelha ME, Biasi N. Vestibular vocal fold behavior during phonation in unilateral vocal fold paralysis. *J Voice.* 1999;13(1):36-42.

68. Smith ME, Berke GS, Gerratt BR, et al. Laryngeal paralyses: theoretical considerations and effects of laryngeal vibration. *J Speech Hear Res.* 1992;35:545-554.

69. Hirano M, Bless DM. *Videostroboscopic Examination of the Larynx.* San Diego, CA: Singular Publishing Group; 1993:167-169.

70. Isshiki N, Ishikawa T. Diagnostic value of tomography in unilateral vocal cord paralysis. *Laryngoscope.* 1976;86:1573-1578.

71. Dedo HH. The paralyzed larynx: an electromyographic study in dogs and humans. *Laryngoscope.* 1970;80:1455-1517.

72. Woodson GE. Configuration of the glottis in laryngeal paralysis. II: animal experiments. *Laryngoscope.* 1993;103:1235-1241.

73. Woodson GE. Configuration of the glottis in laryngeal paralysis. I: clinical study. *Laryngoscope.* 1993;103:1227-1234.

74. Hirano M, Nozoe I, Shin T, Maeyama T. Electromyography for laryngeal paralysis. In: Hirano, M, Kirchner JA, Bless DM, eds. *Neurolaryngology: Recent Advances.* Boston, MA: College-Hill; 1987:232-248.

75. Koufman JA, Walker FO, Joharji GM. The cricothyroid muscle does not influence vocal fold position in laryngeal paralysis. *Laryngoscope.* 1995;105:368-372.

76. Heuer RJ, Sataloff RT, Emerich K, et al. Unilateral recurrent laryngeal nerve paralysis: the importance of "preoperative" voice therapy. *J Voice.* 1997;11(1):88-94.

77. Ward PH, Berci G, Calcaterra TC. Superior laryngeal nerve paralysis: an often overlooked entity. *Trans Am Acad Ophthalmol Otolaryngol.* 1977;84:78-89.

78. Adour KK, Schneider GD, Hilsinger RL. Acute superior laryngeal nerve palsy: analysis of 78 cases. *Otolaryngol Head Neck Surg.* 1980;88:418-424.

79. Tanaka S, Hirano M, Umeno H. Laryngeal behavior in unilateral superior laryngeal nerve paralysis. *Ann Otol Rhinol Laryngol.* 1994;103:93-97.

80. Sataloff RT, Mandel S, Rosen DC. Neurologic disorders affecting the voice in performance. In: Sataloff RT, ed. *Professional Voice: Science and Art of Clinical Care.* 2nd ed. San Diego, CA: Singular Publishing Group; 1997;479-498.

81. Koufman JA. Approach to the patient with a voice disorder. *Otolaryngol Clin North Am.* 1991;24:989-998.

82. Isshiki N, Tanabe M, Ishizaka K, et al. Clinical significance of asymmetrical vocal cord tension. *Ann Otol Rhinol Laryngol.* 1977;86:58-66.

83. Berke G, Moore D, Hantke D, et al. Laryngeal modeling: theoretical, in-vitro, in-vivo. *Laryngoscope.* 1987;97:871-881.

84. Hornykiewicz O. Metabolism of brain dopamine in human parkinsonism: neurochemical and clinical aspects. In: Costa E, Cote L, Yahr M, eds. New York, NY: Raven Press; 1966.

85. Stewart C, Winfield L, Hunt A, et al. Speech dysfunction in early Parkinson's disease. *Mov Disord.* 1995;10: 562-565.

86. Ho AK, Bradshaw JL, Iansek T. Volume perception in parkinsonian speech. *Mov Disord.* 2000;15:1125-1131.

87. Fox C, Ramig L. Speech and voice characteristics of men and women who are elderly and have idiopathic Parkinson disease. *Am J Speech Lang Pathol.* 1997;6, 85-94.

88. Ramig L. Dromey C. Aerodynamic mechanisms underlying treatment related changes in SPL in

patients with Parkinson disease. *J Speech Hear Res.* 1996;39:798-807.

89. Hirose H, Joshita Y. Laryngeal behavior in patients with disorders of the central nervous system. In: Hirano M, Kirchner JA, Bless DM, eds. *Neurolaryngology: Recent Advances.* Boston, MA: Little, Brown, and Co; 1987;258-266.

90. Larson K, Ramig L, Scherer R. Preliminary speech and voice analysis during drug-related fluctuations in Parkinson's disease. *J Med Speech-Lang Pathol.* 1994;2:211-226.

91. Freed C, Breeze R, Rosenberg N, et al. Survival of implanted fetal dopamine cells and neurologic improvement 12 to 46 months after transplantation for Parkinson disease. *New Engl J Med.* 1993;327:1549-1555.

92. Schultz G, Peterson T, Sapienza C, et al. Voice and speech characteristics of persons with Parkinson's disease pre- and post-pallidotomy surgery: preliminary findings. *J Speech Lang Hear Res.* 1999;42:1176-1194.

93. Baker K, Ramig L, Johnson A, Freed C. Preliminary speech and voice analysis following fetal dopamine transplants in five individuals with Parkinson disease, *J Speech Lang Hear Res.* 1997;40:615-626.

94. Sarno MT. Speech impairment in Parkinson's disease. *Arch Phys Med Rehab.* 1968;49:269-275.

95. Weiner WJ, Singer C. Parkinson's disease and non-pharmacologic treatment programs. *J Am Geriatr Soc.* 1989;37:359-363.

96. Ramig LO, Bonitati C, Lemke J, et al. Voice treatment for patients with Parkinson disease: development of an approach and preliminary efficacy data. *J Med Speech-Lang Pathol.* 1994;2(3):191-210.

97. Dromey C, Ramig L, Johnson A. Phonatory and articulatory changes associated with increased vocal intensity in Parkinson disease: a case study. *J Speech Lang Hear Res.* 1995;38:751-764.

98. Ramig LO, Dromey C: Aerodynamic mechanisms underlying treatment related changes in SPL in patients with Parkinson disease. *J Speech Lang Hear Res.* 1996;39:798-807.

99. Ramig L, Sapir S, Countryman S, et al. Intensive voice treatment (LSVT) for individuals with Parkinson disease: a two-year follow-up. *J Neurol, Neurosurg Psychiatry.* In review.

100. El Sharwaki A, Ramig L, Logemann J, et al. Swallowing and voice effects of Lee Silverman Voice Treatment (LSVT): a pilot study. *J Neurol, Neurosurg Psychiatry.* In review.

101. Liotti M, Vogel D, New P, et al. *A PET study of functional reorganization of premotor regions in Parkinson's disease following intensive speech and voice treatment (LSVT).* A paper presented to the Academy of Neurology. Toronto, Canada; November, 1998.

102. Ramig L, Pawlas A, Countryman S. *The Lee Silverman Voice Treatment: A Practical Guide for Treating the Voice and Speech Disorders in Parkinson Disease.* The National Center for Voice and Speech (NCVS) and The LSVT Foundation; Louisville, CO: 1995.

103. McHenry M. Acoustic characteristics of voice after severe traumatic brain injury. *Laryngoscope.* 2000;110(7):1157-1161.

104. Brin MF, Fahn S, Blitzer A, et al. Movement disorders of the larynx. In: Blitzer A, Brin MF, Sasaki CT, et al, eds. *Neurologic Disorders of the Larynx.* New York, NY: Thieme Medical Publishers; 1992;248-278.

105. Glick TH. *Neurologic Skills: Examination and Diagnosis.* Boston, MA: Blackwell Scientific Publications; 1993.

106. Duffy J. *Motor Speech Disorders.* St. Louis, MO: Mosby; 1995.

107. Duffy J, Folger W. *Dysarthria in unilateral central nervous system lesions.* Paper presented at the annual convention of the America Speech-Language Hearing Association. Detroit, MI; 1986.

108. Aring CD. Supranuclear (pseudobulbar) palsy. *Arch Int Med.* 1965;115;19.

109. Penney JB, Young AB, Shoulson I, et al. Huntington's disease in Venezuela: 7 years of follow-up on symptomatic and asymptomatic individuals. *Mov Disord.* 1990;5:93-99.

110. Ramig LA. Acoustic analyses of phonation in patients with Huntington's disease: preliminary report. *Ann Otol Rhinol Laryngol.* 1986;95:288-293.

111. Rosenfield DB, Donovan DT, Sulek M, et al. Neurologic aspects of spasmodic dysphonia. *J Otolaryngol.* 1990;19:231-236.

112. Izdebski K. Symptomatology of adductor spasmodic dysphonia: a physiologic model. *J Voice.* 1992;6:306-319.

113. Cannito M, Johnson H. Spastic dysphonia: a continuum disorder. *J Commun Disord.* 1981;14:215-223.

114. Blitzer A, Lovelace RE, Brin MF, et al. Electromyographic findings in focal laryngeal dystonia (spastic dysphonia). *Ann Otol Rhinol Laryngol.* 1985;94:591-594.

115. Blitzer A, Brin MF, Fahn S, et al. Clinical and laboratory characteristics of focal laryngeal dystonia: study of 110 cases. *Laryngoscope.* 1988;98:636-640.

116. Freeman FJ, Cannito M, Finitzo-Hieber T. Classification of spasmodic dysphonia by visual perceptual and acoustic means. In: Gates GA, ed. *Spastic Dysphonia: State of the Art.* New York, NY: The Voice Foundation; 1985:5-18.

117. Finitzo T, Freeman F. Spasmodic dysphonia: whether and where: results of seven years of research. *J Speech Hear Res.* 1989;32:541-555.

118. Blitzer A, Brin MF. The dystonic larynx. *J Voice.* 1992;6:294-297.

119. Hanson DG, Logemann JA, Hain T. Differential diagnosis of spasmodic dysphonia: a kinematic perspective. *J Voice.* 1992;6:325-337.

120. Cannito MP, Kondraske GV, Johns DF. Oral-facial sensorimotor function in spasmodic dysphonia. In: Moore CA, Yorkston KM, eds. *Dysarthria and Apraxia of Speech: Perspectives on Management.* Baltimore, MD: Paul H. Brookes Publishing Co; 1991;205-225.

121. Jacome DE, Yanez GF. Spastic dysphonia and Meigs disease [letter]. *Neurology.* 1980;30:349.

122. Robe E, Brumlik J, Moore P. A study of spastic dysphonia (neurologic and electroencephalic abnormalities). *Laryngoscope.* 1960;70:219-245.

123. Finitzo-Hieber T, Freeman FJ, Gerling IJ, et al. Auditory brainstem response abnormalities in adductor spasmodic dysphonia. *Am J Otolaryngol.* 1982;3:26-30.

124. Tolosa E, Montserrat L, Bayes A. Blink reflex studies in focal dystonias: enhanced excitability of brainstem interneurons in cranial dystonia and spasmodic torticollis. *Mov Disord.* 1988;3:61-69.

125. Cohen LG, Ludlow CL, Warden BS, et al. Blink reflex excitability recovery curves in patients with spasmodic dysphonia. *Neurology.* 1989;39:572-577.

126. Devous MD, Pool KD, Finitzo T, et al. Evidence for cortical dysfunction in spasmodic dysphonia: regional cerebral blood flow and quantitative electrophysiology. *Brain Lang.* 1990;39:331-344.

127. Schaefer SD, Freeman FJ, Finitzo T, et al. Magnetic resonance imaging findings and correlations in spasmodic dysphonia patients. *Ann Otol Rhinol Laryngol.* 1985;94:595-601.

128. Lee MS, Lee SB, Kim WC. Spasmodic dysphonia associated with a left ventrolateral putaminal lesion. *Neurology.* 1996; 47:827-828.

129. Pool KD, Freeman FJ, Finitzo T, et al. Heterogeneity in spasmodic dysphonia: neurologic and voice findings. *Arch Neurol.* 1991;48:305-309.

130. Davis PJ, Bartlett D, Luschei E, Berke GS. Coordination of the respiratory and laryngeal systems in breathing and vocalization. In: Titze IR, ed. *Vocal Fold Physiology: Frontiers in Basic Science.* San Diego, CA: Singular Publishing Group; 1993:189-226.

131. Ludlow CL, VanPelt F, Koda J. Characteristics of late responses to superior laryngeal nerve stimulation in humans. *Ann Otol Rhinol Laryngol.* 1992;101:127-134.

132. Ludlow CL, Schulz GM, Yamashita T, Deleyiannis FW. Abnormalities in long latency responses to superior laryngeal nerve stimulation in adductor spasmodic dysphonia. *Ann Otol Rhinol Laryngol.* 1995;104:928-935.

133. Bielamowicz S, Ludlow CL. Effects of botulinum toxin on pathophysiology in spasmodic dysphonia. *Ann Otol Rhinol Laryngol.* 2000;109:194-203.

134. Bloch CS, Hirano M, Gould WJ. Symptom improvement of spastic dysphonia in response to phonatory tasks. *Ann Otol Rhinol Laryngol.* 1985;94:51-54.

135. Ginsberg BI, Wallack JJ, Srain JJ, et al. Defining the psychiatric role in spastic dysphonia. *Gen Hosp Psychiatry.* 1988;10:132-137.

136. Murry T, Cannito MP, Woodson GE. Spasmodic dysphonia: emotional status and botulinum toxin treatment. *Arch Otolaryngol Head Neck Surg.* 1994;120:310-316.

137. Roy N, Bless DM, Heisey D. Personality and voice disorders: a superfactor trait analysis. *J Speech Lang Hear Res.* 2000;43:749-768.

138. Ludlow CL, Sedory SE, Fujita M. Neurophysiological control of vocal fold adduction and abduction for phonation onset and offset during speech. In: Gauffin J, Hammarberg B, eds. *Vocal Fold Physiology: Acoustic, Perceptual, and Physiological Aspects of Voice Mechanisms.* San Diego, CA: Singular Publishing Group; 1991:197-206.

139. Woodson GE, Zwirner P, Murry T, et al. Functional assessment of patients with spasmodic dysphonia. *J Voice.* 1992;6:338-343.

140. Woodson GE, Zwirner P, Murry T, et al. Use of flexible fiberoptic laryngoscopy to assess patient with spasmodic dysphonia. *J Voice.* 1991;5:85-91.

141. Koufman JA, Blalock PD. Classification of laryngeal dystonias. *The Visible Voice.* 1992;1(3):4-5,19-23.

142. Zwirner P, Murry T, Swenson M, et al. Effects of botulinum toxin therapy in patients with adductor spasmodic dysphonia: acoustic, aerodynamic, and videoendoscopic findings. *Laryngoscope* 1992; 102:400-406.

143. Hartman DE, Aronson AE. Clinical investigations of intermittent breathy dysphonia. *J Speech Hear Disord.* 1981;46:428-432.

144. Merson RM, Ginsberg AP. Spasmodic dysphonia: abductor type. a clinical report of acoustic, aerodynamic, and perceptual characteristics. *Laryngoscope.* 1979;89:129-139.

145. Wolfe VI, Bacon M. Spectrographic comparison of two types of spastic dysphonia. *J Speech Hear Disord.* 1976;41:325-332.

146. Zwitman DH. Bilateral cord dysfunctions: abductor type spastic dysphonia. *J Speech Hear Disord.* 1979;44:373-378.

147. Koufman JA, Blalock PD. Diagnosis of spasmodic dysphonia by spectral analysis. *The Visible Voice.* 1992;1(3):6-7,15-18.

148. Watson BC, Schaefer SD, Freeman FJ, et al. Laryngeal electromyographic activity in adductor and abductor spasmodic dysphonia. *J Speech Hear Res.* 1991;34:473-482.

149. Van Pelt F, Ludlow CL, Smith PJ. Comparison of muscle activation patterns in adductor and abductor spasmodic dysphonia. *Ann Otol Rhinol Laryngol.* 1994;103:192-200.

150. Ludlow CL, Naunton RF, Terada S, et al. Successful treatment of selected cases of abductor spasmodic dysphonia using botulinum toxin. *Otolaryngol Head Neck Surg.* 1991;104:849-855.

151. Deleyiannis FW, Gillespie M, Bielamowicz S, Yamashita T, Ludlow CL. Laryngeal long latency response conditioning in abductor spasmodic dysphonia. *Ann Otol Rhinol Laryngol.* 1999;108:612-619.

152. Rontal M, Rontal E, Rolnick M, et al. A method for the treatment of abductor spasmodic dysphonia with botulinum toxin injections: a preliminary report. *Laryngoscope.* 1991;101:911-914.

153. Blitzer A, Brin MF, Stewart C, et al. Abductor laryngeal dystonia: a series treated with botulinum toxin. *Laryngoscope.* 1992;102:163-167.

154. Bidus KA, Thomas GR, Ludlow CL. Effects of adductor muscle stimulation on speech in abductor spasmodic dysphonia. *Laryngoscope.* 2000; 110:1943-1949.

155. Titze IR. *Principles of Voice Production.* Upper Saddle River, NJ: Prentice Hall; 1994.

156. Titze IR. Measurements for the assessment of voice disorders. In: Cooper JA, ed. *Assessment of Speech and Voice Production: Research and Clinical Applications.* NIDCD Monograph. Vol 1. 1991;42-49.

157. Giovanni A, Ouaknine M, Guelfucci R, Yu T, Zanaret M, Triglia JM. Nonlinear behavior of vocal fold vibration: the role of coupling between the vocal folds. *J Voice.* 1999:13:465-476.

158. Larson C, Kempster G, Kistler M. Changes in voice fundamental frequency following discharge of single motor units in cricothyroid and thyroarytenoid muscles. *J Speech Hear Res.* 1987;30:552-558.

159. Titze IR. A model for neurologic sources of aperiodicity in vocal fold vibration. *J Speech Hear Res.* 1991;34:460-472.

160. Davies P, McGowan R, Shadel C, Scherer R. Practical flow duct acoustics applied to the vocal tract. In: Titze IR, ed. *Vocal Fold Physiology: Frontiers in Basic Science.* San Diego, CA: Singular Publishing Group; 1993:93-142.

161. Rothenberg M. Acoustic interaction between the glottal source and the vocal tract. In: Stevens KN, Hirano M, eds. *Vocal Fold Physiology.* Tokyo, Japan: University of Tokyo Press; 1979:305-328.

162. Orlikoff RF, Baken RJ. The effect of the heartbeat on fundamental frequency perturbation. *J Speech Hear Res.* 1989;32:576-583.

163. Orlikoff RF. Vowel amplitude variation associated with the heart cycle. *J Acoust Soc Am.* 1990;88:2091-2098.

164. Titze IR, Baken RJ, Herzel H. Evidence of chaos in vocal fold vibration. In: Titze IR, ed. *Vocal Fold Physiology: Frontiers in Basic Science.* San Diego, CA: Singular Publishing Group; 1993:143-188.

165. Scherer RC, Gould WJ, Titze IR, et al. Preliminary evaluation of selected acoustic and glottographic

measures for clinical phonatory function analysis. *J Voice*. 1988;2:230-244.

166. Heiberger VL, Horii Y. Jitter and shimmer in sustained phonation. In: Lass NJ, ed. *Speech and Language: Advances in Basic Research and Practice*. Vol. 7. New York, NY: Academic Press; 1982:299-332.

167. Ramig LA, Ringel RL. The effects of physiological aging on selected acoustic characteristics of voice. *J Speech Hear Res*. 1983;26:22-30.

168. Linville SE. Intraspeaker variability in fundamental frequency stability: an age-related phenomenon? *J Acoust Soc Am*. 1988;83:741-745.

169. Wilcox K, Horii Y. Age and changes in vocal jitter. *J Gerontol*. 1980;35:194-198.

170. Horii Y. Jitter and shimmer differences among sustained vowel phonations. *J Speech Hear Res*. 1982;25:12-14.

171. Ramig LA, Scherer RC, Titze IR, et al. Acoustic analysis of voices of patients with neurologic disease: rationale and preliminary data. *Ann Otol Rhinol Laryngol*. 1988;97:164-172.

172. Ludlow C, Coulter D, Gentges F. The differential sensitivity of frequency perturbation to laryngeal neoplasms and neuropathologies. In: Bless DM, Abbs JH, eds. *Vocal Fold Physiology: Contemporary Research and Clinical Issues*. San Diego, CA: College-Hill Press; 1983:381-392.

173. Zwirner P, Murry T, Woodson GE. Phonatory function in neurologically impaired patients. *J Commun Disord*. 1991;24:287-300.

174. Baken RJ. Irregularity of vocal period and amplitude: a first approach to the fractal analysis of voice. *J Voice*. 1990;4:185-197.

175. Herzel H, Steinecke I, Mende W, et al. Chaos and bifurcations during voiced speech. In: Mosekilde E, ed. *Complexity, Chaos and Biological Evolution*. New York, NY: Plenum Press; 1991:41-50.

176. Gleick J. *Chaos: Making a New Science*. New York, NY: Viking Penguin; 1987.

177. Herzel H, Berry D, Titze IR, Saleh M. Analysis of vocal disorders with methods from nonlinear dynamics. *J Speech Hear Res*. 1994;37:1008-1019.

178. Matassini L, Hegger R, Kantz H, Manfredi C. Analysis of vocal disorders in a feature space. *Med Eng Phys*. 2000;22:413-418.

179. Hertrich I, Ackermann H. Gender-specific vocal dysfunctions in Parkinson's disease: electroglotto-graphic and acoustic analyses. *Ann Otol Rhinol Laryngol*. 1995;104:197–202.

180. Hertrich I, Lutzenberger W, Spieker S, Ackermann H. Fractal dimension of sustained vowel productions in neurological dysphonias: an acoustic and electroglottographic analysis. *J Acoust Soc Am*. 1997;102:652-654.

181. Ramig LA, Shipp T. Comparative measures of vocal tremor and vocal vibrato. *J Voice*. 1987;2:162-167.

182. Horii Y. Acoustic analysis of vocal vibrato: a theoretical interpretation of data. *J Voice*. 1989;3:36-43.

183. Jankovic J. Tremors: pathophysiology, differential diagnosis and pharmacology. *Neuro Cons*. 1984;2:1-8.

184. Brown JR, Simonson J. Organic voice tremor: a tremor of phonation. *Neurology*. 1963;13:520-525.

185. Hachinski VC, Thomsen IV, Buch NH. The nature of primary vocal tremor. *Can J Neurol Sci*. 1975;2:195-197.

186. Hartman DE, Overholt SL, Vishwanat B. A case of vocal cord nodules making essential (vocal) tremor. *Arch Otolaryngol*. 1982;108:52-53.

187. Massey EW, Paulson GW. Essential vocal tremor: clinical characteristics and response to therapy. *South Med J*. 1985;78:316-317.

188. Ludlow CL, Bassich CJ, Connor NP, et al. Phonatory characteristics of vocal fold tremor. *J Phonetics*. 1986;14:509-515.

189. Philippbar SA, Robin DA, Luschei ES. Limb, jaw and vocal tremor in Parkinson's patients. In: Yorkston K, Beukelman D, eds. *Recent Advances in Clinical Dysarthria*. San Diego, CA: College-Hill Press; 1991.

190. Hartman DE, Abbs JH, Vishwanat B. Clinical investigations of adductor spastic dysphonia. *Ann Otol Rhinol Laryngol*. 1988;97:247-252.

191. Jiang J, Lin E, Wu J, Gener C, Hanson DG. Effects of simulated source of tremor on acoustic and airflow voice measures. *J Voice*. 2000;14:47-57.

192. Aronson AE, Ramig LO, Winholtz WS, et al. Rapid voice tremor, or "flutter," in amyotrophic lateral sclerosis. *Ann Otol Rhinol Laryngol*. 1992;101:511-518.

193. Murray TJ. Essential tremor. *Can Med Assoc J*. 1981;124:1559-1570.

194. Findley LJ. Epidemiology and genetics of essential tremor. *Neurology*. 2000;54(suppl 4):S8-S13.

195. Deuschl G, Elble RJ. The pathophysiology of essential tremor. *Neurology.* 2000;54(suppl 4):S14-S20.

196. Jenkins IH, Bain PG, Colebatch JG, et al. A positron emission tomography study of essential tremor: evidence for overactivity of cerebellar connections. *Ann Neurol.* 1993;34:82-90.

197. Lou JS, Jankovic J. Essential tremor: clinical correlates in 350 patients. *Neurology.* 1991;41:234-238.

198. Aronson AE, Hartman DE. Adductor spastic dysphonia as a sign of essential (voice) tremor. *J Speech Hear Disord.* 1981;46:52-58.

199. Lebrun Y, Devreux F, Jean-Jaques R, et al. Tremulous speech. *Folia Phoniat.* 1982;34:134-142.

200. Koda J, Ludlow CL. An evaluation of laryngeal muscle activation in patients with voice tremor. *Otolaryngol Head Neck Surg.* 1992;107:684-696.

201. Koller WC, Hristova A, Brin M. Pharmacological treatment of essential tremor. *Neurology.* 2000;54(suppl 4):S30-S38.

202. Hartman DE, Vishanat B. Spastic dysphonia and essential (voice) tremor treated with primidone. *Arch Otolaryngol.* 1984;110:394-397.

203. Stager SV, Ludlow CL. Responses of stutterers and vocal tremor patients to treatment with botulinum toxin. In: Jankovic J, Hallett M, eds. *Therapy with Botulinum Toxin.* New York, NY: Marcel Dekker; 1994:481-490.

204. Hertegård S, Granqvist S, Lindestad P. Botulinum toxin injections for essential voice tremor. *Ann Otol Rhinol Laryngol.* 2000;109:204-209.

205. Warrick P, Dromey C, Irish J, et al. Botulinum toxin for essential tremor of the voice with multiple anatomical sites of tremor: a crossover design study of unilateral versus bilateral injection: *Laryngoscope.* 2000;110:1366-1374.

206. Finnegan EM, Luschei ES, Gordon JD, Barkmeier JM, Hoffman HT. Increased stability of airflow following botulinum toxin injection. *Laryngoscope.* 1999;109:1300-1306.

207. Goldman MS, Ahlskog JE, Kelly PJ. The symptomatic and functional outcome of stereotactic thalamotomy for medically intractable essential tremor. *J Neurosurg.* 1992;76:924-928.

208. Carpenter MA, Pahwa R, Miyawaki LK, Wilkinson SB, Searl JP, Koller WC. Reduction in voice tremor under thalamic stimulation. *Neurology.* 1998;50:796-798.

209. Taha JM, Janszen MA, Favre J. Thalamic deep brain stimulation for the treatment of head, voice, and bilateral limb tremor. *J Neurosurg.* 1999;91:68-72.

210. Obwegeser AA, Uitti RJ, Turk MF, Strongosky AJ, Wharen RE. Thalamic stimulation for the treatment of midline tremors in essential tremor patients. *Neurology.* 2000;54:2342-2344.

211. Yoon MS, Munz M, Sataloff RT, Spiegel JR, Heuer RJ. Vocal tremor reduction with deep brain stimulation. *Stereotact Funct Neurosurg.* 1999;72:241-244.

212. Dromey C, Kumar R, Lang AE, Lozano AM. An investigation of the effects of subthalamic nucleus stimulation on acoustic measures of voice. *Mov Disord.* 2000;15:1132-1138.

213. Holmes RJ, Oates JM, Phyland DJ, Hughes AJ. Voice characteristics in the progression of Parkinson's disease. *Int J Lang Commun Disord.* 2000;35:407-418.

214. Perez K, Ramig L, Smith M, Dromey C. The Parkinson larynx: tremor and videolaryngostroboscopic findings. *J Voice.* 1996;10:354-361.

215. Deuschl G, Toro C, Valls-Sole J, Zeffiro T, Zee DS, Hallett M. Symptomatic and essential palatal tremor. 1. Clinical, physiological and MRI analysis. *Brain.* 1994;117:775-788.

216. `Deuschl G, Löhle E, Toro C, Hallett M, Lebovics RS. Botulinum toxin treatment of palatal tremor (myoclonus). In: Jankovic J, Hallett M, eds. *Therapy with Botulinum Toxin.* New York, NY: Marcel Dekker; 1994:567-576.

217. Lapresle J. Palatal myoclonus. *Adv Neurol.* 1986;43:265-273.

218. Doody RS, Rosenfield DB. Spasmodic dysphonia associated with palatal myoclonus. *Ear Nose Throat J.* 1990;69:829-832.

219. Toland AD, Porubsky ES, Coker NJ, et al. Velopharyngo-laryngeal myoclonus: evaluation of objective tinnitus and extrathoracic airway obstruction. *Laryngoscope.* 1984;94:691-695.

220. Drysdale AJ, Ansell J, Adeley J. Palato-pharyngo-laryngeal myoclonus: an unusual cause of dysphagia and dysarthria. *J Laryngol Otol.* 1993;107:746-747.

221. Hartelius L, Buder E, Strand E. Long-term phonatory instability in individuals with multiple sclerosis. *J Speech Lang Hear Res.* 1997;40:1056-1072.

222. Kent RD, Netsell R, Abbs JH. Acoustic characteristics of dysarthria associated with cerebellar disease. *J Speech Hear Res.* 1979;22:627-648.

223. Aronson AE, Brown JR, Litin EM, et al. Spastic dysphonia II. Comparison with essential (voice) tremor and other neurologic and pychogenic dysphonias. *J Speech Hear Disord.* 1968;33:220-231.

224. Ackermann H, Ziegler W. Acoustic analysis of vocal instability in cerebellar dysfunctions. *Ann Otol Rhinol Laryngol.* 1994;103:98-104.

225. Carpenter RJ, McDonald TJ, Howard FM. The otolaryngologic presentation of amyotrophic lateral sclerosis. *Trans Am Acad Ophthalmol Otolaryngol.* 1978;86:479-484.

226. Carrow E, Rivera V, Mauldin M, et al. Deviant speech characteristics in motor neuron disease. *Arch Otolaryngol.* 1974;100;212-218.

227. Strand EA, Buder KM, Yorkston KM, et al. Differential phonatory characteristics of four women with amyotrophic lateral sclerosis. *J Voice.* 1994;8:327-339.

228. Silbergleit AK, Johnson AF, Jacobson BH. Acoustic analysis of voice in individuals with amyotrophic lateral sclerosis and perceptually normal vocal quality. *J Voice.* 1997;11:222-231.

229. Garfinkle TJ, Kimmelman CP. Neurologic disorders: amyotrophic lateral sclerosis, myasthenia gravis, multiple sclerosis, poliomyelitis. *Am J Otolaryngol.* 1982;3:204-212.

230. Beukelman DR, Kraft GH, Freal J. Expressive communication disorders in persons with multiple sclerosis: a survey. *Arch Phys Med Rehab.* 1985;66:675-677.

231. Darley FL, Brown JR, Goldstein N. Dysarthria in multiple sclerosis. *J Speech Hear Res.* 1972;15:229-245.

232. Farmakides MN, Boone DK. Speech problems of patients with multiple sclerosis. *J Speech Hear Disord.* 1960;25:385-390.

233. Stacy M, Jankovic J. Differential diagnosis of Parkinson's disease and the parkinsonism plus syndromes. *Neurol Clin.* 1992;10:341-359.

234. Bawa R, Ramadan HH, Wetmore SJ. Bilateral vocal cord paralysis in Shy-Drager syndrome. *Otolaryngol Head Neck Surg.* 1993;109:911-914.

235. Hanson DG, Ludlow C, Bassich C. Vocal fold paresis in Shy-Drager syndrome. *Ann Otol Rhinol Laryngol.* 1984;92:85-90.

236. Williams AJ, Hanson D, Calne D. Vocal cord paralysis in Shy-Drager syndrome. *J Neurol Neurosurg Psychiatry.* 1979;42:151-153.

237. Countryman S, Ramig LO, Pawlas AA. Speech and voice deficits in parkinsonian plus syndromes: can they be treated? *J Med Speech-Lang Pathol.* 1994;2:211-225.

238. Guidi AM, Bannister R, Gibson WPR, et al. Laryngeal electromyography in multiple system atrophy with autonomic failure. *J Neurol Neurosurg Psychiatry.* 1981;44:49-53.

239. Steele JC, Richardson JC, Olszewski J. Progressive supranuclear palsy. *Arch Neurol.* 1964;10:333-359.

240. Kluin KJ, Foster NL, Berent S, et al. Perceptual analysis of speech disorders in progressive supranuclear palsy. *Neurology.* 1993;43:563-566.

241. Metter EJ, Hanson WR. Dysarthria in progressive supranuclear palsy. In: Moore CA, Yorkston KM, eds. *Dysarthria and Apraxia of Speech: Perspectives on Management.* Baltimore, MD: Paul H. Brookes Publishing Co; 1991:127-136.

242. Tolosa E, Peña J. Involuntary vocalizations in movement disorders. *Adv Neurol.* 1988;49:343-363.

243. Salloway S, Stewart CF, Israeli L, et al. Botulinum toxin for refractory vocal tics. *Mov Disord.* 1996;11:746-748.

244. Trimble MR, Whurr R, Brookes G, Robertson MM. Vocal tics in Gilles de la Tourette syndrome treated with botulinum toxin injections. *Mov Disord.* 1998;13:617-619.

245. Kwak CH, Hanna PA, Jankovic J. Botulinum toxin in the treatment of tics. *Arch Neurol.* 2000;57:1190-1193.

246. Hillel A, Dray T, Miller R, et al. Presentation of ALS to the otolaryngologist/head and neck surgeon: getting to the neurologist. *Neurology.* 1999;53(8 suppl 5):S22-25; discussion S35-36.

247. Rosenfield DB. Neurolaryngology. *Ear Nose Throat J.* 1987;66:323-326.

248. Sataloff RT. The physical examination. In: Sataloff RT, ed. *Professional Voice: Science and Art of Clinical Care.* 2nd ed. San Diego, CA: Singular Publishing Group; 1997:207-213.

249. Yorkston KM, Beukelman DR, Bell KR; Laryngeal function. In: *Clinical Management of Dysarthric Speakers.* Boston, MA: College-Hill Press, Little, Brown, and Co; 1988:241-267.

250. Miller RH, Rosenfield DB. The role of electromyography in clinical laryngology. *Otolaryngol Head Neck Surg.* 1984;92:287-291.

251. Parnes SM, Satya-Murti S. Predictive value of laryngeal electromyography in patients with vocal cord paralysis of neurogenic origin. *Laryngoscope.* 1985:95:1323-1326.

252. Lovelace RE, Blitzer A, Ludlow CL. Clinical laryngeal electromyography. In: Blitzer A, et al, eds. *Neurologic Disorders of the Larynx.* New York, NY: Thieme Medical Publishers; 1992:66-81.

253. Munin MC, Murry T, Rosen CA. Laryngeal electromyography: diagnostic and prognostic applications. *Otolaryngol Clin North Am.* 2000;33:759-770.

254. Yin SG, Qiu WW, Stucker FJ, Batchelor BM. Critical evaluation of neurolaryngological disorders. *Ann Otol Rhinol Laryngol.* 2000;109:832-838.

255. Swenson MR, Zwirner P, Murry T, et al. Medical evaluation of patients with spasmodic dysphonia. *J Voice.* 1992;6:320-324.

CHAPTER 27

Vocal Fold Paralysis

Glendon M. Gardner, MD

Michael S. Benninger, MD

This chapter discusses the presentation, evaluation, and treatment of patients with unilateral or bilateral vocal fold immobility or hypomobility. Some of the surgical procedures will be described in detail, while others are covered more completely in other chapters. The chapter begins with a discussion of vocal fold position, then addresses the clinical assessment and treatment of unilateral, and then bilateral vocal fold paralysis.

POSITION OF THE VOCAL FOLDS FOLLOWING LARYNGEAL PARALYSIS

Vocal fold position following motor nerve paralysis has been a subject of some controversy. Classic teaching has stated that one can determine the site of the neurologic injury based on the position of the vocal fold. The position of vocal folds as traditionally described with various neural injuries are shown in Figure 27-1. With the advent of laryngeal electromyography, recent studies have demonstrated that there is poor correlation between specific injuries and vocal fold position.[1] Therefore, clinical determination of site of lesion based upon vocal fold position alone is often difficult. The following section presents some of the arguments in this controversy.

Unilateral Superior Laryngeal Nerve Paralysis

The superior laryngeal nerve (SLN) provides supraglottic sensation via its internal branch, and motor innervation to the cricothyroid muscle (CT) via its external branch.[2,3] Paralysis of the SLN affects vocal fold position by altering CT function. The CT is described traditionally as containing two bellies: the more medial pars recta, which originates on the anterior inferior cricoid cartilage and inserts on the inferior cornua of the thyroid cartilage; and the more lateral pars oblique, which runs obliquely to insert on the inferior border of the thyroid cartilage.[3,4] The action of the CT muscle in an intact larynx is to "tilt the cricoid lamina backward through the cricothyroid joint, thus lengthening, tensing, and adducting the vocal cords."[3] The effect of isolated SLN paralysis upon vocal fold positioning has long been the subject of debate, owing in part to imprecise and confusing terminology. Recently, however, a consensus has been evolving in the literature regarding position of the vocal folds following SLN lesion. Canine and human electromyographic and videostroboscopic studies show that following local anesthesia and/or sectioning of the SLN, the true vocal fold (TVF) on the affected side appears normal at rest. During phonation, because of the unopposed action of the contralateral cricothyroid muscle, the anterior portion of the cricoid cartilage is pulled upward and laterally, toward the intact side. This rocking motion results in deviation of the posterior portion of the larynx to the paralyzed side.[2] Other authors feel that if the cricothyroid joints are intact, the thyroid cartilage can only move in its natural direction regard-

FIGURE 27-1. *Vocal fold position following right-sided laryngeal nerve injury as traditionally described. Position during phonation. (A) Paramedian position, seen with compensated unilateral RLN injury. (B) Lateral (cadaveric) position, seen with combined SLN and RLN injury. (C) Intermediate position, seen with poorly compensated RLN injury or well-compensated combined SLN and RLN injury. (D) Isolated SLN injury with shift of posterior commissure to the right and bowing of false vocal fold.*

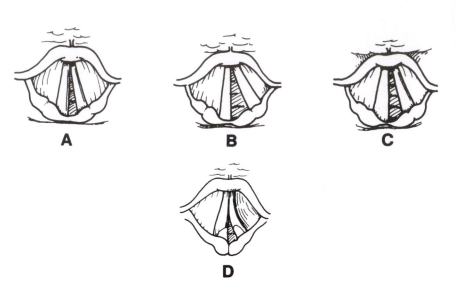

less of whether one CT muscle is paralyzed or not, and that no deviation of the thyroid cartilage relative to the cricoid cartilage is possible.[5] The proposed rocking motion is also thought to lengthen the aryepiglottic fold on the intact side and shorten the aryepiglottic fold on the paralyzed side. As a result of the loss of tension on the affected side, the ipsilateral vocal fold may appear wavy during phonation. It may also appear to be at a lower level during inspiration and at a higher level during expiration.[2,4,6,7] Ipsilateral bowing of the true vocal fold, prolapse of the false vocal fold, and altered waveform on videostroboscopy have been reported in a canine study (Elizabeth Ransom, personal communication, 1993) and is also seen in humans shortly after injury (Figures 27-1 and 27-2).[8] Videostroboscopic analysis after lidocaine injection of the SLN in humans reveals moderate traveling wave asymmetry, decreased velocity and excursion of the involved side, and decreased tension of the vocal fold on the involved side.[9]

Clinically, patients with unilateral SLN paralysis are said to be at higher risk of aspiration because of their sensory deficit. Patients with unilateral SLN injury have been reported to suffer from lower pitched, weak, monotonous, and easily tired voice.[6] (Elizabeth Ransom, personal communication, 1993.)

Koufman reported on 26 patients with unilateral vocal fold paralysis and demonstrated with laryngeal EMG that the status of the cricothyroid muscle did not influence the vocal fold position.[10]

Bilateral Superior Laryngeal Nerve Paralysis

Not often described, this lesion is said to cause no change in vocal fold positioning because of the symmetric loss of movement with phonation. However, close scrutiny usually reveals a "floppy" epiglottis, and vocal

folds that are bowed and lower than usual in the membranous portion. An increased risk of aspiration has been suggested, presumably secondary to a loss of supraglottic sensory innervation.[2]

Unilateral Recurrent Laryngeal Nerve Paralysis

The recurrent laryngeal nerve innervates the lateral cricoarytenoid, thyroarytenoid, vocalis and aryepiglottic muscles via its anterior branch, and the posterior cricoarytenoid and interarytenoid muscles via its poste-

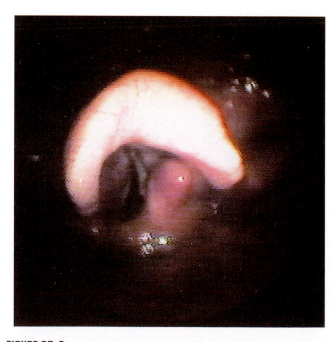

FIGURE 27-2. *Isolated left superior laryngeal nerve paralysis. Note shift of posterior commissure to left and prominence of left false vocal fold.*

rior branch.[3] Innervation of the interarytenoid muscle is classically described as bilateral, being the only intrinsic laryngeal muscle to receive bilateral innervation. One study suggests that not only does the interarytenoid muscle receive bilateral innervation via the RLN, but that the SLN also contributes to interarytenoid innervation.[8] Unilateral paralysis of the RLN results in nonfunction of all intrinsic laryngeal muscles with the exception of the interarytenoid and cricothyroid muscles. The vocal fold has classically been described as assuming a paramedian position (Figures 27-1 and 27-3). Upon phonation, the true vocal fold may display apparent active adduction caused by the unopposed action of the cricothyroid muscle or the interarytenoid muscle.[2] Vocal fold waveform is often seen on the involved side by videostroboscopic analysis but marked wave asymmetry, lower velocity, and later onset of vibration are seen on the paralyzed side.[9] Breathiness, rapid air escape, and diplophonia are characteristic vocal findings.[4,6,9]

Despite these well-described positions related to unilateral recurrent laryngeal nerve paralysis, it is again noted that clinical determination of site of lesion based on vocal fold position alone is often difficult. Electromyography may be necessary to isolate the site of lesion.

Bilateral Recurrent Laryngeal Nerve Paralysis

With bilateral RLN paralysis, occasionally encountered following thyroid surgery, both vocal folds assume the median to paramedian position. Here too, apparent active adduction results from the unopposed action of

the cricothyroid muscles. Symmetric movement is expected and, although incomplete closure may occur, no shifting of the posterior portion of the larynx is seen because of the action of bilateral cricothyroid muscles.

The position of the vocal folds in bilateral paralysis depends somewhat on the site of lesion. Because, typically, this is secondary to injury to the two RLNs, the unopposed action of the cricothyroid muscles can result in good approximation and vibration with adduction resulting in good voice. Even if the vocal folds are in a paramedian position, the myoelastic and aerodynamic forces can result in good vocal fold waveform, which is usually symmetric as viewed by videostroboscopy. The lack of activity of either posterior cricoarytenoid muscle results in inadequate glottic chink for respiration. The rare high vagal bilateral paralysis (usually central paralysis) results in poor closure and a poor airway (Figures 27-4 and 27-5). Infants with Arnold-Chiari malformation will present with airway compromise.

Complete Vagal Section (Superior and Inferior Laryngeal Nerve Paralysis)

In instances of complete loss of vagal motor input, the vocal folds have been reported to assume an intermediate or "cadaveric" position.[11] The folds are more lateral than with isolated RLN injury because of the loss of adduction otherwise provided by the cricothyroid muscle when the SLN is intact.[2,9] (Elizabeth Ransom, personal communication, 1993.) Our recent studies in dogs have shown that immediately following sectioning of the SLN and RLN on the same side, the vocal fold assumes a paramedian position at rest but with adduc-

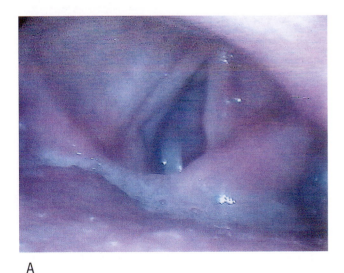

A

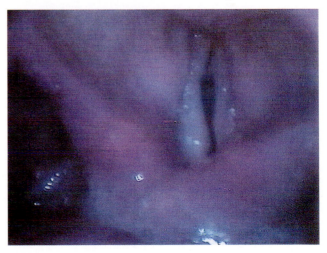

B

FIGURE 27-3. *Right recurrent laryngeal nerve paralysis. (A) Abduction. (B) Adduction—note vocal fold in paramedian position. Vocal fold excursion is greater on uninvolved (left) side.*

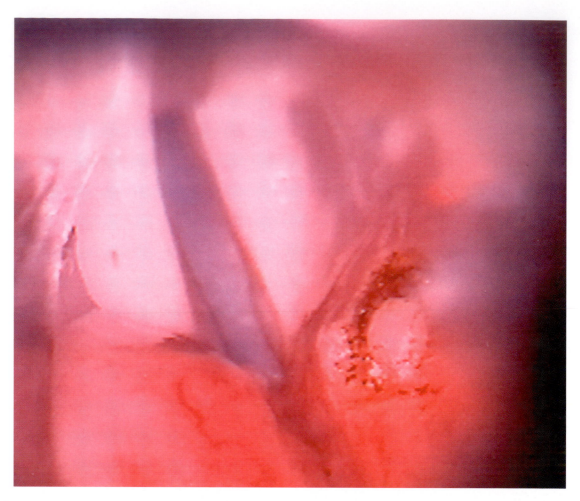

FIGURE 27-4. *Patient with bilateral vocal fold paralysis due to diabetic neuropathy at beginning of right CO_2 laser arytenoidectomy showing initial incision.*

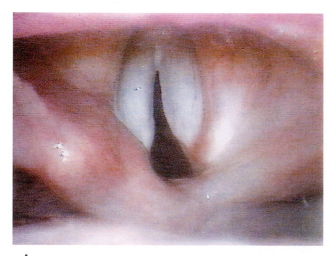

A

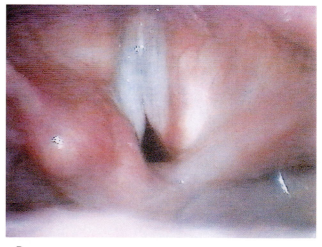

B

FIGURE 27-5. *A patient with bilateral vocal fold paralysis following thyroidectomy. Patient is status post right laser arytenoidectomy and temporary stitch lateralization. She had been tracheostomy-dependent because of airway insufficiency and is now decannulated. (A) Quiet respiration. (B) Phonation.*

tion during phonation, the characteristic findings of a shift of the posterior portion of the larynx to the side of lesion and fullness of the false vocal fold noted with a SLN injury are also seen (Elizabeth Ransom, personal communication, 1993). It is possible that the lateralized position that has been described is caused by the long-term effects of a sustained paralysis unlike the more acute effects immediately following injury. When a SLN injury is induced on one side while a RLN injury occurs on the other, the individual effects of the two separate lesions are seen immediately following denervation: the vocal fold assumes a paramedian position on the side of the RLN lysis and posterior shifting is noted toward the side of the SLN lysis with attempts at phonation. Long-term effects may, however, differ (Figures 27-6 and 27-7). Videostroboscopy may show the vocal folds vibrating at different levels with profound asymmetry of the traveling wave. Loss of vocal fold tension on the involved side with decreased traveling wave velocity and excursion is seen. The uninvolved vocal fold may be positioned higher than the paralyzed fold.[9]

THE EVALUATION OF VOCAL FOLD PARALYSIS

The evaluation of vocal fold paralysis is aimed at determining the cause of the immobility and the severity of the symptoms in order to guide treatment. Often, the cause is obvious, such as a known transection of the nerve with trauma, or during surgery for a malignancy involving the recurrent laryngeal nerve. Frequently the etiology is not readily apparent as in the case of idiopathic paralysis. Furthermore, immobile vocal folds may not be paralyzed.

We will address the presentation for unilateral and bilateral vocal fold immobility in separate sections, focusing on the many different etiologies for these conditions.

Presentation of Unilateral Vocal Fold Immobility

Dysphonia is by far the most common presenting complaint for patients with a unilateral immobile vocal fold, followed by aspiration and weak cough.[12] The voice is usually characterized as weak and breathy, hoarse or rough. Onset can be noted immediately after extubation following iatrogenic injury to the recurrent laryngeal nerve or after external trauma. Patients with idiopathic vocal fold paralysis often report awakening with a dysphonic voice with a normal voice just the previous day. Other patients will report a slow (days to weeks) gradual onset. These are often found to have an enlarging neoplasm (usually malignant) impinging on the RLN or vagus nerve. Patients with SLN motor dysfunction (extrinsic branch) note difficulty with high pitch, and aspiration if it is primarily a sensory problem (intrinsic branch).

If the etiology is obvious from the history (thyroidectomy) and the physical examination is consistent (not suggestive of arytenoid dislocation) then no further workup is necessary.

A review of previously reported studies suggests that thyroid surgery was once the most common cause of unilateral and bilateral vocal fold paralysis.[13,14] Recently, extralaryngeal malignancies have been found to be the most common cause.[15,16] A review of 251 consecutive cases of vocal fold paralysis (159 unilateral and 92 bilateral) at Henry Ford Hospital has shown that nonlaryngeal malignancies, primarily pulmonary, are

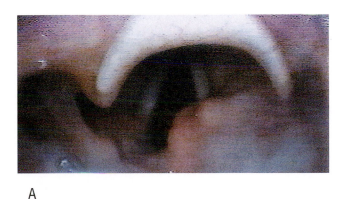

A

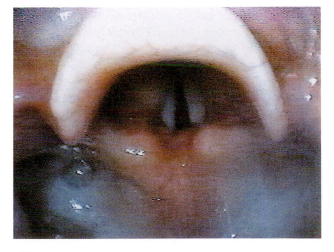

B

FIGURE 27-6. *Poorly compensated right vocal fold paralysis 6 months following resection of vagus nerve during skull base surgery. Note lateralized position. (A) Abduction. (B) Adduction.*

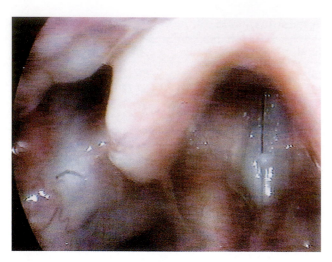

FIGURE 27-7. *Well-compensated left vocal fold paralysis 12 months following resection of vagus nerve during skull base surgery. Note prominence of left false vocal fold, which is also seen in isolated superior laryngeal nerve (SLN) paralysis (adduction).*

the cause of the majority of unilateral paralysis, accounting for 25%, and for a large percentage of bilateral paralyses (Table 27-1).[17] Treating these underlying causes will occasionally result in return of motion of the vocal fold.

Surgical Trauma

As noted in most early studies, surgery of the thyroid or parathyroid glands was the most common cause of unilateral vocal fold paralysis. This was because of the intimate relationship of the thyroid vessels and the RLN and SLN. Some other surgical procedures have become more often performed and have resulted in unilateral vocal fold paralysis. The anterior approach to the cervical spine is a very popular approach to the anterior vertebral bodies from C3 to T1 and results in unilateral vocal fold paralysis in 2% to 7% of cases.[18] Interestingly, the right RLN is injured more often during these cases than the left. This may be caused by the shorter course of the right RLN and the resultant less slack in the nerve, making it more prone to stretch-induced trauma from retraction.[18]

An increasingly aggressive surgical approach to pulmonary malignancies has made this an increasingly common cause of unilateral vocal fold paralysis. The left RLN is at higher risk because of its more intrathoracic course.

Nonneoplastic pulmonary processes, such as invasive aspergillosis have also been reported to cause unilateral vocal fold paralysis. While this is more common in immunocompromised patients, it can occur in otherwise healthy individuals.[19]

Etiology	Unilateral	Bilateral	Total
Non-laryngeal malignancy	39 (25)	17 (19)	56 (23)
Idiopathic	37 (23)	14 (15)	51 (20)
Thyroidectomy	16 (10)	16 (17)	32 (12)
Neurologic	14 (9)	12 (13)	26 (11)
Trauma	17 (10)	14 (16)	31 (13)
Iatrogenic (non-thyroidectomy)	19 (12)	5 (5)	24 (9)
Post-intubation	6 (4)	11 (12)	17 (7)
Cardiomegaly/thoracic aneurysm	8 (5)	0 (0)	8 (3)
Mediastinal adenopathy/TB	3 (2)	0 (0)	3 (1)
Rheumatoid arthritis	0 (0)	3 (3)	3 (1)
TOTAL	**159**	**92**	**251**

Legend: ( ) = %

TABLE 27-1. *Vocal Fold Immobility—Henry Ford Hospital 1987–1991*

Other Anatomic Causes of Unilateral Vocal Fold Paralysis

Ortner's syndrome is also known as cardiovocal syndrome and consists of a left recurrent laryngeal nerve palsy secondary to cardiac disease such as a dilated left atrium in the case of mitral valve stenosis compressing the RLN against the aortic arch. Other causes include aneurysms of the large intrathoracic vessels.[20]

The high incidence of extralaryngeal malignancies, cardiomegaly, and mediastinal adenopathy as possible etiologies implies that unless the cause is readily apparent, close vigilance to rule out these causes is necessary. We have found that a thorough history, office laryngoscopy, careful head and neck examination, chest x-ray, and CT scan or MRI scan from the skull base through the superior mediastinum is a sufficient workup to identify these tumors. MRI or CT of the chest has not revealed unsuspected neoplasms, nor is the routine cost of these procedures justified. Of the 251 patients discussed above, no pulmonary or mediastinal neoplasm was identified which was not noted on CXR, while all surviving patients have had at least one year of follow-up.[17] Conceivably, this is because a neoplasm would have to be of sufficient size to be identified by CXR in order to cause enough external compression of the RLN to result in a paralysis. Some, however, do advocate routine chest CT and esophagram for all idiopathic vocal fold paralyses.[21]

As described earlier, immobility and paralysis are not necessarily synonymous. An immobile fold may be secondary to paralysis or cricoarytenoid joint fixation, while at times a paralysis of the recurrent laryngeal nerve may not result in immobility of the vocal fold because of the actions of the uninvolved intrinsic and extrinsic laryngeal muscles. A mechanically immobile arytenoid should be suspected when the problem arises immediately after extubation when the surgery was not likely to injure the laryngeal nerves, after external trauma to the neck, or in the case of severe rheumatoid arthritis. Palpation of the joint in the office or under anesthesia may be necessary. If direct laryngoscopy is done, a dislocated arytenoid can be reduced at the time of endoscopy.[22] Endotracheal intubation can cause true vocal fold paralysis.[23] It is thought that the endotracheal tube cuff in the subglottis (rather than in the trachea) can compress the anterior branch of the recurrent laryngeal nerve where it enters the larynx between the cricoid and thyroid cartilages.[23] Following long-standing unilateral paralysis, some joint fixation may occur.

A unilateral immobile vocal fold caused by central neurologic disease is unlikely to be an isolated finding. A complete history and physical examination should reveal other neurologic dysfunction.

The next issue to consider is whether the immobility is permanent or only a temporary paresis or paralysis. Fortunately, laryngeal electromyography has been helpful in assessing the innervation of laryngeal muscles. The EMG can be conveniently used to assess the thyroarytenoid and posterior cricoarytenoid muscles innervated by the RLN and the cricothyroid muscle innervated by the SLN. Koufman has developed a workable scale for interpretation of laryngeal EMG in vocal fold paralysis (Table 27-2).[1] Laryngeal muscles do have some dissimilarities to splanchnic muscles and experience is necessary to be able to make an appropriate evaluation. Furthermore, reinnervation potentials do not necessarily mean that normal vocal fold movement will occur, nor does denervation imply that reinnervation will not take place. However, our experience has shown that the absence of significant recruitment despite signs of rein-

Class	Spontaneous Activity	Recruitment	Individual Motor Unit Morphology	Interpretation
I	Absent	Normal	Normal	Normal
II	Absent	Reduced	Polyphasic units	Old injury
III	Present	Reduced	Polyphasic units	Equivocal*
IV	Present	Absent	Fibs, myokimea, etc.	Denervation

*In this situation, the EMG may indicate either ongoing denervation or early recovery.

TABLE 27-2. *Interpretation of Laryngeal EMG in Vocal Fold Paralysis*

nervation (polyphasic motor units) at 6 months invariably results in permanent immobility or severe hypomobility probably caused by synkinesis.

The quality of voice with unilateral vocal fold immobility should be assessed and can help in treatment planning. The most important parameter is the patient's perception of his/her own voice quality, which can be assessed using the Voice Handicap Index (VHI) questionnaire.[24,25] (See Chapter 18.) The otolaryngologist's and the speech-language pathologist's perceptions are also critical and can be measured systematically for research purposes. Tape-recording helps to assess changes in voice quality over time or with treatment. Objective evaluations that assess voice are numerous and are beyond the scope of this chapter. Nonetheless, certain basic determinations are valuable in the assessment of any voice disorder: perceptual assessment, determination of pitch, range, and perturbation, evaluation of vibration with videostroboscopy, and airflow rates.

The ability to examine the larynx directly with a laryngeal mirror is helpful for a global assessment of the larynx. Flexible fiberoptic nasopharyngolaryngoscopy allows for more specialized evaluation of laryngeal function, particularly during running speech. It allows for sniffing, which maximally stimulates the posterior cricoarytenoid muscles demonstrating the best airway in cases of bilateral vocal fold immobility. Videostrobo-scopy may help to determine whether normal vocal fold vibration is present, to assess the character, quality, symmetry, and excursion of the traveling wave and, most importantly, to assess closure. It is closure that is most affected by the various procedures which medialize the immobile vocal fold. In some cases videostroboscopy can be useful to rule out other pathologies or to help assess for hyperfunctional voice behaviors, and it is critical in the evaluation of post-treatment results. Occasionally, patients with unilateral paralysis without treatment accommodate sufficiently to achieve complete closure and allow return of normal vocal fold vibration, as viewed by videostroboscopy. Airflow rates can be indirectly measured utilizing maximum phonation time (MPT), which can be performed in any office setting with a stopwatch or more directly assessed with the aid of spirometry or sophisticated airflow instruments, such as the Nagashima Phonatory Function Analyzer. Increased airflow rates and shortened phonation times are expected with unilateral vocal fold paralysis while normal values may be seen with bilateral vocal fold paralysis. Fundamental frequency and pitch range decrease with unilateral vocal fold paralysis but may be within normal ranges in bilateral vocal fold paralysis. Caution must be exercised when using such tasks in that compensatory behaviors have frequently developed as a result of the disorder making objective tests difficult to interpret. Compensatory (often hyperfunctional) voice behaviors may persist after surgical intervention and interfere with accurate assessment of treatment results. Retesting following voice rehabilitation will give more accurate determinations of ultimate voice function. Despite these limitations, we feel that the combination of practitioner and patient perceptual assessment (Voice Handicap Index, VHI), evaluation of pitch range, vocal fold vibratory characteristics (stroboscopy), and airflow rates are all valuable in evaluating a patient with vocal fold immobility and judging the results of therapy. Frequency and intensity perturbations are generally assessed but may be difficult to interpret, although they have been found to be helpful in some patients.

A further difficulty is determining which patients will compensate for their paralysis even if the immobility is permanent. Despite electromyography showing denervation and in situations where reinnervation is not likely or possible, many patients will compensate satisfactorily for their occupational, social, or avocational needs. This is particularly true in young, otherwise healthy patients with good vocal fold bulk. In such patients, waiting to see if sufficient accommodation will take place under the care and instruction of a skilled speech-language pathologist is indicated. Usually, a 6 to 12-month interval is sufficient although we have seen return of function up to 18 months after injury. In patients with near-aphonia or those having difficulty with aspiration, early intervention is often indicated. Some now proceed with intervention at the time or shortly after major neurologic, base of skull, or pulmonary surgery where significant aspiration and subsequent sequelae are expected.[26] We now recommend such early intervention in selected cases and some authors advocate voice therapy in virtually all cases of vocal fold paralysis or paresis.[27]

Idiopathic vocal fold immobility presents many difficulties in treatment planning. Is recovery likely to occur? Will return of function be normal or synkinetic, or will the patient accommodate sufficiently? Although the general sense is that idiopathic vocal fold paralyses tend to recover spontaneously, the literature suggests that this may not be the case.[17] In the Henry Ford Hospital series, only 13.5% of unilateral and 21% of bilateral idiopathic paralyses recovered spontaneously. It is likely that both the true rate of idiopathic paralysis and recovery from these insults is greater than would be gleaned from these reports. Havas reported a 75% recovery rate among patients with idiopathic palsies, while Ramadan et al reported only a 19% recovery rate in the same population.[28,29] Many temporary idiopathic pareses result in either mild or quickly resolving dysphonias, and the patient does not seek general medical or otolaryngologic care.

The real challenge in idiopathic vocal fold paralysis may be in early identification resulting in earlier intervention, which may prevent prolonged or permanent sequelae. It is well accepted that herpetic involvement in cranial nerve injury (such as occurs in herpes zoster oticus) is often polyneuropathic. In otologic/facial nerve herpes infection, systemic steroids and/or an anti-herpetic medication may be offered. Such approaches may be applicable to idiopathic vocal fold paralysis if identified early. Anecdotal use of Acyclovir has been reported in the literature.[30] Large, multi-institutional studies may be needed to determine if any efficacy or indication exists.

Once the etiology is determined and recovery is not expected, then decisions about potential intervention can be made. At the time of patient presentation, counseling and conservative treatment, such as voice therapy, should begin despite not knowing the etiology.

TREATMENT OF UNILATERAL VOCAL FOLD PARALYSIS

Treatment of unilateral vocal fold paralysis aims at improving voice quality and preventing aspiration. The site of injury (RLN or combined SLN plus RLN), the bulk of the vocal fold, the degree of compensation (Figure 27-6), the general health and pulmonary status of the patient, and degree of proprioceptive integrity will all play a role in the quality of voice after unilateral vocal fold paralysis. The surgeon must evaluate carefully all these parameters and discuss potential options while weighing the benefits, simplicity, and risks of surgery with the patient and should consult with other members of the voice team prior to proceeding.

The Role of Voice Therapy

Voice therapy is very important in the general treatment of patients with a unilateral vocal fold paralysis. Assessment can help determine the degree or likelihood of accommodation and can assess whether there are any compensatory behaviors which have developed that will inhibit rehabilitation. Many patients may develop hyperfunctional voice behaviors in an attempt to compensate. Such behaviors will be counterproductive to effective vocalization alone or after surgical treatment. Voice therapy alone may provide sufficient improvement in many patients. If surgical intervention is planned, voice therapy preoperatively will facilitate rehabilitation postoperatively.[27]

Surgical Treatment of Unilateral Vocal Fold Paralysis

Many different techniques are available for treatment of unilateral vocal fold paralysis. In an effort to standardize nomenclature for laryngoplastic procedures, a classification has been developed by the Speech, Voice, and Swallowing Disorders Committee of the American Academy of Otolaryngology—Head and Neck Surgery (AAO-HNS) and adopted by the Board of the AAO-HNS (Table 27-3).

The goal of all surgical approaches to unilateral vocal fold paralysis is to improve closure. We may think of these different procedures as being static, dynamic, permanent, or temporary. The static procedures put the immobile vocal fold in the midline so that the mobile vocal fold may approximate it, while the dynamic procedures attempt to restore the motion of the immobile vocal fold, hopefully restoring the glottis to as near-normal a situation as possible. The dynamic procedures all involve reinnervation or electrical pacing of the immobile vocal fold, and the static procedures consist of using some substance to better position the vocal fold. These substances include Teflon, Gelfoam, fat, fascia, silastic, collagen, hydroxylapatite, Gore-Tex, tissue expanders, and others.

Injection Laryngoplasty (IL)

In the not too distant past, certainly the most commonly performed procedure for the treatment of a paralyzed unilateral vocal fold was Teflon injection into the immobile vocal fold. This may still be the most common procedure performed by general otolaryngologists. Teflon was introduced as a supposedly inert substance which can medialize the vocal fold and can be injected either transorally[31] or transcutaneously.[32] Proper placement is lateral to the vocal process of the arytenoid, deep in the thyroarytenoid muscle in the midportion (on the vertical axis). In experienced hands, Teflon is a quick and effective way of improving voice.[33,34] It has significant drawbacks, which may have prompted interest in other methods of medialization. These include improper amount (too much) or site of placement (too superficial, too inferior, too anterior), which can result in bolus shifting and/or granuloma formation. Granulomas may occur even with proper injection as Teflon does promote a foreign body reaction.[35,36] The result is often a very stiff, non-vibrating vocal fold and a less than acceptable voice.[37] The surgical removal of Teflon is difficult because of its infiltration into the muscle fibers, and is generally ungratifying.[38] Finally, although experienced laryngologists find the results to be predictable, many find that the results are suboptimal. Although other modalities of treatment have preempted the use of Teflon, for some it remains an important treatment option. Its ease of use and transoral approach provide effective medialization for those with significant systemic disease, incurable neoplasms

A. Laryngeal Framework Surgery (LFS) with

Arytenoid adduction (AA)

Medialization (M)

Lateralization (L)

Anterior Commissure

        Retrusion—(relaxation) (ACR)

        Protrusion—(tensing) (ACP)

Cricothyroid Approximation (CTA)

Medialization laryngoplasty can be qualified by method of medialization

    —Medialization laryngoplasty with

        s—silastic

        c—cartilage

        e—expander

        o—other

B. Injection Laryngoplasty (IL)

    D—Direct

    I—Indirect

    —Injection laryngoplasty with

        t—Teflon

        g—Gelfoam

        col—collagen

        f—fat

        o—other

Abbreviations may be used, ie:

Laryngeal framework surgery with medialization—silastic (LFS-M-s)

Laryngeal framework surgery with arytenoid adduction (LFS-AA)

Injection laryngoplasty—direct—Teflon (IL-D-t)

TABLE 27-3. *Laryngoplastic Phonosurgery Classification*

affecting the recurrent laryngeal nerve in individuals where aspiration is the primary problem, or those not requiring subtle voice changes.[12]

Gelfoam, a temporary injectable substance, has been used in patients with acute needs for medialization where vocal fold movement may return and a permanent procedure is not necessarily indicated. It can also be used to help predict results from other permanent injected substances.

Recently, autologous fat has been advocated as an alternative to Teflon.[39,40] The advantage is that it is abundant in supply and is a homograft. The unpredictability of the degree of reabsorption, concerns over the best methods to harvest and process the fat, and lack of long-term results have prevented more widespread acceptance. Studies in cats suggest that the fat does not last more than 12 months, while other studies in dogs show that it remains viable longer.[41-43] All authors recommend overinjection of the fat. The expected reabsorption is seen as a drawback for permanent correction of this problem, but may make fat an ideal substance for short-term (6-12 months) improvement when recovery is possible.[44]

Collagen is a bioimplant substance that is integrated into host tissues. It is used to provide bulk and soften scars.[45] It has been advocated as a method to medialize vocal fold paralysis, particularly in the face of small defects.[45] It also can be injected at multiple sites to smooth out irregular vocal folds and can allow the chronic scarred vocal fold to soften and become more supple. This substance is still investigational for this indication in the United States but may have an important role in the treatment of the unilateral vocal fold paralysis in the future. Bovine collagen is commercially available but may induce a foreign body reaction, while autologous collagen can be processed from a sample of the patient's skin.

Another biomaterial which has been injected into the vocal fold is fascia. Preliminary results in 18 patients demonstrated excellent voice recovery, but long-term follow-up is not yet available.[46]

Laryngeal Reinnervation

Loss of neuronal input to the vocal fold has led to natural attempts to reinnervate the vocal fold to restore movement. Following denervation of the unilateral vocal fold, reinnervation occurs in many patients over time. Even if this reinnervation is via the originally injured nerve, normal motion often does not result, most likely because of synkinesis and simultaneous activity of both the adductors and abductors of the vocal fold. This may prevent atrophy, but otherwise is not clinically significant. In the face of known transection, immediate anastomosis of the nerve at the time of injury is recommended.[47] In recurrent laryngeal nerve paralysis, different techniques have been advocated. All have the potential advantages of prevention of denervation muscle atrophy, return of some vocal fold mobility, and can be used in cases in which there is potential for recovery of vocal fold function or with other static procedures to medialize the vocal fold.[48]

Tucker[49] described a nerve muscle pedicle utilizing a small muscle pedicle from the omohyoid muscle innervated through the ansa system to the posterior cricoarytenoid muscle in bilateral vocal fold paralysis or the thyroarytenoid muscle in unilateral vocal fold paralysis. Although animal studies have shown that reinnervation occurs and some of his patients have had satisfactory return of mobility, results have been unpredictable. More recently, Crumley[50] has proposed direct anastomosis of the ansa cervicalis nerve to the recurrent laryngeal nerve. This can stabilize the arytenoid cartilage by reinnervating the intrinsic laryngeal muscles, rotating the cartilage into a more stable position, and resulting in more normal tension and symmetry with the opposite fold. Better voice outcome may occur. A specific ansa cervicalis to adductor branch of the RLN has also shown promise.[51] A more complete discussion of this topic is found in Chapter 38.

Medialization Laryngoplasty With Implant

Non-injection medialization of vocal folds has gained much recent popularity because of its relative simplicity, potential for reversibility, and the predictability of outcome. Initial efforts at surgical vocal fold medialization, using an implantable substance such as thyroid cartilage or rib, were described by Isshiki.[52,53] Later, Koufman used silastic and he and others have verified the efficacy of this procedure.[37,54,55] Silastic medialization can be used with other procedures such as reinnervation or arytenoid adduction and may be done at the time of major skull base or pulmonary surgery where sacrifice of laryngeal nerves is expected and the significant sequelae of unilateral paralysis such as aspiration pneumonia especially need to be avoided.[54]

The results of silastic medialization are dependent on the position of the vocal fold at the time of treatment, the skill and experience of the surgeon, and the rapidity with which the implant can be placed. Large posterior glottic chinks are difficult to close satisfactorily with silastic medialization alone and may also require an arytenoid adduction procedure. Once the cartilaginous window is opened, the size and shape of the necessary implant should be determined with relative rapidity to prevent intraoperative edema from interfering with measurements. In the hands of experienced laryngologic surgeons, the results of silastic medialization are excellent and have been confirmed by both perceptual and objective assessments.[52,54] Return of normal or almost normal vocal fold vibration is expected in the majority of patients.[37] One of the drawbacks to silastic medialization is the required skill of the surgeon. Initial attempts should be performed in a controlled setting such as the cadaver laboratory or instruction hands-on courses. Extrusions have rarely been observed. Unsatisfactory outcomes are usually caused by improper size or placement (usually too superior) of the implant. Such limitations tend to be minor in experienced hands, which have resulted in silastic medialization becoming the workhorse of treatment for unilateral vocal fold paralysis at this time among laryngologists. Premade silastic and hydroxylapatite implants are now available.[56,57] Gore-Tex has also been used for medialization laryngoplasty.[58] For a more thorough discussion of this subject, see Chapter 37 by Zeitels.

Arytenoid Adduction

As mentioned above, it may, at times, be difficult to achieve satisfactory glottic closure by either injection or implantation techniques alone in patients with large posterior glottic gaps, particularly when associated with combined superior laryngeal nerve and recurrent laryngeal nerve paralyses. In such cases, arytenoid adduction has been advocated as the best technique for medialization. This procedure is accomplished by traditionally placing a permanent suture through or around the muscular process of the arytenoid cartilage and then suturing this to the thyroid cartilage anteriorly and somewhat laterally, thereby resulting in medial rotation of the vocal process of the arytenoid with posterior glottic closure. This simulates activity of the lateral cricoarytenoid muscle in a static manner. Arytenoid adduction may be used with other procedures such as reinnervation and is usually performed either simultaneously with, or after silastic medialization.[26,55,59] Arytenoid adduction is a difficult procedure and requires significant experience. Its role is now limited because of the success of other methods of medialization. It is an important adjunctive procedure where medialization has been unsuccessful with standard approaches because overlarge silastic implants or excessive Teflon used in an attempt to close large posterior gaps usually result in worse results and more complications. Some authors now advocate performing arytenoid adduction with all silastic medialization procedures rather than in selective cases (James Netterville, personal communication, 1998).

Arytenoidopexy has been introduced recently as an alternative to classical arytenoid adduction/rotation[60] and is described in Chapter 37 by Zeitels.

EVALUATION OF PATIENTS WITH BILATERAL VOCAL FOLD IMMOBILITY (BVFI)[61]

Presentation

Patients with BVFI present with airway-related complaints. They range from dyspnea and mild inspiratory stridor only with exertion to severe respiratory distress and biphasic stridor at rest. The severity of symptoms depends, of course, on the degree of obstruction, but also on the rapidity of the development of the obstruction. In fact, a patient may be surprisingly comfortable with a distressingly small airway if that airway compromise has developed slowly over years.

Depending on the etiology, dyspnea may develop rapidly, over weeks or months, or slowly, over years. Often, in the more chronic cases, patients will give a history of having been diagnosed with asthma and then treated for years for that condition. The "wheezing" they experienced was always stridor and they did not always respond to bronchodilators as expected. A flow volume loop demonstrating an extrathoracic obstruction, or bronchoscopy revealing the glottic narrowing, prompts a referral from the pulmonologist to the otolaryngologist.

Voice complaints rarely are the primary reason a patient with BVFI will seek medical attention. If the onset is slow and gradual, the voice is usually considered normal by the patient and other observers although more specific questioning will often reveal problems with vocal fatigue and some decrease in range and loudness.

Presentation and History Based on Etiology

Iatrogenic Trauma

BVFI caused by endotracheal (ET) intubation trauma is uncommon, but presents immediately or within hours after extubation. It is thought that during a difficult or overly rough intubation, anterior motion of the thyroid cartilage relative to the cricoid cartilage may compress the recurrent laryngeal nerves (RLNs) and cause BVFI. Another theory is that high endotracheal tube cuff pressure with the cuff placed at the infraglottis may compress the RLNs as they enter the larynx.[62-65] It is also possible that hyperextension of the neck can cause stretching of the vagus nerves and a resultant BVFI.[62] Unilateral arytenoid subluxation is an unusual occurrence, and bilateral is even more so. As of 1996, only two cases of bilateral arytenoid subluxation caused by intubation injury were in the literature.[66,67] Transient BVFI was reported after use of a laryngeal mask airway, although the mechanism was unclear.[68]

Surgery of the Neck and Chest

While unilateral vocal fold paralysis is not uncommon following many open procedures of the neck, the likelihood of simultaneous injury to both recurrent laryngeal or vagus nerves is small. This may occur during surgery of the thyroid gland, trachea, esophagus, or brain stem. In these cases, the patient will experience airway obstruction immediately or soon after extubation. Completion thyroidectomy or second contralateral carotid endarterectomy can cause BVFI if an earlier unilateral vocal fold paralysis has gone unrecognized. Laryngeal examination should always be done prior to these procedures. Again, if BVFI results from such surgery, the patient will be symptomatic soon after extubation.

Radiation Therapy

External beam radiation therapy for laryngeal malignancies induces an expected inflammatory response. As the tissues then recover, fibrosis may occur. The resultant scar may affect the soft tissue of the vocal folds or the cricoarytenoid joint(s) resulting in BVFI.[11,17,69] Airway obstruction and symptoms can present very late, eg, months or years after treatment. In such cases recurrent tumor must be ruled out. Chondronecrosis may also be responsible for these changes in laryngeal function and is more likely to occur if repeated biopsies to rule out recurrence are performed. The altered tissue may make surgical repair much more difficult as poor healing is the rule in these cases.

External Laryngeal Trauma

Blunt or penetrating trauma to the neck can cause immediate BVFI if both recurrent laryngeal nerves are injured. Bilateral arytenoid cartilage subluxation or dislocation may also occur from severe blunt trauma leading to BVFI, although only unilateral cases have been reported in the literature.[70] In these cases, the patient would present immediately with airway obstruction.

Arthritis of Cricoarytenoid Joint

Arthritis involving the cricoarytenoid joints may impair the motion of the arytenoid cartilages eventually resulting in BVFI. This has been estimated to occur in as many as 25% of patients with rheumatoid arthritis.[71] Onset is gradual and other signs of arthritis are usually evident elsewhere in the body. Other conditions that have been associated with cricoarytenoid arthritis include gout, Tietze's syndrome, ankylosing spondylitis, Reiter's syndrome, Crohn's disease, mumps, and collagen vascular disease.[71,72]

Two cases of BVFI caused by bilateral RLN paralysis in systemic lupus erythematosus (SLE) have been reported.[73,74] These patients had other signs of connective tissue disease and both responded to systemic steroids. Other cranial neuropathies have been reported in SLE.[75]

Neoplasms

The most common neoplasm of the larynx, squamous cell carcinoma, is unlikely to cause BVFI or posterior glottic stenosis (PGS) without first presenting with dysphonia and being obvious on examination.

Chondromas or chondrosarcomas of the larynx usually arise in the posterior lamina of the cricoid cartilage. In this location, one or both cricoarytenoid joints may be involved, leading to BVFI. Patients present with gradual onset of dysphonia and dyspnea.[76] Excision of the tumor via laryngofissure may result in restoration of the arytenoid mobility. The excision and reconstructive methods will depend on the exact size and location of the tumor.

Malignancies of the thyroid gland rarely cause unilateral vocal fold paralysis and even less commonly BVFI. Esophageal cancer is also unlikely to cause BVFI without first causing dysphagia severe enough to lead to a medical evaluation. A tracheal malignancy arising from the posterior wall could cause BVFI before the tumor itself obstructs the airway. In each of these situations, one vocal fold would most likely be paralyzed first, causing dysphonia, and one would hope lead to an evaluation that would reveal the tumor.

Arnold-Chiari Malformation, Meningomyelocele

Congenital causes of BVFI include Arnold-Chiari malformation and meningomyelocele and other causes of hydrocephalus that may cause herniation of the brain stem and compression of the vagus nerves. This possibility must always be evaluated in young children noted to have BVFI.[77]

Diabetes Mellitus

While the peripheral neuropathy of diabetes mellitus is more likely to affect the upper cranial nerves, it may also affect the vagus or recurrent laryngeal nerves resulting in BVFI. The onset of dysphonia and stridor is slow and gradual. Evidence of other neuropathies may not be present.[78]

Insecticide Poisoning

Three types of organophosphate toxicity syndromes have been described: acute (instantaneous), intermediate (hours to days), and delayed (weeks to months). Thompson and Stocks described the case of a 2-year-old boy who developed BVFI shortly after ingesting a substance contaminated with the insecticide. The problem resolved after 2 days of ventilatory support.[79] An acute cholinergic crisis is followed by a respiratory paresis, cranial nerve paresis, and decreased deep tendon reflexes. Recognition of the cause is crucial to appropriate care.

Amyotrophic Lateral Sclerosis (ALS)

ALS is a degenerative disease that eventually involves both upper and lower motor neurons, although a patient may present first with signs of one or the other or both. As the lower motor neurons become more affected, the vocal folds gradually weaken and drift to the midline, causing airway compromise. The upper motor neuron lesion may also cause hyperreflexia and laryngospasm with stridor.[80] Considering the progressive and eventually fatal course of ALS, treatment of the airway obstruction is medical, in the case of laryngospasm, and tracheotomy for BVFI. In the author's experience, however, most patients succumb before needing tracheotomy.

Closed Head Injury, Cerebrovascular Accident

Closed head injuries and strokes can cause a variety of upper and lower motor neuron injuries. To affect both vagus nerves, the injury must involve the medulla, which is often incompatible with life. BVFI has been noted after these events.[81] As mentation and articulation are often also affected, it may not initially be apparent that there is laryngeal dysfunction.

Myasthenia Gravis

Myasthenia gravis is an autoimmune disease in which antibodies attack the acetylcholine receptors on motor endplates of muscle fibers. This usually first manifests itself with bulbar involvement and affects both pharyngeal and laryngeal function, more commonly bilaterally than unilaterally. There is fatigue with use. Diagnosis is made by observing an improvement in function with the edrophonium (Tensilon) test or with neostigmine, which allows more time.[82-84]

Other Neurologic Disorders

BVFI has been described in at least one patient with postpolio syndrome.[85] In this study of nine patients, two had unilateral vocal fold immobility, but abnormal EMG activity bilaterally. One had previously undergone tracheotomy for BVFI, which apparently had improved. This suggests that these patients may have fluctuation in their laryngeal activity and those with prior bulbar polio are at risk for development of BVFI.

Charcot-Marie-Tooth disease has also presented with BVFI along with deafness, diaphragmatic weakness, and cerebellopontine weakness.[86] Leigh disease, an uncommon neurodegenerative disorder also known as subacute necrotizing encephalomyopathy, causes BVFI as well as ophthalmoplegia, nystagmus, ataxia, hypotonia spasticity, and other neurologic deficits.[87]

A family history of BVFI suggests that the patient may have an autosomal dominant hereditary motor and sensory neuropathy. The severity of the laryngeal paralysis and the other manifestations of the disease vary considerably, even within one affected family.[88,89]

Radiologic Evaluation

The history will direct the workup. If there is no apparent cause, CT scanning of the neck including the skull base and thoracic inlet is indicated as described above for unilateral vocal fold immobility. If a central neurologic disorder is suspected, an MRI may be more appropriate than a CT.

Pulmonary Function Tests

Abnormal pulmonary function test results, specifically an abnormal flow-volume loop, often prompt a referral from the internist or pulmonologist to the otolaryngologist. While the area of obstruction is visible to the otolaryngologist and the diagnosis is obvious, pulmonary function tests are helpful in documenting the severity of the obstruction and the improvement after treatment.

TREATMENT FOR BILATERAL VOCAL FOLD PARALYSIS

Bilateral vocal fold paralysis results in respiratory obstruction in most patients. Although occasional patients with gradual onset of paralysis or those with a paramedian position of the vocal folds may have an adequate airway for respiration, it is only the rare individual who does not have activity restriction. Furthermore, a simple viral illness may result in edema that may convert an adequate to a compromised airway. Bilateral vocal fold paralyses, therefore, almost always require intervention although there are many patients who will delay treatment until they get into trouble or succumb from their underlying disease. Patients frequently have a tracheotomy early in the course of their disease and most patients will have a tracheotomy at some time during their treatment, although some surgeons perform the definitive airway expanding procedure without doing a tracheotomy. Most surgeons, however, prefer to first secure the airway with tracheotomy and then consider treatment options to improve breathing and allow for decannulation. One of the difficulties with treating bilateral vocal fold paralysis is that the better the airway, the worse the voice and the greater the risk for aspiration. Thorough preoperative counseling is advisable to prevent unrealistic expectations on the part of the patient. It may be necessary to perform conservative surgery initially so that over-eager vocal fold lateralization does not result in significant dysphonia. The patient needs to be cautioned that more than one operation may be necessary to allow both decannulation and quality voice production.

Medical Treatment

Treatment of inflammatory conditions may or may not improve the mobility of the vocal folds.[73,74,90] Therapy will, however, create a more favorable environment for healing with less scarring after surgical repair has been performed. This treatment should be instituted before the surgery takes place.

Systemic steroids will reduce mucosal edema, which can improve the airway short-term, but are unlikely to provide a definitive solution, unless the etiology is a connective tissue disorder. If that is the case, long-term steroids may be the treatment of choice and at least one month of steroids should be used: Start with one week of prednisone 1 mg/kg/day and then taper; reassess at the end of the month for a beneficial effect.

Indications for Surgical Intervention

The goal of surgery is to improve the posterior glottic airway. Surgical procedures can be categorized as: dynamic, in which the normal mobility of the vocal folds is restored; static conservative, in which the airway is enlarged without irreversibly destroying tissue; and static destructive, in which normal tissue is removed to improve the airway in a static manner. While the first two methods are preferable, it is the last category that most consistently yields adequate airway results, but may adversely affect voice and swallowing. Tracheotomy bypasses the problem entirely.

Not all stenotic airways should be treated surgically. Some patients are only mildly symptomatic. Some are dyspneic only with strenuous exertion. Some are too ill to tolerate surgery or do not have the pulmonary reserve to tolerate any aspiration, which may occur postoperatively. The advantages and potential complications of each procedure must be discussed thoroughly with the patient preoperatively. With several surgical techniques the voice result is very unpredictable, as is the effect on swallowing. While we consider the need for tracheotomy to be a failure in these situations, there are those patients who would rather keep a tracheotomy than risk any change in voice or dysphagia. The patient must always be advised that keeping or undergoing a tracheotomy is a viable option.

History

Tracheotomy is the oldest surgical treatment of BVFI or PGS. In 1922, Chevalier Jackson removed the entire vocal fold and ventricle which, while it provided an excellent airway, caused severely breathy dysphonia and aspiration.[91] The King procedure is an open operation in which a mobilized arytenoid is fixed laterally.[92] Kelly and Woodman provided further modifications of King's procedure.[93,94]

Thornell described the first endoscopic arytenoidectomy in 1948.[95] Whicker and Devine reported an initial success rate of 82% in a series of 147 patients treated with Thornell's technique, which improved to 92% when some of the failures underwent a contralateral procedure. They reported a 96% voice preservation rate,[96] although this does not imply a completely normal voice.

Endoscopic Surgery

There are various endoscopic techniques for enlarging the posterior glottic airway in a static manner. These procedures involve excision of tissue at or anterior to the arytenoid so as to gain as much cross-sectional area as possible without disturbing the majority of the membranous vocal folds, which are crucial for voice production.

Ossoff et al described the classic CO_2 laser arytenoidectomy and partial cordectomy in 1983.[97] This procedure involves vaporization of the mucosa overlying the arytenoid cartilage, the cartilage itself, and a portion of the posterior aspect of the membranous vocal fold. The defect must be flush with the inner aspect of the cricoid cartilage. At least the anterior half of the membranous vocal fold remains intact to make contact with the unoperated side. At the end of the procedure, the defect is quite large. Initially the voice is breathy and the patient may aspirate liquids. As the wound heals, however, the defect contracts considerably and the voice and swallowing improve. The airway decreases in area, but in most cases remains adequate for decannulation or relief of symptoms. In 1990, Ossoff et al reported an 86% rate of decannulation in a series of 28 patients.[98]

There have been many modifications of the technique described above. Remacle et al preserve a shell of the posterior aspect of the arytenoid cartilage. They feel that this stabilizes the posterior aspect of the airway, preventing prolapse of the mucosa into the glottic gap. They report excellent airway results in 40 of 41 patients with only one posterior synechia and 2 granulomas, which resolved spontaneously. A good or normal voice resulted in 39 of the 41 patients.[69]

Others, including the author, have modified Ossoff's technique by preserving the mucosa along the medial aspect of the arytenoid cartilage.[99] (L. Arick Forrest, MD, personal communication, 1995.) This may be sutured laterally after resection of the arytenoid cartilage and a portion of the posterior vocalis muscle and vocal ligament is complete. The final airway result also seems more predictable with this submucosal technique. Some investigators have resected varying portions of the arytenoid cartilage while preserving the mucosa and suturing it laterally.[100,101]

Dennis and Kashima utilize a more conservative procedure for enlarging the posterior airway. A C-shaped portion of the membranous vocal fold is removed with the CO_2 laser just anterior to the vocal process without exposing cartilage. This can be done unilaterally, bilaterally, or in a stepwise manner as need dictates.[102] Eckel et al compared Kashima's technique with Ossoff's and found that both procedures were equally effective at achieving an adequate airway and both affected voice to an unpredictable degree. Partial cordectomy was faster and easier to perform and arytenoidectomy was more likely to cause subclinical aspiration as seen on flexible endoscopic evaluation of swallow (FEES).[103]

Suture lateralization of one immobile vocal fold in BVFI was described by Ejnell as an alternative to tracheotomy in cases where the prognosis is favorable for recovery of activity of at least one vocal fold or as a long-term solution. He and other authors have reported results comparable to those described above.[104-107] The procedure is quite easy to perform. While one surgeon observes the larynx via direct laryngoscopy, a second surgeon passes a 16-gauge needle through the thyroid cartilage aiming for just superior to the vocal process of the arytenoid cartilage and an O nylon suture is passed through the needle. The needle is then passed just inferior to the vocal process and the suture threaded by the endoscopist out the needle, taking care not to sever the suture on the needle. The suture is tied tightly enough to achieve the desired airway with the arytenoid rotated to a paramedian position. Voice is minimally affected if the vocal fold is not lateralized too far.[104-107] A lateral position results in a very breathy voice and re-operation with loosening of the suture may be required. No complications are reported. The procedure is reversible should the activity of either vocal fold return.

Suture lateralization has also been combined with standard arytenoidectomy and partial cordectomy procedures.[108] Lichtenberger designed an endo-extralaryngeal needle carrier to facilitate this procedure.

Variations on endoscopic approaches to BVFI are numerous. Linder and Lindholm create a groove along the lateral superior aspect of the true vocal fold, including the vocal process with the CO_2 laser. Fibrin glue is injected into the groove to hold the medial aspect of the fold laterally. They report a success rate of 5/9 after one procedure and 8/9 after several. Patients who required bilateral procedures had "breathy but still intelligible voices."[109]

Rontal and Rontal describe a precise lysis of the interarytenoid and thyroarytenoid attachments to the arytenoid cartilage, as well as removal of the vocal process to allow the arytenoid cartilage to move laterally, thereby improving the airway in 8 patients with BVFI. They report 100% success regarding airway and excellent postoperative voices.[110]

Open Surgery

The posterior glottis may be approached via anterior laryngofissure. This provides excellent exposure from the inferior aspect of the cricoid ring to the superior aspect of the arytenoid cartilages. The anterior thyroid cartilage must be divided exactly in the midline at the anterior commissure to avoid disruption of the anterior vocal folds.

Arytenoidectomy may be done via an external approach, either anterior laryngofissure or a lateral approach, with resection of the posterior aspect of the thyroid cartilage and elevation of the pyriform sinus mucosa to gain access to the arytenoid cartilage.

Reinnervation

For BVFI caused by paralysis of both recurrent laryngeal or vagus nerves, reinnervation of one or both posterior cricoarytenoid (PCA) muscles would be the

ideal solution to open the posterior glottis. This would restore laryngeal function with glottic opening on inspiration, without destroying intrinsic laryngeal structures. For the technique to be successful, at least one arytenoid must be passively mobile.

Reinnervation for BVFI was first described by Tucker in 1976 when he mobilized a branch of the ansa hypoglossi and a small block of muscle from the anterior belly of the omohyoid and sutured it to the PCA. His first series of five patients was initially 100% successful and in 1989 he reported a 74% success rate in 214 patients with BVFI with a minimum of 2-year follow-up.[111,112] Baldissera et al and Doyle et al reported success in the cat model when using phrenic nerve. Baldissera's group performed two anastamoses involving the phrenic nerve and RLNs to reinnervate both PCA muscles. Reinnervation with restoration of motion was successful in 6/6 cats unilaterally and 5/6 contralaterally.[113] Doyle et al transplanted the phrenic nerve directly into the PCA of cats and achieved inspiratory abduction of the paralyzed vocal fold in 9/12 subjects.[114] Crumley first transferred the phrenic nerve to the omohyoid muscle in 3 monkeys and then transferred the muscle to denervated PCA muscles achieving success in all 3 animals. This study demonstrated the possibility of replacing the PCA if necessary.[115]

Maniglia has investigated reinnervation of the posterior cricoarytenoid muscle with the motor branch of the superior laryngeal nerve and reported good results in an animal model.[116] These procedures are attractive in that they do not prevent other treatments and may be reasonable first-line approaches in infants and small children.

Laryngeal Pacing

Laryngeal electrical pacing involves implanting a pacing device similar to a cardiac pacemaker with the electrode inserted in or laid on the PCA muscle. The device triggers with inspiration. One arytenoid must be passively mobile, as with laryngeal reinnervation procedures. The first report of electrical pacing in the human larynx was by Zealear et al in 1996.[117] This patient has also received injections of botulinum toxin A to the thyroarytenoid muscles to improve the airway and has been successful (Mark Courey, MD, personal communication, June 1999).

Botulinum Toxin A

Cohen and Thompson injected botulinum toxin A (Botox) into the cricothyroid muscles of dogs in whom the recurrent laryngeal nerves had been sectioned.[118] They noted that the vocal folds lateralized after injection with an improved airway and this effect lasted the expected time based on the different doses given.

SUMMARY

The treatment of vocal fold paralysis relies on satisfactory history and voice evaluation, determination of etiology of paralysis, and assessment of compensation and expected recovery. Many patients with unilateral vocal fold paralysis will accommodate satisfactorily for their own voice needs either independently or more usually with the aid of an experienced voice pathologist. In those patients where compensation is not sufficient, interventional treatment is necessary. Bilateral vocal fold paralysis presents different problems and requires different solutions.

The type of treatment should be based on the patient's needs, the experience of the physician, and the cost and ease of the procedure. As this is a rapidly evolving area, the clinician should be aware of the advantages and disadvantages of new techniques as they develop. He or she should be experienced in more than one technique as different situations may require different approaches. Finally, the clinician should evaluate the pre- and postoperative voice and airway results of the procedures used so that he/she can modify approaches based on personal experience and the developments within the field.

REFERENCES

1. Koufman JA. Laryngeal electromyography (EMG): clinical applications. *Vis Voice.* 1993;2:49-53.

2. Levine H, Tucker H. *Surgical Management of the Paralyzed Larynx.* Philadelphia, PA: Saunders; 1975.

3. Hollingshead W. *Anatomy for Surgeons.* 3rd ed. Philadelphia, PA: Harper and Row; 1982.

4. Bevan K, Griffiths M, Morgan M. Cricothyroid muscle paralysis: its recognition and diagnosis. *J Laryngol Otol.* 1989;103:191-195.

5. Woodson GE. Laryngeal neurophysiology and its clinical uses. (Review; 60 refs). *Head Neck.* 1996;18:78-86.

6. Abelson T, Tucker H. Laryngeal findings in superior laryngeal nerve paralysis: a controversy. *Otolaryngol Head Neck Surg.* 1981;89:463-470.

7. Hirano M. Surgical anatomy and physiology of the vocal folds. In: Gould W, Sataloff R, Spiegel J, eds. *Voice Surgery.* St. Louis, MO: Mosby Inc; 1993: 135-158.

8. Liancai M, Sanders I, Wu B, et al. The intramuscular innervation of the human interarytenoid muscle. *Laryngoscope.* 1994;104:33-38.

9. Sercarz J, Berke G, Gerratt B, et al. Videostroboscopy of human vocal fold paralysis. *Ann Otol Rhinol Laryngol.* 1992;101:567-576.

10. Koufman JA, Walker FO, Joharji GM. The cricothyroid muscle does not influence vocal fold position in laryngeal paralysis. *Laryngoscope.* 1995;105: 368-372.

11. Pressman, K. (rev. by Kirchner J). *Physiology of the Larynx.* Washington, DC: AAO-HNS Foundation; 1986.

12. Gardner GM, Shaari CM, Parnes SM. Long-term morbidity and mortality in patients undergoing surgery for unilateral vocal cord paralysis. *Laryngoscope.* 1992;102:501-508.

13. Maisel R, Ogura J. Evaluation and treatment of vocal cord paralysis. *Laryngoscope.* 1974;84:302-316.

14. Tucker H. Vocal cord paralysis—1979: etiology and management. *Laryngoscope.* 1979;90:585-590.

15. Parnell F, Brandenburg J. Vocal cord paralysis. A review of 100 cases. *Laryngoscope.* 1970;80: 1036-1045.

16. Barondess J, Pompei P, Schley W. A study of vocal cord palsy. *Trans Am Clin Climatol Assoc.* 1985;97:141-148.

17. Benninger MS, Gillen JB, Altman JS. Changing etiology of vocal fold immobility. (Review; 15 refs). *Laryngoscope.* 1998;108:1346-1350.

18. Weisberg NK, Spengler DM, Netterville JL. Stretch-induced nerve injury as a cause of paralysis secondary to the anterior cervical approach. *Otolaryngol Head Neck Surg.* 1997;116:317-326.

19. Nakahira M, Saito H, Miyagi T. Left vocal cord paralysis as a primary manifestation of invasive pulmonary aspergillosis in a nonimmunocompromised host. (Review; 6 refs). *Arch Otolaryngol Head Neck Surg.* 1999;125:691-693.

20. Thirlwall AS. Ortner's syndrome: a centenary review of unilateral recurrent laryngeal nerve palsy secondary to cardiothoracic disease. *J Laryngol Otol.* 1997;111:869-871.

21. Altman JS, Benninger MS. The evaluation of unilateral vocal fold immobility: is chest X-ray enough? *J Voice.* 1997;11:364-367.

22. Sataloff RT. Arytenoid dislocation: techniques of surgical reduction. *Op Tech Otolaryngol Head Neck Surg.* 1998;9:196-202.

23. Laursen RJ, Larsen KM, Molgaard J, Kolze V. Unilateral vocal cord paralysis following endotracheal intubation. *Acta Anaesthesiol Scand.* 1998;42:131-132.

24. Jacobson B, Johnson A, Grywalski C, et al. The Voice Handicap Index (VHI): development and validation. *J Speech Lang Pathol.* 1997;6:66-70.

25. Benninger MS, Ahuja AS, Gardner G, Grywalski C. Assessing outcomes for dysphonic patients. *J Voice.* 1998;12:540-550.

26. Netterville JL, Stone RE, Luken ES, Civantos FJ, Ossoff RH. Silastic medialization and arytenoid adduction: the Vanderbilt experience. A review of 116 phonosurgical procedures. *Ann Otol Rhinol Laryngol.* 1993;102:413-424.

27. Heuer R, Sataloff R, Emerich K, et al. Unilateral recurrent laryngeal nerve paralysis: the importance of "preoperative" voice therapy. *J Voice.* 1997;11:88-94.

28. Havas T, Lowinger D, Priestley J. Unilateral vocal fold paralysis: causes, options and outcomes. *Aust N Z J Surg.* 1999;69:509-513.

29. Ramadan HH, Wax MK, Avery S. Outcome and changing cause of unilateral vocal cord paralysis. *Otolaryngol Head Neck Surg.* 1998;118:199-202.

30. Benninger MS. Acyclovir for the treatment of idiopathic vocal cord paralysis. *Ear Nose Throat.* 1992;71:207-208.

31. Dedo H. Injection and removal of Teflon for unilateral vocal cord paralysis. *Ann Otol Rhinol Laryngol.* 1992;101:81-85.

32. Strasnick B, Berke G, Ward P. Transcutaneous Teflon injection for unilateral vocal cord paralysis. *Laryngoscope.* 1991;101:785-787.

33. Livesey JR, Carding PN. An analysis of vocal cord paralysis before and after Teflon injection using combined glottography. *Clin Otolaryngol Allied Sci.* 1995;20:423-427.

34. Harries ML, Morrison M. Management of unilateral vocal cord paralysis by injection medialization with teflon paste. Quantitative results. *Ann Otol Rhinol Laryngol.* 1998;107:332-336.

35. Dedo H, Carlsoo B. Histologic evaluation of teflon granulomas of human vocal cords. *Acta Otolaryngol.* 1982;93:475-484.

36. Lewy R. Responses of laryngeal tissue to granular teflon in situ. *Arch Otolaryngol Head Neck Surg.* 1966;83:355-359.

37. Gardner GM, Parnes SM. Status of the mucosal wave post vocal cord injection versus thyroplasty. *J Voice.* 1991;5:64-73.

38. Netterville JL, Coleman JR Jr, Chang S, Rainey CL, Reinisch L, Ossoff, RH. Lateral laryngotomy for the removal of Teflon granuloma. *Ann Otol Rhinol Laryngol.* 1998;107:735-744.

39. Mikaelian D, Lowry L, Sataloff R. Lipoinjection for unilateral vocal fold paralysis. *Laryngoscope.* 1991;101:465-468.

40. Brandenburg J, Kirkham W, Koshkee D. Vocal cord augmentation with autogenous fat. *Laryngoscope.* 1992;102:495-500.

41. Saccogna PW, Werning JW, Setrakian S, Strauss M. Lipoinjection in the paralyzed feline vocal fold: study of graft survival. *Otolaryngol Head Neck Surg.* 1997;117:465-470.

42. Wexler D, Gray S, Jiang J, et al. Phonosurgical studies: fat-graft reconstruction of injured canine vocal cords. *Ann Otol Rhinol Laryngol.* 1989;98:668-673.

43. Archer SM, Banks ER. Intracordal injection of autologous fat for augmentation of the mucosally damaged canine vocal fold: a long-term histological study. Paper presented at: The Second World Congress on Laryngeal Cancer. Sydney, Australia; 1994.

44. Laccourreye O, Crevier-Buchman L, Pimpec-Barthes F, Garcia D, Riquet M, Brasnu D. Recovery of function after intracordal autologous fat injection for unilateral recurrent laryngeal nerve paralysis. *J Laryngol Otol.* 1998;112:1082-1084.

45. Bless D, Ford C, Loftus J. Role of injectable collagen in the treatment of glottic insufficiency: a study of 199 patients. *Ann Otol Rhinol Laryngol.* 1992;101:237-246.

46. Rihkanen H. Vocal fold augmentation by injection of autologous fascia. *Laryngoscope.* 1998;108:51-54.

47. Green D, Ward P. The management of the divided recurrent laryngeal nerve. *Laryngoscope.* 1977;100:779-794.

48. Chhetri DK, Gerratt BR, Kreiman J, Berke GS. Combined arytenoid adduction and laryngeal reinnervation in the treatment of vocal fold paralysis. *Laryngoscope.* 1999;109:1928-1936.

49. Tucker HM. Reinnervation of the unilaterally paralyzed larynx. *Ann Otol Rhinol Laryngol.* 1977;86:789-794.

50. Crumley R. Update: ansa cervicalis to recurrent laryngeal nerve anastomosis for unilateral laryngeal paralysis. *Laryngoscope.* 1991;101:384-387.

51. Sercarz JA, Nguyen L, Nasri S, Graves MC, Wenokur R, Berke GS. Physiologic motion after laryngeal nerve reinnervation: a new method. *Otolaryngol Head Neck Surg.* 1997;116:466-474.

52. Isshiki N, Morita H, Okamura H, et al. Thyroplasty as a new phonosurgical technique. *Acta Otolaryngol.* 1974;78:451-456.

53. Isshiki N. Recent advances in phonosurgery. *Folia Phoniatr (Basel).* 1980;32:119-124.

54. Koufman JA. Laryngoplasty for vocal cord medialization: an alternative to Teflon. *Laryngoscope.* 1986;96:726-731.

55. Slavitt D, Maragos N. Physiologic assessment of arytenoid adduction. *Ann Otol Rhinol Laryngol.* 1992;101:321-326.

56. Montgomery WW, Montgomery SK. Montgomery thyroplasty implant system. *Ann Otol Rhinol Laryngol (Suppl).* 1997:170:1-16.

57. Cummings C, Purcell L, Flint P. Hydroxylapatite laryngeal implants for medialization: preliminary report. *Laryngoscope.* 1993;102:843-851.

58. McCulloch TM, Hoffman HT. Medialization laryngoplasty with expanded polytetrafluoroethylene. Surgical technique and preliminary results. *Ann Otol Rhinol Laryngol.* 1998;107:427-432.

59. Kraus DH, Orlikoff RF, Rizk SS, Rosenberg DB. Arytenoid adduction as an adjunct to type I thyroplasty for unilateral vocal cord paralysis. *Head Neck.* 1999;21:52-59.

60. Zeitels SM, Hochman I, Hillman RE. Adduction arytenopexy: a new procedure for paralytic dysphonia with implications for implant medialization. (Review; 110 refs). *Ann Otol Rhinol Laryngol (Suppl).* 1998;173:2-24.

61. Gardner G. Posterior glottic stenosis and bilateral vocal fold immobility. *Otolaryngol Clin North Am.* 2000;33:855-877.

62. Cavo J Jr. True vocal cord paralysis following intubation. *Laryngoscope.* 1985;95:1352-1359.

63. Holley H, Gildea J. Vocal cord paralysis after tracheal intubation. *JAMA.* 1971;215:281-284.

64. Minuck M. Unilateral vocal cord paralysis following endotracheal intubation. *Anesthesiology.* 1976;45:448-449.

65. Nuutinen J, Karaja J. Bilateral vocal cord paralysis following general anaesthesia. *Laryngoscope.* 1981;91:83-86.

66. Talmi YP, Wolf M, Bar-Ziv J, Nusem-Horowitz S, Kronenberg J. Postintubation arytenoid subluxation. *Ann Otol Rhinol Laryngol.* 1996;105:384-390.

67. Chatterji S, Gupta N, Mishra T. Valvular glottic obstruction following extubation. *Anesthesia.* 1984;39:246-247.

68. Inomata S, Nishikawa T, Suga A, Yamashita S. Transient bilateral vocal cord paralysis after insertion of a laryngeal mask airway. *Anesthesiology.* 1995;82:787-788.

69. Remacle M, Lawson G, Mayne A, Jamart J. Subtotal carbon dioxide laser arytenoidectomy by endoscopic approach for treatment of bilateral cord immobility in adduction. *Ann Otol Rhinol Laryngol.* 1996;105:438-445.

70. Stack B, Ridley M. Arytenoid subluxation from blunt laryngeal trauma. *Am J Otolaryngol.* 1994;15:68-73.

71. Miller F, Wanamaker J, Hicks D, et al. Cricoarytenoid arthritis and ankylosing spondylitis. *Arch Otolaryngol Head Neck Surg.* 1994;120:214-216.

72. Hussain M. Relapsing polychondritis presenting with stridor from bilateral vocal cord palsy. *J Laryngol Otol.* 1991;105:961-964.

73. Saluja S, Singh RR, Misra AK, et al. Bilateral recurrent laryngeal nerve palsy in systemic lupus erythematosus. *Clin Exp Rheumatol.* 1989;7:81-83.

74. Teitel A, MacKenzie C, Stern R, et al. Laryngeal involvement in systemic lupus erythematosus. *Semin Arthritis Rheum.* 1992;22:203-214.

75. Zvaifler N. Neurologic manifestations. In: Schur P, ed. *The Clinical Management of Systemic Lupus Erythematosus.* New York, NY: Grune & Stratton; 1983:167-188.

76. Lewis J, Olsen K, Inwards C. Cartilaginous tumors of the larynx: clinicopathologic review of 47 cases. *Ann Otol Rhinol Laryngol.* 1997;106:94-100.

77. Holinger L, Holinger P, Holinger P. Etiology of bilateral abductor vocal cord paralysis. *Ann Otol Rhinol Laryngol.* 1976;85:428-436.

78. Sommer D, Freeman J. Bilateral vocal cord paralysis associated with diabetes mellitus: case reports. *J Otolaryngol.* 1994;23:169-171.

79. Thompson JW, Stocks RM. Brief bilateral vocal cord paralysis after insecticide poisoning. A new variant of toxicity syndrome [Comments]. *Arch Otolaryngol Head Neck Surg.* 1997;123:93-96.

80. Newman DS, Gardner GM, Jacobson B. *Management of laryngospasm in amyotrophic lateral sclerosis.* Paper presented at: 9th Annual Symposium on ALS/MND; 1998.

81. Aronson A. Laryngeal-phonatory dysfunction in closed-head injury. *Brain Inj.* 1994;8:663-665.

82. Griffiths C, Bough D. Neurologic diseases and their effect on voice. *J Voice.* 1989;3:148-156.

83. Job A, Raman M, Gnanmuthu C. Laryngeal stridor in myasthenia gravis. *J Laryngol Otol.* 1992;106: 633-634.

84. Tyler H. Neurologic disorders. In: Fried M, ed. *The Larynx: A Multidisciplinary Approach.* Boston, MA: Little, Brown; 1988:173-178.

85. Driscoll BP, Gracco C, Coelho C, et al. Laryngeal function in post-polio patients. *Laryngoscope.* 1995;105:35-41.

86. Fukuda H, Kitani M, Imaoka K. A case of hereditary motor and sensory neuropathy with vocal cords palsy and diaphragmatic weakness. *Rinsho Shinkeigaku.* 1993;33:175-181.

87. Lin YC, Lee WT, Wang PJ, Shen YZ. Vocal cord paralysis and hypoventilation in a patient with suspected Leigh disease. *Pediatr Neurol.* 1999;20:223-225.

88. Donaghy M, Kennett R. Varying occurrence of vocal cord paralysis in a family with autosomal dominant hereditary motor and sensory neuropathy. *J Neurol.* 1999;246:552-555.

89. Manaligod JM, Smith RJ. Familial laryngeal paralysis. *Am J Med Genet.* 1998;77:277-280.

90. Smith G, Ward P, Berci G. Laryngeal involvement by systemic lupus erythematosus. *Trans Am Acad Ophthalmol Otol.* 1977;84:124-128.

91. Jackson C. Ventriculocordectomy: a new operation for the cure of goitrous glottic stenosis. *Arch Surg.* 1922;4:257-274.

92. King B. A new and function restoring operation for bilateral abductor cord paralysis. *JAMA.* 1939; 112:814-823.

93. Woodman D. A modification of the extralaryngeal approach to arytenoidectomy for bilateral abductor paralysis. *Arch Otolaryngol.* 1946;43:63-71.

94. Kelly J. Surgical treatment of bilateral paralysis of the abductor muscles. *Arch Otolaryngol Head Neck Surg.* 1941;33:293-304.

95. Thornell W. Intralaryngeal approach for arytenoidectomy in bilateral abductor vocal cord paralysis. *Arch Otolaryngol Head Neck Surg.* 1948;47:505-508.

96. Whicker J, Devine K. Long-term results of Thornell arytenoidectomy in bilateral vocal cord paralysis. *Laryngoscope.* 1972;82:1331-1336.

97. Ossoff RH, Karlan MS, Sisson GA. Endoscopic laser arytenoidectomy. *Lasers Surg Med.* 1983; 2:293-299.

98. Ossoff RH, Duncavage JA, Shapshay SM, Krespi YP, Sisson GA Sr. Endoscopic laser arytenoidectomy revisited. *Ann Otol Rhinol Laryngol.* 1990; 99:764-771.

99. el Chazly M, Rifai M, el Ezz AA. Arytenoidectomy and posterior cordectomy for bilateral abductor paralysis. *J Laryngol Otol.* 1991;105:454-455.

100. Benninger M, Bhattacharya N, Fried M. Surgical management for bilateral vocal fold immobility. *Op Tech Otolaryngol Head Neck Surg.* 1998;9:1-8.

101. Rontal M, Rontal E. Endoscopic laryngeal surgery for bilateral midline vocal cord obstruction. *Ann Otol Rhinol Laryngol.* 1990;99:605-610.

102. Dennis DP, Kashima H. Carbon dioxide laser posterior cordectomy for treatment of bilateral vocal cord paralysis. *Ann Otol Rhinol Laryngol.* 1989; 98:930-934.

103. Eckel HE, Thumfart M, Wassermann K, Vossing M, Thumfart WF. Cordectomy versus arytenoidectomy in the management of bilateral vocal cord paralysis [published erratum appears in *Ann Otol Rhinol Laryngol.* 1995;104(2):119]. *Ann Otol Rhinol Laryngol.* 1994;103:852-857.

104. Ejnell H, Tisell LE. Acute temporary laterofixation for treatment of bilateral vocal cord paralyses after surgery for advanced thyroid carcinoma. *World J Surg.* 1993;17:277-281.

105. Geterud A, Ejnell H, Stenborg R, Bake B. Long-term results with a simple surgical treatment of bilateral vocal cord paralysis. *Laryngoscope.* 1990;100:1005-1008.

106. Hawthorne MR, Nunez DA. Bilateral vocal cord palsy: the alternative to tracheostomy. *J Otolaryngol.* 1992;21:364-365.

107. Moustafa H, el Guindy A, el Sherief S, Targam A. The role of endoscopic laterofixation of the vocal cord in the treatment of bilateral abductor paralysis. *J Laryngol Otol.* 1992;106:31-34.

108. Lichtenberger G, Toohill RJ. Technique of endo-extralaryngeal suture lateralization for bilateral abductor vocal cord paralysis. *Laryngoscope.* 1997;107:1281-1283.

109. Linder A, Lindholm CE. Vocal fold lateralization using carbon dioxide laser and fibrin glue. *J Laryngol Otol.* 1992;106:226-230.

110. Rontal M, Rontal E. Use of laryngeal muscular tenotomy for bilateral midline vocal cord fixation. *Ann Otol Rhinol Laryngol.* 1994;103:583-589.

111. Tucker HM. Human laryngeal reinnervation: long-term experience with the nerve-muscle pedicle technique. *Laryngoscope.* 1978;88:598-604.

112. Tucker HM. Long-term results of nerve-muscle pedicle reinnervation for laryngeal paralysis. *Ann Otol Rhinol Laryngol.* 1989;98:674-676.

113. Baldissera F, Cantarella G, Marini G, et al. Recovery of inspiratory abduction of the paralyzed vocal cords after bilateral reinnervation of the cricoarytenoid muscles by one single branch of the phrenic nerve. *Laryngoscope.* 1989;99:1286-1292.

114. O'Grady KF, Irish JC, Doyle DJ, Gullane P, Butany J. Effects of medialization laryngoplasty on airway resistance: a pilot study. *Laryngoscope.* 1999;109:419-424.

115. Crumley R. Muscle transfer for laryngeal paralysis: restoration of inspiratory vocal cord abduction by phrenic-omohyoid transfer. *Arch Otolaryngol Head Neck Surg.* 1991;117:1113-1117.

116. Maniglia A, Dodds B, Sorenson K, et al. Newer techniques of laryngeal reinnervation: superior laryngeal nerve (motor branch) as a driver of the posterior cricoarytenoid muscle. *Ann Otol Rhinol Laryngol.* 1989;98:907-909.

117. Zealear DL, Rainey CL, Herzon GD, Netterville JL, Ossoff RH. Electrical pacing of the paralyzed human larynx. *Ann Otol Rhinol Laryngol.* 1996;105:689-693.

118. Cohen S, Thompson J. Use of botulinum toxin to lateralize true vocal cords: a biomedical method to relieve bilateral abductor vocal cord paralysis. *Ann Otol Rhinol Laryngol.* 1987;96:534-541.

CHAPTER 28

Management of the Spasmodic Dysphonias

Christy L. Ludlow, PhD, CCC-Speech

Eric A. Mann, MD, PhD

CHARACTERISTICS OF FOCAL DYSTONIAS

The spasmodic dysphonias (SDs) are currently understood to be focal dystonias affecting only the laryngeal muscles during speech.[1-3] Other focal dystonias include torticollis, blepharospasm, oral mandibular dystonia, and writer's cramp.[4-9] Each is a chronic, adult-onset, motor control disorder with abnormal levels of muscle tone. These abnormal contractions can occur at any time that the patient is awake (eg, torticollis[10]), can be exacerbated by other movements involving the cranial musculature (eg, speaking can increase blepharospasm[7,11]), and may occur only during performance of a particular task (eg, writer's cramp[9]). In each form, certain muscles are affected, which become exacerbated or triggered during volitional movement. In some forms, long periods of hyperactivity can be observed in a muscle while the patient is at rest.[4,12]

Focal dystonias are those involving abnormal activity in only a few muscles. The degree to which the disorder is focal determines the severity of the disorder, with only a few muscles being affected in the milder forms of the disorder. This is also predictive of treatment benefit. If only a few muscles are affected, then botulinum toxin injections can be selective to the particular muscles disturbing movement. However, in more severe forms with more muscles involved, botulinum toxin injections may be less effective because not all the muscles involved can be injected without producing significant side effects such as swallowing or airway problems in the treatment of SD.

The focal dystonias are often task specific,[13] that is, muscle tone abnormalities occur only during certain task(s). In oromandibular dystonia, for example, a patient may have jaw opening dystonia during speech, but not during chewing.[14] Similarly, speech is usually affected in the SDs while singing, laughter, and crying may not be affected.[15] These characteristics have contributed to considerable misunderstanding of such patients[13,16] who were previously thought to have a psychiatric disorder. With progression of the disorder, usually within the first two years, additional muscles and/or tasks may become affected.

The degree to which the disorder is task specific also affects management decisions. If only one of several laryngeal functions is affected, the aim would be to reduce the level of muscle tone during that particular task without disrupting function during other tasks. When botulinum toxin injection is being used for treatment and the muscles are spasmodic or tremorous during only one activity, the dosage should be small so as not to paralyze the entire muscle and interfere with other functions.

DIAGNOSIS OF SPASMODIC DYSPHONIA

Diagnosis of the SDs is based on symptoms.[17] Patients often first notice their symptoms during a period of increased stress, following an upper respiratory infection, or during a speech performance. Sometimes the onset is gradual with symptoms first occurring only in certain situations, and waxing and waning depending upon stress or speaking demands. In others, the symptoms may remain chronic at the initial severity level. Diagnosis is based on the particular type of voice symptoms in speech and the exclusion of other neurologic movement disorders that could account for laryngeal movement control abnormalities. Table 28-1 summarizes the usual speech symptom characteristics of each type of SD.

SD is an idiopathic disorder, that is, the cause and risk factors for the development of the disorder are unknown. Recent genetic studies have identified the genetic abnormality for idiopathic torsion dystonia,[18] which usually begins in childhood. Some of the family members have only SD,[19] indicating that SD may be related to idiopathic torsion dystonia. Cases of familial spasmodic dysphonia are rare, however, and no associated genetic locus for SD has been found at the present time, as is the case for other focal dystonias.[20] Current thinking is that the pathogenesis of some focal dystonias are the result of a genetic predisposition interacting with acquired factors later in life. Some of the acquired factors may include head injury, chronic drug exposure, or peripheral injuries.[21] Some factors reported as associated with the onset of other focal dystonias include overuse in hand cramps,[13] pain following injury,[22] or extensive dental work in oral mandibular dystonia.[23] Many patients with SD report an upper respiratory infection associated with the onset of symptoms, and we have seen some patients who report onset following laryngeal surgery, although the presence of SD prior to surgery could not be eliminated.

Type	Voice Symptoms	Speech Materials Used to Test
Adductor Spasmodic Dysphonia	Voice breaks in vowels	All voiced sentences, eg, "We mow our lawn all year," "We rode along Rhode Island Avenue."
Abductor Spasmodic Dysphonia	Prolonged voiceless consonants	Sentences or syllables containing voiceless consonants, eg, "The puppy bit the tape," "When he comes home, we'll feed him," repetitions of the syllables, "see," "key," "he," "tea,"and "pea."
Vocal Tremor: adductor	Regular voice breaks or frequency and intensity modulation at around 5 Hz.	Prolonged vowel ("ah" or "ee") using a speaking voice in the habitual pitch range.
Vocal Tremor: abductor	Regular breathy breaks resulting in loss of volume during vowels.	Prolonged vowel ("ah" or "ee") using a speaking voice in the habitual pitch range.
Hyperfunctional Voice Muscular Tension Dysphonia Severe Adductor Spasmodic Dysphonia	Constantly tight, strained effortful voice with glottal fry or harsh voice.	Constant voicing tasks are difficult with less difficulty on sentences with frequent voiceless consonants.
Breathy Dysphonia/ Psychogenic Dysphonia/ Severe Abductor Spasmodic Dysphonia	Constantly breathy voice, increased airflow on voiceless consonants.	All voicing tasks are difficult with more difficulty on sentences with frequent voiceless consonants.

TABLE 28-1. *Speech Symptoms Characteristic of Each of the Spasmodic Dysphonias*

Adductor Spasmodic Dysphonia

Speech is characterized by intermittent voice breaks in the middle of vowels. It is effortful, with strain and sometimes hoarseness, although the essential symptom is voice breaks. These are heard most often in continually voiced sentences, particularly when glottal stops mark word boundaries such as in "we_eat," or when two voiced sounds occur in sequence within a word such as "ye_ar" or "d_og." In the sentences, "We eat eels every day," "We mow our lawn all year," and "A dog dug a new bone," the voice breaks are caused by rapid hyperadductions of the folds which interrupt phonation and can be seen on fiberoptic nasolaryngoscopy.[24] During a break there is a rapid shortening and squeezing of the vocal folds resulting in a quick glottic closure, which interrupts airflow through the glottis.

Specialists in this field are in agreement that patients with hyperadduction voice breaks in vowels have adductor SD. However, there is disagreement on whether patients with constant strain and strangle without intermittent voice breaks also have SD. Constantly strained patients without voice breaks may be diagnosed with muscular tension dysphonia.[25] During fiberoptic videolaryngoscopy these patients have anterior-posterior squeezing of the laryngeal inlet and hyperconstriction of the ventricular (or false) vocal folds resulting in a "pinhole" appearance during speech. Their constantly tight voice is extremely effortful, causing such patients to often appear more severely affected than those with only the intermittent spasmodic breaks.

A diagnosis of muscular tension dysphonia suggests that such patients do not have a neurologic motor control disorder, but a functional voice production disorder caused by excessive laryngeal tension.[26] A holistic treatment approach to such a patient is often used, combining voice therapy and psychologic counseling. To date, no neurophysiologic studies have determined whether these patients have neurophysiologic abnormalities similar to SD patients.

Others feel that patients with constant strain-strangled voice have a variant of SD, perhaps a more severe form, and should be managed using botulinum toxin injections in a fashion similar to patients with adductor voice breaks. At present, until some objective methods become available for identifying the focal dystonias, which are not dependent upon voice symptoms, it is best to make decisions based on individual patient characteristics. Some patients with constantly tight voices benefit from botulinum toxin injections, while some do not. Patients who do not benefit from voice therapy for hyperfunctional voice may have no discernible differences from patients with SD on reports of stress or psychosocial difficulties. When such patients' voice symptoms are improved by botulinum toxin injection, their level of anxiety may improve as well.[27] In general, however, the presence of voice breaks in speech should be the diagnostic criterion for adductor SD and administering botulinum toxin injections.

Abductor Spasmodic Dysphonia

Abductor SD is rare and accounts for only 15% of patients with spasmodic dysphonia. As in adductor SD, diagnosis of abductor SD is based on speech symptoms. These patients have prolonged voiceless consonants caused by difficulties with voice onset following such voiceless sounds as /h/, /s/, /f/, /p/, /t/, and /k/. Additional symptoms, which may occur in some but not all abductor SD patients, include: pitch or phonatory breaks during vowels, and a breathy voice quality. On fiberoptic laryngoscopy, these patients have excessive and prolonged abduction during voiceless consonants. Vocal fold abduction interferes with closure for the following vowel. Patients with abductor SD, however, rarely have difficulties with vocal fold adduction for voice onset at the beginning of speech, except when speech begins with a voiceless consonant. Sustained prolonged vowels are usually normal, except in very severe patients who may present with a breathy voice quality. The laryngeal gesture of producing partial glottal opening for a voiceless consonant with airflow (such as for /h/), followed by adduction for a vowel, is particularly difficult for these patients.

To examine for symptoms of abductor SD, the patient's speech should be compared during voiced sentences such as "We mow our lawn all year" which should contain few abnormalities, with sentences containing a high proportion of voiceless consonants such as "The puppy bit the tape" and "When he comes home we'll feed him." Syllable repetitions can also be used comparing repetitions of "ee-ee-ee-ee-ee" with the vowel separated by glottal stops, which is relatively unaffected in abductor SD, with repetitions of "pea," "tea," "key," or "see' which are more likely to be affected. In more severe cases, patients with abductor SD may have a breathy voice quality along with voiceless consonant prolongations.

Difficulties and disagreements can occur, however, concerning patients with constant breathiness or whispering dysphonia. Some patients with whispering dysphonia have a psychogenic dysphonia and are most appropriately managed using voice therapy.[28-30] These patients whisper constantly and do not have any greater difficulty with sentences that contain a high proportion of voiceless consonants than with those containing all voiced segments. Referral to a social worker, psychologist, or psychiatrist to examine the patients for any emotional explanations for the voice disorder can sometimes be helpful. Some individuals, however, also have emotional stresses that are unrelated to their disorder.

Another confounding diagnosis may be neurologic diseases that affect vocal fold movement control. We have had patients who initially were diagnosed as having abductor spasmodic dysphonia who later developed additional neurologic problems and were subsequently diagnosed as having Parkinson's disease. It is difficult to know whether the voice symptoms were an early manifestation of Parkinson's disease or a separate disorder.

Although our voice team involves a neurologist, psychiatrist, and social worker as well as a speech-language pathologist and otolaryngologist, in most instances the final consensus regarding diagnosis depends mainly on the voice symptoms. We have found that intermittent symptoms, that is, where patients report that they have intervals when they are completely symptom free, are often associated with psychogenic dysphonias. Although symptoms in the SDs usually vary in severity dependent upon stress and fatigue, the symptoms rarely disappear entirely without intervention.[31] Patients with psychogenic dysphonia may also exhibit pitch switching; that is, their voice may become high-pitched for several minutes or hours at a time, and then return to normal.

A typical patient profile in psychogenic voice disorders may include: 1) indifference to voice symptoms; 2) referral to one's different voices as independent of one's self with statements like, "See, it came again"; 3) dependence upon someone else to speak for them; and 4) a history of abuse or emotional crises in their childhood which they were unable to resolve. Voice therapy aimed at teaching the patient how to produce a normal voice in a supportive, nonthreatening manner can be effective.[32]

However, none of these observations is without exceptions. Some patients with adductor or abductor SD report that after they first experienced symptoms, these abated for a year or two, then returned, and progressed. Further, many patients with SD have family and life events as devastating as those of patients with psychogenic dysphonia. Some patients with SD develop anxiety as a result of having a voice disorder, which then abates with treatment.[27] On the other hand, some patients may have an unrelated psychiatric disturbance which should be treated concurrently with their voice disorder.[33]

Compensatory Speech Patterns

Patients with SD sometimes use compensatory techniques to communicate with less effort. Patients with adductor SD, for example, may speak in a whisper to have greater control with less effort. When a patient presents with a whispering aphonia, therefore, it is important to ask him/her to attempt to speak with voice. The more typical symptoms of adductor or abductor SD may then emerge. Others speak on inhalation, which opens the glottis, to overcome the hyperadduction and produce voice more easily. During testing, such patients should be encouraged to speak on exhalation to allow symptom evaluation. Some adductor SD patients learn to initiate speech with an /h/ to avoid hyperadduction of the folds. Similarly, patients with abductor SD may initiate voice with a glottal stop or anterior-posterior squeeze of the ventricular folds to prevent breathy interruptions. During evaluation, patients with mixed adductor and abductor symptoms should be asked to describe which techniques they were taught in therapy, or strategies they have developed to manage their symptoms when they are in situations where intelligible speech is essential.

Compensatory techniques can also interfere with symptom management, particularly when botulinum toxin, total or selective recurrent nerve section, or recurrent nerve avulsion is selected. Patients may continue to use their compensatory techniques after treatment, which may interfere with the treatment result. Speaking on inhalation is a compensatory technique that often requires voice therapy to reverse when a patient has been using it for many years.

Mixed Adductor and Abductor Spasmodic Dysphonia

Although extremely rare, a few patients have symptoms of both adductor and abductor SD. Such patients are difficult to treat as botulinum toxin injections usually produce side effects with no benefit. In our experience, thyroarytenoid injections produce breathiness that exacerbate the disorder while posterior cricoarytenoid injections provide no benefit.

Voice Tremor

Voice tremor can occur in combination with adductor or abductor SD, or in isolation. It can best be detected on prolonged vowels when regularly spaced voice breaks or modulations in frequency and intensity are heard. This disorder affects women more often than men and may be a familial form of benign essential tremor. It can occasionally appear in younger women in their twenties and remain a chronic disorder throughout life without progression. Frequently, however, it first appears in late middle age. Like the dystonias, tremor can be focal, affecting the muscles only in the vocal folds, and task specific, occurring only during voicing. Treatment with botulinum toxin injections into the thyroarytenoid muscles is most effective when the disorder is both focal and task specific. In one series, 60% of patients received benefit.[34] When the patient also has head tremor, laryngeal injections have limited effect. When many regions of the vocal tract are affected such as the ventricular folds, posterior pharynx, or soft palate, botulinum toxin injections may not noticeably benefit the voice but the patient may experience reduced effort when speaking. Beta-blockers, such as propanolol, also can be used in these patients in conjunction with botulinum toxin injection but have little measurable voice effect. A trial of methazolamide was disappointing in patients with vocal tremor.[35] Thus far, no pharmacologic trials have reported benefits in a series of voice tremor patients.

Recent reports of deep brain stimulation in the thalamus have benefited a few patients with vocal tremor.[36,37] These are only preliminary reports, however, in patients with tremor affecting many body regions. It is encouraging, however, that some benefit was found for the voice. These reports may also provide some insight into the mechanisms involved in tremor pathophysiology, at least in some patients.

Adductor SD With Tremor

Often patients with adductor SD have an associated tremor producing regular voice offsets, intermittent reductions in voice amplitude, or variations in fundamental frequency. Tremor often is most evident in the speaking range and may disappear at higher pitch ranges. Sometimes a voice tremor patient is thought to have adductor SD because the tremor causes voice breaks in vowels during speech. However, when the patient is asked to produce a prolonged vowel, the regularity of the glottal stops or frequency and amplitude variations can be heard, usually around 5 Hz.[38]

The identification of adductor tremor when mixed with adductor SD is important for predicting treatment results following either laryngeal nerve surgery or botulinum toxin injection. Frequently these treatments will reduce the adductor spasms but not control tremor, which then becomes more evident.[39] This may be caused by differences in pathophysiology underlying these two types of symptoms; that is, reducing muscle activation seems to have a role in the reduction of adductor spasms but may have little effect on adductor tremor.

Abductor Tremor

Although much more rare, abductor tremor produces periodic breathy breaks in phonation and can be easily detected in prolonged phonation. This can occur in association with abductor spasmodic dysphonia or in isolation. On fiberoptic nasolaryngoscopy during prolonged vowels, the vocal folds have regular abductions during phonation, producing either regular reductions in amplitude and/or increases in fundamental frequency. This disorder is probably the most difficult to manage; botulinum toxin into the posterior cricoarytenoid muscle is usually of limited benefit and recurrent nerve surgery would not be appropriate. We have seen patients who have undergone bilateral thyroplasty with limited benefit.

PATHOPHYSIOLOGY

For many years, spasmodic dysphonia was considered to be a psychologic disorder. This idea was reinforced by the absence of symptoms in many SD patients while laughing, singing, or following sedation with barbiturates.[15,40] Furthermore, many SD patients who underwent psychologic evaluation were thought to have an underlying emotional conflict or psychologic disorder as the cause of their symptoms.[41] In recent years, however, abnormalities in various neurologic reflex responses in SD patients[42,43] and the association of SD with other focal dystonias suggest that SD is, in fact, a neurologic disorder.[1] Psychologic disorders such as depression, anxiety, and somatization appear to be more common in SD patients when compared to control subjects.[44] However, these disorders may be a response to the debilitating voice effects of SD on social interactions and job performance, because these often resolve following successful treatment for SD.[44,45]

The name of the spasmodic dysphonias was changed in the early 1980s from spastic dysphonia to spasmodic dysphonia when bursts were observed in the laryngeal muscles during interruptions in phonation in an SD patient.[46] Systematic studies of patient groups with SD, however, did not show the expected pattern of muscle tone abnormalities of increased thyroarytenoid activity in adductor SD and increased posterior cricoarytenoid activity in abductor SD. Schaefer et al[47] found greater variation of muscle activity in adductor SD patients than in controls but no clear pattern of activation abnormality. The results differed across speech tasks with the greatest variation in thyroarytenoid levels found in the patients on repeated word and sentence tasks. To further investigate physiologic differences in laryngeal muscle activity in adductor and abductor SD, Watson et al[48] examined thyroarytenoid and posterior cricoarytenoid muscles during sustained /i/ and /s/ productions. Some adductor SD patients had normal levels of thyroarytenoid (TA) activity while some abductor SD patients had higher levels of thyroarytenoid activity than the adductor SD patients or the controls. Another study examined untreated adductor and abductor SD patients,[49] during repetition of syllables which were particularly difficult for SD patients: "ee" repetition with glottal stops between vowels (for adductor SD) and the syllable "see" (for abductor SD). Intrinsic (thyroarytenoid, cricothyroid, and posterior cricoarytenoid) and extrinsic (thyrohyoid and sternothyroid) laryngeal muscles were measured while the patients produced the syllables, albeit with considerable difficulty. None of the EMG measures differed from normal in either patient group. The results suggested that the patients were using a normal pattern of muscle activation for speech and that voice breaks were caused by the *intrusion* of spasmodic bursts overlaid upon a normal muscle activation pattern.

Adductor Spasmodic Dysphonia

Nash and Ludlow[50] compared laryngeal muscle activity during speech with and without voice breaks and found increased levels of thyroarytenoid activity during breaks in adductor spasmodic dysphonia. A nonsignificant trend for an increase in the cricothyroid muscle during speech breaks was also found. Thus, the abnormality in SD was not an overall abnormal level of muscle tone but rather the intrusion of spasmodic muscle bursts on an otherwise normal pattern of muscle recruitment.

In another electromyographic study of adductor SD patients before and after botulinum toxin injection,[51] the number of spasmodic bursts were counted from unidentified electromyographic recordings in the thyroarytenoid and cricothyroid muscles in normal controls and adductor SD patients before and after treatment. The number of bursts was greater in the thyroarytenoid muscles in the patients. After treatment, the number of bursts were reduced both in the treated and untreated muscles. Furthermore, the initial numbers of bursts and the change in bursts correlated well with the frequency of voice breaks pretreatment and their reduction after treatment. The problem in SD, then, is the intrusion of involuntary muscle bursts which account for the numbers of voice breaks before and after injection of botulinum toxin.

Neurophysiologic studies have addressed what mechanisms could be involved in the generation of spasmodic muscle bursts. The laryngeal adductor reflex is elicited by electrical stimulation of the superior laryngeal nerve.[52] An ipsilateral R1 response in the thyroarytenoid muscle is followed by a later bilateral response, the R2. This reflex can be elicited by a single stimulus but when stimuli are presented in pairs with short intervals between them, responses to the second stimulus

are reduced in amplitude. This is known as a conditioning effect, and demonstrates the presence of normal inhibitory mechanisms responsible for the control of these reflex responses.[53] Studies of patients with adductor spasmodic dysphonia have demonstrated that these conditioning effects are absent or reduced in most adductor SD patients.[53] In a later study of abductor SD, similar abnormalities were found for a group of patients with abductor SD, although the abnormality was not quite as consistent as in adductor SD.[54]

Abductor Spasmodic Dysphonia

Only a few studies have examined the pathophysiology of this rare type of SD. In a clinical study of 10 abductor SD patients,[55] spasmodic bursts were found in a variety of muscles associated with prolonged voice offsets. Six of the patients had spasmodic bursts in the cricothyroid muscle, while only a few had spasms in the posterior cricoarytenoid muscle. Many had simultaneous spasms in several muscles, the thyroarytenoid, posterior cricoarytenoid, and cricothyroid. One patient did not have spasmodic bursts in any muscle but rather a lack of activity was noted during phonation in the thyroarytenoid muscle. In another study,[48] an abductor patient had higher levels of thyroarytenoid activation than either the controls or the adductor SD patients.

The results to date, therefore, have been much less clear-cut in abductor SD than in adductor SD. Difficulties have included the lack of a clear-cut diagnosis, rarity of patients, and difficulty accessing the posterior cricoarytenoid muscle. A recent report[56] compared thyroarytenoid, cricothyroid, and posterior cricoarytenoid muscle activity in patients with abductor SD with controls during speech breaks and in similar speech without breaks. Abnormal levels of muscle tone were found between the two sides with increased levels of activity on the right side in the patients. These seem to have corresponded to reduced left-sided movement during speech. This is a controversial finding, but suggests that the voice is unstable both for initiating and sustaining phonation because of tension differences between the two sides of the larynx.

Vocal Tremor

Only a few studies have examined laryngeal muscle activity in voice tremor. Tomoda et al[57] studied the thyroarytenoid muscle in two patients and found tremor bursts associated with exhalation and phonation. They proposed that the tremor was activated during the expiratory part of the respiratory cycle. Koda and Ludlow[38] examined laryngeal muscle tremor in both intrinsic and extrinsic laryngeal musculature during inspiration, expiration, phonation, and whisper. A variety of muscles were affected with tremor bursts in the patients studied. Tremor occurred most frequently during phonation and less during inspiration. Although tremor was correlated between muscles on the right and left sides of the larynx, the sides were often out of phase by as much as 20 ms. The mechanism responsible for tremor generation is unknown but the recent results with thalamic stimulation suggest that the thalamus may be one part of the circuit.[36,37]

MANAGEMENT

Several treatment approaches have been employed aiming at controlling or reducing the speech symptoms of these patients. Botulinum toxin injection is currently the treatment of choice for controlling symptoms in adductor SD. Until more is known about the pathophysiology causing these disorders, treatments cannot be expected to reverse the disorder. Although these various treatment techniques have different success rates, none benefit all patients with these disorders (Table 28-2).

A careful evaluation of patients by a multidisciplinary team is needed before the best type of treatment for that patient can be selected. The patient should be counseled on the advantages and disadvantages of each management approach and the expected result with each. The following treatment options are currently available: botulinum toxin muscle injection, recurrent nerve section or avulsion, traditional voice therapy, inhalation therapy, respiratory control therapy, neuropharmacologic management, and experimental surgical approaches.

Botulinum Toxin Injection

The injection of small amounts of botulinum toxin into muscles produces a chemical denervation of muscle fibers by blocking the release of acetylcholine at neuromuscular junctions. The first therapeutic use of botulinum toxin was by Dr. Alan Scott, an ophthalmologist, who reported benefit following injection of the extraocular muscles for the treatment of strabismus.[58,59] It was found that abnormalities caused by muscle imbalances could be corrected for up to 3 months. Because of subsequent reinnervation of endplates, the denervation is only temporary, and the symptoms return when muscle function returns. In 1985, successful treatment of patients with blepharospasm[60] and torticollis[61] demonstrated the potential for use in treatment of focal dystonias. The first reports in spasmodic dysphonia were in 1987 by Miller et al[62] and by Blitzer et al.[63] Miller and his associates used large unilateral injections (35 mouse units) into the thyroarytenoid muscle while

Blitzer et al used much smaller bilateral thyroarytenoid injections of between 2.5 and 3.5 mouse units.[63]

Of note, there are currently two commercially available formulations of botulinum toxin worldwide. BOTOX is marketed in the United States, while Dysport is more commonly used in Europe and the United Kingdom. Clinical studies in humans indicate that BOTOX is more potent than Dysport on a per unit basis. However, there is no consensus in the literature regarding the relative potencies of the two formulations, with reported BOTOX: Dysport conversion factors ranging from 1:5 to 1:2.41.[64] All further references to botulinum toxin dosages in this chapter refer to the BOTOX formulation.

Both Miller et al and Blitzer et al use the percutaneous approach for the administration of the botulinum toxin. A hollow, Teflon-coated hypodermic needle with a bared tip and hub is used as a monopolar electromyographic electrode. The hub is connected as one pole of a physiologic amplifier. The patient is grounded, and a reference electrode is placed on the neck and connected to the other pole of the amplifier. The hypodermic needle is connected to a syringe containing a solution of 2.5 mouse units of botulinum toxin in 0.1 ml of saline. The needle is inserted through the cricothyroid membrane between the cartilages and angled superiorly and slightly laterally into the body of the fold following the procedures described by Hirano and Ohala for locating and verifying placement in the thyroarytenoid muscle.[65] The physiologic amplifier is connected to an oscilloscope and an audio speaker for visual and auditory feedback to demonstrate when the electrode is in muscle. Once the electrode is thought to be in muscle, the patient is asked to phonate and if a noticeable increase in muscle activity is observed, then it is assumed that the electrode is in the appropriate location for injection of botulinum toxin. In bilateral injections, usually 2.5 units are injected into one location on each side. In unilateral injections, usually 5 units are injected into each of two or three locations, resulting in a total dosage of 10 to 15 units on one side. Generally subsequent treatment dosages can be somewhat reduced because some physiologic effects of botulinum toxin on the muscle last for up to 36 months.[66] Both the bilateral and unilateral injection approaches have been used successfully for the treatment of adductor spasmodic dysphonia with somewhat similar results.[66-68] The bilateral injection approach is used more frequently, probably because less toxin is used, reducing the cost of treatment.

Advantages of Treatment With Botulinum Toxin

Botulinum toxin injection has become the treatment of choice for adductor SD, mainly because it is transient and less costly than surgery[69] (Table 28-2). If a particu-

Therapeutic Approach	Advantages	Disadvantages	Patient Types Benefited
Botulinum toxin injection of laryngeal muscles	Temporary effects No permanent injury Temporary side effects	Temporary symptom control Reinjection required approx. every 3-4 months with breathy voice and dysphagia side effects	Moderate to severe adductor SD Focal vocal tremor Selected patients with abductor SD
Recurrent laryngeal nerve section or avulsion	Potential long-term benefit Can be managed with botulinum toxin injections if symptoms return	Unpredictable side effects Return of symptoms in 40% of patients Permanent unilateral paralysis	Focal severe adductor SD
Voice therapy	No permanent injury to the larynx Assists patient with greater insight into voice problem	Poor carryover Limited long-term benefit Best combined with other approaches	Mild adductor SD Mild abductor SD Psychogenic voice disorders Hyperfunctional voice disorders
Inhalation voice therapy	No permanent injury to the larynx	Not yet studied Limited voice change in some patients Poor carryover	Severe constantly tight voice Constantly breathy voice
Respiratory control training	No permanent injury to the larynx	Not yet studied in SD Limited voice change in some patients Poor carryover	Hyperfunctional voice disorders Abductor SD
Neuropharmacologic intervention	No permanent injury to the larynx	Not yet studied in SD Limited voice change in some patients	Inderal for voice tremor Artane for abductor SD Liorsel for adductor SD
Experimental surgery: neural stimulation	Possible long-term use	Potential nerve injury Only 6 patients studied Limited information on type of voice disorder or symptom change	Perhaps abductor SD

TABLE 28-2. *Management Approaches for the Spasmodic Dysphonias (Continues)*

Therapeutic Approach	Advantages	Disadvantages	Patient Types Benefited
Type III thyroplasty	Long-term change	Structural injury to larynx with pitch lowering	Not recommended
		Increased vocal fold adduction, failures may be frequent	

TABLE 28-2. *Management Approaches for the Spasmodic Dysphonias (Continued)*

lar injection regimen does not benefit a patient, other injection approaches may be tried or the patient can then be considered for other treatments. Rather than surgical approaches that permanently alter the larynx and produce neural or structural injury, patients can select botulinum toxin treatment without risk of a permanent alteration to their larynx. This is also a disadvantage of this treatment. The patient will benefit during the denervation phase but will have symptoms return following reinnervation caused by motor nerve sprouting. Reinjection is usually required every 4 to 5 months, making treatment costly in the long run.

Dosages and Treatment Regimens

For patients with adductor spasmodic dysphonia, using the percutaneous approach, the dosage is usually 12-15 mouse units for a unilateral thyroarytenoid injection[69] or 2-2.5 units for a bilateral thyroarytenoid injection[69] (Table 28-3). Others have reported using a peroral or indirect approach with similar bilateral dosages.[70] Using a transcartilaginous approach to the thyroarytenoid muscle with anatomic landmarks, smaller dosages of 2 units may have been used on each side.[71] Neither the peroral or transcartilaginous approaches use electromyographic verification to ensure that the needle is in muscle tissue. Therefore, both require visual monitoring of the needle location. The smaller effective dosage using the transcartilaginous approach may be because the anterior portion of the thyroarytenoid muscle is injected. The anterior portion of this muscle seems to have a greater role in vocal fold adduction than the more posterior portion, which is usually injected by the percutaneous method.[72]

A change in symptoms is usually noticed within 3 days following injection. Often patients report some reductions in voice breaks by 48 hours and sometimes a reduction in effort as early as 6 to 12 hours after injection. The effects of the toxin can continue to increase up to 7 days after injection, probably because of diffusion of the toxin through the muscle. This is why some patients report that their voice is best 3 days after an injection followed by the onset of breathiness and other side effects by 5 days. The usual side effects include 3 to 5 days of difficulty swallowing liquids. Patients should be advised to sip through a straw and to avoid swallowing liquids quickly. Breathiness can last between 7 and 20 days and may sometimes be more pronounced following bilateral injections, particularly in males with mild to moderate symptom severity.

Larger dosages (20-25 units unilaterally, 4 units bilaterally) can sometimes be administered in more severely affected women without the risk of significant side effects such as swallowing difficulties for liquids and breathiness. However, caution is advised in treating men. Often dosages greater than 15 units unilaterally or 2 or 2.5 units bilaterally can result in significant side effects, aspiration of liquids and prolonged voice loss for several weeks in men. This may be because the larger cartilages in the male larynx have different biomechanical effects following muscle denervation.

Development of Resistance to Treatment With Botulinum Toxin

Patients with torticollis who are receiving large dosages, often greater than 100 units per treatment, may develop antibodies to botulinum toxin type A.[73] Generally, the frequency of reinjection rather than the total dosage is thought to play a role in the development of antibodies. Because there is no cross-reactivity between the various botulinum toxin types[74] they can then be treated with other types such as Type F[75] or Type B. There are very few reports of antibody resistance developing following laryngeal injections, presumably because the injection dosages are small. One case was reported in 1991 following a series of laryngeal injections for the treatment of stuttering.[76] The patient then responded to Type F injections that produced the expected reduction in movement following unilateral laryngeal injection. Two other cases of resistance to laryngeal botulinum toxin injections for SD have recently been reported in patients receiving cumulative doses of approximately 70 to 80 units over several years.[77]

Type of SD	Muscle	Approach	Side(s)	Dosage (Mouse Units)
Adductor	Thyroarytenoid	Percutaneous	Bilateral	2-2.5 each side
			Unilateral	10-15
		Peroral	Bilateral	2-5 each side
			Unilateral	10
		Transcartilaginous	Bilateral	2 each side
			Unilateral	10
Adductor post-RLN section	Thyroarytenoid	Percutaneous	Unilateral (surgical side)	15
			Bilateral	2.5 each side
Abductor SD	Posterior cricoarytenoid	Percutaneous	Unilateral	10-12
			Bilateral	5 each side, sequentially
	Cricothyroid	Percutaneous	Bilateral	3-5 each side
Vocal tremor	Thyroarytenoid	Percutaneous	Unilateral	12-15
			Bilateral	2.5 each side
	Thyrohyoid	Percutaneous	Bilateral	3-5 each side
	Sternothyroid	Percutaneous	Bilateral	3-5 each side

TABLE 28-3. *Dosages for Treatment of Various Types of Spasmodic Dysphonia Using Botulinum Toxin Type A*

One demonstrated systemic resistance, the other did not, but failed to respond to a unilateral injection of the forehead on one side. By injecting 10 units on one side of the forehead, an asymmetry in forehead wrinkling will be seen if the patient still responds to botulinum toxin. Surprisingly, not all patients who have become resistant to treatment with botulinum toxin are found to have circulating antibodies.[78]

Injection Types for Different Types of SD Patients

Thyroarytenoid injections have been demonstrated to be beneficial in most patients with adductor spasmodic dysphonia.[3,79-83] Few failures have been reported. These occur mainly in male patients with mild adductor SD symptoms who have prolonged breathiness. Their side effects may negate any benefits they may

experience. On the other hand, patients with extensive dystonia, affecting additional structures such as the head or pharyngeal musculature, often receive only partial benefit following laryngeal injections. In our series of over 200 patients, we have had only a few adductor SD patients who did not show some benefit from botulinum toxin injections. One was a primary nonresponder to botulinum toxin type A, although she tested negative for antibodies to the toxin. The others had mixed symptoms of both adductor SD and abductor SD. Some others have only received a partial benefit because of extensive dystonia and a few milder patients have not returned for reinjection because the side effects outweighed the benefits.

Adductor SD patients with symptom return following recurrent nerve section have been treated using similar methods to those used with adductor patients who have not undergone surgery.[84] Either a unilateral injection on the side of the paralysis can be effective in controlling symptoms, or in more severe cases of this type, a bilateral injection can be used.

Treatment with botulinum toxin injections is more difficult in patients who have previously undergone unsuccessful type III thyroplasty. First, because of severe scarring and changes in the thyroid cartilage, these patients are best injected using a peroral or indirect approach. In addition, some attempt at surgical reversal is often necessary before these patients can benefit significantly. Patients who have not benefited from a thyroplasty should be advised that the prognosis is guarded for a significant improvement with botulinum toxin injections.

Treatment of Abductor Spasmodic Dysphonia by Botulinum Toxin Injection

Several reports are currently available regarding the use of botulinum toxin treatment for patients with the abductor type. Injections of the cricothyroid and, more commonly, the posterior cricoarytenoid muscles have been used in abductor SD patients. Unfortunately, the success has been limited and more unpredictable than in adductor SD.

One group[55] selected 10 patients who had cricothyroid spasms on clinical electromyography and injected 5 units into each of the cricothyroid muscles. Speech was improved on objective measures of speech in 6 patients. Patients with constant breathiness and other muscle abnormalities did not receive benefit. In another series,[85] 32 patients with abductor SD were treated using the percutaneous approach to the posterior cricoarytenoid. The posterior cricoarytenoid, on the posterior cricoid cartilage, is accessed by rotating the larynx and passing the needle posterior to the thyroid lamina. Both the patients and the experimenters used unblinded rating scales. None of the patients' speech reached the normal range; the greatest improvement was to a level 70% of normal and the average percent improvement was 39%. Of the 32 patients, 20 improved with posterior cricoarytenoid injections, 9 required both posterior cricoarytenoid and cricothyroid injections, and 3 required a Type I thyroplasty with posterior cricoarytenoid injections. In another study,[86] five patients were injected in the region of the posterior cricoarytenoid by passing the needle through the cricothyroid membrane, through the glottis between the two arytenoids medially and into the interarytenoid muscle. Caution is needed with this approach as the cricoarytenoid joint could be impaled and joint motion reduced, as happened in one of their five patients who had no benefit.

In a recent study,[87] although 60% of patients reported some benefit similar to previous studies,[85] an independent blinded assessment of voice symptoms failed to show a benefit for either the percutaneous[85] or the peroral[88] approaches to muscle injection. Overall, the severity of side effects are greater and the duration of benefits are less following injection in abductor SD than in adductor SD.[89] Alternative treatment approaches that are more effective are needed for patients with abductor SD.

Treatment of Vocal Tremor With Botulinum Toxin Injection

Vocal tremor can occur in association with adductor SD or in isolation. Some patients with adductor tremor of the vocal folds, without tremor involvement of other regions of the vocal tract, respond reasonably well to botulinum toxin injections into the thyroarytenoid muscle. A recent series[34] found that botulinum toxin injection was beneficial in 50% of patients on objective measures. The authors concluded that this treatment is much less effective in treating tremor than adductor SD. Either unilateral or bilateral thyroarytenoid injections can be used in adductor voice tremor (Tables 28-2 and 28-3) and larger dosages are sometimes more effective.[34]

Remaining Questions Regarding the Use of Botulinum Toxin in Spasmodic Dysphonia

With one exception, none of the studies of botulinum toxin in SD were blinded trials with random assignment to treatment. One study compared botulinum toxin injection with saline placebo injections in a controlled trial with 13 patients. Significant improvements were found in the botulinum toxin injected group in comparison with the saline injected group. Larger controlled trials are still needed.

At present botulinum toxin type A is an accepted, effective, and safe treatment for adductor SD. It is much less effective in abductor SD and tremor. Although over 1,000 patients are currently being treated,[90] no long-term follow-up of a cohort of patients has been conducted to determine whether they remain in treatment. Some patients seem to be opting for more long-lasting symptom control rather than a lifetime of laryngeal injections[91,92] while others may be deciding to forego treatment because of cost or other factors. The extent to which patients are making these choices is not known.

One of the problems with botulinum toxin therapy for spasmodic dysphonia has been the poor predictability of patients' responses. This result was illustrated in a report by Aronson and his colleagues[93] who compared patients' responses on three subsequent injections. The placement of the toxin in the laryngeal muscles may vary because of the difficulties with the percutaneous injection technique. Even with an attempt to angle the injection needle superiorly after passing through the cricothyroid membrane, usually the needle tip will be in the posterior inferior portion of the thyroarytenoid at the confluence of the thyroarytenoid, lateral cricoarytenoid, and the medial portion of the cricothyroid muscles.[94] The indirect approach to the thyroarytenoid may yield more consistent results because the thyroarytenoid muscle alone is more likely to be affected using this approach.[70] The selection of which technique might be most accurate will depend largely upon the physician's skill and experience in using a particular technique.

Another reason for the variability of responses to injection is that when a patient returns three months after an injection, the most active muscle fibers are going to be those unaffected by the previous injection. The pattern of reinnervation and location of the previous injection will determine which regions of the muscle are most active at the time of reinjection. Because the dennervation effects of an injection are most prominent for one year,[66] the location of the dennervated and remaining active fibers will vary with each injection regardless of the skill of the physician. Therefore, it is doubtful that the variation in result from one injection to the next will be reduced in the future.

Many centers are now using smaller dosages of toxin for injections than were first used. This may be because of a cumulative effect of treatments over time, thus requiring a smaller dosage to receive the same benefit.[95] In blepharospasm patients, who have been treated for a longer period of time and studied more intensively, authors have reported that some patients who initially had a good response had a decrease in duration or intensity of benefits on multiple subsequent injections.[96,97] Thus far this has not been found to be the case in SD, although individual patients have not been followed over time.

Physiologic and structural changes take place in a muscle as a result of botulinum toxin treatment.[98-101] Following chemical denervation, both motor nerve sprouting as well as reinnervation provide the return of symptoms. Some reports have not found the expected results of motor nerve sprouting in patients with repeated treatment with botulinum toxin for blepharospasm.[98,100,101] A more recent report of a study of motor axons in the obicularis oculi of 9 blepharospasm patients found some differences from untreated control muscles. The treated muscles had 1) thin, unmyelinated axonal collaterals to end plates, 2) increased number of muscle fibers innervated by more than one motor axon, 3) a profusion of unmyelinated axonal sprouts, 4) increased range of end plate sizes, and 5) multiple end plates on individual fibers.

Another issue that has not yet been addressed is the possible effects of repeated needle damage in muscles being repeatedly injected, independent of the botulinum toxin effects. The effects of scarring and possible fibrosis as a result of repeated needle insertions needs to be determined.[102] This is particularly important, given the small size of the laryngeal muscles in comparison with neck muscles being treated in torticollis patients.

In summary, although botulinum toxin is currently the most beneficial approach, this treatment is most helpful in patients with adductor SD with focal involvement, that is, with spasmodic bursts affecting only the thyroarytenoid muscle. Other types of SD patients may not benefit to the same degree. These include patients with extensive tremor involvement, milder adductor SD patients, and some patients with abductor spasmodic dysphonia. Therefore, accurate diagnosis is important before treatment is begun.

Surgical Management

Recurrent Laryngeal Nerve Section

Dedo[103] first introduced recurrent laryngeal nerve section as a treatment for adductor SD in 1976. Noting improvement in voice symptoms following temporary unilateral RLN paralysis with lidocaine injection, he subsequently removed a 1-cm segment of the RLN below the inferior pole of the thyroid gland in 34 patients. All patients demonstrated a reduction or elimination in voice breaks and associated facial and neck grimaces or tics. Although all were pleased with their voice improvement, several patients developed the breathiness, pitch control problems, and hoarseness that are characteristic of unilateral vocal fold paralysis.

Early enthusiasm for the procedure[104-106] was quickly tempered by reports of recurrent voice symptoms in some patients.[107-109] Aronson and DeSanto[110] noted an alarming 64% recurrence rate in 33 patients at 3 years following surgery, and 48% of failed patients had a worse voice than before surgery. Interestingly, the authors observed a higher failure rate in females compared to males (77% vs 36%). They attributed the recurrent symptoms in these patients to intensified activity of the contralateral innervated vocal fold and/or other surrounding muscles because return of vocal fold movement was not observed on the operated side. However, other studies have demonstrated reinnervation of the vocal fold on the operated side in cases of recurrence by electromyography[84,107] and histology.[111,112] Furthermore, patients with recurrent symptoms have responded well to revision surgery[107,109,113] or Botox injections[84] to the previously operated side, suggesting that reinnervation is the most likely cause of postsurgical recurrences.

Dedo reported recurrent symptoms in approximately 10-15% of his patients[114,115] and has maintained that his results are better than those of others for two reasons. First, he resects a portion of the nerve, turns back each stump, and ligates each end. Second, prior to and immediately following surgery, Dedo and his colleagues provide some voice training so that the patients gain more insight into preventing overpressure and making the best use of their voice postsurgery. He has also suggested that laser thinning of the body of the vocal fold, to achieve lateralization of the vocal fold edge, can be helpful in reducing the overpressure seen in patients with recurrent symptoms.[115]

One obvious advantage of the recurrent nerve section is that, even using the conservative estimate of Aronson,[110] a minimum of 30-40% of patients could have a long-term benefit and may not need additional treatment. Furthermore, those patients who fail surgery can be treated using botulinum toxin injections with somewhat similar results to those obtained in patients without prior surgical intervention.[84]

There are several disadvantages with this approach. The patients will have a longstanding paralysis even when there has been reinnervation. This can produce respiratory difficulties and an increased risk of laryngospasm.[91,116] The patient also has a greater risk of developing a bilateral paralysis in the future if there is injury to the opposite nerve, because one side is already paralyzed. In addition, if the patient develops an excessively breathy voice, additional vocal fold medialization procedures may be required, which can result in symptom recurrence.[115] Finally, the timing of reinnervation is difficult to predict. Some patients have undergone vocal fold medialization for treatment of excessive breathiness one year following nerve section, only to have SD symptoms return at 3 years following the nerve section. Overall, the inability to predict if the patient will have a positive result before surgery, the difficulties with SD diagnosis, and the controversy over long-term success rates make the nerve section less preferred to botulinum toxin injection at the present time. However, several patients who have benefitted from botulinum toxin injections, but found the need for regularly repeated injections tiresome and costly, have eventually elected to have the recurrent nerve resection.

Recurrent Nerve Avulsion

Because of the reports of reinnervation following recurrent nerve section,[107,113] Netterville and his colleagues[111] developed a more radical approach to nerve resection, termed recurrent laryngeal nerve avulsion. This more extensive removal of the recurrent nerve is an effort to reduce the risk of reinnervation of the sectioned recurrent laryngeal nerve. After mobilization of the ipsilateral thyroid lobe, all branches of the RLN are identified, traced, and avulsed from their muscular insertions deep to the cricopharyngeus muscle. The proximal end of the nerve is then dissected for 3-4 cm beneath the clavicle where it is suture ligated and divided. The total length of RLN removed averages 9 cm, in contrast to an average of 2 cm reported in previous RLN section studies. Intermediate follow-up on 12 patients averaging 1.5 years following the procedure showed no recurrence of symptoms.[111] The authors subsequently reported long-term follow-up of 3 to 7 years on 18 patients following recurrent laryngeal nerve avulsion.[112] Sixteen patients (89%) were free of SD symptoms at 3-year follow-up, although two of these patients later developed recurrent spasms following medialization laryngoplasty for treatment of weak voice. Thus, an overall recurrence rate of 22% (4/18) was reported for the series, which compares favorably to long-term recurrence rates for RLN section.[110,113] Of note, perceptual analysis of postoperative voices revealed some degree of abnormality (pitch, intensity, and/or quality) in all patients, consistent with the effects of unilateral vocal fold paralysis. Patients should be counseled regarding these potential effects preoperatively. Weed et al[91] recommend that nerve avulsion be reserved for patients who do not benefit from or do not tolerate Botox injections, and for patients who have failed prior RLN section.

Experimental Surgical Approaches

Some experimental surgical approaches have been used in SD, usually by one investigator on a small number of patients.[117,118] Because many of these techniques permanently alter the laryngeal structure,[118] or can injure the recurrent laryngeal nerve,[119] accurate diagnosis and objective symptom assessment need to be employed when such procedures are used. Diagnosis is presently based on symptoms; thus, the need to exclude patients with a psychogenic or functional dysphonia is of great importance. These patients could undergo spontaneous recovery.[31] Structural or neural alterations as a result of surgical intervention could interfere with their ability to regain a normal voice.

Selective Laryngeal Adductor Denervation-Reinnervation

Berke et al[92] recently presented preliminary results with selective denervation of the laryngeal adductor muscles in an attempt to achieve a permanent bilateral adductor weakness that mimics the transient effects of Botox. Although unilateral selective denervation of laryngeal adductor muscles has been previously proposed[120] for the treatment of SD, the new procedure involves bilateral section of the adductor RLN branches to the thyroarytenoid and lateral cricoarytenoid muscles with intentional reinnervation of the proximal thyroarytenoid branches using branches of the ansa cervicalis nerve. The aim of this directed reinnervation is to prevent unwanted reinnervation by RLN efferents and to preserve adductor muscle tone.

The study presented one to five-year follow-up on 21 patients with adductor SD who underwent the procedure. In general, symptoms and overall severity of SD improved from moderate to severe ratings preoperatively to mild to absent ratings postoperatively. All patients experienced severe vocal fold bowing and breathiness in the early postoperative period that improved after 3 to 6 months. Aspiration of greater than two weeks' duration was noted in two patients, one of whom required hospitalization for aspiration pneumonia. Additional treatments (Botox, voice therapy, collagen injection, thyroarytenoid myotomy) were also performed in several patients to enhance the postoperative voice result. As noted by the authors, long-term follow-up in a larger patient population will be required to define the role of this procedure in the treatment of adductor SD. In particular, the effects of bilateral denervation on airway protection and fine motor control of the larynx for speech (pitch variability, loudness range, and voice onset timing) require further careful assessment. Because the procedure is technically difficult and produces permanent structural and functional changes in the larynx, it should be reserved for patients with relatively severe disease. However, the authors report promising results with normal conversational voice intensity and good inflection in most adductor SD patients treated thus far.

Nerve Stimulation

Friedman has reported using a recurrent nerve stimulator in patients with spasmodic dysphonia.[117,119] Initially, the stimulator was implanted unilaterally in one abductor spasmodic dysphonia patient using a cuff electrode around the recurrent laryngeal nerve. Close postoperative monitoring showed no stimulation-induced alterations in respiratory or cardiac rate and no cardiac arrhythmias. When the stimulator was set at rates between 10 and 25 Hz, the vocal fold on the side of the stimulator moved toward the midline. Stimulation under these conditions was associated with improvement in voice quality as assessed by the patient and the investigators.

Subsequently, Friedman et al[119] reported follow-up on 5 SD patients implanted with the recurrent laryngeal nerve stimulator. Global assessment of voice quality by the patients and investigators generally ranged between minimal change and marked improvement in all cases,

but none achieved a near-normal voice. The authors did not specify whether the patients had adductor or abductor SD. Although no effects of stimulation on cardiac or respiratory function were observed, one patient developed a permanent vocal fold paralysis from the procedure. In the same study, the authors reported additional safety experience in 113 patients that they had implanted with a vagus nerve stimulator to control epilepsy. The system and implantation technique were similar to that described for the SD patients except that a spiral electrode was placed around the vagus nerve. The most common adverse events associated with stimulation were hoarseness, throat pain, and cough. An additional patient developed a vocal fold paralysis as a result of sustained stimulation from a system malfunction. Based on the established safety profile and greater ease of electrode placement, the authors recommended future study of vagal rather than recurrent nerve stimulator implantation for treatment of SD.

The stimulator may act by blocking or overriding any neural impulses that usually produce spontaneous muscle bursts resulting in the voice breaks. Thus, the neural stimulation may replace abnormal uncontrolled muscle spasms with tonic contractions. However, nerve stimulators can often produce nerve injury either because of compression reducing blood supply to the nerve, or if there is movement, producing twisting or pressure directly on the nerve. As noted by the authors, this approach is currently experimental, and further well-controlled studies are required to establish the long-term safety, effectiveness, and practicality of nerve stimulation in the treatment of SD.

Thyroplasty

Type III thyroplasty was reported by Tucker[118] in a series of 18 patients with SD. This procedure was first recommended by Isshiki[121] who proposed that it should help patients with spasmodic dysphonia because it would reduce vocal fold tension. The procedure involves sectioning the thyroid cartilage by a superior-inferior cut on either side of the thyroid keel. The keel is then repositioned into the larynx, which shortens, thickens, and medializes the vocal folds. The result is a lower fundamental frequency[122] and some reduction in the airway. Because the vocal folds become more medialized, this procedure could increase hyperadduction. Tucker[118] reported short-term relief of spasms in 9 out of 16 patients. No long-term assessment of results was provided to determine whether there is any sustained benefit in this subset of patients.

As mentioned previously, some patients with persistent symptoms following thyroplasty have been referred for botulinum toxin injection because of their poor result following the procedure. These patients have poorer results than others treated by botulinum toxin injection who had not had prior surgery.[123] The ability to reverse the surgery is limited because of the difficulty in protruding and anchoring the thyroid keel. Furthermore, the lowering of the fundamental frequency in female patients may add to their voice abnormalities. Finally, this procedure may exacerbate vocal fold hyperadduction in adductor SD patients. At present, Type III thyroplasty is not recommended for treatment of adductor SD.

Blitzer et al[85] reported using Type I thyroplasty to increase medialization on one side in three patients with abductor SD. This was used as a last resort when botulinum toxin injections into the posterior cricoarytenoid and the cricothyroid were not effective. Long-term follow-up is needed to determine if the partial benefits were maintained over time. Type I thyroplasty may also be helpful in reducing breathiness following RLN section or avulsion,[112] although medialization may increase the risk of SD symptom recurrence in these patients.

Isshiki et al[124] recently described the use of Type II midline lateralization thyroplasty in one female patient with presumed adductor spasmodic dysphonia. Following midline division of the thyroid cartilage, the thyroid alae were retracted laterally and a 2×3 mm perforation was made in the anterior commissure to widen it. After closing the perforation with a free composite cartilage graft, the thyroid alae were anchored in the lateralized position using silicone shims. Approximately 17 months postoperatively, the authors report no signs of recurrence and no perceptible voice strain. One possible advantage of this technique is that it allows a wide range of lateralization of the anterior vocal folds to relieve overpressure and voice spasms. Revision procedures, if required, would be theoretically possible by simply adjusting the size of the silicone shim. Furthermore, the procedure damages neither muscle nor nerve, and its success is not jeopardized by reinnervation as seen with other currently used procedures. Contamination of the operative field following perforation of the anterior commissure increases the possibility of wound infection, but this was not observed in the case reported. As with all other surgical procedures proposed for SD, long-term control of voice symptoms will be key in evaluating the usefulness of Type II thyroplasty for this indication.

Preclinical Studies

Genack et al[125] described a myectomy in rabbits that might have application for spasmodic dysphonia patients. Partial unilateral thyroarytenoid myectomy was performed in the rabbit model through a thyroplas-ty cartilage window. Follow-up electromyography on the myectomy side three months postoperatively revealed reduced compound muscle action potentials compared to the control side. Histologic studies on the operated side demonstrated replacement of excised muscle fibers with loose areolar connective tissue without evidence of muscle regeneration. The obvious benefit of this procedure over RLN section or avulsion is that it is not dependent on denervation for its therapeutic effect. The lack of muscle regeneration following partial myectomy in this study holds promise for a sustained therapeutic effect in SD patients. The authors note that this procedure could be performed bilaterally to maintain adductor balance between the thyroarytenoid muscles. Further preclinical studies in this area are warranted and should include longer follow-up for assessment of muscle regeneration and electromyographic findings.

Voice Therapy

Traditional Voice Therapy

Voice therapy has not yet been demonstrated to be effective for patients with adductor SD. However, there are three reasons to recommend a trial of voice therapy for some SD patients. First, voice therapy may aid in diagnosis in the event that a psychogenic voice disorder or symptom exaggeration is suspected. Sometimes patients may unconsciously exaggerate their symptoms because of the difficulties they have in getting others to recognize the significance of their problem. The exaggerated symptoms may confound the diagnosis. Voice therapy may aid in removing these added voice production difficulties and unmask the SD symptoms to allow for accurate diagnosis and treatment. Laryngeal musculoskeletal tension reduction techniques have recently been advocated for muscular tension dysphonia[126] and may be helpful as an initial therapeutic trial for differentiating between muscular tension dysphonia and SD.[126] Some patients may derive secondary gains from their voice disorder, such as time off from work or more attention from a spouse. Voice therapy, which is aimed at symptom management, can teach some such patients how to produce a normal voice. A trial of six sessions of voice therapy is usually adequate to determine if patients could benefit from this type of therapy. If an initial benefit is found, then patients should be encouraged to continue until they have reached a plateau or can fully control their symptoms for their everyday communication needs.

Second, voice therapy is recommended to provide support for patients unlikely to benefit from other treatment approaches such as botulinum toxin or recurrent nerve avulsion. Patients with mild and/or inconsistent symptoms and only occasional overpressure spasms, but otherwise normal voice production, often have little benefit from botulinum toxin. The severity of the side effects of breathiness and dysphagia often override any benefit they derive. This is particularly the case for males with mild adductor SD symptoms, who often have breathiness and dysphagia for over a month following injection. When their voice returns, their symptoms are reduced for only a short period before symptoms return at three months.

Third, some patients report using voice therapy techniques following botulinum toxin injection to prolong the period during which they are symptom free. Murry and his colleagues, determined that the duration of benefit was extended significantly when patients were administered voice therapy before injection and during the post-injection period.[127] They concluded that a combined regimen of botulinum toxin and voice therapy was beneficial in not only controlling the symptoms of SD but also in reducing the hyperfunctional voice production behaviors.

Traditional voice therapy approaches for adductor SD employ techniques for avoiding over-pressure. Breathy voice onsets, reduced speech emphasis, using a head focus, and laryngeal manipulation are aimed at reducing laryngeal tension.[32,128] Some adductor SD patients also have glottal fry and can benefit from pitch elevation, and increasing pitch variation for intonation. In addition, relaxation training[129] and respiratory training emphasizing controlled breathing and coordination with speech onset,[128,130,131] often help patients gain greater insight into the control of laryngeal tension during speech.

Inhalation Voice Therapy

Inhalation voice therapy incorporates a technique developed by Susan Shulman, a speech-language pathologist in Dallas, Texas. Shulman employs a gradual therapeutic regimen of teaching patients to phonate on inhalation. As patients become more skilled in coordinating inhalation with speech, they can gradually employ a mixture of speaking on both inhalation and exhalation. Shulman explains that, "It is necessary to remember that voicing on inhalation is an alternate method that is designed to provide the patients with a voice when it is not possible to obtain acceptable voicing on exhalation; speaking on exhalation is always the original goal. It is important that the clinician first attempt to utilize voicing on inhalation as a means of relaxation for improving voice on exhalation" (personal communication).

This therapy also includes many other techniques used by most voice therapists for patients with hyperfunctional voice or muscular tension dyspho-

nia,[26,32,128-131] such as laryngeal massage and relaxation exercises, including yawn-sigh and relaxed breathing.

One explanation as to why this approach may be beneficial is that inspiration activates the posterior cricoarytenoid to enhance vocal fold abduction.[132,133] Perhaps when adductor SD patients use inhalation during speech onset, the abduction muscle activation pattern associated with inspiration occurs during speech onset, and hyperadduction is reduced. However, this approach cannot be used successfully by all patients and sometimes one movement abnormality is replaced by another. Objective studies are needed to evaluate the efficacy of this and other voice therapies for SD.

Summary: Voice Therapy for Spasmodic Dysphonia

Clinicians have found limited benefit with voice therapy for SD patients in general; thus, controlled trials have to date seemed unnecessary. Dr. Morton Cooper has suggested that voice therapy can be beneficial,[134] but others have suggested that this may be because he is seeing patients with psychogenic overlay.[135] Voice therapy, however, might be beneficial to SD patients in gaining greater insight into their voice production control difficulties. At present, we recommend a trial of voice therapy for the following types of SD patients:

1. patients with mild intermittent symptoms of adductor SD;
2. patients with a psychogenic dysphonia, psychogenic overlay or symptom exaggeration;
3. patients requesting assistance with increasing benefit duration following botulinum toxin injection; and
4. abductor SD patients receiving limited benefit from botulinum toxin injections.

We currently do not recommend voice therapy for:

1. patients with voice tremor; or
2. previously untreated patients with moderate to severe adductor SD without compensatory overlay.

Usually, moderate to severely affected SD patients are not able to benefit from voice therapy. Until they have had some symptom reduction by botulinum toxin injection, voice therapy is only frustrating and could produce a negative attitude towards therapy postinjection when they might be able to benefit.

One of the greatest difficulties with voice therapy for SD patients is the difficulty with compliance. Many SD patients do not complete a trial of six sessions, making it difficult to determine if they can or cannot benefit. Of course, poor participation in trial therapy is an outcome measure in itself; the patients find little benefit and therefore drop out. Furthermore, with treatment alternatives such as botulinum toxin injection or surgery that offer immediate symptom control, voice therapy can be an unattractive alternative.

Neuropharmacologic Therapy

There are no controlled studies to date demonstrating effective symptom control in SD or vocal tremor using neuropharmacologic agents. However, often clinicians have individual patients who have reported or evidenced significant symptom relief in an unblinded trial. Propranolol (Inderal), a beta-blocker, has been used in treating voice tremor patients to "blunt" the tremor but not significantly reduce it. Trihexyphenidyl HCL (Artane), an anticholinergic, has some benefit when patients have a severe dystonia. Benzotropine mesylate (Cogentin), also an anticholinergic, has provided some patient benefit but little symptom change. Baclofen (Liorsel), a muscle relaxant, has provided some relief in a few individuals but has not significantly eliminated symptoms in patients with SD. Many patients are prescribed diazepam (Valium), a CNS depressant with muscle relaxant effects, or alprazolam (Xanax), a benzodiazepam, to reduce stress resulting from the effects the disorder has on their daily lives.

In general, the role of neuropharmacologic agents in SD has been to provide some patient relief without any demonstrable symptom reduction. Often positive responses are idiosyncratic to a few patients, while most do not report any benefit. Perhaps some patient benefits are caused by suggestion, the presence of psychogenic overlay, or symptom exaggeration. To date, no controlled neuropharmacologic studies have demonstrated significant symptom reduction in SD patients. At present, the role of these medications in the management of SD is only an adjunct to other approaches.

SUMMARY

At present, management techniques for spasmodic dysphonia are only aimed at peripheral control of the voice symptoms. Botulinum toxin and recurrent nerve section have been studied more frequently, and the results with botulinum toxin seem most predictable in adductor SD. However, this treatment is costly and usually requires continued reinjection as long as the patient has the disorder. Improved treatments are needed for vocal tremor and abductor SD. Improved understanding of the etiology and pathophysiology of these disorders are needed to develop long-term and effective treatment alternatives.

REFERENCES

1. Blitzer A, Brin MF, Fahn S, Lovelace RE. Clinical and laboratory characteristics of focal laryngeal dystonia: study of 110 cases. *Laryngoscope.* 1988;98:636-640.

2. Blitzer A, Lovelace RE, Brin MF, Fahn S, Fink ME. Electromyographic findings in focal laryngeal dystonia (spastic dysphonia). *Ann Otol Rhinol Laryngol.* 1985;94:591-594.

3. Blitzer A, Brin MF. Laryngeal dystonia: a series with botulinum toxin therapy. *Ann Otol Rhinol Laryngol.* 1991;100:85-89.

4. Fahn S. Concept and classification of dystonia. Fahn S, ed. *Advances in Neurology: Dystonia.* Vol 50. New York, NY: Raven Press; 1988:1-8.

5. Golper LAC, Nutt JG, Rau MT, Coleman RO. Focal cranial dystonia. *J Speech Hear Disord.* 1983;48:128-134.

6. Jankovic J. Etiology and differential diagnosis of blepharospasm and oromandibular dystonia. Jankovic J, Tolosa E, eds. *Advances in Neurology: Facial Dyskinesias.* Vol 49. New York, NY: Raven Press; 1988:103-117.

7. Jankovic J, Nutt JG. Blepharospasm cranial-cervical dystonia (Meige's syndrome): familial occurrence. Jankovic J, Tolosa E, ed. *Advances in Neurology: Facial Dyskinesias.* Vol 49. New York, NY: Raven Press; 1988:117-123.

8. Lagueny A, Deliac MM, Julien J, Demotes-Mainard J, Ferrer X. Jaw closing spasms—a form of focal dystonia? An electrophysiological study. *J Neurol Neurosurg Psychiatry.* 1989;52:652-655.

9. Sheehy MP, Rothwell JC, Marsden CD. Writer's cramp. Fahn S, ed. *Advances in Neurology: Dystonia.* Vol 50. New York, NY: Raven Press; 1988:457-472.

10. Chan J, Brin MF, Fahn S. Idiopathic cervical dystonia: clinical characteristics. *Movement Dis.* 1991;6:119-126.

11. Tolosa E, Marti MJ. Blepharospasm-oromandibular dystonia syndrome (Meige's syndrome): clinical aspects. Jankovic J, Tolosa E, eds. *Advances in Neurology: Facial Dyskinesias.* Vol 49. New York, NY: Raven Press; 1988:225-237.

12. Berardelli A, Rothwell JC, Day BL, Marsden CD. The pathophysiology of cranial dystonia. Fahn S, ed. *Advances in Neurology: Dystonia.* Vol 50. New York, NY: Raven Press; 1988:525-535.

13. Rosenbaum F, Jankovic J. Task-specific focal tremor and dystonia: categorization of occupational movement disorders. *Neurology.* 1988;38:522-527.

14. Paulson GW, Barnes J. Oral facial dystonia triggered by speech. *Psychosomatics.* 1988;29:236-238.

15. Bloch CS, Hirano M, Gould WJ. Symptom improvement of spastic dysphonia in response to phonatory tasks. *Ann Otol Rhinol Laryngol.* 1985;94:51-54.

16. Golper LE, Nutt JG, Rau MT, Coleman RO. Focal cranial dystonia. *J Speech Hear Disord.* 1983;48:128-134.

17. Gates G. Introduction. *J Voice.* 1992;6.

18. Kramer PL, Heiman GA, Gasser T, et al. The DYT1 gene on 9q34 is responsible for most cases of early limb-onset idiopathic torsion dystonia in non-Jews. *Am J Hum Genet.* 1994;55:468-475.

19. Brin MF, Blitzer A, Stewart C. Laryngeal dystonia (spasmodic dysphonia): observations of 901 patients and treatment with botulinum toxin. *Adv Neurol.* 1998;78:237-52:237-252.

20. Bressman SB, Warner TT, Almasy L, et al. Exclusion of the DYT1 locus in familial torticollis. *Ann Neurol.* 1996;40:681-684.

21. Jankovic J. Post-traumatic movement disorders: central and peripheral mechanisms. *Neurology.* 1994;44:2006-2014.

22. Berry DA, Herzel H, Titze IR, Krischer K. Interpretation of biomechanical simulations of normal and chaotic vocal fold oscillations with empirical eigenfunctions. *J Acoust Soc Am.* 1994;95:3595-3604.

23. Sankhla C, Lai EC, Jankovic J. Peripherally induced oromandibular dystonia. *J Neurol Neurosurg Psychiatry.* 1998;65:722-728.

24. Parnes SM, Lavorato AS, Myers EN. Study of spastic dysphonia using videofiberoptic laryngoscopy. *Ann Otol.* 1978;87:322-326.

25. Morrison MD, Rammage LA. Muscle misuse voice disorders: description and classification. *Acta Otolaryngol (Stockh).* 1993;113:428-434.

26. Morrison MD, Nichol H, Rammage RA. Diagnostic criteria in functional dysphonia. *Laryngoscope.* 1986;96:1-8.

27. Murry T, Cannito MP, Woodson GE. Spasmodic dysphonia. Emotional status and botulinum toxin treatment. *Arch Otolaryngol Head Neck Surg.* 1994;120:310-316.

28. Aronson AE. Importance of the psychosocial interview in the diagnosis and treatment of "functional" voice disorders. *J Voice.* 1990;4:287-289.

29. Aronson AE, Brown JR, Litin EM, Pearson JS. Spastic dysphonia: II. Comparison with essential (voice) tremor and other neurologic and psychogenic dysphonias. *J Speech Hear Disord.* 1968;33:219-231.

30. Aronson AE, Peterson HW, Litin EM. Psychiatric symptomatology in functional dysphonia and aphonia. *J Speech Hear Disord.* 1966;31:115-127.

31. Chevrie-Muller C, Arabia-Guidet C, Pfauwadel MC. Can one recover from spasmodic dysphonia? *Br J Disord Commun.* 1987;22(2)117-128.

32. Aronson AE. *Clinical Voice Disorders: An Interdisciplinary Approach.* 2nd ed. New York, NY: Thieme-Stratton; 1985.

33. Morrison M, Rammage L, Nichol H, Pullan B, May P, Salkeld L. *The Management of Voice Disorders.* San Diego, CA: Singular Publishing Group; 1994.

34. Hertegard S, Granqvist S, Lindestad PA. Botulinum toxin injections for essential voice tremor. *Ann Otol Rhinol Laryngol.* 2000;109:204-209.

35. Busenbark K, Ramig L, Dromey C, Koller WC. Methazolamide for essential voice tremor. *Neurology.* 1996;47:1331-1332.

36. Yoon MS, Munz M, Sataloff RT, Spiegel JR, Heuer RJ. Vocal tremor reduction with deep brain stimulation. *Stereotact Funct Neurosurg.* 1999;72:241-244.

37. Carpenter MA, Pahwa R, Miyawaki KL, Wilkinson SB, Searl JP, Koller WC. Reduction in voice tremor under thalamic stimulation. *Neurology.* 1998;50:796-798.

38. Koda J, Ludlow CL. An evaluation of laryngeal muscle activation in patients with voice tremor. *Otolaryngol Head Neck Surg.* 1992;107:684-696.

39. Izdebski K, Shipp T, Dedo HH. Predicting postoperative voice characteristics of spastic dysphonia patients. *Otolaryngol Head Neck Surg.* 1979;87:428-434.

40. Brodnitz FS. Spastic dysphonia. *Ann Otol Rhinol Laryngol.* 1976;85:210-214.

41. Barton R. The whispering syndrome of hysterical dysphonia. *Ann Otol Rhinol Laryngol.* 1960;69:156-165.

42. Ludlow CL, Schulz GM, Yamashita T, Deleyiannis FW. Abnormalities in long latency responses to superior laryngeal nerve stimulation in adductor spasmodic dysphonia. *Ann Otol Rhinol Laryngol.* 1995;104:928-935.

43. Deleyiannis FW, Gillespie M, Bielamowicz S, Yamashita T, Ludlow CL. Laryngeal long latency response conditioning in abductor spasmodic dysphonia. *Ann Otol Rhinol Laryngol.* 1999;108:612-619.

44. Liu C, Wang N, Chen R, et al. Emotional symptoms are secondary to the voice disorder in patients with spasmodic dysphonia. *General Hospital Psychiatry.* 1998;20:255-259.

45. Murry T, Cannito MP, Woodson GE. Spasmodic dysphonia. Emotional status and botulinum toxin treatment. *Arch Otolaryngol Head Neck Surg.* 1994;120:310-316.

46. Shipp T, Izdebski K, Reed C, Morrissey P. Intrinsic laryngeal muscle activity in a spastic dysphonic patient. *J Speech Hear Disord.* 1985;50:54-59.

47. Schaefer SD, Roark RM, Watson BC, et al. Multichannel electromyographic observations in spasmodic dysphonia patients and normal control subjects. *Ann Otol Rhinol Laryngol.* 1992;101:67-75.

48. Watson BC, Schaefer SD, Freeman FJ, Dembowski J, Kondraske G, Roark R. Laryngeal electromyographic activity in adductor and abductor spasmodic dysphonia. *J Speech Hear Res.* 1991;34:473-482.

49. Van Pelt F, Ludlow CL, Smith PJ. Comparison of muscle activation patterns in adductor and abductor spasmodic dysphonia. *Ann Otol Rhinol Laryngol.* 1994;103:192-200.

50. Nash EA, Ludlow CL. Laryngeal muscle activity during speech breaks in adductor spasmodic dysphonia. *Laryngoscope.* 1996;106:484-489.

51. Bielamowicz S, Ludlow CL. Effects of botulinum toxin on pathophysiology in spasmodic dysphonia. *Ann Otol Rhinol Laryngol.* 2000;109:194-203.

52. Ludlow CL, Van Pelt F, Koda J. Characteristics of late responses to superior laryngeal nerve stimulation in humans. *Ann Otol Rhinol Laryngol.* 1992;101:127-134.

53. Ludlow CL, Schulz GM, Yamashita T, Deleyiannis FWB. Long latency response abnormalities to superior laryngeal nerve stimulation in adductor spasmodic dysphonia. *Ann Otol Rhinol Laryngol.* 1995;104:928-935.

54. Deleyiannis F, Gillespie M, Yamashita T, Bielamowicz S, Ludlow CL. Laryngeal long-latency response conditioning in abductor spasmodic dysphonia. *Ann Otol Rhinol Laryngol.* 1999;108:612-619.

55. Ludlow CL, Naunton RF, Terada S, Anderson BJ. Successful treatment of selected cases of abductor spasmodic dysphonia using botulinum toxin injection. *Otolaryngol Head Neck Surg.* 1991;104:849-855.

56. Cyrus CB, Bielamowicz S, Evans FJ, Ludlow CL. *Adductor muscle activity abnormalities in abductor spasmodic dysphonia.* Presented at the American Academy of Otolaryngology—Head and Neck Surgery, 1999.

57. Tomoda H, Shibasaki H, Kuroda Y, Shin T. Voice tremor: dysregulation of voluntary expiratory muscles. *Neurology.* 1987;37:117-122.

58. Scott AB. Botulinum toxin injection into extraocular muscles as an alternative to strabismus surgery. *Ophthalmology.* 1980;87:10:1044-1049.

59. Scott AB. Botulinum toxin injection of eye muscles to correct strabismus. *Trans Am Ophthalmol Soc.* 1981;LXXIX:734-770.

60. Scott AB, Kennedy RA, Stubbs HA. Botulinum A toxin injection as a treatment for blepharospasm. *Arch Ophthalmol.* 1985;103:347-350.

61. Tsui JK, Eisen LA, Mak E, Carruthers J, Scott A, Calne DB. A pilot study on the use of botulinum toxin in spasmodic torticollis. *Can J Neurol Sci.* 1985;12:314-316.

62. Miller RH, Woodson GE, Jankovic J. Botulinum toxin injection of the vocal fold for spasmodic dysphonia. *Arch Otolaryngol Head Neck Surg.* 1987;113:603-605.

63. Blitzer A, Brin MF, Fahn S, Lovelace RE. Localized injections of botulinum toxin for the treatment of focal laryngeal dystonia (spastic dysphonia). *Laryngoscope.* 1988;98:193-197.

64. Dressler D, Rothwell JC, Marsden CD. Comparing biological potencies of Botox and Dysport with a mouse diaphragm model may mislead. *J Neurology.* 1998;245:332.

65. Hirano M, Ohala J. Use of hooked-wire electrodes for electromyography of the intrinsic laryngeal muscles. *J Speech Hear Res.* 1969;12:362-373.

66. Davidson B, Ludlow CL. Long-term effects of botulinum toxin injections in spasmodic dysphonia. *Otolaryngol Head Neck Surg.* 1996;105:33-42.

67. Adams SG, Hunt EJ, Charles DA, Lang AE. Unilateral versus bilateral botulinum toxin injections in spasmodic dysphonia: acoustic and perceptual results. *J Otolaryngol.* 1993;22:171-175.

68. Maloney AP, Morrison MD. A comparison of the efficacy of unilateral versus bilateral botulinum toxin injections in the treatment of adductor spasmodic dysphonia. *J Otolaryngol.* 1994;23:160-164.

69. NIH consensus development conference statement: clinical use of botulinum toxin. *Arch Neurol.* 1991;48:1294-1298.

70. Ford CN, Bless DM, Lowery JD. Indirect laryngoscopic approach for injection of botulinum toxin in spasmodic dysphonia. *Otolaryngol Head Neck Surg.* 1990;103:752-758.

71. Green DC, Berke GS, Ward PH, Gerratt BR. Point-touch technique of botulinum toxin injection for the treatment of spasmodic dysphonia. *Ann Otol Rhinol Laryngol.* 1992;101:883-887.

72. Castellanos PF, Gates GA, Esselman G, Song F, Vannier MW, Kuo M. Anatomic considerations in botulinum toxin type A therapy for spasmodic dysphonia. *Laryngoscope.* 1994;104:656-662.

73. Greene P, Fahn S, Diamond B. Development of resistance to botulinum toxin A in patients with torticollis. *Mov Disord.* 1994;9:213-217.

74. Siegel LS. Evaluation of neutralizing antibodies to type A, B, E, F botulinum toxins in sera from human recipients of botulinum pentavalent (ABCDE) toxoid. *J Clin Microbiol.* 1989;27:1906-1908.

75. King RB, Ludlow CL, Hallett M. A comparison of neurologic findings in spasmodic dysphonia and voice tremor. *Neurology.* 1991;submitted.

76. Ludlow CL, Hallett M, Rhew K, et al. Therapeutic use of type F botulinum toxin. *New Engl J Med.* 1992;326:349-350.

77. Smith ME, Ford CN. Resistance to botulinum toxin injections for spasmodic dysphonia. *Arch Otolaryngol Head Neck Surg.* 2000;126:533-535.

78. Chen R, Karp BI, Hallett M. Botulinum toxin type F for treatment of dystonia: long-term experience. *Neurology.* 1998;51:1494-1496.

79. Jankovic J, Schwartz K, Donovan DT. Botulinum toxin treatment of cranial-cervical dystonia, spasmodic dysphonia, other focal dystonias and hemifacial spasm. *J Neurol Neurosurg Psychiatry.* 1990;53:633-639.

80. Ludlow CL. Treatment of speech and voice disorders with botulinum toxin. *JAMA.* 1990;264:2671-2675.

81. Ludlow CL, Naunton RF, Sedory SE, Schulz GM, Hallet M. Effects of botulinum toxin injections on speech in adductor spasmodic dysphonia. *Neurology.* 1988;38:1220-1225.

82. Zwirner P, Murry T, Swenson M, Woodson GE. Effects of botulinum toxin therapy in patients with adductor spasmodic dysphonia: acoustic, aerodynamic, and videoscopic findings. *Laryngoscope.* 1992;102:400-406.

83. Truong DD, Rontal M, Rolnick M, Aronson AE, Mistura K. Double-blind controlled study of botulinum toxin in adductor spasmodic dysphonia. *Laryngoscope.* 1991;101:630-634.

84. Ludlow CL, Naunton RF, Fujita M, Sedory SE. Spasmodic dysphonia: botulinum toxin injection after recurrent nerve surgery. *Otolaryngol Head Neck Surg.* 1990;102:122-131.

85. Blitzer A, Brin M, Stewart C, Aviv JE, Fahn S. Abductor laryngeal dystonia: a series treated with botulinum toxin. *Laryngoscope.* 1992;102:163-167.

86. Rontal M, Rontal E, Rolnick M, Merson R, Silverman B, Truong DD. A method for the treatment of abductor spasmodic dysphonia with botulinum toxin injections: a preliminary report. *Laryngoscope.* 1991;101:911-914.

87. Bielamowicz S, Squire S, Bidus K, Ludlow CL. Assessment of posterior cricoarytenoid botulinum toxin injections in patients with abductor spasmodic dysphonia. *Ann Otol Rhinol Laryngol.* In press.

88. Rhew K, Fiedler DA, Ludlow CL. Technique for injection of botulinum toxin through the flexible nasolaryngoscope. *Otolaryngol Head Neck Surg.* 1994;111:787-794.

89. Ludlow CL. Treating the spasmodic dysphonias with botulinum toxin: a comparison of results with adductor and abductor spasmodic dysphonia and vocal tremor. Tsui J, Calne D, eds. *The Dystonias.* New York, NY: Marcel Dekker, Inc; 1995:431-446.

90. Blitzer A, Brin MF, Stewart CF. Botulinum toxin management of spasmodic dysphonia (laryngeal dystonia): a 12-year experience in more than 900 patients. *Laryngoscope.* 1998;108:1435-1441.

91. Weed DT, Jewett BS, Rainey C, et al. Long-term follow-up of recurrent laryngeal nerve avulsion for

the treatment of spastic dysphonia. *Ann Otol Rhinol Laryngol.* 1996;105:592-601.

92. Berke GS, Blackwell KE, Gerratt BR, Verneil A, Jackson KS, Sercarz JA. Selective laryngeal adductor denervation-reinnervation: a new surgical treatment for adductor spasmodic dysphonia. *Ann Otol Rhinol Laryngol.* 1999;108:227-231.

93. Aronson AE, McCaffrey TV, Litchy WJ, Lipton RJ. Botulinum toxin injection for adductor spastic dysphonia: patients' self-ratings of voice and phonatory effort after three successive injections. *Laryngoscope.* 1993;103:683-692.

94. Ludlow CL, Yeh J, Cohen LG, Van Pelt F, Rhew K, Hallett M. Limitations of laryngeal electromyography and magnetic stimulation for assessing laryngeal muscle control. *Ann Otol Rhinol Laryngol.* 1994;103:16-27.

95. Ludlow CL, Bagley JA, Yin SG, Koda J. A comparison of different injection techniques in the treatment of spasmodic dysphonia with botulinum toxin. *J Voice.* 1992;6:380-386.

96. Holds JB, Fogg SG, Anderson RL. Botulinum A toxin injection: failures in clinical practice and a biomechanical system for the study of toxin-induced paralysis. *Ophthal Plast Reconstruct Surg.* 1990;6:252-259.

97. Freuh BR, Felt DP, Wojno TH, Musch DC. Treatment of blepharospasm with botulinum toxin: a preliminary report. *Arch Ophthalmol.* 1984;102:1464-1468.

98. Holds JB, Alderson K, Fogg SG, Anderson RL. Motor nerve sprouting in human orbicularis muscle after botulinum A injection. *Invest Ophthalmol Vis Sci.* 1990;31:964-967.

99. Alderson K, Holds JB, Anderson RL. Botulinum-induced alteration of nerve-muscle interactions in the human orbicularis oculi following treatment for blepharospasm. *Neurology.* 1991;41:1800-1805.

100. Harris CP, Alderson K, Nebeker J, Holds JB, Anderson RL. Histologic features of human orbicularis oculi treated with botulinum A toxin. *Arch Ophthalmol.* 1991;109:393-395.

101. Borodic GE, Ferrante R. Effects of repeated botulinum toxin injections on orbicularis oculi muscle. *J Clin Neuro-Opthalmol.* 1992;12:121-127.

102. Jaffe DM, Solomon NP, Robinson RA, Hoffman HT, Luschei ES. Comparison of concentric needle versus hooked-wire electrodes in the canine larynx. *Otolaryngol Head Neck Surg.* 1998;118:655-662.

103. Dedo HH. Recurrent laryngeal nerve section for spastic dysphonia. *Ann Otol Rhinol Laryngol.* 1976;85:451-459.

104. Levine HL, Wood BG, Batza E, Rusnov M, Tucker HM. Recurrent layngeal nerve section for spasmodic dysphonia. *Ann Otol Rhinol Laryngol.* 1979;88:527-530.

105. Bocchino JV, Tucker HM. Recurrent laryngeal nerve pathology in spasmodic dysphonia. *Laryngoscope.* 1978;88:1274-1278.

106. Barton RT. Treatment of spastic dysphonia by recurrent laryngeal nerve section. *Laryngoscope.* 1979;89:244-249.

107. Fritzell B, Feuer E, Knutsson E, Shiratzki H. Experiences with recurrent laryngeal nerve section for spastic dysphonia. *Folia Phoniat.* 1982;34:160-167.

108. Aronson AE, DeSanto LW. Adductor spastic dysphonia: 1 1/2 years after recurrent laryngeal nerve resection. *Ann Otol Rhinol Laryngol.* 1981;90:2-6.

109. Wilson FB, Oldring DJ, Mueller K. Recurrent laryngeal nerve dissection: a case report involving return of spastic dysphonia after initial surgery. *J Speech Hear Disord.* 1980;45:112-118.

110. Aronson AE, DeSanto LW. Adductor spasmodic dysphonia: three years after recurrent nerve section. *Laryngoscope.* 1983;93:1-8.

111. Netterville JL, Stone RF, Rainey C, Zealear DL, Ossoff RH. Recurrent laryngeal nerve avulsion for treatment of spastic dysphonia. *Ann Otol Rhinol Laryngol.* 1991;100:10-14.

112. Banoub M, Rao U, Motta P, Tetzlaff JE, Eliachar I, Blitzer A. Recurrent postoperative stridor requiring tracheostomy in a patient with spasmodic dysphonia. *Anesthesiology.* 2000;92:893-895.

113. Fritzell B, Hammarberg B, Schiratzki H, Haglund S, Knutsson E, Martensson A. Long-term results of recurrent laryngeal nerve resection for adductor spasmodic dysphonia. *J Voice.* 1993;7:172-178.

114. Dedo HH, Izdebski K. Intermediate results of 306 recurrent laryngeal nerve sections for spastic dysphonia. *Laryngoscope.* 1983;93:9-16.

115. Dedo HH, Izdebski K. Problems with surgical (RLN section) treatment of spasmodic dysphonia. *Laryngoscope.* 1983;93:268-271.

116. Salassa JR, DeSanto LW, Aronson AE. Respiratory distress after recurrent laryngeal nerve section for spastic dysphonia. *Laryngoscope.* 1982;92:240-245.

117. Friedman M, Toriumi DM, Grybauskas VT, Applebaum EL. Implantation of a recurrent laryngeal nerve stimulator for the treatment of spastic dysphonia. *Ann Otol Rhinol Laryngol.* 1989;98:130-134.

118. Tucker HM. Laryngeal framework surgery in the management of spasmodic dysphonia: preliminary report. *Ann Otol Rhinol Laryngol.* 1989;98:52-54.

119. Friedman M, Wernicke JF, Caldarelli DD. Safety and tolerability of the implantable recurrent laryngeal nerve stimulator. *Ann Otol Rhinol Laryngol.* 1994;104:1240-1244.

120. Carpenter RJ, Henley-Cohn JL, Snyder GG. Spastic dysphonia: treatment by selective section of the recurrent laryngeal nerve. *Laryngoscope.* 1979;89:2000-2003.

121. Isshiki N. Recent advances in phonosurgery. *Folia Phoniat.* 1980;32:119-154.

122. Slavit DH, Maragos NE, Lipton RJ. Physiologic assessment of Isshiki type III thyroplasty. *Laryngoscope.* 1990;100:844-848.

123. Rhew K, Ludlow CL. Botulinum toxin injection after type III thyroplasty in spasmodic dysphonia. Unpublished.

124. Isshiki N, Tsuji DH, Yamamoto Y, Iizuka Y. Midline lateralization thyroplasty for adductor spasmodic dysphonia. *Ann Otol Rhinol Laryngol.* 2000;109:187-193.

125. Genack SH, Woo P, Colton RH, Goyette D. Partial thyroarytenoid myectomy: an animal study investigating a proposed new treatment for adductor spasmodic dysphonia. *Otolaryngol Head Neck Surg.* 1993;108:256-264.

126. Roy N, Ford CN, Bless DM. Muscle tension dysphonia and spasmodic dysphonia: the role of manual laryngeal tension reduction in diagnosis and management. *Ann Otol Rhinol Laryngol.* 1996;105:851-856.

127. Murry T, Woodson GE. Combined-modality treatment of adductor spasmodic dysphonia with botulinum toxin and voice therapy. *J Voice.* 1995;9:460-465.

128. Colton RH, Casper JK. *Understanding Voice Problems: A Physiological Perspective for Diagnosis and Treatment.* Baltimore, MD: Williams & Wilkins; 1991.

129. Berstein DA, Borkovec TD. *Progressive Relaxation Training: A Manual for the Helping Professions.* Champaign, IL: Research Press; 1973.

130. Boone DR. Respiratory training in voice therapy. *J Voice.* 1988;2:20-25.

131. Blood G. Efficacy of a computer-assisted voice treatment protocol. *Am J Speech-Lang Pathol.* 1994;3:57-66.

132. Fujita M, Ludlow CL, Woodson GE, Naunton RF. A new surface electrode for recording from the posterior cricoarytenoid muscle. *Laryngoscope.* 1989;99:316-320.

133. Kuna ST, Smickly JS, Insalaco G. Posterior cricoarytenoid muscle activity during wakefulness and sleep in normal adults. *J Appl Physiol.* 1990;68:1746-1754.

134. Cooper M. Stop committing voice suicide. Los Angeles, CA: Voice & Speech Company of America; 1996.

135. Fox S, Trace R. Role of voice therapy varies in SD treatment. *Adv SLP Aud.* 1993;December 20:11-12.

CHAPTER 29

Psychologic Aspects of Voice Disorders

Deborah Caputo Rosen, RN, PhD

Reinhardt J. Heuer, PhD

Steven H. Levy, MD

Robert T. Sataloff, MD, DMA, FACS

The first task of the otolaryngologist treating any patient with a voice complaint is to establish an accurate diagnosis and its etiology. Only as a result of a thorough, comprehensive history and physical examination (including state-of-the-art technology) can the organic and psychologic components of the voice complaint be elucidated. All treatment planning and subsequent intervention depend on this process. However, even minor voice injuries or health problems can be very disturbing for many patients and devastating to some professional voice users. In some cases, they even trigger responses that delay return of normal voice. Such stress, and fear of the evaluation procedures themselves, often heighten the problem and may cloud diagnostic assessment. Moreover, some voice disorders may be entirely psychogenic, and professional psychologic assessment may be required to complete a thorough evaluation.

Although "voice," the newest subspecialty of otolaryngology, now provides a greatly improved standard of care for all patients with voice disorders, most of the advances in this field resulted from interest in and the study of voice professionals. Professional performers are not only demanding, but also remarkably self-analytic. Like athletes, performers have forced health care providers to change our definition of normalcy. Ordinarily, physicians, psychotherapists, and other professionals are granted great latitude in the definition of "normal." For example, if a microsurgeon injures his or her finger, and the hand surgeon restores 95% of function, the surgeon-patient is likely to be satisfied. If the same result occurs in a world class violinist, that last 5% (or 1%) may mean the difference between renown and obscurity. Traditionally, we have not been trained to recognize, let alone quantify and restore, these degrees of physical perfection. Arts medicine practitioners have learned to do so, including those in the field of voice. The process has required advances in scientific knowledge, clinical management, technology for voice assessment, voice therapy, and surgical technique. The drive to expand our knowledge has also led to unprecedented teamwork and interdisciplinary collaboration. As a result, voice care professionals have come to recognize important psychologic problems commonly found in patients with voice disorders. Such problems were ignored in past years. Now they are looked for diligently throughout evaluation and treatment. When identified, they often require intervention by a psychological professional with special knowledge about voice disorders, as well as by a speech-language pathologist (SLP) and other voice team members.

Arts medicine psychologists specializing in the management of performance anxiety are becoming more common, but there are still very few psychological professionals with extensive experience in diagnosing and treating other psychologic concomitants of voice disorders. It is important for the physician and all other members of the voice care team to recognize the importance of psychologic factors in patients with voice disorders and to be familiar with mental health professionals in various disciplines in order to build a multidisciplinary team, generate appropriate referrals, and coordinate optimal patient care.

Psychiatrists are licensed physicians who have completed medical training, residency in psychiatry, and often additional training. They are qualified not only to establish medical and psychiatric diagnoses and provide therapy, but also to prescribe medications. Psychologists make mental health diagnoses, administer psychologic tests, and provide therapy. They do not prescribe medications, but often work closely with a physician (usually a psychiatrist) who may prescribe and help manage psychotropic medications during the course of psychotherapy. Clinical psychologists have a Masters or Doctoral degree in psychology and may have subspecialty training. Other clinical disciplines (ie, social work, nursing, counseling) license graduate-level practitioners to provide psychotherapy. Laryngologists, phoniatrists, and speech-language pathologists are not formally mental health professionals, although all have at least limited training in psychologic diagnosis. Specialty definitions vary from country to country. In the United States, laryngologists are responsible for medical diagnosis and treatment, and voice surgery. They also prescribe any medications needed to treat organic voice problems and occasionally take responsibility for prescribing psychoactive medications. Speech-language pathologists are responsible for behavioral therapy for speech, language, and swallowing disorders. In many other countries, phoniatrists perform behavioral therapy in addition to making diagnoses. Phoniatrists are physicians. Traditionally, in some countries they have been members of an independent specialty that does not include laryngeal surgery. In other countries, they have been subspecialists of otolaryngology. The European Union has recently determined that in the future, in member countries, phoniatry will be a subspecialty of otolaryngology. Both speech-language pathologists and phoniatrists include at least some psychologic assessment and support in their therapeutic paradigms. However, they are not fully trained mental health professionals and must be constantly vigilant to recognize significant psychopathology and recommend appropriate referral for treatment by a psychologist or psychiatrist. Finding a mental health professional familiar with the special needs and problems of voice patients, especially singers and actors, is not easy. Arts medicine psychology is a relatively new field, as was voice care in the early 1980s. Nevertheless, it is usually possible to find a psychological professional who is either knowledgeable or at least interested enough to become knowledgeable. Resources are available in the literature to assist the interested mental health professional,[1] and incorporating such a colleague into the voice care team is extremely beneficial.

PSYCHOLOGY AND VOICE DISORDERS: AN OVERVIEW

Patients seeking medical care for voice disorders come from the general population. Consequently, a normal distribution of comorbid psychopathology can be expected in a laryngology practice. Psychologic factors can be causally related to a voice disorder and/or consequences of vocal dysfunction. In practice, they are usually interwoven.

The essential role of the voice in communication of the "self" creates special potential for psychologic impact. Severe psychologic consequences of voice dysfunction are especially common in individuals in whom the voice is pathologically perceived to be the self, such as professional voice users. However, the sensitive clinician will recognize varying degrees of similar reaction among most voice patients who are confronted with voice change or loss.

Our work with professional voice users has provided insight into the special intensification of psychologic distress they experience in association with lapses in vocal health. This has proved helpful in treating all patients with voice disorders, and has permitted recognition of psychologic problems that may delay recovery following vocal injury or surgery.

Self-esteem comprises not only who we believe we are, but also what we have chosen to do as our life's work. A psychologic double-exposure exists for performers who experience difficulty separating the two elements. The voice is in, is therefore of, indeed, is the self. Aronson's extensive review of the literature supports the maxim that the "voice is the mirror of the personality"—both normal and abnormal. Parameters such as voice quality, pitch, loudness, stress pattern, rate, pauses, articulation, vocabulary, syntax, and content are described as they reflect life stressors, psychopathology, and discrete emotions.[2] Sundberg describes Fonagy's research on the effects of various states of emotion on phonation. These studies revealed specific alterations in articulatory and laryngeal structures and in respiratory muscular activity patterns related to ten different emotional states.[3] Vogel and Carter include descriptive summaries of the features, symptoms, and signs of communication impairment in their text on neurologic and psychiatric disorders.[4] The mind and body are inextricably linked. Thoughts and feelings generate neurochemical transmissions that affect all organ systems. Therefore, not only can disturbances of physical function have profound emotional effects, disturbances of emotion can have profound bodily and artistic effects.

PROFESSIONAL VOICE USERS: SPECIAL CASE

It is useful to understand in greater depth the problems experienced by professional voice users who suffer vocal injuries. Most of our observations in this population occur among singers and actors. However, it must be remembered that, although they are the most obvious and demanding professional voice users, many other professionals are classified as professional voice users. These include: politicians, attorneys, clergy, teachers, salespeople, broadcasters, shop foremen (who speak over noise), football quarterbacks, secretaries, telephone operators, and others. Although we are likely to expect profound emotional reactions to voice problems among singers and actors, many other patients may also demonstrate similar reactions. If we do not recognize these reactions as such, they may be misinterpreted as anger, malingering, or other difficult patient behavior. Some patients are unconsciously afraid that their voices are lost forever and are psychologically unable to make a full effort at vocal recovery after injury or surgery. This blocking of the frightening possibilities by rationalization ("I haven't made a maximum attempt so I don't know yet if my voice will be satisfactory") can result in prolonged or incomplete recovery after technically flawless surgery. It is incumbent upon the laryngologist and other members of the voice team to understand the psychologic consequences of voice disturbance and to recognize them not only in extreme cases, but even in their more subtle manifestations.[1]

Typically, successful professional voice users (especially actors, singers, and politicians) may fall into a personality subtype that is ambitious, driven, perfectionistic, and tightly controlled. Externally, they present themselves as confident, competitive, and self-assured. Internally, self-esteem, the product of personality development, is often far more fragile. Children and adolescents do the best they can to survive and integrate their life experiences, utilizing psychologic defense strategies that develop early in childhood. All psychologic defense mechanisms are means to that end. Most of these defenses are not under conscious control. They are an habitual element of the fabric of one's response to life, especially in stressful or psychologically threatening situations.

All psychologic adjustment expresses itself through the personality of the patient, and it is essential to focus on the personality style of every performer who seeks psychologic help. This can best be done during psychologic assessment and evaluation by exploring daily activities, especially those pertaining to the performer's involvement with his/her art, the patient's growth and personality development as an artist, and relationships with people both within and outside his/her performing environment. Each developmental phase carries inherent coping tasks and responsibilities, which can play an important part in the patient's emotional response to vocal dysfunction. Learning about, valuing highly, and managing our unique, individual psychologic vulnerabilities are critical to adaptive psychologic function throughout life.

Research into body image theory provides a theoretical basis for understanding the special impact of stress or injuries to the voice in vocal performers. The body is essential to perception, learning, and memory and the body serves as a sensory register and processor of sensory information.[5] Body experience is deeply personal and constitutes a private world typically shared with others only under conditions of closest intimacy. Moreover, the body is an expressive instrument, the medium through which individuality is communicated verbally and nonverbally.[5] It is therefore possible to anticipate direct correspondence between certain physical illness or injury and body and self-image. Among these are psychosomatic conditions and/or body states with high levels of involvement of personality factors. In these cases, body illness or injury may reactivate psychopathologic processes that began in early childhood or induce an emotional disorder such as denial or inappropriately prolonged depression.[5] Psychologic reactions to a physical injury are not uniformly disturbing or distressing and do not necessarily result in maladjustment. However, Shontz[5] notes that reactions to body injury are more a function of how much anxiety is generated by the experience than by the actual location, severity, or type of injury itself.

Human beings are remarkably adaptive and capable of living with most types of difficulties, injuries, or disabilities if they feel there is a good reason for doing so. If one's life has broad meaning and purpose, any given disorder takes on less significance. When a physical disability or any given body part becomes the main focus of concern or has been the main source of self-esteem in a person's life, that life becomes narrowed and constricted. Patients adapt satisfactorily to a personal medical condition when the problems of living related to the injury cease to be the dominant element in their total psychologic life.

A unique closeness exists between one's body and one's identity; this body-self is a central part of self-concept. The interdependence of body image and self-esteem means that distortion of one will affect the other. The cognitive-behavioral model for understanding body image includes the perceptual and affective components, as well as attitudinal ones. From the cognitive perspective, any body image producing dysphonia results from irrational thoughts, unrealistic expectations, and faulty explanations.[6] Body-image constructs and their affective and cognitive outcomes relate to personality types and cognitive styles. For example, depressive personality types chronically interpret events in terms of deficiencies and are trapped by habitual self-defeating thoughts. Anxious personality types chronically overestimate risks and become hypervigilant. These types of cognitive errors generate automatic thoughts which intensify body-image-related psychopathology.[1]

It is the task of personality theorists to explain the process of the genesis of the self. There are numerous coherent personality theories, all substantially interrelated. The framework of Karen Horney (1885-1952) is particularly useful in attempting to understand the creative personality and its vulnerabilities. In simplification, she formulated a "holistic notion of the personality as an individual unit functioning within a social framework and continually interacting with its environment."[7] In Horney's model, there are three selves. The actual self is the sum total of the individual's experience; the real self is responsible for harmonious integration; and the idealized self sets up unrealistically high expectations which, in the face of disappointment, result in self-hatred and self-alienation. We have chosen Horney's theory as a working model in evolving therapeutic approaches to the special patient population of professional voice users. They are the laryngologist's most demanding consumers of voice care and cling to their physician's explanations with dependency.[1,8]

It may be useful, for theoretical clarity, to divide the experience of vocal injury into several phases. In practice, however, these often overlap or recur and the emotional responses are not entirely linear.

- The phase of problem recognition. The patient feels that something is wrong, but may not be able to clearly define the problem, especially if the onset has been gradual or masked by a coexisting illness. Usually, personal "first aid" measures will be tried, and when they fail, the performer will manifest some level of panic. This is often followed by feelings of guilt when the distress is turned inward against the self, or rage or blame when externalized.

- The phase of diagnosis. This may be a protracted period if an injured performer does not have immediate access to a laryngologist experienced in the assessment of vocal injury. He or she may have already consulted with voice teachers, family physicians, allergists, nutritionists, peers, or otolaryngologists and speech-language pathologists without specialized training in caring for professional voice users. There may have been several, possibly contradictory, diagnoses and treatment protocols. The vocal dysfunction persists, and the patient grows more fearful and discouraged. If attempts to perform are continued, they may exacerbate the injury and/or produce embarrassing performances. The fear is of the unknown, but it is intuitively perceived as significant.

- The phase of treatment: acute/rehabilitative. Now, fear of the unknown becomes fear of the known, and of its outcome. The performer, now in the sick role, initially feels overwhelmed and powerless. There is frequently a strong component of blame that may be turned inward. "Why me, why now?" is the operant, recurrent thought. Vocal rehabilitation is an exquisitely slow, carefully monitored, frustrating process, and many patients become fearful and impatient. Some will meet the criteria for major depression, which is discussed in additional detail, as is the impact of vocal fold surgery.

- The phase of acceptance. When the acute and rehabilitative treatment protocol is complete, the final prognosis is clearer. When there are significant lasting changes in the voice, the patient will experience mourning. Even when there is full return of vocal function, a sense of vulnerability lingers. These individuals are likely to adhere strictly, even ritualistically, to preventive vocal hygiene habits and may be anxious enough to become hypochondriacal.[1,8,9]

The psychological professional providing care to this special population must be well versed in developmental psychology, be experienced in the world of the performer, and retain an unshakable empathy for the patient who has experienced the psychologically disorganizing impact of vocal injury. It is critical to harken back to one of the earliest lessons taught to all psychotherapists in training. That is, the therapist must, through accurate empathy, earn the right to make interpretations and interventions. When this type of insightful and accurate support is available to the professional voice user, the psychotherapist may well be the patient's rudder in the rough seas of diagnosis, treatment, and rehabilitation.

PSYCHOGENIC VOICE DISORDERS

Voice disorders are divided into organic and non-organic etiologies. Various terms have been used interchangeably (but imprecisely) to label observable vocal dysfunction in the presence of emotional factors which cause or perpetuate the symptoms. Aronson argues convincingly for the term *psychogenic*, which is "broadly synonymous with functional, but has the advantage of stating positively, based on an exploration of its causes, that the voice disorder is a manifestation of one or more types of psychological disequilibrium, such as anxiety, depression, conversion reaction, or personality disorder, that interfere with normal volitional control over phonation."[2]

Psychogenic disorders include a variety of discrete presentations. There is disagreement over classification among speech-language pathologists, with some excluding musculoskeletal tension disorders from this heading. Aronson and Butcher et al conclude that the hypercontraction of extrinsic and intrinsic laryngeal muscles, in response to emotional stress, is the "common denominator" behind the dysphonia or aphonia in these disorders.[2,10] In addition, the extent of pathology visible on laryngeal examination is inconsistent with the severity of the abnormal voice. They cite four categories:

1. *Musculoskeletal tension disorders*: including vocal abuse, vocal nodules, contact ulcers, and ventricular phonation

2. *Conversion voice disorders*: including conversion muteness and aphonia, conversion dysphonia, and psychogenic adductor spastic dysphonia

3. *Mutational falsetto* (puberphonia)

4. *Childlike speech in adults*

Psychogenic dysphonia often presents as total inability to speak, whispered speech, extremely strained or strangled speech, interrupted speech rhythm, or speech in an abnormal register (such as falsetto in a male). Usually, involuntary vocalizations during laughing and coughing are normal. The vocal folds are often difficult to examine because of supraglottic hyperfunction. There may be apparent bowing of both vocal folds consistent with severe muscular tension dysphonia, creating anterior-posterior "squeeze" during phonation. Long-standing attempts to produce voice in the presence of this pattern may even result in traumatic lesions associated with vocal abuse patterns, such as vocal fold nodules. Normal abduction and adduction of the vocal folds may be visualized during flexible fiberoptic laryngoscopy by instructing the patient to perform maneuvers that decrease supraglottic load, such as whistling or sniffing. In addition, the singing voice is often more easily produced than the speaking voice in these patients. Tongue protrusion and stabilization during the rigid telescopic portion of the examination will often result in clear voice. The severe muscular tension dysphonia associated with psychogenic dysphonia can often be eliminated by behavioral interventions by the speech-language pathologist, sometimes in one session. In many instances moments of successful voice have been restored during stroboscopic examination.

Electromyography may be helpful in confirming the diagnosis by revealing simultaneous firing of abductors and adductors. Psychogenic dysphonia has been frequently misdiagnosed as spasmodic dysphonia, partially explaining the excellent spasmodic dysphonia cure rates in some series.

Psychogenic voice disorders are not merely the absence of observable neurolaryngeal abnormalities. This psychiatric diagnosis cannot be made with accuracy without the presence of a psychodynamic formulation based on understanding of the personality, motivations, conflicts, and primary as well as secondary gain associated with the symptoms.[1,11,12]

Conversion disorders are a special classification of psychogenic symptomatology and reflect loss of voluntary control over striated muscle or the sensory systems as a reflection of stress or psychologic conflict. They may occur in any organ system, but the target organ is often symbolically related to the specifics of the unconsciously perceived threat. The term was first used by Freud to describe a defense mechanism that rendered an intolerable wish or drive innocuous by translating its energy into a physical symptom. The presence of an ego-syntonic physical illness offers primary gain: relief from the anxiety, depression, or rage by maintaining the emotional conflict in the unconscious. Secondary gain often occurs by virtue of the sick role.

Classic descriptions of findings in these patients include indifference to the symptoms, chronic stress, suppressed anger, immaturity and dependency, moderate depression, and poor sex role identification.[12,13] Conversion voice disorders also reflect a breakdown in communication with some of the emotional significance in the patient's life; wanting but blocking the verbal expression of anger, fear, or remorse, and significant feelings of shame.[1,2]

Confirmed neurologic disease and psychogenic voice disorders do coexist and are known as somatic compliance.[14,15] Of course, potential organic causes of psychiatric disorders must always be thoroughly ruled out. Insidious onset of depression, personality changes, anxiety, or presumed conversion symptoms may be the first presentation of central nervous system (CNS) disease.[16]

THE SPEECH-LANGUAGE PATHOLOGIST'S ROLE IN TREATING PSYCHOLOGIC DISTURBANCES IN PATIENTS WITH VOICE DISORDERS

Speech-language pathology is a relatively new profession in the United States. Its roots are in psychology. The original members of the field came primarily from a psychology background. Early interest in the psychologic aspects of voicing are evidenced in texts such as *The Voice of Neurosis.*[17] Luchsinger and Arnold present an excellent review of the early literature in their text, *Voice-Speech-Language.*[18] At the present time, speech-language pathologists need to be familiar with models of treatment from the psychological tradition, the medical tradition, and the educational tradition. When discussing the speech-language pathologist's role in managing functional voice problems, it must be made clear at the outset that the speech-language pathologist does not work in isolation but as part of a team, including, at a minimum, a laryngologist and speech-language pathologist. Singing instructors, acting instructors, stress specialists, psychologists, neurologists, and psychiatrists must be readily available and cognizant of the special needs of voice patients.

Psychology is defined as the study of human behavior, and the speech-language pathologist's role in treating voice-disordered patients is normalizing the patient's speaking and communication behavior. In this sense, all the activities of speech-language pathologists with voice-disordered patients are psychologic. The purpose of this chapter is not to present a full description of the role of the speech-language pathologist but to describe those areas in which the speech-language pathologist must deal with issues not directly related to the physical vocal mechanism. However, a brief overview of the activities engaged in by the speech-language pathologist and the voice patient help set the groundwork for a discussion of psychologic issues. A more detailed description has been published elsewhere.[19]

Preparation for Treatment

The speech-language pathologist must be aware of, and able to, interpret the findings of the laryngologist, including strobovideolaryngoscopy. Particular attention should be paid to findings demonstrating muscle tension or lack of glottic closure not associated with organic or physical changes. The perceptions of the laryngologist regarding organic and functional aspects of the patient need to be known.

A case history is taken, reviewing and amplifying the case history reported by the laryngologist. The case history should include but not be limited to the topics summarized in Table 29-1.

Subjective and objective measures of the patient's vocal mechanism and communication skills need to be obtained, including, but not limited to, the parameters listed in Table 29-2.

The speech-language pathologist should be able to develop a plan of behavioral changes. The case history provides an adequate sample of the patient's voice use in an interview situation. It is important to note how the patient's voice changes when talking about certain topics and to note evidence of improvement or fatigue as the interview proceeds. It provides data on what speaking activities are most important to the patient and which may need to be addressed initially in therapy. It provides information of the patient's willingness to talk about stressful issues or needs beyond direct focus on voicing and speech skills, which may be important regarding referral to other specialists dealing with stress and emotional or physical health. It establishes an initial rapport, or lack of it, with the clinician that may predict success, or failure, in therapeutic intervention. It also provides the speech-language pathologist with a sample of the patient's communication style and verbosity.

The physical assessment provides the speech-language clinician with objective support for what the clinician has heard and information about how the patient is producing the voice. As behavioral change instituted during the therapy is based on eradication of symptoms of maladaptive voice or communication, to list and evaluate confirmed symptoms at this stage lead to the development of an overall therapeutic plan. Focus should be initially on identification of the underlying behavior or behaviors responsible for maintaining the current voice. Early attention to these underlying behaviors reduces the length of therapy and should predict improvement of voicing.

Therapeutic Stage

Information giving is essential at the beginning and throughout the course of therapy. Patients need to know the reason(s) for the activities in which they are engaging and why these activities are important in changing their current voice problem. Without a thorough understanding of the reasons for changing behavior the probabilities of behavioral change are reduced.

The patient needs to know that a voice disorder is not usually caused by a single agent, but is rather a combination of physical changes, such as communication demands on the voice, the patient's skills in producing speech, and the patient's attempts to compensate for

1. Circumstances surrounding the onset, development, and progress of the voice disorder, including:

   • illnesses of the patient
   • recent changes in employment
   • speaking responsibilities associated with the patient's employment
   • effects of the voice disorder on employment
   • employment environment
   • speaking activities outside of employment
   • environment in which social speaking activities occur
   • effects of the voice disorder on social exchange and social activities
   • activities the patient has had to give up because of voice disorder
   • illness or difficulty among family members or friends
   • stress factors at work and at home
   • methods of dealing with stress

2. Exploration of the social structure of the patient and environment, including:

   • family and living arrangements
   • friends and social gathering places
   • relationships with co-workers and superiors

3. The patient's response to the voice disorder needs to be explored as follows:

   • what bothers the patient most about the voice disorder?
   • what has the patient done to change voicing and how effective have these attempts been?
   • estimates of the speaking times at work and socially, now and before the voice disorder.
   • how does the patient feel about speaking at the present time—stressed, indifferent, depressed, challenged?

4. General health issues should be addressed:

   • chronic illness, including asthma, allergies, diabetes, thyroid dysfunction, chronic fatigue
   • head and neck trauma, including whiplash, concussion, spinal degeneration, temporomandibular joint disease, facial injury
   • surgery
   • high fevers
   • nonvocal symptoms, including swallowing difficulty, pain on speaking or swallowing, numbness, neck stiffness or reduced range of motion, voice quality, speaking rate, movement limitations of the articulators, nasal regurgitation, tremor or shakiness

5. Medications

   • prescription medications
   • over-the-counter drugs, including nonsteroidal anti-inflammatory drugs (NSAIDs), cough drops, decongestants, antihistamines, mouthwash, vitamins, alcohol, tobacco and caffeine products, and water intake.

TABLE 29-1. *The History*

1. Average fundamental frequency and loudness of the patient's conversational voice.

2. Average fundamental frequency, loudness, and speaking rate during a selected reading passage, both in normal reading and in the professional voice (if a professional speaker).

3. Acoustic and aerodynamic measures of sustained vowels, including:

   • measures of perturbation

   • measures of breathiness and noise

   • measures of vocal breaks and quality change

   • measures of airflow

   • measures of glottic pressure

4. Preferred breathing patterns for speech:

   • shallow, deep, appropriate for phrase length

   • clavicular, thoracic, abdominal, or mixed

   • coordination with voicing—exhalation initiated before voicing, glottic closure prior to initiation of exhalation

   • coordinated breath/voicing

5. Neck and laryngeal use:

   • positioning of the larynx during speech—high, low, inflexible

   • tension in the extralaryngeal muscles, particularly the omohyoid

   • laryngeal/hyoid space—present, reduced

   • position of the hyoid—tipped, tense, discomfort on palpation of the cornu

6. Use of the articulators:

   • Oral examination, including lip movements and symmetry, tongue movements and symmetry, palatal sufficiency in nonspeech contexts, diadochokinetic rates

   • ability to separate jaw and anterior tongue activity during the production of /l/, /t/, /d/, /n/

   • tongue tension during speech

   • jaw tension and jaw jutting during speech

   • looseness of temporomandibular joint during speech movements

TABLE 29-2. *Vocal Function Assessment*

vocal changes. The initial goal in therapy is to manage communicative demands and improve the patient's ability to produce more normal voice. Reassessment of the need for medical/surgical interventions for physical changes is planned with the patient. Reassurance is provided that the goal of therapy is not to change personality or limit communication opportunities, but to return these at least to the level of communication enjoyed prior to the onset of the voice problem.

Patients need to be educated regarding their current breathing pattern. It may be insufficient for the demands placed on the patient's voice or a contributor to increased tension in the vocal mechanism. Abdominal breathing is the natural and preferred method of breathing by the body. Abdominal breathing is not a new skill. Patients engage in abdominal breathing when they are relaxed and when they are sleeping.

Patients need to be informed that predominately clavicular or thoracic breathing is usually the product of stress, a societal preference toward tight clothing, and/or demands by parents, teachers, and society in maintaining a tight tucked-in stomach. All these factors lead to a reduction of abdominal release during inhalation that leads to restriction in diaphragmatic downward motion and maximal inflation of the lungs. Suggested techniques for teaching effective, relaxed breathing may be found in Appendix 29-1.

Instruction in behavior is provided so that the patient understands that the vocal folds are opened by the flow of air from the lungs and closed because of their own elasticity and Bernoulli's principle. The vocal folds are vibrating much too rapidly to be manipulated by laryngeal effort, and patients need to comprehend that the emotional system and the conscious speech system share control of voicing, which varies with emotional context. The patient needs to know that laryngeal control is primarily automatic and that efforts to produce voice are counterproductive. The quality of the patient's voice during physiologic sound-making, such as laughter, and a gentle cough can predict the quality of sound when extra effort is removed. Humming and sighing are also effective means of demonstrating the effect of reduced effort. Modeling by the clinician of easy, well-supported, well-resonated voice during these conversations can be a highly effective means of modifying the patient's vocal production in the therapy setting. Suggested techniques for teaching these aspects of efficient, relaxed voice production are included in Appendix 29-1.

A pattern of frequent tension checks needs to be established with the cooperation of the client. These need not be elaborate warm-up exercises or cool-down practice. The patient may decide to practice abdominal breathing in the shower, blowing the water away from his/her face, or humming with a relaxed jaw while inhaling the warm steamy air. The patient may be able to stroke the face, jaw, or neck at each stop light while driving to or from work or take an easy belly breath followed by a relaxed sigh. The patient may check his/her jaw tension before picking up the telephone to say "hello." A brief reminding note can be taped to the inside of the telephone receiver.

Abdominal breathing can be practiced leaning over the desk while reading memos or correcting examination papers. A sip of water between tasks can help the patient focus on relaxation of the jaw or throat and can be preceded by a deep abdominal inhalation. The patient can be very creative and very helpful in identifying times when correct vocal behavior can be practiced. Multiple reminders during the busy day can be more effective than a half-hour practice in the isolation of the patient's home and more likely to be done.

All these exercises are helpful in aiding the patient to become aware of the subtle nature of tension in the speaking mechanism, but may be overwhelmed by overriding tension not associated directly with speaking behavior in the face and neck. A decision must be made as to whether the speech-language pathologist has the skill to develop a more stringent relaxation regimen or if the patient needs, and is amenable to, a referral to an expert in stress management.

A discussion of relevant and irrelevant talking is necessary if the patient talks excessively. The patient needs to know that total vocal rest, if extended past a week, can lead to muscle atrophy and additional voice problems. The concept of vocal naps during the day and the possibility of reducing talking, or more positively, becoming a better listener in noisy environments, should be introduced. The patient is more knowledgeable than the therapist as to when and how long these quiet times can be inserted into the daily schedule.

Patients under stress will bring their "job-voice" home with them. The patient will often complain that family members nag about the use of too loud a voice, of being too demanding, or of using too many directions. A vocal nap during the ride home with an added cool-down protocol can be helpful in providing a positive transition. The patient should be reminded that singing in the car over the noise of traffic and radio and engine noises can be abusive.

The patient needs to know that most people utilize visual cues (lip read) in noisy environments. If the patient has been successful in developing open oral resonance and articulation patterns, the ability of the patient's listeners to understand in noisy situations is enhanced. A slower rate of talking is also helpful in improving comprehension. The patient should be instructed in the effective use of light to highlight his/her face during such conversations.

Voice patients under stress often violate the rules of conversation, including rules of relevance, brevity, and turn taking. A discussion of these rules may lead to an awareness of inappropriate communication patterns or the revelation of an underlying personality difficulty that may lead to a referral to a psychological professional. Often persons with difficulty in personal relationships and/or coping with their circumstances can admit to a voice disorder, but not the underlying personal difficulties. The experience of voice therapy, especially supportive rather than prescriptive voice therapy, may lead to the acceptance of a referral to a professional trained in dealing with these underlying difficulties that might have been rejected at initial interview. The combination of an inability to relax following focal voice exercises, an inability to modify communication behaviors, a tendency for the patient to revert to discussions of personal problems rather than focus on the process on communication, all assist the therapist in reinforcing the idea that the patient's problem lies outside the realm of traditional voice therapy. A statement by the therapist such as, "You have very real problems, but I am not trained to deal with them. I know someone who can help you," can be the beginning of a successful referral.

Finally, the patient needs to know that voice therapy is short term and finite. The goal of therapy is to identify underlying behavioral, emotional, and physical factors, modify current vocal behaviors, and develop better communication skills. The therapist must be aware that the stressed patient can develop inappropriate dependence upon the therapist. If therapy sessions begin to focus more on the patient's day-to-day personal problems than on voice, the time for psychologic referral is long past. Patients need to know that voice therapy usually is successful in only a few sessions, unless there are other problems that maintain the maladaptive vocal behavior. The therapeutic goal in these cases is to identify the underlying problems and make the appropriate referrals. This is a difficult concept for some patients, particularly singers, who are used to taking singing lessons most of their life.

Patients often respond to a voice change by struggling to continue to use their voices in their daily jobs. Teachers will continue to teach, preachers will continue to preach, and sales personnel will continue to sell. The fear of losing their livelihood drives them to modify their speaking techniques, usually applying extra effort, which results in fatigue, pain, and progressive voice loss. They will stop doing enjoyable leisure activities that involve talking and begin to feel impoverished both personally and socially. Feelings of self-worth are also diminished. They feel as though they are not doing their job as well as possible and often consider job changes that do not suit their training or skills.

The speech-language pathologist (SLP) can be very helpful in reducing these feelings by focusing on a plan to return the patient to comfortable functioning in his/her current occupation. If the patient is successful in modifying the effortful and compromised voice using the techniques described above, these reactions subside. The SLP should develop a therapeutic program that will provide the most rapid return of better voicing. The patient needs to be evaluated for the key elements producing vocal fatigue and vocal quality changes. A program of vocal hygiene that can alleviate environmental and behavioral stresses in the workplace, a program of reasonable vocal rest during the workday, and the initiation of a program which will reinstate the balance between respiratory, voicing, and resonance effort in vocal technique are very important. A timetable of when the patient can resume specific activities or when the treatment program will be reviewed to assess alternate treatment options gives the patient something to work

toward. Selected practical aspects of voice therapy are reviewed in Appendix 29-1.

EXAMPLES OF PSYCHOLOGIC ASPECTS OF VOICE DISORDERS

Case 1

Case 1 had been a fifth-grade schoolteacher for 20 years. She denied having any previous voice problems, other than vocal fatigue by the end of the week at the end of the school year. She also assisted her husband, a pediatrician, as his receptionist during evening office hours. However, she now presented with progressive hoarseness. She was diagnosed with vocal fold swelling, gastroesophageal reflux laryngitis, and pinpoint vocal nodules by a laryngologist. She was seen by a speech-language pathologist one month prior to the end of the school year.

Case history revealed important life differences. The previous summer the regular receptionist at her husband's office had taken a maternity leave, and she had volunteered her services over the summer months. It was a busy office, and she spent many hours on the telephone and talking with patients. Her voice did not feel rested at the beginning of the school year.

Because of her excellent teaching record she had been assigned a student teacher who required a great deal of counseling, typically after school hours. She found herself rushing from school to her husband's office without time to eat. She began eating after office hours, experiencing heartburn and disrupted sleep. Her voice was worse in the morning and even more fatigued after the school day. She was physically tired before the day began. She had been given a prescription for ranitidine (Zantac), but did not believe it was helping her.

She noted that her students, her husband, and the patients at her husband's office complained that she was "yelling at them." She was very worried about her ability to continue teaching with "no voice." She was worried about the status of her marriage. She was seriously considering quitting teaching but was ambivalent because she really enjoyed teaching and felt she had a great deal to give both to her students and student teachers. She felt that engaging in voice therapy would only complicate her already busy schedule. She stated: "The harder I try, the worse things seem to get." She then cried.

Evaluation of her voice revealed a shallow thoracic breathing pattern. She had developed a pattern of taking a quick breath and holding it prior to initiation of voicing, resulting in glottal attack rates of 54% (normal 15%). Her voice was loud, low pitched, and rough. She was using a tense jaw, jutting forward during speech. These characteristics were even worse when demonstrating her current teaching voice. She felt her voice was very different in the classroom now than before her voice problems began.

The following therapeutic plan was developed. Direct voice therapy was deferred until July following the end of school and a brief vacation. In the meantime she was urged to continue using the ranitidine and to institute a more rigorous program to control her reflux. The matter of paperwork was discussed. She decided not to take a new student teacher in the fall, but to try to teach.

Therapy in July focused on reducing vocal effort, reestablishing abdominal breathing, reducing glottal stopping, jaw relaxation, and open oral resonance for loudness. Classroom teaching materials were used for exercises. She was able to modify her vocal behaviors easily, although she continued to voice concern about her ability to use them in the classroom. A probable set of voice rests during the school day was discussed and cool-down procedures to implement on the trip to the office were planned. At the end of the therapy, review by the laryngologist demonstrated a reduction in the size of the vocal nodules, resolution of vocal swelling, and reduced reflux findings. She decided to try teaching but was still worried. A plan was developed to see her for therapeutic review two weeks into the school year, then, as needed, mid-fall, at winter break, at spring break, and at the end of the school year. If she felt she did not need to come in, she would call and report how her voice was progressing.

At the meeting two weeks into the school year, she reported that she was "surviving." She was still concerned about whether she was using her voice correctly. Through discussion, she decided she would enlist her students as monitors, particularly for loudness. During the fall, she called to say she was doing well. Her voice was strong and she was much less tired. She reported that her class had taken their role in monitoring her voice very enthusiastically and seriously. Her admission of voice problems and need for help had become an advantage for noise control in her classroom and in student/teacher interactions. She was planning to develop a vocal hygiene section in her curriculum.

At winter break, she reported her voice was not as fatigued and she was eagerly looking forward to return to teaching after the break.

At spring break, she no longer experienced vocal fatigue. Glottal attack remained under 10%. She was sleeping all night. Her reflux appeared to be under control. She was dismissed from therapy but reminded to contact the therapist if she experienced any problems.

Some patients appear to react to life stresses by overuse of their voices and excessive tension focused in the speaking mechanism. They may consider themselves talkative and congenial persons but actually talk constantly, rapidly, or in an excessively loud voice. They appear to be afraid of silence or afraid that if they give up their turn to talk they will not be able to talk again. They often complain of pain and tension in the neck and jaw or of a feeling of breathlessness. They may seek treatment when their inappropriate speaking patterns lead to benign lesions of the larynx or when some other organic change in the vocal mechanism causes their voice to break down. Modeling slower, softer voicing and turn-taking during therapeutic sessions can be very helpful in reducing these vocal faults and providing a more reasonable speaking pattern. The development of relaxation programs for the face and neck to be used frequently during the day is useful. Discussions of the rules of discourse (how to behave and interact during discussions) may be helpful.

Some patients bring with them a severe overall body reaction to the stresses of their life. They complain of fatigue, sleeplessness, tension, and pain. They are unable to turn off their "work voice" at home. They complain of lack of time to complete all the activities with which they are engaged. Standard therapeutic procedures often are ineffective because they are unable to distinguish the subtle changes in support, voicing, or resonation caused by the overriding levels of general tension. They appear to be out of harmony with their body. Focal relaxation of the vocal mechanism is unsuccessful. They usually deny having emotional problems and have difficulty dealing with daily stress, but continue to return to nonvocal issues during the course of therapy. The SLP can be helpful in allowing these patients to experience a supportive one-on-one relationship as a prelude to referral to a psychologic professional. Often after several sessions with the SLP protesting that, "We are talking about issues I am not able to help you with, but Dr. X can," the patient is receptive to referral. Often referral to a stress manager or professional trained in Feldenkreis or Alexander technique or some other relaxation/body awareness method can be useful. The patient may return to the SLP following resolution of some of these issues. The SLP needs to be careful not to continue the therapeutic relationship so long as the patient becomes dependent on an ineffectual but sympathetic ear.

Case 2

Case 2 presented with a large hemorrhagic cyst on one vocal fold and a reactive lesion directly opposite the cyst on the other vocal fold. She was married and had an adopted son. She was a grade school teacher. She had been forced to take a sabbatical because her voice had deteriorated. On evaluation she presented with a loud, hoarse voice with frequent glottal attacks and frequent aphonic breaks. She was extremely verbal with frequent run-on sentences and sentence revisions. She demonstrated a pattern of taking a rapid, large chest breath followed by holding the breath with her larynx at the end of inhalation. She demonstrated excessive tension in the speech musculature. Her conversational style was repetitious. Interestingly, her teacher's voice was better controlled. She admitted that yelling at a sporting event probably caused the cyst. She was seen prior to surgery. Therapy consisted in promoting a softer, more breathy voice. The combination of being relieved from teaching duties and modifying voicing behaviors was successful in eliminating the reactive lesion. Surgery for the hemorrhagic cyst was planned and carried out successfully. She was able to complete a week of voice rest following the surgery. The following weeks of gradual increased voice use were difficult for her. Therapy focused on reducing glottal attacks, improving breath support, and monitoring loudness. Materials included readings and repeated sentences and phrases. Materials from her classroom texts were used in preparation for her return to the classroom. She made excellent progress. However, when therapy moved to monitoring her new skills in general conversation, it became clear that she was unable to recognize her loudness level, control her excessive talking, or identify hard glottal attack.

She returned to school and was seen on a limited schedule similar to that used with the previously described patient. She complained of continued vocal fatigue and hoarseness. She developed a pattern of bringing small gifts. She had limited success in developing self-monitoring skills outside of controlled materials or classroom activities. She successfully completed the school year with no return of vocal fold masses. However, her monitoring skills and general levels of tension remained unchanged. The termination of therapy was discussed. She was very anxious about the termination, citing the continued fatigue and difficulties in monitoring her speech outside the classroom. It was suggested that emotional factors might play a role in her lack of success in changing these behaviors and that she might wish to begin seeing the psychologist associated with the practice. At this point, she admitted to a long history of both physical and verbal abuse, first from her father and then from her husband. It became clear that her failures in therapy led to criticism by the therapist that satisfied her unconscious need for abuse.

PATIENTS WITH APHONIA

As illustrated in the following case, there appear to be four categories of patients who have little voicing capability in the absence of structural or neurologic etiology. These include: whispered voice; tense aphonia with intermittent squeaky, high-pitched syllables or words (often misdiagnosed as spasmodic dysphonia); low-pitched, rough, strangled voice quality; and voluntary muteness.

Cases 3 and 4 describe patients with whispered voice without vocal paralysis, vocal injury, or other pathology. Usually the vocal folds of such patients appear to be normal. Initial case history may or may not reveal psychologic trauma associated with the onset of the aphonia. Nonspeech sounds such as cough, laugh, cry, and throat clearing are present and normal. These sounds can often be extended gradually into speech with the help of a therapist. If the patient is ready to give up the aphonic behavior, therapy is relatively brief, often obtaining normal voice within one session.

Case 3

Case 3 presented with a loud strained whispered voice. The laryngologist had found no laryngeal pathology. Case history revealed no changes in lifestyle, or environment, at the time of onset. However, the voice problem began about one year after her husband's retirement as owner and manager of a large grocery store. The family lived in a small town some distance from any cultural area. She felt the voice loss was related to a bad cold and allergy she had experienced at the time of onset. Normal voice was observed during throat clearing, coughing, and laughter. When asked "what bothered her about her voice loss," she answered, "I can't talk to my friends!"

Therapy consisted of extending the throat clear to "ah" to "hum" to longer and longer "hum-m-m-m" sounds. She was then able to produce the "hum" which was extended into single "m" words. At this point, she reverted to a whisper. The process was repeated with additional focus on relaxed production. This time she was able to extend to days of the week, counting, short phrases, sentences and, finally, conversation. It is not unusual to have to start at the beginning several times with these patients. She was very relieved and thankful to be able to talk again. During the ensuing conversation, she said: "Now, maybe he will let me rejoin my bridge club." When re-questioned about changes in her lifestyle, she admitted that since her husband's retirement her life had changed extensively. She had thought, however, that it was only part of what to expect when one's spouse retired. He had begun to criticize her housekeeping in the same managerial style he used with his employees at the store. He had always done this, but now that he was retired and home it became almost constant. She was resentful because he did not volunteer to help. After about a year, he became more and more concerned with expenses and living on a fixed income. He complained about her extravagance in entertaining her bridge club every other month, even though he continued to golf regularly and attend his bowling team matches. He finally forbade her to entertain her bridge club and essentially took away her only source of pleasure and enjoyment. It was at this point her voice deteriorated.

The mechanism of conversion reaction was then discussed in terms of the conflict between anger, resentment, and frustration versus maintenance of a loving relationship that might suffer irreparable damage if feelings were verbalized. She agreed that this was what had happened. These matters were discussed with her husband and the couple consented to marriage counseling on their return to their local community.

Some patients achieve secondary gain from a voice disorder, as illustrated in case 4. Often these patients come to the voice pathologist at the insistence of others. There frequently is a lack of affect surrounding the patient's feeling about his/her voice problem.

Case 4

Case 4 was a very wealthy widowed woman. She was brought to the voice center at the insistence of her unmarried sister who had come to live with her after the death of her husband. The onset of her voice problem had been gradual, beginning with speech within the home. The laryngologist reported normal vocal folds with no evidence of structural or neurologic pathology. The patient demonstrated little concern about her voice problem other than an inconvenience. When asked how her voice interfered with her life, she stated, with a little smile: "Well, when I am at parties, everyone has to come up to me to converse, and of course, I cannot reprimand or manage the servants, and I can't do the grocery shopping, my sister has to do that." Although physiologic sounds were present in involuntary voice such as coughing and "fuller" sounds like "uh-huh," she was unable to extend them into any semblance of speech voicing. The effect was a modified form of a whisper. She took umbrage at the suggestion of counseling or any emotional etiology for her voice problem and terminated contact. She refused to have her case discussed with her sister. It appeared to be clear that her voice problem would not improve until her sister and friends stopped reinforcing the positive impact of her voice problem.

Cases 5 and 6 exemplify a second group of aphonic patients who present with tense aphonic speech with intermittent squeaky, high-pitched syllables or words. They are often misdiagnosed with spasmodic dysphonia, currently thought to be a neurologic disorder. Careful differential diagnosis is important. However, initial evaluation and treatment are similar regardless of the diagnosis.

These patients may present with a history of emotional disorder or severe stress, reflux, asthma, and/or chemical sensitivity resulting in laryngospasm. Strobovideolaryngoscopy usually reveals severe muscle tension with anterior-posterior constriction, elevated laryngeal position, reduced abduction and adduction and, in many cases, evidence of reflux laryngitis. Evaluation of the vocal mechanism finds the larynx held high in the neck. There is tension in the jaw, tongue, and extralaryngeal muscles. Breathing is high in the chest with excessive inspiratory effort. Therapy includes Aronson's digital manipulation,[2] yawn-sigh, swallow and gargling activities to lower and relax the larynx. Tongue and jaw must be relaxed, using techniques described previously. Good abdominal breathing must be developed. Therapy needs to be intensive, on a daily basis. Appointments on a weekly basis allow too much time for the tension reactions to reestablish themselves, reducing the effectiveness of therapeutic intervention. Referral to a stress manager or psychologist is sometimes necessary. If voice therapy is successful in establishing normally pitched voice with little evidence of tension, but spasmodic aphonic breaks persist, the patient should be reevaluated for the presence of spasmodic dysphonia.

Case 5

Case 5 presented with a high-pitched squeaky voice with frequent aphonic breaks. He felt his voice problem was directly related to his work situation. He was a middle manager in a utility company. He felt his company was in the process of downsizing, but instead of firing employees, the company designated some employees as eligible for upgrade training. The training consisted of EST-like sessions with no bathroom or food breaks and constant berating of the employee. Several of his fellow employees quit. He vowed to fight the system. However, at this point he lost his voice. He was transferred within the company from sales to a computer-intensive position. His voice returned to the presenting squeaky quality. He felt the stress of his treatment at work and resulting stress at home were directly related to his problem. Evaluation revealed high, tense laryngeal position, pain on palpation of the hyoid bone supporting the tongue, and "chest heave" breathing pattern. He was seen for a period of three days. Initially he was unable to maintain a relaxed lowered laryngeal position. He was able to monitor his larynx position digitally and was aware of the mechanism. When his larynx was lowered he produced normally pitched but breathy voice. Cues to make his voice louder improved voice quality but tended to introduce laryngeal tension and lifting of the larynx. Continued therapy, to relax the tongue and jaw and to develop abdominal breathing, were effective in producing normal voice. He refused suggestions for referral to the voice team psychologist. He contacts the therapist on occasion and continues to be symptom-free.

Case 6

Case 6 was a teacher's assistant in a preschool program. She came to school early one day and found the janitor cleaning the floors with a strong disinfectant liquid cleaner. Excessive cleaning fluid had spilled from the container and had spread across the floor. She was unable to breathe and was sent to the hospital emergency room where she received muscle relaxants and oxygen to restore breathing. Her breathing improved but her voice became high pitched and squeaky. She experienced two other incidents of breathing difficulties associated with the smells in a new store and when buying carpet. She was unable to use commercial cleaning products in her home without experiencing shortness of breath. She was diagnosed with laryngospasm. Strobovideolaryngoscopy revealed severe muscle tension and elevated larynx, but normal laryngeal function. Voice evaluation revealed high laryngeal positioning, extreme tension in the neck and extralaryngeal muscles, and a rapid, shallow, thoracic breathing pattern. The patient was convinced that her voice problem was related to "damage while hospitalized" and was considering suing the hospital. Gentle digital massage and head and neck relaxation exercises restored her voice to normal. Therapy then focused on reducing fears of breathing and voicing. She was given strategies, including slow, deep, abdominal breathing and jaw and throat relaxation patterns to counteract the return of the laryngeal spasms. She consented to referral to a stress management/psychology professional. Therapy with the psychologist focused on deep relaxation and hypnotic suggestion to reduce fears and anxiety. She was able to return to work. She still avoided areas with strong smells but was able to utilize her compensation techniques. She has not required hospitalization for breathing difficulties since.

A third group of aphonic patients present with aphonia accompanied with a low-pitched, rough, strangled voice quality, such as case 7. Strobovideolaryngoscopy reveals extreme supralaryngeal tension with both ante-

rior/posterior and medial compression of supralaryngeal structures. Often laryngeal examination is discontinued and voice therapy pursued because of the difficulty in viewing the vocal folds beneath the extreme supralaryngeal closure. Emotional trauma is usually present in these cases. Again, these patients are often misdiagnosed as having spasmodic dysphonia. Frequently, the same techniques utilized with whispering patients are helpful in modifying the vocal behavior towards normal. In addition, inhalation speech can be helpful in breaking the supraglottic tension.

Case 7

Case 7 lost her voice following the death of her grandson. Her voice was low, rough, strangled, and intermittently aphonic. Voice evaluation demonstrated generalized reduction of movement in the respiratory and articulatory systems with excessive tension in the extralaryngeal musculature. During the history, she described the death of her grandson. Her daughter and son-in-law went out to dinner, leaving their son with her and her husband. During the evening, the child suffered a severe asthma attack and died in her arms despite CPR. During the telling of the story her voice became more and more strangled. The therapist commented that she sounded like she wanted to cry and offered a tissue. At this, she burst into tears and great sobbing. She began to cry in a normal voice: "I am so angry." The therapist asked if she was angry because of the death of her grandson. She replied: "No, I am angry because I have not had a chance to grieve." Continuing in a normal voice, she related that her husband, daughter, and son-in-law were devastated by the death, which left her to make all arrangements for the autopsy, funeral, and burial. Her anger was especially directed toward her husband, who did not help, nor give her any expression of sympathy or sensitivity to the depth of her feelings and about the death and its aftermath. At the end of this revelation, the therapist gently brought her attention to the fact that her voice had become quite normal. She said: "Yes, but that's not the problem." She agreed to and was immediately referred to the voice team psychologist. She was followed periodically by speech therapy. Her voice remained stable. The psychologist reported that her problems with her family were much more extensive than those she had related to the speech-language pathologist.

Case 8

Case 8 was referred from his local speech-language pathologist to be evaluated for possible spasmodic dysphonia. He had been unable to obtain any normal speech after several months of therapy. His therapy had focused on relaxation techniques and breathing.

The patient presented with severe muscle tension dysphonia and low-pitched rough voice with a predominating whisper. Laryngoscopy could not be completed because of the severe supraglottic constriction. He denied any emotional trauma associated with the onset of his voice problem. His wife, however, felt it might be related to the death of his mother, followed within a month by the death of his father. He was also in the process of beginning retirement. All direct attempts at relaxing his voice, including inhalation speech, were ineffective or caused his voice to become worse. During instruction episodes and general conversation, he produced an occasional normal word or phrase. The therapist decided that direct therapy was not effective and began modeling normal easy voicing in conversation. Normal words and phrases were pointed out, and he was asked to reproduce the same vocal feeling and style in further conversation. Conversation focused on positive experiences and pleasurable activities. Over the course of four sessions, the frequency of normal voice continued to increase. His wife reported episodes of normal voice at home. By the fifth session, his voice was consistently normal except for a reduction in vocal loudness. There was no evidence of spasm. At this point, strobovideolaryngoscopy was completed and was within normal limits. At the next session, the subject of his parent's deaths was broached. He denied that this was a problem "that a good man should not let it bother him. A man should be strong enough to deal with such an inevitable occurrence." He felt it had been inappropriate for his previous female therapist to focus on that problem and found it difficult to cooperate with her in relaxation and breathing tasks. He was not ready to discuss his reaction. At the next session, he maintained his voicing. He also was able to begin to modify his breathing pattern to increase support and loudness. At the next session, he announced that he felt his voice had returned to normal and terminated therapy. He was seen six months follow-up with the laryngologist and continued to maintain relatively normal voice.

Case 9 describes a fourth form of aphonia, voluntary muteness. Voluntary muteness in the absence of severe laryngeal pathology, developmental language delay, or severe hearing loss is very rare. In over 35 years of experience with voice patients, we have seen only one such case.

Case 9

Case 9 was a 12-year-old boy. His mother, a loquacious and verbal woman, brought him to the voice center. She was concerned about his preparation for bar mitzvah. She was planning a large ceremony and big party, which she thought he would enjoy. However, he would not talk to her about the event or talk to the cantor or rabbi during training lessons. She had taken him to a psychologist, but he would not talk to her either. He was doing well in school although she did not know how much talking he did there. She reported that his father was a soft spoken man of few words. She felt that voice therapy might be helpful in increasing his loudness and ability to perform at his bar mitzvah.

Strobovideolaryngoscopy demonstrated a normal larynx. However, the laryngologist was unable to get him to vocalize with any strength. The therapist agreed to attempt short-term therapy, but felt that the boy had found a powerful tool to control his mother.

He reluctantly participated in breathing exercises and better oral resonance. He would practice portions of the readings required at the bar mitzvah service, but only in exchange for a turn at a computer game.

He arrived at the third session more animated than he had ever been before. His teacher had given the class a book report assignment. Each student was to read a book and then report orally to the class about the story from the point of view of one of the characters in the book. The report could only be five minutes long. He had chosen Tom Sawyer and wanted to report in the guise of that character. He discussed in detail his plans for a costume and asked for help in presenting an already prepared presentation. We worked on appropriate breath support and phrasing, projection and open oral resonance, and editing for length. He asked for an additional session to give us more time prior to his presentation. It was hoped that a breakthrough had occurred. He was working as hard as any aspiring actor, reporting that he received an A+ on his presentation. However, when the work resumed on his bar mitzvah readings, the old reluctance returned. He was able to demonstrate his skills if rewarded, but continued to be silent at home. His mother reported that he would at least mumble to the cantor. Plans for a large bar mitzvah were canceled. His mother was reluctant to re-engage in psychotherapy, and the patient discontinued voice therapy.

VOICE PROBLEMS ASSOCIATED WITH PSYCHOSIS

Rarely does the voice of the psychotic patient present as the most prevalent symptom. Several studies have been published characterizing the speech of the schizophrenic. These characteristics are considered to be the by-product of affect, aura, and relational disturbances. Speech therapy for those voice characteristics is rarely considered. However, occasionally such a patient will be encountered in a voice center, as illustrated by case 10.

Case 10

Case 10 had a successful career in a medical subspecialty. However, she aspired to a career in opera. She had taken many lessons, but had been discouraged by her family and teachers to pursue this professionally. She had been highly unsuccessful while auditioning for roles. She came to the voice center to have her singing/speaking voice evaluated. Strobovideolaryngoscopy revealed normal laryngeal structures. She revealed, during history-taking, that her voice was fine at work, because of the lead shielding at the hospital. However, at home, her voice was disrupted and changed in quality, particularly when she was practicing singing and acting and at auditions. When asked why, she reported that "they" were shooting laser beams at her and shocking her, which disrupted her voice and made her voicing very tense. When asked, "Who they were" she replied, "Certain others who are jealous of my talents and want to thwart my career in singing." She also reported that the beams "they" were using burned her and produced changes in her skin color around her neck and shoulders.

When reading a passage, she winced, dodged, and several times cried out in pain. When this behavior was questioned, she reported calmly that "they" had followed her to the center and were shooting laser beams and using electric shock on her. She was reluctant to work on her speaking voice because the problems of tension that she had were caused by an external force and not by her.

Her evaluation by our singing specialist was similar. She was urged by the entire team to submit to evaluation by a psychiatrist, but would not do so.

VOICE PROBLEMS ASSOCIATED WITH ADOLESCENCE

Mutational falsetto is high-falsetto voicing, often with frequent pitch breaks. The voice is thin and high pitched. Falsetto voice requires a different shaping of the glottis and different breath support than typical voicing. The larynx must ride high in the neck to produce falsetto. It is a normal phenomenon; most males can produce it. It is used frequently in singing by rock and roll singers and developed extensively by classical countertenors, but is not a preferred means of speech communication. It occurs in some young men following the onset of laryngeal growth associated with adolescence. The techniques described above for use with patients with squeaky voices are useful in this group. Usually, normal voicing is easily achieved during the evaluation and trial therapy sessions. Often the patient has both falsetto and normal voice, but prefers the falsetto for

various personal reasons. Most of these patients are nonmuscular young men with little self-confidence. It has often been misdiagnosed as spasmodic dysphonia because of the pitch breaks.

Case 11

Case 11 was a 23-year-old auto body repairman. He was concerned about laryngeal cancer. His girlfriend and parents accompanied him to the voice clinic. Strobovideolaryngoscopy revealed normal larynx and the presence of falsetto voicing. During the voice evaluation, he was asked if he had any other voices. In a normal deep baritone he answered "Yes." He used the deep voice around his colleagues at the auto body shop. He used the falsetto voice with his girlfriend, his family, and his high school friends. His life was organized around the premise that the two groups of people were never present at the same time. When asked why he needed the dichotomy of voice, he answered that he was afraid his girlfriend and family would not like this other voice. He was asked if he would be willing to try. His girlfriend was brought into the room and he used his deep voice. She, of course, was thrilled. He was relieved, and his voice problem was solved.

Case 12

Case 12 was a 19-year-old college student. He had just completed his freshman year at a religious college. He had attended a choir school during his primary school years and had sung many soprano solos. His best singing occurred just prior to adolescent voice change. He continued to sing soprano although his voice became thin and he had difficulty keeping his voice from cracking following vocal mutation. His speaking voice continued to be high, breathy, and characterized by pitch breaks.

When he arrived at college, he enrolled in the religious music department, hoping to continue a career in choral singing. His singing teacher, instead of being impressed by his high voice, referred him to a local speech-language pathologist. He was diagnosed with spasmodic dysphonia, presumably because of the numerous pitch breaks. He was referred for neurologic workup and Botox injections. His singing teacher was not convinced of this diagnosis and referred him to our voice center.

Strobovideolaryngoscopy revealed a normal larynx with falsetto voice patterning. He was convinced that "spasmodic dysphonia had destroyed his singing voice." He was counseled on the effects of adolescent voice change. We explored the large size and angular shape of his larynx, comparing it to the much smaller, rounded larynx of a child. The symptoms of spasmodic dysphonia were described and tapes of spasmodic dysphonic voices were played for him.

Attempts at producing low-pitched normal voice extending from cough and throat-clearing sounds were successful but transition into speech sounds was difficult. He was asked to put his finger across his "Adam's apple" and tuck his chin down toward his chest. This maneuver made falsetto voicing impossible. Normal low-pitched voicing was achieved and transferred to syllables, words, phrases, question/answers, and monologue. The positioning cues were gradually replaced by gentle downward tactile cues. He was engaged in conversation using the "new" voice for at least 30 minutes. He was asked to use his new voice with other personnel, his family (who had accompanied him to the center), and on the telephone to his singing teacher. His family was relieved that Botox injections were not necessary. Breath support was practiced in context of his speech. By the end of the evaluation and trial therapy session, he was convinced that he was a baritone and could continue singing in that role. He no longer felt he had spasmodic dysphonia. The singing specialist at the voice center saw him and it was reported that he was able to maintain his speaking voice and begin some singing exercises focusing on lower range extension and breath support. He was asked to call the center the following day to report on continued use of the "new" voice. During that call, the patient reported that he had retained his lower voice. He was looking forward to returning to college and working with his singing teacher on developing his baritone voice.

Occasionally, males with mutational falsetto demonstrate personal conflicts with their fathers, attachment problems with their mothers, or gender confusion. These patients tend to produce normal voice reluctantly and fail to maintain it, often complaining that such a voice is not appropriate for them. Counseling and referral to a psychological professional to focus on these difficulties is necessary.

Young women do not present with mutational falsetto. Rarely, a young postpubescent girl will present with immature voice. This is characterized by high pitch and melody, inflection, articulation, and word choice more reminiscent of a preschool child than a postpubertal young adult. Usually, strong dependent behaviors are described in the history.

Case 13

Case 13 was a 17-year-old high school student who aspired to a career in musical theater. She had been highly successful in obtaining roles as a child in productions of *Annie*. She had been thwarted lately in winning any role because of her voice. She was close to tears and appeared to be very depressed. Laryngologic examination demonstrated normal structures but muscle tension associated with high pitch. Her voice was very high pitched and immature with a mild lisp and "r" sound distortions. She was seen in therapy and made progress in controlled contexts. However, she was unable to transfer her more mature voice to home and school environments. She was very unhappy about this and felt that something was blocking her ability to use her more mature voice outside the office. She readily accepted referral to psychologic services. However, because of travel distance she was seen by someone closer to her home.

SUMMARY

In summary, speech-language pathologists provide many services in the context of a team approach to functional voice disorders. The speech-language pathologist's task is to modify disordered voices into serviceable voices with sufficient stamina to endure the demands of lifestyle and environment. The speech-language pathologist provides a caring and supportive environment that allows patients to explore possible underlying causes. Speech-language pathologists assist in the differential diagnosis of functional from organic disorders. He or she must be able to discern the difference between functional voice patterns and those that require medical/surgical treatment, and to share such insights with the laryngologist responsible for making medical diagnoses. Sensitivity to the fact that the voice is the mirror of emotions is essential. Each speech-language pathologist must be aware of his/her own limitations and be prepared to provide prudent and appropriate referral to other professionals trained in dealing with the psychologic and emotional issues as necessary. Above all, each speech-language pathologist must develop strong and cooperative relationships with other professionals who care for patients with voice disorders.

THE MENTAL HEALTH PROFESSIONAL'S ROLE IN TREATING PSYCHOLOGIC DISTURBANCES IN PATIENTS WITH VOICE DISORDERS

Role of the Psychological Professional

Both psychologists and psychiatrists specialize in attending to emotional needs and problems. Psychiatrists, as physicians, focus on the neurologic and biologic causes and treatment of psychopathology. Psychologists have advanced graduate training in psychologic function and therapy. They concern themselves with cognitive processes such as thinking, behavior, and memory; the experiencing and expression of emotions; significant inner conflict, characteristic modes of defense in coping with stress; and personality style and perception of self and others, including their expression in interpersonal behavior. Other mental health professionals also provide psychotherapy to performers. In the author's (RTS) practice, clinical psychologists and a psychiatrist serve as members of the voice team, along with SLPs, singing voice specialists, and others. They work directly with some patients and offer consultation to the physician and other professionals.

Assessment of patients is done throughout the physician's history-taking and physical examinations, as well as in a formal psychiatric interview when appropriate in our center. Personality assessment, screening for or evaluating known psychopathology, and assessing potential surgical candidates is performed. Occasionally, psychometric instruments are added to the diagnostic interview. Confidentiality of content is extended to the treatment team to maximize interdisciplinary care. Because of their special interest in voicing parameters, the voice team psychologists are especially attuned to the therapeutic use of their own voices for intensifying rapport and pacing/leading the patient's emotional state during interventions.[20-22]

Psychotherapeutic treatment is offered on a short-term, diagnosis-related basis. Treatment is designed to identify and alleviate emotional distress and to increase the individual's resources for adaptive functioning. Individual psychotherapeutic approaches include brief insight-oriented therapies, cognitive/behavioral techniques, gestalt interventions, stress management, skill building, and clinical hypnosis.

After any indicated acute intervention is provided, and in patients whose coping repertoire is clearly adequate to the stressors, a psycho-educational model is used. The therapy session focuses on a prospective discussion of personal, inherent life stressors, and predictable illnesses. Stress management skills are taught and audiotapes are provided. These offer portable skills and supplemental sessions may be scheduled by mutual decision during appointments at the center for medical examinations and speech or singing voice therapy. A group therapy model, facilitated by the psychologist, has also been used to provide a forum for discussion of patient responses during the various phases of treatment. Participants benefit from the perspective and progress of other patients, the opportunity to decrease their experience of isolation, and the sharing of resources.

Long-term psychodynamic psychotherapy, chronic psychiatric conditions, and patients requiring psychopharmacologic management are referred to other consultant mental health professionals with special interest and insight in voice-related psychologic problems, or to the psychiatrist on our team. The voice team's psychologists also serve in a liaison role when patients already in treatment come to our center for voice care. In addition, the psychologist participates in professional education activities in the medical practice. These include writing, lecturing, and serving as a preceptor for visiting professionals. Specially trained psychologists have proven to be an invaluable addition to the voice team, and close collaboration with team members has proven to be valuable and stimulating for psychologists interested in the care of professional voice users.

General Psychopathologic Presentations

Otolaryngologists and all other health care providers involved with patients with voice disorders should recognize significant comorbid psychopathology and should be prepared to consult an appropriate mental health professional. Psychologists and psychiatrists are responsible for psychologic diagnosis and treatment, but it is important to select mental health professionals with advanced understanding of the special problems associated with voice disorders (especially, but not exclusively, in professional voice users). Patterns of voice use may provide clues to the presence of psychopathology, although voice disturbance is certainly not the principal feature of major psychiatric illness. Nevertheless, failure to recognize serious psychopathology in voice patients may result not only in errors in voice diagnosis and failures of therapy, but, more importantly, in serious injury to the patient, sometimes even death.

Although a full depressive syndrome, including melancholia, can occur as a result of loss, it fulfills the criteria for a major depressive episode only when the individual becomes preoccupied with feelings of worthlessness and guilt, demonstrates marked psychomotor retardation and other biologic markers, and becomes impaired in both social and occupational functioning.[23] Careful listening during the taking of a history will reveal a flat affect, including slowed rate of speech, decreased length of utterance, lengthy pauses, decreased pitch variability, monoloudness, and frequent use of vocal fry.[1] Author William Styron described his speech during his depressive illness as "slowed to the vocal equivalent of a shuffle."[24]

Major depression may be part of the patient's past medical history, may be a comorbid illness, or may be a result of the presenting problem. The essential feature is a prominent, persistent despondent mood characterized by a loss of pleasure in nearly all activities. Appetite and sleep are disturbed and there may be marked weight gain or loss, hypersomnia, or one of three insomnia patterns. Psychomotor agitation or retardation may be present. Patients may be distracted easily and demonstrate memory disturbances and difficulty concentrating. Feelings of worthlessness, helplessness, and hopelessness are a classic triad. Suicidal ideation, with or without plan, and/or concomitant psychotic features, may necessitate emergency intervention.

Major affective disorders are classified as unipolar or bipolar. In bipolar disorder, the patient will also experience periods of mania, which is a recurrent elated state first occurring in young adulthood. First manic episodes in patients over 50 should alert the clinician to medical or CNS illness, or to the effects of drugs. The presentation of the illness includes the following major characteristics on a continuum of severity: elevated mood, irritability/hostility, distractibility, inflated self-concept, grandiosity, physical and sexual overactivity, flight of ideas, decreased need for sleep, social intrusiveness, buying sprees, and inappropriate collections of possessions. Manic patients demonstrate impaired social and familial behavior patterns. They are manipulative, alienate family members, and tend to have a very high divorce rate.[10,25] Vocal presentation will manifest flight of ideas (content), rapid-paced, pressured speech, and often increased pitch and volume. There may be dysfluency related to the rate of speech, breathlessness, and difficulty in interrupting the language stream. Three major theories, based on neuroanatomy, neuroendocrinology, and neuropharmacology, are the most currently promulgated explanations for these disease states, but they are beyond the scope of this chapter.[20,25-33]

Treatment of affective disorders includes psychotherapy. Diagnosis and short-term treatment of reactive depressive states may be performed by the psychologist on the voice team, utilizing individual or group therapy modalities. Longer-term treatment necessitates a referral to a community-based psychotherapist, ideally one whose skills, training, and understanding of the medical and artistic components of the illness are well known to the referring laryngologist. The use of psychopharmacologic agents is a risk/benefit decision. When the patient's symptom severity meets the criteria for major affective disorder, the physiologic effects of the disease, as well as the potential for self-destructive behavior, must be carefully considered.

Anxiety is an expected response in reaction to any medical diagnosis and the required treatment. However, anxiety disorders are seen with increasing incidence. Vocal presentations of anxiety vary with the continuum of psychiatric symptoms, ranging from depression to agitation and including impairment of concentration. Psychotherapy, including desensitization, cognitive/behavioral techniques, stress management, hypnosis, and insight-oriented approaches are helpful. Patients must learn to tolerate their distress and identify factors that precipitate or intensify their symptoms. Medication may be used to treat the neurotransmitter disturbances and decrease the frequency of episodes. However, it may leave the underlying conflict unresolved and negatively affect artistic quality.[1,8,27] Some medical conditions are commonly associated with a presenting symptom of anxiety. These include CNS disease, Cushing's syndrome, hyperthyroidism, hypoglycemia, the consequences of minor head trauma, premenstrual syndrome, and cardiac disease such as mitral valve prolapse and various arrhythmias. Medications prescribed for other conditions may have anxiety as a side effect. These include such drugs as amphetamines, corticosteroids, caffeine, decongestants, cocaine, and the asthma armamentarium.[4]

Although psychotic behavior may be observed with major affective disorders, organic CNS disease, or drug toxicity, schizophrenia occurs in only 1-2% of the general population.[32] Its onset is most prominent in mid to late adolescence through the late 20s. Incidence is approximately equal for males and females and schizophrenia has been described in all cultures and socioeconomic classes. This is a group of mental disorders in which massive disruptions in cognition or perception, such as delusions, hallucinations, or thought disorders, are present. The fundamental causes of schizophrenia are unknown but the disease involves excessive amounts of neurotransmitters, chiefly dopamine. There is a genetic predisposition. Somatic delusions may present as voice complaints. However, flattening or inappropriateness of affect, a diagnostic characteristic of schizophrenia, will produce voice changes similar to those described for depression and mania. Where hallucinatory material creates fear, characteristics of anxiety and agitation will be audible. Perseveration, repetition, and neologisms may be present. The signs and symptoms also include clear indications of deterioration in social or occupational functioning, personal hygiene, changes in behavior and movement, an altered sense of self, and the presence of blunted or inappropriate affect.[4,23,32] The disease is chronic and control requires consistent use of antipsychotic medications for symptoms management. Social support in regulating activities of daily living is crucial in maintaining emotional control. Family counseling and support groups offer the opportunity to share experiences and resources in the care of individuals with this difficult disease.

Psychoactive Medications

All psychoactive agents have effects that can interfere with vocal tract physiology. Treatment requires frequent, open collaboration between the laryngologist and the psychiatrist. The patient and physician need to carefully weigh the benefits and side effects of available medications. Patients must be informed of the relative probability of experiencing any known side effect. This is especially critical to the professional voice user and plays an important role in developing a treatment plan when there is no imminent serious psychiatric risk. An overview of psychoactive medications is provided in Appendix 29-2.

Ongoing psychiatric treatment of patients with voice disorders mandates a careful evaluation of current and prior psychoactive drug therapy. In addition, numerous psychoactive substances are used in the medical management of neurologic conditions such as Tourette's syndrome (haloperidol), chronic pain syndromes (carbamazepine), and vertigo (diazepam, clonazepam).

The laryngologist must thus identify symptoms that may be causally related to drug side effects and avoid drug interactions. It is appropriate (with the patient's consent) to consult with the prescribing physician directly to advocate the use of the psychoactive drug least likely to produce adverse effects on the voice while adequately controlling the psychiatric illness. Patients with major psychiatric disorders should be under the care of a psychiatrist. The voice team should be guided by his or her recommendations. The psychiatric disease is most likely to be the highest priority in terms of risk to the patient.[28]

Eating Disorders and Substance Abuse

The rapport of the laryngologist and voice team may also allow patients to reveal other self-defeating disorders. Among the most common in arts medicine are body dysmorphic (eating) disorders and substance abuse problems. Comprehensive discussion of these subjects is beyond the scope of this chapter but it is important for the laryngologist to recognize such conditions, not only because of their effects on the voice, but also because of their potentially serious general medical and psychiatric implications. In addition to posterior laryngitis and pharyngitis, laryngeal findings associated with bulimia include subepithelial vocal fold hemorrhages, superficial telangiectasia of the vocal fold mucosa, and vocal fold scarring.[27]

Bulimia is a disorder associated with self-induced vomiting following episodes of binge eating. It may occur sporadically, or it may be a chronic problem. Vomiting produces signs and symptoms similar to severe chronic reflux as well as thinning of tooth enamel. Bulimia nervosa can be a serious disorder and may be associated with anorexia nervosa. Bulimia may be more prevalent than is commonly realized. It has been estimated to occur in as many as 2-4% of female adolescents and female young adults, and this number is rising. Laryngologists must be attentive to the potential for anorexia and exercise addiction in the maintenance of a desirable body appearance in performers.

Appetite Suppressants

There is enormous popular interest in the use of appetite suppressants in weight management. Many myths persist about proper weight management approaches in singers and the value and/or risk of weight loss. The availability and popularity of appetite suppressant drugs, and marketing approaches which included making them available in franchised weight loss centers, led many Americans to explore the use of "Fen-Phen" (phentermine [Ionamine and others] and fenfluramine [Pondomin]). Another drug that gained popularity is dexfenfluramine hydrochloride (Redux). These medications have limited efficacy in changing metabolism and limiting cravings. Many patients took these drugs in combinations that were never approved for concomitant use. Laryngologists and psychologic professionals caring for singers and other performers should be certain to investigate the potential use of these medications, which were voluntarily withdrawn from the market by their manufacturer in 1997 because of a significant correlation with cardiac valve damage and with pulmonary hypertension. The laryngologist should question patients about the use of OTC and "herbal" products such as ephedra and "Metabolife." These too are potentially harmful because of sympathomimetic effects.

Alcohol, benzodiazepines, stimulants, cocaine, and narcotics are notoriously readily available in the performing community and on the streets. Patients who demonstrate signs and symptoms, or who admit that these areas of their lives are out of control, have taken the first step to regaining control, and this should be acknowledged while efficiently arranging treatment for them. The window of opportunity is often remarkably narrow. The physician should establish close ties to excellent treatment facilities where specialized clinicians can offer confidential outpatient management, with inpatient care available when required for safety.[1]

Neurogenic Dysphonia

Patients with neurologic disease are likely to experience psychiatric symptoms, especially depression and anxiety. These disorders cause physiologic changes that may exacerbate or mask the underlying neurologic presentation. Metcalfe and colleagues cite the incidence of severe depression and/or anxiety in neurologic patients at one-third.[34] Site of lesion affects the incidence, with lesions of the left cerebral hemisphere, basal ganglia, limbic system, thalamus, and anterior frontal lobe more likely to produce depression and anxiety.[35] These same structures are important in voice, speech, and language production, so depression and anxiety logically coexist with voice and language disorders resulting from CNS pathology.[35,36] Dystonias and stuttering are also associated with both neurologic and psychogenic etiologies, and must be carefully distinguished by the laryngologist before instituting interdisciplinary treatment.[37]

Stress Management

Stress pervades virtually all professions in today's fast-moving society. A singer preparing for a series of concerts, a teacher preparing for presentation of lectures, a lawyer anticipating a major trial, a businessperson negotiating an important contract, or a member of any other goal-oriented profession, each must deal with a myriad of demands on his or her time and talents. In 1971, Brodnitz reported on 2,286 cases of all forms of voice disorders and classified 80% of the disorders as attributable to voice abuse or psychogenic factors resulting in vocal dysfunction.[38] However, regardless of the incidence, it is clear that stress-related problems are important and common in professional voice users. Stress may be physical or psychologic and it often involves a combination of both. Either may interfere with performance. Stress represents a special problem for singers, because its physiologic manifestations may interfere with the delicate mechanisms of voice production.[1]

Stress is recognized as a factor in illness and disease and is probably implicated in almost every type of human problem. It is estimated that 50-70% of all physicians' visits involve complaints of stress-related illness.[39] Stress is a psychologic experience that has physiologic consequences. A brief review of some terminology may be useful. *Stress* is a term that is used broadly. Our working definition is emotional, cognitive, and physiologic reactions to psychologic demands and challenges. The term *stress level* reflects the degree of stress experienced. Stress is not an all-or-none phenomenon. The psychologic effects of stress range from mild to severely incapacitating. The term *stress*

response refers to the physiologic reaction of an organism to stress. A stressor is an external stimulus or internal thought, perception, image, or emotion that creates stress.[40] Two other concepts are important in a contemporary discussion of stress: coping and adaptation. Lazarus has defined coping as "the process of managing demands (external and internal) that are appraised as taxing or exceeding the resources of the person."[41] In the early 1930s, Hans Selye, an endocrinologist, discovered a generalized response to stressors in research animals. He described their responses using the term *general adaptation syndrome*. Selye (cited in Green and Snellenberger[40]) postulated that the physiology of the research animals was trying to adapt to the challenges of noxious stimuli. The process of adaptation to chronic and severe stressors was harmful over time. There were three phases to the observed response: alarm, adaptation, and exhaustion. These phases were named for physiologic responses during a sequence of events. The alarm phase is the characteristic fight or flight response. If the stressor continued, the animal appeared to adapt. In the adaptation phase, the physiologic responses were less extreme but the animal eventually became more exhausted. In the exhaustion phase, the animal's adaptation energy was spent, physical symptoms occurred, and some animals died.[40]

Stress responses occur in part through the autonomic nervous system. A stressor triggers particular brain centers, which in turn affect target organs through nerve connections. The brain has two primary pathways for the stress response, neuronal and hormonal, and these pathways overlap. The body initiates a stress response through one of three pathways: through sympathetic nervous system efferents which terminate on target organs such as the heart and blood vessels; via the release of epinephrine and norepinephrine from the adrenal medulla; and through the release of various other catecholamines.[40] A full description of the various processes involved is beyond the scope of this chapter. However, stress has numerous physical consequences. Through the autonomic nervous system, it may alter oral and vocal fold secretions, heart rate, and gastric acid production. Under acute, anxiety-producing circumstances, such changes are to be expected. When frightened, a normal person's palms become cold and sweaty, the mouth becomes dry, heart rate increases, his or her pupils change size, and stomach acid secretions may increase. These phenomena are objective signs that may be observed by a physician and their symptoms may be recognized by the performer as dry mouth and voice fatigue, heart palpitations, and "heartburn." More severe, prolonged stress is also commonly associated with increased muscle tension throughout the body (but particularly in the head and neck), headaches, decreased ability to concentrate, and insomnia. Chronic fatigue is also a common symptom. These physiologic alterations may lead not only to altered vocal quality, but also to physical pathology. Increased gastric acid secretion is associated with ulcers, as well as reflux laryngitis and arytenoid irritation. Other gastrointestinal manifestations, such as colitis, irritable bowel syndrome, and dysphagia are also described. Chronic stress and tension may cause numerous pain syndromes although headaches, particularly migraines in vulnerable individuals, are most common. Stress is also associated with more serious physical problems such as myocardial infarction, asthma, and depression of the immune system.[27,40] Thus, the constant pressure under which many performers live may be more than an inconvenience. Stress factors should be recognized, and appropriate modifications should be made to ameliorate them.

Stressors may be physical or psychologic and often involve a combination of both. Either may interfere with performance. There are several situations in which physical stress is common and important. Generalized fatigue is seen frequently in hard-working singers, especially in the frantic few weeks preceding major performances. In order to maintain normal mucosal secretions, a strong immune system to fight infection, and the ability of muscles to recover from heavy use, rest, proper nutrition, and hydration are required. When the body is stressed through deprivation of these essentials, illness such as upper respiratory infection, voice fatigue, hoarseness, and other vocal dysfunctions may supervene.

Lack of physical conditioning undermines the power source of the voice. A person who becomes short of breath while climbing a flight of stairs hardly has the abdominal and respiratory endurance needed to sustain him or her optimally through the rigors of performance. The stress of attempting to perform under such circumstances often results in voice dysfunction.

Over-singing is another common physical stress. As with running, swimming, or any other athletic activity that depends upon sustained, coordinated muscle activity, singing requires conditioning to build up strength and endurance. Rest periods are also essential for muscle recovery. Singers who are accustomed to singing for one or two hours a day stress their physical voice-producing mechanism severely when they suddenly begin rehearsing for 14 hours daily immediately prior to performance.

Medical treatment of stress depends upon the specific circumstances. When the diagnosis is appropriate but poorly controlled anxiety, the singer can usually be helped by assurance that his or her voice complaint is related to anxiety and not to any physical problem. Under ordinary circumstances, once the singer's mind is put to rest regarding the questions of nodules, vocal fold injury, or other serious problems, his or her training usually allows compensation for vocal manifestations of anxiety, especially when the vocal complaint is minor. Slight alterations in quality or increased vocal fatigue are seen most frequently. These are often associated with lack of sleep, over-singing, and dehydration associated with the stress-producing commitment. The singer or actor should be advised to modify these and to consult his or her voice teacher. The voice teacher should ensure that good vocal technique is being used under performance and rehearsal circumstances. Frequently, young singers are not trained sufficiently in how and when to "mark." For example, many singers whistle to rest their voices, not realizing that active vocalization and potentially fatiguing vocal fold contact occur when whistling. Technical proficiency and a plan for voice conservation during rehearsals and performances are essentials under these circumstances. A manageable stressful situation may become unmanageable if real physical vocal problems develop.

Several additional modalities may be helpful in selected circumstances. Relative voice rest (using the voice only when necessary) may be important not only to voice conservation but also to psychologic relaxation. Under stressful circumstances, a singer needs as much peace and quiet as possible, not hectic socializing, parties with heavy voice use in noisy environments, and press appearances. The importance of adequate sleep and fluid intake cannot be overemphasized. Local therapy such as steam inhalation and neck muscle massage may be helpful in some people and certainly do no harm. The doctor may be very helpful in alleviating the singer's exogenous stress by conveying "doctor's orders" directly to theater management. This will save the singer the discomfort of having to personally confront an authority and violate his or her "show must go on" ethic. A short telephone call by the physician can be highly therapeutic.

When stress is chronic and incapacitating, more comprehensive measures are required. If psychologic stress manifestations become so severe as to impair performance or necessitate the use of drugs to allow performance, psychotherapy is indicated. The goals of psychotherapeutic approaches to stress management include:

- changing external and internal stressors;
- changing affective and cognitive reactions to stressors;
- changing physiologic reactions to stress; and
- changing stress behaviors.

A psycho-educational model is customarily used. Initially, the psychotherapist will assist the patient in identifying and evaluating stressor characteristics. A variety of assessment tools are available for this purpose. Interventions designed to increase a sense of efficacy and personal control are designed. Perceived control over the stressor directly affects stress level and it changes one's experience of the stressor. Laboratory and human research has determined a sense of control to be one of the most potent elements in the modulation of stress responses. Concrete exercises that impose time management are taught and practiced. Patients are urged to identify and expand their network of support as well. Psychologic intervention requires evaluation of the patient's cognitive model. Cognitive restructuring exercises as well as classical behavioral conditioning responses are useful, practical tools that patients easily learn and utilize effectively with practice. Cognitive skills include the use of monitored perception, thought, and internal dialogue to regulate emotional and physiologic responses. A variety of relaxation techniques are available and are ordinarily taught in the course of stress-management treatment. These include progressive relaxation, hypnosis, autogenic training and imagery, and biofeedback training. Underlying all these approaches is the premise that making conscious normally unconscious processes leads to control and self-efficacy.[1]

As with all medical conditions, the best treatment for stress in singers is prevention. Awareness of the conditions that lead to stress and its potential adverse effect on voice production often allows the singer to anticipate and avoid these problems. Stress is inevitable in performance and in life. Performers must learn to recognize it, compensate for it when necessary, and incorporate it into their singing as emotion and excitement—the "edge." Stress should be controlled, not pharmacologically eliminated. Used well, stress should be just one more tool of the singer's trade.

Performance Anxiety

Psychologic stress is intrinsic to vocal performance. For most people, sharing emotions is stressful even in the privacy of home, let alone under spotlights in front of a room full of people. Under ordinary circumstances, during training, a singer or actor learns to recognize his or her customary anxiety about performing, to accept it as part of his or her instrument, and to compensate for it. When psychologic pressures become severe enough to impair or prohibit performance, careful treatment is required. Such occurrences usually are temporary and happen because of a particular situation such as short notice for a critically important performance, a recent

family death, and so forth. Chronic disabling psychologic stress in the face of performance is a more serious problem. In its most extreme forms, performance anxiety actually disrupts the skills of performers; in its milder form it lessens the enjoyment of appearing in public.[1]

Virtually all performers have experienced at least some symptoms of hyperarousal during their performance history and all fear their reemergence. Some fortunate people seem to bypass this type of trauma, exhibiting only mild symptoms of nervousness ahead of performance, which disappear the moment they walk on stage.[42] In these individuals, personal physiology works consistently for instead of against them.[1] The human nervous system functions exquisitely for the great majority of our needs, but in performance anxiety it begins to work against the performer in those very circumstances when he or she wants most to do well. Human autonomic arousal continues to be under the sway of primal survival mechanisms, which are the basic lines of defense against physical danger: they prepare the individual to fight or flee in response to the perception of threat.[1] They are essential to our survival in situations of physical danger. The dangers that threaten performers are not physical in nature, but the human nervous system cannot differentiate between physical and psychologic dangers, producing physiologic responses that are the same. When the physical symptoms associated with extreme arousal are enumerated, it is easy to understand why they can be major impediments to skilled performance and may even be disabling. They include rapid heart rate, dry mouth, sweating palms, palpitations, tremor, high blood pressure, restricted breathing, frequency of urination, and impaired memory.[1]

This process is cognitive, and Beck and Emery[42] describe the development of cognitive sets using an analogy to photography. The individual scans the relevant environment and then determines which aspect, if any, on which to focus. Cognitive processing reduces the number of dimensions in a situation, sacrifices a great deal of information, and induces distortion into the "picture." Certain aspects of the situation are highlighted at the expense of others, the relative magnitudes and prominence of various features are distorted, and there is loss of perspective. In addition, they describe blurring and loss of important detail. These are the decisive influences upon what the individual sees. They describe how the cognitive set influences the picture that is perceived. The existing cognitive sets determine which aspects of the scene will be highlighted, which glossed over, and which excluded. The individual's first impressions of an event provide information that either reinforces or modifies the preexisting cognitive set. The initial impression is critical because it determines whether the situation directly affects the patient's vital interest. It also sets the course of subsequent steps in conceptualization and the total response to a situation.[42] According to the cognitive model, at the same time the individual is evaluating the nature of the threat, he or she is also assessing the availability and effectiveness of internal resources for dealing with it and deflecting potential damage. The balance between potential danger and available coping responses determines the nature and intensity of the patient's stress response. Two major behavioral systems are activated, either separately or together, in response to the threat: those mediated by the sympathetic branch of the autonomic nervous system, "the fight or flight response," and those related to the parasympathetic branch, "the freeze or faint response."

A major feature of performance anxiety is that the actual fear prior to entering the situation appears plausible. A complex web of factors in this situation may aggravate the patient's fears. These may include the relative status of the performer and of the evaluator, the performer's skill, his or her confidence in the ability to perform adequately in a given "threatening situation," and the appraisal of the degree of threat (including the severity of potential damage to one's career and self-esteem). The individual's threshold of automatic defenses that undermine performance and the rigidity of the rules relevant to the performance in question are also factored into the intensity of the response. Unfortunately, the experience also increases the likelihood of the undesirable consequences. A vicious cycle is created in which the anticipation of an absolute, extreme, irreversible outcome makes the performer more fearful of the effects and inhibited when entering the situation.[42] Negative evaluation by judges or audiences is the common psychic threat. The individual suffering from performance anxiety believes that he or she is being scrutinized and judged. Components under observation include fluency, artistry, self-assurance, and technique.

Although most fears tend to decline with continued exposure and expertise, Caine notes that even highly skilled performers do not always experience lessening of performance anxiety over time.[43] Indeed, she describes a dilemma for the expert performer in which a potentially humiliating and frightening mistake is less and less tolerable. A behavioral feedback loop becomes established. The act of performance becomes the stimulus perceived as a threat. In situations of danger, the individual's physiology primes him or her to become more alert and sensitive to all potential threats in the surrounding environment. Anticipating mistakes increases arousal, which further enhances access to memories of mistakes and feelings of humiliation, which activates more fears and more arousal. This process is linked by catastrophic thoughts, physiologic manifestations of anxiety, and imagery. Unfortunately, this process is often initiated very early in a young performer's training.[1] This process can also be seen in other highly driven and perfectionistic groups of individuals, for example, many surgeons.

A variety of psychotherapeutic treatment approaches to performance anxiety have been described in the literature. The most effective of these are cognitive and behavioral strategies, which assist performers in modulating levels of arousal to more optimal levels. Cognitive therapy addresses the essential mechanism sustaining performance anxiety: the cognitive set a performer brings to the performance situation. The autonomic nervous system is merely responding to the threat as it is perceived, and the intensity of the response correlates to the degree of threat generated by the sufferer's catastrophic expectations and negative self-talk. Cognitive restructuring techniques are extremely effective in producing the necessary adjustments. Monitoring internal self-dialogue comprises the first step in recognizing the dimension of the problem. These excessively self-critical attitudes enhance the probability of mistakes. Homework exercises designed to monitor critical thoughts are assigned. In the second step of cognitive treatment, adaptive, realistic self-statements are substituted. Behaviorally based treatment approaches such as thought-stopping, paired relaxation responses and "prescribing the symptom" are also utilized. Hypnosis is efficacious, providing relaxation techniques and introducing positive, satisfying, and joyful imagery.[1]

Brief psychotherapeutic approaches produce effective outcomes, but some proponents of the psychodynamic approach argue that the underlying conflicts will resurface in some form of symptom substitution. This author's (DCR) clinical approach includes an exploration for secondary gain offered by disabling performance anxiety. The performer's unconscious fear must be addressed for these treatments to remain effective and to avoid eventual symptom substitution. Patients are asked: "What does this symptom accomplish for you?" The question may sound unsympathetic, and the patient may need to search deeply for the answer. This search requires significant courage. If the patient makes effective use of the treatment strategies, what might be expected of him or her? Where might success lead? Is he or she ready to go on to the next phase in a performance career, or does it remain safer to be immobilized? Which problem is honestly more terrifying: the symptom of performance anxiety or the possibility of success? What would be the consequences of resolving the immobilizing performance anxiety? The patient is asked to imagine life in which the problem is no longer present. This exploration is often conducted using the relaxation and enhanced perception available in hypnosis.[1] Most of these questions are painful ones to answer. For some performers, success beckons with one hand and signals caution with the other. Eloise Ristad describes this with extraordinarily pragmatic wisdom.[44]

> The part of us that holds back knows that change involves challenges-losses as well as gains. Change always means dying a little; leaving behind something old and tattered and no longer useful to us even though comfortably familiar.

A successful psychotherapeutic response to disabling performance anxiety requires a thorough explanation of the personal meaning of the symptom to the patient as well as an extensive and exciting repertoire of strategies for affecting personal change.

Reactive Responses

Reaction to illness is a major source of psychiatric disturbance in patients with significant voice dysfunction. Loss of communicative function is an experience of alienation that threatens human self-definition and independence. Catastrophic fears of loss of productivity, economic and social status and, in professional voice users, creative artistry, contribute to rising anxiety. Anxiety is known to worsen existing communication disorders, and the disturbances in memory, concentration, and synaptic transmission secondary to depression may intensify other voice symptoms and interfere with rehabilitation.

The self-concept is an essential construct of Carl Rodgers' theories of counseling. Rodgers described self-concept as composed of perceptions of the characteristics of the self and the relationships of the self to various aspects of life, as well as the values attached to the perceptions. Rodgers suggested that equilibrium requires that patients' self-concepts be congruent with their life experiences. It follows, then, that it is not the disability per se, that psychologically influences the person, but rather the subjective meaning and feelings attached to the disability. According to Rodgers, the two major psychologic defenses which operate to maintain consistent self-concept are denial and distortion.[45]

Families of patients are affected as well. They are often confused about the diagnosis and poorly prepared to support the patient's coping responses. The resulting stress may negatively influence family dynamics and intensify the patient's depressive illness.[46] As the voice-

injured patient experiences the process of grieving, the psychologist may assume a more prominent role in his or her care. Essentially, the voice-injured patient goes through a grieving process similar to patients who mourn other losses such as the death of a loved one. In some cases, especially among voice professionals, the patients actually mourn the loss of their self as they perceive it.

The psychologist is responsible for facilitating the tasks of mourning and monitoring the individual's formal mental status for clinically significant changes.[1,8,9] There are a number of models for tracking this process. The most easily understood is that of Worden,[47] as adapted by the author (DCR). Initially, the task is to accept the reality of the loss. The need for and distress of accepting this is vestigial during the phase of diagnosis, and is held consciously in abeyance during the acute and rehabilitative phases of treatment, but it is reinforced with accumulating data measuring the patient's vocal function. As the reality becomes undeniable, the mourner must be helped to express the full range of grieving affect. The rate of accomplishing this is variable and individual. Generally, it will occur in the style with which the person usually copes with crisis and may be florid or tightly constricted. All responses must be invited and normalized. The psychologist facilitates the process and stays particularly attuned to unacceptable, divergent responses or to the failure to move through any particular response.

As attempts to deny the loss take place and fail, the mourner gradually encounters the next task: beginning to live and cope in a world in which the lost object is absent. This is the psychoanalytic process of decathexis; it requires the withdrawal of life energies from the lost object and the reinvesting of them in the self. For some professional voice users, this may be a temporary state as they make adjustments required by their rehabilitation demands. In other cases, the need for change will be lasting: change in fach, change in repertoire, need for amplification, altered performance schedule or, occasionally, change in career.[1,8,9]

As the patient so injured seeks to heal his or her life, another task looms. Known as recathexis, it involves reinvesting life energies in other relationships, interests, talents, and life goals. The individual is assisted in redefining and revaluing the self as apart from the voice. The voice is then seen as the product of the self, rather than as the equivalent of the self. For many performers this is painfully difficult.[1,8,9,47] Rosen and Sataloff have described in detail research applying the various theoretical models of grief resolution to the perception of vocal injury in professional voice users.[8]

The Surgical Experience

When vocal fold surgery is indicated, many individuals will demonstrate hospital-related phobias or self-destructive responses to pain. Adamson et al describe the importance of understanding how the patient's occupational identity will be affected by surgical intervention.[48] Vocal fold surgery has an impact on the major mode of communication that all human beings utilize; the impact is extraordinarily anxiety-producing in professional voice users. Even temporary periods of absolute voice restriction may induce feelings of insecurity, helplessness, and dissociation from the verbal world. Carpenter details the value of an early therapy session to focus on the fears, fantasies, misconceptions, and regression that frequently accompany a decision to undergo surgery.[49]

Surgical discussion usually highlights vocal fold surgery as elective for benign disease. The patient chooses surgery as the best or only remaining means to regaining the previously "normal" voice, or a different but desirable voice. The standard of care includes a thorough preoperative discussion of the limits and complications of surgery, with recognition by the surgeon that anxiety affects both understanding and retention of information about undesirable outcomes. Personality psychopathology or unrealistic expectations of the impact of surgery on their lives are factors for which surgical candidates can be screened.[5,50,51] Recognizing such problems preoperatively allows preoperative counseling and obviates many postoperative difficulties.

Although a thorough discussion is outside the scope of this chapter, surgically treated voice patients include those undergoing laryngectomy, with or without a voice prosthesis. The laryngectomized individual must make major psychologic and social adjustments. These include not only those adjustments related to a diagnosis of cancer, but also to a sudden disability: loss of voice. With the improvement in prognosis, research has begun to focus on the individual's quality of life after the laryngectomy. There is wide variability in the quality of preoperative and postoperative psychologic support reported by patients during each phase of care. Special psychologic issues in professional voice users diagnosed with laryngeal cancer are discussed in detail in other works.[1] Providing this support is a crucial role for the voice team's psychologist.[21,24,52]

SUMMARY

Psychophysiologic research informs our treatment and maximizes the benefits of medical interactions in every specialty. This is the rightful role of the arts medicine psychologist: to possess mastery of the knowledge bases of psychology and medicine and also an experiential understanding of the performing arts so that he or she may stand in alliance with the injured performer on the journey to explore, understand, and modify the psychologic impact of performance-related injuries. The speech-language pathologist must understand the psychologic factors that may cause, or be caused by, voice disorders. The speech-language pathologist must also recognize his/her limits as a psychologic counselor and know when to refer to and collaborate with a mental health professional while maintaining responsibility for voice modification and some degree of psychologic support. The laryngologist must recognize the need for therapy in individual patients, accurately diagnose the presence of organic and/or functional disorders, select and coordinate the therapy team, and retain overall responsibility for the therapeutic process and the patient's outcome. Those who are privileged to care for that uniquely human capability—the voice—quickly come to understand the essential role of psychologic awareness in our treatment failures and successes.

REFERENCES

1. Rosen DC, Sataloff RT. *Psychology of Voice Disorders*. San Diego, CA: Singular Publishing Group; 1997.

2. Aronson A. *Clinical Voice Disorders*. 3rd ed. New York, NY: Thieme Medical Publishers; 1990:117-145, 314-315.

3. Sundberg J. *The Science of the Singing Voice*. DeKalb, IL: Northern Illinois University Press; 1985:146-156.

4. Vogel D, Carter J. *The Effects of Drugs on Communication Disorders*. San Diego, CA: Singular Publishing Group; 1995:31-143.

5. Shontz F. Body image and physical disability. In: Cash T, Pruzinsky T, eds. *Body Images: Development, Deviance and Change*. New York, NY: Guilford Press; 1990:149-169.

6. Freedman R. Cognitive behavioral perspectives on body image change. In: Cash TF, Pruzinsky T, eds. *Body Images: Development, Deviance and Change*. New York, NY: Guilford Press; 1990:273-295.

7. Horney K. Cited by: Meissner W. Theories of personality. In: Nicholi A, ed. *The New Harvard Guide to Psychiatry*. Cambridge, MA: Harvard University Press; 1988:177-199.

8. Rosen DC, Sataloff RT. Psychological aspects of voice disorders. In: Rubin JS, Sataloff RT, Korovin G, Gould WJ, eds. *Diagnosis and Treatment of Voice Disorders*. New York, NY: Igaku-Shoin Medical Publishers; 1995:491-501.

9. Rosen DC, Sataloff RT, Evans H, Hawkshaw M. Self-esteem in singers: singing healthy, singing hurt. *NATS J*. 1993;49:32-35.

10. Butcher P, Elias A, Raven R. *Psychogenic Voice Disorders and Cognitive-Behavior Therapy*. San Diego, CA: Singular Publishing Group; 1993;3-22.

11. Ostwald P, Avery M, Ostwald LD. Psychiatric problems of performing artists. In: Sataloff RT, Brandfonbrenner A, Lederman R, eds. *Performing Arts Medicine*. San Diego, CA: Singular Publishing Group; 1997:337-348.

12. Nemiah J. Psychoneurotic disorders. In: Nicholi A, ed. *The New Harvard Guide to Psychiatry*. Cambridge, MA: Harvard University Press; 1988:234-258.

13. Ziegler FS, Imboden JB. Contemporary conversion reactions: II conceptual model. *Arch Gen Psychiatry*. 1962;6:279-287.

14. Hartman DE, Daily WW, Morin KN. A case of superior laryngeal nerve paresis and psychogenic dysphonia. *J Speech Hear Disord*. 1989;54:526-529.

15. Sapir S, Aronson AE. Coexisting psychogenic and neurogenic dysphonia: a source of diagnostic confusion. *Br J Disord Commun*. 1987;22:73-80.

16. Cummings JL, Benson DF, Houlihan JP, Gosenfield LF. Mutism: loss of neocortical and limbic vocalization. *J Nerv Ment Dis*. 1983;171:255-259.

17. Moses PJ. *The Voice of Neurosis*. New York, NY: Grune and Stratton; 1954.

18. Luchsinger R, Arnold E. *Voice-Speech-Language— Clinical Communicology: Its Physiology and Pathology*. Belmont, CA: Wadsworth; 1965.

19. Rulnick RK, Heuer RJ, Perez KS, Emerich KA, Sataloff RT. Voice therapy. In: Sataloff RT, ed. *Professional Voice: Science and Art of Clinical Care*. 2nd ed. San Diego, CA: Singular Publishing Group; 1997:699-720.

20. Weissman MM. The psychological treatment of depression. Evidence for the efficacy of psychotherapy alone, in comparison with, and in combination with pharmacotherapy. *Arch Gen Psychiatry*. 1979;38:1261-1269.

21. Gardner WH. Adjustment problems of laryngectomized women. *Arch Otolaryngol*. 1966;83:31-42.

22. Lankton S. *Practical Magic: A Translation of Neuro-Linguistic Programming into Clinical Psychotherapy*. Cupertino, CA: Meta Publications; 1980:174.

23. American Psychiatric Association. *Diagnostic and Statistical Manual of Mental Disorders III*. Washington, DC: American Psychiatric Association; 1987:206-210.

24. Styron W. *Darkness Visible: A Memoir of Madness*. New York, NY: Random House; 1990:27.

25. Klerman G. Depression and related disorders of mood. In: Nicholi A, ed. *The New Harvard Guide to Psychiatry*. Cambridge, MA: Harvard University Press; 1988:309-336.

26. Ross E. Rush A. Diagnosis and neuroanatomical correlates of depression in brain-damaged patients: implications for a neurology of depression. *Arch Gen Psychiatry*. 1981;38:1344-1354.

27. Sataloff RT. Stress, anxiety and psychogenic dysphonia. In: Sataloff RT, ed. *Professional Voice: The Science and Art of Clinical Care*. 2nd ed. San Diego, CA: Singular Publishing Group; 1997:195-200.

28. Sataloff RT, Lawrence VL, Hawkshaw M, Rosen DC. Medications and their effects on the voice. In: Benninger MS, Jacobson BH, Johnson AF, eds. *Vocal Arts Medicine: The Care and Prevention of Professional Voice Disorders*. New York, NY: Thieme Medical Publishers; 1994:216-225.

29. Schatzberg A, Cole J. *Manual of Clinical Psychopharmacology*. 2nd ed. Washington, DC: American Psychiatric Press; 1991:40, 50, 55, 58, 66, 68, 69, 72-77, 110-125, 158-165, 169-177, 185-227, 343-348.

30. Stam H, Koopmans J, Mathieson C. The psychological impact of a laryngectomy: comprehensive assessment. *J Psychosoc Oncol*. 1991;9:37-58.

31. Stroudmire A. *Psychological Factors Affecting Medication Conditions*. Washington, DC: American Psychiatric Press; 1995:187-192.

32. Tsuang M, Faraone S, Day M. Schizophrenic disorders. In: Nicholi A, ed. *The New Harvard Guide to Psychiatry*. Cambridge, MA: Harvard University Press; 1988:259-295.

33. Watkins J. *Hypnotherapeutic Techniques*. New York, NY: Irvington Publishers; 1987:114.

34. Metcalfe R, Firth D, Pollock S. Creed F. Psychiatric morbidity and illness behaviour in female neurological in-patients. *J Neurol Neurosurg Psychiatry*. 1988;51:1387-1390.

35. Gianotti G. Emotional behavior and hemispheric side of lesion. *Cortex*. 1972;8:41-55.

36. Alexander MP, LoVerne SR Jr. Aphasia after left hemispheric intracerebral hemorrhage. *Neurology*. 1980;30:1193-1202.

37. Mahr G, Leith W. Psychogenic stuttering of adult onset. *J Speech Hear Res*. 1992;35:283-286.

38. Brodnitz FS. Hormones and the human voice. *Bull NY Acad Med*. 1971;47:183-191.

39. Everly GS. *A Clinical Guide to the Treatment of Human Stress Response*. New York, NY: Plenum Press; 1989:40-43.

40. Green J, Snellenberger R. *The Dynamics of Health and Wellness. A Biopsychosocial Approach*. Fort Worth, TX: Holt, Reinhardt and Winston; 1991:61-64, 92, 98, 101-136.

41. Lazarus RS, Folkman S. *Stress Appraisal and Coping*. New York, NY: Springer-Verlag; 1984;283.

42. Beck A, Emery G. *Anxiety Disorders and Phobias: A Cognitive Perspective*. New York, NY: Basic Books; 1985:38-50, 151.

43. Caine JB. Understanding and treating performance anxiety from a cognitive-behavior therapy perspective. *NATS J*. 1991;47:27-51.

44. Ristad E. *A Soprano on Her Head: Right Side Up Reflections on Life and Other Performances*. Moab, UT: Real People Press; 1982:154, 155.

45. Rodgers CA. A theory of personality and interpersonal relationships as developed in a client centered framework. In: Koch S, ed. *Psychology: A Study of a Science*. New York, NY: McGraw-Hill, 1959:184-256.

46. Zraick RJ, Boone DR. Spouse attitudes toward the person with aphasia. *J Speech Hear Res*. 1991;34:123-128.

47. Worden W. *Grief Counseling and Grief Therapy*. New York, NY: Springer-Verlag; 1982:7-18.

48. Adamson JD, Hersuberg D, Shane I. The psychic significance of parts of the body in surgery. In: Howells JG, ed. *Modern Perspectives in the Psychiatric Aspects of Surgery*. New York, NY: Brunner Mazel; 1976:20-45.

49. Carpenter B. Psychological aspects of vocal fold surgery. In: Gould WJ, Sataloff RT, Spiegel JR, eds. *Voice Surgery*. St Louis, MO: Mosby; 1993:339-343.

50. Macgregor FC. Patient dissatisfaction with results of technically satisfactory surgery. *Aesthetic Plast Surg*. 1981;5:27-32.

51. Ray CJ, Fitzgibbon G. The socially mediated reduction of stress in surgical patients. In: Obourne DJ, Grunberg M, Eisner JR, eds. *Research and Psychology in Medicine*. Vol 2. Oxford, England: Pergamon Press; 1979:521-527.

52. Berkowitz JF, Lucente FF. Counseling before laryngectomy. *Laryngoscope*. 1985;95:1332-1336.

53. Cole JO, Bodkin JA. Antidepressant drug side-effects. *J Clin Psychiatry*. 1990;51:521-526.

54. *Physician's Desk Reference*. Oradell, NJ: Medical Economics Data; 1994:2000-2003, 2267-2270.

55. *Physician's Desk Reference*. Oradell, NJ: Medical Economics Data; 1996:B20.

56. *Physician's Desk Reference*. Oradell, NJ: Medical Economics Data. 2000:3237, 1073, 3070, 562, 2209, 1649.

57. *Physician's Desk Reference*. Oradell, NJ: Medical Economics Data. 1997:1615, 1878, 2239.

58. Janitec P, Davis J, Prescorn F, Ab S. *Principles and Practice of Psychopharmacology*. Baltimore, MD: Williams and Wilkins; 1998:164-184, 230-289, 433-439.

APPENDIX 29-1
Suggested Voice Therapy Techniques

BREATHING

Patients are taught that taking a deep, high-chest breath increases air pressure in the lungs greatly, triggering a Valsalva response with closure of the glottis and laryngeal and chest muscle tension. The kind of breath the patient takes may influence tension in other parts of the vocal mechanism. High-chest breathing can contribute to a feeling of breathiness and tightness in the chest. Abdominal breathing produces lesser increases of lung air pressure and removes the tension from the neck and larynx. The patient needs to know what he/she is about to say before he/she inhales the breath to say it, and this concept is discussed and practiced. This simple construct eliminates respiratory/laryngeal incoordination, reduces revisions and struggle during speaking, and allows the patient to focus on how he/she is saying something rather than on the content of what is being said. Speech should be a continuous breath event, beginning with inhalation of the appropriate amount of air, through easy transition to exhalation and voicing, to the end of the utterance. Instruction and discussion of these matters prior to the initiation of a program of breath-support exercises increases the patient's willingness to change and turns the reluctant patient into an active participant in the process of change. Specific breathing exercises to incorporate abdominal breathing are available in many other publications.

Similarly, the patient needs to know that modification of articulation postures and open, relaxed jaw positioning improve loudness and acuity in noisy environments and can be invaluable in improving communication without effort and fatigue in most speaking circumstances. Tongue tension or pulling the tongue back in the mouth leads to tension in the hyoid and larynx region. These effects can easily be demonstrated and discussed by having the patient tense the tongue or retract the tongue while digitally monitoring tension under the chin and at the sides of the larynx. The same effects can be demonstrated during talking activities. Patients need to learn to explore the feelings associated with tension and extra speaking effort.

RELAX JAW MOVEMENT AND ARTICULATION

Closed, tense jaw articulation and substitution of jaw movement for tongue and lip movements increase tension and fatigue in the face and increase the amount of pulling on the temporomandibular joint capsule. These same methods of speaking reduce lip reading and loudness in noisy speaking situations. Patients learn that in American English only six sounds, /s/, /z/, /ʃ/, /ʒ/, /tʃ/, and /dʒ/ require closure of the jaw. All other consonants and all vowels can be produced by modifying the position of the lips and tongue with no, or minor, jaw adjustment. Most of speech can be produced with the jaw in a relaxed, partially open neutral position. This can be demonstrated by monitoring tension in the masseter muscle, placing the fingers of both hands in front of the ears and alternately clenching and opening the jaw. The patient will be able to feel the bulking of the masseter during clenching and the stretching of the masseter muscle fibers when the jaw is wide open. The neutral speaking position is identifiable by the absence of muscle bulk or stretched fibers. The patient needs to experience the feeling of relaxation associated with this speaking position. The patient can then be instructed in producing the syllable /la/ by simply lifting the tongue and touching the roof of the mouth behind the upper front teeth and then dropping the tongue to a relaxed position behind, but touching, the lower front teeth. This is extended to other consonants (/ta/, /da/, /na/, /ka/, and /ga/). When the patient is proficient in eliminating jaw tension in these contexts, the effect of lip movement in addition to relaxed jaw and tongue by producing words such as, too, due, coo, load, coat, etc, is practical. Lip consonants without tensing the jaw are then added. The sounds /f/, /v/, /th/, /o/, and voiced th, (/ð/) need to be monitored for jaw jutting. Open relaxed jaw with improved oral resonance and relaxed tongue can then be practiced in words and phrases. Then the patient can practice in sentences. Practice should initially be done monitoring jaw position and movement with fingers between the posterior molars and with a mirror. As the patient begins to feel comfortable with a relaxed jaw, the tactile monitoring and then the visual monitoring can be eliminated. At this point, the patient should identify phrases and sentences he/she uses frequently, such as; "Hello"; "Put them away"; "I don't like that behavior," and so forth, which can be used as frequent daily reminders in their normal speech of more normal oral resonance and speech production. This assists in carry-over. Practice continues with sentences including jaw closure sounds and open vowels, such as: "He is going"; "Let me have a piece of pie"; "I chose two friends to go with me," and so forth. The open relaxed jaw can then be extended into question and answer activities, monologue, and dialogue.

APPENDIX 29-2
Psychoactive Medications

ANTIDEPRESSANTS

Antidepressant medications include compounds from several different classes. Tri- and tetracyclic antidepressants (TCAs) block the reuptake of norepinephrine and serotonin and have secondary effects on pre- and post-synaptic receptors.[29] An H1-H2-receptor blockade has also been demonstrated.

Schatzberg and Cole summarize the side effects of TCAs as

- anticholinergic (dry mouth and nasal mucosa, constipation, urinary hesitancy, gastro-esophageal reflux),
- autonomic (orthostatic hypotension, palpitations, increased cardiac conduction intervals, diaphoresis, hypertension, tremor),
- allergic (skin rashes),
- CNS (stimulation, sedation, delirium, twitching, nausea, speech delay, seizures, extrapyramidal symptoms), and
- other (weight gain, impotence).[29]

These may be dose related and agent specific.

Monoamine oxidase inhibitors (MAOIs) are useful in depression that is refractory to tricyclics. The mode of action involves inhibiting monoamine oxidase (MAO), which allows a buildup of norepinephrine. The full restoration of enzyme activity may take two weeks after the drug is discontinued.

The side effects of MAOIs may be extremely serious and troublesome. The one most commonly reported is dizziness secondary to orthostatic hypotension. When MAOIs are taken, hypertensive crisis with violent headache and potential cerebrovascular accident, or hyperpyrexic crisis with monoclonus and coma, may be produced by ingesting foods rich in tyramine, or by many medications, including meperidine (Demerol), epinephrine, local anesthetics containing sympathomimetics, decongestants, selective serotonin reuptake inhibitors (SSRIs), venlafaxine HCl, and surgical anesthetics. Other side effects include sexual dysfunction, sedation, insomnia, overstimulation, myositis-like reactions, myoclonic twitches, and a small incidence of dry mouth, constipation, and urinary hesitancy.[29]

A few antidepressants have been developed with different chemical structures and side effect profiles. Trazodone (Desyrel) is pharmacologically complex. It blocks serotonin reuptake, has antihistamine properties, has alpha-1 and serotonin-2 antagonism. It is helpful in depression associated with insomnia. Three side effects are particularly noteworthy: sedation, acute dizziness with fainting (especially when taken on an empty stomach), and priapism.[1,53-55] Effexor (venlafaxine HCl) is a potent reuptake inhibitor of serotonin and norepinephrine and a weak reuptake inhibitor of dopamine. It is useful in both major depression and generalized anxiety disorder.[56]

Nefazodone hydrochloride (Serzone) is another antidepressant. Its chemical structure is different from the SSRIs, tri/tetracyclics, and MAOIs. It appears to inhibit neuronal reuptake of serotonin and has serotonin-2 antagonism. It has been advertised as useful in depressions characterized by anxiety. Side effects include significant orthostasis, potential activation of mania, and a questionable potential for priapism. Decreased cognitive and motor performance, dry mouth, nausea, and dizziness, are also noted as well as other frequently recurring side effects. This drug has notable medication interactions with Halcion, Xanax, and Propulsid. It is not recommended for patients with unstable heart disease.[57]

Bupropion (Wellbutrin) was released in 1989. It blocks the reuptake of norepinephrine and dopamine. It is not anticholinergic. The most commonly reported complaint is nausea. However, a potential risk of seizures exists, and the drug is not recommended in patients with a history of seizures, head trauma, or anorexia or bulimia.[29,53]

A group of antidepressant drugs that selectively inhibit the reuptake of serotonin are most likely to be selected as first pharmacologic agents. These include fluoxetine (Prozac), sertraline (Zoloft), paroxetine (Paxil), and citalopram (Celexa). They appear to be effective in typical episodic depression and for some chronic refractory presentations.[29,53] Major side effects are significant degrees of nausea, sweating, headache, mouth dryness, tremor, nervousness, dizziness, insomnia, somnolence, constipation, and sexual dysfunction. There are drug interactions with the concomitant administration of tryptophan, MAOIs, warfarin, cimetidine, phenobarbital, and phenytoin. Clearance of citalopram may be reduced by concomittant administration of omeprazole, metoprolol, or macrolide antibiotics.[53,56,57]

MOOD STABILIZING

Mood-stabilizing drugs are those that are effective in manic episodes and prevent manic and depressive recurrences in patients with bipolar disorder. These include lithium salts and several anticonvulsants. Lithium is available in multiple formulations, and prescribing is guided by both symptom index and blood levels. Lithium side effects are apparent in diverse organ systems. The most commonly noted is fine tremor, especially noticeable in the fingers. With toxic lithium levels, gross tremulousness, ataxia, dysarthria, and confusion or delirium may develop. Some patients describe slowed mentation, measurable memory deficit, and impaired

creativity. Chronic nausea and diarrhea are usually related to gastrointestinal tract mucosal irritation, but may be signs of toxicity. Some patients gain weight progressively and may demonstrate edema or increased appetite. Lithium therapy affects thyroid function. In some cases it is transitory, but there may be goiter with normal T3 and T4 but elevated TSH levels.[29]

Polyuria and secondary polydipsia are complications of lithium and may progress to diabetes insipidus. In most cases, discontinuing the medication reverses the renal effects. Prescribed thiazide diuretics can double the lithium level and lead to sudden lithium toxicity. Non steroidal anti-inflammatory drugs (NSAIDs) decrease lithium excretion. Cardiovascular effects include the rare induction of sick sinus syndrome. The aggravation of psoriasis, allergic skin rashes, and reversible alopecia are associated with lithium therapy, as are teratogenic effects.[29]

ANTICONVULSANT

Three anticonvulsant compounds appear to act preferentially on the temporal lobe and the limbic system. Carbamazepine (Tegretol) carries a risk of agranulocytosis or aplastic anemia, and is monitored by complete blood counts and symptoms of bone marrow depression. Care must be taken to avoid the numerous drug interactions that accelerate the metabolism of some drugs or raise carbamazepine levels.[29]

Valproic acid (Depakote, Depakene) is especially useful when there is a rapid-cycling pattern. The major side effect is hepatocellular toxicity and pancreatitis. Thrombocytopenia and platelet dysfunction have been reported. Sedation is common, and tremor, ataxia, weight gain, alopecia, and fetal neural tube defects are all side effects that patients must comprehend.[29,58] Newer anticonvulsants (Topamax) as well as gabapentin (Neurontin) are also used as mood-stabilizing agents.[58]

ANXIOLYTICS

Anxiolytics are the psychotropic drugs most commonly prescribed, usually by nonpsychiatric specialists, for somatic disorders. It behooves the laryngologist to probe for a history of past or current drug therapy in markedly anxious or somatically focused patients with vocal complaints. Benzodiazepines produce effective relief of anxiety but have a high addictive potential that includes physical symptoms of withdrawal, including potential seizures, if the drug is stopped abruptly. It is important to remember that this class of drugs is commonly available on the streets and from colleagues. The most common benzodiazepine side effect is dose-related sedation, followed by dizziness, weakness, ataxia, decreased motor performance, and mild hypotension. Clonazepam (Klonopin) is a benzodiazepine and may produce sedation, ataxia, and malcoordination, as well as (rarely) disinhibition, agitation, or asituational anger.[29] Alterations of sensory input, either by CNS stimulants (cocaine, amphetamines, and over-the-counter vasoconstrictors) or depressants, are potentially dangerous in a voice professional. The patient who is unaware of these effects should be apprised of them promptly by the laryngologist.[1,28]

Phenobarbital and meprobamate are no longer commonly used as anxiolytics in the United States. Clomipramine (Anafranil) and fluvoxamine (Luvox) are useful in the anxiety evident in an obsessive-compulsive disorder. The side effects are similar to those of the tricyclic antidepressants: dry mouth, hypotension, constipation, tachycardia, sweating, tremor, and anorgasmia.[29] Fluoxetine (Prozac) has also proved effective for some patients with obsessive-compulsive disorder, and appears better tolerated.[29]

Hydroxyzine, an antihistamine, is occasionally prescribed for mild anxiety and/or pruritus. It does not produce physical dependence but does potentiate the CNS effects of alcohol, narcotics, CNS depressants, and tricyclic antidepressants. Side effects include notable mucous membrane dryness and drowsiness.[29]

Buspirone (BuSpar) is not sedating at its usual dosage levels, and it has little addictive potential. Side effects include mild degrees of headache, nausea, and dizziness. However, it is poorly tolerated in patients accustomed to the more immediate relief of benzodiazepines.[29]

Beta-blockers are used by some clinicians to mask physiologic symptoms of sympathetic arousal in performance anxiety. Their side effects are serious and may include bradycardia, hypotension, weakness, fatigue, clouded sensorium, impotence, and bronchospasm. There is controversy regarding their potential to induce depression.[29] Although the problem of upper respiratory tract secretion dryness was diminished and other symptoms of performance anxiety were lessened in two studies,[27] the drugs are potentially dangerous. Moreover, they leave the underlying conflict unresolved and negatively affect artistic quality.[27] Some authors still prefer them, especially in those patients who may be at risk for drug dependency.

ANTIPSYCHOTIC DRUGS

Various antipsychotic drugs (haloperidol [Haldol], chlorpromazine HCl [Thorazine], perphenazine [Trilafon], molindone [Moban], loxapine HCl [Loxitane], and clozapine [Clozaril] have a mode of action that involves dopamine antagonism, probably in the mesolimbic or mesocortical areas. They also have endocrine effects through dopamine receptors in the hypothalamic-pituitary axis.[29] These potent agents have very significant side effects. Sedation, accompanied by fatigue during early dosing and akinesia with chronic administration, is frequently described. Anticholinergic effects include postural hypotension, dry mouth, nasal congestion, and constipation. The endocrine system is also affected, with a direct increase in blood prolactin levels. Breast enlargement and galactorrhea are seen in men and women and correlate with impotence and amenorrhea. Weight gain is often excessive and frequently leads to noncompliance. Skin complications such as rash, retinal pigmentation, and photosensitivity can occur. Rare but serious complications include agranulocytosis, allergic obstructive hepatitis, seizures, and sudden death secondary to ventricular fibrillation.[29] A drug recently marketed which selectively blocks dopamine receptors without blocking receptors in the basal ganglia is risperidone (Risperdal).[54] Additional new antipsychotics useful in some psychotic patients include olanzapine (Zyprexa) and quetiapine (Seroquel).[56]

Approximately 14% of patients receiving long-term (greater than 7 years) treatment with antipsychotic agents develop tardive dyskinesia ranging from minimal tongue restlessness to incapacitating, disfiguring choreiform and/or athetoid movements, especially of the head, neck, and hands. Unfortunately, there is no cure for the condition once it develops, nor are there accurate predictors for which patients will be affected.[29]

The mode of action in neurologic side effects of the neuroleptics is primarily cholinergic-dopaminergic blockade. Dystonia usually involves tonic spasm of the tongue, jaw, and neck but may range from mild tongue stiffness to opisthotonos.[29] Pseudoparkinsonism may occur very early in treatment and is evidenced by muscle stiffness, cogwheel rigidity, stooped posture, and mask-like facies with loss of salivary control. Pill-rolling tremor is rare. Akathisia, an inner-driven muscular restlessness with rhythmic leg jiggling, hand wringing, and pacing, is extremely unpleasant. Multiple drug regimens are employed to diminish these symptoms.[29]

Neuroleptic malignant syndrome is a potentially fatal complication of these drugs. Patients manifest hyperthermia, severe extrapyramidal signs, and autonomic hyperarousal. Neuroleptics also affect temperature regulation generally and can predispose to heat stroke.[29]

CHAPTER 30

Medications and the Voice

Thomas M. Harris, FRCS

John S. Rubin, MD, FACS, FRCS

Voice is the primary means of human communication, and the sound signals that we make are used to communicate not only intellectual processes but also emotional, aspirational, and spiritual content. The means given us to communicate all these messages is a biomechanical system governed by complex neurochemistry both centrally within the central nervous system and peripherally. It is potentially affected by all the body's humoral biofeedback mechanisms.

One problem encountered when trying to treat a biomechanical system with systemically applied medications is that drugs do act systemically, and all will have some degree of unwanted side effects. The drawback is specificity. Even with the advent of increasingly specific receptor binding of drugs, there is still no answer to the problem of how to treat a small part of a single anatomic entity on the one hand, while also wishing to treat a single defined problem of dysfunction involving several different systems on the other.

Voicing is an activity superimposed on other older systems essential for the maintenance of life, and our ability to treat voice problems pharmacologically reflects this. Most pharmacologically active medications used in the management of voice problems have a temporary and reversible activity, although the physician should be wary of medications whose effects may be permanent. Unfortunately, many of the drugs used to treat other unrelated medical conditions may have an adverse effect on the voice, and it is not always possible to learn about them adequately by cross-checking in the *Formulary* under "side effects." There have been several overviews of the subject over the last twelve years, all with a similar story to tell.[1-5]

Patients do not, in general, complain of problems specifically relating to inappropriate autonomic function, to the histamine inflammatory cascade, or to gastroesophageal reflux. The few who already "know all the answers" can be exceedingly difficult to treat. Mostly patients complain of vocal dysfunction, and the symptoms that may relate to that dysfunction. Sometimes they may also attribute inflammatory features to the problem.

For example, the patient with dysphonia is likely to complain of (at least) one of the following symptoms, which they will relate to their dysphonia: thick mucus, cough, throat clearing, vocal fatigue/loss of stamina, problems with the *passaggio*, loss of vocal range, loss of vocal timbre, coarsening vibrato, pitch and register instability, sudden reduction in voice, gradual reduction/loss of voice, lowering or rising of pitch, breathy or rough voice quality.

It is incumbent upon the treating physician to determine the cause of these complaints. Etiology could range from inflammatory or mechanical problems directly having an impact at the vocal fold level (for example, acute laryngitis), or having an impact on other elements of the vocal tract (for example, asthma or chronic obstructive pulmonary disease); endocrinopathies (for example, thyroid axis dysfunction), central nervous system pathology (eg, Parkinson's disease), psychologic disorders, and so forth. This list is almost endless. Many of these are further described in other chapters of this book. Medications, used for related or unrelated medical problems (for example, high blood pressure, depression, etc), may also have an impact upon the vocal tract in a deleterious manner.

It is clear from the above brief discussion that it is not appropriate to prescribe any medication for a voice problem without taking a very thorough history of the problem as well as performing a detailed examination of the subject's entire vocal tract. An accurate determination as to the etiology has to be made before recommending therapy, weighing the pharmacologic benefits of any particular medication against their unavoidable side effects. To this end, the physician must have at his or her disposal, accurate knowledge not only of the activity of classes of drugs but the variation between different members of those classes. A side effect that may be inevitable and endurable in the treatment of serious or life-threatening disease may be intolerable in the medical treatment of a voice disorder. In this chapter we review the types and classes of drugs used most commonly in laryngologic practice together with their associated problems.

AUTONOMIC NERVOUS SYSTEM

First, we briefly review the autonomic system. The autonomic nervous system is the motor system regulating the organs of the body, including smooth (involuntary) muscles, cardiac muscles, and glands. It is composed of two systems, the sympathetic (thoracolumbar) and parasympathetic (craniosacral). On the whole, these systems are antagonistic to each other, frequently travel together, and innervate many of the same organs. The primary neurotransmitter of the sympathetic (adrenergic) system is norepinephrine and that of the parasympathetic system, acetylcholine.[6]

In the sympathetic system the chemical mediator released at the synaptic terminal of preganglionic sympathetic fibers is acetylcholine and these fibers are termed "cholinergic." The chemical mediator of postganglionic fibers to smooth muscle and piloerector muscles is epinephrine or norepinephrine. Such fibers are called adrenergic fibers. Postganglionic fibers to sweat glands are cholinergic.

Cholinergic fibers can be blocked at the synapse by atropine and by anticholinergic drugs (such as methaneline bromide, propantheline bromide, and methscopolamine bromide). They can be stimulated by cholinergic drugs such as acetylcholine and pilocarpine. Pilocarpine also promotes sweating. Agents that inhibit the enzyme cholinesterase, which normally hydrolyzes acetylcholine at the synapse, will mimic the action of acetylcholine, an example being physostigmine.

Postganglionic sympathetic fibers to the viscera are adrenergic. However, the response of smooth muscle depends on the local type of receptor. Thus, stimulation of bronchial and coronary musculature causes dilation while stimulation of the vessels usually causes contraction. Postganglionic adrenergic fibers can be stimulated or mimicked by epinephrine or norepinephrine, or blocked by drugs such as dibenamine.

The parasympathetic system is divided into two outflow components, the cranial and the sacral. The cranial supplies the head and neck, as well as the foregut and midgut derivatives (including the pharynx, larynx, esophagus, lungs, and stomach). Both preganglionic and postganglionic synapses of the paraganglionic system are cholinergic. Thus, they are stimulated by cholinergic drugs (acetylcholine, physostigmine, pilocarpine) and blocked by anticholinergic drugs (atropine, banthine).

Stimulation of cholinergic fibers will cause hypermotility of visceral muscle and promote secretions rich in water and enzymes. Blockade causes reduction of motility and of secretions, decreased hypochloric acid in the stomach and dryness of the mouth.[7]

In summary, when the sympathetic system is stimulated, the "fight, flight, fright" syndrome occurs with elevation of heart rate, blood pressure, shift of blood flow from the skin and gut to skeletal muscles. The face becomes pale, palms sweat, vocal tract dries, pupils and bronchioles dilate. When the parasympathetic system is stimulated, saliva increases, heart rate slows, and skin flushes.[8]

RESPIRATORY SECRETIONS AND MEDICATIONS

All air-breathing animals depend on a large surface area of mucous membrane covered with a thin blanket of mucus which is mainly water-containing, but also has glycoproteins linked by disulfide bonds.[4] This blanket permits the exchange of gases with the atmosphere. Without this thin lubricating layer of fluid with its surfactant properties lying on top, exchange of respiratory gases cannot take place and death will result. The mucus blanket is a dynamic structure requiring constant clearance and renewal, and any conditions, disease, or medication that slows this process is necessarily going to produce adverse effects. The list of pharmacologic agents that may be used with benefit is short.

Cough

Cough and/or swallow are the mechanisms employed to propel mucus out of the chest through the larynx. The vocal folds are devoid of ciliary mucosa, and, therefore, periodic clearance of mucus from the subglottis is normal. If, for any reason, there is overproduction of mucus within the chest, then a productive cough may be generated. Drying of the increased flow of mucus is contraindicated; the aim being simply to remove the offending tracheobronchial deposits of spent mucus. A nonproductive cough or "dry" cough has no physiologic function and may, therefore, be treated symptomatically.

The oldest and still in many ways most satisfactory primary treatment for cough remains steam inhalation. The steam soothes laryngeal irritation and reduces the drying out of the thickened mucus deposits. While not strictly a medication, the authors believe that this should remain a mainstay of treatment for cough. We do not prescribe any aromatic compounds to be added to the steamed water. One which is widely available but which we oppose is menthol, an agent that stimulates cold receptors in mucosa. This produces a pleasant but illusory sensation of clear airways while the subject is inhaling the compound, but this sensation is promptly lost when the inhalation is terminated.

When irritation is principally supralaryngeal, a simple "over-the-counter" demulcent of linctus is soothing. A demulcent functions in a similar manner to saliva substitutes (eg, Xerolube, Salivart, Saliva Orthana) or tear substitutes (eg, Hypromellose, Liquifilm, or Ilube), the aim being to coat the dry, irritated membrane with a soothing, low-viscosity, hydrophilic layer. In appropriate doses, there appear to be no significant side effects in clinical practice. It must be recalled that the principal function of the larynx is to protect the lower airway; thus, none of this linctus will actually reach the vocal folds or below, when swallowed or placed in the nose or mouth. On the other hand, 5% propylene glycol in a physiologically balanced salt solution, delivered by large particle mist, has been described to provide helpful lubrication to the larynx in dry climates; the authors have no experience with its use, however.[5]

At times, the physician may feel that the clinical situation warrants prescription of a cough suppressant, and there may be occasions when a cough is so severe that it may produce damage to the vocal folds or elsewhere. In these relatively limited circumstances a cough suppressant may be used with benefit. This group of medications falls into two broad classes: the opiate-based preparations, which act chiefly within the medulla and higher cortical centers as a tranquilizer, and antihistamine (H1 receptor) suppressants, which are used for their anticholinergic rather than strictly antihistaminic effects. Neither class of medication is ideal in the treatment of a voice disorder, because both are sedating and both tend to dry the mucus blanket. In addition, many proprietary cough suppressants contain the nonspecific alpha-sympathomimetic agent, pseudoephedrine, which produces a drying effect on vocal tract secretions, as well as tachycardia, insomnia, and cardiac irritability. Under most circumstances there are products with fewer side effects that may be used in their stead. For example, Sataloff feels that frequently, preparations containing dextromethorphan together with a wetting agent work well in voice professionals.[5]

Thick Mucus

During the course of an uncomplicated upper respiratory infection, the phase of hypersecretion is followed by a period of reduced secretions of the mucus blanket, with potential drying of the mucosa. The use of wetting agents to limit the associated symptoms is both logical and effective. Although saline spray cannot be strictly considered to be a medication, as its mode of action is largely physical, it should nonetheless remain high on the list of useful treatments for conditions causing dysphonia. Patients may be asked to make up their own saline solution, but several products now exist which produce an instant, highly portable, means of providing an aerosol of saline under pressure (eg, Stérimar). Care should be taken to use only products that do not contain any potentially irritating propellant. It is also logical and moderately effective to try to increase the production of as thin and nonviscous a layer of mucus as possible.

Expectorants are available over-the-counter and are commonly used to increase mucus production. Most increase mucus production in low dosages, but in higher dosage may have marked emetic properties (eg, guaifenesin containing products [Humibid]), iodinated glycerol (which is effective but no longer generally available in some countries [Organidin], benylin expectorant and many others).

Inflamed mucosa is much more permeable to plasma components than normal mucosa. Respiratory mucosa secretes glycoproteins that polymerize into the mucus by producing disulfide cross-bonding.[4] After a viral upper respiratory infection there will be leakage of inflammatory fluid across the membrane, and this fluid will contain proteins which do not have the same physical properties as respiratory mucosal glycoproteins. Unfortunately, these too can cross-bond with glycoproteins to produce the viscous mucus plugs and secretions that are troublesome to voice users.

Mucus-Splitting Agents

Agents which can split the disulfide cross-bonds are available. Acetylcysteine[8] (Mucomist) and carbocisteine (Mucodyne) have been demonstrated to be effective in "normalizing" the thick mucus produced in conditions such as bronchitis. In addition, the manufacturers claim that there is an objective reduction in goblet cell hyperplasia in certain animal models. Their use in phoniatric practice is uncommon, however, and the authors are not aware of any peer-reviewed articles objectively demonstrating their value in this area.

Although not pharmacologically "active," the importance of steam and water aerosols in the management of thick mucus in the presence of bronchial irritation needs to be stressed. Humidity is essential to keep viscous mucus mixed with inflammatory exudate on the move. Water droplet size in steam from boiled water is ideal for even distribution throughout the larynx, trachea, and bronchi. Theoretically, ultrasonically generated water vapor may have a droplet size that is smaller, possibly causing a disproportionate amount of water to end in the alveoli. The authors are not aware of any problems with such a technique as reported in the literature, however.

MEDICATIONS MODIFYING ALLERGIC OR ASTHMATIC SYMPTOMS

Patients exhibiting dysphonic symptoms will not infrequently complain of nasal blockage. Blockage may be actual or perceived. If actual, and bone or cartilage is causing the obstruction, then the management is surgical. If the obstruction is from soft tissue, and is caused by a pathologic process in the tissue or to rhinosinusitis, the management may also include surgery. There is a gray area between obvious medical and surgical management which we encounter frequently in conditions such as nasal polyposis.

By contrast, acute allergic rhinitis is clearly a medical problem. This condition is more fully described as an anaphylactoid (Type 1) allergy. The nasal mucous membrane reacts to noxious stimuli or immunoglobulin (IgE) release by allergens, by releasing histamines and other slower acting inflammatory mediators such as kinins (a class of peptides), leukotrienes, and prostaglandins (both arachidonic acid derivatives). Histamine is the mediator which causes the most rapid biochemical changes that we see. It is found widely distributed in the surface membranes of the body, mostly in bound form within mast cells. The nose and respiratory tract are ideally suited for deposition of particles of allergenic material, and it is for this reason that the res-

piratory tract demonstrates the most common forms of allergic reaction.

Antihistamines

Ideal management of allergic rhinitis and allergic asthma remains avoidance to exposure to the allergen. However, this is frequently impossible to achieve and the fall-back situation generally includes the systemic or topical use of antihistamines and/or steroids, the former usually administered systemically and the latter topically. Certain new classes of antihistamines are now becoming available that also have anti-inflammatory potential (eg, Neoclarityn) and may in the future change this equation.

Antihistamines (H1 receptor antagonists) are widely used in clinical practice often without clearly defined clinical indications. They act as competitive inhibitors at receptor sites and are therefore most useful when administered prior to exposure to allergens.

Generally, antihistamines have associated anticholinergic side effects. While they may restrict the effects of histamine release, and reduce the acute features of onset of anaphylaxis, they will commonly produce unwanted side effects such as:

1. an increase in viscosity of the mucosal blanket;
2. a drying effect in the mucosa of the aerodigestive tract;
3. gastrointestinal motility changes;
4. some sedation.[5,8]

Although the design of modern antihistamines has greatly increased receptor specificity and reduced crossing of the blood-brain barrier by the medication, the end product is still less than perfect. Nonetheless, useful examples of these more recent developments include: acrivastine, cetirizine hydrochloride, fexofenadine, loratadine, and mizolastine. It is therefore suggested that the use of antihistamines be restricted primarily to the prophylactic or early treatment of definite Type 1 allergic conditions, and that they not be used as part of a general package of treatment to "reduce inflammation."

Mast Cell Stabilizers

Other medications with fewer associated problems may also be considered, especially for prophylaxis and for treating children. Mast cell stabilizers such as sodium cromoglicate and nedocromil inhibit the release of mediators from sensitized mast cells. This class of medication is useful in the prevention of performance-related bronchial hyperreactivity and exercise-induced asthma. The problems associated with this class of drug predominantly relate to the fact that the sensitized mucosa has to be kept covered with the medication for it to be effective, and this demands frequent application. In addition, the powder form in which sodium cromoglicate is commonly supplied seems to thicken the mucus blanket somewhat, and performers may find this troublesome. Sodium cromoglicate is of no value in the treatment of acute asthma and is not very effective in the management of food allergies.

Inhaled Corticosteroids

Corticosteroids are potent anti-inflammatory agents. Used in topical form, they are frequently prescribed for a number of chronic inflammatory conditions such as allergic rhinitis, rhinosinusitis, asthma, chronic obstructive airway disease, and relapsing conditions such as bronchial hyperactivity.

Systemic absorption from inhaled corticosteroids in commercially available sprays does occur and the recent warnings of possible systemic effects by the Committee on Safety of Medicines[9] has prompted a reexamination of their use, particularly in children. First-generation topical corticosteroids such as betamethasone and dexamethasone may have clinically significant systemic absorption, and certain recent papers have pointed out their potential for causing systemic problems.[10,11] Therefore, only brief use of such agents should be routinely recommended, particularly in children.[12]

Gastrointestinal absorption of all inhaled steroids (that reach the GI tract) is significant. Certain intranasal steroids, for example, mometasone furoate and fluticasone propionate have been found to have very low oral bioavailability.[12,13]

In general, inhaled corticosteroids are well tolerated, often over prolonged periods of time. Because of concerns with long-term effects on growth, however, the manufacturers warn against using such agents in young children. The prescribing physician should also recall that atrophic side effects, although localized, are similar to the systemically prescribed medications. Unfortunately, these compounds tend to concentrate and deposit on parts of the airway where there is cross-sectional narrowing (eg, the vocal folds). Damage to the larynx especially by steroid inhalations intended for the chest, can be reduced by good inhalation technique, the use of spacers or similar devices, post-inhalation breath-holding, and rinsing and swallowing with water following inhalation.[14-18] Damage to the larynx from nasal use of corticosteroids can be markedly reduced by the simple expedient of not sniffing when spraying (personal communication from Glenis Scadding, 2001).

In general, as with all treatments, the benefits must outweigh the risks and common sense must be used.

With inhaled nasal steroids, risks, while present, are relatively small and can be reduced by careful and appropriate use.

Sympathomimetics

There are several commercially available nasal and systemic preparations with a sympathomimetic as one of the active agents. These cause marked vasoconstriction of the nasal mucosa and may assist the voice professional to perform during the active rhinorrhea phase of an upper respiratory infection. Used topically (intranasally) they should be used with caution and for no more than 3 days. Topical sympathomimetics are well absorbed and do have systemic effects as described above for adrenergic agents. Among other side effects, drying of the vocal tract is identifiable from both topical and systemic applications. Prolonged use intranasally can lead to a syndrome entitled "rhinitis medicamentosa" wherein the local vasoconstrictive effects of the medication work for shorter time periods and the nose becomes paradoxically blocked, potentially leading to an addictive state of use.

Sympathomimetics are available by inhalation, particularly for the brochodilator effect in asthmatics (eg, salbutamol). Xanthines (for example, aminophylline) may also be administered systemically for reversible airway disorders, particularly acute exacerbations of asthma.

Administration of sympathomimetic agents is associated with many side effects, not the least being fine tremor, nervous tension, headache, palpitations, tachycardia, muscle cramps, hypokalemia after high doses, and hypersensitivity reactions, including paradoxical bronchospasm.[19]

Recent or Still Experimental Therapy

There may prove to be a role for leukotriene receptor antagonists (eg, montelukast or zafirlukast) as useful adjunctive therapy in the prophylaxis of allergic rhinitis or asthma not adequately controlled by inhaled corticosteroids and/or beta-agonists. It must be noted, however, that Churg-Strauss syndrome (characterized by asthma, rhinosinusitis, systemic vasculitis, and eosinophilia) has been reported in the United Kingdom in association with use of these drugs, especially where there has been a rapid withdrawal of steroids. Careful monitoring is advised.

SYSTEMIC CORTICOSTEROIDS FOR ACUTE LARYNGEAL INFLAMMATION

Acute allergic reactions produce an inflammatory response by the body, with increased secretions, increased membrane and capillary permeability, and a brisk aggregation of inflammatory exudates. Affected tissues rapidly become edematous and stiffen because of the increase in extracellular fluid and inflammatory cellular components. Diuretics cannot easily reduce the resulting edema as the water content is protein-bound.[20] This acute inflammatory reaction is reduced by the natural production of corticosteroids.

Management of acute laryngitis as well as inflammation elsewhere in the vocal tract may include treatment with synthetic corticosteroids such as methylprednisolone and its more potent relative dexamethasone. Treatment of acute inflammation using systemic steroids may produce a rapid reduction (never resolution) of the inflammation, and so their use among laryngologists is popular.

Treatment dosages and duration varies considerably. In general, laryngologists tend to prescribe systemic corticosteroids for laryngeal inflammatory conditions for shorter periods of time than pulmonologists do for inflammatory conditions of the chest. One of the authors (JSR) prefers to prescribe relatively low dose methylprednisolone in descending doses (typically 15-25 mg in one dose on the first day with descending doses by 5 mg daily to 0 mg). Other authors have found a higher dosage regimen (prednisolone 60 mg or dexamethasone 6 mg) intramuscularly followed by an oral tapering dose over 3-6 days to be more beneficial.[5]

Physicians who prescribe such agents must be familiar not only with the dose/potency relationships between the different glucocorticoids, but also with the possible side effects, which are considerable. Side effects are generally not noted with the short-term use which is appropriate for acute laryngitis. Nonetheless, side effects from short-term use of systemic corticosteroids can include insomnia, mood change (usually euphoria, although psychosis has been reported), irritability, gastric irritation (including possible ulcer or hemorrhage and increase in reflux), blurred vision, mild vocal tract dryness, membrane and capillary fragility.

Longer-term steroids have been associated with side effects such as tissue atrophy, muscle weakness, dyskinesia, fat redistribution, and wasting. Exogenous steroids will disrupt endogenous steroid production and may cause a Cushingoid state; precipitous discontinuation can lead to Addisonian-like crises.

Systemic steroids should be used with particular care in patients with diabetes on the basis that: 1) they will depress the immune system generally and thus may mask infection, which diabetics are particularly prone to, and 2) steroid use will increase circulating glucose and could precipitate dangerously elevated levels of glucose.

That said, when used in appropriate dosages for appropriate indications in well-selected patients, systemic corticosteroids have a significant and useful role.

GASTROESOPHAGEAL REFLUX AND LARYNGOPHARYNGEAL REFLUX

The symptoms of gastroesophageal reflux (GER) and laryngopharyngeal reflux (LPR) appear to be misunderstood by many afflicted individuals and treating physicians, and are not uncommonly ascribed to the "sinuses," "post-nasal drip," or nonspecific allergies. This contrasts dramatically with the findings of authors such as Koufman and Cummins.[21] They found 50% of 132 patients with laryngeal and voice disorders to have objective evidence of LPR, of which only a third of the LPR positive group were actually aware of heartburn as a symptom. This problem is pervasive among dysphonic patients; thus, it is dealt with in detail in its own chapter. (See Chapter 24 by Koufman.)

Depending on the clinical evidence of supine versus upright reflux, effective medical management may only require physical elevation of the head of the patient's bed by about four inches, coupled with dietary and lifestyle modifications. More persistent symptoms will require medical management or, at times, surgery. Medical management can be broken into antacids, histamine H2 receptor blockers, and proton pump inhibitors.[22]

Antacids

The principal ingredients of antacids fall into three categories:

1. aluminum and magnesium-containing compounds;
2. sodium bicarbonate and calcium carbonate;
3. alginate-containing preparations.

The first two groups directly neutralize acid; the third provides a glutinous raft that floats on the surface of stomach contents and, to some extent, corks the gastroesophageal sphincter and coats irritated esophageal mucosa. There are numerous proprietary, non-prescription compounds containing combinations and variations of these substances available over-the-counter from pharmacies.

Antacids do have a drying effect on the vocal tract and in some individuals may cause constipation, diarrhea, or bloating.[5] There have been some concerns expressed in the popular press over long-term usage of aluminum containing compounds although the authors have not, to date, identified any objective evidence supporting these contentions. There may also be some concerns regarding long-term usage of compounds with significant quantities of bismuth.

Histamine H2 Receptor Antagonists

For symptoms of GER not satisfactorily managed by the above measures, especially for performers in whom abdominal support for voicing produces brisk upright reflux, medical management may require the use of a histamine H2 receptor antagonist (eg, cimetidine, famotidine, nizatidine, ranitidine). This group of antihistamines selectively blocks histamine-mediated production of gastric acid and is almost entirely free of the hypnotic side effects of their nonspecific cousins. Dryness of the vocal tract has been reported as have liver function alteration, gastrointestinal disturbance, headache, dizziness, rashes, confusion, and very occasional hypersensitivity reactions.

Proton Pump Inhibitors

The most recent group of drugs used to reduce gastric acid secretion is the proton pump inhibitors (eg, omeprazole, lansoprazole, pantoprazole, rabeprazole). These highly effective medications now appear to be the treatment of choice in the acute medical management of GER, especially where there is evidence of esophagitis. No other medication is as effective in hydrogen ion transfer blockade. It is also the drug of choice in the maintenance management of LPR-related conditions such as posterior laryngitis and arytenoid granuloma. Although biochemically different, the range of side effects is not dissimilar to those of the H2 receptor antagonists, for example, GI disturbance, headache, hypersensitivity reactions, liver enzyme, and hematologic changes.

Prokinetic Agents

As adjunctive treatment to acid-reducing medications, a prokinetic agent (eg, metoclopramide) may be considered in order to improve gastroesophageal sphincter function, and to speed gastric emptying. Until recently another drug in this category, cisapride, was proving very effective; however, it has recently been withdrawn on both sides of the Atlantic because of potentially hazardous cardiac side effects. As a result, at the time of writing, there are a significant number of patients with symptoms previously controlled by this drug who now require a careful reappraisal of their anti-reflux maintenance.

Caveat: Medications that modify symptoms of gastritis, GER, and LPR may also mask the early signs of malignant gastroesophageal disease. It is not uncom-

mon clinical practice at the time of writing for a laryngologist to institute short-term treatment with one of the agents described above. It is recommended that the treating physician consider, in patients in whom long-term management is being suggested, a referral to a gastrointestinal physician.

HORMONES

The larynx has been shown to have a significant number of receptors for estrogens and androgens.[23-25] Timonen found 15.6% of women treated for voice disturbances to have endocrinologic causation.[26] Hormone medications may affect voice quality by alterations in fluid content or structural changes, the latter being particularly seen following administration of androgens.[27]

Sex Hormones

Androgen-containing agents have been used or recommended for such conditions as endometriosis, fibrocystic breast disease, postmenopausal sexual dysfunction, and as part of some chemotherapeutic regimens for cancer. Such medicines can have as side effects hirsutism, alopecia, and permanent lowering of the fundamental frequency of the voice. They should only be used when absolutely indicated and following a frank discussion of risk-benefits.[5,28-30]

Similarly, estrogen-containing compounds have been used in males as part of some chemotherapeutic regimens for cancer of the prostate or during trans-sexual procedures. There is less information available regarding the long-term effects of such medications upon the voice.

Birth control pills with relatively high progesterone content may produce androgen-like changes in the voice.[5,31] Most oral contraceptives currently prescribed in the western world have a better estrogen-progesterone balance, and voice changes are uncommon (less than 5%) and tend to abate following discontinuation.[5]

At menopause there is a 10-20 fold drop in estradiol levels but the ovaries continue to secrete androgens.[32] As such the voice tends to lower in fundamental frequency.[33]

In recent years, hormone replacement therapy has become widespread throughout the western world. There are many reasons for giving a patient long-term replacement, and the cardiologic, skeletal, and emotional consequences of this are now becoming comprehensively documented. What are much less widely covered are the vocal consequences of hormone replacement therapy (HRT). Work relating to the measurable effects of HRT on postmenopausal women, for example, that of

Lindholm et al[34] is scarce in the literature. Notwithstanding this gap in the evidence base, HRT is not infrequently prescribed in the hope of delaying age-related vocal changes, frequently with little prior knowledge of the estrogenic/progestegenic/androgenic capacity of the medication prescribed. Unforeseen problems, such as difficulty in pitch matching, register breaks and other symptoms, may occur. Empirically there is little doubt that HRT, if used appropriately, can help an aging voice. However caution is advised, and it is the authors' feeling that this is best done in conjunction with a gynecologic opinion.

Thyroid

Thyroid axis abnormalities can have an impact upon the larynx, frequently producing significant changes in vocal quality. Hypothyroidism causes accumulation of mucopolysaccharides throughout the body. It can cause the vocal folds to thicken. It is associated with loss of range, efficiency, and a "muffling" of the voice.[35] Medical correction of the hypothyroid state with thyroxine will frequently improve voicing parameters. Hyperthyroidism can also affect vocal quality.

BETA-BLOCKERS

Beta-blockers are a class of antihypertensive medication that lower heart rate and blood pressure. These agents have also been noted to reduce anxiety during performance and have been used by snooker players, musicians, singers, and others.[36,37] They also produce an increase in salivation.[37] They are potentially dangerous in individuals with underlying pulmonary problems and may induce asthma attacks. Gates[38] has concluded that in doses sufficient to reduce stage fright, beta-blockers may also cause a lackluster performance. Most laryngologists recommend against their use in performers. Individuals with crescendoing preperformance anxiety may be better advised to seek counseling (See Chapter 29 by Sataloff, Psychologic Aspects of Voice Disorders.)

MEDICATIONS WITH POTENTIAL ADVERSE EFFECTS

Many medications, when administered systemically, can have a deleterious impact upon vocal performance either directly, through their effects on the vocal tract, or indirectly, through CNS or other manifestations. Psychotropic agents represent a typical example. The numbers of drugs available are legion and cannot possibly be discussed in full. A table is addended discussing certain side effects of many of these classes of drugs

(Table 30-1). It is by nature incomplete but may prove helpful to the prescribing physician or the patient.

SUMMARY

Caring for professional voice users is rewarding but, at the same time, can be quite demanding. It is incumbent upon the physician or caregiver that they understand the potential effects of medications that they may prescribe upon the patient's vocal tract. As noted, the most notable effects of medications upon the vocal tract occur through the autonomic nervous system, an understanding of which is important. A thorough history of medications being taken, both prescription and nonprescription, is essential, as is monitoring while treatment is in progress.

REFERENCES

1. Lawrence VL. Common medications with laryngeal effects. *Ear Nose Throat J.* 1987;66: 23-28.

2. Martin FG. Drugs and vocal function. *J Voice.* 1988;2:338-344.

3. Harris TM. The pharmacological treatment of voice disorders. *Folia Phoniatr (Basel).* 1992;44:3-4;143-154.

4. Thompson AR. Pharmacological agents with effects on voice. *Am J Otol.* 1995;16:12-18.

5. Sataloff RT, Hawkshaw M, Rosen DC. Medications: Effects and side effects in professional voice users. In: Sataloff RT, ed. *Professional Voice: Science and Art of Clinical Care.* 2nd ed. San Diego, CA: Singular Publishing Group; 1997:457-469.

6. Sooy CD, Boles R. Neuroanatomy for the otolaryngology head and neck surgeon. In: Paparella MM, Shumrick DA, Gluckman JL, Meyerhoff WL, eds. *Otolaryngology.* 3rd ed. Philadelphia, PA: W B Saunders Co; 1991:107-142.

7. Davies J, Duckert L. Embryology and anatomy of the head, neck, face, palate, nose and paranasal sinuses. In: Paparella MM, Shumrick DA, Gluckman JL, Meyerhoff WL, eds. *Otolaryngology.* 3rd ed. Philadelphia, PA: W B Saunders Co; 1991:59-106.

8. Goodman U, Rall T, Nies AS, et al. *Goodman and Gilman's The Pharmacologic Basis of Therapeutics.* New York, NY: Pergamon Press; 1990:658.

9. The safety of inhaled nasal corticosteroids. *Curr Prob Pharmacol Care.* 1999;24:8.

General	More Specific	Potential Adverse Symptoms and Comments
Analgesics/Anti-Inflammatants	Aspirin	• Platelet dysfunction • Increased likelihood of submucosal hemorrhage • GI upset • Be wary of aspirin in other over-the-counter compounds
	Narcotic-containing	• CNS depression
	Nonsteroidal Anti-Inflammatants	• GI side effects • Some minor clotting abnormalities
	Paracetamol	• Potential for liver irritation at high dosages
Antibiotics		• GI disturbance • Increased likelihood of candida • Possibility of superinfection
Anticholinergics		• Dry vocal tract • Blurred vision
Antihistamines (H1 receptor blockers)		• Sedation • Dryness • Be wary of combinations with sympathomimetics
Antihypertensives		• Many with parasympathomimetic effects
	Diuretics	• Dry mucous membrane • Thickened secretions
	Reserpine and methyldopa	• Dryness
	Alpha-adrenergic agonists	• Dryness • Reduced secretions
	ACE inhibitors	• Cough
Anti-Parkinson's Agents		• Many with anticholinergic side effects
	L-dopa	• GI disturbance • Oral dryness • Blurred vision • CNS changes
	Amantadine	• Anticholinergic side effects

TABLE 30-1. *Partial List of Medications with Potential Adverse Effects on the Vocal Tract (Continues)*

General	More Specific	Potential Adverse Symptoms and Comments
	Dopamine receptor agonists	• GI disturbance • CNS changes
	Monoamine Oxidase Inhibitors	See Psychotropic section
Antitussive Medications		• Be wary of combination agents and vehicle(eg, H1 receptor antagonists, sympathomimetics, alcohol)
	Opiate-containing	• Sedation • Constipation • Dryness
Antiviral Medications		• Agitation • Tachycardia • Xerostomia • Xerophonia
Corticosteroids		• Suppress immune system (increased risk of infection) • Suppress endogenous steroid production • GI disturbance • CNS irritability • Muscle wasting • Fluid redistribution • Increased glucose
GI Medications		
	Antacids	• Dryness of vocal tract • Constipation
	H2 receptor blockers	• Occasional dryness of vocal tract
	Proton Pump Inhibitors	• Bloating, • Abdominal pain • Nausea
Psychotropic Agents		• All have effects that can interfere with vocal tract physiology

	Tricyclic and Tetracyclic Antidepressants	• Anticholinergic side effects:
		  Dry vocal tract
		  GER

TABLE 30-1. *Partial List of Medications with Potential Adverse Effects on the Vocal Tract (Continues)*

General	More Specific	Potential Adverse Symptoms and Comments

		• Autonomic side effects:
		    Palpitations
		    Sweating
		• Allergic:
		    Skin rashes
		• CNS:
		    Stimulation or sedation
		    Nausea
		    Seizures

	Monoamine Oxidase Inhibitors	• Dizziness • Hypertension from certain foods and medications • Sedation • Insomnia • Small incidence of dry mouth • Small incidence of constipation
	Serotonin Reuptake Inhibitors	• Weakly cholinergic but do cause some mucosal drying • Sedation • GI disturbance • Blurred vision
	Phenothiazines	• Strong H1 receptor antagonists • Dryness of vocal tract always seen
	Benzodiazepines	• High addictive potential • No anticholinergic effects • May affect speech production by action on CNS
	Lithium	• Nausea • Diarrhea • May affect mentation • May alter thyroid function
Sprays/Inhalants (laryngeal)	Anesthetic (Lidocaine)	• Not recommended • Increased likelihood of vocal fold injury/hemorrhage
	Vasoconstrictor	• Generally not recommended • Use only under emergent extreme circumstances

TABLE 30-1. *Partial List of Medications with Potential Adverse Effects on the Vocal Tract (Continues)*

General	More Specific	Potential Adverse Symptoms and Comments
	Diphenhydramine	• Has anesthetic effect and may increase likelihood of vocal fold injury
	Oxymetazoline	• No anesthetic effect
	Corticosteroids	• Dryness • Affects mucosal blanket • Questionable atrophy • Increased candida
Sympathomimetics		• Increased dryness of vocal tract • Thickened secretions • Xanthines reduce lower esophageal sphincter pressure and may increase reflux

TABLE 30-1. *Partial List of Medications with Potential Adverse Effects on the Vocal Tract*

10. Findlay CA, MacDonald JF, Wallace AM, Geddes N, et al. Lesson of the week: childhood Cushing's syndrome induced by betamethasone oral drops and repeat prescriptions. *Br Med J.* 1998;Vol 317; No 7160:739-740.

11. Homer JJ, Gazis TG. Cushing's syndrome induced by betamethasone nose drops (12). *Br Med J.* 1999;Vol 318; No 7194:1355-1356.

12. Scadding G. Effects of intranasal steroids on childhood growth. *ENT News.* November/December, 1999; Vol 8 (pt 5):27-28.

13. Schenkel EJ, Skoner DP, Bronsky EA. *One Year of Treatment With Mometasone Furoate Aqueous Nasal Spray (MFNS) Does Not Suppress Growth in Children.* Poster 31B, EAACI; Brussels, Belgium; July 1999.

14. Moren F. Drug deposition of pressurised inhalation aerosols. I. Influence of actuator tube design. *Int J Pharmacol.* 1978;1:205-212.

15. Dolovich M, Ruffin R, Newhouse MT. Clinical evaluation of a simple demand inhalation device: MDI aerosol delivery device. *Chest.* 1983;84:36-41.

16. Newman SP, Pavia D, Garland N. Effects of various inhalation modes on the deposition of radioactive pressurised aerosols. *Eur J Respir Dis.* 1982;119(suppl):57-65, 1982.

17. Berkowitz R, Rachelefsky G, Harris AG, Chen R. A comparison of triamcinolone acetonide MDI with a built-in tube extender and beclomethasone dipropionate MDI in adult asthmatics. *Chest.* 1998;114:757-765.

18. Lavy JA, Wood G, Rubin JS, Harries M. Dysphonia associated with inhaled steroids. *J Voice.* 2000;14:581-588.

19. *British National Formulary.* British Medical Association and the Royal Pharmaceutical Society of Great Britain.

20. Koufman JA. Infectious and inflammatory diseases of the larynx. In: Ballenger JJ, Snow JB, eds. *Otorhinolaryngology.* 15th ed. Philadelphia, PA: Williams and Wilkins (Lea & Febiger); 1996:535-555.

21. Koufman JA, Cummins M. The prevalence and spectrum of reflux in laryngology: a prospective study of 132 consecutive patients with laryngeal and voice disorders. Available at: wfubmc.edu/voice/reflux_prev_study.html; 2002.

22. Sataloff RT, Castell DO, Katz PO, Sataloff DM. *Reflux Laryngitis and Related Disorders.* San Diego, CA: Singular Publishing Group; 1999.

23. Abramson AL, Steinberg BM, Gould WJ, et al. Estrogen receptors in the human larynx. Clinical

study of the singing voice. *Transcripts of the 13th Symposium on Care of the Professional Voice.* 1984;2:409-413.

24. Virolainen E, Tuohiman P, Aitasato A, et al. Steroid hormone receptors in laryngeal carcinoma. *Otolaryngol Head Neck Surg.* 1986;4:512-517.

25. Newman S-R, Butler J, Hammond EH, Gray SD. Preliminary report on hormone receptors in the human vocal fold. *J Voice.* 2000;14:72-81.

26. Timonen S, Sonninen A, Wichmann K. Endocrinological laryngopathy. In: Follio KE, Vara P, eds. *Annales Chirurgiae et Gynaecologiae Fenniae.* 1962;51:3-29.

27. Damste PH. Virilization of the voice due to anabolic steroids. *Folia Phoniat.* 1968;16:10-18.

28. Baker J. A report on alterations to the speaking voices of four women following hormonal therapy with virilising agents. *J Voice.* 1999;13:496-507.

29. Pattie MA, Murdoch B, Theodoros D, Forbes K. Voice changes in women treated for endometriosis and related conditions: the need for comprehensive vocal assessment. *J Voice.* 1998;12:366-371.

30. Gerritsma EJ, Brocaar MP, Hakkesteegt MM, Birkenhager JC. Virilization of the voice in post-menopausal women due to the androgenic steroid nandrolone decanoate (Decadurabolin). The effects of medication for one year. *Clin Otolaryngol.* 1994;19:79-84.

31. Krahulec I, Urbanova O, Simko S. Voice changes during hormonal contraception. *Cesk Otolaryngol.* 1977;26:234-237.

32. Khaw K. The menopause and hormone replacement therapy. *Post-graduate Med J.* 1992;68:615-623.

33. Boulet MJ, Oddens BJ. Female voice change around and after the menopause: an initial investigation. *Maturitas.* 1996;23:15-21.

34. Lindholm P, Vilkman E, Raudaskoski T, Suvanto-Lukkonen E, Kauppila A. The effect of post-menopause and postmenopausal HRT on measured voice values and vocal symptoms. *Maturitas.* 1997;28:47-53.

35. Sataloff RT, Spiegel JR, Rosen DC. The effects of age on the voice. In: Sataloff, RT, ed. *Professional Voice: Science and Art of Clinical Care.* 2nd ed. San Diego, CA: Singular Publishing Group; 1997:259-267.

36. James IM. The effects of oxprenolol on stage fright in musicians. *Lancet.* 1977;2:952-954.

37. Brantigan CD. The effect of beta blockage and beta stimulation on stage fright. *Am J Med.* 1982;72:88-94.

38. Gates GA, Saegert J, Wilson N, et al. Effects of beta-blockade on singing performance. *Ann Otol Rhinol Laryngol.* 1985;94:570-574.

CHAPTER 31

The Role of the Speech-Language Pathologist in the Treatment of Voice Disorders

Thomas Murry, PhD
Clark A. Rosen, MD, FACS

Treatment of voice disorders by speech-language pathologists has steadily advanced over the past 25 years. The vast expansion of research in vocal fold physiology and voice disorders has increased the understanding of techniques and methods for behavioral management of voice disorders. More importantly, these advances have resulted in increased use of voice therapy to avoid surgery, to prepare patients for voice surgery, and to maximize vocal rehabilitation following surgery. Laryngology and speech-language pathology have melded a treatment rationale that combines the expertise of these two disciplines in order to maximize voice rehabilitation.

The modern speech-language pathologist brings essential vocal mechanics, voice physiology information, and behavior management skills to the evaluation and treatment process. The speech-language pathologist uses behavioral techniques to reduce traumatic voice use, increase vocal efficiency, and produce a clearer tone. The speech-language pathologist develops and applies perceptual cues for the patient to identify and monitor changes in phonation. Voice therapy methods also include the application of cognitive strategies to complement acquisition of new motor skills. The therapeutic process requires the speech-language pathologist to have a keen sense of observational and interventional treatment methods.

Successful voice therapy is grounded in an understanding of laryngeal anatomy, physiology of the respiratory, laryngeal, and articulatory systems, knowledge of physiologic phonetics, and excellent auditory discrimination. These skills develop as the speech-language pathologist works in a voice care setting. Listening to a variety of voice samples is an integral part of this training. Continuously challenging one's listening acuity, coupled with observation of posture and breathing, contribute to the treatment of voice disorders with voice therapy.

The professional singer presents with a specific set of needs that the speech-language pathologist must take into consideration. Vocal difficulty in any individual is significant; however, for performers, voice loss may mean career changes, loss of income, or other significant changes in life. Thus, the speech-language pathologist must establish appropriate goals for the voice performer that account for a return to full voice use if appropriate. They must have the necessary knowledge to achieve the highest and best voice use for the patient.

The role of the speech-language pathologist in the treatment of voice disorders complements the role of the laryngologist. The speech-language pathologist (SLP) is an essential member of the voice care team, and his/her role in the treatment of voice disorders extends from the time of the first visit until such time as the patient has achieved the highest and best use of the voice. This chapter reviews the key aspects of treatment and focuses on the role of the speech language pathologist in caring for those with a voice disorder.

THE VOICE EVALUATION

Ultimately, the goals of the voice evaluation are to establish a set of parameters that describe voice quality and voice usage and to relate these parameters to a well-designed treatment program. Figure 31-1 presents a typical algorithm for the voice evaluation process from evaluation to treatment. The model is a combined approach by the laryngologist and speech-language pathologist.

The role of the SLP in the evaluation process is significant because treatment is related not only to the pathology of the disorder, but also to the associated pathophysiology (often compensatory). The SLP should understand the medical and surgical issues regarding the patient's voice problem and treatment. Patients often ask questions regarding pending or future voice surgery. It is common to discuss surgical options with the patient; however, these discussions should be kept at a minimum, and the SLP should refer most questions back to the surgeon. The SLP should know the surgical alternatives but focus on behavioral issues during the diagnostic process.

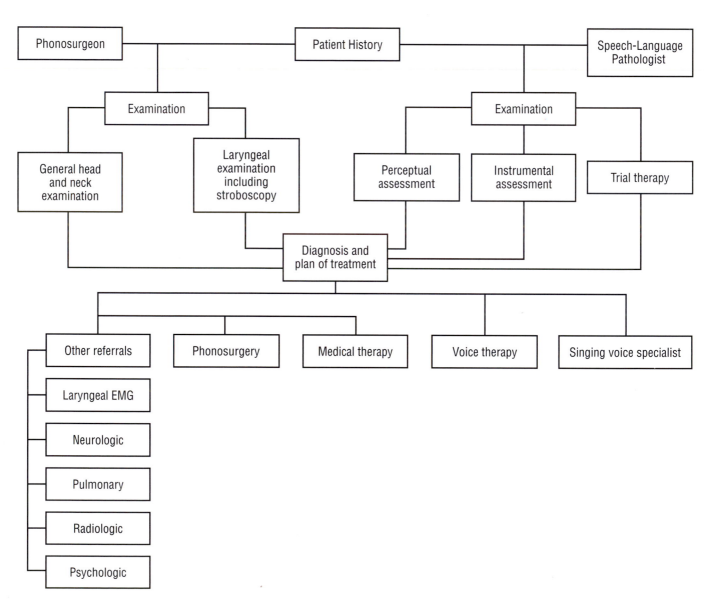

FIGURE 31-1. *Voice Evaluation and Treatment Algorithm*

The voice evaluation consists of a detailed patient history relating previous voice use and training to current voice limitations. This may be done using a case history questionnaire[1] or simply through a discussion of the voice changes since their inception. Regardless of whether or not a questionnaire is used, the evaluation process focuses on voice use, both past and present, medical history, and changes in both speaking and singing. The history should identify the chief complaint, length of time of the problem, circumstances surrounding the onset of the problem, previous voice problems and treatments, and how the voice problem affects the patient's current and future work and social status.

A perceptual assessment of the voice quality should also be done. This includes a perceptual rating of the appropriateness of pitch and loudness, voice qualities, and rate of speech.[2] It may also include singing range and the effects of vocal fatigue. If the patient has already completed surgery prior to his or her first visit to the speech-language pathologist, then the history should include a detailed description of the preoperative voice and the patient's comparisons of the preoperative with the postoperative voice. All diagnostic sessions should include perceptual judgments by the SLP regarding voice quality, loudness, and pitch range. This can be done during the interview, as well as by using controlled stimuli. The current approach to diagnosis of the voice disorder involves instrumental assessment; however, the informal and formal perceptual assessment provides a significant lead as to how the voice is used by the patient and a preliminary insight into the nature and severity of the voice disorder.

The use of rating scales may be valuable. Rating scales, either those used by the clinician[2] or those used by the patient, provide an indication of the severity of the voice disorder. Patient self-rating scales give the voice care team an understanding of how the patient views his/her voice handicap.[3] Rating scales used by the clinician allow a record of perceptual variation that may be documented from time to time. Ratings may be done using sustained phonation or standardized voice tasks (sustained and connected speech). Previous investigations indicate that both are reliable when the patient is asked to produce the samples at his or her comfortable effort level.[4,5] The GRBAS scale developed by Hirano[2] provides a consistent and efficient method for perceptual rating by the clinician. The *Voice Handicap Index*[3] is a valid and reliable scale for the patient's self-perception of severity. These are the two scales that should be part of the initial assessment.

Additional aspects of the voice evaluation include the patient's posture and alignment during his or her normal speaking activities. The importance of a well-supported speaking voice cannot be underestimated. This begins with posture and how the individual uses the body to deliver the voice. The correct erect posture is standing upright with the feet slightly apart and the knees unlocked. The shoulders should be loose, and the head should be over the shoulders and not extended out from the shoulders. Thus, if one were evaluating a university professor, it would be appropriate to observe and listen to a short segment of his or her lecture. For those who sit much of the time at their job, posture should be an erect back with shoulders relaxed and the feet flat on the floor. Thus, for secretaries or others who sit at their job most of the day, it is appropriate to ask them to demonstrate their posture and alignment at a desk and observe the speech in this simulated setting. In some cases, it may be particularly helpful for the therapist to go to the patient's work environment and observe conditions and behaviors first hand.

Special attention should be given to situations such as stage performances, the coach's bench voice, courtroom voice use, or the elementary teacher who often is bending at children's desks. All these postures may contribute to poor alignment, and, therefore, poor support of the vocal mechanism.

Instrumental Assessment

The use of instrumental assessment procedures for voice care is now common. Acoustic analysis provides an objective measure of the patient's voice under controlled conditions. Common measures include: frequency range, intensity range, and mean speaking fundamental frequency. These measures are done quite simply when the voice is not severely dysphonic. However, as the dysphonia increases, the reliability of acoustic measures decreases.[6] The use of the voice range profile provides a dynamic assessment of the range of voice capable in the patient. The voice range profile is a valuable measure not only for singers but also for all patients with voice disorders undergoing treatment.[7] It should be mentioned, however, that if there is a suspicion of a lesion, the therapist must be sure that performing a voice range profile would not cause additional damage to the vocal folds. In our practice, the Kay Computerized Speech Laboratory (CSL) (Englewood, New Jersey) and the multidimensional voice profile acoustic analyses systems are the primary acoustic tools. However, numerous other systems are now available.

A physiologic analysis of the interaction between pulmonary function and laryngeal function should also be done during the diagnostic process. Instrumentation is available to obtain mean airflow rate, estimates of subglottic air pressure, and the resultant laryngeal airway resistance value during voice production. These measures provide an objective assessment of the interaction of respiratory and phonatory components (ie, laryngeal valving efficiency).

Compliance

A third aspect of the voice evaluation is to determine through observation, as well as assessment, the patient's compliance or possible compliance with treatment programs. Whether the patient is to undergo surgery and voice therapy or voice therapy only, the issue of compliance is extremely important. One often gets a feel for the level of compliance as a result of questions regarding the importance of voice use by the patient. One or two trial sessions of voice therapy should also be considered at this time as a measure of assessing overall compliance with the treatment program. This is sometimes referred to as "unloading" and includes therapeutic procedures to determine the patient's ability to modify vocal function. It is at this point that communication among the SLP, the surgeon, and the patient is particularly important. Without an understanding of the need for compliance and the issues related to compliance, treatment is not likely to be successful. Communication between the SLP and the surgeon will help to formulate the treatment plan. For example, a patient with Reinke's edema is not likely to show much long-term improvement with surgery or voice therapy if she or he continues to smoke cigarettes and maintain the forceful, low-pitched voice usually seen in these patients. A behavioral management program of voice use, along with modification of personal habits related to smoking, should be integrated into an intensive treatment of these patients.[8]

Review of Results: Establishing the Diagnosis

When the medical and speech-language pathology evaluations have been completed, the voice care team establishes a medical diagnosis, and, with the patient, a plan of treatment is developed. Once the patient knows the diagnosis, a reasonable explanation as to how the vocal injury or voice disorder occurred is important. This often comes about as a result of an in-depth review of the case history by the speech-language pathologist. An explanation of relevant issues in each individual's case is often necessary so that the patient understands that it was not his or her singing teacher or a mysterious virus that caused the problem. If the patient understands the behavioral implications and their relationship to the voice disorder, he or she will be more likely to accept the voice therapy component of treatment. Moreover, he or she will be less likely to want a "magic

pill" to correct the condition. Thorough understanding of how a vocal injury occurred is the first step toward prevention of another injury in the future.

The goals of treatment should address behavioral concerns, medication if necessary, and the role and timing of phonosurgery (if needed). An appropriate model for patients with benign vocal fold lesions is one in which the laryngologist supports the need for behavioral modification and the speech-language pathologist supports the possible need for phonomicrosurgery. *Both of these treatment modalities should be presented to the patient (when indicated) at the same time so that the patient understands that the comprehensive management of this disorder is the most successful approach to recovery.*

TREATMENT

Once the diagnosis and plan of treatment are determined, the major role of the speech-language pathologist is to provide voice therapy. Table 31-1 lists the most common voice disorders for which voice therapy is usually the initial treatment modality. This may be done in conjunction with surgical procedures that precede or (preferably) follow the therapy, or it may be the sole treatment modality. In some cases, voice therapy is also done in conjunction with psychotherapy to maximize

---

Vocal Fold Nodules

Vocal Fold Cyst

Vocal Fold Polyp

Reinke's Edema*

Muscle Tension Dysphonia

Paradoxical Vocal Fold Motion Disorder

Vocal Fold Paresis

Vocal Fold Paralysis**

Neurogenic Voice Disorders

Functional Dysphonia

Vocal Fold Granuloma

---

* Unless significant airway restriction is present.

** Unless the patient is at high risk for aspiration.

TABLE 31-1. *Common Voice Disorders for Which Voice Therapy is the Initial Treatment of Choice*

the control of behavioral issues that coexist with the voice disorder.

Although voice therapy is a prominent treatment modality for treating many kinds of voice disorders, there is little agreement among speech-language pathologists regarding the specific techniques to be used. Moreover, in the past, "voice experts" advanced ideas that worked for them, but were never tested for efficacy or outcomes. Nonetheless, the contributions by the so-called experts appear to be the primary basis for treatment even to this day. That is not to say that these treatments do not work. Rather, it is to say that the treatment of voice disorders remains ripe for studies of efficacy and outcome.

The medical referral process and the service delivery systems now in force in the United States govern voice therapy. Treatment often relies on third-party payors who limit the number of treatment sessions. Thus, the modern-day speech-language pathologist must use existing information about the disorder, its pathophysiology, function, and objective measurements to guide the therapy within the number of sessions allowed. In the current health delivery system, there is little or no room for extraneous sessions to work for long periods of time on unitary aspects of voice production. The voice therapist incorporates breathing techniques with postural adjustments, muscle relaxation, and specific phonatory exercises targeted at the underlying cause of the dysphonia. The patient should be given a series of breathing and relaxation exercises to practice at home. It is important that the patient begin an active daily treatment program from the first therapy visit. The importance of home practice of therapy skills cannot be overemphasized. While some patients may show significant improvement in the time allotted to therapy by insurance plans, behavioral changes may require more time than originally allowed. The physician and the therapist should take a proactive stand and provide information to the insurer documenting improvement and the rationale for further voice therapy. Follow-up instrumental assessments, laryngostroboscopic examination (with photos), or other indications such as reduced/lost work time should be used to justify additional treatment coverage. It is important for the speech pathologist and laryngologist to provide documentation and objective measures to demonstrate the efficacy of voice therapy as a viable treatment for voice disorders.

General Treatment Guidelines

Recently, Casper and Murry provided guidelines or general concepts essential to the success of any voice therapy program.[9] These concepts must be implemented in all treatment programs, regardless of the specific therapeutic techniques employed. The universal uses of these concepts underlie all voice therapy programs and should be included during each treatment session.

Patient education is the first step in all voice therapy treatment. A thorough understanding of normal voice production will help to educate the patient about the dysphonic voice. Diagrams may be useful. A review of the videolaryngoscopic examination may be helpful to point out lesions, movement disorders, or other aspects of the examination that are related to the dysphonia. Along with this type of education, the patient should also have an understanding of the voice therapy process. This is not a long and extended process but rather a behavior-oriented approach to targeting specific behaviors that contribute to the dysphonia.

Once the patient has an understanding of the goals of voice therapy and the methods to achieve the goals, specific exercises and behavioral modifications are designed to reach the goals. The patient should also understand that voice therapy does not eliminate such things as vocal fold paralysis, vocal fold cyst, or a vocal fold polyp in most cases. Voice therapy, however, provides the most efficient use of the voice given the conditions of the voice and leads to improvement in voice quality. For vocal nodules, however, it is expected that proper voice therapy with adequate compliance will reduce or eliminate the nodules in greater than 95% of the cases. This is similar to taking proper care of a callus, which disappears following the reduction of trauma to the callused area. Once the patient understands the process, basic vocal fold anatomy and physiology, and the goals of treatment, the therapy process may begin with both the therapist and the patient well aware of the goals and the methods needed to reach them.

Vocal Hygiene

Vocal hygiene is another universal essential component to treatment. In some cases, vocal hygiene may be the only form of treatment. Vocal hygiene encompasses three major areas. This includes: 1) the knowledge of what is traumatic or stressful to the vocal folds themselves; 2) techniques to improve or expedite recovery such as the use of steam or other hydration, the reduction of inhaled medications (if possible); and 3) the reduction or elimination of throat clearing. The awareness of noxious stimuli, such as cigarette smoke, strong chemicals, or alcohol must also be pointed out and monitored during the therapy program. For the singer or actor, specific reference must be made to the importance of voice rest before and after a performance, the avoidance of excessive speaking (especially before a performance such as for interviews, telephone calls, or visits from well-wishers). Other aspects of vocal hygiene include the understanding of the effects of loud laughing, excessive coughing, or crying. All of these can lead to further vocal damage, and a program to monitor this behavior must be implemented at the start of therapy. Patients with voice disorders that involve the lack of or poor vocal fold closure must also be aware that the attempts to produce long phrases in loud or noisy conditions must be eliminated. This in itself will help to regulate the use of breathing more appropriately.

Vocal hygiene focuses on healthy use of the vocal organs. Such things as increased hydration, elimination of throat clearing, and others that are noted in Table 31-2 must be spelled out to the patient in detail. A clear understanding of how the vocal mechanism works, and the many ways in which it can be injured, is also part of the vocal hygiene program.

A proper vocal hygiene program coupled with voice therapy can change behavior so that the vocal folds are not damaged further and a reactive lesion, if present, may be reduced. The patient must use his auditory and kinesthetic awareness to detect easier voice usage,

improved voice quality, and less voice effort as part of the vocal hygiene program.

Voice Therapy (Direct)

For many voice disorders, voice therapy is the treatment of choice. It is a treatment based on behavioral methods that allows the patient to correct faulty vocal habits, develop an awareness for good and bad voice quality, and understand the nature of healthy voice use, both for the speaking and singing voice. A comprehensive program of voice care may include: 1) initial treatment and, if necessary, preparation for surgery; 2) an acute postoperative period and/or; 3) postoperative rehabilitation.

In some cases, the preoperative treatment will be sufficient, and the patient may not require surgical treatment for the disorder.

The ultimate goals of voice therapy are:

1. To return the voice to optimal use;

2. To improve voice quality and increase vocal efficiency with minimal vocal effort;

3. To establish a vocal hygiene program that will be useful not only immediately but also following surgery. It should also be one that is capable of being applied over long periods of time to establish a healthy vocal lifestyle.

Vocal rehabilitation must be planned and executed properly in order to ensure that the goals are met. The specific means to achieve the goals of therapy must be structured to the patient's needs. If surgery is involved, the timing of surgery must be selected based on voice requirements, performance requirements, or other job-related speaking and singing demands. Once the surgery date is scheduled, the voice therapist assists with establishing a preoperative voice use schedule, a postoperative voice rest schedule, and a coordinated follow-up treatment schedule to take advantage of the postoperative laryngeal examination and interaction with the laryngologist. Although voice care and rehabilitation are primarily done by the voice therapist, other disciplines such as psychiatry, gastroenterology, physical therapy, singing instruction and pediatrics may be asked to play a role in the pre- and postoperative care of the patient on an as-needed basis.

The Treatment Period

Voice therapy may be extensive if vocal habits are poor and the goal is to establish healthy voice use that includes lifestyle adjustments. This is especially true for patients with Reinke's edema who often have a history of excessive cigarette smoking, loud voice use, and

---

1. Eliminate smoking

2. Avoid singing when sick

3. Control gastroesophageal reflux

4. Reduce or eliminate throat clearing

5. Maintain adequate hydration

6. Eat a balanced diet

7. Use warm up and cool down period before and after singing

8. Exercise to maintain good overall body condition

9. Know the effects of medications, over-the-counter preparations, alternative medicines, and prescription medicines on the voice

10. Avoid loud talking in the presence of background noise

11. Avoid inhaling of second-hand smoke and other irritants

12. Avoid extensive strained whispering

TABLE 31-2. *Critical Aspects of a Vocal Hygiene Program*

episodes of vocal misuse. Preoperative voice therapy programs should involve a course of vocal hygiene.

A comprehensive voice therapy program includes exercises for muscle relaxation, posture and alignment, and breathing, as well as preparation for recovery after surgery if surgery is planned. The preoperative time becomes important because it provides the voice care team with an indication of the patient's level of compliance. If a patient is not compliant with the preoperative voice therapy, then phonosurgery may be best delayed or cancelled.

Muscle relaxation exercises are useful to scale down the force of voice onset and perhaps the overall loudness of the voice as well. A program of general body relaxation provided by a physical therapist may be helpful, along with specific exercises to the head and neck muscles. Specific exercises for the lips, tongue, jaw, and neck selected by the speech-language pathologist should also be included in the program.[10-12] Direct laryngeal massage has also been shown to have a positive benefit to relax muscles of the neck area and to alter laryngeal posture. With a relaxed laryngeal posture, the onset of phonation may be less forceful.[13]

Preoperative Voice Therapy

Patients undergoing surgery for vocal fold cyst and granuloma are routinely placed on complete voice rest after surgery for three to seven days, as well as those having surgery for vocal polyps or Reinke's edema. While there are a number of opposing thoughts regarding complete voice rest, it is generally a good idea to plan several days of complete voice rest following surgery. The surgical treatments for vocal fold paresis and paralysis may involve some voice rest, but it need not be as extensive as it is following the removal of benign vocal fold lesions. Of specific importance in the voice rest period is the avoidance of whispering and coughing. Patients should be asked not to whisper but rather to use a pencil and paper during complete voice rest. Voice rest should always be used judiciously as it does involve a significant hardship on most patients. Voice rest should be monitored, as the psychologic strain of not talking sometimes is more difficult to tolerate than attempting to talk in a soft, breathy voice. It should be remembered that voice rest alone does not help a person return to healthy voice use if the person has not been treated for excessive traumatic vocal behavior or poor vocal habits that led to the disorder in the first place.

Postoperative Rehabilitation

The role of the speech-language pathologist immediately after surgery is to make sure the patient understands the reason for the voice rest period and to begin vocal exercises once the voice rest is completed. The acute voice rest period should end with the laryngologist and speech pathologist starting the patient on easy vocalization. The exercises may include using the consonants /n/, /w/, /y/, /h/. With easy voice onsets using these consonants connected to vowels, the patient begins to sense the notion of easy voice onset and reduction of force. For patients with long-standing Reinke's edema, these exercises should be initiated above the patient's preoperative speaking pitch. It is important at the outset of the therapy to refocus the voice to proper pitch range with low-effort level.

The acute postoperative period is also an excellent time to initiate voiceless muscle relaxation exercises or review the muscle relaxation and breathing exercises that were taught in the preoperative voice therapy sessions. Exercises for the lips, tongue, jaw, neck, and shoulders are appropriate at this time. Specifically, in a standing as well as sitting position, the patient should be asked to take away the pressure from the upper part of the chest near the top of the sternum by using slow exhalations followed by inhalations. These may be accompanied by breathy vowels during the end of the voice rest. Once voice rest is complete, the patient should focus the vowels forward in the oral cavity and concentrate on ease of onset and the auditory perception of voice quality. Clearly, the acute postoperative period offers the patient a time to tune into his support systems for phonation and to prepare for easy voicing.

The first postoperative visit to the speech-language pathologist is extremely important. If the plan of treatment is not explained well, and if the rationale is not sound, patients may be reluctant to return for therapy, feeling that surgery corrected the problem. It is often a good idea to tell the patient to think of his voice much like a football player thinks of his knee or shoulder, that recovery is slow and requires limited and controlled use. As recovery of the voice improves, the use increases. It is important for the patient not to overdo voice use or voice practice in the first days of recovery. Slow and controlled reacquisition of voice, especially pitch range and voice quality, helps to develop confidence in voice use and prevents the opportunity for overuse and strain to reoccur.

Specific Voice Therapy Techniques

Confidential Voice

Casper and Murry described some of the more frequently used therapeutic techniques for voice therapy.[9] One technique is the use of the confidential voice. The confidential voice is used most often to reduce or eliminate excessive vocal fold contact, thereby decreasing the force of vocal fold collision. This also helps to reduce hyperfunctional behaviors such as false vocal fold adduction. The treatment is described as confidential voice because it typically sounds like the voice that one uses to describe things in a quiet setting and almost in a breathy voice. It is produced with the vocal folds slightly abducted, which results in increased airflow and reduced loudness.[14] When produced correctly, the confidential voice results in the reduction of excessive muscle tension and the reduction of supraglottal constriction. The addition of tension to increase loudness may result in a vocal harshness that is readily identifiable to the patient.

Reduced vocal intensity is one positive feature of the confidential voice. Although it may be difficult for patients to use this voice throughout the day, it often can be employed at least part of the day. The intent of this technique is to eliminate hyperfunctional or traumatic behaviors to allow lesions such as vocal nodules to heal as a result of reduced excessive vocal contact in the area of the nodules and to help reduce muscle tension and vocal fatigue.[15] The patient should be aware that use of the confidential voice is not the endpoint of therapy and that it is only a temporary means of promoting healing, especially when there are bilateral midfold lesions.

The confidential voice technique is useful for treating muscle tension dysphonias, hyperfunctional dysphonia, vocal fatigue and, as an early postoperative voice therapy technique, to reduce strong glottal attack. If the patient continues to report excessive fatigue during this phase of the treatment, further examination should be done, and the patient should be observed using the technique in conversational speech in order to verify that he or she is using it appropriately. It is important that the SLP and patient understand that whispering is not acceptable as it puts excessive tension on the vocal folds and is not a long-term solution to communication.

Resonant Voice Therapy

Resonant voice therapy, or a voice with a frontal focus, usually refers to an easy voice associated with vibratory sensations felt in the facial area.[16] The focus in resonant therapy is on the production of the voice primarily through feeling and hearing. The feeling is specific both in terms of vibratory sensation and in terms of the use of onset of phonation. The patient is required to listen to changes in voice quality in order to achieve maximum ease of voice with the least amount of effort. This treatment method historically derives from the work of Lessac,[17] who used this approach to improve the voices of students in theatrical training. The goal is

to place the voice high in the head so that resonance is achieved easily through all the resonators from the supraglottic area up through the face. A variety of flexibility exercises related to pitch and intonation should be used once the placement is obtained. Initially, placement of the voice is obtained with the humming of the /m/ phoneme. It should be noted that patients often reject the more forward placement as it often leads to a higher pitch, and they do not sound like themselves.

Laryngeal Massage

In this technique, the SLP massages or manipulates the laryngeal area. Roy and his colleagues[13,19] have reported on this, as has Morrison.[18] Circumlaryngeal massage is used primarily in the treatment of patients with hyperfunctional dysphonias. This may include patients with benign lesions, as well as those without specific lesions, but who present with extreme false vocal fold closure, high laryngeal position in the neck, or supraglottic anterior-posterior compression during phonation. These patients are best examined with flexible endoscopy and, in fact, may be treated with a flexible endoscope coupled to a video camera as feedback for monitoring the supraglottic constrictions. The specific exercises include hyoid massage in which the hyoid bone is encircled using the thumb and index finger and the tips of the posterior horns are identified and massaged in a circular motion with gentle downward pressure. Other exercises include starting at the thyroid notch and working posteriorly. In addition, with the fingers along the superior border of the thyroid cartilage, the larynx is gently moved downward and occasionally laterally. The patient is instructed to hum or prolong a vowel during this procedure.

Vocal Function Exercises

Vocal function exercises date back to the middle of the twentieth century when Briess described a series of specific muscle dysfunctions that could be alleviated by "rebalancing" various laryngeal postures. Recently, Stemple formalized this series of exercises.[16] Again, it should be pointed out that no significant research supports the value of these exercises. However, there is some evidence that singers, as well as normal speakers, produce improved voice after the exercises are completed.

The exercises are centered around four distinct phases. These include: muscle warm-up, muscle stretching, muscle contracting, and muscle power building. The exercises are recommended for many types of dysphonias, especially those in which early midvocal fold contact occurs. The vocal function exercises include sustained phonation, generally at a pitch level higher than that in which the person usually speaks, and graduation from soft voice to moderate volume and pitch gliding from lowest to highest pitch on certain words. Stemple has provided guidelines for these exercises. When done according to the guidelines, there is a general improvement in voice quality, and patients report an easier mode of phonation.

Miscellaneous Techniques

The Lee Silverman Voice Treatment (LSVT) is a specialized program developed for patients with dysphonia associated with Parkinson's disease.[20] This intensive four-week, four-session-per-week program is geared to counteract the communication disorders associated with Parkinson's disease and to increase the strength of the phonatory mechanism through focusing on loudness. It is well known that Parkinson's patients have poor perception of their overall level of loudness. In essence, what this treatment approach attempts to do is to "recalibrate" the speaker's ear so that his/her perception of loudness is similar to that of the listener and that his/her phrasing is maintained at a certain loudness level throughout the entire phrase. During treatment, the focus is on increasing the effort phonation to reach this "recalibration" goal. By repetitive productions of loud, sustained vowels, the patient learns to realign his or her auditory perception of his or her phonation level to that of a normal hearing listener.

This program has seen significant research, which demonstrates its efficacy with Parkinson's disease patients. Moreover, this treatment program has also demonstrated that by focusing on a single factor, loudness, patients also improve in clarity of speech and overall speech intelligibility. The LSVT program has been used extensively for Parkinson's patients over the past five years with proven long-term positive effects.[20] It is now being tried with patients who present with vocal fold atrophy, unilateral vocal fold paralysis, and other problems in which loudness may provide enhancement to communication difficulties.

The Accent Method originally developed by Sven Smith[21] has been used in the treatment of many types of dysphonias for the last 50 to 60 years. This method has been adopted more in other countries than in the United States. The accent method focuses on breathing as the underlying control mechanism of voice production. Accentuated and rhythmic movements of the body and then of voicing produce an awareness of voice change in the patient. Easy voice production is stressed with an open throat, and attention is given primarily to the lower abdominal structures in breathing. Smith believes that the training of new motor patterns is based on the rhythmic nature of the patterns and that the accent method allows for the patient to focus on "music-like" rhythms.

Accent method therapy revolves around dialogue in which the therapist asks a question, and the patient gives a rhythmic answer such as "What is your NAME?" and "My NAME is Mona." This rhythm is then modified with accents on various syllables. The accents are produced using strong contracting of the abdominal musculature. Eventually, the accented rhythms are maintained, but the body movements are extinguished. Kotby[22] has formalized the accent method of Smith and demonstrated its usefulness with vocal fold lesions, vocal fold atrophy, and muscle tension dysphonias.

Treatment of voice disorders in transgender individuals has become more prominent in recent years. The most common transgender voice need is for the biologic male patient to produce a higher pitch and a more feminine intonation pattern. Vocal exercises for these patients are generally initiated early in the transgender process. The focus is on gradually raising pitch through intonation patterns so that the speaking fundamental frequency increases to approximately a mean of 180 Hz (for male to female). Attempts to change pitch should be structured over a fairly long period of four to eight months so as not to produce strain in the individual. In addition to pitch-changing exercises using inflection practice, patterns that focus on soft initiation, slightly increased breathiness and vowel prolongation are typically used to achieve the feminine characteristics of phonation.

SUMMARY

The speech-language pathologist plays a crucial role in the diagnosis and treatment of voice disorders. Perceptual assessment of vocal production, instrumental assessment in order to monitor change, and the ability to obtain proper case history are the key factors in the diagnostic phase of the speech-language pathologist's role. Treatment of voice disorders by the SLP must be focused on changing the physiology of phonation and educating the patient on the need to change vocal function. Treatment is done in conjunction with the other voice care team's activities (medical treatment, surgery, singing). Preoperative voice therapy provides an avenue in which the voice care team may develop an impression of the patient's ability to change vocal habits, the ability to comply with the changes, and the motivational level. Postoperative voice therapy provides the continuation of rehabilitation after surgical care has been completed. In most cases, rehabilitation is not a lengthy process and involves no more than 12 sessions of voice therapy. The successful voice therapist will recognize when changes are not occurring and look for reasons such as incorrect diagnosis, poor patient compliance, or poor therapeutic techniques. In these cases, changes must be made, and the voice care team must work together to achieve optimal vocal rehabilitation.

REFERENCES

1. Sataloff RT. *Vocal Health and Pedagogy*. San Diego; CA: Singular Publishing Group; 1998:391-397.

2. Hirano M. *Clinical Examination of Voice*. Wien/New York, NY: Springer Verlag Co; 1981.

3. Jacobson BH, Johnson A, Gryzwalsky C, Benninger M. The Voice Handicap Index (VHI): development and validation. *J Voice*. 1998;12(4):540-550.

4. Brown WS, Morris RJ, Murry T. Comfortable effort level revisited. *J Voice*. 1996;10(3):299-305.

5. Murry T, Brown WS, Morris RJ. Patterns of fundamental frequency for three types of voice samples. *J Voice*. 1995;9:282-289.

6. Titze J. *Workshop on Acoustic Voice Analysis*. Denver, CO: National Center for Voice and Speech; 1995:18-23.

7. Titze IR. Acoustic interpretation of the voice range profile. *J Speech Hearing Res*. 1992;35:21-34.

8. Sataloff RT. Introduction to treating vocal hygiene. In: Sataloff RT, ed. *Vocal Health and Pedagogy*. San Diego, CA: Singular Publishing Group; 1998:257-264.

9. Casper J, Murry T. Voice therapy methods in dysphonia. *Otolaryngology Clinics of North America*. Philadelphia, PA: W. B. Saunders; 2000.

10. Rulnick RK, Heuer RJ, Perez KS, Emerich KA, Sataloff RT. Voice therapy. In: Sataloff RT, ed. *Vocal Health and Pedagogy*. San Diego, CA: Singular Publishing Group; 1998:265-296.

11. Colton RH, Casper JK. *Understanding Voice Problems: A Physiological Perspective for Diagnosis and Treatment*. Baltimore, MD: Williams and Wilkins; 1996.

12. Andrews M. *Manual of Voice Treatment: Pediatrics Through Geriatrics*. San Diego, CA: Singular Publishing Group; 1995:110-139.

13. Roy N, Bless DM, Heisey D, et al. Manual circumlaryngeal therapy for functional dysphonia: an evaluation of short and long-term treatment outcomes. *J Voice*. 1997;11:321-331.

14. Verdolini K, Ramig LO, Jacobson B. Outcome measurement in voice disorders. In: Frattali C, ed. *Measuring Outcomes in Speech-Language Pathology*. New York, NY: Thieme-Medical Publishers; 1998.

15. Verdolini-Marston K, Burke MK, Lessac A, et al. A preliminary study on two methods of treatment for laryngeal nodules. *J Voice*. 1995;9:74-85.

16. Stemple JC, Glaze LE, Gerdeman BK. *Clinical Voice Pathology: Theory and Management*. 2nd ed. San Diego, CA: Singular Publishing Group; 1995.

17. Lessac A. *The Use and Training of the Human Voice: A Biodynamic Approach to Vocal Life*. Mountain View, CA: Mayfield Publishing Co; 1997.

18. Morrison MD, Rammage LA, Belisle G, Nichol H, Pullan B. Muscular tension dysphonia. *J Otolaryngologica*. 1983;12:302-306.

19. Roy N, Leeper HA. Effects of manual laryngeal musculoskeletal tension reduction technique as a treatment for functional voice disorders: Perceptual and acoustic measures. *J Voice*. 1993;7:242-249.

20. Mead C, Ramig LO, Beck J. Parkinson's disease with severe dementia: effectiveness of intensive voice therapy. *ASHA*. 1989;31:118.

21. Smith S, Thyme K. Statistic research on changes in speech due to pedagogic treatment (The Accent Method). *Folia Phoniatr*. 1976;28:98-103.

22. Kotby N, El-Sady S, Basiouny S, et al. Efficacy of the accent method of voice therapy. *J Voice*. 1991;5:316-320.

CHAPTER 32

The Role of the Voice Specialist in the Non-medical Management of Benign Voice Disorders

Linda M. Carroll, PhD, CCC-SLP

Therapeutic management of vocal fold pathology has long been the domain of speech-language pathologists and phoniatrists. However, with the emergence of broader fields of study within the umbrella of speech-language pathology, few clinicians have extensive coursework or experience in voice disorders. Laryngologists are often faced with a dilemma: select a speech-language pathologist who has done some voice therapy and hope that he/she makes the right decisions on the rehabilitation management of patients with pathology, or select a voice teacher/trainer who is interested in the diagnostic aspects of vocal technique and hope that he/she correctly analyzes the multiple factors encompassed in voice disorders and plans (with the laryngologist's input) a successful treatment strategy for recovery of vocal function. Both have distinct disadvantages. On the one hand, speech-language pathologists may make presumptions that singing or professional use of the voice is inherently abusive and dangerous. Additionally, they may lack the expertise to discriminate between good, excellent, and exceptional vocal technique and quality, and they frequently lack in-depth knowledge of repertoire, performance demands, or career demands. On the other hand, most voice teachers and trainers lack comprehensive training in voice disorders, syndromes, comprehensive assessment, clinical documentation, and medical management.[1]

During the past 10 years, a new "crop" of multidisciplinary speech-language pathologists has emerged: the vocologists. Vocologists are speech-language pathologists (individuals with a Master's or Doctorate in speech-language pathology) with prior experience in the performing arts (singing or theater), and additional training in voice research and interdisciplinary clinical management. Vocologists are trained to pay attention to the fine details of professional voice use while establishing an overview perspective on the best management of voice disorders. Because vocologists are few in number, many laryngologists have expanded their voice team to include a *voice specialist* (specialized voice teacher or specialized acting trainer) to address the needs of the vocal athlete during the rehabilitation process, and as an adjunct to traditional voice therapy in the nonprofessional voice user. The voice specialist is in addition to the speech-language pathologist in the rehabilitation team, who is also ideally a specialist in voice care.

Assessment and treatment of the vocal athlete (professional speaker or professional singer) require a different set of standards and often require additional exercises. Because the livelihood of voice professionals often demand fine-tuned accuracy and predictability of vocal function, they have higher demands regarding vocal function and a greater expectancy of vocal finesse. Singing and theater arts exercises have been used for decades as adjuncts to traditional speech exercises for vocal improvement.[2-8] The great speakers from Nero to Churchill to Kennedy have been assisted by voice trainers and singing teachers. The voice care team should, therefore, investigate all factors and treatments that ultimately influence the long-term success of intervention, allowing the patient to achieve the goal of not merely a normal voice, but an *exceptional* voice.

WHO NEEDS SPECIAL ATTENTION?

Although not every individual is blessed with remarkably pleasant vocal quality, most speakers are capable of excellent communication skills. Individuals who depend on professional voice use (singing or speaking) for their livelihood should be referred to the comprehensive voice team: speech-language pathologist, singing voice specialist, and acting voice trainer. Individuals who participate avocationally in the performing arts also should be referred to the comprehensive voice care team. Lastly, any patient who has not responded adequately to traditional speech therapy also should be referred to the voice care team because of the specialized assessment and training these individuals provide. The voice care team guides the patient first to optimum vocal quality and, second, to excellent communication skills with an underlying excellent vocal technique.

Disorders that may benefit from evaluation and intervention include vocal fold edema, masses, paresis, musculoskeletal tension dysphonia, and others. Vocal fold cysts, polyps, nodules, granulomas, and Reinke's edema often regress or resolve with the reduction of vocally abusive habits through the use of voice production exercises. Improved function can also be found with sulcus vocalis and scar. Commonplace vocal hyperfunction and hypofunction are addressed easily through vocal retraining from the singing and speaking voice specialists. Vocal pathologies that historically have been treated surgically may benefit from a trial of voice modification guided by the voice specialist, or voice technique modification may be a component of preoperative and postoperative care if surgical management is deemed necessary.[4,5,9]

If possible, the laryngologist and patient should avoid unnecessary surgical intervention. They should initially consider nonsurgical approaches even though the "quick fix" may seem attractive to both. The mere presence of pathology on the vocal folds does not warrant surgery.[5,10-12] If the patient is able to function successfully in a career and the pathologic lesion is deemed benign by an experienced laryngologist, there may be no need to remove an asymptomatic lesion. There are numerous vocal superstars among all styles of singing (including opera) who perform with unobtrusive pathologic lesions and speak and sing effectively despite the lesion. Ideally, this is accomplished with consistent monitoring by an experienced voice care team. If laryngeal surgery does become necessary, it is important that the voice user have the best possible technique prior to surgery. Preoperative voice training may reduce unnecessary edema, allowing more exact analysis of the critical region to be dissected by the phonosurgeon, thereby minimizing the removal of vocal fold tissue.

Vocal retraining is important following phonosurgery or surgery of the supraglottic structures or other portions of the vocal tract (such as tonsillectomy) to facilitate efficient coordination of the respiratory, articulatory, and resonatory systems in order to reduce habitual dependency on phonatory strain in communication during the critical postoperative period. Following tonsillectomy in the professional voice user, the patient needs special guidance by the voice care team to gradually stretch the oropharyngeal tissues for optimum resonance balance, and to learn new muscle memory patterns for the more open vocal tract.

Cases involving mucosal disruption of the vocal folds (such as a mucosal tear) or a vocal fold hemorrhage need referral to the voice specialist after a period of voice rest.[10,13] Rehabilitation following such an injury should include a speech-language pathologist (for general speaking voice use), singing voice specialist (to improve mucosal wave propagation and return to full vocal range), and acting voice trainer (to optimize projection of the speaking voice). Total voice rest for several weeks or months is no longer considered an appropriate treatment. This strategy of protracted silence has been tried unsuccessfully in the past, often resulting in either hypofunctional voice patterns including a fear of any vocal use, or hyperfunction upon return to voice use, resulting in re-injury. Prolonged voice rest may also elicit a period of discoordination of the voice.

THE EVALUATION

Professional voice users require fine control of the respiratory, phonatory, articulatory, and resonatory subsystems. Singers require greater control of these subsystems because of the musical and stylistic demands of their occupation. Changes in laryngeal control, whether caused by edema, lesion, or nerve paresis, invariably cause inefficient compensations in vocal technique. Minor disturbances secondary to a cold or allergy may cause the patients to use compensatory gestures that become a problem more serious than the original condition. The singing and speaking voice trainer's knowledge of the concepts of voice production can provide a viable methodology to reorient the control and balance of the vocal subsystems.

Detailed assessment of the vocal subsystems includes general posture and athleticism, general coordination, respiratory control and flexibility, source (laryngeal) control and flexibility, filter (resonance) control and flexibility, clarity of speech, quality of voice during speaking and singing tasks, stress management skills, appropriateness of current repertoire and performance schedule, and the psychologic ramifications of a vocal disorder. Much of the nature of vocal injury is linked to explosive or abusive onsets of phonation in speech. These may occur for vowel-initiated words ("hard glottal attacks") in speech and singing or for the conversational filler words such as "um-hum, alright, okay, sure, yes, no." It is imperative that vocal patterns be monitored in both modes of phonation as excessive use of hard glottal attacks and abrupt "filler words" can predispose to injuries of the larynx.

The patient may exhibit inefficient function in any of the assessment areas. It is important to note, however, that observed function may be influenced strongly by knowledge of vocal fold pathology, and that the patient's typical voice use pattern may have been altered in the recent past as a self-management strategy. The voice patient may want the voice specialist to assess only a specific area of technical deficit, but all team members have an obligation to be more thorough (objectively and subjectively) and to assess overall coordination and compensation.

The thorough assessment begins with objective assessment of aerodynamic and acoustic function using calibrated laboratory instrumentation for standard measures. Objective measures can cue the voice specialist toward a specific set of exercises, thereby shortening the rehabilitation process. Deficits in objective respiratory measures may indicate the need for more thorough subjective respiratory management and downstream compensation, even if the presenting complaint did not specifically mention breathing problems. This may also trigger referral to a pulmonologist. Deficits in laryngeal aerodynamic measurement (mean transglottal flow rate, subglottal pressure, estimated laryngeal airway resistance) would indicate the need for greater attention to laryngeal breath management and laryngeal tension. Weak transfer function of the source signal (as indicated by reduced amplitude of singer's formant and wide bandwidths of formants) indicates the need for greater attention to the resonance aspects of vocal production, even if vocal clarity or projection were not mentioned in the original complaint. Although objective testing is generally prescribed by the laryngologist, these measures can be invaluable in prioritizing the specific goals that the voice care team establishes for the individual.

Objective Evaluation

Objective evaluation and documentation are important facets of any rehabilitation program and of voice training in general. The most accessible objective instrumentation available to the voice specialist is a piano or keyboard. The patient's physiologic fundamental frequency range of phonation (total pitch range) may be approximated easily using the piano. Conversion charts of fundamental frequency equivalency to pitch or note names may be found in a number of sources.[5,7,14-17] Starting at midrange, the patient should be instructed to sing (either in stepwise fashion or sliding) downward to the patient's lowest tone (excluding vocal fry). Measurement of the highest tone (including falsetto and flageolet) may be measured in similar fashion. Once recorded, this becomes a permanent record in the patient's file, listed under laryngeal function measurement. The normal range of phonation for adults is about 35 semitones.[18] If intensity range on each tone is also measured (generally at 30 cm from the mouth) with a sound level meter (easily purchased at electronic stores), a voice range profile or phonetogram is the resultant graph.[19,20] The voice range profile yields useful information on specific weaknesses and technical adjustments by the injured voice user and can illustrate register transitions.

Other objective measures of laryngeal function include jitter (fundamental frequency perturbation), shimmer (amplitude perturbation), maximum flow declination rate, vibrato characteristics (frequency and amplitude) and the electroglottographic measures of duty cycle (opening phase, closing phase) and closed phase. A patient with increased jitter should be given exercises that involve cricothyroid muscle function (sliding scales, arpeggio scales), whereas a patient with increased shimmer should be given exercises that involve the thyroarytenoid muscle function (messa di voce). A standard laryngeal/aerodynamic test for hypofunction and hyperfunction is the s/z ratio. Calculation of the s/z ratio (maximum phonation on /s/ divided by maximum phonation on /z/) yields a vocal efficiency index (normal s/z ratio is 1.0).[21] Significantly reduced s/z ratio is indicative of hyperfunction, while significantly elevated s/z ratio is associated with hypofunction.

Hyperfunction is also indicated by significantly reduced mean transglottal flow rate and high laryngeal airway resistance values. Subjectively, these patients often present with symptoms of musculoskeletal tension dysphonia that may have precipitated symptoms and/or laryngeal lesions associated with voice abuse and misuse. Hyperfunctional patients need thorough assessment of pulmonary function to determine causal relationships for their behaviors. Reduced pulmonary strength may lead to laryngeal hyperfunction in an effort to compensate downstream. The underlying respiratory deficiency should be addressed through referral to a pulmonologist.

Although the vast majority of normative data for laryngeal function measures has been established on untrained (or minimally trained) voice users, more studies are now being published on vocal athletes such as trained speakers and singers.

The use of video documentation is also important. Audiovisual recording allows the patient to see any postural adjustments or tensions that may adversely affect the accessibility of efficient vocal production. It is important to note that many hyperfunctional gestures are related to unnecessary skeletal adjustments, especially protrusion and elevation of the head and neck with pitch (F_0) changes, excessive tongue or jaw tension, and adjustments of the clavicle in crescendo gestures. Arranging a video monitor for the patient to use for biofeedback during the training session is generally helpful. Positioning the video camera for a side view can be especially helpful in revealing to the patient his/her skeletal adjustments.

Visual biofeedback has also been found to be beneficial for restoring efficient use of the phonatory system, utilizing videostroboscopy, electroglottography, spectrography, and vibrato characteristics (through use of the Vocal Demodulator).[22] Acoustically, a delayed auditory feedback system (set at 100-400 ms delay) can be helpful for allowing patients to sense the sound production and hear the resultant quality. Kinesthetic feedback may help the patient to sense the subtle postural consequences during vocal production.

Use of biofeedback is often helpful in determining clarity of vocal projection. Through use of spectrum analysis (such as with Kay Elemetrics [Lincoln Park, NJ] VisiPitch model 3300 Sona-Match), bandwidth information for formants can be examined for efficiency. Efficiency of filtering and clarity of sound is evident by a narrow bandwidth for the formants. Inefficient filtering and "muddy" speech or singing is evident with wider formant bandwidths. With biofeedback, the patient can improve awareness of those sensations and adjustments for focused resonance and improved vocal quality. Without biofeedback, some patients may have difficulty tuning into the subtle, yet important, aspects of resonance.

Subjective Evaluation

The subjective evaluation process is an assessment of the voice user's choice of strategies and decision-making skills with the voice. The following issues in vocal technique must be addressed:

How well does the patient use the voice?

Does the patient have a consistent and predictable vocal technique?

Is the patient's breath management efficient and consistent?

How is the patient's posture while standing and while sitting?

Does the patient use resonance optimally?

Are there sites of tension that are interfering with voice use and vocal finesse?

Does the patient make the kinds of decisions that increase or reduce tension?

Does the patient make the kinds of decisions that exacerbate the pathology?

Does the patient depend on skillful vocal technique or rely solely on "tricks"?

Is the patient able to self-correct to more efficient, healthy use of the voice?

How malleable is the patient's muscle memory?

Is vocal energy well directed or misdirected?

A sample evaluation form used by the author is provided in Table 32-1.

The intellectual recognition of a faulty action is only the first step toward correction of a muscular habit. Issues of tactile and muscle memory, muscle behavior, and the interaction between the psyche and physiology of the patient must be addressed in the athletic retraining of the injured voice. Appropriate exercises may be of great benefit in correcting inefficiencies that led to the vocal injury, avoiding re-injury while promoting recovery of necessary skills.

General Posture

Posture should be athletic, energized, and flexible. Good posture does not include a stiff back or shoulders drawn back. Posture of the lower torso should include knees relaxed (but not overtly bent) and the weight evenly distributed over both hips. The upper torso is best managed through the orientation of the shoulder blades. If the shoulder blades rest slightly close together, the upper chest cavity (thoracic cavity) will not migrate to a "collapsed" position. The resulting rib cage position reduces both slumping and clavicular breathing

Date of Evaluation: Linda M. Carroll, Ph.D. CCC/SLP
Otolaryngologist/Referring Physician: Vocologist/Speech Pathologist
Medical Diagnosis: 424 West 49th Street, Suite 1
Speech Pathologist: New York, NY 10019
Send reports to: tel: 212.459.3929

Subjective Evaluation: Voice

Patient Name: Tape: ❏ Mini Disk ❏ Cassette ❏ Video
Address: ❏ Prof voice user ❏ Nonprof voice user
City/State/Zip   ❏ Singer ❏ Actor
Age: DOB: Performance Style:
Sex: ❏ M   ❏ F
Brief background history:

Presenting complaints, symptoms:

Perceptual analysis:
(0 = WNL, 3 = severe) Grade __ Roughness __ Breathiness __ Asthenic __ Strain __

Subjective evaluation: **Treatment Probes/Exercises**
Source Characteristics
Quality:

WNL	Hoarse	Breathy	Tremor
F_0 Breaks	Vocal fry	Diplophonia	
Strident/Strained	Glottal Attacks	Aphonic	

F_0:

WNL	↓ range	↓ F_0 variability
F_0 breaks	↓ / ↑ F_0	

Intensity:

WNL	↓ control	↓ / ↑ db

Rate:

WNL	Short, closed syllables

General Source comments:
Singing skill:
        F_0 range:
        Vibrato characteristics:
        Comments:
Acting/Dramatic Text skill:
Filter Characteristics:
Resonance:

WNL	Low tone focus	Thin/weak	Hyper/Hyponasal
Nasal Emission	↓ loft	↓ ring	

        Comments:
Power Characteristics:
Respiratory/Aerodynamic:

Effective	Thoracic	Clavicular	↓ coordination
Effortful	Stridor	Lengthy breath pausing	
Holds breath	↓ skill	Excessive abdominal movement/tension	

        Comments:
General Posture: Comments
Tension Management: Sites of tension:
Summary/Recommendations:
Goals:

TABLE 32-1. *Subjective Voice Evaluation Form*

and may feel unusual at first to the patient (it should not, however, be painful). The efficient "position of rest" is found easily from the "posture finders" exercise from Directed Energy Vocal Technique (DEVT).[4,13] The patient should stand, extending arms out to each side with palms down as he/she observes the orientation of the shoulder blades; then the patient should rotate his/her palms up as he/she senses movement of the shoulder blades lower and closer together (see Figures 32-1 and 32-2).

The shoulders should not be raised. The upper chest should remain relatively expanded in the front. The clavicles should not drop significantly on expiration, and the shoulders should not lift on inspiration. The knees should be relaxed and the lower back should be released, not hyperextended, with a loose position in the pelvis (neither too far tilted nor contracted). Care must be taken to determine that this posture is based simply on skeletal orientation, and not muscular holding (more in-depth alignment exercises may be found in the works of F. M. Feldenkrais[23] and Moshe Alexander).[24] This simple exercise helps the patient improve efficiency of posture, allowing free movement of the lower rib structures and abdominal musculature, which then leads to improved efficiency of breath management during inspiration and exhalation.

Head and neck position should be assessed carefully for elevation or protrusion. Invariably, the posture of the upper torso is the leading culprit in inefficient head and neck position. It is not uncommon to see long-term difficulty with efficient posture in women who have large breasts or have had breast reduction surgery. Their upper torso memory pattern is typically ingrained to include the (former) physique, which was often associated with rounded shoulders (or slumped posture). Men who overly develop the rectus abdominus muscle (through excessive "crunches" at the gym) develop excess bulking and difficulty with an efficient "position of rest."

Some performers have occupational hazards that may lead to inefficient posture unless they are monitored carefully. These include choral singers (singing "over" the music folder), Broadway performers (because of the raked stage and the desire to get closer to their audiences), singer/guitarists (who often choose weak postures while holding the guitar, and lean into the microphone), club entertainers (who play piano while leaning into a microphone), and radio announcers (who lean into microphones). Performers need to be counseled that efficient posture on and off the stage is essential. Particularly hazardous posture may be found at social gatherings (as people lean forward in an effort to hear others), when seated in a car, when watching television/computer monitor, or when talking on the telephone.

Posture Exercises

Goal: *To reduce excessive tension in the upper torso, allowing ease of inspiration and expiration.*

Exercise 1: "Elbow kiss": With the patient standing, have him/her bring the hands to each shoulder, raising elbows parallel to shoulders. Alternately bring elbows together in

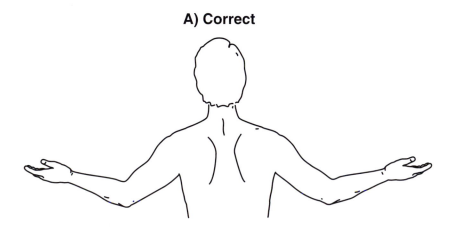
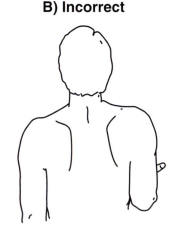

A) Correct   **B) Incorrect**

FIGURE 32-1. *(A) Alignment of the shoulder blades; shoulder blades are relaxed but in close proximity, with the upper chest remaining expanded. (B) Incorrect alignment. Tensions of expressivity may pull the shoulders upward and/or forward, compromising breath efficiency.*

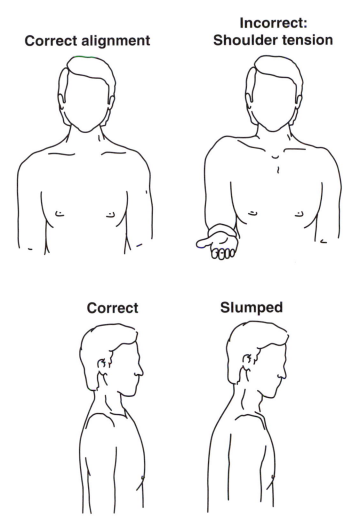

Correct alignment

Incorrect: Shoulder tension

Correct

Slumped

FIGURE 32-2. *Correct and incorrect alignment of the upper torso. Excessive physical expressivity may result in lifted shoulders or slumped chest positions.*

the front and try to have them touch behind the back. Maintain regular breathing pattern during the exercise.

Exercise 2:   "Ceiling touch": Have the patient reach for the ceiling with one arm alternately extended above head. Breathe during arm extension.

Exercise 3:   "Trapezius release": Instruct the patient to clasp his/her hands together and place them behind the fullest part of the back of the head. The elbows should be brought forward. The patient should then isometrically push the head back into the clasped hands and pull the head forward with the hands/arms, feeling the pull against the back and sides of the neck. The patient should breathe comfortably while maintaining this isometric exercise for approximately 20-30 seconds. Then he/she should suddenly release the clasped hands, allowing the head to move freely on the now-loosened neck. The patient should feel a reduction in neck/shoulder tensions, which may lead to improved access of lower breathing patterns (caused by reduced muscle tension of the upper torso).

Exercise 4:   "Figure 8s": With the patient standing, have him/her bring the hands to each shoulder, and raise the elbows (parallel to shoulder). Using the elbows as "paintbrushes," he/she is asked to attempt to paint the number 8 from the ceiling to the floor, bending the knees and moving the torso as necessary, maintaining a regular breathing pattern as the torso contorts to form the figure 8s. (Note: This is hard to do.) Repeat, with elbows facing the back. (Note: This is even harder to do!)

General Coordination

Trunk stability and general coordination are traditionally assessed in young children with a speech or language issue. Because the professional voice user with a vocal disorder is typically an adult, it is easy to overlook general coordination and stability of physical function. It is important to note carefully and bring to the patient's attention any observed episodes of slight hip swaying (while standing), particularly if it occurs during phonation. Instability of the lower trunk impairs respiratory control. Upon identification, many patients have difficulty controlling swaying movements of the torso. Many performers incorrectly add tension to avoid body swaying (which has significant ramifications for respiratory control). This may be redirected easily into energized, intention movement found in tai chi, for example. Many performers have also found this form of exercise helpful for stress management, in addition to the improved support and trunk stability.

Other issues of general coordination include eye movements/blinking (which are often associated with the swallow reflex, which would entrap the larynx during phonation) at the beginning of high notes, and arm or hand tension during speech and singing. Video documentation and analysis are usually sufficient to reinforce verbal comment by the voice specialist.

One standard vocal exercise that assesses respiratory-laryngeal-resonance coordination is a /β/ lip flutter (vibration therapy). This phoneme (a voiced bilabial fricative) tests the ability of the patient to balance the power, source, and filter subsystems during pitch change (see Figure 32-3).

It is, in effect, a test of the patient's general tendency to cheat in vocal technique. If the patient locks his/her support or fails to use adequate support, the lip flutter (a "raspberry" sound) will stop or fade away. If the patient uses hyperfunction at the source, the sound will stop. If the patient uses excess tension in the filter subsystem (usually at the lips), the sound will stop. If the lip flutter is tested in a *messa di voce* (crescendo-diminuendo) task (see Figures 32-4A, 32-4B), more detailed analysis is possible of the singer's strategy for use of hypofunction and hyperfunction. Initially, some patients may need to reduce lip tension by placing their hands gently on the corners of the mouth. Other patients may need to use a tongue flutter (with tongue extended over the lower lip) or a rolled "r" (/r/) to achieve balanced coordination.

A more difficult vocal exercise to test coordination of the subsystems is a panting exercise. The DEVT panting exercise examines the patient's ability to coordinate the alternation between a delicate vocal task (*messa di voce* on vowels) and a dynamic respiratory task (panting) (see Figures 32-5A, B, C, and D).

This exercise may be done throughout the entire vocal range, and should begin on a medium low note for the patient, and at a moderately slow tempo. After each short *messa di voce,* the patient exhales and inhales three times. After completing the given vowels, the patient then executes a staccato (short, bouncy singing), legato (smooth, fluid singing) and then marcato (detached but still connected singing), diatonic scale. Most singers can accomplish the diatonic scales on one breath. Many singers typically view panting exercises as a repeated exhalatory exercise. It should be viewed as a *quiet inhalatory exercise* first and foremost. The panting exercise should not be repeated exhalations; it should be exhalation followed by inhalation.

While phonating and panting, the patient should slowly rotate the head from side to side to identify and reduce any neck and trapezius tensions (particularly in the more complex versions of the panting exercise). The preliminary goals of therapeutic work should be oriented primarily toward finding a reasonably good vocal technique, and the development of the extreme high range should be deferred until freedom is achieved in the comfortable middle range of the voice. Likewise, the patient who wants to increase the power of an injured voice should wait until an easy flexibility of the voice (as demonstrated with *messa di voce* exercises) has been restored. Patients with nerve paresis may find this exercise difficult initially, but will ultimately find it a most valuable exercise for coordination of the weakened larynx. In a healthy voice, the vocal folds lengthen in the diminuendo maneuver (loud to soft change in dynamics), as well as in light staccato exercises and ascending fun-

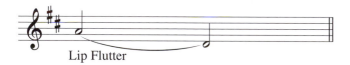

Lip Flutter

FIGURE 32-3. *Descending lip flutter (vibration therapy exercise) to coordinate the subsystems.*

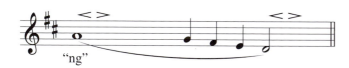

"ng"

FIGURE 32-4A. *Descending slide on lip flutter (vibration therapy)* with messa di voce.

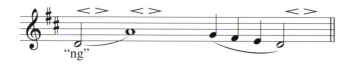

"ng"

FIGURE 32-4B. *Lip flutter (vibration therapy)* with messa di voce *and change in fundamental frequency and descending scale.*

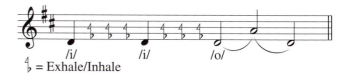

/i/   /i/   /o/

♩ = Exhale/Inhale

FIGURE 32-5A. *Simple panting exercise (exhale-inhale) on "ee" (/i/) sound with slide on "oh" (/o/). The patient should begin with this simplest version of the panting exercise, and then advance on to the more complicated versions.*

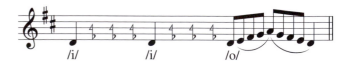

/i/   /i/   /o/

FIGURE 32-5B. *Simple panting exercise on "ee" (/i/) with ascending-descending scale on "oh" (/o/).*

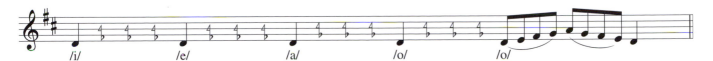

FIGURE 32-5C. *Panting exercise with changing vowels (to address resonance skill) and ascending-descending scale.*

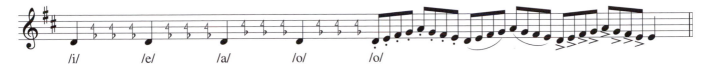

FIGURE 32-5D. *Complex panting exercise with changing vowels and ascending-descending scales sung staccato, legato, and marcato.*

damental frequency. In all patients, the panting exercise may induce dryness and/or wooziness, and the patient should be counseled to sip water moderately and rest as needed. The woozy feeling typically subsides in successive days as a higher level of training is accomplished. Occasional sighs to release physical tension and redirect stress are advised. Shaking of the hands may also facilitate the marcato portion of exercise 32-5D.

Power (Respiratory) Control and Flexibility

Vocal athletes (and patients in general) are usually more concerned with support of the breath stream (or pressure head) than control of the inhalatory aspect of the respiratory cycle. This may lead to rigid support strategies rather than flexible, energized, and fluid support. Failure to recognize the importance of inhalation control often leads to clavicular or thoracic breathing patterns. The old adage of "what goes in, comes out" is true for control and flexibility of respiration. If the inhalatory aspect of respiration is poor (tense, rigid, late, stridor, etc), the ability of the vocal athlete to execute a well-directed breath stream for phonation is markedly impaired.

Breathing Exercises

Goal: *To improve access to lower rib expansion for improved abdominal-diaphragmatic breathing.*

Exercise 1: Lower rib expansion. With the patient standing, have him/her bend forward at the waist and place hands on the lower rib cage (thumbs forward, fingers on the low ribs of the back). He/she should breathe in to feel symmetric expansion of lower ribs during inhalation (the voice specialist should have hands placed over patient's hands to sense breathing skill). The

patient then exhales slowly, feeling gentle, continuous inward movement of low rib cage. He/she should repeat the exercise twice, then the patient should hold his/her breath briefly between inhalation and exhalation and change posture to a more erect position. The rib cage movement should not change appreciably. The patient continues until standing erect. The breath should now be "centered" in the lower rib cage, rather than high in the torso. (Note: The voice specialist may need to assist the patient in the exhalatory process, using some hand pressure to define further the inspiratory and expiratory movements.) If the patient has had a lower respiratory infection (pneumonia, bronchitis) in the past six months, additional attention should be paid to symmetry of respiratory movements, and ability to both slowly and suddenly exhale and inhale.

Exercise 2: Rib and intercostals stretch. While standing, the patient extends one arm over the opposite shoulder, bends the torso to "drape" over that side, and breathes three times, feeling rib expansion. This exercise is repeated on the opposite side.

Goal: *Improve awareness of abdominal and rib cage contribution to support.*

Exercise 1: "Wh-exercise": Instruct the patient to exhale using a gentle, long "wh" sound, unvoiced, with relaxed, pursed lips for as long as he/she can comfortably exhale. The patient should sense the slow, inward movement of the lower torso musculature coordinating with rib cage movement. This exercise may also be done on /ʃ, ʒ, θ, ð, s, z, v, f/, or with the patient leaning into a flat surface (wall or door), arms straight, feet approximately 2 feet from the wall.

Goal: *Improve respiratory preparedness and planning.*

Exercise 1:   "Candle-blowing": Instruct the patient to exhale gently with two short "wh" puffs (similar to blowing out a small candle on a cupcake), breathe in, and then blow out for one long, slow exhalation (similar to blowing out candles on a large cake). The exercise is repeated with two short "wh" puffs followed by one long "wh" puff. Note: This exercise also trains respiratory preparedness. The patient should plan the breath for the task ahead, rather than as a recovery event. It is important that the patient's breath management be such that a short breath is taken before the short respiratory task, and a long breath is taken before the long respiratory task. There is often a great desire to "rebound" after the long respiratory task, which would lead to breath mismanagement for the repeat candle-blowing exercise. Inefficient respiratory skill would be a big breath after the long exhalation and a short breath after the short exhalations. Efficient breath management is a long breath after the short task (to plan for the long task), and a short breath after the long task (to plan for the upcoming short task).

Exercise 2:   "Progressive counting exercise": The patient is instructed to count aloud from 1-10 at a regular rhythmic pace (approximately 92 metronomic beats per minute), using flexible pitch and loudness changes. The first two recitations of the rote task are begun with 4 metronomic beats for the inhalation phase, with the patient instructed to use all the breath during the 1-10 rote task. The next two recitations of the rote task are given 3 metronomic beats, then 2 beats, then 1 beat and then only a catch-breath between the 10 and next 1-10 count. Breathing pattern should be monitored to ensure smooth inhalation over the inhalatory beat pattern, with no appreciable shoulder movement. This exer-

cise is particularly helpful in not only training respiratory preparedness, but also allowing the patient to trust lower rib cage involvement in respiration.

Exercise 3:   Tadoma: If excessive breath flow is noted (such as with nodules, polyps, paralysis), the Tadoma technique may be helpful in normalizing the flow of breath. The Tadoma technique is based on increased sensory awareness of breath.[25] Tadoma requires the patient to place the back of the hand (which is more sensitive to breath) very close to the front of the mouth (~1/2") during phonation. Although originally designed for speech therapy with the severely hearing-impaired, Tadoma has been translated into the field of stuttering and voice to monitor sudden changes in breath flow from vowel to vowel.

The last segment of respiratory assessment should be during conversational speech. Many patients hold their breath (unconsciously) when listening, particularly to questions. This creates physical tensions which can affect the voice adversely. Patients should be counseled to breathe as they listen.

Source (Laryngeal) Control and Flexibility

Matching pitch is rarely a problem for a singer. Following general pitch contours is rarely a problem with non-singers. The greater difficulty comes in controlling minute changes in pitch.

Goal: *Improved control and coordination of the intrinsic laryngeal muscles.*

Exercise 1:   Vocal slide: The task of a slow vocal slide (see Figure 32-6) is particularly helpful in reducing vocal fold edema (nodules, polyps) and improving control within the vocal range (paresis, paralysis, scar, reduced amplitude, sulcus vocalis). The exercise is designed to very slowly change from a lower pitch to a higher pitch and then back to a lower pitch to test the patient's control over the thyroarytenoid and cricothyroid muscles. Loudness should not change when pitch is being changed and breath pressure should not change appreciably. The exercise should be done primarily in modal voice, with extension up to the higher passaggio.

Many patients have difficulty initially in executing a smooth, slow change in pitch because of the presence of

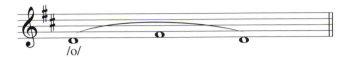

FIGURE 32-6. *Sliding third exercise, with gradual change of fundamental frequency, on "oh" (/o/) vowel.*

pathology. It is *essential* that they learn to execute this smooth maneuver without compensatory hyperfunction in an effort to gain control of and strengthen the intrinsic laryngeal muscles. If the sliding interval is too large (greater than a fourth), the breath supply may be inadequate and the task may result in a gross assessment of source function rather than a fine assessment of source function. The interval of a major third is generally best. When a weak area of source function is observed with the sliding scale, it should be repeated slowly until no "glitches" or sudden pitch changes are audible with proper technique. Ideally, the slide should be a slow glissando slide (or vocal moan) rather than artistically sung. Inability to control fundamental frequency in minute increments after an appropriate course of voice therapy may be an important factor in surgical decision-making.

Exercise 2: "Ng-sniff": An extension of the sliding third exercise is the "ng-sniff" exercise from DEVT (see Figure 32-7). This exercise requires control of the thyroarytenoid muscle and resonance changes for the diminuendo, with contrasting cricothyroid function for accomplishing the ascending fundamental frequency.

The "ng-sniff" exercise should be limited to the modal voice, with extension up through the upper passaggio, but not exclusively in loft register.

A moderate diminuendo should be accomplished on the lower tone and completed before the change in F_0. Many singers erroneously view the diminuendo aspect as a reduction of vocal energy and a weaker voice quality. If the diminuendo is accompanied by a reduction in overall energy (which should not be the case in a well-directed voice), the voice fails to project in the diminuendo and loses quality and source control. In the accomplished performer, moderately soft tones are usually

accompanied by more overall coordination than moderately loud tones. As fundamental frequency is increased during the slide, there should not be a significant increase in mean breath flow or an appreciable elevation of the vertical laryngeal position (VLP). Changes in VLP may be attributed to excessive extrinsic laryngeal muscle activity or excessive diaphragmatic relaxation during phonation. As a rise in VLP shortens the vocal tract length, the vocal production becomes thin in timbre, which generally is not desired.

It is important to remember the role of the diaphragm in source control. Aside from the diaphragm's primary role as the muscle of inspiration, it may have a secondary effect in that it can provide a resistance to premature compression of the column of air against the underside of the vocal folds.[26,27] It is probably this antagonistic relationship between the abdominal viscera and the diaphragm that helps fine-tune subglottal pressure, resulting in stable VLP and reduced hyperfunctional behaviors.

Exercise 3: Coloratura scales: Source flexibility is typically assessed through coloratura (fast sequential scales) and arpeggios (changing interval scales). Typically, the patient begins with rapid 5-note ascending/descending scales and then advances to 9-tone ascending/descending scales. There is some evidence[28] that the speed of coloratura and arpeggios may be dependent on the patient's vibrato speed.

Exercise 4: Descending scale with trill: A descending 5-tone scale (beginning midrange) with a trill on the lowest note is particularly helpful in improving source control of both the low and extreme low range. During the exercise, the vocal folds are gradually slackened and then required to minimally adjust cricothyroid length during a 2-tone trill (see Figure 32-8). Although the exercise is only done in the mid to lower range of the vocal range, it translates skill to high voice access and control.

Additionally, many patients exhibit improved focus of the speaking voice following this exercise, with fewer

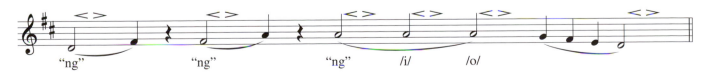

FIGURE 32-7. *"Ng-sniff" (/ŋ/) exercise with messa di voce on long notes.*

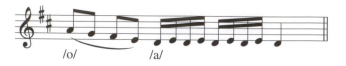

FIGURE 32-8. *Descending 5-tone scale with trill, designed to improve extreme low and extreme high source control.*

episodes of vocal fry.

Exercise 5: "Buckingham Exercise": This exercise (see Figure 32-9) is particularly helpful for Reinke's edema (polypoid corditis) and paralysis. The rationale for this source exercise is to control transition from aperiodic vibrations (vocal fry) to periodic vibrations in loft register using a loft-dominant vowel (connected scales on /o/).

This exercise increases the patient's ability to compensate for the aperiodic vibrations encountered at the source level from these pathologies. Yodeling also improves control of the source.

Exercise 4: "Calling": An extension of Arthur Lessac's "call" exercise,[29] calling is done with a wide variety of pitch changes. The patient is instructed to sigh gently, then sigh while saying "hello" softly (repeat 5 times), and then extend to an elongated fuller "calling" quality extending into the higher frequency range of the voice (avoiding yelling or screaming). The first syllable of the "hello" begins in the medium-low range of the voice and then ascends into the higher range of the voice for the final syllable, which is then carried down in a glissando pattern to the lower frequency range (see Figure 32-10).

The phrases "away," "for me," "for you," and "at home" are also used in the calling exercise, as well as other daily phrases (okay, not now). "Calling" is accomplished through a conscious monitoring of the use of

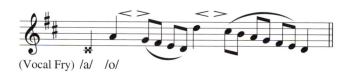

FIGURE 32-9. *"Buckingham" exercise coordinating aperiodic voice source (vocal fry) with periodic voice source (clear tone).*

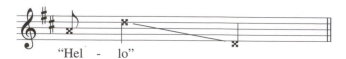

FIGURE 32-10. *"Calling" exercise to coordinate resonance with pitch change. This exercise also works well as a beginning transfer exercise from sustained phonation to conversational speech.*

optimum oral-nasal resonance ("ring" and "loft" resonance) while gently exercising the intrinsic laryngeal muscles. Pressed phonation should be avoided. Flow phonation is desired.

Filter Control and Flexibility

Filtering of the source signal is the most important aspect of the voice because it yields much of the vocal signature. Unless a radical permanent change has occurred at the source level (such as would be the case with severe hormonal effects on the voice), the vocal signature is predominantly the domain of the filter system. Improved skill of filtering the source signal should reduce demand on the larynx.

Efficient filtering is the product of a balance of "ring" resonance and "loft" resonance (DEVT). Ring resonance is that aspect of resonance that has a sensation of buzzing on the facial bones. The concept of ring and loft resonance is important for speakers and singers. An imbalance of filter control may predispose the voice user to vocal injury or inefficiency, and may perpetuate or aggravate pathology. Examples of someone with ring-dominant production include Ross Perot and Jean Stapleton portraying the television character "Edith Bunker." Examples of someone with loft-dominant production include Julia Child and James Earl Jones as the movie character "Darth Vader." Examples of good balance of ring and loft resonance would be Martin Luther King, Walter Cronkite, James Earl Jones (using his typical voice), Carol Burnett, and Hillary Rodham Clinton.

Ring resonance (and Y-buzz, as described below) affords projection of the voice, and gives brightness to the timbre. Ring resonance is felt to be the dominant sensation when singing in chest voice. Loft resonance is that aspect of resonance that has a sensation of height or space in the cranium. This is felt easiest with a descending slide on "oh" beginning on a medium high pitch. Loft resonance helps protect the voice from injury, and gives richness to the timbre. Loft resonance is felt to be associated with loft register. Aerodynamically, ring resonant productions have been found to have less mean transglottal airflow than loft resonant productions.[30] A healthy voice has a balance of ring and loft resonance in both speech and singing modes.

Tonal placement is often discussed in traditional speech therapy. Essentially, tonal placement is efficient when more "work" for phonation and voice quality is being done in the filter subsystem than at the voice source, and the patient does not sense a great deal of effort or contribution to the voice quality from the larynx. There are a variety of approaches to improve resonance for efficient tonal placement. The concept of tonal placement, and resonance in general, can be difficult for some patients because it requires attention to subtle sensations and vibrations downstream.

Goal: *Improve awareness of resonance.*

Exercise 1:   Instruct the patient to massage his/her face for 30-45 seconds, with specific attention to the nose, cheeks, upper lip area, and forehead (massage should reduce facial tension and improve circulation, promoting easier recognition of resonance sensations). Following the massage, instruct the patient to place his/her hands on the nose/cheek area and hum gently, feeling the buzz created by the hum. Encourage the patient to verbalize the sensations, even if the sensations are slight (verbalization improves the patient's memory for resonance areas).

Exercise 2:   Instruct the patient to hum gently while standing in a corner, facing the corner, with his/her face approximately 2 inches from the surface. The patient should feel the reflection of sound waves on the facial bones, reinforcing awareness of resonance areas for vocal projection.

Goal: *Improve access to forwarding resonance.*

Exercise 1:   "Child's taunt": Designed to isolate ring resonance, the child's taunt [næ-næ-næ-næ-næ-næ] (see Figure 32-11) should be done with specific attention to the vibrations along the hard palate and nose. The sound should not be "anchored" to the larynx, but should be quite focused, rather brassy in timbre, and noisy. If it is too nasal, it can develop a "twang" quality. Subtleties of producing ring resonance may vary from day to day for the individual, depending on fluid loading, congestion, and so forth.

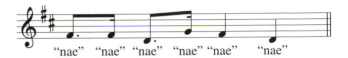

"nae" "nae" "nae" "nae" "nae"   "nae"

FIGURE 32-11. *"Child's taunt" exercise to increase awareness of ring resonance.*

Exercise 2:   "Ng-sniff": This exercise, described above in "Source control" improves the patient's awareness of ring resonance during the "ng" (/ŋ/) sound, and further exercises the patient's ability to change resonance from forward ring resonance (for the crescendo) to back loft resonance (for the diminuendo). These changes are intrinsic to this exercise. The resonance sensations between crescendo and diminuendo may not be so apparent during routine singing. Change of vowel (or filtering) allows the patient to transfer the sensations of resonance from the nasal phoneme into vowels that are ring dominant /i/, and loft dominant (/o/). The "ng-sniff" exercise should be limited to the modal voice, with extension up through the upper passaggio, but not into exclusive loft register.

Exercise 3:   "Y-buzz": An exercise by Arthur Lessac and outlined in great detail in his text *The Use and Training of the Human Voice,*[29] the Y-buzz addresses the sensations of forward resonance during sustained "y" for words containing the /j/ phoneme (yes, yellow, you, computer, unusual, future). During the Y-buzz (sustained /j/ production), the patient is instructed to sense the focused forward resonance "on the forward gum-ridge section of the hard palate and in the nasal bone, traveling toward the bridge of the nose and the connecting forehead."[29(p122)] For this exercise, words that use the "y" sound are elongated during the /j/ portion as the patient slowly moves the contact of the tongue against the hard palate typical of /j/ to a more anterior release that increases the patient's awareness of a focused sound. Words are then shortened and transferred into conversation. Lessac summarizes the efficient forward resonance as "when your voice functions solely as in inner vibrating current, never pushed and never impeded, you will experience it as a bone-conducted vibratory feeling that uses energy without abusing it … a feeling that transmits its bone-conducted vibrations to the farthest rows and corners of the theatre or concert hall."[29(p124)]

Goal: *Improve access to back resonance.*

Exercise 1:   "Hoot-owl": Designed to isolate the sensations associated with loft resonance, the patient is instructed to imitate a hoot-owl ("hoo-hoo") descending from medium high frequency range of the voice, using slightly pursed lips with an open jaw space, while focusing on the sensations of open space in the back of the cranium (which is sensory only, not physiologic).

Exercise 2:   Yawn-sigh: The patient is instructed to yawn and allow voicing to escape during the exhalatory phase, while sensing the increased oral-pharyngeal space created during the yawn.

Exercise 3:   Diminuendo: The patient is instructed to sustain a comfortable note (or a note within a scale passage) and slowly diminish the intensity, maintaining energy and focus in the sound, with the diminuendo accomplished through an increased awareness of loft resonance.

Goal: *Improved balance of resonance.*

Exercise 1:   Vowel variation: During the simple vowel variation, the patient is instructed to slowly change vowels (progressing through the vowel quadrangle) while maintaining a steady fundamental frequency and loudness (see Figure 32-12). There should not be an appreciable change of breath flow as the vowel changes.

Exercise 2:   Progressive vowel variation: This exercise is an extension of the sliding third exercise (see above under Source control), but

requires the vocalist to maintain vocal control while slowly changing vowels in the vowel quadrangle. The vowel quadrangle is the organization of the American vowels, written in International Phonetic Alphabet, whereby vowels are organized by their articulatory and resonance characteristics (see Table 32-2).

The forward vowels (ring dominant) use the tongue as the primary articulator, whereas the back vowels (loft dominant) use the lips as the primary articulator. The adapted vowel variation begins with the ring dominant tongue vowel /i/ and gradually arrives at loft dominant lip vowel /u/ (see Figure 32-13). The jaw should not change position (degree of openness, closed) significantly as the tongue and lips shape the vowels. In addition, airflow should not change appreciably during the vowel variation.

The exercise repeats the same interval progressing from /ɪ/ to /e/, /e/ to /ɛ/, /ɛ/ to /æ/, /æ/ to /a/, /a/ to /ɑ/, /ɑ/ to /ɔ/, /ɔ/ to /o/, /o/ to /ʊ/, and /ʊ/ to /u/. (Note: this exercise should not be done for longer than 5 minutes.)

Exercise 3:   *Messa di voce:* Touted for centuries as the ultimate vocal gesture, the gradual

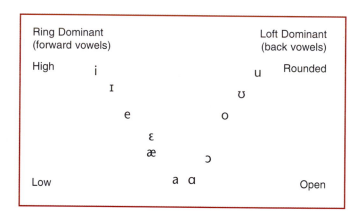

TABLE 32-2. *Vowel Quadralateral (in International Phonetic Alphabet) for Progressive Vowel Variation Exercise*

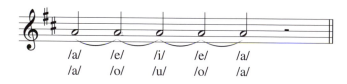

FIGURE 32-12. *Simple vowel variation exercise designed to target consistency of resonance and quality as the vowel changes.*

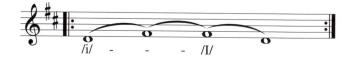

FIGURE 32-13. *Progressive vowel variation exercise. The patient should begin the sliding third scale on the vowel /i/, change to /ɪ/ during the sustained higher note and then descend to the original note, continuing to progress through the vowel quadralateral.*

crescendo-diminuendo (without appreciable change in fundamental frequency) is now receiving attention by voice scientists for investigation of its respiratory, laryngeal, and resonance effects. *Messa di voce* exercises are helpful for a variety of voice disorders (nodules, polyps, Reinke's edema, polypoid corditis, cysts, paresis, paralysis, sulcus vocalis) because of the physiologic demands on the respiratory management, intrinsic laryngeal muscles, and resonance balance. *Messa di voce* trains a skill that is found in all vocal styles. Although the exercise appears easy, it is a complex vocal task. The more difficult portion of the exercise (or phrase gesture) is the diminuendo (lessening of the intensity). For speakers, the *messa di voce* exercise may be elicited in an imitation of race cars in the famed "Indianapolis 500" race, as the cars zoom around the curved racetrack (verbalized as "nee-auh").

Clarity of Speech

Dysarthria is rarely an issue with professional voice users. It is important to note, however, that small changes in clarity or quality of speech may be an indicator of onset of a systemic disease. Multiple sclerosis and Parkinson's disease may be manifested first as a speech or vocal complaint. Although the comprehensive oral-peripheral examination of the speech structures is typically performed by the speech pathologist, the voice trainer should be familiar with the key areas of assessment for symmetry in function, strength, and dexterity.

Phonemically loaded phrases and sentences are a helpful supplement for optimizing communication skills (through articulatory dexterity) in the voice-disordered patient. Sample sentences that target specific articulatory dexterity include:

labial movements:

> "We watched wily weasels in the wonderful Wyoming wilderness."

coarticulation:

> "Unique New York, unique New York, unique New York."

> "The sixth sheiks's sixth sheep's sick."

In the theater arts world, Edith Skinner's approach to articulatory clarity is familiar to many, with proponents advocating her approach and exercises for "good American speech." Others reject her teaching of optimum placement for the individual phonemes as too mechanical and too affected. Nevertheless, Skinner's text *Speak With Distinction* (1990) has a plethora of exercises geared for specific phonemic awareness and clarity.[31]

Ultimately, the patient should be aware of the importance of clear, energized consonants, focused vowels, and reduced phonatory effort. During singing and professional speaking, the consonants should be used as "springboards" for the vowels, taking advantage of the focused energy of well-placed articulatory resistance of consonants to reduce laryngeal effort. The importance of the patient understanding the effects of phonemic placement, such as incorporation of Y-buzz exercise into "thank you" and the focused resonance of the /n/ for "no," should not be dismissed in patients with laryngeal pathology.

Quality of Voice During Colloquial Mode

The voice trainer needs to assess vocal quality and tonal placement across modes of speech and singing, from professional to colloquial. Singers often disregard the need for excellent vocal quality and technique in simple songs and in hymns. They should be coached to use their best possible technique and artistry while singing these seemingly innocuous melodies.

The most common abuse of quality and tone focus in speech is during "filler words." Filler words are essentially the communication conjunctors used to indicate continued attention while listening. Although they may vary somewhat from speaker to speaker, the most common filler words are "um-hum," "okay," "yes," "no," "all right," and "sure." If the filler words are spoken abruptly, with little pitch change, or with passive vocal energy, there is greater demand on the source subsystem. If, in contrast, the filler words become a more conscious aspect of the patient's communicative style and are resonated and elongated with a slight melodic pattern, there is greater demand on the filter subsystem and a release of "work" (or tension) at the source (laryngeal) level. In essence, filler words act as a "reboot" for the voice throughout the day. Changing an automatic speech pattern (such as filler words) into a conscious vocal exercise also allows the patient to practice throughout the day on other people, thereby optimizing practice time by not having to create as much dedicated practice time per day. Another advantage to more fluid filler word production is the perception by the listener that the patient is more agreeable, more thoughtful, and in a better mood. Anecdotal studies on frequency of filler word use indicate an average of 200 per day. That could translate into 200 episodes of vocal abuse, or 200 episodes of well-directed vocal massage and vocal exercise.

Patients often reduce their prosodic variability in colloquial speech when they suspect they have injured their voices, or upon hearing a definitive diagnosis, fearing that vocal excursions might have a negative impact on vocal quality and healing. This is not true. Reduced prosody (change of pitch, loudness, rate, varied pause time) acts somewhat like repetitive motion injury to the larynx. Increased prosody, especially of pitch and loudness, allows vocal freedom (particularly of the cricothyroid muscle) and creates more natural speech (provided that the prosodic variability is not excessive) and provides a "vocal massage" throughout the day.

A helpful exercise for prosodic variability is the concept of "Text to song, song to speech." In this exercise, patients sing (not chant) an arbitrary melody (with changing rhythms) for the target text, and then speak the same text. Usually, the patient has greater vocal flexibility and greater access to resonance following this exploration. Another flexibility exercise is the "counting exercise." This exercise uses rote counting (1,2,3,4,5) beginning at medium pitch and is repeated at successively lower pitches, with the targeted pitch close to the sung pitch, with pitch inflections used for each spoken number (see Figure 32-14).

Vocal quality may be affected adversely by physical tensions and/or psychologic impediments, particularly in the injured voice. Perhaps the most familiar approach to balancing the forces of physical, psychologic, and textual demands for theater is that of Kristin Linklater.[32] Linklater's work focused on connecting sound to the breath, releasing the breath easily.

PSYCHOLOGICAL RAMIFICATIONS OF VOCAL DISORDER

The greatest obstacle patients have is a fear of loss of personal identity. Professional vocal athletes are by nature identified through their vocal attributes first. They are identified as "Judy, the singer" or "Mark, the tenor" or "John, the great actor." When a vocal problem arises, they may not be able to function in part (or whole) as the professional vocal athlete they perceive as their identity. This is particularly true if the vocal athlete requires phonosurgery. They fear temporary or permanent loss of range, quality, flexibility, sensation, or

laryngeal appearance. In essence, they have lost their trust of the voice. The voice care team must recognize these concerns.[33] Referral to a psychotherapist who specializes in performers may be necessary.

PSYCHOLOGIC AND PHYSIOLOGIC ISSUES OF STRESS

Performance anxiety is commonplace among performers and public speakers and is considered normal behavior in high-level performance. Performers with voice disorders can benefit from a team that includes professions for counseling, hypnotherapy, and other professional psychologic services. The voice specialist must handle referrals to other professionals through the referring physician in order to maintain integrity in the chain of referrals, avoid interfering inadvertently with medical care, and continue the successful team management process.

From the voice trainer's perspective, perhaps the most important strategy in stress reduction is attention to the interaction between the physiology of respiration and the psychology of stress. Public speakers tend to hold the breath while listening to a questioning reporter and then reply without refreshing the breath. Singers and actors may also fall into this trap, which can also increase laryngeal tension. The habit of holding one's breath is often seen prior to musical entrances or stage dialogue. Three deep breaths can make a significant difference in calming the nervous body and voice and preparing for efficient phonations physically and psychologically.

Physical exercise is a second important strategy in reducing overall stress. The choice of exercise should be carefully considered as the activity should reduce body tension and effort, rather than overindulgence in "strength training." Swimming, cross-country skiing, fencing, racquetball, and basketball are all good choices, depending on the needs and likes of the patient.

Meditative and hypnotic exercises are practiced regularly, either intentionally or unintentionally, by most great performers. Mesmerizing the audience with one's level of self occurs when techniques similar to those of meditation and self-hypnosis are implemented. Collecting energies and focusing concentration on the

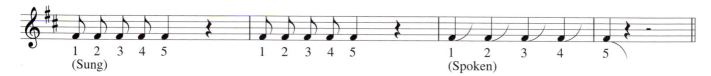

FIGURE 32-14. *"Counting exercise" using rote speech task with transition from singing mode to speech mode with pitch inflections for speech mode.*

ultimate goal allow confidence in performance. Just as an Olympic athlete practices visualization of success, these strategies, both physical and mental, can be valuable to the vocal athlete.

The excitement of performance releases adrenaline in the body. This sudden surge of adrenaline may be unnerving to the performer, but should be channeled into "directed energy" rather than masked with medications or alcohol. Although many performers request beta-blockers, this practice is usually not recommended. These medications usually lead to dull lackluster performances. The voice trainer must help the voice user learn to perform with confidence.

DESIGNING AN EXERCISE PROGRAM

Vocal exercises should be prescribed in an organized manner, with rationales and expected results (or gains) for each exercise. If the patient does not understand the specific need for an exercise, he/she may misjudge when to use the exercise, or may misjudge the production found during the exercise.

All patients should be able to demonstrate good posture and be able to execute a *messa di voce* that is based on filter contributions rather than overt source or power supply contributions. Exercises should be designed to bring the higher registers (falsetto, loft register) down to the lower register (modal/chest). Register integration and balanced resonance are essential for all voices and vocal styles.

Perhaps the single most important education for the patient with a voice disorder is vocal warm-up prior to heavy voice use (such as a rehearsal, conference meeting, social meeting, or concert), followed by a vocal cool-down immediately after the heavy voice use. Much of the work on exercise physiology as applied to voice is contained in a text by Saxon and Schneider *Vocal Exercise Physiology*,[34] and it is worth reading to understand the basics of exercise physiology (although they are not well tested on voice). Essentially, the vocalist must adequately prepare and readjust the body and the voice for marathon vocal control, quality, and endurance. Marathon runners would develop muscle spasms if they suddenly stopped at the finish line, but with continuation of ever-gentler activity, eventually slow walk, and finishing with stretches, the runner may avoid or reduce the possibility of injuries. The vocal warm-up consists of physical stretches, followed by specific exercises designed to optimize control and finesse of respiration, phonation, resonance, and articulation. Vocal exercises begin in midrange and gradually encompass the entire physiologic range. Exercises should be selected based on the needs of the voice that day, rather than a mechanical series of exercises.

A simple cool-down is the opposite of a warm-up and should proceed from the middle-high voice into the lower-middle voice. Descending scales, long, expressive tones, or a soulful expressive melody (humming "Amazing Grace," "Mary had a little lamb" or the Brahms "Lullaby") acts as a massage, encouraging blood circulation to the muscle of heavy use, evacuating lactic acid, and restoring oxygen debt incurred in anaerobic activity. After a strenuous performance or a difficult rehearsal, many performers instinctively want to be quiet or want to desist immediately from any vocal activity. Cool-down exercises are preferable. With use of vocal cool-down, the vocal muscles begin to recover and many vocalists report that their voice is more readily available the next day.

Many performers feel a sense of elation following a successful performance, and they often segue too soon into a party environment, carrying their elated and boisterous vocal tones with them. A few moments of descending hums (which can begin with the audience applause) to readjust the voice into a comfortably normal speech mode moderate the potential for injury at a noisy party or smoky restaurant.

In the development of an appropriate vocal exercise routine, simplicity is an important element. An exercise routine should take the typical injured voice user between 5 and 15 minutes and should not be excessively complex. In fact, a 5-minute routine of three simple exercises is often sufficient initially. This exercise routine should be accomplished in a program of 4 to 5 brief exercise sessions per day for optimal benefit.

It is vitally important that the issue of proper hydration during exercise be addressed simultaneously to avoid the effects of excessive friction on the vocal folds. Sipping room temperature water is recommended. Gulping large quantities of water (ie, a large glass) may exacerbate gastroesophageal reflux disease, especially when one is engaging in breathing and singing exercises. Moderation is recommended.

Physical Exercise

Overall body conditioning plays an important role in the rehabilitation of the voice. A healthy voice is usually accompanied by a healthy body. Aerobic exercise that is geared toward efficient use and coordination of muscles, without forceful or abrupt movements that could induce laryngeal tension (ie, avoiding a strenuous Valsalva maneuver) is recommended. Although some well-known singers are overweight, their success is from their efficiency of vocal production, despite the adverse effects their weight may have had on the body. Although an impressive masculine physique has launched more than a few careers, strenuous bodybuilding that includes serious weight lifting is discouraged. Exercises such as basketball, rowing, tennis, fencing, and swimming, which require upper body coordination without excess tension, are advocated.

Patients should be cautioned on their use of strenuously aerobic exercise when experiencing a cold or upper respiratory infection. Rapid, full inhalations which occur with physical exercise (and with the "panting exercise" above) increase exacerbation of infection, including increased risk for myocarditis.[35]

Issues of Chronologic Age

The effects of age and general body conditioning on the voice have been researched in depth by Chodzko-Zajko and Ringel[36] and Hollien[37], and more recently reviewed by Linville.[38] A body maintained in good physical condition facilitates a younger-sounding voice. Likewise, vocal muscles that are abused or misused for a long period of time tend to maintain those behavior patterns and make voices sound "old" prematurely. It was once felt that older voices wobble naturally. However, any voice, young or old, may wobble (or weaken) when there is inefficient connection of the respiratory, phonatory, resonatory, and articulatory subsystems. The majority of "wobbly old voices" respond with new youthful capabilities when effective coordination of the voice is reestablished.

Training of the voice can be undertaken at an early age with the understanding that the goals of training are to optimize the efficiency of the changing voice and reduce the vocal patterns of abuse and misuse often found in young speakers and singers. Many children enjoy the community involvement that participation in the theater affords. The projection of the young voice, however, may overdevelop the heavy (modal voice) mechanism to the detriment or total exclusion of the light (loft register) mechanism. Maintaining flexibility in vocal color, range, and dynamics has long been the goal of high-quality children's choral programs. It is strongly recommended that children who wish to excel in theater concurrently maintain their skills in choral ensemble singing. This helps avoid the habit of always singing too loudly (provided that the choral direction is appropriate). Likewise, extending the vocal fundamental frequency range should not be a primary goal with prepubescent or pubescent voices. If extension of the range of frequency and power is desired, it is best to wait until the effects of puberty have subsided. Efficient use of the entire vocal range is desirable for all ages.

HYDRATION

Dryness is an important issue in the continuing care of the voice. Simply drinking more water may be an important strategy in recovering from a voice disorder. The voice trainer may be helpful in educating the patient about issues which may adversely affect lubrication and, if necessary, bring them to the attention of the physician. Salivary flow is important: stimulating salivary flow with non-medicated lozenges, lemon drops, and so forth, is prudent. Drinking lemon juice or vinegar, however, may not be prudent especially in patients with GERD. Foods and drugs that induce dryness should be avoided when possible. The voice trainer should encourage the professional voice user to ask his/her laryngologist about medications, whether over-the-counter or prescription. Alcohol is a vasodilator; its consumption causes drying and reduces fine motor control and sensations of tension or pain from inappropriate or potentially damaging vocal behaviors. (For the same reason, any lozenge that anesthetizes the pain of a sore throat should be avoided.) Alcohol dulls the sensorium and should be avoided if professional voice use is scheduled. Many commercial (alcohol-based) mouthwashes also induce dryness. Another drying agent may be silica–based toothpaste, which can leave behind a microscopic silica gel (used as an abrasive to clean teeth). On days of performances, it may be more prudent for some singers or actors to brush with commercially available isotonic baking soda toothpaste. Microscopic food particles will continue to stimulate salivary flow, contributing to "moister" voice use. The voice trainer helps ensure that the patient is aware of the importance of these and other vocal hygiene and lifestyle issues.

On the topic of baking soda and salt, the author would be remiss not to mention Dr. Wilbur James Gould's non-medicated gargle recipe:

> 1/2 teaspoon salt
>
> 1/2 teaspoon baking soda
>
> 1/2 teaspoon corn syrup (Karo)
> (or honey or other syrup)
>
> 6 ounces of warm water
>
> Gargle quietly and gently for 2 long, boring minutes. Do not rinse.

Although there has been some discussion on the remotely abusive effects of gargling, if it is done quietly and conservatively, or if the mouth is simple rinsed thoroughly (without swallowing), this folk remedy is generally recommended as an adjunct for preserving (or reacquiring) the sensation of a moist, fresh voice.

To maintain the proper level of laryngeal lubrication, the voice user should remember the old adages of Van Lawrence.[39] "Keep moist," and "mucus is our friend." The kidneys are the body's "computers" for adjusting the level of systemic hydration. If more fluid is needed, the kidneys conserve water, causing urine to be darker. Clear urine indicates adequate levels of hydration. The amount of water necessary varies by the individual and environmental conditions. Drinking 1 ounce for every 2 pounds of body weight is recommended by some, while others recommend 8 to 10 glasses of water per day for adequate hydration. To avoid systemic dehydration, the voice user should drink enough water to "pee pale." Medications to assist in maintaining desirable lubrication may be helpful in some cases, as discussed elsewhere in this book.

The blanket of thin, runny mucus covering the entire mucous membrane is swept along by cilia (microscopic cytoplasmic hairs). Maintaining a high level of moist blanket keeps the mucus thin and runny. Failure of the mucus glands to secrete enough serous fluid results in a thicker blanket of mucus; secretions and foreign matter accumulate, and phlegm thickens. Further, in a performance situation, adrenaline attenuates the salivary flow in the mouth, thickening and decreasing the total fluid available in the vocal tract, and results in a failure to lubricate the vocal folds. The voice trainer helps ensure that the patient is aware of these normal phenomena and has effective coping strategies. In a performance the voice user can simply bite the tip of the tongue just to the point of pain, allowing an instantaneous flow of saliva in the oral cavity.

LIFESTYLE ISSUES FOR THE VOICE PATIENT

Being a professional voice user is comparable to being a violinist who carries a Stradivarius at all times. Everywhere a voice user goes, the instrument goes too. It is logical that voice conservation should be observed. The voice user should obviously avoid certain activities such as yelling at noisy sports events, speaking over noise at raucous nightclubs, and being in irritating, smoky environments. There are many other behaviors that a professional voice user may need to regard with care, including use of ingested substances.

LIFESTYLES AND LIFELONG VOCAL PREPAREDNESS

Poor technique is often blamed for vocal failures. Although poor technique is possible, especially when combined with other difficulties such as infection or injury, it is important not to discount the level of technique attained by many self-trained performers. Sound vocal training may be learned through formal or informal study. Although many acquire their muscle memory through formal training, others have stronger influence from performing experiences and mentors, and some are naturally good technicians. Singers such as Ella Fitzgerald and Mabel Mercer have developed incredibly complex and predictable vocal techniques based on years of experience and hard-learned lessons. Good vocal habits should be established early in the career, but when the voice continues to develop, a voice specialist can be a valuable helper for the predominantly self-trained voice. Although it is possible to develop a sound, reliable technique later in life, many patients fear that they will lose their vocal identity. They often do not understand that they will, instead, be expanding vocal skill while maintaining the critical personality aspects of their vocal style. Patient motivation is a key issue in adapting motor patterns and behavioral decisions. The assistance of an experienced voice specialist can be invaluable in dealing with the issues of compensation especially in light of moderate or major injuries. There is no substitute for someone else's experienced ears and eyes.

Each style of performance has its own demands. Technique is technique, however. Style is primarily an issue of interpretation. Although cross-specialization is possible among various vocal performance styles, it is not commonplace. A solid vocal technique and acting technique, however, can utilize the same sets of muscular strategies in the coordination of resonance, articulation, and respiration while reducing the risk to the phonatory mechanism. Healthy, efficient use of the voice is possible with all styles of voice use. People with certain vocal styles and occupations have traditionally had shorter careers. It is rare to see a commodities trader "in the pit" for more than a few years, primarily because of the extreme level of vocal misuse that pervades that industry. It may be rare to have the lead singer of a heavy metal band continue to heavily abuse the voice for more than a few years without noticeable vocal changes. It is not unusual for classical singers and classic actors to have significantly longer careers. This may be caused in part by the consistent reliance on skilled voice teachers, acting teachers, and coaches in that segment of the industry. Well-trained voice users usually take only well-calculated risks. They do not take extraordinary risks daily, and they tend to pamper their voices more than the untrained or nonprofessional voice user.

CANCELLATION OF APPEARANCES

When should a performance be canceled? If the voice user is technically strong enough to sing by sensation, not sound, it is generally safe to perform with those instructions after medical evaluation and clearance. The voice trainer can be invaluable in reconfirming vocal hygiene and ensuring good vocal technique. It is wise to note the admonition by Punt that performers should not "say an unnecessary word unless they are paid for it."[40] If there is a sudden and dramatic voice change, the performer should cancel, even if the voice change happens in the middle of the concert. Sudden voice change may indicate a hemorrhage or mucosal tear, and continued use of the voice may permanently impair normal healing of the membranes. The performer should seek an examination by a physician as soon as possible. Vocal trainers can help patients understand the importance of such precautions, and their professional acceptability.

If the performer's abdominal strength is compromised by illness or muscle cramping, the performer should not risk the voice. Inaccessibility of reliable, well-supported breath management imposes risks for vocal injury as support may be inadequate, and this may result in compensation by inappropriate muscles. When the performance is not critical, the performer should not risk the career. Judgment calls are never easy to make, however, and decisions should be made jointly by the patient, voice teacher/trainer, physician, and the performer's management. Officials who insist that the indisposed performer continue a performance obligation at the risk of permanent vocal injury should be advised that they must take responsibility for lifelong damage incurred because of their insistence.

AUDITORY FEEDBACK IN PERFORMANCE

Performing conditions and performance spaces vary considerably among the vocal arts forms. If microphones are used (which for singers—and ideally also for professional speakers—should always be a microphone designed for singing amplification rather than speech), the performer should be skilled in the proper use of the amplification system. Separate monitor speakers for the voice user are essential when amplification is used, particularly for singers. There are new in-the-ear monitors that are being used by nonclassical and classical performers in large theaters. They are individually molded and require supervision by an audiologist or otologist. They often require numerous readjustments to optimize function and preserve the hearing of the user. These monitors avoid the pitfalls of the monitor feedback squeal encountered in public address systems, but they are not foolproof. A backup monitor system must be available in the event of failure of the ear mold monitors.

Good hearing is as important as a good voice for the voice professional. The preservation of hearing is an important issue, especially with the commonplace use of portable stereos with headphones. Headphones allow a very high level of sound to be transmitted directly to the ear. Users typically listen to stereos, especially portable stereos and radios, at significantly higher levels of intensity than they realize. These higher levels may cause permanent hearing threshold changes. The Occupational Safety and Health Administration regulations state that prolonged exposure to noise (8 hours at 90 dBA) is unsafe and hearing protection is necessary.[41] The risk of temporary (and potentially permanent) hearing loss increases as intensity and duration increase. Hearing loss in singers and actors creates a special problem and may be the root of some inappropriate technical adjustments.

PARTNERSHIP OF THE VOICE SPECIALIST WITH THE SPEECH-LANGUAGE PATHOLOGIST

The voice specialist and speech-language pathologist share the common goal of optimizing vocal production but do so using different techniques. The experienced voice specialist has invaluable practical voice skills, as well as personal experience in professional voice use. The speech-language pathologist has stronger scientific and medically related training for speech and language development and disorders, but typically has only rudimentary to intermediate training in voice. Speech therapy focuses on maximizing efficiency of the colloquial speaking voice. Specialized voice training maintains a higher level of overall skill of vocal efficiency throughout the entire physiologic fundamental frequency range of phonation and critically examines the choices for transmitting that phonation in a variety of acoustic environments. Terminology may differ between the two specialties. Training methods to achieve vocal efficiency may differ. Although some voice specialists tend to stay "married" to one intervention method, the more successful approach is generally eclectic in nature, designed specifically for the individual patient. This is important because of the muscle memory patterns for each individual.

Traditional speech therapy addresses adjustments in behavior (such as yelling, level of hydration), then breath management, easy vocal onset, awareness of resonance, and connected speech patterns. Optimizing oral-nasal resonance is typically done by the voice specialist. Attention to habitual, abusive speech patterns (including excessive throat clearing and harsh glottal onsets) and language disorders is the primary province of a speech-language pathologist. In behavior modification, any addictive trait is given a substitute rather than an admonition of restraint. Whereas much of the literature in speech-language pathology recommends telling the patient, "Don't yell," the voice specialist teaches the voice user to substitute a rather high energy sound production that is based on elongation of the sound (gentle "calling"). Although earlier speech-language pathology texts reported singing (and acting) as "abusive," efficient vocalization is not abusive. The voice specialist and speech-language pathologist can work together very effectively as a team.

Locating a voice specialist can sometimes be problematic. In the past, many voice teachers and theater coaches were reluctant to collaborate with a medical team on the care of injured voices. Excellent voice teachers and theater coaches are highly skillful in detecting inefficient breath patterns, poor resonance choices, and instances of vocal strain. These professionals are excellent candidates for clinical training as voice specialists and, if they can afford the time for completing additional graduate education in speech-language pathology, to become vocologists. Advanced study in speech-language pathology and the resulting certification (CCC/SLP) are advocated and would enable those individuals to practice privately in the area of voice therapy as well as maintain their private voice training studios. Voice specialists who do not hold licensure (and in most states the Certificate of Clinical Competence from the American Speech-Language-Hearing Association) can participate in the rehabilitation process (generally as a speech aide) under the direct supervision of a physician or licensed speech-language pathologist, but cannot legally provide voice therapy independently.

Voice trainers who specialize in singing may be found in the community, or through local and national singing teacher associations (such as the National Association of Teachers of Singing). The New York Singing Teachers Association (which was a parent organization for the National Association of Teachers of Singing) is currently developing a program for certification of voice teachers, testing their knowledge base in a variety of areas, including medical/therapeutic management. Voice trainers who specialize in acting voice may be located through local colleges, community theaters, or through the national organization Voice and Speech Trainers Association (VASTA). Speech-language pathologists who specialize in voice disorders may be found by contacting the American Speech, Language and Hearing Association (ASHA). ASHA has a variety of subspecialty divisions members may join, with voice (Special Interest Division 3) as one of the specialty areas.

Perhaps the most compelling rationale for use of specialized voice exercises as adjuncts to more traditional voice therapy exercises is access to a mode of phonation (singing or elocutionary speech) which may not have as many compensatory behaviors established, and the development of higher skill level (singing and elocutionary voice/acting voice) for lesser demanding tasks (colloquial speech).

SUMMARY

Vocal rehabilitation is a simple yet complex process. It is simple in that it requires basic coordination of three main subsystems: respiration, source, and filter. Yet it is complex because of the many factors influencing the efficiency of each of those subsystems, particularly in the voice professional. A vocal disorder rarely emerges or resolves because of one facet of vocal production. The many nuances of phonatory control and compensation are best addressed through a combination of traditional and specialized therapy. Because singing and professional speaking require greater control of the nuances of vocal quality and coordination across subsystems, it is logical to use select vocal exercises to improve vocal control and assist in resolution of the pathology. The voice specialist, with his/her additional training and experience in vocal production, is an invaluable asset to the voice care team.

FOR FURTHER INFORMATION, CONTACT:

The Voice Foundation: 1721 Pine Street, Philadelphia, PA, 19103 USA. [www.voicefoundation.org]

The New York Singing Teachers Association: c/o Janet Pranschke, 153 Johnson Avenue, Staten Island, NY 10307, USA. [www.nyst.org]

The National Association of Teachers of Singing: 2800 University Blvd North, JU Station, Jacksonville, FL 32211, USA. [www.nats.org]

Voice and Speech Trainers Association: c/o Lisa Wilson, 1535 S. Florence Avenue, Tulsa, OK 74104, USA. [www.VASTA.org]

National Center for Voice and Speech: c/o Ingo R. Titze, Ph.D., Department of Speech Pathology and Audiology, The University of Iowa, Iowa City, IA 52242 [www.ncvs.org]

American Speech-Language-Hearing Association: 10801 Rockville Pike, Rockville, MD 20852, USA. [www.asha.org]

REFERENCES

1. Carroll LM: Application of singing techniques for the treatment of dysphonia. In: Rosen C, Murray T, eds. *Otolaryngologic Clinics of North America: Voice Disorders and Phonosurgery II*. Philadelphia, PA: WB Saunders Co; 2000.

2. Benninger MS, Jacobson BH, Johnson AF. *Vocal Arts Medicine: The Care and Prevention of Professional Voice Disorders*. New York, NY: Thieme Medical Publishers; 1994.

3. Peacher G. H*ow to Improve Your Speaking Voice.* New York, NY: Fell Publishers; 1966.

4. Riley WD, Carroll LM. The role of the singing-voice specialist in non-medical management of benign voice disorders. In: Rubin JS, Sataloff RT, Korovin GS, Gould WJ, eds. *Diagnosis and Treatment of Voice Disorders*. New York, NY: Igaku-Shoin; 1995:405-423.

5. Sataloff RT. *Professional Voice: The Science and Art of Clinical Care*. 1st ed. New York, NY: Raven Press; 1991.

6. Sataloff RT. Training teachers to work with injured voices. *NATS J.* 1992;49(1):2-26.

7. Sataloff RT. *Professional Voice: The Science and Art of Clinical Care*. 2nd ed. San Diego, CA: Singular Publishing Group; 1997.

8. Sataloff RT. *Vocal Health and Pedagogy*. San Diego, CA: Singular Publishing Group; 1998.

9. Brodnitz FS. *Vocal Rehabilitation: A Manual*. Rochester, MN: American Academy of Ophthalmology and Otolaryngology;1971.

10. Gould WJ, Sataloff RT, Spiegel JR. *Voice Surgery*. St. Louis, MO: Mosby; 1993.

11. Lawrence V. Singers and surgery. Part II; Vocal tract surgery. *NATS Bull.* 1982;38(5):20-21.

12. Spiegel JR, Sataloff RT, Hawkshaw MJ. Surgery for the voice. *NATS J.* 1990;46(5):28-30.

13. Riley WD, Korovin GS, Gould WJ. Directed energy in vocal technique: a preliminary study of clinical application. Presented at: The Voice Foundation Symposium: Care of the Professional Voice; 1990; Philadelphia, PA.

14. Hirano M. *Clinical Examination of Voice*. New York, NY: Springer-Verlag; 1981.

15. Prater RJ, Swift RW. *Manual of Voice Therapy*. Boston, MA: Little, Brown & Co; 1984.

16. Culver CA. *Musical Acoustics*. New York, NY: Blakiston; 1951.

17. Titze IR. *Principles of Voice Production*. Englewood Cliffs, NJ: Prentice-Hall; 1994.

18. Hollien H, Dew D, Philips P. Phonational frequency range of adults. *J Speech Hear Res.* 1971;14: 755-760.

19. Coleman RF. Sources of variation in phonetograms. *J Voice.* 1993;7(1):1-14.

20. Schute HK, Seidner W. Recommendations by the Union of European Phoniatricians (UEP): standardizing voice area measurement/phonetography. *Folia Phoniatr.* 1983;35:286-288.

21. Kent RD. *Reference Manual for Communicative Sciences and Disorders*. Austin, TX: Pro-Ed; 1994.

22. Winholtz WS, Ramig LO. Vocal tremor analysis with the vocal demodulator. *J Speech Hear Res.* 1992;35(3):562-573.

23. Feldenkrais M. *Body and Mature Behavior*. New York, NY: International University; 1949.

24. Alexander FM. *The Use of Self*. London, England: Methuen; 1932.

25. Reed CM, Rabinowitz WM, Durlach NI, et al. Research on the Tadoma method of speech communication. *J Acoust Soc.* 1985;77:247-257.

26. Leanderson R, Sundberg J, von Euler C. Role of diaphragmatic activity during singing: a study of transdiaphragmatic pressures. *J App Physiol.* 1987;62:259-270.

27. Sundberg J. Breathing behavior during singing. *NATS J.* 1993;January/February, 4-9:49-51.

28. Titze IR, Solomon NP, Luschei ES, et al. Interference between normal vibrato and artificial stimulation of laryngeal muscles at near-vibrato rates. *J Voice.* 1994;8(3):215-223,.

29. Lessac A. *The Use and Training of the Human Voice*. 3rd ed. Mountain View, CA: Mayfield Publishing Co; 1977:122-159.

30. Carroll LM. Interaction of laryngeal and velopharyngeal mechanics: a look at resonance in singers. Presented at: American Speech-Language-Hearing Association Annual Convention; 1999; San Francisco, CA.

31. Skinner E. *Speak with Distinction*. New York, NY: Applause Theatre Book Publishers; 1990.

32. Linklater K. *Freeing the Natural Voice*. New York, NY: Drama Book Publishers; 1976.

33. Rosen DC, Sataloff RT. *Psychology of Voice Disorders*. San Diego, CA: Singular Publishing Group; 1997.

34. Saxon KG, Schneider CM. *Vocal Exercise Physiology.* San Diego, CA: Singular Publishing Group; 1995.

35. Friman G, Ilback NG. Acute infection: metabolic responses, effects on performance, interaction with exercise, and myocarditis. *Int J Sports Med.* 1998;19(suppl 3):S172-S182.

36. Chodzko-Zajko WJ, Ringel RL. Physiological aspects of aging. *J Voice.* 1987;1(1):18-26.

37. Hollien H. "Old voice": what do we really know about them? *J Voice.* 1987;1(1):2-17.

38. Linville SE. The sound of senescence. *J Voice.* 1996;10(2):190-200.

39. Sataloff RT, Titze IR. V*ocal Health and Science: A Compilation of Articles for the NATS Bulletin and the NATS Journal.* Jacksonville, FL: The National Association of Teachers of Singing; 1991.

40. Punt NA. Applied laryngology—singers and actors. *Proc R Soc Med.* 1968;61:1152-1156.

41. Sataloff RT, Sataloff J. *Occupational Hearing Loss.* New York, NY: Marcel Dekker, Inc; 1987.

CHAPTER 33

Laryngeal Manipulation

Jacob Lieberman, DO, MA

John S. Rubin, MD, FACS, FRCS

Thomas M. Harris, FRCS

Adrian Fourcin, PhD

This chapter, written by an osteopath, two laryngologists, and a speech scientist, is on manipulation of the larynx and the perilaryngeal structures. This is a young science, perhaps still more of an art than a science, but which takes as its predecessors, principles from anatomy, physiology, osteopathy, and physical therapy. In this chapter we present a synopsis of the role that laryngeal manipulation plays in our clinical practice. Concepts presented in this chapter are fresh and still undergoing change. Many come out of an ongoing collaboration with the Sidcup Voice Unit.

Certain aspects of manipulation, for example, side-to-side movement of the larynx, have been used by physicians as a part of the routine clinical examination for well over a century, and by performers for centuries. One or two quick side-to-side movements of the larynx to help relax the larynx are part of many performers' routine preparations.

Recently, manipulation of the larynx has been reported on by practitioners as one form of treatment in patients presenting with functional voice disorders,[1-7] and more generally in patients with muscular tension dysphonia (Murray Morrison, Instructional Course, Annual Meeting of the American Academy of Otolaryngology Head and Neck Surgery, September 1999; Murray Morrison, Laryngology Research meeting, AAOHNS annual meeting, San Antonio 1998; John Rubin, Laryngology Research meeting, AAOHNS annual meeting, San Antonio 1998).

Currently, the core team of the voice clinic at Sidcup consists of laryngologist(s), speech and language pathologist(s), an osteopath, and a singing teacher. The osteopath is also a certified child, family, and adolescent psychodynamic psychotherapist; similarly, the speech and language pathologist has taken extra training in counseling. There is also immediate access to a psychiatrist, other singing teachers, and coaches.

The role of the osteopath is to examine the relationship of posture, breathing mechanics, and the function of the larynx to voice production. In the Sidcup clinic the osteopath is frequently called upon to assist in the diagnosis, as well as to assist at an early stage in the rehabilitative management (Table 33-1).

In this chapter we discuss laryngeal manipulation from an osteopathic perspective. Anatomy and physiology, indications for manipulation, the osteopathic examination, tenets of basic manipulation and advanced manipulation, treatment outcomes, and our current hypotheses for the underlying mechanisms involved are presented.

BIOMECHANICS OF THE LARYNX

The larynx is a complex structure consisting of cartilages, muscles, ligaments, joints, and mucous membranes, all interacting in highly precise and timed functions, that is, synergetically. Given the sphincteric nature of laryngeal closure, it is our view that it is over-

Assessment of Posture and Laryngeal Apparatus (Joints and Muscles) in Hyperfunctional Dysphonia

This protocol is a nonexhaustive reference for the assessment of posture and the laryngeal apparatus. It is designed to accompany the instructional course on the detailed anatomy of the larynx, its palpatory assessment, and the assessment of posture-related aspects of voice dysfunction. It can be used in multidisciplinary voice clinics as part of the overall assessment of voice patients to provide a framework for practitioner agreement and research.

1.   POSTURE and LARYNGEAL ACTIVITY

1.1   OBSERVATIONS:

Sitting: (while patient is providing history):   (tick as appropriate)

Anterior neck compartment:

Observation				
Signs of increased muscular activity:	Smooth		Conspicuous Rt	Conspicuous Lt
Static (patient is silent)	Normal	High	Low	Deviated
Level and position of thyroid lamina				
Bulging omohoid muscle activity in speech	Dynamic (talking)	Absent	Present Rt	Present Lt
Skin crease asymmetry		Absent	Present Rt	Present Lt
Head position in the sagittal plane	Tilt	Absent	Present Rt	Present Lt
Head gestures (head nodding in speech/swallowing)		Absent	Present Rt	Present Lt
Jaw movement (vertical and lateral plane)*	Asymmetric	Absent	Present Rt	Present Lt

Standing: (lateral view):   (tick as appropriate)

1.1.2

Weight bearing (sagittal plane, observed from the side):	Normal	Anterior sway	Posterior sway

TABLE 33-1. *Lieberman's Protocol (Revised)(Reproduced with permission from Lieberman J. Principles and techniques of manual therapy. In: Harris T, Harris S, Rubin JS, Howard DM, eds. The Voice Clinic Handbook. Whurr Medical Publishers, London, 1998, appendices 6.1 and 6.2: 132-137.)*

		Normal		
Spinal curve (exaggerated: hyper-hypolordosis):	Lumbar	Normal lordosis	Decreased lordosis	Increased lordosis
	Thoracic	Normal kyphosis	Decreased kyphosis	Increased kyphosis
	Cervical	Normal lordosis	Decreased lordosis	Increased lordosis
Rib cage:	Flexibility	Normal	Decreased	
	Function	Normal	Raised	Held
Breathing patterns:	Diaphragmatic	Normal	Decreased	Paradoxical
	Upper chest	Absent	Present	Increased
	Clavicular	Absent	Present	Increased
Head position (cervical translation):	Anterior	Absent	Present	
	Cervical thoracic hump	Absent	Present	Cervical level

1.1.3   Spinal Curves

Standing: (anterior/posterior view):

	Normal		
Lumbar-thoracic (including scoliosis)	Normal	Asymmetry Rt	Asymmetry Lt
Scapular level	Normal	Raised Rt	Raised Lt
Head level	Normal	Tilt Rt	Tilt Lt

1.1.4   Spinal Curves

Standing: (vertical axis):

NOTE: the normal larynx moves with the torso

	Normal		
Torso rotation	Normal	Clockwise	Counterclockwise
Pelvis rotation	Normal	Clockwise	Counterclockwise

TABLE 33-1. *Lieberman's Protocol (Revised) (Reproduced with permission from Lieberman J. Principles and techniques of manual therapy. In: Harris T, Harris S, Rubin JS, Howard DM, eds. The Voice Clinic Handbook. Whurr Medical Publishers, London, 1998, appendices 6.1 and 6.2: 132-137.)*

	Head rotation	Normal	Clockwise	Counterclockwise
2.1 PALPATION:	(tick as appropriate)			
Cervical spinous processes:	Palpable	No	Yes	Cervical level
Suboccipital musculature (above C2):	Tonus	Normal	Increased Rt	Increased Lt
	Symmetry	Normal	Increased Rt	Increased Lt
	Tenderness	No	Increased Rt	Increased Lt
Cervical musculature (other):	Tonus	Normal	Increased Rt	Increased Lt
	Symmetry	Normal	Increased Rt	Increased Lt
	Tenderness	No	Increased Rt	Increased Lt
TMJ:	Movement	Normal	Asymmetry Rt	Asymmetry Lt
	Opening	Normal	Asymmetry Rt	Asymmetry Lt
	Tenderness	No	Increased Rt	Increased Lt
Sternocleidomastoid muscle:	Tonus	Normal	Increased Rt	Increased Lt
	Symmetry	Normal	Increased Rt	Increased Lt
	Tenderness	No	Increased Rt	Increased Lt
3.1 The LARYNGEAL APPARATUS:	(tick as appropriate)			
OBSERVATION:				
Superior suspensory muscles	Tone	Normal	Low	High

TABLE 33-1. *Lieberman's Protocol (Revised)(Reproduced with permission from Lieberman J. Principles and techniques of manual therapy. In: Harris T, Harris S, Rubin JS, Howard DM, eds. The Voice Clinic Handbook. Whurr Medical Publishers, London, 1998, appendices 6.1 and 6.2: 132-137.)*

	Normal	Increased	Decreased
Laryngeal range of movement (in speech and swallowing):	Normal	Increased	Decreased
Inferior suspensory muscles: Tone	Normal	Asymmetric Rt	Asymmetric Lt
4.1 The LARYNGEAL APPARATUS: PALPATION (tick as appropriate)			
Palpate for position, tone, symmetry, tenderness both in static (passive) and dynamic (swallowing, speech singing):			
Hyoid	Normal	High	Low
Geniohyoid: static — Tone	Normal	Asymmetric	Asymmetric
Tenderness:	None	Present	
Geniohyoid: dynamic	Normal	Asymmetric	
Superior suspensory muscles: static — Tone	Normal	Asymmetric Rt	Asymmetric Lt
Tenderness:	None	Rt	Lt
Superior suspensory muscles: dynamic	Normal	Asymmetric Rt	Asymmetric Lt
Inferior suspensory muscles: static — Tone	Normal	Asymmetric Rt	Asymmetric Lt
Tenderness:	None	Rt	Lt
Inferior suspensory muscles: dynamic	Normal	Asymmetric Rt	Asymmetric Lt
Thyrohyoid apparatus: static — Coronal: attitude hyoid to thyroid	Parallel	Tilt Lt	Tilt Rt
Size of gap:	None	Diminished Rt	Diminished Lt
Tenderness:	None	Rt	Lt
Symmetry:	Normal	Asymmetric Rt	Asymmetric Lt
Thyrohyoid apparatus: dynamic (movement)	Normal	Rotation Rt	Rotation Lt

TABLE 33-1. *Lieberman's Protocol (Revised) (Reproduced with permission from Lieberman J. Principles and techniques of manual therapy. In: Harris T, Harris S, Rubin JS, Howard DM, eds. The Voice Clinic Handbook. Whurr Medical Publishers, London, 1998, appendices 6.1 and 6.2: 132-137.)*

Cricothyroid muscles: static			
Tone	Normal	Asymmetric Rt	Asymmetric Lt
Tenderness:	None	Rt	Lt
Cricothyroid visor (joint) (head neutral): static			
Resting state:	Closed	Mid position open	Open
Cricothyroid joint: dynamic			
Anterior arch:	None	Present	
Changes with siren:	No change	Closes	
Changes with yawn:	No change	Opens	
Posterior glide of arch with pitch rise:	No change	Diminishes	
Constrictor muscles: (perform lateral shift test):			
Mobility:	Absent	Present Rt	Present Lt
Tenderness:	None	Asymmetric Rt	Asymmetric Lt
Internal laryngeal structures (for experienced therapists only):			
Accessible:	No	Rt	Lt
Tenderness:	None	Rt	Lt
Movement:	None	Rt	Lt

TABLE 33-1. *Lieberman's Protocol (Revised)(Reproduced with permission from Lieberman J. Principles and techniques of manual therapy. In: Harris T, Harris S, Rubin JS, Howard DM, eds. The Voice Clinic Handbook. Whurr Medical Publishers, London, 1998, appendices 6.1 and 6.2: 132-137.)*

ly simplistic to argue that any given phonatory behavior occurs on the basis of a single muscular activity. The relative pull of each muscle is balanced by the activities of other muscles. The overall vectors of pull and joint axes determine the actual position of the arytenoids and, hence, of the vocal folds.[8] This is particularly apt when discussing the various muscles (interarytenoid, lateral cricoarytenoid, and so forth), which have direct attachment to the muscular process of the arytenoid cartilages and are involved in medial positioning of the vocal fold.

Furthermore, the larynx is suspended from the basicranium, not by direct bony attachment, but by a series of muscular and ligamentous attachments. If posture could, in one sense, be considered to be a constant battleground, balancing activity between the deep extensor and flexor groups of muscles, then the larynx could be viewed as a potential victim in this struggle, in part because of its location in the anterior neck, in part by its dense muscular attachments to the prevertebral fascia, and in part because of its attachments to the basicranium above and the trachea below.

The larynx can be considered to be an "intrusion" into the pharynx. Its major role is that of airway protection, and this is critical to life itself. The larynx protects the lower airway biomechanically both by creating a diversion for the food particles around the endolarynx and by closing sphincterically and moving in an upward and forward fashion with each swallow.

Another critical role is pressure-valving. Pressure-valving prevents ingress or egress of air and allows sudden increases in intrathoracic and intra-abdominal pressures to occur. This permits activities such as coughing, defecation, and weight-lifting.[9]

Phonation has been considered as a more recent activity and has been related to the lowering of the larynx from the basicranium.[10] Scherer has noted that phonation only occurs in a narrow range of overall vocal fold movement, approximately 10-15% that brings the vocal folds nearest to one another.[11]

Hast published his study on the physiology of the cricothyroid muscle over 30 years ago,[12] yet biomechanics of the larynx remain poorly understood. That said, investigators have correlated laryngeal injury with inefficient or abnormal laryngeal function or have identified vocal improvement through reduction in mechanical strain via voice therapy or other techniques.[12-15]

More specific techniques involving manual circumlaryngeal therapy have been espoused for such conditions as functional dysphonia[1-4] and more generally for hyperfunctional conditions (Murray Morrison, Instructional Course, Annual Meeting of the American Academy of Otolaryngology Head and Neck Surgery, September

1999; Murray Morrison, Laryngology Research meeting, AAOHNS annual meeting, San Antonio 1998; John Rubin, Laryngology Research meeting, AAOHNS annual meeting, San Antonio 1998).

Much further investigation is needed, emphasizing the development of methods to recognize and quantify biomechanical dysfunction and restoration.[15] For the physical therapist who is attempting to improve muscular or joint efficiency or position and thereby improve the voice, the entire vocal tract needs to be considered. This should include the deep and superficial postural muscles as well as the muscles, joints, and ligaments directly related to the sound source. In that regard, the importance of posture has been identified by individuals such as Alexander, Pilates, Feldenkrais, Rolf, and others.[16-19] While physical therapy has become integrated into rehabilitation of sports injuries, it is only recently that these fields have been applied to voice research or rehabilitation.

LARYNGEAL JOINTS

There are two pairs of joints of particular importance to the position and configuration of the vocal folds, the cricothyroid and the cricoarytenoid.

The Cricothyroid Joint

The cricothyroid joint is a synovial joint that consists of a circular facet on the medial aspect of the inferior horn of the thyroid cartilage, articulating with an articular facet on the side of the lamina of the cricoid. This articular facet lies at the junction of the arch and the body of the cricoid, and faces in a dorsolateral and superior manner. Of note, the two cricoid facets are often asymmetric.[20] The joint is stabilized by its capsule as well as by a posterior and a lateral ligament. The posterior ligament is said to control movement of the inferior horn of the thyroid, while the lateral ligament limits posterior displacement of the thyroid, with respect to the cricoid.[21]

The cricothyroid joint is considered by Lieberman to be a key element in the tensioning mechanism of the vocal ligament.[14,22] The radiating fibers that moor the lower horn of the thyroid to the cricoid permit rotation about a (predominantly) transverse axis, and allow it to "rotate up and down like the visor of a helmet."[21,p.699] This is turn leads, indirectly, to stretching and tightening of the vocal ligament with a corresponding increase in fundamental frequency of the voice. In a study of fresh cadavers, this was found to correspond to a stretch of 25% in the length of the vocal ligament.[20,23]

Lieberman and Harris[8] (Jacob Lieberman, unpublished data, 2000) have also identified, through palpation, some movement of the cricoid in an anterior-posterior (A-P) direction in relation to the thyroid during phonation. This movement has also been identified by Boileau Grant.[21] By pulling the thyroid cartilage anteriorly with respect to the cricoid cartilage, such movement increases tension in the vocal ligament. It lacks the mechanical advantage that the lever mechanism provides through rotation about the cricothyroid joint, however (Tom Harris, personal observation, 2002).

A-P movement in the cricothyroid joint is observed in many young female singers who perform in musical theatre. It is worth noting that the dorso-lateral orientation of the facets is designed to stop such a movement. It is therefore quite possible that the flexibility of the inferior horns of the thyroid cartilage, as well as stretched ligament, allow such a movement to take place. While such A-P movement seems to increase the vocal range, for instance in belting, it may also render the joint to be less stable.

The Cricoarytenoid Joint

The cricoarytenoid is a synovial joint of the saddle type. Each arytenoid has a deeply grooved base with a facet that articulates with an elliptical joint facet in the posterior aspect of the upper cricoid. Each cricoid facet is a raised structure, convexly curved and measuring approximately 6 mm along its major, longitudinal axis. This axis runs as (very nearly) an arc with its center based at the anterior commissure along the posterior, lateral, and superior margin of the cricoid cartilage. As this axis exceeds the transverse diameter of the corresponding arytenoid articular surface, a degree (only a few millimeters) of sliding along the axis is made possible.[9,15,21,23,24] It may be utilized during forceful laryngeal closure.

The primary motion, however, is forward and backward gliding along the minor axis of the cricoid facet[23,24] (or looked at from a different perspective, revolving about the long axis [Tom Harris, personal observation, 2002]). This bidirectional movement results in changes not only anterior and posterior, but also vertical, because of the oblique setting of the long axis. It resembles the movement of a rocking chair, thus "rocking" is a common description. "Rotation" is also described, but by and large ignores the vertical displacement, which is significant. Letson notes that for each "unit" of vertical displacement, there are two units of medial-lateral displacement.[24]

To summarize, arytenoid motion occurs in three directions. Anterior and posterior movements and vertical movements are caused by "revolving" or "pitch-like" motion along the minor axis of the cricoid. The medial and lateral motion is determined by the orientation of the cricoarytenoid facet. During adduction, the outward angulation of the vocal process away from the body of the arytenoid permits the length of the vocal process to approximate at the proper vertical height.[24-26]

LIGAMENTS OF THE CRICOARYTENOID JOINT

There are a fibrous articular capsule and two ligaments that stabilize and limit movement of the cricoarytenoid joint. The posterior cricoarytenoid ligament attaches to the superior rim of the cricoid lamina between the two cricoarytenoid facets, and extends anteriorly to the medial surface of the arytenoid cartilage.[20,23] Together with the articular capsule, its primary function is, most likely, prevention of lateral dislocation of the arytenoid on forced abduction of the vocal folds.[20,23]

The anterior ligament of the cricoarytenoid joint is the vocal ligament.[23] It extends from the vocal process of the arytenoid and then condenses to form Broyle's ligament and insert into the thyroid cartilage just inferior to the thyro-epiglottic ligament. It stabilizes the arytenoid and maintains the positional integrity of the true vocal fold, thereby allowing the vocal fold to be acted upon by the intrinsic laryngeal muscles.

The vocal ligament forms the upper border of the triangular membrane (also known as the cricothyroid ligament and the conus elasticus). This membrane attaches below to the whole length of the upper border of the arch of the cricoid; in front it blends into the median cricothyroid ligament. After curving medial to the lower border of the thyroid cartilage it ends above in the free upper border, the vocal ligament.[9,21,23]

The quadrangular membrane is a fibroelastic sheath, more delicate than the cricothyroid ligament. It extends bilaterally from either side of the epiglottis and curves backward to the lateral border of the arytenoid cartilage. Its free upper edge condenses slightly to form the aryepiglottic ligament. Its free lower border condenses to form the vestibular ligament, the basis of the false vocal fold.

INTRINSIC AND EXTRINSIC LARYNGEAL MUSCLES

From the standpoint of manipulation of the larynx, it is helpful to think in terms of groups of muscles, phonatory function, and overall activity. The laryngeal muscles are definable in this manner. Useful groupings include:

1. "Special muscles" of phonation: the thyroarytenoid and cricothyroid;

2. Intrinsic muscles that insert into the epiglottis and/or quadrangular membrane;

3. Intrinsic muscles that insert into the muscular process of the arytenoids;

4. Extrinsic muscles that elevate the larynx: the suprahyoid suspensory group;

5. Extrinsic muscles that depress the larynx: the infrahyoid suspensory group;

6. The constrictor muscles which elevate and pull the larynx backward against the deep cervical fascia and the cervical spine.

Special Phonatory Muscles

The *vocalis muscle* is the medial body of the thyroarytenoid muscle. It travels in an anterior-posterior (AP) fashion with the vocal ligament forming the substance of the true vocal fold. Contraction of the vocalis causes bulking and shortening of the free edge of the vocal fold and stiffening of the muscle. It acts to help control pitch production, thereby causing lowering of the fundamental frequency, at least during soft phonation.[9,27-31] While it is not possible to access this muscle digitally, it can be manipulated through the articulation of the cricothyroid joint.

The *cricothyroid muscle* is readily accessible to manipulation. Although often considered to be an intrinsic laryngeal muscle because of its impact upon pitch, the cricothyroid is really an extrinsic laryngeal muscle. Unlike the other intrinsic laryngeal muscles (innervated by the recurrent laryngeal nerve) its innervation is from the external branch of the superior laryngeal nerve. The cricothyroid originates on the anterior surface of the arch of the cricoid. It divides into two parts, the pars recta (anterior or oblique part) that passes upwards to the ala of the thyroid, and the pars oblique (posterior or horizontal part) that passes more outward to the inferior cornu of the thyroid. Contraction, particularly of its vertical belly, causes increased tension and stretch on the vocal ligament, thereby affecting pitch.[32-34] The oblique part of the cricothyroid muscle is probably responsible for the AP movement described above.

Harris and Lieberman have named the opening and closing action of the cricothyroid joint on the anterior thyroid and cricoid cartilages the "cricothyroid visor."[8,14] The resting state, and contraction, of the cricothyroid muscle has a marked impact on the "cricothyroid visor," and is believed by them to be significant in voice production. Furthermore, they postulate that abnormal patterns of muscular activity can occur in the cricothyroid muscle and in the "visor" mechanism leading to voice problems, and that manipulation of this muscle and joint can markedly improve these problems.[8,14]

Intrinsic Muscles That Insert Into the Epiglottis and/or Quadrangular Membrane

Intrinsic muscles that insert into the quadrangular membrane are recognizable by having the name "epiglottis" as part of their title: for example, aryepiglotticus. Such muscles have as one of their actions the drawing down of the epiglottic cartilage over the larynx. They work as part of the swallowing mechanism, helping to protect the endolarynx from food particles. They act in synchrony, one with another, in a vegetative fashion under reflexogenic control.[35,36]

It is unclear if these muscles participate significantly in patterns of voicing or voice disorders. Estill has postulated that one vocal quality, "twang," may be associated with constriction of the epiglottis in association with aryepiglottic contraction.[37] More research is required to confirm these suggestions. While these muscles are difficult to access via basic laryngeal manipulation, it appears that they relax subsequent to general relaxation of the laryngeal musculature.

Intrinsic Muscles That Insert Into the Muscular Process of the Arytenoids

Muscles that insert into the muscular process of the arytenoid cartilage (and thereby have "arytenoid" as part of their name) are invariably linked to movement and/or tensioning of the true vocal fold. All these muscles are true intrinsic laryngeal muscles and are innervated by the recurrent laryngeal nerve.

During swallowing the true vocal folds are brought and held tightly together by several of these muscles acting in synchrony. The posterior cricoarytenoid has been generally posited to be the one intrinsic laryngeal muscle that causes the vocal folds to abduct. That said, it is clear that the laryngeal intrinsic muscles do not act in a vacuum. There are patterns of muscular movements that bring the vocal folds to the desired position or level of stretch or tension (and we postulate that the vector for maximum abduction involves the lateral cricoarytenoid as well as the posterior cricoarytenoid[8]).

These muscles are accessible to the experienced practitioner in laryngeal manipulation. However, it is rarely appropriate to manipulate them directly as they are so intricately linked to fundamental reflexogenic activities. Attempts at such manipulation, unless the patient is adequately prepared, are likely to lead to throat discomfort, and are not recommended for the beginner.

Extrinsic Muscles That Elevate the Larynx: the Suprahyoid Suspensory Group

The suprahyoid suspensory muscle group are powerful muscles that play an important role in the act of swallowing. These muscles extend upward from the hyoid bone into the base of the tongue, and skull base. It is not at all uncommon for patients to present to the voice clinic with a "raised" larynx, and "held" suprahyoid musculature. There are many potential reasons for this to occur.

From a physiologic perspective, one understandable cause is as follows: muscular imbalances between the deep flexors and the deep extensors of the neck are commonplace, with the almost inevitable outcome being the deep extensors "triumphing." The end result of this (and associated muscular imbalances) is recognizable to all of us: "slumped" posture, rounded shoulders, head held forward, and chin tilted up. Chin tilt can be exacerbated by the necessity of performing on a raked stage. As the head translates further forward, there is a tendency for adaptive "shortening" of the stylohyoid muscle, one of the suprahyoid suspensory muscles (E. Blake, personal observation, 2001).

Other causes might typically include performing with laryngeal edema or with nodules on the vocal folds, and, in an attempt to obtain vocal fold closure, recruiting extrinsic laryngeal muscles and thereby raising the larynx.

Lieberman has also found an association between a tight and foreshortened thyrohyoid muscle (with the clinical correlate of a foreshortened and "held" thyrohyoid membrane) and unresolved emotional issues.[22]

This group of muscles is readily accessible to laryngeal manipulation.

Extrinsic Muscles That Depress the Larynx: the Infrahyoid Suspensory Group

The sternothyroid, sternohyoid, and omohyoid muscles are a part of the muscles known as "strap" muscles or "ribbon" muscles. They are involved in the swallowing mechanism to lower the larynx and assist in "resetting" the mechanism.[35,38] These muscles are readily accessible to the beginner in laryngeal manipulation.

Although not strictly relevant to this section, note that the geniohyoid and strap muscles working synchronously tend to pull the larynx in an anterior direction, and thereby act in an antagonistic fashion to the constrictors.[8,39,40]

The Constrictor Muscles

The constrictor muscles form a muscular sling that defines the posterior and lateral parts of the pharynx.

There are three constrictors, superior, middle, and inferior, one overlapping the other, extending from the basicranium to the cervical esophagus. Each is fan-shaped, attaching to its counterpart via a tough raphe of fibrous tissue just anterior to the prevertebral fascia. The middle constrictor is the only muscle of the constrictor group which "anchors" the hyoid bone; the inferior constrictor "anchors" the thyroid cartilage, with attachments from the upper border of the thyroid cartilage to the lower border of the cricoid cartilage.[21]

In our view, the constrictors are involved in many presentations of hyperfunctional voice disorders. The patient's ability or failure to relax these muscles, with or without manipulation, is a useful indicator of prognosis for treatment outcome (J. Lieberman, personal observation, 2002).

DEEP MUSCLES OF THE NECK

The deep muscles of the neck can be divided into the posterior extensors, the suboccipital muscle group, the deep anterior neck flexors, and the superficial anterior neck flexors. We shall not spend much time on these important groups of muscles as they are outside the scope of the chapter, but discuss them briefly as problems therein can lead to foreshortening of muscles involved with voicing (as described above).

The Posterior Extensors

The key group of muscles here are the erector spinae muscles. They span the vertebrae, give support, establish, and maintain appropriate extension of the vertebral column. The muscles attached to the skull produce extension, lateral flexion, and rotation of the head.

The erector spinae includes, superficially, the iliocostalis, longissimus, and the spinalis. Deeper muscles include the semispinalis, the deep short muscles, the multifidis, and cervicis.[41]

Suboccipital Muscle Group

These muscles extend the skull at the atlanto-occipital joint and rotate it at the atlanto-axial joint. They are important for stereoscopic vision. Muscles include the rectus capitis posterior major and minor, and the obliquus capitis superior and inferior.

Deep Anterior Neck Flexors

These include the three scalene muscles and the prevertebral muscles (the longus colli, longus capitis, rectus capitis anterior and lateralis). Their actions include: scalenes—weak neck flexion, and lifting and stabilizing the upper two ribs; prevertebral muscles—twisting the head on the neck and flexing the neck.

Superficial Anterior Neck Muscles

These include the sternocleidomastoid, levator scapulae, trapezius, and splenius. The sternocleidomastoid turns the head obliquely to the other side. When working with its opposite member it pulls the head downward and forward. The levator scapulae raises and helps rotate the scapula. The trapezius holds the shoulder back and up, steadies and raises the scapula, draws the head backward and to one side. The splenius supports the spine.[41]

These muscles are readily accessible to osteopathic manipulation and often held in a contracted state in patients with voice disorders (also in individuals with musculoskeletal related headache). As previously noted the deep extensors frequently are found to be held in a contracted state. Another common finding is for various fibers of the trapezius to be contracted and tender in patients with voice disorders (E. Blake, personal observation, 2002).

It is facile to believe that any one muscle works in isolation in the larynx or elsewhere, but this is generally not the case. Several muscles work together both synergistically and antagonistically in the same reflex arc. For example, the tensor fascia lata is an extensor of the hip when the knee is flexed less than 20 degrees, and acts as a flexor of the hip when the knee is flexed beyond 20 degrees (J. Lieberman, personal observation, 1999). In the larynx, as elsewhere, muscles work together, the net pull leading to movement or to stability.[8]

INDICATIONS FOR LARYNGEAL MANIPULATION IN VOICE PATIENTS

As we have worked together over time as a team, we have identified more indications for referral to an individual specially trained in laryngeal manipulation. There are two basic indications for such as referral. The first is when the otolaryngologist has identified abnormal musculoskeletal patterns in a patient presenting with a voice problem. This indication is predominantly for treatment from the therapist. The second general indication is for assessment when the laryngologist is uncertain as to the cause of the dysphonia, for example, in the absence of obvious vocal fold mucosal pathology. Let us review these instances.

1. The otolaryngologist is reasonably certain that a musculoskeletal problem exists and is affecting voice production. Typical instances for referral might include:

   a. The patient with the high-held larynx and tightly held base of tongue musculature, with or without mucosal pathology of the true vocal folds. This type of referral is likely to lead to rapid improvement over one or two sessions. This pattern also responds quickly to Roy's or Mathieson's circumhyoid manipulation.[1-3]

   b. The patient with a forward-held (hyperlordotic) neck with a palpable "shelf" on palpation of the posterior spinous processes at, typically, C4/C5 or C5/C6, and a forward-held cricoid in relationship to the anterior thyroid. This, with or without mucosal pathology of the true vocal folds, is likely to represent a long-standing postural pattern. It is likely to respond to laryngeal manipulation but to take several sessions and possibly to require intermittent follow-up (J. Rubin, personal observation, 2002).

   c. The patient with reduced range of motion of the cricothyroid visor, with a voice that tires easily. This pattern, with or without mucosal pathology at the level of the vocal folds, is likely to be an end result of "guarding" the larynx, but responds rapidly to laryngeal manipulation.

   d. The patient with the low-held larynx, in association with tightly held sternocleidomastoid muscles; the phoniatric correlate being a gravelly voice with a marked amount of "creak" in the voice quality. This is likely to respond well to laryngeal manipulation, or to Mathieson's combination of manipulation and speech therapy.[2]

   e. The patient with the exquisitely tender and tightly held thyrohyoid membrane, usually unilaterally. This is likely to respond to manipulation; however, gentle investigation into possible unresolved emotional issues would not be amiss. Lieberman finds the combination of manipulation and application of psychodynamic models extremely beneficial in the management of such cases whose symptoms are considered as a physical manifestation of emotional state of mind (J. Lieberman, personal observation, 2002).

2. The otolaryngologist is uncertain as to the cause of the dysphonia. In this circumstance, the osteopathic assessment is likely to be of benefit in demonstrating whether or not there is any underlying muscular or joint pathology.

There are certain caveats. (1) A traditional course of therapy with a speech-language pathologist (SLP) may well successfully treat some or all of the patients treated by the physical therapist. Management is not exclusive; we frequently obtain opinions and/or management protocols from both SLP and osteopath. (2) In the patients with secondary hyperfunction, caused by, for example, a partial palsy, a sulcus, chronic pharyngolaryngeal reflex, and so forth, the underlying cause needs to be identified and treated appropriately. (3) Much as with speech therapy, any new pattern of musculoskeletal positioning needs to be internalized by the patient if it is to be long-lasting. This may require several sessions (see research section in this chapter).

Case histories follow, demonstrating some of the authors' indications for manipulation.

Case History 1: Acute Management

One of the authors was contacted only hours prior to performance by a performer suffering from increasing vocal difficulties.

He saw the performer and concluded that the performer was suffering from mild laryngeal edema, which could be managed medically with a single dose of prednisone. However, there were also significant musculoskeletal issues identified, thus, an osteopath was contacted and came backstage to see the performer.

After explaining the process, the osteopath proceeded to perform a ten-minute period of general relaxation manipulation to the performer's neck, followed by a five-to-ten-minute period of manipulation directed specifically at the tender, held region. Ten to fifteen minutes post-therapy the performer found that the laryngeal discomfort had eased markedly. The performer was then able to perform credibly in the role.

Case History 2: Subacute Management

A performer presented to one of the otolaryngologists following the acute onset of hoarseness brought on by an episode of violent coughing and retching. One vocal fold was noted to be discolored, consistent with a vocal fold hemorrhage. Judicious voice rest led to improvement to baseline from the standpoint of laryngeal appearance and stroboscopic function, but the performer continued to suffer from vocal fatigue. It was postulated that the performer had developed new musculoskeletal "habits" involving the perilaryngeal musculature because of (unconscious) protection of the larynx. Osteopathic consultation was requested together with consultation with the performer's singing voice teacher. Following two or three sessions of basic manipulation procedures of the perilaryngeal musculature and neck,

as well as work with the singing voice teacher over a few weeks, the performer felt to be back at baseline.

OSTEOPATHIC EVALUATION

The history and assessment of the patient by the osteopath should result in a functional diagnosis as well as a treatment plan. Much as with the otolaryngologist, history taking begins the moment the patient presents to the office. Body movements, both voluntary and involuntary, and general body positioning while the patient is absorbed in presenting his history, frequently give subtle or obvious clues to the underlying musculoskeletal pathology. A conventional medical history is taken, with emphasis on problems affecting the gastrointestinal tract, respiratory system, central nervous system, or psyche. Sleep patterns, gynecologic issues, and the musculoskeletal system are all reviewed. For greater detail on the history see the chapter by Sataloff on the History and Physical Examination of Patients With Voice Disorders (Chapter 11).

OSTEOPATHIC ASSESSMENT

The osteopathic assessment (see Table 33-1) begins with visual observation and then proceeds to palpation. Palpation is performed to assess the resting muscle tone, contracted muscle tone, resting joint position, range of motion, and ease of mobility.

If failure to relax a muscle following activity leads to hyperfunctional muscular behavior, and voice and swallow require repetitive, complex muscular activity, then it is hardly surprising that both the laryngeal and perilaryngeal musculature are at risk for hyperfunctional patterns. These patterns are identifiable by tight, tender, and contracted muscles. This results in loss of full joint range of movement and loss of movement pattern. It is experienced as stiffness.[42]

It should be recalled that, although the patient presents with a hoarse voice, the osteopath is interested in far more than the larynx; he needs to evaluate the entire vocal tract. Specifically, he will need to assess (1) general posture; (2) head position; (3) integrity of the deep and more superficial muscles of the neck; (4) integrity of the muscles, joints, and ligaments supporting breathing; (5) integrity of the muscles, joints, and ligaments of the pharynx and larynx; (6) position of the laryngeal cartilages and hyoid bone.

General Posture

The general posture of an individual plays a significant role in the development or perpetuation of voice problems. As noted above, there is a steady state between the extensors and the flexors of the body. In our society this balance is frequently abrogated. There is often peer pressure leading children to assume a "slumped" position. Adults spend much of their working day and evening seated in front of computer screens or televisions, often in unhealthy postural positions. Unfortunately, the media has paid much attention to bulging abdominal muscles (the "six pack" appearance) in individuals with flat stomachs. This has led to an emphasis in adults' sports time, on exercises designed to pull the lower rib cage down toward the pelvis. Thus, even during exercise, adults tend to develop muscles that promote abnormal postural patterns.

These postural patterns lead to a cascade of compensatory postural changes with a resultant hyperlordotic neck. This in turn places the suprahyoid suspensory muscles at significant risk for the development of chronic spasm, and can lead to inefficient muscular patterns of voicing.

There are many other causes of general postural problems relating to spinal curvatures and asymmetries, injuries, or congenital problems affecting the pelvis, hips, legs, and feet, all of which can ultimately affect voice production.

Head Position

Head position has a direct effect on voice production. The adult head weighs 14 to 16 pounds. Position of the head can affect the resting length of the suspensory muscles. Hyperlordosis has already been discussed above. Head tilt or anterior-posterior displacement can affect voice. Examples of individuals with head tilt might include: teachers who work from a piano, with their students always singing from the same side of the piano; many instrumentalists (for example, some woodwind players, guitarists, violinists), and so forth.

Integrity of the Deep Muscles of the Neck

These muscles have been reviewed above briefly. All are involved in head, neck, or upper spine positioning or stability. Abnormalities in any of these muscles ultimately can lead to voice problems.

Integrity of the Muscles, Joints, and Ligaments Supporting Breathing

The mechanisms inherent to the "bellows" are crucial to voice production.[43] Limitation of motion, caused by injury, inflammation, infection, aging, and so forth, can decrease efficiency of these mechanisms. Examples might include: limitation of rib cage movement, for example, as caused by ankylosing spondylitis; reduction

of efficiency of the muscles and ligaments supporting expiration, for example, stretching of the rectus abdominis muscles during pregnancy. Of note, at times the emotional state of the patient may also influence abdominal support or pattern of breathing.

Integrity of the Muscles, Joints, and Ligaments of the Pharynx and Larynx

These have been reviewed in some depth above. Palpation of these structures gives the osteopath insights into the voicing mechanism at the level of the sound source. Examples might include: (1) increased tension, tenderness, or guarding in the suspensory musculature; (2) a held cricothyroid visor with decreased range of motion of the cricothyroid joint, both changes often being found in prolonged voice misuse patterns.[22]

Much emphasis recently has been placed on the Morrison muscular tension dysphonia patterns, type 1 through 4[44,45]; however, they primarily have been identified by the patterns of visualized vocal fold closure. Harris has attempted to go one step further and characterize the specific muscular misuse patterns that have led to the observed vocal fold closure patterns.[46]

The relative size of the thyrohyoid space (and the thyrohyoid muscles) should be assessed. Lieberman notes that in individuals with hyperfunctional voicing disorders, the space is much reduced in surface area.[22]

Position and Mobility of the Laryngeal Cartilages and Hyoid Bone

1. Thyroid cartilage position. This can be observed readily as well as palpated. Deviation of the thyroid cartilage from center is frequently accompanied by major underlying postural changes. Examples might include rotation of the torso to one side, scoliosis, abnormal unilateral hypertrophy of the superficial muscles of the neck (for example, unilateral torticollis), surgery (for example, following a unilateral radical neck dissection), unilateral hyperostosis of the cervical spine, and so forth.

2. Limitation of movement of the thyroid cartilage on side-to-side movement (rotation). This finding may be associated with aging, hyperostosis of the cervical spine, or a tumor of the larynx or neck. In young, otherwise healthy performers, the most common cause of this limitation of movement, however, is increased resting muscular tone in the "strap" muscles. This is generally indicative of a musculoskeletal pattern associated with increased "holding" or "guarding" of

these muscles. It is often associated with voice changes, including lowering of the fundamental frequency of the speaking voice and a gravelly quality to the voice. This muscular pattern is readily amenable to laryngeal manipulation.

3. Hyoid position. The hyoid bone is the principal structure below which the remainder of the larynx is suspended. It should lie in a horizontal plane, and be located just below the mandible. Typically it lies approximately 1/2 inch caudal to the body of the mandible. Angulation of either side towards the mandible suggests unilateral tight posterior hyoglossus or stylohyoid muscles or anterior thyrohyoid ligaments.[22] Such angulation may also be associated with inflammatory lymphadenopathy in zone two (the jugulo-digastric region) of the neck (J. Rubin, personal observation, 2002). Lateral tilting of the hyoid bone may be associated with unilateral tightness of the superior suspensory muscles or to the unilateral pull of a tight thyrohyoid muscle. When the hyoid bone appears to be pulled forward anteriorly, a tight geniohyoid muscle should be suspected.[22] The reverse may occur should the middle constrictor muscle be hypertonic (J. Lieberman, personal observation, 2002).

In patients with a "held" larynx, or a posteriorly backed larynx, consideration should be given to the possibility of unresolved emotional issues. Aronson has noted that one common denominator of psychogenic voice disorders is a hypercontractile state of the intrinsic and extrinsic laryngeal musculature.[6] These considerations are very important to successful long-term intervention, but are outside the scope of this chapter (see Chapter 29, Psychologic Aspects of Voice Disorders, for further insights).

The superior suspensory muscles consist of the stylohyoid, geniohyoid, hyoglossus, mylohyoid, and anterior and posterior bellies of the digastric muscles. As noted, excessively tight suprahyoid musculature in association with a high-held larynx signifies marked muscular hyperactivity often in association with unresolved emotional issues.[22] One example of such a clinical scenario is that not uncommonly found in mutational dysphonias.

The inferior suspensory muscles should be palpated. These include the sternothyroid, sternohyoid, and omohyoid muscles. These muscles are long, with thin bellies and are thus difficult to assess by direct palpation. Their quality can be inferred by assessing the resting level of the larynx and by stretching it upward and laterally (see below). An extremely low-held, or "anchored" larynx should be checked for. Koufman has classified one type

of speaking-voice abuse pattern as the "Bogart-Bacall" syndrome, in which the patient speaks with a very low-pitched fundamental frequency. This is associated with a low-held larynx.[47,48]

ENDOLARYNGEAL EXAMINATION

Prior to laryngeal manipulation by an osteopath, the larynx should be examined by an otolaryngologist with a flexible or rigid endoscope, preferably with an attached stroboscope, and the results relayed to the osteopath. Particular attention should be paid to the characteristic appearance of any known patterns of dysphonia. Typically these include muscular tension dysphonia, as described by authors such as Morrison, Koufman, or Harris,[44-46,48] or bowing. There may also be evidence of asymmetry of vocal fold movement or of arytenoid position (see below).

The otolaryngologic examination should include evaluation for evidence of extra-esophageal reflux (posterior interarytenoid "heaping," piriform pooling, posterior laryngeal edema or redness, and so forth), and for subtle laryngeal mucosal pathology that may be the source of the abnormal muscular behavior. The stroboscope will be of critical importance here, as subtle asynchrony of the mucosal wave, areas of adynamism, and so forth may lead the examiner to infer the possibility of such pathologies as a partially resolved vocal fold palsy, a small cyst, sulcus, or scar, all of which could be the source of the muscular dyskinesia.

The arytenoid cartilages and the cricoarytenoid joints are accessible to palpation by the osteopathic practitioner with adequate experience, particularly in long, thin-necked individuals. Similarly, the posterior cricoarytenoid muscles and interarytenoid muscles can be palpated and compared for tenderness and hypertonicity. These maneuvers require considerable skill and can be very uncomfortable to the patient, however. Thus, they should be considered to be outside the scope of this chapter. It is worth noting that the patient's response to such an examination can assist in the diagnosis, one example being the irritable larynx (Murray Morrison, Instructional Course, Annual Meeting of the American Academy of Otolaryngology Head and Neck Surgery, September 1999).

BASIC LARYNGEAL MANIPULATION

Generally speaking, common sense needs to be used when considering performance of laryngeal manipulation. For example, laryngeal manipulation is not advisable in patients with laryngeal or thyroid malignancies, or in instances of Graves' disease. In the presence of other anterior neck pathologies, the techniques should be modified appropriately to avoid unnecessary discomfort. Prior to manipulation, a thorough explanation of the proposed procedure, its risks and benefits, should be given to the patient, and his or her permission sought.

Particular care must be exercised when working in the area overlying the carotid artery and especially around the carotid body and sinus.

Prior to any manipulation, the osteopath gently palpates for any deviation from "normal" anatomic structures, for example, an unusually enlarged or prominent carotid sinus in relation to the hyoid bone and its attachments. Imaging has not been found to be necessary, as direct hands-on palpation is very sensitive to such abnormalities. While laryngeal manipulation proves to be a highly safe treatment in experienced hands, we teach that energetic or inadvertent manipulation should not be performed near the carotid; it can lead to rapid changes in blood pressure and/or pulse rate; it can also lead to loosening of atheromatous plaques in elderly patients.

Similarly, care should be exercised in instances of previous laryngeal trauma, surgery, or radiation where normal anatomy may be altered.

General

In cases of soft tissue damage caused by repetitive strain injury, similar to certain orthopedic problems, the muscles will be chronically shortened, fibrotic or scarred, and tender to touch. By working on the muscles, the osteopath is able to stretch scar contractures, lengthen the muscle belly, increase blood flow, and improve lymphatic drainage. The osteopath probably also affects the neuromuscular pattern of outflow locally and centrally, although this requires further clarification through research.[22]

Limitation of joint movement can also be addressed by direct joint manipulation, as well as by soft tissue techniques to surrounding musculature. In addition to reducing muscle spasm, the practitioner also attempts to alter head position, reduce hyperlordotic spinal curve, and improve mobility in the thoracic spine.

Treatment aims include restoration of joint mobility and muscle function. Perhaps as important is bringing to the conscious level the unconscious and habitual abnormal postural patterns that need to be corrected.[42]

General concepts of manipulation to attain these goals include those of:

1. Identification of the indicated muscle or structure to work on.

2. Stabilization of indicated muscle against a known, more fixed structure (for example, the cricoid cartilage).

3. Passive stretch where two structures (for example, hyoid bone and mandible) are held apart under gentle stretch for a period of time.

4. Dynamic stretch (the patient activates a muscle that the osteopath wishes to manipulate, and the osteopath works with or against the patient's own force).

5. Muscle kneading.

6. Working beyond guarding (the osteopath maintains stretch beyond the point at which the patient holds back).

BASIC MANIPULATION: GENERAL TECHNIQUE

Much of basic manipulation involves general soft tissue work on the posterior neck, shoulders, and upper back. The patient is treated while lying supine on a firm table or gurney with a moveable head support.

First the cervical and upper thoracic spinous processes are carefully assessed for evidence of abnormal alignment, tenderness and integrity or laxity of interspinous ligaments. The cervical and upper thoracic spine is gently investigated for range of motion. This will give the osteopath information as to what can be safely accomplished.

The erector spinae muscles are then palpated and gently placed under stretch, during which time the osteopath checks for focal or point tenderness or guarding. Similar procedures are performed on the other posterior extensors and suboccipital group of muscles. Focal areas of spasm are identified and stretched to relax the hypertonic muscle, increase blood flow, and break the spasm.[22]

Not uncommonly the superficial anterior neck muscles are addressed next. The levator scapulae and splenius are frequent sources of neck pain and often require specific work. The trapezius is another muscle frequently found to be tight or in spasm. Often certain fibers of the trapezius may be found to be contracted and others stretched, given the size of this muscle and its broad insertions.

Frequently the anterior neck, larynx, and laryngeal and pharyngeal muscles are next addressed. Areas particularly relevant to voice problems include: suprahyoid suspensory muscles, cricothyroid visor, scalenes, sternocleidomastoids, and lower strap muscles.

Suprahyoid Suspensory Muscles

As previously noted these muscles are at particular risk for chronic shortening, thereby causing the laryngeal complex to be elevated and effecting a change in resonatory pattern.

These are large powerful muscles and can be addressed individually. When using soft tissue techniques it is best to stabilize the hand against the mandible or the hyoid bone and work from this solid base.

The patient can actively assist by attempting to initiate a swallow (but not a full swallow) while the osteopath gently presses down against the hyoid. This type of combined patient/practitioner activity is termed "dynamic stretch."

Cricothyroid Visor

This "keystone" area has been anatomically characterized above. The osteopath can relax both cricothyroid muscles individually, applying soft tissue stretch techniques, working against the cricoid cartilage as his solid base. He can also work directly on each cricothyroid joint. Dynamic stretch, in this instance would involve the patient "sirening" the pitch up from low to high, thereby actively placing the cricothyroid muscle into contraction, while the osteopath stretches this muscle.

Scalenes, Sternocleidomastoids, and Lower Strap Muscles

The larynx frequently is found to be held in an abnormally low position, a typical correlate being tightly held and tender lower bellies of the SCM, scalenes, and lower strap muscles.

This is a common problem noted in 26% of Koufman's patients with "functional" voice problems,[48] but must be differentiated from a chronically high-held rib cage (as seen in some patients with severe emphysema).

These muscles can be stretched against the solid base of the upper sternum and medial clavicles, and are readily accessible to manipulation.

SUCCESSFUL OUTCOME AFTER LARYNGEAL MANIPULATION

In our clinical experience, albeit anecdotal, the following are comments frequently made by patients immediately following laryngeal manipulation: immediate change in pitch, audible to patient and practitioner; increased resonance; increased ease of swallowing associated with a sense of "openness"; decreased hoarseness; decreased "wobble"; decreased pain and discomfort.

In the longer term, it is not uncommon for there to be reported an increase in stamina, vocal flexibility and range, better negotiation of the passaggio, and shorter duration of recovery time following laryngeal exertions. Research to confirm these anecdotal impressions is needed, as discussed below.

There is often resolution of the laryngeal "click" (that is caused by anterior movement of the hyoid bone over the thyroid cartilage and is frequently associated with chronically shortened and tightly held thyrohyoid muscles) and a decreased need to clear the throat. Finally, JL finds in many of his patients acknowledgment of underlying emotional issues related to the laryngeal pathology (Jacob Lieberman, unpublished data, 1999).

Because of the relaxed laryngeal musculature and the small alteration in laryngeal position, professional voice users occasionally experience what they call a "wild voice," momentarily. Warming-up type exercises are required to allow the performer to get used to the changes.

In the pilot study assessing the efficiency of manipulation versus conventional speech therapy, the two modalities were found to be dissimilar but complementary.[7] Manipulation was found to excel at rapidly reducing tension in muscles that were tightly held in the "unaware" patient. With manipulation, early vocal fatigue was found to be reduced as was laryngeal discomfort. While conventional speech therapy was found to address these problems as well, the progress was slower. Speech therapy, however, was found to be better at substituting more efficient voicing patterns over the pretreatment dysphonic patterns.

ADVANCED MANIPULATION

Advanced manipulation is designed for instances in which the laryngeal intrinsic muscles require direct address. This might include times when the laryngeal "set" needs to be altered. For example, Lieberman has directly manipulated the intrinsic muscles of certain patients with granulomas who have failed traditional therapy, the aim being to reduce the hard prephonatory gesture and resultant impact of the arytenoid cartilages. In Lieberman's practice, advanced manipulation is not uncommonly combined with elements of psychotherapy that focus on unresolved emotional issues.

It must be remembered that manipulation of the intrinsic muscles of the larynx involves working on the posterior aspect of the larynx on muscles that are designed for mainly reflexogenic activities. Such manipulation requires considerable palpatory skill, as well as great sensitivity in working with patients.

ONGOING RESEARCH

Laryngeal manipulation has been developed, and practiced in Queen Mary's Hospital Sidcup, Kent, for the last fourteen years. Initially the team looked at the relationship of head position, shoulder girdle, and hyperfunctional voice disorders.[7]

The clinic has developed a research protocol with Professor A. Fourcin using the laryngograph to record vocal parameters prior to and immediately following manipulation, in an attempt to validate the anecdotal findings described above. Preliminary laryngographic data have often confirmed clinical findings, including: immediate change in fundamental frequency of the speaking voice, better control, and wider vocal range. As an example, a patient with spasmodic dysphonia treated with manipulation is presented (Figure 33-1). The project is ongoing.

Other research projects in planning involve assessing cricothyroid joint activity, diaphragmatic breathing, and the function of the thyrohyoid mechanism.

SUMMARY

We have presented a synopsis of the role that laryngeal manipulation plays in our practice. Certainly in our voice clinics, the more we have considered the possibility of musculoskeletal issues in patients with voice disorders, the more reasons we have found for referring such patients for diagnostic investigation and treatment by a physical therapist, osteopath, or by practitioners with similar skills. The critical issue is for the therapist to participate actively in the voice clinic so that he or she will develop sensitivity to the needs of the patient.

That said, muscles do not work in isolation. The musculoskeletal system is driven by thoughts and affects. The effects of physical therapy, passive and active manipulation in particular, are immediate and frequently effective in (at least temporarily) breaking through unconscious neuromuscular pathways (habits). To be long-lasting, the "new" musculoskeletal behavior must be internalized by the patient. Many or most of our patients require refresher sessions to reinforce the beneficial behavior patterns.

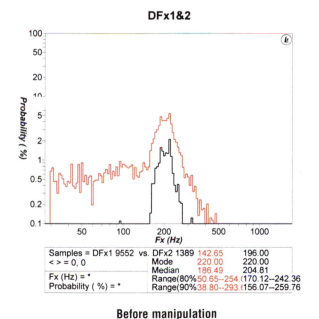

Before manipulation

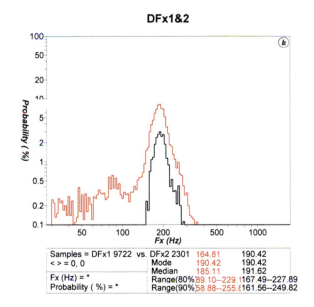

After manipulation

FIGURE 33-1. *Laryngographic data taken from a patient with spasmodic dysphonia before and after one treatment with laryngeal manipulation. (Courtesy of Professor Adrian Fourcin) (A) Plot 1A shows range, before and after one manipulation. Range as defined herein refers to the range of frequencies contained within the speaking voice, while reading from a standard text. Note the reduction in spread of the first order distribution (in red), and the slight improvement in range definition shown by the second order distribution (in black), both following manipulation. (Continues)*

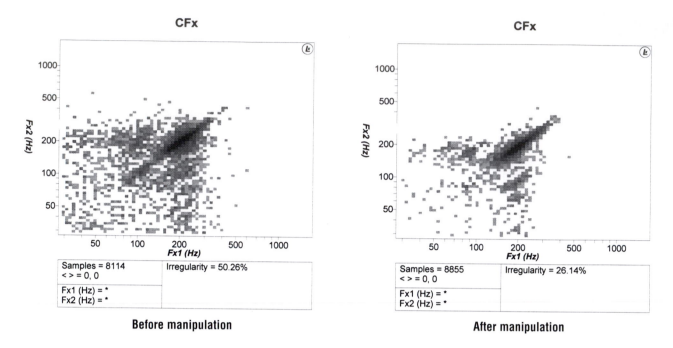

FIGURE 33-1. *(B) Plot 1B shows regularity, before and after one manipulation. Regularity as defined herein refers to the extent to which successive vocal fold periods are comparable, while reading from a standard text. Note the reduction in irregularity in the post manipulation distribution. (Continues)*

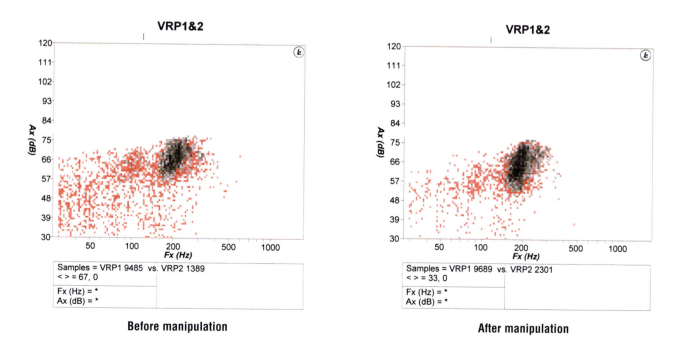

FIGURE 33-1. *(C) Plot 1C shows a phonetogram before and after one manipulation. The phonetogram as defined herein refers to the distribution of loudness against pitch, while reading from a standard text. Note that the post manipulation plot demonstrates a more compact control of loudness (less dispersion).(Continues)*

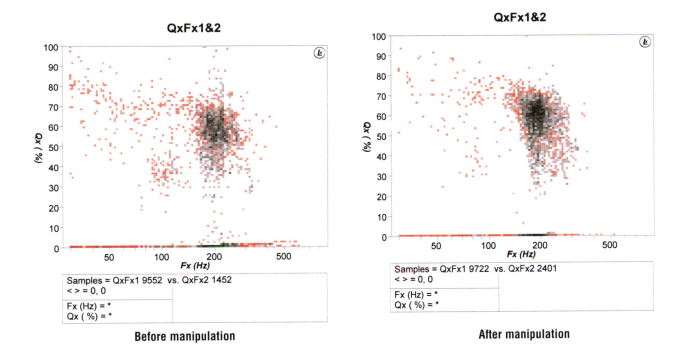

Before manipulation

After manipulation

FIGURE 33-1. *(D) Plot 1D shows "quality" before and after one manipulation. "Quality" as defined herein refers to the extent to which the closed phase percentage of the total period is well defined in the speaking voice, while reading from a standard text. Note that there is a (somewhat) better definition of the closed phase in the post manipulation plot.(Continued)*

Manipulation is a potent treatment modality, but it does not resolve underlying emotional conflicts. Hence, a small proportion of our patients will benefit from a short course of supportive counseling, or from more formal psychotherapy.

REFERENCES

1. Mathieson L. Vocal tract discomfort in hyperfunctional dysphonia. *Voice*. 1993;2:40-48.

2. Mathieson L. *Greene and Mathieson's The Voice and Its Disorders*. 6th ed. London, England: Whurr Publishers Limited; 2001.

3. Roy N, Leeper HA. Effects of the manual laryngeal musculoskeletal tension reduction technique as a treatment for functional voice disorders: perceptual and acoustic measures. *J Voice*. 1993;7:242-249.

4. Roy N, Bless DM, Heisey D, Ford CN. Manual circumlaryngeal therapy for functional dysphonia: an evaluation of short- and long-term treatment outcomes. *J Voice*. 1997;11:321-331.

5. Aronson AE. *Clinical Voice Disorders: an Interdisciplinary Approach*. 2nd ed. New York, NY: Georg Thieme Verlag; 1985.

6. Aronson A. *Clinical Voice Disorders*. 3rd ed. New York, NY: Thieme Medical Publishers; 1991:117-145.

7. Harris S, Harris T, Lieberman J, Harris D. The multidisciplinary voice clinic. In: Freeman M, Fawcus M, eds. *Voice Disorders and Their Management*. London, England: Whurr Publishers; 2000:313-332.

8. Harris T, Laryngeal mechanisms in normal function and dysfunction. In: Harris T, Harris S, Rubin JS, Howard DM, eds. *The Voice Clinic Handbook*. London, England: Whurr Publishers; 1998:64-90.

9. Rubin JS. The structural anatomy of the larynx and supraglottic vocal tract: a review. In: Harris T, Harris S, Rubin JS, Howard DM, eds. *The Voice Clinic Handbook*. London, England: Whurr Publishers; 1998:15-33.

10. Laitman JT, Noden DM, Van de Water TR. Formation of the larynx: from homeobox genes to critical periods. In: Rubin JS, Sataloff RT, Korovin GS, Gould WJ, eds. *Diagnosis and Treatment of Voice Disorders*. New York, NY: Igaku-Shoin Medical Publishers; 1995:9-23.

11. Scherer RC. Laryngeal function during phonation. In: Rubin JS, Sataloff RT, Korovin G, Gould WJ, eds. *Diagnosis and Treatment of Voice Disorders.* New York, NY: Igaku-Shoin Publishers; 1995:86-104.

12. Hast MH. Mechanical properties of the cricothyroid muscle. *Laryngoscope.* 1966;76:537-548.

13. Cooper DS, Partridge LD, Alipour-Haghighi F. Muscle energetics, vocal efficiency, and laryngeal biomechanics. In: Titze IR, ed. *Vocal Fold Physiology: Frontiers in Basic Science.* San Diego, CA: Singular Publishing Group; 1993:37-92.

14. Harris T, Lieberman J. The cricothyroid mechanism, its relationship to vocal fatigue and vocal dysfunction. *Voice.* 1993;2:89-96.

15. Rubin JS, Sataloff RT. Voice: new horizons. In: Sataloff RT, ed. *Professional Voice: The Science and Art of Clinical Care.* 2nd ed. San Diego, CA: Singular Publishing Group; 1997.

16. Fisher K. Early experience of a multidisciplinary pain management programme. *Hol Med.* 1988;3:47-56.

17. Robinson L, Fisher H, Knox J, Thomson G. *The Official Body Control Pilates Manual.* London, England: Macmillan Publishers; 2000.

18. Feldenkrais M. *Awareness Through Movement.* New York, NY: Harper & Row; 1972.

19. Rolf IP. *Rolfing: Reestablishing the Natural Alignment and Structural Integration of the Human Body for Vitality and Well-being.* Rochester, VT: Healing Arts Press; 1989.

20. Dickson D, Dickson W. Functional anatomy of the human larynx. *Proc Penn Acad Ophthalmol.* 1971;29.

21. Boileau Grant JC. *Grant's Atlas of Anatomy.* 6th ed. Baltimore, MD: Williams & Wilkins; 1972.

22. Lieberman J. Principles and techniques of manual therapy: application in the management of dysphonia. In: Harris T, Harris S, Rubin JS, Howard DM, eds. *The Voice Clinical Handbook.* London, England: Whurr Publishers; 1998:91-138.

23. Dickson DR, Maue-Dickson W. *Anatomical and Physiological Basis of Speech.* Boston, MA: Little, Brown & Co; 1982.

24. Letson JA Jr, Tatchell R. Arytenoid movement. In: Sataloff RT, ed. *Professional Voice: The Science and Art of Clinical Care.* San Diego, CA: Singular Publishing Group; 1997:131-145.

25. Baken RJ, Isshiki N. Arytenoid displacement by simulated intrinsic muscle contraction. *Folia Phoniatr.* 1977;29:206-216.

26. Von Leden H. The mechanics of the cricoarytenoid joint. *Arch Otolaryngol.* 1961;73:63-72.

27. Arnold GE. Physiology and pathology of the cricothyroid muscle. *Laryngoscope.* 1961;71:687-753.

28. Choi HS, Berke GS, Ye M, Kreiman J. Function of the thyroarytenoid muscle in a canine laryngeal model. *Ann Otol Rhinol Laryngol.* 1993;102:769-776.

29. Fujimura O. Body-cover theory of the vocal fold and its phonetic implications. In: Stevens KN, Hirano M, eds. *Vocal Fold Physiology.* Tokyo, Japan: University of Tokyo Press; 1981:271-288.

30. Titze IR, Jiang J, Drucker DG. Preliminaries to the body-cover theory of pitch control. *J Voice.* 1988;1(4):314-319.

31. Vilkman E, Alku P, Laukkanen A. Vocal-fold collision mass as a differentiator between registers in the low-pitch range. *J Voice.* 1995;9:66-73.

32. Alipour-Haghighi F, Perlman Al, Titze IR. Tetanic response of the cricothyroid muscle. *Ann Otol Rhinol Laryngol.* 1991;100:626-631.

33. Alipour-Haghighi F, Titze IR, Perlman AL. Tetanic contraction in vocal fold muscle. *J Speech Hear Res.* 1989;32:226-231.

34. Titze IR, Durham PL. Passive mechanisms influencing fundamental frequency control. In: Baer T, Sasaki C, Harris KS, eds. *Laryngeal Function in Phonation and Respiration.* San Diego, CA: College-Hill Press; 1987:304-319.

35. Broniatowski M, Sonies BC, Rubin JS, et al. Current evaluation and treatment of patients with swallowing disorders. *Otolaryngol Head Neck Surg.* 1999;120:464-473.

36. Hellemans J, Agg HO, Pelemans W, et al. Pharyngoesophageal swallowing disorders and the pharyngoesophageal sphincter. *Med Clin North Am.* 1981;65:1149-1171.

37. Estill J. *Voicecraft: A User's Guide to Voice Quality. Vol 2, Some Basic Voice Qualities.* Santa Rosa, CA: Estill Voice Training Systems; 1995.

38. Rubin JS. The physiologic anatomy of swallowing. In: Rubin JS, Broniatowski M, Kelly J, eds. *The Swallowing Handbook.* San Diego, CA: Singular Publishing Group; 2000:1-20.

39. Sonninen A. The role of the external laryngeal muscles in the length-adjustment of the vocal cords in singing. *Acta Otolaryngol.* 1956;118:218-231.

40. Vilkman E, Sonninen A, Hurme P, Korkko P. External laryngeal frame function in voice production revisited: a review. *J Voice.* 1996;10:78-92.

41. Lumley JSP, Craven JL, Aitken JT. *Essential Anatomy.* Edinburgh, Scotland: Churchill Livingstone; 1973.

42. Rubin JS, Lieberman J, Harris TM. Laryngeal manipulation. *Otolaryngol Clin North Am.* 2000;33:1017-1034.

43. Rubin JS. Mechanisms of respiration (the bellows). In: Harris T, Harris S, Rubin JS, Howard DM, eds. *The Voice Clinic Handbook.* London, England: Whurr Publishers; 1998:49-63.

44. Morrison MD, Rammage LA, Gilles M, et al. Muscular tension dysphonia. *J Otolaryngol.* 1983;12:302-306.

45. Morrison M, Rammage L, Nichol H, et al. *The Management of Voice Disorders.* San Diego, CA: Singular Publishing Group; 1994.

46. Harris S. Speech therapy for dysphonia. In: Harris T, Harris S, Rubin JS, Howard DM, eds. *The Voice Clinic Handbook.* London, England: Whurr Publishers; 1998:186-195.

47. Gould WJ, Rubin JS. Special considerations for the professional voice user. In: Rubin JS, Sataloff RT, Korovin G, Gould WJ, eds. *Diagnosis and Treatment of Voice Disorders.* New York, NY: Igako-Shoin Press; 1995:424-435.

48. Koufman J, Blalock O. Functional voice disorders. *Otolaryngol Clin North Am.* 1991;24:1059-1073.

CHAPTER 34

Special Considerations for the Professional Voice User

John S. Rubin, MD, FACS, FRCS

Gwen S. Korovin, MD, FACS

Ruth Epstein, PhD, MRCSLT

A professional voice user may be defined as someone who uses the voice as a primary means of occupational communication. The crucial aspects of the definition revolve around: 1) a requirement of communication by means of the voice, and 2) the production of a desirable and dependable vocal sound, which carries its own message and which is, in many cases, compelling. Under this umbrella falls a large portion of the working population. Singers, actors, broadcasters and announcers, public speakers, politicians, and talk show hosts are immediately evident. Other important groups for whom the voice is critical include barristers and trial lawyers, lay preachers, clergy, teachers and coaches, telephone operators, receptionists, salespeople, stock and bond traders, exercise instructors; the list is almost indeterminable.

Within these groups, the voice is used in many differing ways: The salesperson uses the voice to convince others, and, frequently, to be "earnest" or "sincere." The trial lawyer's voice can cajole, soothe, or threaten, often within the same time frame. On radio and at sporting events, "vocal signature" of the broadcaster assumes great importance, in many instances allowing for immediate recognition by the public. Many broadcasters' and performers' voices are so well known to the public that even the slightest vocal change caused by illness or emotion is immediately apparent.[1] The voices of politicians and statesmen have probably affected significant changes in history as we know it. Franklin Delano Roosevelt's fireside chats gave the United States a collective will to carry on during the Depression. Winston Spencer Churchill's vocal presentation powerfully reinforced the image of the battling bulldog keeping all foes at bay. John Fitzgerald Kennedy's voice quite possibly won the presidential debate of 1960 and hence the presidency.

With some exceptions, a professional singer generally specializes in a particular musical style, be that classical, popular, rock, musical theater, rap, and so forth, each style with its own requirements. For the classical singer, clarity of sound is necessary; harshness or hoarseness is immediately perceptible and undesirable. The rock singer may purposefully "color" the voice with harshness or graininess. Unlike the classical performer, who is generally comfortably balanced while performing, the rock singer may have developed a reputation for singing on the move. Problems associated therein include maintenance of sufficient breath control to sustain the required power and pitch of the voice. Problems may be exacerbated in musical theater where singing requirements may include a harness or trapeze or skates, a weighty head costume, or a constricting belt or sheath. This places a range of potential challenges in the path of satisfactory voice production.

Professional voice users as a group have the highest of work ethics and an unusually good appreciation of their state of health. They generally will not seek out the help of a laryngologist unless they are certain that something specific is wrong with their vocal tract; their level of anxiety as to its ramifications on their career will be great, and they will be likely to downplay the extent of the ailment and its duration.

LARYNGOLOGIST'S ROLE

What then is the laryngologist's role? As with all patients, when seeing a professional voice user, the laryngologist must assess the general medical condition of the patient as well as the specific vocal complaint. A holistic approach is necessary. A comprehensive, detailed patient history is essential, or else the laryngologist may well miss a vital clue.

The laryngologist must differentiate professional voice users from all his/her other patients; it is the voice that is crucial to the professional's career and in many instances the career is the driving force and top priority of the professional's life. Some may even have difficulty in differentiating their voices from themselves as individuals. While the health of the patient and his/her vocal apparatus is the laryngologist's foremost responsibility, the laryngologist needs to always consider the professional voice user's unique immediate and career requirements.

This chapter focuses on care of the singer, actor, and public speaker; however, principles discussed herein will also apply to the other groups that fall within our definition of a professional voice user. For the sake of simplicity the text will use the male gender throughout; however, it applies equally to women.

ANATOMY: THE DRIVING FORCE OF THE VOICE

To care successfully for someone who relies on his voice, a critical understanding of how the voice is generated is necessary. Voice is produced through the function of three main mechanisms which, together, encompass a large portion of the body: the breathing apparatus or "bellows," the true vocal folds or "oscillator," and the upper airway and oral cavity or "resonator." Mention should also be made of neural control both on a brain stem/cerebellar level, inter-relating the respiratory apparatus and laryngeal musculature, and on a cortical level, with complex inter-relationships allowing minor changes in emotional state to have an impact upon vocal quality. In addition, the body's musculature as it affects posture will have an impact upon the vocal mechanism and voice production. Effectively, therefore, one should consider the entire body as the vocal organ.

PRODUCTION OF VOICE

For the production of voice, there must be a power source. This source, or "bellows," consists of the rib cage and pleurae, the diaphragm and intercostal muscles, the abdominal and back musculature, and the lungs. The back and thoracic musculature lift and stabilize the rib cage. The lungs expand and contract in association with the movements of the rib cage and pleurae. The diaphragm (and to a lesser extent the external intercostal muscles) is the major muscle involved in inspiration. The abdominal muscles and intercostals assume a greater and greater role as the demands on the expiratory system increase from simple reflexive expulsion to prolonged and controlled release of breath for phonation. The orientation of the ribs determines the range through which they can move, that of the upper ribs permitting more of a "pump handle" type of motion and that of the lower ribs a "bucket handle" movement.

Many problems therein can deleteriously affect the efficiency of the system. These might include intrinsic problems of the lungs and pleura, for example, asthma, chronic obstructive pulmonary disease, tuberculosis, or pleurisy. Musculoskeletal problems also can cause difficulties with the power source. Examples might include diastasis recti secondary to multiple parity, umbilical or inguinal hernia, muscle spasm of the shoulder girdle or paraspinous musculature, or age-induced calcifications of the costal cartilages.[2-5]

At the level of the glottis (the "oscillator"), expiration causes alternative buildup and release of air pressure at the vocal folds, which mechanically open and close in a caudad to cephalad direction. The pressure differential created by virtue of a large volume of compressed air streaming through the small glottal space initiates vocal fold vibration, partially through the Bernoulli effect, (but only when the vocal folds are within the nearest 14% of their adductory range).[6] This effect is activated when an object prevents a flowing substance, such as air, from streaming freely, thus creating layers of stream. In the glottis, the middle layer of stream goes through undisturbed while the lateral layers are deflected by the vocal folds; the negative pressure thus created draws the folds together.

This pulsatile stream is translated into sound, the fundamental frequency (F_0) being dependent upon the number of oscillations per second. The sound wave can vibrate at a wide frequency range. Modal register in untrained speakers has been demonstrated to vary from 75 to 450 Hz in men and 130 to 520 Hz in women.[7,8] In primary school teachers it has been postulated that the vocal folds may vibrate up to 1 million times per day (Erkki Vilkman, unpublished observation, 1999).

Pitch correlates nonlinearly with the physical measure of fundamental frequency.[6] It depends on the vocal fold length and tension. In a string model, pitch is directly related to tension and inversely related to mass (or thickness) and length of the string. Researchers have attempted to apply this model to the vocal folds, with varying degrees of success, recognizing that the vocal folds do not function like vibrating strings.[9] Tension changes, both lateral and longitudinal, have been related to pitch variation. Increasing vocal fold length in modal register has been found to correlate to increased F_0; in falsetto, however, the vibrating length shortens as frequency increases. Vocal fold thickness or mass has been found to be of particular importance in modal range; an increase in length correlates with a decrease in mass and higher vibrating frequencies.[9-14] Colton relates this to the stretch of a rubber band; after certain stretch, the thickness remains the same.[9] Stretch is caused by contraction of the intrinsic laryngeal muscles.

The sound created at the level of the vocal folds is a buzz tone and contains a complete set of harmonic partials. It is then damped, amplified, and shaped by the "resonators," which consist of the soft tissues of the supraglottic larynx, pharynx, vault of the nasopharynx, and oral cavity, finally to be shaped into recognizable sound and language by the articulators, particularly the tongue, palate, and lips.[15-17] Certain frequencies are amplified. These are the formants. The adult male vocal tract is approximately 17-20 cm in length with formants at roughly 500, 1500, 2500, and 3500 Hz. The adult female formants are about 15% higher. The second formant is particularly sensitive to the tongue shape and the third to the position of its tip.[17]

To summarize, voice is produced by a power source causing the oscillator to vibrate, thereby producing a sound that is subsequently shaped by the resonators and articulators.

HISTORY

Detailed history-taking is essential. It must incorporate ailments affecting the entire body, as well as those specific to the vocal tract. The history should be unrushed and detailed. Most professional voice users, when faced with what they perceive as a potentially career-ending vocal illness, will be extremely fearful when they come into the office.[18] A gentle and sympathetic approach will go a long way in obtaining an accurate history, which is essential to adequate treatment.

In many centers the voice professional completes a questionnaire while in the waiting room. Some centers also incorporate questions which provide a psychologic profile. This allows the patient to focus on the problem,

makes him more receptive to questioning and, in a sense, begins the relaxation or unburdening process.

The taking of the history has already been elegantly described elsewhere in this book. In this chapter, we relate further information on history-taking in the singer/professional voice user on the basis that it is critical to formulation of any treatment strategy. Even if a cyst or other discrete vocal fold pathology is found during the examination, the question that the laryngologist needs to ascertain is what has caused the performer to fall from his performance plateau.

We present the history-taking in terms of: 1) the current voice problem; 2) non-medical events or stressors that may have caused or led to the voice problems; 3) medical problems that may have caused or led to the voice problems. Recall that a general medical history must evaluate overall health. Many problems, including asthma, emphysema, chronic bronchitis, endocrinopathies, many central nervous system disorders, and so forth can affect the vocal mechanisms directly. Although important to the professional voice user, a detailed description is outside the scope of this chapter.

The Current Voice Problem

This includes an overview by the patient as to what he perceives the problem to be and what has led to the problem. Vocal and career goals are investigated. Then a detailed vocal history is taken. This should include any history of vocal training both for the speaking and singing voice. The number and type of rehearsals or performances over the previous several months is important.

It is useful to know exactly when the performer noted the problem and in what context. For example, one performer was having intermittent voice problems in between a successful rehearsal and the actual performance, often with just hours between them. We discovered that he was regularly eating copious amounts of "junk" types of food in-between. When he stopped this activity, the problems ceased.

Information regarding length and timing of warm-up and of rehearsals is important. Singers and actors frequently over-rehearse, especially in the period just before a major performance.

Date of the next performance is an essential piece of information. Management may well vary, depending on the timing therein. Usually, however, the laryngologist does not have the luxury of prolonged investigations, as the performer may seek care within hours or days of an important performance.[19]

The laryngologist needs to clarify exactly what the performer feels is wrong with his voice. This often gives the vital clue as to the etiology. A well-trained singer can generally sing for over an hour without developing vocal fatigue. Fatigue suggests musculoskeletal issues and may point to over-singing or overuse of the voice, although serious neurologic problems may also present with this complaint. Prolonged warm-up time is frequently associated with reflux.[19] Pain while singing is often the result of vocal abuse, as are choking or coughing in rarer situations.

A harsh voice with loss of dynamic range may be associated with vocal polyps, Reinke's edema, or other mass lesions.[20,21] Difficulty with the passaggio and loss of the upper range could well indicate prenodular edema. Breathiness may be indicative of vocal fold palsy, or other problems preventing closure of the vocal folds.[22] Post-viral partial paresis is probably much more common than previously appreciated.[23] A voice weakening with use, especially in association with increased nasality and ptosis, could be indicative of myasthenia gravis.[24] Although other pathologies often are associated with these symptoms, the ones mentioned here must be included in the differential diagnosis.

Non-medical Events

These might include any of the following:

- Troubles in the family, home, or friends
- Interpersonal difficulties in the production or activity
- Difficulties with the acoustics, including the actual space or venue, difficulty with the microphones or with feedback, and so forth.
- Difficulties with the role or activity, part of which may be inappropriate for the performer's range. Furthermore, the role/part may require intensive learning and rehearsing, or may have the potential to be abusive to the voice. Examples might include occupations such as aerobics instruction or primary school teaching; performances such as cartoon character voiceovers or a staged scream; operatic death scenes sung while lying down, and so forth. Also, nonoccupational activities may be abusive, such as yelling at sporting events, cheerleading, and so forth.

Medical Problems or Issues

These are extremely diverse and are well-covered elsewhere in this book. In synopsis, they may include (among others):

- Infection

    Upper respiratory infection, laryngitis, bronchitis, sinusitis, and so forth.

- Inflammation/Irritation

    Cigarette or passive smoke, reflux, pollution, stage effects, bulimia, cough, and so forth.

- Allergy and asthma
- Hormonal issues
- Neurologic issues
- Physical injuries and or musculoskeletal issues
- Medications and recreational drugs
- Stress and anxiety

PHYSICAL EXAMINATION

The physical examination is well-presented elsewhere in this book. We limit ourselves to what we see as critical issues in the examination for the performer. These include: 1) the examination philosophy; 2) musculoskeletal and postural issues; 3) the general ear, nose, and throat (ENT) examination; 4) the laryngeal examination.

The Examination Philosophy

In general, every effort should be made to allow the patient to feel at ease. Unlike many general busy ENT clinics, enough time should be allotted. We generally allow for 30 minutes when scheduling a new patient who is a performer, and frequently find that the examination runs to 45 minutes or longer.

The examination begins the moment the patient walks into the examining room. Observation of the patient's posture and ease of movements can often give clues to the overall picture. Poor posture can lead to poor breath control and poor performance. Bruxism or jaw clenching is often associated with a functional disorder.

The patient must be listened to carefully, not only for what he is saying but also for how he is saying it. Listen for length of phrases and length of pauses. Even well-trained singers may have poorly trained speaking voices or hard glottal attacks with obvious faulty vocal habits.[25] No matter how sophisticated the equipment available for laboratory analysis, the evaluation begins by listening to the patient during phonation. Breathiness, harshness, dynamic range, and pitch can all be evaluated grossly even by a relatively inexperienced observer.

The laryngologist should not hesitate to have the singer sing a glissando or scale while standing; similarly, the public speaker should read a passage. Posture, abdominal support, and breath control can all be investigated in this manner.[19,26,27]

Musculoskeletal and Postural Issues

These will be evident in a considerable percentage of the performers seen by the laryngologist. Musculoskeletal and postural issues may be either the primary cause of the voice disorder, or may occur secondary to other causes. Examples of primary musculoskeletal causes for dysphonia might include such issues as scoliosis, age-related calcification of the laryngeal and costal cartilages, or muscular spasm caused by a whiplash type of injury or a prolapsed cervical disc or just poor posture. These may all lead to abnormal or inefficient voicing techniques.

Examples of secondary musculoskeletal issues identified in the examination might include a high held larynx with tight suprahyoid musculature in certain patients with emotional issues; supraglottic hyperfunction and laryngeal guarding may be evident in certain patients with gastroesophageal reflux; and supraglottic hyperfunction in patients with vocal fold pathologies including palsy, bowing, and sulcus vocalis.

Considerable information can be gleaned from the manner in which the neck is held, the level and range of motion of the laryngeal cartilages, and the range of motion of the cricothyroid joint.[28] Limitation or restriction of movement can have a direct impact on performance and is discussed in greater detail elsewhere in this book. The thyroid gland should be palpated carefully for evidence of masses. Previous neck surgery could cause scar bands limiting laryngeal motion and thus have an impact upon the voice. This also needs investigation.[27]

The General ENT Examination

The ears, nose, and throat are examined routinely. This is well-covered elsewhere, but certainly, as with other patients, hearing loss should be looked for because of the danger of alteration of the perception of vocal production. A nasal examination will provide vital clues to the presence of allergy or rhinosinusitis, both of which can have an impact upon the voice. Similarly, a significant deviation of the septum can cause nasal obstruction and excessive dryness, affecting the laryngopharyngeal tract.

Examination of the mouth, oral cavity, and pharynx is directed toward investigation of the state of the mucous membranes. Dry mucous membranes could be a sign of dehydration, underlying systemic disorders (Sjogren's, etc.), or use of various drugs (antidepressants, diuretics, etc.). All these could have an impact upon the voice. The teeth should be examined for signs of wear facets suggestive of bruxism, an indication of excessive musculoskeletal tension.[27,29] The condition of the tongue is extremely important. Vitamin and mineral deficiencies, monilia, endocrinopathies, and so forth can all cause glossitis. The tonsils, pharynx, and palate need investigation for infectious processes, but also for more subtle abnormalities such as submucous cleft palate, post-tonsillectomy tethering, or various neurologic conditions. Findings in the nasopharynx such as adenoid obstruction or inflammation, Thornwaldt's cyst, postnasal drip, and so forth can all have an impact upon resonation of the voice.

The Laryngeal Examination

The laryngeal examination is well-covered elsewhere in this book. From the perspective of most performers, it will be expected that some type of permanent laryngeal recording will be made and that they will be able to review it with the laryngologist. At the time of this writing, we still find stroboscopy with a rigid 70° telescope to be satisfactory for viewing the larynx in most performers; the flexible fiberoptic nasendoscope is available for those with active gag reflex and/or severe supraglottic hyperfunction, or when dynamic voice evaluation is indicated to assess vocal fold motion and laryngeal and vocal tract posture during speech and song.

We find the review of the video with the performer to be extremely useful on the following levels:

1. Educational. It allows the performer to better understand the anatomy of his larynx and the effects of the pathology on it.

2. Assurance. It allows the performer to see that there is or is not any obvious pathology (both of which at times can be reassuring), and to see the effects that the nonsurgical or surgical treatment plan has had.

3. Involvement. It helps the performer to feel that he is becoming involved in his treatment plan, while at the same time helping him to focus on the mucosal or musculoskeletal issue(s) that have been identified by the laryngologist.

LABORATORY ANALYSIS

This is well-covered in another chapter of this book. It should include measures of aerodynamics and of acoustics. These objective findings can then be used during voice therapy or after surgery as markers of improvement.

SPECIAL CONSIDERATIONS

Environmental Factors

The modern performer or public speaker finds himself going from city to city usually by jet plane, often with climatic changes in humidity and temperature, and then staying in air-conditioned rooms. The humidity in most airplanes is around 8%[8] and the air is recirculated, unavoidably containing irritants. Finkelhor, et al have demonstrated in an in vitro model, that vocal folds that are dehydrated have a higher threshold of oscillation.[30] Furthermore, dry vocal folds are incapable of fine glottic approximation.[25]

The locale itself can be problematic. A performer used to low altitudes may have considerable difficulties in cities at very high altitudes, such as Mexico City or Denver. The smog in Los Angeles could act as a further irritant.

Popular music performers, stand-up comics, and so forth, frequently find themselves in smoke-filled rooms with poor acoustics and considerable background noise. This can be particularly problematic if the performer does not have adequate feedback and has difficulty monitoring the level of his voice. This latter problem is exacerbated in an outdoor arena without acoustic reverberation. It is possible for singers to train themselves to appreciate the loudness of their voice from internal vibrations and signals. This can be voice-saving in many circumstances and should be encouraged.

In order to maintain humidification when traveling, the performer should carry with him a humidifier, take long showers, or run hot water to create steam. The professional voice user must also make an effort to drink enough water and adequately hydrate; special care should be taken on long plane trips. A good rule of thumb is that adequate hydration is attained when the urine is consistently pale in color.

Allergy

Allergy is a common problem worldwide. About 20% of the population of the United States suffer from allergic disease.[31] The topic is too complex to go into in any depth in the context of this chapter; however, it is of great importance to the performer. Even mild allergies can be problematic for professional voice users because of their effect on mucous and the mucosal cover layer. Symptoms may include lower respiratory manifestations, including the worsening of asthma. Upper respiratory manifestations might include blocked nose, rhinorrhea (watery nasal discharge), watery and itchy eyes, and a scratchy throat with the tendency to throat clear.

They may cause vocal fatigue or voice breaks. Swollen nasal turbinates could also have an adverse impact on resonation, creating a blocked hypernasal sound.[31]

A recent study has also incriminated allergy as a potential cofactor in the development of laryngeal pathologies. It appears that hypersensitivity to different inhalatory and nutritional allergies may make the laryngeal mucosa more susceptible to the adverse effects of other factors, including vocal misuse, smoking, gastroesophageal reflux, and environmental irritants.[32]

Infectious Disorders

Professional voice users tend, as a group, to interact frequently with the general public. Thus, they are exposed repeatedly to viral exanthems. During the prodromal phase of a viral upper respiratory infection, with symptoms of malaise, congestion, and irritation, the performer can usually continue to work, provided there is no laryngeal involvement. Once the viral syndrome progresses to laryngeal inflammation, or swelling of the vocal folds with associated hoarseness, cancellation of the performance should be considered. Use of a local nasal decongestant sprayed through the mouth onto the vocal folds to facilitate an essential performance in a public speaker or an actor has been suggested.[8] We are opposed to this, because of the drying effects of the sympathomimetic on the laryngeal surface and the supplying glands. Cortisone should be used in the acute course of a viral illness only under extreme circumstances.

Severe influenza associated with fevers and chills is an obvious reason to cancel a performance. Air travel can exacerbate the condition, leading to hemorrhage into a sinus or middle ear space; it must be closely monitored. Prolongation of nasal symptoms must be aggressively investigated for sinusitis and treated as appropriate.

Exudative pharyngitis or bronchitis should be treated with a course of antibiotics. A culture should be taken prior to beginning treatment.

All cases of upper respiratory infection require lubrication of the laryngopharynx, including increased fluid intake, mucus thinning, and the maintenance of appropriate levels of humidification.

A prolonged postviral cough is not uncommon and can be damaging to the epithelium of the vocal folds. A nonsedating cough suppressant may well be appropriate.

Medications

This chapter only outlines this enormous problem as there is a comprehensive description of medications and their effects on the voice elsewhere in this book.

Commonly Abused Medications

Use of over-the-counter medication or prescription-only medication without adequate medical supervision is common among vocal performers. Among the medications most commonly overused, aspirin and non-steroidal anti-inflammatories undoubtedly lead the list. Overuse of either can lead to gastritis and increase the likelihood of vocal fold hemorrhage in the stressed performer who is over-rehearsing or performing. This can be a problem of particular significance in the immediate premenstrual and early menstrual period because of increased capillary fragility. Frequently the performer will not even be aware that the product being used (for example Alka Seltzer Plus) contains aspirin. Patient education is essential.

Corticosteroids

Corticosteroids have the potential for abuse. Among the majority of professional voice users, there is a general lack of understanding of some of the potential side effects, including immunosuppression, elevation in blood sugar, adrenal suppression, loss of bone density, and so forth.

However, there is a place for systemic steroids in the armamentarium of the laryngologist. A short course, in the face of laryngeal edema brought on by voice abuse, can save a performance. When prescribed in pill form, it can be given in descending dosages through a medrol (methylprednisone) dose pack or low dose prednisone (5 tablets of 5 mg each) decreased daily by 5 mg decrements.[8] When administered in such a manner, the course is generally well tolerated with few side effects (it should not be administered during pregnancy except under very extenuating circumstances, following a frank discussion of risk/benefit with the patient and in consultation with the patient's obstetrician). The most commonly reported side effect is mild insomnia. We generally prescribe an antacid concomitantly, as prednisone can also irritate the stomach lining.

Antibiotics

Performers believe that "the show must go on," and consequently are apt to perform while ill. They will often seek medical attention, however, from physicians who are unaware of their medical history, but aware that much is riding on the performance. Thus, they may rapidly develop a small pharmacopeia including a variety of antibiotics.

Antibiotics can cause serious side effects, not the least being nausea, gastritis, vaginitis, and fungal pharyngitis. While there are clear indications for antibiotics, they should only be prescribed if an appropriate culture is obtained and, most importantly, if appropriate follow-up is arranged.

Antihistamines

Antihistamines are necessary in the treatment of severe environmental allergies, but they tend to be over-prescribed and can have side effects, several of which affect voice production. Many cause sleepiness and/or decrease alertness. Some of the agents that do not cross the blood-brain barrier have other cardio-sensitizing effects with the possibility of arrhythmias. The side effect that does relate to voice production is the thickening of mucous secretions. The laryngopharyngeal tract can suffer from excessive drying, especially if the agent is used in association with an alpha-adrenergic agent.

Sprays and Gargles

Nasal sprays must be used with caution. Alpha-adrenergic sprays all have the potential for rebound stuffiness. They should only be used for a maximum of three days.

Steroid-containing nasal sprays can be helpful in breaking up the rebound effect of alpha-adrenergic sprays or in the treatment of allergic rhinitis. The addition of cromolyn as a mast cell stabilizer may be efficacious. The cortisone nasal sprays can dry the nasal membranes possibly leading to epistaxis. Saline nasal spray is also helpful in cleansing purulent or tenacious postnasal drip.

Over-the-counter throat lozenges are frequently used by the voice patient. The laryngologist should recommend lozenges without medication. Lozenges that are gelatinous without medication will help lubricate the throat.

All laryngeal sprays can cause dangerous reactions; oily glycerine sprays can lead to lipoid pneumonia. Corticosteroid containing sprays have a well-researched and accepted role in management of asthma in children and adults. They have also been used by performers in the form of an aerosol in order to reduce laryngeal edema. We are opposed to such an application. Inhaled steroid use can be associated with the development of fungal pharyngitis. It is also conceivable that cortisone aerosols may alter the viscosity of the mucus secreted onto the vocal folds and thereby have a deleterious effect on the voice or, over time, they may cause vocal fold changes and/or atrophy.[33]

Anesthetic sprays and gargles are not infrequently passed from one cast member to another on opening night. The problem with these agents is that, to be effective, they must anesthetize the vocal apparatus. When this occurs, the singer (or public speaker) loses vital neural feedback and has a tendency to overuse the voice with the potential for damage and even vocal hemorrhage.

Agents that have been used to increase or thin mucus flow include guaifenesin, products containing iodine or potassium, mists with propylene glycol, and so forth, but we only recommend the former. Adequate hydration is the surest and safest way to decrease tenacious secretions. Even this has certain risks: large quantities of water drunk rapidly can increase the likelihood of reflux or even cause hyponatremia. Common sense is necessary.

Stress and Anxiety

The voice has an essential role in communication of the "self."[34] It has been called the mirror of the soul.[35] In many ways, it is the barometer of the emotions; it changes with every emotion such that a single spoken word or phrase can express joy, love, happiness, fear, hatred, or misery. In the singer, performance anxiety sometimes presents in the form of increased vibrato. In the public speaker, it can present as sudden dryness of the throat, a need to clear the throat, tightness of the throat with pitch breaks, and loss of dynamic range.

Almost all performers suffer from performance anxiety. Thus, a variety of remedies many of which have already been alluded to, have been attempted. Anxiolytics are mentioned only to be condemned; the risks of anesthetic sprays outweigh the benefits.

Beta-blockers will prevent many of the signs of preperformance anxiety, including maintenance of a slow regular pulse. Most voice specialists do not recommend the use of these agents on the basis that: 1) they have many potential complications, including hypotension, thrombocytopenic purpura, depression, exacerbation of certain pulmonary conditions, and so forth; 2) they can be dangerous, causing rebound hypertension if stopped precipitously; and 3) many performers use their anxiety to produce a world class performance, whereas with beta-blockers they would have a steady but lackluster performance.

Antacids taken about 1/2 hour prior to performance may prevent some of the concomitant hyperacidity associated with preperformance anxiety. They may, however, also cause a slight dryness of the mouth, which could be deleterious.

In some individuals, there is a tendency toward shallow or decreased respirations as part of preperformance anxiety. In these instances, two or three voiced yawn-sighs can prove beneficial. Not only will they (slightly) raise oxygen saturation and lower CO_2 levels, the act of yawning will also help release tightened and held muscles in the neck and lower the level of the larynx. However, it must be emphasized that repetitive deep breathing could

bring about hyperventilation and carry with it its own side effects. Again, common sense is required.

Overall, regular coaching, adequate preparation, and appropriate warm-up exercises remain the cornerstone to manage this problem.

The laryngologist must determine how much of a problem the anxiety is. Crescendoing anxiety or inability to perform in public without the benefit of medications, in a professional who spends most of his life in the public eye, could be a sign of an underlying psychologic disturbance, which requires professional guidance.[29]

Reflux Pharyngolaryngitis

Reflux is another problem commonplace among professional voice users. The reader is referred to the chapter by Koufman in this book (Chapter 24) for detailed information. In 1991, Sataloff reported reflux laryngitis in 45% of consecutive professional voice users.[36] Generalized symptoms include chronic cough, belching, throat clearing, throat pain, catarrh, and intermittent hoarseness, often improving as the day progresses. Frequently in the performer the condition is so chronic that he is totally unaware of the symptoms. It is also not uncommon for the performer to suffer from reflux only while singing and particularly while performing.

Symptoms may be brought on or exacerbated by weight lifting or abdominal workouts, or by a change in diet.

Should the laryngologist have his/her suspicions aroused to the possibility of reflux during the examination (arytenoid edema, etc), a course of H2 blockers, or proton pump inhibitors could be commenced without definitive proof. Apples, red wine, caffeine, chocolate, and highly spiced food should be stopped and an anti-reflux regimen begun. Modified barium swallow, cine-esophagram or endoscopy may be useful to identify reflux and/or related pathology. At the time of this writing, the gold standard in quantification of laryngo-pharyngeal reflux is pH monitoring, but its sensitivity and specificity are not 100%.[37]

Patient education in relation to diet and lifestyle and participation in the management of this disorder is of particular importance.

Vocal Abuse/Misuse

Vocal abuse, either of the singing or of the speaking voice, is not uncommon in the performer.

Vocal Abuse/Misuse When Singing

Vocal abuse/misuse in professional singers can occur in many forms. Singers in the two extremes of their careers have a tendency to try to overextend their vocal limits. There is a particular problem in choral masters asking children to perform work too difficult for their vocal ages.[38,39] The older performer is susceptible to the risk of accepting roles no longer suited for his voice. In all performers, there is always the possibility of inadequate time for preparation for a particular role. To make up for this, the performer is likely to over-rehearse just before the performance.

Professional performers generally have very high work ethic. This can lead to the unwise decision by the performer to perform when not at peak, when suffering from an upper respiratory ailment, and so forth. Among popular music singers, there is a tendency to color the voice. This vocal coloration may become a part of the performer's signature and be necessary for vocal recognition by the public, but may well lead to chronic irritation of the vocal folds. Musical theater has become the mainstay of Broadway and the West End. Belting is perhaps more effortful than operatic style, and may be required while on skates, in the air, and so forth. Performing in eight shows a week can represent a significant stressor for the performer's larynx, particularly if the performer is not at peak.

The role of the laryngologist is to diagnose the underlying problem, and determine how serious it is with relation not only to any upcoming performance but also to the performer's career. The laryngologist must make up his/her own mind on a case by case basis as to whether the performer can perform as is, or needs to cancel. He/she must also make certain that the performer is working closely with an appropriate singing and/or voice teacher. A close working relationship with a speech-language pathologist with a special interest in voice may be of great benefit to the performer.

Regarding general guidelines, the laryngologist should have a relatively low index for suggesting cancellation for an established performer. It is the crucial or critical performance, especially in the young or not-yet-established performer, which requires the greatest deliberation. If there is sufficient time (several days) prior to the performance, voice rest in association with aggressive humidification and medical management may save the performance. It is not sufficient to let the performer state that he will "mark" the rehearsals, as what "marking" means can vary extensively from performer to performer; and some forms of "marking" (for example, whispering) may actually be detrimental. It must be recalled that it is the overall health of the performer and his future professional life that must be considered first and foremost.

Vocal Abuse/Misuse When Speaking

It is not uncommon for a professional trained in singing to have no training in speaking. Similarly, it is the rule rather than the exception for public speakers to have little or no formal training in speaking. Often a public speaker such as a political candidate on the campaign trail will assume that he can project his voice or shout without proper training. Such public speakers may get away with the abuse for a time, but it will eventually catch up with them. For an actor, however, the most common cause of voice abuse is too much rehearsal, frequently in a dry environment.

Koufman classified one type of speaking-voice abuse seen among professional voice users as the "Bogart-Bacall" syndrome; he found it in 26% of his patients with functional voice disorders.[40] The patient speaks with a very low fundamental frequency, frequently at the lowest note of his pitch range. The use of an unnaturally low fundamental frequency for too long or at high intensities can lead to the formation of vocal fold nodules.

The laryngologist needs to have close interaction with a singing-voice teacher or speech-language pathologist in these conditions. Refer to the chapters by Murry and Rosen or Carroll (Chapters 31, 32) in this book for further information.

Musculoskeletal Pathologies

Musculoskeletal and postural issues are frequently part of the process leading to voice disorders. A neck held in a hyperextended hyperlordotic position, a cervicodorsal shelf, or head tilt are commonplace among the general population. Limitation of motion of the cricothyroid joints with contraction of the cricothyroid muscle, or tenderness of the muscles that attach to the lateral body of the hyoid bone may also be found during the examination. These are amenable to intervention by an osteopath or physical therapist.

Tension Fatigue

This is one type of musculoskeletal voice disorder that is seen particularly in the hard-driving vocal professional. The patient presents with dysphonia, vocal fatigue, and pain upon phonation. This was the most common finding among patients with functional voice disorders in Koufman's series.[40] It is somewhat less common among trained singers and actors, but more common among other professional voice users.

The condition is characterized by poor breath control and excessive muscular tension in the neck and base of tongue musculature.[40] The jaw is frequently held in a rigid position, the sternocleidomastoid and trapezius muscles are tight, and the base of tongue musculature is contracted and frequently in spasm. These patients also suffer from other musculoskeletal tension syndromes, for example, tension headache, temporal mandibular joint syndrome, bruxism, and so forth. The vocal quality is often strained and harsh and pitch range is limited. There are frequently hard glottal attacks.

As most of these patients will not have voice coaches, a speaking-voice teacher will need to be consulted and relaxation techniques instituted (see the chapter by Carroll).

DISCRETE VOCAL FOLD PATHOLOGY

These pathologic conditions are well-covered elsewhere in this book and we will not belabor them. From the standpoint of the professional voice user, the key issues surrounding management of these vocal abuse pathologies include:

1. The etiology of the pathology
2. The effect on the voice
3. The risks versus benefits of the treatment plan chosen (particularly from the standpoint of time off work and upcoming commitments)
4. The effects on the professional voice user's career

The Etiology of the Pathology

If prenodular edema or early nodules have been identified in the performer working in eight shows per week over the last six months, and the performer anticipates being in the production for the forseeable future, the treatment plan may well need to differ from a performer who has been over rehearsing for a single upcoming performance.

An example of the latter is as follows: a young professional voice user who was preparing for a singing competition presented to one of the authors six days prior to the competition, with the ultimate diagnosis of prenodular edema, secondary to over-rehearsing and reflux. The treatment plan included relative voice rest and an anti-reflux program. The performer went on to perform credibly in the competition.

The Effect of the Pathology on the Voice

The effects of prenodular edema or early Reinke's edema may well be devastating to the voice of a performer specializing in early music. In a performer specializing in Country and Western, "R & B," or rap, it may actually be contributory to that performer's vocal signature.

An example of the latter is a self-trained "rap" singer. He was currently preparing a recording and the recording company was concerned about an increase in the gravelly quality of his voice. A previous recording confirmed the characteristics of his vocal signature.

Laryngeal examination demonstrated Reinke's edema, supraglottic hyperfunction, and reflux. The laryngologist referred him to a speech-language pathologist and commenced an anti-reflux program. The performer felt that his voice returned to its previous state, without change in his underlying vocal signature, enabling him to fulfill his contractual obligations and finish the recording.

The Risks Versus Benefits of the Treatment Plan Chosen (particularly from the standpoint of time off work and upcoming commitments)

As an example, one of the authors treated a performer in a musical theater production who was found to have a vocal polyp, which was causing some difficulty with his upper range, but which he was more or less able to "sing around." At the time of assessment he only had a few more weeks in his current role, but was to start in a new production two months thereafter. The treatment plan, after considerable discussion with him, was for the performer to start working with a speech-language pathologist immediately, and once the production completed to undergo surgical removal of the polyp followed by close and careful rehabilitation. His larynx was stabilized and his voice was fine by the beginning of the next production.

The Effect of the Pathology and its Management on the Professional Voice User's Career

This is, of course, the ultimate consideration and is not always straightforward to answer.

One of the authors saw a professional voice user who presented with a granuloma of the arytenoid process, which had recurred following surgery. It was having an impact upon vocal stamina, and thus placed the patient's career in jeopardy. Reflux management in combination with intensive work with a speech-language pathologist was initiated, but did not bring about significant improvement immediately. The granuloma responded to this therapeutic intervention, but only over a course of several months, during which time the performer's career was placed on hold.

VOCAL FOLD HEMORRHAGE

Vocal fold hemorrhage occurs in the submucosal layer, causing severe hoarseness and swelling. It is frequently precipitated by a cough, shout, or scream, especially in a patient on aspirin or nonsteroidal analgesics. Management is usually medical; it should be considered a laryngologic emergency. Management requires strict voice rest, for up to 2 weeks (or until it resolves), generally with total resorption of the hemorrhage. However, there are exceptions, and early surgical evacuation may be appropriate in rare cases.[41] It is not infrequent for the patient to be left with a prominent vessel on the vocal fold, which could rebleed at a later time, especially during times of vessel fragility. An example of this is at the beginning of the menstrual cycle. If necessary, a decision can be made to treat the vessel surgically if it continues to rebleed.

From the standpoint of the performer, the key issue is to get him to understand the potential risks of continuing to perform with the hemorrhage, and thus to get him to accept the relatively prolonged period of voice rest followed by vocal restriction that is usually necessary.

NON-LARYNGEAL SURGERY

There are certain issues of particular importance in non-laryngeal surgery on performers that shall be presented here. First and foremost, it is important that the surgeon and anesthesiologist be aware that the patient is a performer. This information will generally heighten their level of care for the airway and soft tissues.

Following surgery, the performer should refrain from performing too soon, particularly after any surgery that may affect the production of the voice. This includes abdominal, pelvic, back, and thoracic surgeries.

There may well be a role for the performer to seek rehabilitation from a physiotherapist or voice teacher following such surgery to make certain that he is recovering properly.

Surgery on the neck frequently involves manipulation of the strap muscles. The surgeon should make an effort not to divide or denervate the strap muscles in this patient population because of their importance in controlling vertical laryngeal position and stabilizing the larynx. When operating on the thyroid, he should be aware of the needs of the patient and be particularly careful regarding the superior laryngeal as well as the recurrent laryngeal nerves. When operating on the upper neck, particular caution must be taken with the marginal mandibular nerve and the platysma muscle. Division of the former or imprecise resuture of the latter could affect the ability of the performer to use the depressors of the lower lip with a negative impact on voice production.

Indications for tonsillectomy or uvulopalatopharyngoplasty are the same as for the general public. However, the performer must be aware that both procedures can cause scarring and will change the shape of the pharynx. These changes may affect resonation, with resultant changes of tone. Both these procedures must be considered carefully and thoughtfully by all parties prior to surgery.

Indications for nasal surgery do not differ in the professional voice user from other people. Nasal obstruction caused by deviated nasal septum leading to recurrent episodes of acute sinusitis is such an indication. The voice professional should not expect improvement in the singing voice. An awareness of a possible change in the voice is necessary.

VOICE REST

Voice rest is reserved for cases exhibiting severe mucosal redness and swelling, hemorrhage, or mucosal breaks. It is also prescribed at times for instances of aggravation of previously present vocal pathology. It is rarely necessary to prescribe absolute voice rest for more then three days. Acute vocal hemorrhage is the one instance where it should be extended for up to two weeks. Complete voice rest means, as it suggests, no use of the voice for communication. Whispering may be more traumatic to the larynx than speaking. This differs from restrictive voice use, which may be recommended by certain laryngologists following laryngeal surgery. Others recommend complete voice rest after laryngeal surgery, for up to two weeks.

SUMMARY

Professional voice users as a group have special needs, the foremost being that their voice is crucial to their career. They should be referred to the subspecialist who has been trained in management of the particular ailments from which this group suffers. The laryngologist caring for these patients must be prepared to put aside the requisite time necessary to obtain an adequate history and physical examination. He or she should also have access to a large interdisciplinary body of specialists, including a speech-language pathologist, voice coach, singing voice specialist, osteopath or physiotherapist, gastroenterologist, pulmonologist, neurologist, psychiatrist or psychologist, endocrinologist, and so forth to help in management of the frequently complex problems presented.

The role of the laryngologist is a demanding one. He/she must be able to make the correct diagnosis and initiate an appropriate treatment plan. The laryngologist must also be sensitive to the career needs of this group, but be able to put their health over any immediate performance problem.

REFERENCES

1. Mitchell SA. The professional speaking voice. In: Benninger MS, Jacobson BH, Johnson AF, eds. *Vocal Arts Medicine: The Care and Prevention of Professional Voice Disorders*. New York, NY; Thieme Medical Publishers; 1994:167-176.

2. Rubin JS. Treatment of voice disorders. *Cortlandt Forum*. 1993;6(7):123-126.

3. Dickson DR, Maue-Dickson W. *Anatomical and Physiological Bases of Speech*. Boston, MA: Little, Brown and Co; 1982.

4. Bunch MA. *Dynamics of the Singing Voice*. 3rd ed. Wien: Springer-Verlag; 1995.

5. Rubin JS. Mechanisms of respiration (the bellows). In: Harris T, Harris S, Rubin JS, Howard DM, eds. *The Voice Clinic Handbook*. London, England: Whurr Publishers Ltd; 1998:49-63.

6. Scherer RC. Laryngeal function during phonation. In: Rubin JS, Sataloff RT, Korovin GK, Gould WJ, eds. *Diagnosis and Treatment of Voice Disorders*. New York, NY: Igaku-Shoin; 1995:86-104.

7. Baken RJ. An overview of laryngeal function for voice production. In: Sataloff RT, ed. *Professional Voice, Science and Art of Clinical Care*. 2nd ed. San Diego, CA: Singular Publishing Group; 1997:147-166.

8. Gould WJ. Caring for the vocal professional. In: Paparella MM, Shumrick DA, Gluckman JL, et al, eds. *Otolaryngology*. 3rd ed. Philadelphia, PA: W. B. Saunders; 1991:2273-2288.

9. Colton RH. Physiology of phonation. In: Benninger MS, Jacobson BH, Johnson AF, eds. *Vocal Arts Medicine : The Care and Prevention of Professional Voice Disorders*. New York, NY: Thieme Medical Publishers; 1994:30-60.

10. Perlman AL, Titze IR, Cooper DS. Elasticity of canine vocal fold tissue. *J Speech Hear Res*. 1984;27:212-219.

11. Titze I, Durham P. Passive mechanisms influencing fundamental frequency control. In: Baer T, Sasaki C, Harris K, eds. *Laryngeal Function in Phonation and Respiration*. San Diego, CA: College-Hill Press; 1986:304-319.

12. Hollien H, Colton R: Four laminagraphic studies of vocal fold thickness. *Folia Phoniatr*. 1969;21:179-198.

13. Hollien H. Vocal fold thickness and fundamental frequency of phonation. *J Speech Hear Res*. 1962;5:237-243.

14. Hollien H, Coleman RF. Laryngeal correlates of frequency change: a STROL study. *J Speech Hear Res*. 1970;12:272-278.

15. Titze I. On the mechanics of vocal fold vibration. *J Acoustic Soc Am*. 1976;60:1366-1380.

16. Titze I. Comments on the myoelastic-aerodynamic theory of phonation. *J Speech Hear Res*. 1980;23:495-510.

17. Sundberg J. Vocal tract resonance. In: Sataloff RT, ed. *Professional Voice, Science and Art of Clinical Care*. 2nd ed. San Diego, CA: Singular Publishing Group; 1997:167-184.

18. Carpenter B. Psychological aspects of vocal fold surgery. In: Gould WJ, Sataloff RT, Spiegel JR, eds. *Voice Surgery*. St. Louis, MO: Mosby; 1993:339-343.

19. Sataloff RT, Spiegel JR. Care of the professional voice. *Otolaryngol Clin North Am*. 1991;24:1093-1124.

20. Sanada T, Tanaka S, Hibi S, et al. Relationship between the degree of lesion and that of vocal dysfunction in vocal fold polyp. *Nippon Jibiinkoka Gakkai Kaiho*. 1990;93:388-392.

21. Bennett S, Bishop S, Lumpkin SMM. Phonatory characteristics associated with bilateral diffuse polypoid degeneration. *Laryngoscope*. 1987;97: 446-450.

22. Tucker HM, Lavertu P. Paralysis and paresis of the vocal folds. In: Blitzer A, Brin MF, Sasaki CT, et al. *Neurologic Disorders of the Larynx*. New York, NY: Thieme Medical Publishers; 1992:182-189.

23. Sataloff RT, Mandel S, Rosen DC. Neurologic disorders affecting the voice in performance. In: Sataloff RT, ed. *Professional Voice: Science and Art of Clinical Care*. 2nd ed. San Diego, CA: Singular Publishing Group; 1997:479-498.

24. Colton RH, Jasper JK. Voice problems associated with nervous system involvement. In: *Understanding Voice Problems: A Physiological Perspective for Diagnosis and Treatment*. Baltimore, MD: Williams & Wilkins; 1990:107-150.

25. Jahn AF, Davies, DG. A clinical approach to the professional voice. In: Blitzer A, Brin MF, Sasaki CT, et al. *Neurologic Disorders of the Larynx*. New York, NY: Thieme Medical Publishers; 1992:149-162.

26. Sataloff RT, Spiegel JR, Hawkshaw M. The history. In: Gould WJ, Sataloff RT, Spiegel JR, eds. *Voice Surgery*. St. Louis, MO: Mosby; 1993:173-188.

27. Sataloff RT. Physical examination. In: Sataloff RT, ed. *Professional Voice: Science and Art of Clinical Care*. New York, NY: Raven Press; 1991:91-100.

28. Rubin JS, Lieberman J, Harris TM. Laryngeal manipulation. *Otolaryngol Clin North Am*. 2000;33:1017-1034.

29. Sataloff RT. Stress, anxiety, and psychogenic dysphonia. In: Sataloff RT, ed. *Professional Voice: Science and Art of Clinical Care*. New York, NY: Raven Press; 1991:195-200.

30. Finkelhor BK, Titze IR, Durham PL. The effect of viscosity changes in the vocal folds on the range of oscultation. *J Voice*. 1988;1:320-325.

31. Cohn JR, Spiegel JR, Hawkshaw M, Sataloff RT. Allergy. In: Sataloff RT, ed. *Professional Voice: Science and Art of Clinical Care*. 2nd ed. San Diego, CA: Singular Publishing Group; 1997:369-373.

32. Hocevar-Boltezar I, Radsel Z, Zargi M. The role of allergy in the etiogenesis of laryngeal mucosal lesions. *Acta Otolaryngol (Stockh)*. 1997;527 (suppl):134-137.

33. Lavy JA, Wood G, Rubin JS, Harries M. Dysphonia associated with inhaled steroids. *J Voice*. 2000;14:581-588.

34. Rosen DC, Sataloff RT. Psychological aspects of voice disorders. In: Sataloff RT, ed. *Professional Voice: Science and Art of Clinical Care*. 2nd ed. San Diego, CA: Singular Publishing Group; 1997:305-318.

35. Aronson A. *Clinical Voice Disorders*. 3rd ed. New York, NY: Thieme Medical Publishers; 1990:117-145.

36. Sataloff RT, Spiegel JR, Hawkshaw MJ. Strobovideolaryngoscopy: results and clinical value. *Ann Otol Rhinol Laryngol*. 1991;100:725-727.

37. Sataloff RT, Castell DO, Katz PO, Sataloff DM. *Reflux Laryngitis and Related Disorders*. San Diego, CA: Singular Publishing Group; 1999:55-67.

38. Sataloff RT. The effects of age on the voice. In: Sataloff RT, ed. *Professional Voice: Science and Art of Clinical Care*. New York, NY: Raven Press; 1991:141-151.

39. Sataloff RT, Spiegel J, Rosen DC. The effects of age on the voice. In: Sataloff RT, ed. *Professional Voice: Science and Art of Clinical Care*. 2nd ed. San Diego, CA: Singular Publishing Group; 1997:259-268.

40. Koufman J, Blalock O. Functional voice disorders. *Otolaryngol Clin North Am*. 1991;24(5):1059-1073.

41. Spiegel JR, Sataloff RT, Hawkshaw M, Rosen DC. Vocal fold hemorrhage. In: Sataloff RT, ed. Professional Voice: Science and Art of Clinical Care. 2nd ed. San Diego, CA: Singular Publication Group; 1997:541-554.

CHAPTER 35

Laryngotracheal Trauma

Yolanda D. Heman-Ackah, MD

Vijay Rao, MD

George S. Goding, Jr., MD

The incidence of laryngotracheal trauma is estimated to be 1 in 14,000-30,000 emergency department visits in the United States.[1,2] Trauma to the laryngotracheal complex can be classified as blunt, penetrating, caustic, thermal, and iatrogenic injuries. The morbidity associated with these injuries ranges from chronic airway obstruction to voice compromise, with complication rates as high as 15-25%.[3-5] Because of their potential for airway compromise, these injuries can be lethal, with mortality rates of 2-15%.[3,5] Injuries to the larynx and trachea often accompany other severe injuries, and the neck can appear to be deceptively normal even in cases of serious laryngotracheal disruption.

BLUNT INJURY

Blunt injury to the larynx and trachea is the most common cause of laryngotracheal injury in the United States today, accounting for 60% of all injuries to the laryngotracheal complex.[2,4] These injuries result from motor vehicle collisions in the adult population and from accidents involving all-terrain vehicles, bicycles, contact sports, and hanging type injuries in the young adult, adolescent, and pediatric populations. Adults and children differ not only in the mechanisms of injury, but also in the types of injuries experienced. These differences can be accounted for, at least in part, by differences in the relative size, position, and degree of calcification of the larynx and trachea.

Adult Framework Injuries From Blunt Trauma

In the adult, the inferior border of the cricoid cartilage sits at the level of the 6th and 7th cervical vertebrae.[6] Thus, in the normal upright position, the larynx is relatively protected from trauma by the overhang of the mandible superiorly, the bony prominence of the clavicles and sternal manubrium inferiorly, and by the mass of the sternocleidomastoid muscles laterally. Laryngeal injuries are relatively rare except when there is a direct blow to the neck. The usual victim of laryngotracheal trauma in a motor vehicle collision is an unbelted front seat passenger or driver in a vehicle without protective airbags. Upon collision, the front seat passenger or driver is propelled forward with the neck in extension, eliminating the mandible as a protective shield. The laryngotracheal complex hits the dashboard or steering wheel with a posterior-superiorly based vector of force, and the thyroid and cricoid cartilages are crushed against the cervical vertebrae (Figure 35-1).[7,8] Direct blows to the larynx can also occur during athletic competition, while falling forward onto a blunt object, or with hanging of the neck from a suspended rope or wire.

A wide spectrum of predictable injuries occurs. The thyroid and cricoid cartilages interact dynamically to protect the airway from blunt injury.[8] Forces to the anterior larynx often are encountered first by the thyroid prominence, which bends against the cervical vertebrae on impact. The thyroid cartilage eventually reaches a

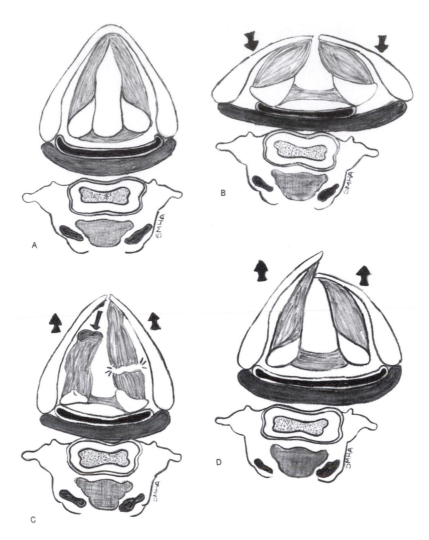

FIGURE 35-1. *Mechanism of blunt laryngeal trauma. (A) Normal laryngeal position; (B) Posteriorly directed force crushing thyroid ala against cervical vertebrae, resulting in a midline fracture; (C) Recovery of larynx from force resulting in detachment of the vocal ligament on the left, tear in the right thyroarytenoid muscle, and bilateral arytenoid dislocation; (D) Recovery of larynx from force resulting in overlapping, displaced thyroid lamina fracture and malposition of the vocal fold. (Courtesy of Yolanda D. Heman-Ackah, MD)*

point of maximal flexibility, and a single median or paramedian fracture occurs (Figure 35-2).

The force then impacts the cricoid ring, which was previously shielded by the anterior projection of the thyroid cartilage. In a patient with a marked laryngeal prominence, multiple fractures of the thyroid cartilage in both the vertical and horizontal planes may occur prior to the distribution of force onto the cricoid cartilage (Figure 35-3).[8] The cricoid has a relatively thin anterior arch that blends laterally into rigidly buttressed tubercles. Lower level impacts result in a single median fracture or multiple paramedian vertical fractures. The

airway is maintained by the lateral buttresses (Figure 35-4). With higher impact forces, secondary lateral arch fractures can occur in the cricoid cartilage, resulting in airway collapse and possible injury to the recurrent laryngeal nerve caused by impingement at the level of the cricothyroid joint (Figures 35-5 and 35-6).

If the force is severe or low in the neck, complete laryngotracheal separation may occur.[9] Separation usually occurs between the cricoid cartilage and the first tracheal ring, resulting in displacement of the trachea inferiorly and soft tissue collapse into the airway, with consequent airway obstruction.[9-12] The strap muscula-

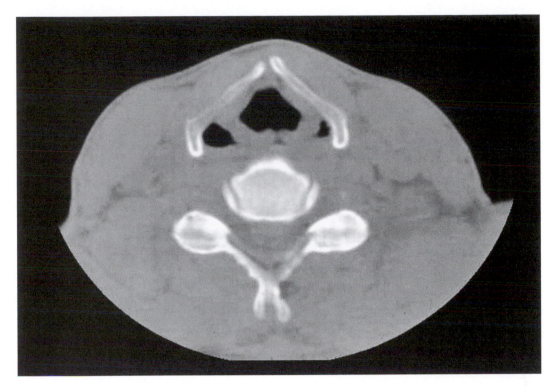

FIGURE 35-2. *Axial CT scan of the thyroid ala. There is a midline thyroid ala fracture with diastasis of fracture segments.*

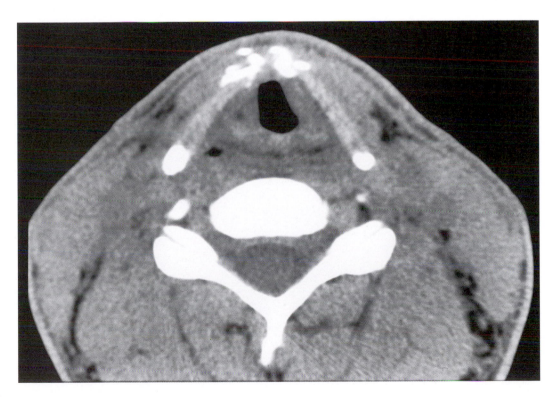

FIGURE 35-3. *Axial CT scan of the thyroid ala demonstrating an anterior comminuted thyroid ala fracture sustained by the patient in a motor vehicle collision.*

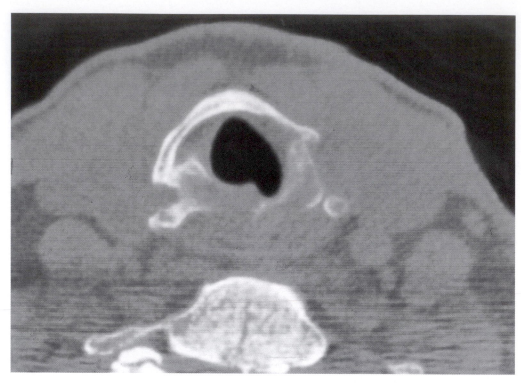

FIGURE 35-4. *Axial CT scan at the level of the thyroid and cricoid cartilages. There is a vertical, displaced posterior cricoid lamina fracture with fusion of the right cricothyroid joint. The airway is maintained by the lateral buttresses.*

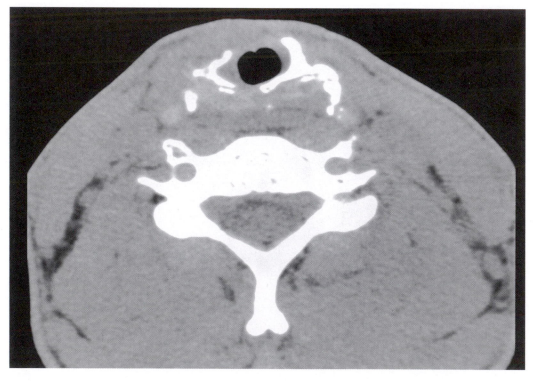

FIGURE 35-5. *Axial CT scan of the cricoid cartilage. The airway is narrowed secondary to anterior and posterior vertical, displaced cricoid lamina fractures.*

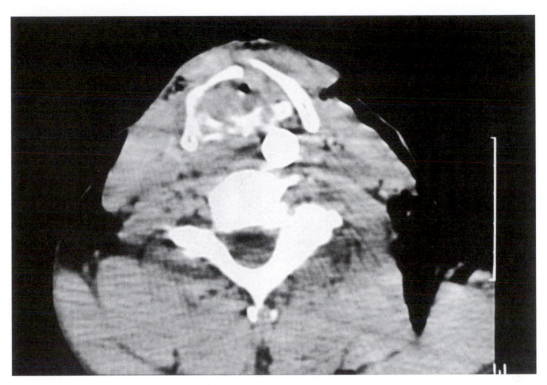

FIGURE 35-6. *Axial CT scan at the level of the thyroid and cricoid cartilages. There are midline and left lateral fractures of the thyroid ala and comminuted fractures of the posterior cricoid lamina with loss of the airway space. The airway was secured below the fracture segments with tracheotomy.*

ture and surrounding cervical fascia can serve as a temporary conduit for air until edema and hematoma formation result in obstruction of this temporary airway.

Pediatric Framework Injuries From Blunt Trauma

Fractures of the thyroid and cricoid cartilage from blunt trauma are uncommon in the pediatric population. The pediatric larynx sits higher in the neck than in the adult, and depending upon the age, can lie between the 2nd and 7th cervical vertebrae. The mandible serves more as a protective shield in the child than it does in the adult.[13] The greater elasticity of the pediatric cartilaginous framework makes it more resilient to external stresses, and the mobility of the supporting tissues tends to protect the laryngotracheal complex more effectively. Children are likely to sustain soft tissue injuries resulting in edema and hematoma formation.[12,13] This is of particular concern in a child because of the relatively smaller diameter of the pediatric airway.

The pediatric patient is more likely than the adult to sustain transection and telescoping injuries. An individual who falls onto the handlebar of the bicycle may suffer a telescoping injury in which the cricoid cartilage is dislocated superiorly underneath the thyroid lamina (Figure 35-7).[12-15] With more forceful blows, complete laryngotracheal separation may occur. The adolescent and young adult riding a snowmobile or an all-terrain vehicle may sustain a "clothes-line" type injury to the neck. Upon collision with the cable or wire, a horizontal, linear force is applied low in the neck, compressing the cricotracheal complex against the anterior cervical vertebrae and resulting in cricotracheal separation.[15] The elasticity of the intercartilaginous ligaments contributes to substernal retraction of the trachea. These are often fatal injuries, but occasionally there is enough fascial stenting to maintain an adequate airway until an artificial airway can be established. There may be an associated injury, and possibly transection of both recurrent laryngeal nerves, which are also compressed against the cervical vertebrae during the injury.[12,15]

Young children may accidentally hang themselves while playing, and adolescents may do so intentionally in suicide attempts. In these instances, the fall to hanging position is usually less than 1-2 feet. The rope around the neck tightens usually in the region of the thyrohyoid membrane, resulting in airway obstruction as the epiglottis closes over the glottis. The distinction between this and the injury that results from intentional

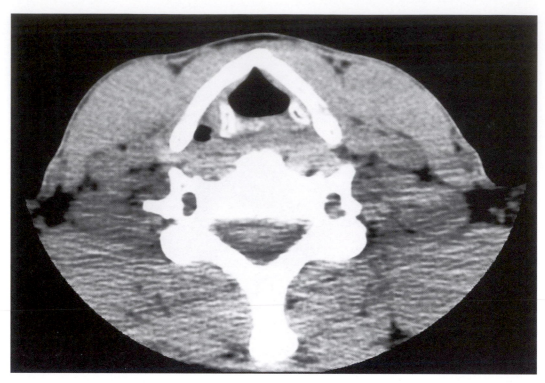

FIGURE 35-7. *Axial CT scan at the level of the thyroid and cricoid cartilages. There is subluxation of the cricoid cartilage under the thyroid ala after the patient sustained an elbow injury to the neck while playing basketball.*

hanging is that in accidental or self-inflicted injuries, death is not necessarily imminent; and, in those who survive, there is usually injury, possibly avulsion, at the level of the thyrohyoid membrane. In intentional hanging, the person is usually dropped a distance of several feet, resulting in death secondary to tracheal transection or spinal cord injury from C_1-C_2 dislocation.[15]

Soft Tissue Injuries From Blunt Trauma

Blunt trauma to the larynx may result in soft tissue injuries with or without associated framework injuries. Rupture of the thyroepiglottic ligament can be associated with either horizontal or vertical fractures of the thyroid cartilage. Narrowing of the laryngeal lumen can occur secondary to herniation of pre-epiglottic tissue or posterior displacement of the epiglottic petiole.[7,11]

Vocal fold injuries result from vertical fractures of the thyroid ala (Figure 35-1). As the thyroid cartilage snaps back from its compression against the cervical vertebrae, the thyroarytenoid muscle and ligament may tear, resulting in a separation at any point along its length. This may be evident as mucosal lacerations or hemorrhage of one or both vocal folds. The mucosa on the arytenoids may be denuded or avulsed. Because of

the traction on the arytenoids from this spring-like motion of the thyroid cartilage, they may also become displaced from the cricoarytenoid joint into a more posterior and lateral or anterior position (Figure 35-8). If one segment of the thyroid cartilage fails to return back to its normal position, an overlapping fracture may occur, resulting in malposition of the vocal fold (Figures 35-9 and 10). Lacerations of the pyriform sinus and upper esophagus may occur as the thyroid cartilage rubs against the cervical vertebrae.[7,11]

Soft tissue injuries associated with cricoid, tracheal, and cricotracheal separation injuries within the cartilaginous framework usually involve crushed or lacerated mucosa. Both recurrent laryngeal nerves are frequently injured and can be severed by blunt trauma that results in cricoid fractures and/or cricotracheal separation. The phrenic nerve can also be injured, especially in cases of cricotracheal separation.[7,9,11,12,15] Associated esophageal lacerations and perforations are common.

Assessment of Blunt Injuries

Initial evaluation and assessment of the blunt trauma patient is similar for adults and children. It is impor-

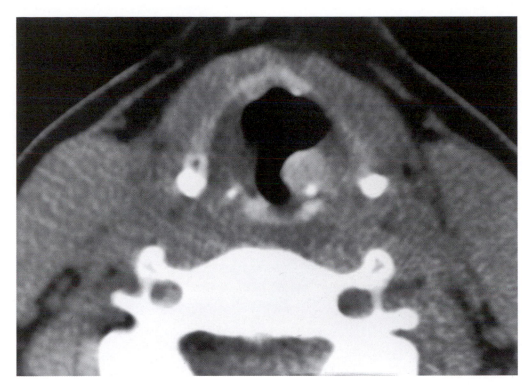

FIGURE 35-8. *Axial CT scan of the larynx at the level of the arytenoids demonstrating anterior dislocation of the right arytenoid cartilage.*

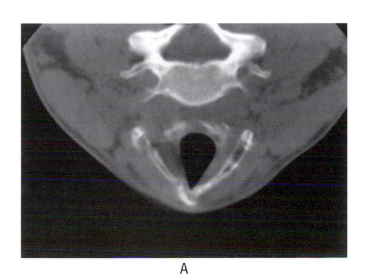

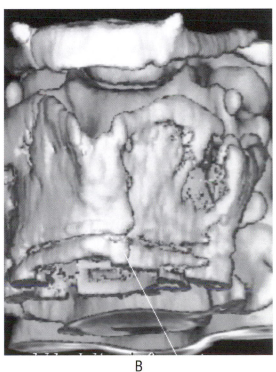

A   B

FIGURE 35-9. *(A) Axial CT scan of the subglottic larynx demonstrating a displaced, paramedian fracture of the left thyroid ala. (B) 3-dimensional CT reconstruction of the left paramedian thyroid ala fracture demonstrating overlapping of the fracture segments.*

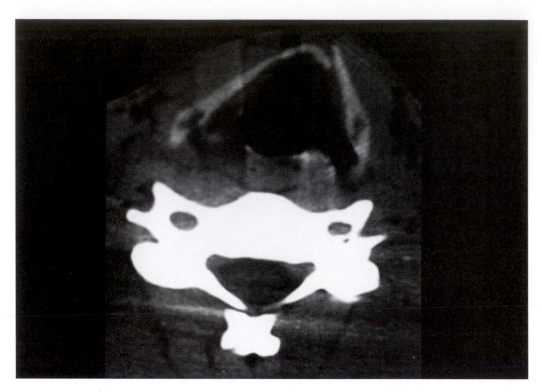

FIGURE 35-10. *Axial CT of the supraglottic larynx. There is a displaced paramedian fracture of the right thyroid ala.*

tant to obtain an understanding of the mechanism of injury. A high index of suspicion for blunt neck injury should be maintained in motor vehicle collisions, even without obvious external signs. Knowledge of the speed of the vehicle at the time of collision, the use of seatbelts by the trauma victim, and the presence and deployment of airbags can also be helpful in estimating the amount of force involved. In the patient with short stature, the force of deceleration against a locking "shoulder" strap that is draped over the neck may also produce significant injury. Assessment of the patient begins with evaluation and stabilization of the airway, paying particular attention to the status of the cervical spine. Assessment then proceeds with evaluation and stabilization of neurologic, cervical spine, cardiovascular, and other emergent organ system injuries. Management of aerodigestive tract injuries varies depending upon the presence of acute airway distress (Figure 35-11).

Evaluation of the Blunt Trauma Patient Without Airway Distress

In the patient without immediate signs of upper airway compromise, the evaluation can proceed with a complete examination, including palpation of the neck, assessment of voice quality, and flexible fiberoptic evaluation of the larynx and upper airway. Fiberoptic laryn-goscopy allows assessment of the mobility of the vocal folds, patency of the upper airway, and integrity of the mucosa. If there is an adequate airway, intubation is not necessary. Because of the potential for the development of worsening laryngeal edema and airway compromise, serial examinations of the airway should be performed during the first 24 to 48 hours after injury if intubation is initially deemed unnecessary.

Management is based on the severity of the initial signs and symptoms.[16]

Patients with any sign of endolaryngeal injury (Table 35-1) should have a thin cut (1 mm) computed tomography (CT) scan of the larynx with bone/cartilage windows to evaluate for possible laryngeal framework injury.[14,16,17] Minimally displaced fractures of the thyroid cartilage can be present with very mild endolaryngeal signs and should be evaluated to determine the likelihood of fracture stability. Table 35-2 lists CT findings that suggest fracture stability and instability.

Fractures that appear to have the potential for instability should be evaluated further with direct laryngoscopy and open exploration for repair. Patients with minimally displaced fractures that are associated with significant endolaryngeal injuries also require direct laryngoscopy, open exploration, and repair of the soft tissue injuries (Table 35-3). Because of the high potential for concomitant cervical spine injuries, assessment

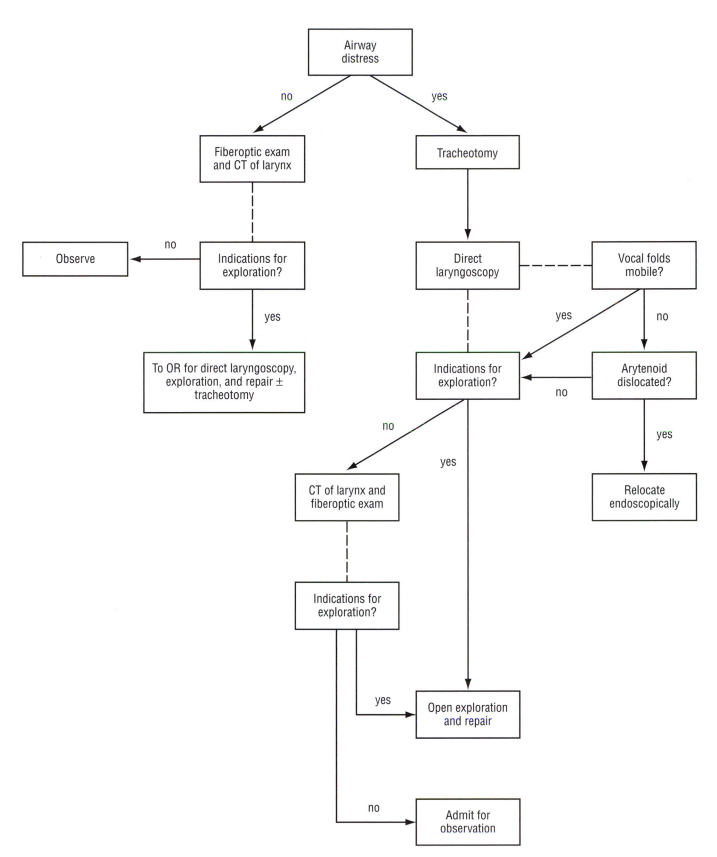

FIGURE 35-11. *Management of blunt laryngeal trauma.*

Hoarseness/dysphonia	Dyspnea
Stridor	Endolaryngeal edema
Endolaryngeal hematoma	Subcutaneous emphysema
Endolaryngeal laceration	Neck pain/point tenderness
Dysphagia	Loss of laryngeal landmarks
Odynophagia	Impaired vocal fold mobility
Hemoptysis	Arytenoid dislocation
Ecchymosis/abrasions of anterior neck	Exposed endolaryngeal cartilage

TABLE 35-1. *Signs and Symptoms of Laryngeal Injury*

Fracture Type	Displacement	Likely Stable	Management
Single Vertical, Unilateral	Nondisplaced	yes	Observe, fixate if symptoms or exam worsen
	Minimally displaced (<1 cartilage width)	yes	Fixate if immediate or delayed voice change, otherwise observe
	Displaced (>1 cartilage width)	no	Reduce and fixate
Single Horizontal, Unilateral	Nondisplaced	yes	Observe, fixate if symptoms or exam worsen
	Minimally displaced	yes	Observe, fixate if symptoms or exam worsen
	Displaced	no	Reduce and fixate
Multiple Unilateral	Nondisplaced	no	Reduce and fixate
	Displaced	no	Reduce and fixate
Multiple Bilateral	Nondisplaced	no	Reduce and fixate
	Displaced	no	Reduce and fixate

TABLE 35-2. *CT Findings That Suggest Fracture Stability*

of the cervical spine is always performed prior to operative intervention of the laryngeal injuries. The presence of a cervical spine injury may preclude the ability to perform a direct laryngoscopy, and repair is begun based on findings on CT scan and flexible endoscopic examination.

Patients without fractures on CT scanning and those with minimally displaced, stable fractures can be observed closely. Soft tissue injuries that consist of isolated mucosal lacerations of the supraglottic larynx, superficial lacerations of the non-vibrating edge of the true vocal fold, small hematomas of the true vocal fold, and/or mild mucosal edema may also be observed. Management of these patients includes the use of antibiotics, anti-reflux medications, reflux precautions, eleva-

| Laceration of vibrating edge of true vocal fold |
| Laceration of anterior commissure |
| Deep laceration of thyroarytenoid muscle |
| Exposed cartilage |
| Impaired vocal fold mobility |
| Arytenoid dislocation |
| Epiglottis displacement |
| Herniation of pre-epiglottic contents |
| Unstable/displaced laryngeal fractures |
| Airway compromise |
| Extensive endolaryngeal edema |

TABLE 35-3. *Indications for Operative Evaluation After Blunt Laryngeal Trauma*

tion of the head of bed, voice rest, and humidity. The use of anti-reflux medications and reflux precautions, including elevation of the head of the bed, helps to limit additional inflammation and delays in wound healing caused by laryngopharyngeal reflux. Humidity helps to keep the vocal folds lubricated, which aids in the re-epithelialization process. The benefit of steroids in this group of patients is controversial. The disadvantage of corticosteroids is that their anti-inflammatory action may interfere with and prolong the natural process of wound healing and result in a prolonged healing phase. The advantage of using steroids is that they may minimize the formation of granulation tissue and decrease laryngeal edema.[2,7,10,16,18,19] In the patient with mild to moderate mucosal edema, high dose steroids are given during the first 24-48 hours to minimize mucosal edema acutely.

Evaluation of the Blunt Trauma Patient With Airway Distress

Signs of upper airway distress include stridor, sternal retraction, and dyspnea. The patient should be examined for signs of upper aerodigestive tract injury. In the presence of immediate post-traumatic airway distress, significant laryngotracheal injury is likely. The neck is stabilized to prevent worsening of unrecognized cervical spine injuries, and the airway is secured with a tracheotomy fashioned at least 2 rings below the injured segments or through the distal transected segment under local anesthesia.[1,2,7,9,12,20-25] Tracheotomy pre-

vents further laryngeal injury, and may expose an unnoticed laryngotracheal separation. Orotracheal and/or nasopharyngeal intubation in the presence of severe laryngotracheal trauma can lead to further laryngeal injury and airway compromise.

In the child with upper airway distress, the airway is secured in the operating room if time permits. General anesthesia is induced using an inhalational agent that is unlikely to cause laryngospasm. During spontaneous respiration, a rigid bronchoscope is passed gently through the injured larynx and trachea to a point distal to the sites of injury. Tracheotomy is performed over the bronchoscope followed by repair of the injuries.[10,13]

Operative evaluation of the larynx with direct laryngoscopy is performed after securing the airway. If direct laryngoscopy reveals significant endolaryngeal injuries (Table 35-3), open exploration and repair are performed. The presence of palpable laryngeal fractures is also an indication for open exploration and repair. If direct laryngoscopy does not reveal a need for open exploration, then a postoperative CT of the larynx is obtained to complete the evaluation.

Surgical Evaluation

Intraoperative evaluation begins with direct laryngoscopy to assess the extent of endolaryngeal injury, esophagoscopy to assess for esophageal lacerations, and bronchoscopy to assess for subglottic and tracheobronchial injuries. The arytenoid cartilages are palpated for possible dislocation. In the patient with isolated cricoarytenoid joint dislocation, reduction can usually be accomplished endoscopically, especially if the dislocation is noted early. With delays in diagnosis beyond even a week, joint ankylosis can begin, making reduction more difficult. Nonetheless, an attempt should be made to relocate the arytenoid cartilage back to its normal position on the cricoid regardless of the interval from the time of injury. In cases of posterior dislocation, this can be accomplished by inserting the anterior lip of an intubating laryngoscope into the posterior aspect of the cricoarytenoid joint while exerting a lifting motion in an anteromedial direction on the cricoid cartilage. Anterior dislocations can be reduced by exerting a posteriorly directed force on the cricoarytenoid joint using the tip of a rigid laryngoscope.[26,27] If no other injuries that require repair are noted on CT scan or on direct laryngoscopy, then open exploration is not necessary.

Open Exploration and Repair

Open exploration is performed to repair mucosal lacerations involving the anterior commissure and/or the vibratory edge of the vocal fold; to repair deep lacerations of the thyroarytenoid muscle; to restore mucosal cover over exposed cartilage; to reposition the vocal ligament and anterior commissure; to reposition a displaced epiglottis or herniated pre-epiglottic contents; to reanastomose separated segments; and to reduce and fixate displaced and/or unstable fractures. If not previously done, tracheotomy is performed to allow intraoperative access to the larynx and postoperative airway management.

Principles of Repair

The basic principles of repair follow the primary principles of wound healing elsewhere in the body. Repair within the first 24 hours after injury is most desirable to prevent granulation tissue formation from occurring prior to closure.[9,16] An attempt should be made to repair all mucosal lacerations and defects in order to promote healing by primary intention. Healing by secondary intention predisposes to a greater deposition of collagen and an increased likelihood of granulation tissue and scar formation, which may result in vibratory dysfunction, stenosis, or webbing of the vocal folds. All de-epithelialized areas that cannot be closed without tension primarily should be covered with local mucosal flaps to minimize scar formation. Free mucosal grafts can be used to cover de-epithelialized areas when local flaps cannot be fashioned; however, these are rarely needed. Fine, absorbable suture on an atraumatic needle seems to help minimize granulation tissue formation.

Exposure

For open exploration, a horizontal neck incision is made and subplatysmal skin flaps are elevated. To expose the thyroid and cricoid cartilages, the strap muscles may be divided in the midline and retracted laterally. When endolaryngeal repair of soft tissue injuries is necessary, entry into the larynx is gained through fractures of the thyroid cartilage that are median or those that are paramedian and less than 0.5 cm from the midline. In patients with lateral or horizontal fractures of the thyroid cartilage, a midline thyrotomy is performed. A midline cut is then made through the anterior commissure under direct visualization, with care not to further disrupt the architecture of the vocal fold. Above the level of the glottis, the endolaryngeal incision is curved lateral to the epiglottis on one side to avoid cutting through its cartilage or mucosa. Care is taken during the exposure to avoid further injury to the recurrent and superior laryngeal nerves.

Endolaryngeal Repair

The functional goal of repair is to realign glottic tissues to their premorbid anteroposterior and transverse planes, beginning posteriorly and proceeding in an ante-

rior direction to maximize exposure (Figure 35-12). The arytenoid is repositioned with meticulous closure of overlying mucoperichondrial defects. If the arytenoid mucosa is damaged badly, local rotation flaps can be developed from the pyriform sinus or postcricoid region. Regardless of the extent of the injuries, an attempt should be made to repair severe unilateral and bilateral arytenoid injuries. Consideration of arytenoidectomy as a secondary procedure can be made at a later date after healing has occurred and the wounds have matured.[7] This approach allows for the possibility of vocalization and respiration if at least one of the arytenoids retains some function.

Lacerations in the thyroarytenoid muscle or mucosa may be repaired with fine absorbable suture. Avascular and crushed mucosal injuries are debrided prior to closure. If primary closure of mucosal disruptions is difficult, local advancement or rotational flaps should be performed. Local advancement or rotational flaps from the pyriform sinus or postcricoid region usually provide adequate coverage of the arytenoid and its vocal process. Adequate mucosa for coverage of the anterior commissure region usually can be obtained from the epiglottis. If an extensive amount of mucosa is needed, the epiglottic mucosa can be elevated off the laryngeal and lingual surfaces of the epiglottis with removal of the cartilage to allow for a large superiorly based epiglottic flap.[28] It is important to ensure meticulous closure and re-epithelialization of the anterior commissure region, as this is the region most likely to develop a web or stenosis as a late complication.

Mucosal defects on the false vocal fold and epiglottis are less likely to pose significant problems with stenosis. If primary repair or a local flap cannot be accomplished, this area can be left open to granulate and mucosalize by secondary intention. A ruptured thyroepiglottic ligament should be re-attached anteriorly to reposition the epiglottis to its more anatomic position. Herniated contents of the pre-epiglottic space should be removed or replaced anterior to the epiglottis and the thyroepiglottic ligament.

The attachment of the vocal ligament at the anterior commissure is inspected. If torn, it is repaired by placing a slow-absorbing monofilament suture through the anterior aspect of the ligament and bringing it through a midline fracture to secure to the thyroid cartilage. If the fracture is paramedian, the suture is brought through the midline of the cartilage and secured. It is important to re-establish the appropriate height of the vocal fold as well as the appropriate midline placement for optimal postoperative voice results. Proper placement of the vocal ligament helps to ensure the proper position of the remainder of the vocal fold.

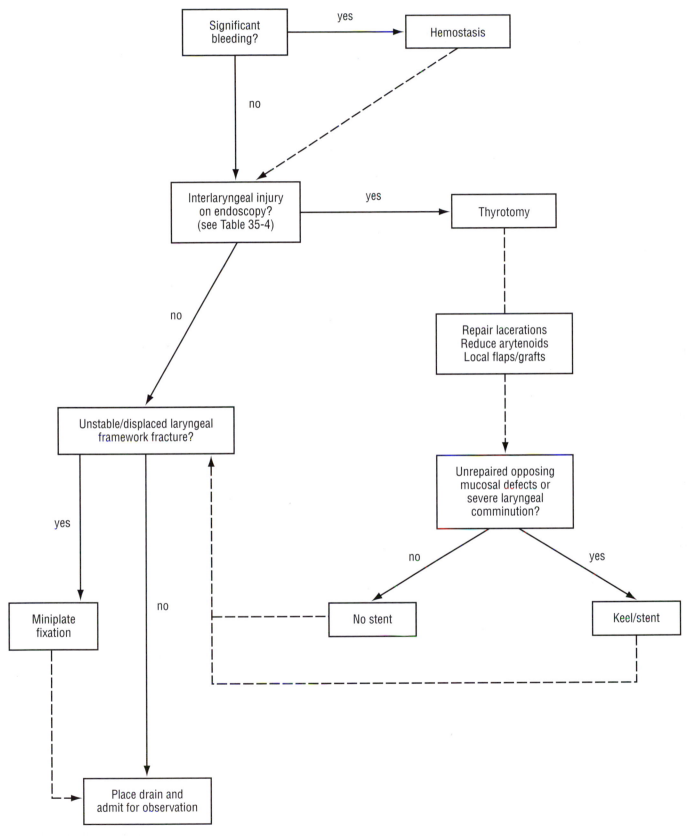

FIGURE 35-12. *Open exploration of laryngeal trauma.*

Endolaryngeal Stenting

After all mucosal injuries are repaired, a decision should be made regarding the necessity of an endolaryngeal stent. Endolaryngeal stents were originally developed to serve as "lumen keepers" and internal fixators. However, these have fallen out of favor for routine use in the last 25 years because of their propensity to move within the larynx. This movement may cause friction on the repaired mucosa, which promotes granulation tissue formation.[29] Endolaryngeal stents and Keels should be reserved for patients with severely comminuted fractures that are not amenable to external fixation, extensive lacerations of opposing mucosa that are not amenable to primary repair of at least one side, and/or mucosal injury in the region of the anterior commissure. In these situations, stenting is helpful in providing internal fixation and in minimizing webbing, especially at the anterior commissure.[16,18] The stent should be soft and pliable so that it does not cause pressure necrosis of the healing mucosal tissue, and it should be secured to prevent mobilization. The anterior commissure region usually can be effectively stented to prevent webbing using a Keel stent. Stents are removed in 7-14 days.

Laryngeal Fixation

Reduction and fixation of the cartilaginous framework is performed after all mucosal injuries have been addressed. If a stent is deemed necessary, it is placed prior to repair of the framework injuries. The fractures are reduced and fixated to ensure a stable reduction. Traditionally, stabilization has been achieved using stainless steel wire or nonabsorbable suture. However, because these provide only two-dimensional fixation, there can be some movement of the laryngeal fragments with head turning, flexion, and swallowing. The recent availability of titanium and absorbable miniplates has allowed more rigid fixation of the laryngeal framework in three-dimensional planes (Figure 35-13). This has the advantage over wire or suture fixation in that it allows for immediate immobility of the fracture segments, can be used effectively in most comminuted fractures, and can decrease the need for endolaryngeal stenting.[30,31] The miniplates can be bent to conform to the geometry of the laryngeal framework, thus preserving the anteroposterior and transverse dimensions of the larynx. Usually, low profile plates in the 1.2 mm to 1.4 mm size range provide adequate fixation of the laryngeal framework and are less prominent than larger profile systems. In patients without significant ossification of the thyroid cartilage, it is often necessary to use drill bits that are two sizes smaller than the screw in order to prevent problems with overdrilling of the soft cartilage.[30-32] For example, if one were to use a 1.3 mm plating system, the

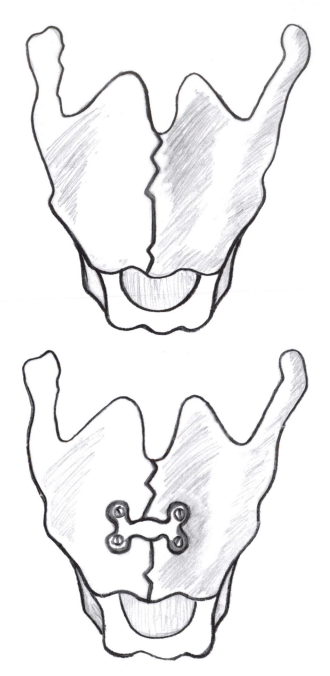

FIGURE 35-13. *Miniplate fixation of a vertical thyroid lamina fracture. (Illustrations courtesy of Sabrina M. Heman-Ackah.)*

hole would be drilled with a 0.8 mm drill bit instead of the usual 1.0 mm drill bit. Alternatively, one may use the 1.0 mm drill bit with the wider threaded "emergency" screws (1.5 mm diameter) from the 1.3 mm plating set or self-drilling screws.

Laryngotracheal Re-anastomosis

In patients with cricotracheal separation, initial intubation is through the distal segment. Any avulsed or badly bruised mucosa or cartilage is resected prior to re-anastomosis to decrease the incidence of granulation tissue formation. Repair is begun with placement of sutures from the posterior tracheal mucosa to the inner cricoid perichondrium using 3-0 absorbable suture or fine wire. The repair then proceeds anteriorly, tying all knots extraluminally. The cricoid and tracheal perichondria and cartilages are then repaired using a 2-0 or 3-0 absorbable suture.[7] The use of absorbable suture decreases the incidence of anastomotic granulation tissue formation and late stenosis.[33] In the presence of cricoid injury and/or in patients in whom postoperative edema seems likely, a T-tube may be placed as a temporary stent. Postoperatively, the neck is kept in flexion for 7-10 days to prevent traction on the anastomotic closure.

Recurrent Laryngeal Nerve Repair

Laryngotracheal separation injuries may be accompanied by bilateral recurrent laryngeal nerve injuries. An attempt should be made to locate the nerves if the vocal folds exhibit evidence of immobility preoperatively. Crushed or otherwise damaged, but intact, nerves should be left alone to regenerate on their own. If a severed nerve is found, the severed ends should be freshened and an attempt should be made to re-anastomose the epineurium using a fine monofilament suture under tension-free closure. If a tension-free closure is unable to be obtained or if the proximal end is unable to be located and the opposite nerve is intact, unilateral ansa cervicalis to recurrent laryngeal nerve transfer is an option. Recurrent laryngeal nerve repair is unlikely to restore full abductor or adductor function to the vocal fold, but they should provide enough tone to the thyroarytenoid muscle for long-term vocalization purposes.[34,35] If soft-tissue injury in the neck is extensive and ansa cervicalis to recurrent laryngeal nerve transfer is unable to be performed, hypoglossal to recurrent laryngeal nerve transfer or cable grafting using a greater auricular or sural nerve graft are other possibilities for nerve repair. In general, better results are obtained with nerve transfer than with cable grafting procedures.

Postoperative Management

The goal of postoperative management is to promote wound healing and limit granulation tissue formation. Patients who undergo mucosal repair of the vocal folds should exercise strict voice rest for the first few days to allow the initial phases of epithelialization to occur. Consideration should be given to the placement of a small flexible nasogastric feeding tube intraoperatively to allow enteral feeding in the early postoperative period. All patients with mucosal injuries are placed on an aggressive anti-reflux protocol, even in the absence of a history of gastroesophageal reflux, to minimize delays in wound healing associated with reflux-induced laryngeal injury.[36] Prophylactic antibiotics are given to patients with open wounds to minimize the risk of chrondritis. Routine tracheotomy care is performed gently to minimize excessive coughing.

PENETRATING INJURIES

Penetrating injuries are the second most common cause of laryngotracheal injuries in the adult and the most common cause in the pediatric population.[1,4,12] These injuries result from accidental or deliberate stab wounds and from gunshot wounds. It is important to understand the mechanism of the injury, the direction of the force, as well as the instrument used to create the injury. If the path has traversed the midline, an injury to the upper aerodigestive tract is likely.

In victims of gunshot wounds, in addition to noting both the entry and exit wounds, it is also helpful to know the caliber and velocity of the weapon used. The kinetic energy ($KE = \frac{1}{2} mv^2$, where KE is kinetic energy, m is mass of the projectile, and v is projectile velocity) released from the bullet on impact determines the degree of tissue damage. Thus, small caliber, high velocity bullets tend to produce greater tissue damage than do the larger caliber, low velocity bullets. The long bullet of the shotgun produces a different type of injury than the short bullet of the pistol or handgun. Because of their shorter length, handgun bullets fly with a straight trajectory, resulting in tissue damage at the site of impact. The bullets of the shotgun are longer and unstable in their trajectory. They, thus, tumble as they leave the barrel of the weapon. This "tumbling" produces significant circumferential "shock wave" damage to surrounding tissue that may extend several centimeters from the site of impact.[37]

In victims of stab wounds, the location and direction of the entrance wound are particularly important to note. Long penetrating objects can create injuries to structures at a significant distance from the entrance wound. As in the blunt trauma patient, victims of penetrating injuries to the larynx and trachea can appear to be comfortable; however, complications from airway compromise, vascular injuries, and esophageal perforations can result in mortality rates as high as 19%.[5,38,39] Therefore, a high index of suspicion coupled with a thorough physical examination is necessary.

Assessment of Penetrating Injuries

The initial concerns in evaluating and treating patients with penetrating injuries are the assessment and establishment of a patent airway and the evaluation and control of vascular and cervical spine injuries, as these are often major contributing factors to early morbidity and mortality in penetrating neck injuries.[38] In patients who require emergent airway control, the decision to perform orotracheal intubation versus tracheotomy must be individualized. The patient with a minor injury is less likely to have an occult laryngotracheal separation, making attempts at intubation less problematic.[38]

Examination of the patient who has sustained a penetrating neck injury involves assessment of all the neck structures. Signs and symptoms of disruption of the upper aerodigestive tract are the same as in the blunt trauma patient (Table 35-1). If they are stable, patients with penetrating neck injuries that cross the midline should have a flexible laryngoscopic examination and CT scan of the neck and larynx to evaluate for possible endolaryngeal injury (Figure 35-14). The patient without any symptoms or signs on flexible endoscopic examination or CT scan or laryngeal injury may be observed closely for development of airway, voice, or esophageal abnormalities. Patients with mild laryngeal inflammation and no other signs of endolaryngeal injury may also be observed. Because of the potential for esophageal injuries, an esophagram with water-soluble contrast should be obtained in patients with minor injuries who do not require rigid endoscopy. The false negative rate with esophagrams has been reported as high as 21%.[40,41] Thus, patients with a negative esophagram who begin to develop odynophagia, fever, or back or chest pain should be evaluated for possible esophageal perforation with flexible or rigid esphagoscopy.

Those patients who are noted to have signs and symptoms of a significant aerodigestive tract injury (Table 35-4) should undergo rigid direct laryngoscopy with consideration for possible open neck exploration and repair.[19,38] Because associated esophageal injuries have been reported in as many as 20-50% of the patients with laryngeal injuries, esophagoscopy should also be performed at the time of rigid endoscopy.[5,38]

Repair of Penetrating Injuries

Repair of penetrating laryngeal injuries and postoperative management is accomplished in a similar fash-

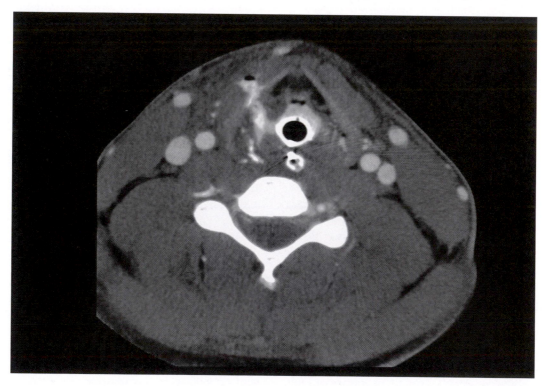

FIGURE 35-14. *Axial CT of the larynx at the level of the false vocal folds after gunshot wound to the left neck. There is shrapnel debris along the trajectory of the bullet from the soft tissues of the left neck anterior to the sternocleidomastoid muscle, through the left thyroid ala, and within the soft tissues of the endolarynx. An endotracheal tube is surrounded by significant endolaryngeal soft tissue edema.*

Endolaryngeal lacerations

Expanding neck hematoma

Subcutaneous emphysema

Audible air leak from neck wound

Hemoptysis

Laryngeal framework disruption

Impaired vocal fold mobility

Endolaryngeal edema

Dysphagia/odynophagia

Stridor/dyspnea

TABLE 35-4. *Indications for Operative Evaluation of Penetrating Laryngeal Injury*

ion as would be done with the blunt trauma patient. In patients with combined esophageal and posterior tracheal wall injuries, consideration should be made for placing a muscle interposition flap between the trachea and esophagus to prevent the formation of a tracheoesophageal fistula. This can be accomplished with the use of a nearby pedicled strap or sternocleidomastoid muscle flap.

CAUSTIC AND THERMAL INJURIES

Caustic and thermal injuries to the larynx can cause significant acute and chronic airway compromise as well as late vocal complications. Caustic injuries occur in both the adult and pediatric populations. Caustic injuries can result from ingestion of bases, acids, or bleaches. The most severe injuries are caused by cases which produce a liquefaction necrosis of muscle, collagen, and lipids with progressively worsening injury over time. Acids cause a coagulation necrosis that occurs more rapidly and tends to damage superficial structures only. In children under age 5, these tend to be accidental ingestions. Adolescent and adult ingestions usually are suicide attempts, and, thus, tend to produce the most severe injuries.[42,43]

Caustic ingestions most often affect the oral cavity, pharynx, and esophagus, but can occasionally contact the larynx and result in edema and mucosal disruption secondary to burn injury. Because the epiglottis and false vocal folds are the initial barriers in preventing aspiration, the laryngeal edema typically seen in caustic ingestions involves the epiglottis and supraglottic lar-

ynx, often sparing the true vocal folds.[42,44] The larynx is examined in all caustic ingestions. Of particular concern is the ingestion of low phosphate or nonphosphate detergents. Ingestions of even small amounts of these may cause severe upper airway edema and airway compromise 1-5 hours after ingestion and warrant admission to the hospital for airway observation even in the absence of other significant injuries.[44] If significant edema or stridor is present, the airway should be stabilized with tracheotomy. Because of the potential for exacerbating the laryngeal injuries, nasotracheal and orotracheal intubation are avoided; tracheotomy is the preferred method of airway stabilization. The mouth, pharynx, and laryngeal inlet should be irrigated with water to remove any remnants of the offending agent. The use of steroids and antibiotics remains common but controversial. Further evaluation and management of esophageal injuries should then proceed. A discussion of the protocol for evaluation and treatment of esophageal injuries is beyond the scope of this chapter but can be found elsewhere.[42,43,45,46]

Thermal laryngeal injuries are usually encountered in patients who have experienced significant burn injuries from closed-space fires.[47] The laryngeal injuries most often result from thermal insult to the supraglottic and glottic larynx.[48] Because inhalational injuries may affect the larynx, tracheobronchial tree, or the lung parenchyma, all patients experiencing significant inhalational injuries should undergo flexible laryngoscopy and bronchoscopy. The diagnosis of laryngeal or tracheal injury is made by the presence of carbonized materials with inflammation, edema, or necrosis.[47] In patients with hypovolemic shock, as commonly occurs in patients with significant burn injuries, there may be severe injury to the larynx or trachea without signs of edema initially. The edema usually ensues with cardiovascular resuscitation.[49] The epiglottis, aryepiglottic folds, and hypopharynx are most prone to edema, which is usually progressive in the first few hours after injury.[49]

The primary concern is protection of the airway. The decision to perform tracheotomy versus endotracheal intubation is controversial. Orotracheal and nasotracheal intubation carry the risk of causing further mucosal injury. There have been several studies to suggest that tracheotomy in the burn patient places the patient at increased risk of long-term sequelae such as tracheal stenosis and sepsis.[48,50,51] In general, tracheotomy is recommended in patients who cannot be endotracheally intubated because of significant laryngeal injury, those who fail extubation, and/or those in whom prolonged respiratory support will be necessary.[47,49,52]

Late complications associated with thermal and caustic injuries include stenosis and webbing. Scar formation may continue for several months following the initial insult.[47] Thus, the larynx and trachea should be serially evaluated over the course of several months. Repair is delayed until scar formation has stabilized. This helps to minimize the incidence of recurrent scar formation and enhances the chances for successful repair.[47,49]

IATROGENIC INJURIES

Iatrogenic injuries to the larynx include radiation injuries and injuries that result from intubation. Doses of radiation used to treat head and neck cancer (6000 cGy-7000 cGy) can result in injury to the mucosa and cartilaginous framework of the larynx if it is included in the radiation field. These injuries are an expected outcome of radiation therapy and can include mucosal drying, soft tissue edema, and laryngeal radionecrosis. The treatment of mucosal drying is symptomatic, encouraging frequent water ingestion. Several preparations are available to minimize xerostomia in patients receiving radiation therapy to the head and neck. These work with variable success. Laryngeal edema from radiation can become problematic, resulting in narrowing of the airway. In some patients, this can be treated effectively with intermittent steroid use. In others, tracheotomy is necessary to help maintain an adequate airway.[53]

The incidence of radionecrosis of the larynx is approximately 1% of patients who receive doses in the range of 6000 cGy to 7000 cGy and increases with larger daily fractions.[54] Patients who continue to smoke or drink alcohol during and after radiation therapy are at increased risk. The presence of laryngopharyngeal reflux may contribute to the development and exacerbation of radionecrosis. Radionecrosis can pose a diagnostic dilemma to the clinician, as the symptoms are similar to the symptoms of recurrent cancer and there is often associated edema and/or ulceration overlying the devitalized tissue. It is often difficult to distinguish between recurrent or persistent tumor and radionecrosis. These patients should undergo direct laryngoscopy and biopsy. Biopsy of radiation-damaged tissue often shows necrotic debris. However, in an inadequately biopsied area, a similar specimen can be obtained in the face of recurrent tumor. Although deep biopsies may exacerbate necrosis, tumor recurrence must be ruled out.[54] Hyperbaric oxygen treatments can be offered to patients with radionecrosis of the larynx, as the increased tissue oxygenation induced by such treatments may promote healing and prevent further damage to the laryngeal framework.[55,56] If the signs and symp-

toms worsen or are not improved with conservative treatment, partial or total laryngectomy should be considered because of the risk of a life-threatening infection with a retained necrotic larynx and because of the high risk of malignancy in this scenario.[54-56]

The most common iatrogenic injury to the larynx results from intubation trauma.[57] Because children are more often subjected to prolonged intubation as premature infants and neonates in the intensive care unit, they are more likely to experience complications as a result of being intubated.[58] The reported incidence of intubation injury in adults and children has decreased in the last 20 years from 18% to 3% because of improved equipment and methods of intubation.[11] The advent of low-pressure cuffed endotracheal tubes of uniform diameter has significantly decreased the incidence of subglottic stenosis. In addition, the development of ventilator adapters to prevent excessive movement of the endotracheal tube has also contributed to a decrease in the incidence of intubation trauma.[11,57]

In neonates, prolonged intubation often leads to circumferential granulation tissue, scarring, and eventual stenosis of the subglottis. This region is most often affected because the cricoid is the narrowest portion of the airway in the neonate and is, thus, most traumatized by the endotracheal tube. The posterior tilt of the cricoid cartilage in neonates likely helps to prevent damage to the interarytenoid region, which is the most common site of injury in the adult.

Subglottic stenosis in the infant from intubation injury can be managed similarly to congenital subglottic stenosis. For stenoses that are less than 50% obstructing, management can consist of observation, dilatation, or CO_2 laser excision. If CO_2 laser is used for a circumferential stenosis, it is done serially with no more than 30% of the circumference resected during any one procedure to prevent restenosis. If the stenosis is 50-70% obstructing, one may consider either endoscopic procedures or open procedures, depending on the location and potential ease of an endoscopic procedure. Stenotic regions that are more than 70% obstructing are best managed using open techniques. Lesions isolated to the subglottic region may be treated with an anterior cricoid split procedure. Longer stenotic regions may be treated with either cartilage grafting or resection with end-to-end anastomosis. Completely stenotic regions require resection and re-anastomosis.[59]

In the adult, the glottis is the narrowest portion of the airway, and the posterior glottis often supports the endotracheal tube in the adult. Movement of the arytenoids against the endotracheal tube with respiration often contributes to ischemic necrosis of the thin mucosa overlying the vocal process. This can be followed by ulceration, chondritis, granulation, and scarring. Often, removal of the endotracheal tube will allow for normal healing in the absence of gastroesophageal reflux, which should be treated presumptively during the healing process.

Scarring of the posterior glottis uncommonly causes problems with airway compromise. Attempts to release posterior glottic scar bands usually should be avoided to prevent worsening stenosis unless substantial symptoms justify the risks. In cases of significant airway compromise and minimal posterior scarring, treatment with microscopic direct laryngoscopy and carbon dioxide laser division of the scar band is usually successful.[60] Care should be taken during these divisions to protect the normal mucosa of the interarytenoid region.[61] Occasionally, repeat microscopic direct laryngoscopy with repeat laser division is needed. In cases with moderate to severe interarytenoid scarring, a laryngofissure with a mucosal advancement flap from the interarytenoid notch or from an aryepiglottic fold or a similar endoscopic procedure can be performed.[62] The value of adjunctive treatment with topical mitomycin-c to prevent restenosis is being studied currently, but preliminary results are encouraging.[63]

SUMMARY

Injury to the laryngotracheal complex can result from blunt, penetrating, caustic, thermal, and iatrogenic insults. The primary concern in the initial management of these injuries is the establishment and maintenance of an adequate airway. Treatment can then address the reconstruction of the normal anatomic relationships of the larynx and trachea in an attempt to restore the normal phonatory, respiratory, and protective functions of the larynx.

REFERENCES

1. Bent JB, Silver JR, Porubsky ES. Acute laryngeal trauma: a review of 77 patients. *Otolaryngol Head Neck Surg.* 1993;109:441-449.

2. Schaefer SD. The treatment of acute external laryngeal injuries. *Arch Otolaryngol Head Neck Surg.* 1991;117:35-39.

3. Jewett BS, Shockley WW, Rutledge R. External laryngeal trauma analysis of 392 patients. *Arch Otolaryngol Head Neck Surg.* 1999;125:877-880.

4. Gussack GS, Jurkovich GJ, Luterman A. Laryngotracheal trauma: a protocol approach to a rare injury. *Laryngoscope.* 1986;96:660-665.

5. Minard G, Kudsk KA, Croce MA, Butts JA, Cicala RS, Fabian TC. Laryngotracheal trauma. *Am Surg.* 1992;58:181-187.

6. Holinger PH, Schild JA. Pharyngeal, laryngeal, and tracheal injuries in the pediatric age group. *Ann Otol Rhinol Laryngol.* 1972;81:538-545.

7. Pennington CL. External trauma of the larynx and trachea: immediate treatment and management. *Ann Otol Rhinol Laryngol.* 1972;81:546-554.

8. Travis LW, Olson NR, Melvin JW, Snyder JG. Static and dynamic impact trauma of the human larynx. *Am Acad Ophthalmol Otolaryngol.* 1975;80:382-390.

9. Ashbaugh DG, Gordon JG. Traumatic avulsion of the trachea associated with cricoid fracture. *J Thorac Cardiovasc Surg.* 1975;69:800-803.

10. Gold SM, Gerber ME, Shott SR, Myer CM 3rd. Blunt laryngotracheal trauma in children. *Arch Otolaryngol Head Neck Surg.* 1997;123:83-87.

11. Bryce DP. Current management of laryngotracheal injury. *Adv Oto-Rhino-Laryngol.* 1983;29:27-38.

12. Ford HR, Gardner MJ, Lynch JM. Laryngotracheal disruption from blunt pediatric neck injuries: impact of early recognition and intervention on outcome. *J Pediatr Surg.* 1995;30:331-334.

13. Myer CM 3rd, Orobello P, Cotton RT, Bratcher GO. Blunt laryngeal trauma in children. *Laryngoscope.* 1987;97:1043-1048.

14. Offia CJ, Endres D. Isolated laryngotracheal separation following blunt trauma to the neck. *J Laryngol Otol.* 1997;111:1079-1081.

15. Alonso WA, Caruso VG, Roncace EA. Minibikes, a new factor in laryngotracheal trauma. *Ann Otol Rhinol Laryngol.* 1973;82:800-804.

16. Schaefer SD, Close LG. Acute management of laryngeal trauma. Update. *Ann Otol Rhinol Laryngol.* 1989;98:98-104.

17. Schild JA, Denneny EC. Evaluation and treatment of acute laryngeal fractures. *Head Neck* 1989;11:491-496.

18. Olson NR. Surgical treatment of acute blunt laryngeal injuries. *Ann Otol Rhinol Laryngol.* 1978;87:716-721.

19. Lucente E, Mitrani M, Sacks SH, Biller HF. Penetrating injuries of the larynx. *Ear Nose Throat J.* 1985;64:406-415.

20. Reece CP, Shatney CH. Blunt injuries to the cervical trachea: review of 51 patients. *South Med J.* 1988;81:1542-1547.

21. Chodosh PL. Cricoid fracture with tracheal avulsion. *Arch Otolaryngol.* 1968;87:461-467.

22. Harris HH. Management of injuries to the larynx and trachea. *Laryngoscope.* 1972;82:1924-1929.

23. Ogura J. Management of traumatic injuries of the larynx and trachea including stenosis. *J Laryngol Otol.* 1971;85:1259-1261.

24. Trone TH, Schaefer SD, Carder HM. Blunt and penetrating laryngeal trauma: a 13 year review. *Otolaryngol Head Neck Surg.* 1980;88:257-261.

25. Fuhrman GM, Stieg FH, Buerk CA. Blunt laryngeal trauma: classification and management protocol. *J Trauma.* 1990;30:87-92.

26. Sataloff RT, Feldman M, Darby KS, Carroll LM, Spiegel JR. Arytenoid dislocation. *J Voice.* 1987;1:368-377.

27. Sataloff RT, Bough ID, Spiegel JR. Arytenoid dislocation: diagnosis and treatment. *Laryngoscope.* 1994;104:1353-1361.

28. Olson NR. Laryngeal suspension and epiglottic flap in laryngopharyngeal trauma. *Ann Otol Rhinol Laryngol.* 1976; 85:533-537.

29. Thomas GK, Stevens MH. Stenting in experimental laryngeal injuries. *Arch Otolaryngol.* 1975;101:217-221.

30. Woo P, Kellman R. Laryngeal framework reconstruction with miniplates: indications and extended indications in 27 cases. *Oper Tech Otolaryngol Head Neck Surg.* 1972;3:159-164.

31. Woo P. Laryngeal framework reconstruction with miniplates. *Ann Otol Rhinol Laryngol.* 1990;99:772-777.

32. Pou AM, Shoemaker DL, Carrau RL, Snyderman CH, Eibling DE. Repair of laryngeal fractures using adaptation plates. *Head Neck.* 1998;20:707-713.

33. Grillo HC, Donahue DM, Mathisen DJ, Wain JC, Wright CD. Postintubation tracheal stenosis: treatment and results. *J Thorac Cardiovasc Surg.* 1994;109:486-493.

34. Crumley RL. Teflon versus thyroplasty versus nerve transfer: a comparison. *Ann Otol Rhinol Laryngol.* 1990;99:759-763.

35. Crumley RL. Update: ansa cervicalis to recurrent laryngeal nerve anastomosis for unilateral laryngeal paralysis. *Laryngoscope.* 1991;101:384-388.

36. Little FB, Koufman JA, Kohut RI, Marshall RB. Effects of gastric acid on the pathogenesis of subglottic stenosis. *Ann Otol Rhinol Laryngol.* 1985;94:516-519.

37. Harrison DF. Bullet wounds of the larynx and trachea. *Arch Otolaryngol.* 1984;110:203-205.

38. Grewal H, Rao PM, Mukerji S, Ivatury RR. Management of penetrating laryngotracheal injuries. *Head Neck.* 1995;17:494-502.

39. Feliciano DV, Bitondo CG, Mattox KL, et al. Combined tracheoesophageal injuries. *Am J Surg.* 1985;150:710-715.

40. Defore WW, Mattox KL, Hansen HA, Garcia-Rinaldi R, Beall AC, DeBakey ME. Surgical management of penetrating injuries to the esophagus. *Am J Surg.* 1977;134:734-737.

41. Glatterer MS Jr, Toon RS, Ellestad C, et al. Management of blunt and penetrating external esophageal trauma. *J Trauma.* 1985;25:784-792.

42. Hawkins DB, Demefer MJ, Barnett TE. Caustic ingestion: controversies in management. A review of 214 cases. *Laryngoscope.* 1980;90:98-109.

43. Schild JA. Caustic ingestion in adult patients. *Laryngoscope.* 1985;95:1199-1201.

44. Einhorn A, Horton L, Altieri M, Ochsenschlager D, Klein B. Serious respiratory consequences of detergent ingestions in children. *Pediatrics.* 1989;84:472-474.

45. Holinger LD. Caustic ingestion, esophageal injury and stricture. In: Holinger LD, Lusk RP, Green CG, eds. *Pediatric Laryngology and Bronchoesophagology.* Philadelphia, PA: Lippincott-Raven Publishers; 1997:295-304.

46. Wijburg FA, Beukers MM, Heymans HS, Bartelsman JF, den Hartog Jager FC. Nasogastric intubation as sole treatment of caustic esophageal lesions. *Ann Otol Rhinol Laryngol.* 1985;94:337-341.

47. Jones JE, Rosenberg D. Management of laryngotracheal thermal trauma in children. *Laryngoscope.* 1995;105:540-542.

48. Moylan J. Smoke inhalation and burn injury. *Surg Clin North Am.* 1980;60:1533-1540.

49. Miller RP, Gray SD, Cotton RT, Myer CM 3rd. Airway reconstruction following laryngotracheal thermal trauma. *Laryngoscope.* 1988;98:826-829.

50. Lund T, Goodwin CW, McManus WF, et al. Upper airway sequelae in burn patient requiring endotracheal intubation or tracheostomy. *Ann Surg.* 1985;201:374-382.

51. Eckhauser FE, Billote J, Burke JF, Quinby WC. Tracheotomy complicating massive burn injury. *Am J Surg.* 1974;127:418-423.

52. Calhoun KH, Deskin RW, Gorza C, et al. Long-term airway sequelae in a pediatric burn population. *Laryngoscope.* 1988;98:721-725.

53. Calcaterra TC, Stern FS, Ward PH. Dilemma of delayed radiation injury of the larynx. *Ann Otol.* 1972;81:501-507.

54. Parsons JT. The effect of radiation on normal tissues of the head and neck. In: Million RR, Cassisi NJ, eds. *Management of Head and Neck Cancer: a Multidisciplinary Approach.* Philadelphia, PA: JB Lippincott Co; 1984:183-184.

55. Feldmeier JJ, Heimback RD, Davold DA, Brakora MJ. Hyperbaric oxygen as an adjunctive treatment for severe laryngeal necrosis: a report of nine consecutive cases. *Undersea Hyperbaric Med.* 1993;20:329-335.

56. Ferguson BJ, Hudson WR, Farmer JC Jr. Hyperbaric oxygen therapy for laryngeal radionecrosis. *Ann Otol Rhinol Laryngol.* 1987;9: 1-6.

57. Richardson MA. Laryngeal anatomy and mechanisms of trauma. *Ear Nose Throat J.* 1981;60:346-351.

58. Cotton RT, Seid AB. Management of the extubation problem in the premature child. *Ann Otol Rhinol Laryngol.* 1980;89:508-511.

59. Lusk RP, Wooley AL, Holinger LD. Laryngotracheal stenosis. In: Holinger LD, Lusk RP, Green CG, eds. *Pediatric Laryngology and Bronchoesophagology.* Philadelphia, PA: Lippincott-Raven Publishers; 1997:172-184.

60. Dedo HH, Rowe LD. Laryngeal reconstruction in acute and chronic injuries. *Otolaryngol Clin North Am.* 1983;16:373-389.

61. Dedo HH, Sooy FA. Endoscopic laser repair of posterior glottic, subglottic, and tracheal stenosis by division or micro-trapdoor flap. *Laryngoscope.* 1984;94:445-450.

62. Dedo HH, Sooy FA. Surgical repair of late glottic stenosis. *Ann Otol Rhinol Laryngol.* 1968;77:435-441.

63. Correa AJ, Reinisch L, Sanders DL, et al. Inhibition of subglottic stenosis with mitomycin-c in the canine model. *Ann Otol Rhinol Laryngol.* 1999;108:1053-1060.

CHAPTER 36

Surgical Management of Benign Voice Disorders

Mark S. Courey, MD

Robert H. Ossoff, DMD, MD

Surgical management of benign voice disorders is predicated on a sound understanding of laryngeal anatomy, histology, physiology, and pathophysiology. It makes no sense to treat an ankle fracture with a foot amputation. Similarly, it seems to make little sense to treat diseases that arise in the subepithelial tissue by stripping normal laryngeal epithelium and cover. This important aspect in the surgical management of benign voice disorders—the preservation of surrounding normal tissue with as little disruption as possible—is crucial to the return of normal laryngeal function postoperatively.[1] To achieve this goal, surgical precision is aided by magnification and delicate laryngeal instrumentation. Furthermore, the timing of surgical intervention to coincide with minimal-surrounding inflammation, whenever possible, needs to be manipulated to the patient's and surgeon's benefit. Patients must be informed of the risks and benefits of surgical intervention. They need to realize that good results from voice surgery rely on adequate preoperative preparation as well as postoperative rehabilitation.[2] Just as orthopedic surgeons would not consider joint replacement until preoperative medical management and physical therapy have been exhausted, laryngologists should not consider vocal fold surgery for benign lesions until this same attention has been given to preoperative voice management. In addition, orthopedic surgeons have found that postoperative rehabilitation is crucial to the success of their surgical procedures, and they initiate therapy as soon as possible during recovery. This same attention to postoperative rehabilitation seems to serve us well when applied to the management of benign voice disorders.

Benign vocal fold abnormalities have been discussed in Chapter 6. In review, they consist of vocal fold nodules or polyps, vocal fold cysts (mucus retention or epidermal inclusion), vascular malformations, sulcus vocalis, polypoid corditis, and others. Knowledge of the initiating site of these lesions is imperative for successful surgical management. Briefly, inflammation and trauma, most commonly from abusive phonation, lead to shearing stress and strain in the superficial portion of the lamina propria. The body's reaction to this repeated trauma leads to the development of lesions such as polypoid corditis, polyps, nodules, and possibly cysts.

The surgical management of these lesions, which arise in the subepithelial tissue is directed at the subepithelial tissue. Many of these lesions, with the exception of nodules and some polyps, arise deeply enough within the superficial layer of the lamina propria (SLLP), that the basement membrane zone (BMZ) of the epithelium and the overlying portion of the SLLP are normal. In these instances, this tissue can and should be preserved. On the other hand, the surgical management of lesions involving the BMZ will require excision of a portion of the BMZ with the overlying epithelium. It is not technically possible to separate the epithelium from the supportive structure of the BMZ,[3] nor would it be necessary as re-epithelialization occurs reliably and rapidly over remaining vocal fold structures.[4] In either case, surgical manipulation of the surrounding normal tissue should be kept to a minimum.

PREOPERATIVE MANAGEMENT

Preoperative management relies on obtaining an accurate history, performing a complete physical examination, and performing and interpreting the videoendostroboscopic examination. These factors aid in diagnosis.[5] Often the diagnosis is not apparent at the first office visit and requires multiple or serial examinations to identify the subtle physical and stroboscopic findings. In addition, because the disorders are benign, and are most commonly caused by inefficient vocal behaviors, the surgeon should allow time to accurately diagnose and assess the effect that the lesion has on both the speaking and the singing voice before the initiation of surgical therapy. For men, periodic interval examinations may take place in 1-, 2-, or 4-week intervals as necessary. In women of childbearing age, however, serial examinations should take place at odd-week intervals, 1, 3, or 5, to assess the effect that menstruation may have on the physical appearance and function of the larynx.

If the diagnosis cannot be established through the interval examination process alone, then therapeutic measures such as voice rest, modification of voice use through speech therapy, and/or voice training may help establish the diagnosis. These measures, which are designed to reduce the causative factors of vocal abuse and misuse, aid in diagnosis by reducing changes and edema in the surrounding tissue. This alters either the initiating or the compensatory vocal behavior. Still, even after vocal modification and serial examination, establishing the diagnosis may not be possible. If the voice disorder is severe, and a suitable voice cannot be achieved and maintained through vocal behavior modification and elimination of other potential sources of trauma, then direct operative microlaryngoscopy with vocal fold palpation and possible exploration is indicated for accurate diagnosis and therapy.

Before surgical intervention, the voice disability must be evaluated in the light of modified vocal behavior. This is necessary to assess the lesion's absolute effect in the life of the patient.[1,6] Surgical therapy is not without risk. Though small, the chance of postoperative scarring from even simple palpation or intubation exists, and the patient should be made aware of this possibility. Therefore, any possible behavior modification that may improve the speaking or singing voice should be employed before surgical intervention.

Initial behavior modification steps are aimed at the identification and elimination of vocal abuse and misuse through vocal abuse reduction programs and the adaptation of methods of efficient voice production. These steps, along with the elimination of harmful substances such as tobacco products, caffeine and high-fat or dairy products, and hydration, improve vocal fold lubrication and promote vocal hygiene.[7] After the abuses have been eliminated, assessment of the vocal mechanism for both the speaking and the singing voice helps identify and correct misuses.

These behavior modification measures have several benefits. First, they aid in diagnosis. Second, proper vocal technique improves function. Third, behavior modification has been shown to reduce the recurrence rate of vocal nodules postoperatively.[8,9] Finally, these measures promote vocal health and may have the added benefit of allowing the patient to continue to function with the pathologic lesion in place.[10] With close observation the patients can then continue their work schedule. Surgery or definitive therapy can be postponed indefinitely or until timing is ideal.

Prior to choosing surgical intervention patients need to understand that postoperative rehabilitation from surgical therapy usually requires between 8 and 12 weeks and that their compliance with these recommendations will have a substantial effect on their overall outcome. This type of postoperative rehabilitation necessitates substantial freedom from work responsibilities and requires considerable effort by the patient and the patient's employer to allow adequate time.

Informed Consent

The risks and benefits of surgery need to be discussed at length with the patient prior to intervention. Surgery is not indicated solely by the presence of a benign-appearing laryngeal lesion, but rather by the troublesome dysphonia that results from the lesion's interference with the normal vibratory patterns. Behavioral and medical intervention may allow patients to develop improved functional capabilities and with these improvements some patients may no longer believe that they require a surgical intervention to fulfill their daily vocal activities. In addition, in spite of improved surgical techniques, healing can still be unpredictable and may lead to worsening of the speaking or singing voice. Patients need to be aware of these possibilities preoperatively and must be willing to accept rare but potentially devastating vocal risks before proceeding. Typically, features that prompt us to recommend surgery include: a failure of the vocal capabilities to improve with medical and/or behavioral management; worsening appearance or enlargement of the vocal fold lesion on interval examination despite medical and/or behavioral management; and the patient's perception and our objective documentation of continued unacceptable limitations in daily vocal activity despite improvement with medical and behavioral therapy. Under these circumstances, the potential benefits of surgery outweigh the possible risks.

The length of the postoperative recuperative period also needs to be discussed with patients preoperatively. Healing of the operative site and resolution of edema need to occur before the resumption of full vocal activity. Heavy use of the vocal mechanism before sufficient healing may result in the development of vocal hyperfunction as the patient uses excess tension to overcome a stiff or edematous vocal fold. The recuperative period may take 8 to 12 weeks or occasionally longer and needs to be tailored to the individual patient based on the physical appearance and characteristics of the healing vocal fold as determined by interval videoendostroboscopic examinations performed during the postoperative rehabilitation period. General guidelines, however, can be discussed with the patient, and the patient can be informed that failure to comply with these restrictions may affect the overall permanent result.

SURGICAL PRINCIPLES—EXPOSURE AND ENDOSCOPES

Endoscopic surgery, like other surgical techniques, relies first on exposure. The largest-caliber laryngoscope that can be comfortably placed in the patient is used. A large variety of laryngoscopes is available, and surgeons should identify several with which they are most comfortable. Preferably, these will permit binocular viewing and be of large enough caliber to allow working space for at least two microlaryngeal instruments simultaneously. For most glottic work, nonhinged microlaryngoscopes of the Holinger or Dedo variety with an upward flair at the distal tip are simple to use and provide adequate exposure of the vocal folds and anterior commissure. The traditional Dedo microlaryngoscope has been enlarged to improve binocular vision and allow greater room for instrumentation (Figure 36-1).[11] Similarly, modifications of the Holinger-type anterior commissure laryngoscope also allow binocular vision and provide enhanced space for instrumentation (Figure 36-2).[12] Other characteristics of useful laryngoscopes include improved lighting for better visualization and photographic documentation and built-in smoke evacuation channels for use with carbon dioxide laser. Finally, some surgeons prefer straight laryngoscopes without an upward flair at the distal tip. In their hands these laryngoscopes provide an unobstructed view of the anterior commissure and allow easier manipulation of this

region.[13] The reader is encouraged to become familiar with several different types of laryngoscopes. Anatomic differences between patients will require dexterity on the part of the surgeon to achieve optimal exposure.

Once the laryngoscope is inserted, the application of a suspension device with complete patient relaxation provides a stable field for inspection, manipulation, and surgical intervention. In delicate microlaryngeal surgery, where precision is of the utmost importance, this is preferable to indirect methods or methods under local anesthesia in which patient movement may be disastrous.[14]

Inspection and documentation are performed with the aid of large-caliber 0º, 30º, and 70º telescopes. These provide excellent monocular optics for visualization and can be coupled with either a video, digital or a 35 mm camera for teaching or documentation purposes.[15] The medial surface of the vocal fold is inspected and the exact extent of the lesion from upper vocal fold lip to lower lip is determined.

Binocular vision is next obtained with the use of an operating microscope. Typically, the 400 mm focal length lens provides good visualization and allows adequate working space. Some surgeons, however, feel more comfortable with a 350 mm focal lens.[16] High magnification with binocular microscope enhances visualization. Typical microscope optics with 1.6 to 2.5 power magnification of the distal lens combined with the 10 or 12.5 magnification of the eyepiece and the focal length of the tube, allow overall magnification of the operative field by at least 6.8 to 12 times.

SURGICAL PRINCIPLES—INSTRUMENTATION

Newer microsurgical techniques are aimed at the preservation of surrounding normal structure. Knowledge of laryngeal anatomy, embryology, and physiology are essential for understanding laryngeal pathologic lesions and theories of their causes. This knowledge will then help direct the surgical approach. For most benign laryngeal lesions, standard cold knife excision techniques are preferable to laser excision techniques.[17] Surgical instrumentation has been improved to provide smaller equipment that is more appropriate for endolaryngeal use. New microscissors, knives, elevators, probes, cup forceps, and suction devices are available in 1- to 4-mm sizes.[18] Instrumentation of this size is essential for delicate and precise excision (Figure 36-3). Currently, several instrument companies produce this microlaryngeal instrumentation. The surgeon is encouraged to work with local representatives to find instruments with which he/she is comfortable and able to obtain reliable outcomes.

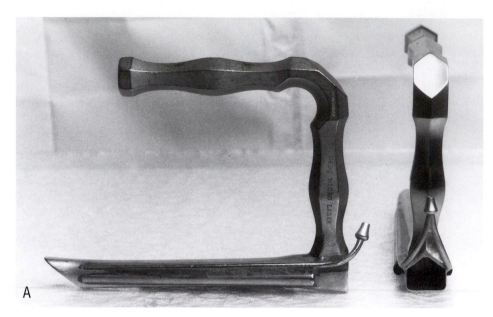

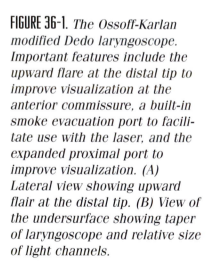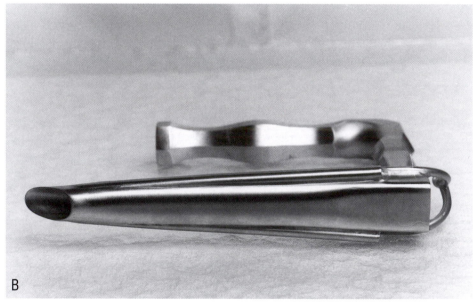

FIGURE 36-1. *The Ossoff-Karlan modified Dedo laryngoscope. Important features include the upward flare at the distal tip to improve visualization at the anterior commissure, a built-in smoke evacuation port to facilitate use with the laser, and the expanded proximal port to improve visualization. (A) Lateral view showing upward flair at the distal tip. (B) View of the undersurface showing taper of laryngoscope and relative size of light channels.*

If the laser is to be used for benign lesion excision, then the carbon dioxide laser is preferable to lasers of other wavelengths.[19-21] The photoabsorptive properties of the carbon dioxide laser wavelength allow adequate laryngeal tissue vaporization with relatively minimal depth penetration. Using the laser in a shuttered or superpulsed mode allows sufficient off-time between laser impacts for thermal relaxation in the tissue being treated. With pulsed mode applications, heat buildup and thermal injury in the surrounding normal tissue is held to a minimum. Laser tissue effects, however, are obtained by delivering energy that causes heating and vaporization. Regardless of technique, a surrounding zone of thermal injury is created for each area of laser impact.[17] This surrounding zone of thermal injury is not present with cold knife excision, and this provides the perceived advantage of cold knife excision techniques over the laser.

If the carbon dioxide laser is to be used, then the newer-generation micromanipulators, which provide a spot size of 250 to 300 µm at a 400 mm focal length, are preferable to the older-generation micromanipulator, which provided an 800-µm spot size at the same working distance. These second generation micromanipulators represent the current standard of care for these cases in which the laser is to be used. The enhanced

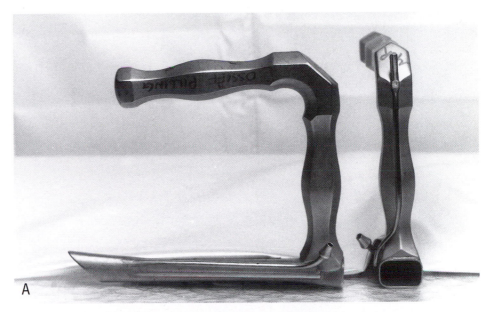

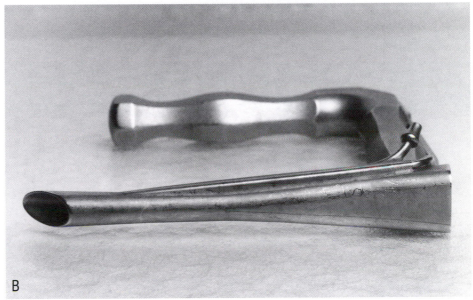

FIGURE 36-2. *The Ossoff-Pilling microlaryngoscope. This maintains the overall dimensions of the Holinger laryngoscope through the distal third to ease insertion in difficult-to-expose patients. (A) Lateral view showing flair at distal end. (B) View of undersurface showing rapid taper through proximal third of laryngoscope.*

precision of the smaller spot size is preferable for most applications and results in a smaller surrounding zone of thermal injury.[17,22]

NODULAR FORMATIONS AND SUBMUCOSAL SCARRING

Perhaps one of the most misunderstood laryngeal disease processes is nodule formation. We reserve the term *nodule* for vocal fold lesions that are most often bilateral and found at the midpoint of the vibrating vocal fold. It is generally agreed upon that nodules are an acquired disorder resulting from chronic vocal abuse and hyperfunction. Nodules, however, appear to repre-

sent a continuum of a disease process. The earliest form is localized submucosal edema followed by a progression of basement membrane changes and submucosal fibrosis leading to eventual submucosal scarring and potential mucosal thickening.[23]

During their earlier stages, nodule formations appear to be reversible by the elimination of vocal abuse. At what point the reversibility is lost, however, is unclear. We recommend surgery for nodules only after strict compliance with a full 12-week course of a vocal abuse reduction program has been unsuccessful at eliminating the nodules in the symptomatic patient. The patient also needs to demonstrate the desire and ability

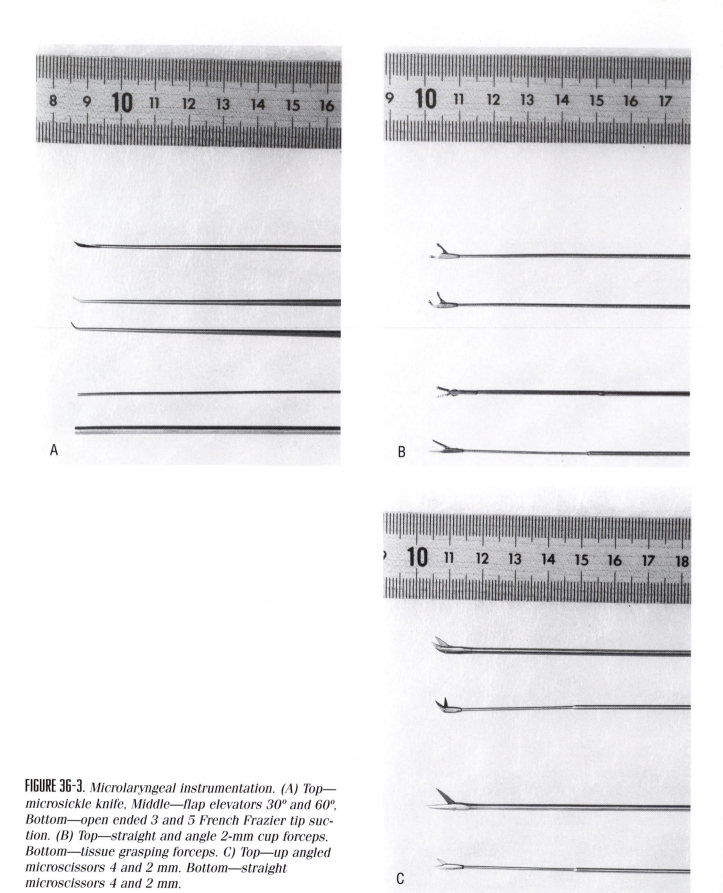

FIGURE 36-3. *Microlaryngeal instrumentation. (A) Top—microsickle knife, Middle—flap elevators 30° and 60°, Bottom—open ended 3 and 5 French Frazier tip suction. (B) Top—straight and angle 2-mm cup forceps. Bottom—tissue grasping forceps. C) Top—up angled microscissors 4 and 2 mm. Bottom—straight microscissors 4 and 2 mm.*

to maintain the new vocal techniques, acquired through the vocal abuse reduction program, postoperatively. In these patients with significant irreversible submucosal fibrosis or significant mucosal thickening, surgical excision appears to be beneficial.

The surgical approach is determined by the preoperative appearance on videostroboscopy and palpation under operative exposure with magnification. For hard nodules that, on palpation, appear to separate from the vocal fold ligament easily, excision is accomplished via a medial microflap technique.[24,25] For disease states with significant submucosal changes and adherence to the vocal ligament, a lateral endoscopic microflap approach that allows identification of the vocal ligament away from the site of the lesion is advisable.

When operative examination reveals relatively minimal submucosal fibrosis and the lesion appears to separate easily from the vocal fold ligament, then a medial microflap excision can be performed. The nodular prominence is retracted with an open-ended suction tip or tissue-grasping forcep. An incision is made over the lesion with a sickle knife (Figure 36-4A). Up-cutting microscissors are then used to separate the lesion from the deeper layers of the lamina propria with as little disruption as possible in the uninvolved SSLP (Figure 36-

4B). The mucosa is elevated laterally over the upper lip region of the vocal fold (Figure 36-4C). The lesion with the involved portion of the epithelium is excised (Figure 36-4D). Finally the preserved mucosa is redraped over the medial surface of the vocal fold (Figure 36-4E). This technique permits excision of the lesion without excessive de-epithelialization of the medial surface of the vocal fold. In addition, it increases the possibilty of saving uninvolved superfical SLLP.

Postoperative voice rest is employed for 1 to 2 weeks until remucosalization and resolution of edema have occurred. Vocal activity is then re-initiated slowly under the guidance of a speech-language pathologist.

When the lesion does not separate easily from the vocal ligament, using a lateral approach and starting dissection in uninvolved regions of the vocal fold facilitates identification of the appropriate plains of dissection. In the lateral microflap procedure,[26] an incision is made in the vocal fold cover on the superior surface of the vocal fold near the ventricle (Figure 36-5A). The anatomy at this point is relatively well-preserved, and this facilitates the identification of the vocal fold ligament. Furthermore, this places the incision well lateral, away from the free edge, and minimizes the possibility of dampening the propagating mucosal wave. A blunt

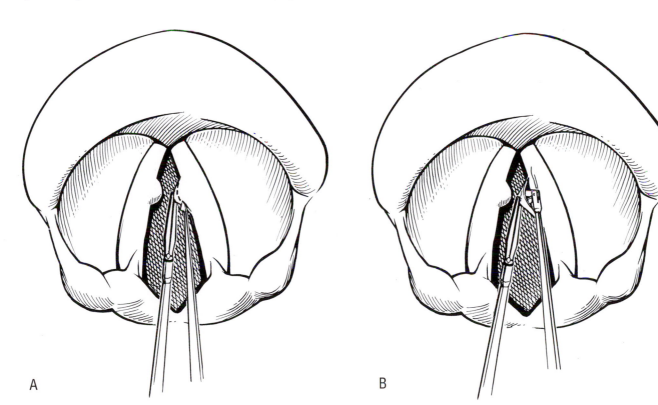

A   B

FIGURE 36-4. *Diagrammatic representation of the medial microflap technique. (A) A microsickle knife incises the mucosa over the lesion. (B) Microscissors are used to separate the lesion from the vocal ligament. (Continues)*

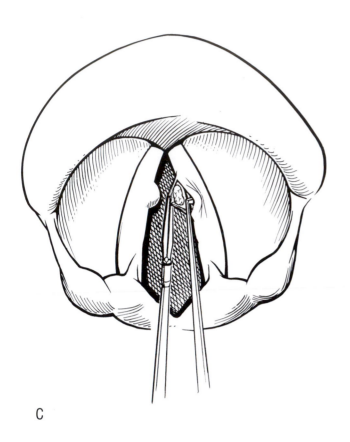

C

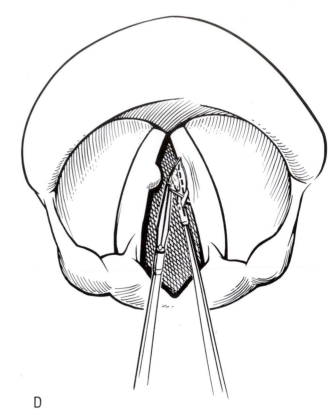

D

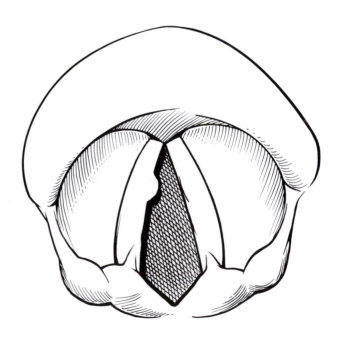

E

FIGURE 36-4. *(C) A flap elevator is used to elevate the mucosa from the vocal ligament to be advanced over the medial surface defect. (D) The lesion is excised with a small portion of the involved overlying cover. (E) The postoperative surgical appearance.*

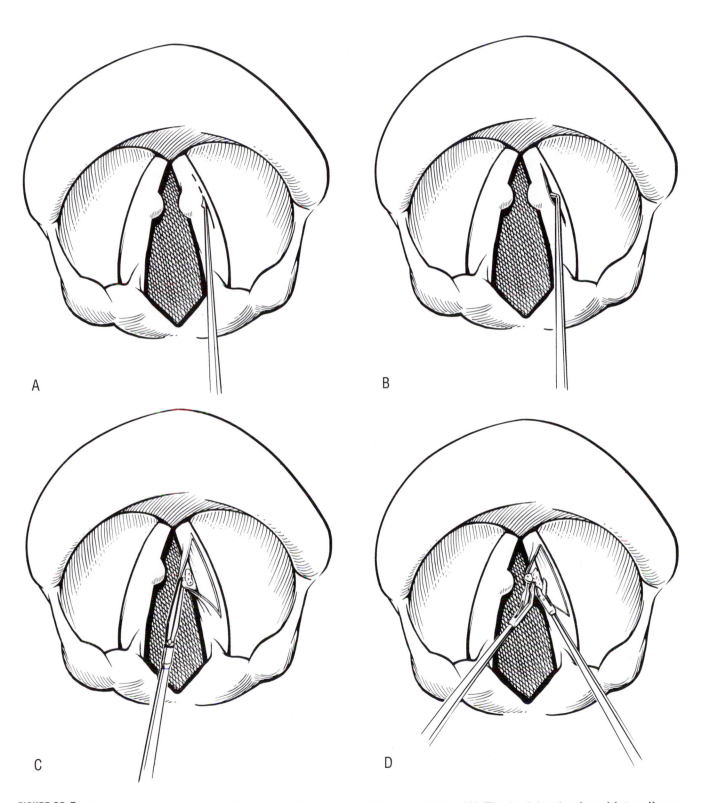

FIGURE 36-5. *Diagrammatic representation of the lateral microflap technique. (A) The incision is placed laterally on the superior surface of the vocal fold near the ventricle. (B) The flap elevator is used to elevate the mucosa and the superficial layer of the lamina propria. (C) The vocal ligament is preserved laterally while the cover and lesion are elevated medially. (D) The lesion is dissected from the mucosal cover. (Continues)*

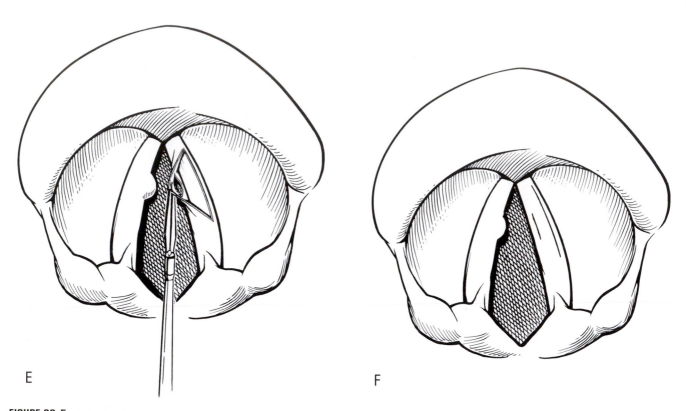

E   F

FIGURE 36-5. *(E) The lesion and involved overlying cover are excised. (F) The cover is redraped in position over the vocal ligament.*

elevator (flap elevator) is inserted and used to elevate the superficial layers of Reinke's space and mucosa from the ligament (Figure 36-5B). Painstakingly, a plane is developed between the lesion and the vocal fold ligament. This may, at times, require sharp dissection. The lesion and cover are then elevated medially while the ligament is preserved laterally (Figure 36-5C). The elevation is carried infraglottically past the lesion. The lesion, attached to the vocal fold cover, is grasped with microcup forceps or an open suction tip and blunt and/or sharp dissection used to separate the lesion from the mucosal cover (Figure 36-5D). If the lesion is too adherent to permit separation, then a small elliptical portion of mucosa may be excised (Figure 36-5E). A butterfly catheter attached to a syringe, or other commercially available endoscopic injection systems are used to inject corticosteroid into the pocket created in the superficial layer of the lamina propria. The cover is redraped over the vocal fold ligament with care being taken to approximate the mucosal edges over the infraglottal surface if a mucosal dehiscence was created (Figure 36-5F). This advancement flap technique is facilitated by previous flap elevation over both the superior vocal fold and the infraglottal surfaces. It permits coverage of the ligament in the infraglottal portion where mucosal wave preservation appears to be the

most important. Currently cohesive forces and vocal rest seem to be adequate to maintain the flap in position postoperatively.

The key to success with the lateral endoscopic microflap technique is to remain superficial within Reinke's space. The surgical plane is actually within the superficial layer of the lamina propria and not immediately deep to the basement membrane zone. With preservation of normal SLLP and minimal disturbance of the intermediate and deep layers of the lamina propria, return of mucosal wave, when it existed preoperatively has been nearly 100%.[24,26] When absent preoperatively, secondary to near total fibrosis of the superficial layer of the lamina propria, return of the mucosal wave postoperatively is not usually evident. These patients, however, appear to gain improved voicing, probably from the creation of a straighter vocal fold margin and improved vocal fold closure as demonstrated on postoperative videostroboscopy.[22]

VOCAL FOLD POLYPS

Polyps, like nodules, appear to be acquired lesions. Unlike nodules, vascular and myxomatous polyps are more common in men. In addition, they are more often unilateral than bilateral. Vascular and myxomatous polyps do not appear to respond to behavioral therapy but require surgical excision for cure.[27] Prior to surgical intervention, however, speech therapy should be undertaken to educate the patients about presumed behavioral causes of polyp formation and to reduce the postoperative recurrence risk. We recommend direct laryngoscopy under general anesthesia with microscopic guidance for curative excision. This method provides greater stability of the operative field over indirect methods and allows more precise excision with less inadvertent risk to the vocal ligament.

Pedunculated polyps, which do not have extensive involvement of the medial surface of the vocal fold, can usually be excised with either knife or microscissors at the base of the pedicle. It is preferable to start with a sickle knife by incising the superior layer of the polyp stalk (Figure 36-6A). The incision is next extended through the top layer of the mucosa with up-cutting scissors (Figure 36-6B), then a flap elevator is used to separate polypoid changes from the normal superficial lamina propria (Figure 36-6C) and the inferior mucosal attachments cut with up-cutting scissors (Figure 36-6D and E).

For sessile polyp-like lesions, however, a medially based microflap technique as described for superficial nodule formation is performed. Microscissors or a sickle knife are used to incise the mucosa on the superior surface of the polyp. As much mucosa as possible is spared on the superior surface to create a superiorly based flap that can be trimmed to cover the defect after excision. A suction tip or blunt elevator is used to separate the myxomatous matrix from the vocal ligament and the previously created superiorly based flap. The scissors are then used to trim the inferior portion of the vocal fold polyp. The superiorly based flap is allowed to cover the created mucosal defect and is trimmed to fit. This technique minimizes the area of mucosal loss along the medial surface of the vocal fold and provides a cover for the vocal ligament which decreases the risk of postoperative scar formation. With this technique, large sessile polyps can be removed without de-epithelializing a significant portion of the vibrating surface of the vocal fold (Figure 36-7A and B).

VASCULAR LESIONS

Vascular lesions can occur anywhere on the superior or infraglottal surface of the vocal fold. They are seen as dilated vessels that run parallel to the free edge of the vocal fold. Often they form an angiomatous cluster

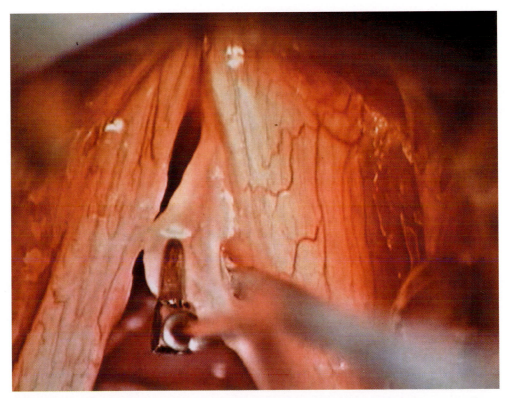

FIGURE 36-6. *This polyp has a short stalk from the inferior to superior direction along the medial surface of the vocal fold. (A) A sickle knife is used to incise the mucosa of the superior aspect of the stalk. (Continues)*

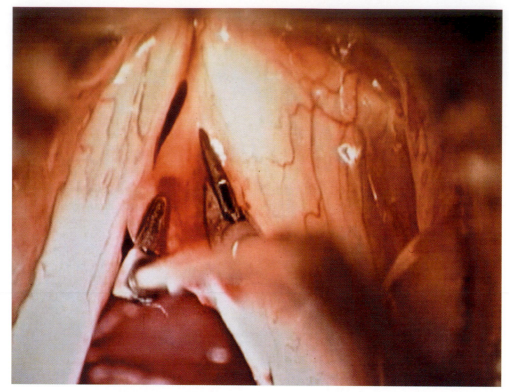

FIGURE 36-6. *(B) The incision is further enlarged with up-cutting microscissors. (Continues)*

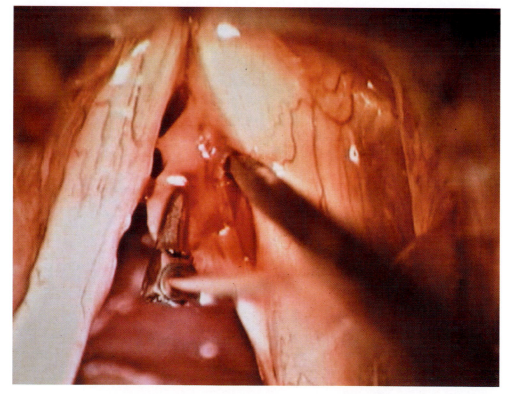

FIGURE 36-6. *(C) The flap elevator is used to dissect the lesion from the underlying normal SLLP. (Continues)*

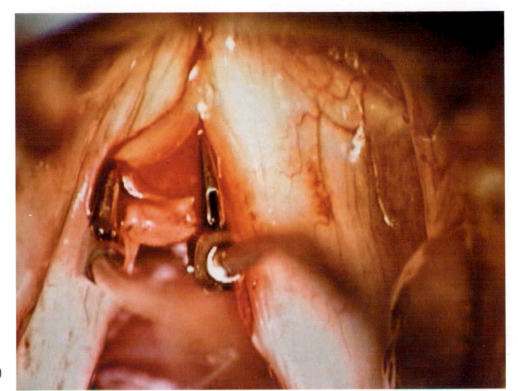

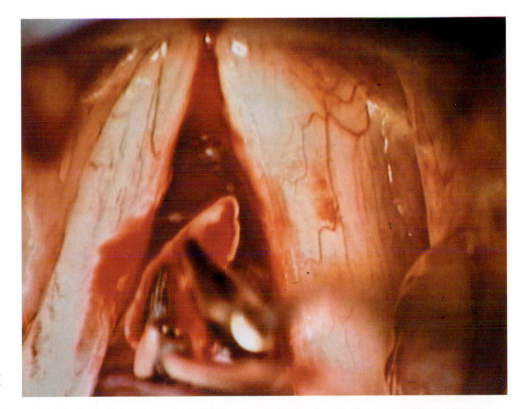

FIGURE 36-6. *(D and E) The inferior mucosal attachments are incised with the up-cutting scissors.*

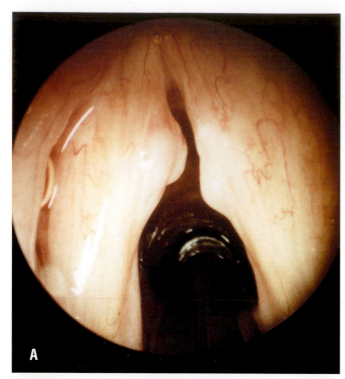

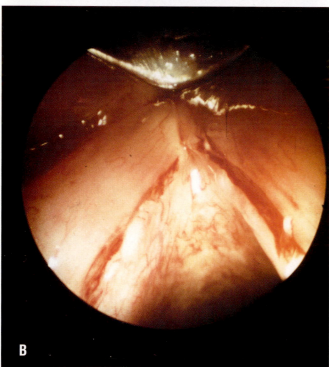

FIGURE 36-7. *Sessile polyps are excised with a medial microflap technique. (A) The preoperative view with the 0° telescope demonstrates the extent of medial surface involvement. (B) After microflap excision, disruption of mucosa along the medial surface has been held to a minimum. This is the view with a 70° telescope.*

near the middle of the vibrating vocal fold.[28-30] The cause of these lesions is unclear. They are more common in female singers, but not unheard of in men. In addition they may occur simultaneously with other benign acquired lesions such as nodules, polyps, and cysts. This may indicate that vascular lesions are acquired, possibly secondary to vocal overuse or hormonal imbalance. Retrospective analysis has shown that the most commonly associated conditions with recurrent hemorrhages are upper respiratory tract infection or hormonal imbalance. Therefore, patients should be observed and treated with hormonal modulation if necessary to prevent repeated hemorrhage.[31]

Isolated microvascular lesions rarely produce vocal symptoms unless they are present on the infraglottal or medial surface and interfere with closure or bleed into the lamina propria. Surgery is indicated if either of these conditions exists. Usually these vascular lesions are found on routine examination. They require observation by serial or interval examination and videostroboscopy to assess their effect on vocal fold vibration and closure. In women, particular attention must be paid to variation in the size of the lesion with menstruation. We have found an increased incidence of hemorrhage during the premenstrual period. If hemorrhage is imminent or recurrent, then photocoagulation with the carbon dioxide laser, or microsurgical excision,[30] may be indicated.

Exposure is obtained (Figure 36-8A). The carbon dioxide laser, in low-power setting (1500 W/cm^2) and in single-pulse focused mode, is used to coagulate the feeding vessel or vessels leading to the angiomatous cluster. Next the draining vessel or vessels are coagulated. Finally, the angiomatous cluster can be excised. Coagulation is achieved by a series of individual laser impacts along the course of the vessel until blanching is observed (Figure 36-8B). The use of chilled saline of the vocal fold prior to photocoagulation is of theoretical benefit. This is achieved using iced saline cottonoids. It may decrease the zone of thermal injury surrounding the area treated with the laser. Other surgeons have advocated microsurgical excision of these lesions to lessen the risks of thermal injury altogether.[30] In this technique the troublesome microvasculature is dissected from the SLLP with a pick-like instrument. Angiomatous clusters are excised with microscissors and knives.

VOCAL FOLD CYSTS

The etiology of vocal fold cysts is uncertain. Vocal fold cysts are either mucosal retention cysts or epidermal inclusion cysts.[32] Mucosal retention cysts are presumed to arise secondary to obstruction of an excretory duct. The wall of the duct consists of cuboidal epithelium. How these excretory ducts come to the lie in the true vocal fold, however, is uncertain, as the vocal fold itself normally has no salivary gland tissue. Presumably these mucosal retention cysts arise from ducts in the subglottis or supraglottis that then, secondary to pressure, migrate or expand into the area of the true glottis. If the cyst is of a presumed congenital nature, then the patient should have a lifelong history of dysphonia. Epidermal inclusion cysts, on the other hand, may be acquired secondary to recurrent vocal fold trauma. This trauma causes an infolding of the mucosa, which then breaks off and forms an inclusion cyst.

In either case the cysts are submucosal and are more frequently unilateral.[16] Their outline may be visualized with steady light examination. Videostroboscopy will enhance their outline and may show a significantly decreased or absent mucosal wave over the area of the cyst.[33] Surgical excision takes place after exposure is achieved. A sickle knife is used to make an incision on the superior surface of the vocal fold laterally, near the ventricle (Figure 36-9A). This place is chosen for the incision site for two reasons. First, the normal anatomy is relatively well-preserved, facilitating identification of the vocal ligament, and second, scarring and contracture on the lateral superior vocal fold have minimal effect on laryngeal vibratory patterns. The incision is finished with

the up-cutting microscissors (Figure 36-9B). As in the case of submucosal scarring, a blunt elevator is inserted and used to separate superficial layers of the lamina propria and mucosal cover from the underlying intermediate and deep layers of the lamina propria (Figure 36-9C). Once the cyst is encountered, the dissection continues between the cyst and vocal fold ligament (Figure 36-9D). This may require either sharp or blunt dissection. Care is taken not to evacuate the contents of the cyst.

Once the lesion is free from the vocal fold ligament, blunt and sharp dissection are used to develop a plane between the lesion and the vocal fold cover (Figure 36-9E). Occasionally these steps can be reversed. The key to surgical success, however, is preservation of the vocal fold ligament and uninvolved SLLP. Thin epithelium may be sacrificed with acceptable results, while vocal ligament and excess SLLP sacrifice will lead to unacceptable voice results. Once the lesion is removed, the operative field is inspected for secondary lesions such as a second cyst. If none is found then corticosteroids are placed into the newly created pocket and the flap is redraped (Figure 36-9F).

Well-circumscribed cysts may be approached through a medial microflap excisional technique if they appear to separate easily from the underlying vocal ligament. Some surgeons prefer this approach even for the

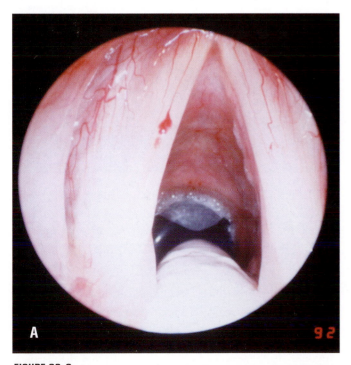
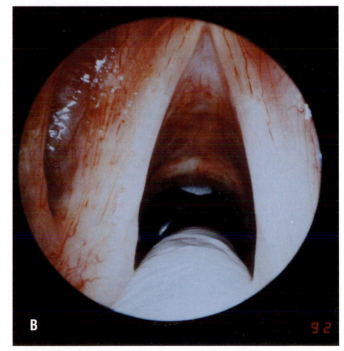

FIGURE 36-8. *A patient with multiple vascular lesions that have been noted to hemorrhage repeatedly. (A) Preoperative appearance. (B) Postoperative appearance immediately following photocoagulation with the CO_2 laser at 1500 W/cm^2.*

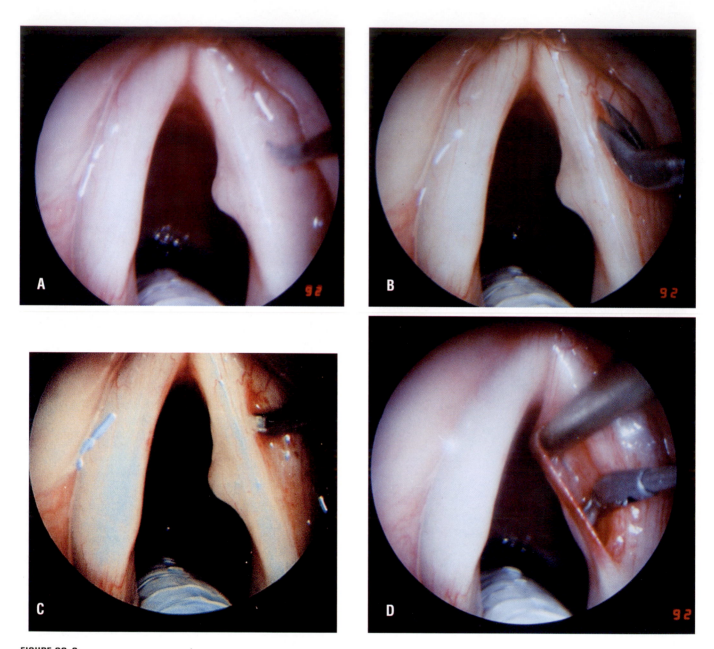

FIGURE 36-9. *A patient with a vocal fold cyst. This was excised using a microflap technique to preserve the overlying, uninvolved mucosal cover. (A) A sickle knife is used to make an incision laterally on the superior surface of the vocal fold. (B) The incision is further defined with up-cutting scissors. (C) A flap elevator is used to elevate the microflap. (D) The lesion is dissected from the vocal ligament. (Continues)*

more challenging cysts described previously.[25] On preoperative stroboscopy these lesions usually result in reduction or absence of mucosal wave. On palpation in the operating room, however, the surgeon can sometimes separate the lesion from the vocal ligament with gentle traction from a small suction. If the lesion appears to separate easily, then a medial microflap will usually allow adequate identification of the vocal liga-

ment, particularly anteriorly and/or posteriorly to the lesion. The lesion can then be freed from the surrounding normal structures with minimal disruption. The surgeon needs to be confident in his or her abilities. Mucosal retention cysts are often larger than they appear on initial observation. As the cysts expand they slowly lateralize the vocal ligament and can make dissection through a medial approach difficult. The cyst is

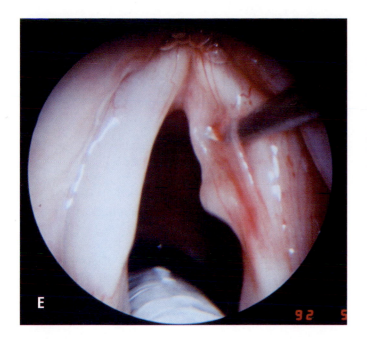

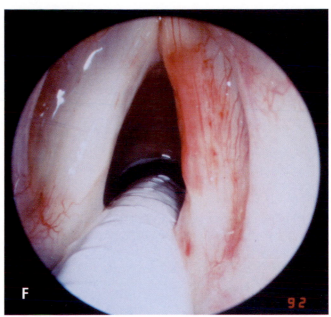

FIGURE 36-9. *(E) The lesion is dissected from the mucosal cover. (F) The mucosal cover is redraped into position.*

more easily punctured through a medial approach. If the cyst is deflated too early in the procedure, then identification of appropriate dissection planes is difficult. If too much tissue is removed scarring will result and if cyst wall remnants are left, then the cyst will reoccur (Figure 36-10A and B).

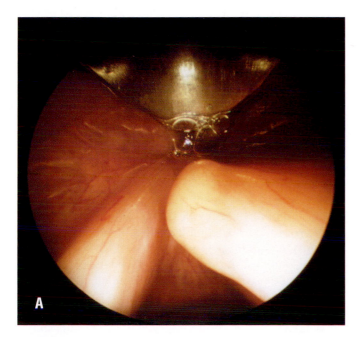

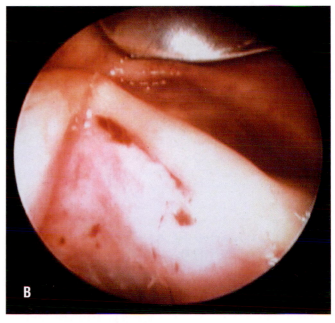

FIGURE 36-10. *Well-circumscribed cysts can be excised with a medial microflap technique. The decision to perform medial versus lateral microflap is made intraoperatively. If the lesion, on palpation, appears to separate easily from the vocal ligament, then a medial approach will allow adequate identification of the appropriate plain within the superficial lamina propria. (A) The 70° telescopic view demonstrates medial surface involvement preoperatively. (B) Postoperatively the same 70° telescope shows a minimal disruption along the vibrating surface.*

SULCUS VOCALIS

Sulcus vocalis is a vocal fold lesion that appears as a furrow running the length of the vocal fold. It actually consists of a fold of mucosa running along the free surface of the vocal fold. The furrowed mucosa may be adherent to the vocal ligament. This adherence disrupts the mucosal wave and leads to increased vocal roughness and fatigue. The etiology of sulcus vocalis, acquired or congenital, is poorly understood. The lesions are, however, more commonly described in men and can be unilateral or bilateral. Sulcus vocalis lesions are occasionally associated with an epidermal inclusion cyst.[34]

Diagnosis relies on physical examination, stroboscopy, and microlaryngoscopy. Videostroboscopy usually shows an altered mucosal wave with incomplete glottal closure in the form of a slit-like or spindle-shaped deficiency between the vibratory portions of the vocal folds. The involved vocal fold may appear bowed on still-light examination. The furrow may or may not be visible on indirect examination. Operative palpation, therefore, is often necessary to confirm the diagnosis.

The treatment of choice when speech therapy does not produce sufficient improvement is surgical excision. One advocated technique involves precise excision of the involved mucosa. A sickle knife is used to incise the mucosa of the upper border. A blunt dissector is then used to dissect the furrow through Reinke's space and to separate it from the vocal ligament. The inferior mucosal border is then incised with either a knife or scissors. Advancement flaps are elevated on either side of the furrow and used to obtain coverage for the medial vibratory surface of the vocal fold. Suturing of the flaps to maintain their position has been advocated by some surgeons. Care must be exercised to avoid overaggressive mucosal resection, which will lead to a dehiscence on the vibratory surface and result in postoperative decreased voicing. Although experience with these lesions has been limited, initial results have been encouraging and have been reported as such by other authors.[35]

Other techniques advocated for surgical management of sulcus include mucosal slicing or fat implantation into the lamina propria. In the mucosal slicing technique originally described by Pontes et al, a surgical plane is created in the deeper layers of the lamina propria, deep to the base of the sulcus. Transverse incisions of variable length are then made in the flap to break the tension created by the lesion. The flap is then redraped and re-epithelialization occurs. This technique has been reported with good results from two separate surgeons.[36,37]

Because of deficiency of normal superfical lamina propria deep to the sulcus, injection of substance into the SLLP to distend this region is difficult. Sataloff

described surgically creating a pocket deep to the sulcus and placing a free-fat graft to help re-create a soft vibratory cushion.[25] Fat implantation techniques have been used successfully by other surgeons as well.[38]

VOCAL FOLD SCARRING

The treatment of vocal fold scarring from previous surgery is an arduous task for any laryngologist. It is often difficult to distinguish whether poor postoperative results are secondary to improper resection or continued vocal misuse. Therefore, before surgical re-exploration, exhaustive speech therapy should be conducted. If no functional improvement is apparent and examination reveals a persisting altered mucosal wave and impaired glottic closure, then surgical exploration may be indicated. The timing of re-exploration should be at least 18 month after the initial procedure. This allows stabilization of healing tissue and provides adequate time for exhaustive speech rehabilitation.

Surgical intervention usually takes the form of an exploratory cordotomy. An incision is made in the mucosal cover near the ventricle. Blunt and sharp dissection are used to find or create a surgical plane in the superficial lamina propria between the mucosal cover and the underlying vocal ligament (intermediate and deep layers of the lamina propria). Corticosteroids are then injected into this newly created pocket and the flap redraped.

Postoperative results with these types of lesions show some improvement in the appearance of the vibratory characteristics of the vocal fold on stroboscopy postoperatively. The main improvement in vocal capabilities, however, appears to result from a straighter vocal fold surface. This improves glottic closure and provides a straighter surface for the normal vocal fold to vibrate against. This improved glottic closure explains the decreased vocal strain, roughness, and vocal fatigue experienced by our patients.

If lysing of scar bands within the lamina propria is unsuccessful at relieving the vocal disorder, then other methods of reconstruction may be indicated. Again, the vibratory abnormality is usually secondary to a loss of normal lamina propria with re-epithelialization occurring directly over the vocal ligament or muscle. Currently, synthetic materials to reconstruct the LP do not exist. In addition, the injection of substances, such as collagen or fat, into this region is difficult if not impossible secondary to scarification and instrumentation. Injected materials will flow from the needle into less dense tissue. Therefore, the scar will remain undisrupted and the softer, more normal tissues, will be infiltrated by the injected material. With regard to the injection of fat into scar tissue, the large size of the needle, 18-gauge, required to transplant viable fat cells, limits placement. The bevel of most 18-gauge needles is 3 to 4 mm. The normal LP is at most 1 to 2 mm in width. Therefore, injection into adherent tissue with a large gauge needle is not possible. For these reasons, some surgeons have attempted LP reconstruction by surgically creating a pocket just deep to existing epithelium. A small piece of fat is then placed into this pocket and the epithelium repositioned over the top of the fat graft.[38] Alternatively, in animal models we have attempted to use synthetic materials of elastin and collagen with limited success.

If reconstruction of the LP is not possible, attempts at reducing the glottal closure defect by medializing the available soft tissue through framework surgery may be employed. Frequently, this can result in some reduction of effort required to phonate. However, because the vibratory structures are not restored, the vocal quality usually remains rough. In addition, if the vocal fold deficiency is in the form of a notch, it is difficult to medialize a small vocal fold segment without over-correction in other regions.

POLYPOID CORDITIS

Polypoid corditis, also termed Reinke's edema or polypoid degeneration, is unlike other vocal fold polyps. It does not appear to be associated with vocal abuse but is intimately associated with cigarette smoking. Kleinsasser reports a 98% association.

Grossly, the vocal folds are sausage-shaped. As the polypoid changes progress, pedunculated lesions develop and involve the entire membranous vocal fold as their base. These lesions prolapse in and out of the glottis and inhibit phonation and, at times, respiration. Portions of the overlying epithelium may become keratotic, but the disease is not associated with an increased risk of cancer. Treatment is, therefore, aimed at excision of the polypoid changes of the superficial layer of the lamina propria with sparing enough mucosal membrane to cover the exposed, and carefully preserved, vocal ligament.

Surgical treatment, with mucosal preservation, allows simultaneous treatment of both vocal folds with minimal risk of web formation. In addition, the microflap excision technique facilitates proper identification of the vocal ligament and minimizes the risk of inadvertent injury. Comparison of surgical techniques indicates that excision via the microflap, or Hirano, technique results in the shortest duration of postoperative dysphonia.[35]

Regardless of the mode of treatment, the superficial layer of the lamina propria is diseased and must be removed. The term *edema* is a misnomer. The superficial layer of the lamina propria is not edematous but is replaced by a myxomatous-appearing stroma. Histologic examination of this stroma reveals relatively minimal increase in vascularity and minimal hyalinization, in contrast to the findings with polyps or nodules. Simple incision of the mucosa does not allow suction evacuation of the tissue, but rather, the tissue needs to be excised. Loss of the normal SLLP through the disease process, and then surgical excision, leads to a reduction in, or loss of, mucosal wave postoperatively. The SLLP does not appear to regenerate, and the mucosa attaches directly to the intermediate layer of the lamina propria. As such, patients need to be counseled with regard to postoperative voice quality. Voice will not return to normal. Reduction of vocal fold mass, however, usually results in an elevation of fundamental frequency and subjective increase in ease of phonation. In addition, patients usually report improved respiration, as the massive polypoid changes can lead to airway obstruction.

The surgical excision technique begins with adequate exposure through a binocular operating microlaryngoscope. A curved sickle knife is used to make an incision on the superior lateral surface of the vocal fold. The flap elevator is used to elevate a flap of mucosal membrane. The myxomatous stroma is then bluntly dissected from the underlying vocal ligament. The mucosa is trimmed with microscissors and redraped to cover the vocal ligament. Care should be taken not to leave excess mucosa as this will lead to an irregular vocal fold margin or increase the chance of recurrence.

POSTOPERATIVE MANAGEMENT

Postoperative management is divided into four phases. Phase 1 consists of 1 to 2 weeks of complete voice rest. Current recommendations regarding the use of voice rest among contemporary laryngologists show considerable variation. Recommendations range from zero to 14 days postoperatively.[1,2] Based on studies of vocal fold remucosalization and wound healing in general, 1 to 2 weeks seems most appropriate.[4] This allows adequate time for the majority of remucosalization to occur. In addition, collagen cross-linking for wound healing is at a point of steady incline. Laryngologists opposed to such lengthy periods of voice rest indicate potential vocal fold atrophy as their reason against use. No objective evidence, however, exists to support this view. In addition, examination of multiple patients after 2-week periods of complete voice rest does not show atrophy.

During phase 1, pharmacotherapy includes the use of antibiotics secondary to the presence of a contaminated surgical wound, pain medication, mucolytic agents, and control of hyperacidity if indicated.

Postoperative phase 2 includes postoperative weeks 2 through 4 and begins with an examination including videostroboscopy. If a microflap technique has been utilized, the operated vocal fold is edematous and stiff. Some evidence of return of the vertical phase difference and mucosal wave exists. The patient is allowed to phonate for 5 minutes the first day off voice rest. The time is then doubled to 10 minutes the second day, then 20 minutes, 40 minutes, 1.5 hours, 3 hours, and so forth. In this manner the patient is back to nearly full conversational speech by the midpoint of the fourth postoperative week.

Good vocal hygiene measures are continued. These include increased water uptake, mucolytic agents, and reflux control if appropriate.[39] The patient is instructed on easy-onset phonation and asked to observe frequent 10-minute periods of vocal rest. Vocal fatigue and strain are signs of over-activity, and the patient is asked to use biofeedback methods for regulating activity.

Postoperative phase 3 includes postoperative weeks 5 through 12 and consists of continued behavior modification and vocal hygiene. Physical examination should show continued resolution of edema with return of the vertical phase difference and the mucosal wave. Frequent examinations and videostroboscopy are performed to assess the effect of continued and increased function on the glottis. Vocal coaching for the singing voice is instituted during phase 3. The vertical phase difference, mucosal wave, and glottic closure should continue to improve with each examination. Should evidence of worsening of these factors develop, then vocal activity is decreased or halted.

Finally, phase 4 consists of weeks 13 and beyond and represents a return to full vocal activity with observation every 6 to 8 weeks. This is carried on for approximately 24 months from the time of surgery. Healing and changes in appearance of mucosal wave and glottic function will continue for up to 2 years postoperatively. Patients will continue to make improvement in their vocal technique and capability. Intermittent vocal re-education or rehabilitation enhances continued vocal hygiene and proper vocal function.

SUMMARY

The surgical management of benign voice disorders relies on accurate history and examination. Videostroboscopy is essential for the examination of glottic vibratory behavior and vocal fold closure. With these tools the accuracy of diagnosis of vocal fold abnormalities is enhanced.[3] However, it is often still not possible to diagnose the exact nature of a vocal fold lesion on the initial examination. In this instance, serial or interval examination is helpful. In addition, behavior modification with vocal abuse reduction and correction of misuses may help to resolve surrounding vocal fold edema and further identify the true lesion. This principle of exhaustive behavioral and medical management before surgical intervention is essential for good surgical results. It is equivalent to the use of physical therapy by the orthopedic surgeon or neurosurgeon prior to definitive joint or disk surgery.

If surgical intervention is deemed necessary, then precise excision of the lesion with minimal disturbance to the surrounding normal tissue is crucial for the return of glottic function postoperatively. Patients who have had overaggressive resection of benign glottic lesions show altered mucosal wave formation and impaired glottic function on postoperative videostroboscopy. These patients have decreased vocal capabilities. To attain this goal of minimal disturbance to the surrounding normal tissues, the surgeon must time the surgical intervention with regard to treatment of the surrounding edema and use precise surgical techniques. Surgeons operating on benign vocal fold lesions should be well-versed in glottic anatomy, histology, and physiology. They should feel comfortable with the use of microlaryngeal instrumentation and in viewing the glottis under high magnification. Currently these techniques are not a standard practice in most residency programs.

After surgical intervention, postoperative rehabilitation with continued behavioral modification and improved vocal hygiene is important for adequate postoperative results. Preoperative physical or speech therapy is beneficial in establishing adequate vocal hygiene habits that can then be applied to the postoperative rehabilitation. Postoperatively patients should expect a 7- to 14-day period of complete voice rest followed by 2.5 months of rehabilitation. Overuse of edematous or stiff vocal fold(s) may result in the acquisition of functional disorders. Therefore, the patient's progress postoperatively needs to be monitored closely with repeat examination and videoendostroboscopy. Activity can be liberalized as the characteristics of vocal fold vibration improve.

REFERENCES

1. Gould WJ. Surgery in professional singers. *Ear Nose Throat J.* 1987;66:327-332.

2. Bouchayer M, Cornut G. Microsurgery for benign lesions of the vocal folds. *Ear Nose Throat J.* 1988;67:446-466.

3. Garrett CG, Coleman JR, Reinisch L. Comparative histology and vibration of the vocal folds: implica-

tions for experimental studies in microlaryngeal surgery. *Laryngoscope.* 2000;110:814-824.

4. Durkin GE, Duncavage JA, Toohil RJ, et al. Wound healing of true vocal cord squamous epithelium following CO_2 laser ablation and cup forceps stripping. *Otolaryngol Head Neck Surg.* 1986;95:273-277.

5. Bastian RW. Factors leading to successful evaluation and management of patients with voice disorders. *Ear Nose Throat J.* 1988;67(6):411-420.

6. Sataloff RT. Surgery for the voice? [editorial]. *Clin Otolaryngol.* 1989;14:185-188.

7. Filter MD, ed. *Phonatory Voice Disorders in Children.* Springfield, IL: Charles C Thomas; 1982:111.

8. Lancer JM, Syder D, Jones AS, et al. Vocal cord nodules: a review. *Clin Otolaryngol.* 1988;13:43-51.

9. Lancer JM, Syder D, Jones AS, et al. The outcome of different management patterns for vocal cord nodules. *J Laryngol Otol.* 1988;102:423-427.

10. McFarlane SC. Treatment of benign laryngeal disorders with traditional methods and techniques of voice therapy. *Ear Nose Throat J.* 1988;67(6):425-435.

11. Ossoff RH, Karpan MS. Instrumentation for microlaryngeal laser surgery. *Otolaryngol Head Neck Surg.* 1983;91(4):456-460.

12. Weed DT, Courey MS, Ossoff RH. Microlaryngeal surgery in the difficult surgical exposure: a new microlaryngoscope. *Otolaryngol Head Neck Surg.* 1994;110(2):247-252.

13. Zeitels SM. Universal modular glotticsurgery system: the evolution of a century of design and technique for direct laryngoscopy. *Ann Otol Rhinol Laryngol Suppl.* 1999;179:2-24.

14. Milutinovic Z. Indirect microsurgery of the vocal folds—videostroboscopy vs microstroboscopy. *Ear Nose Throat.* 1993;72(2):134-141.

15. Kantor E, Berci G, Partlow E, et al. A completely new approach to microlaryngeal surgery. *Laryngoscope.* 1991;101:676-679.

16. Bouchayer M, Cornut G, Loire R, et al. Epidermoid cysts, sulci, and mucosal bridges of the true vocal cord: a report of 157 cases. *Laryngoscope.* 1984;95:1087-1094.

17. Werkhaven J, Ossoff RH. Surgery for benign lesions of the glottis. *Otolaryngol Clin North Am.* 1991;24:1179-1199.

18. Shapshay SM, Healy GB. New microlaryngeal instruments for phonatory surgery and pediatric applications. *Ann Otol Rhinol Laryngol.* 1989;98:821-823.

19. Ossoff RH, Karlan MS. Laser surgery in otolaryngology, In: Ballenger JJ, ed. *Diseases of the Nose, Throat, Ear, Head and Neck, Laser Surgery in Otolaryngology.* 13th ed. Philadelphia, PA: Lea & Febiger; 1991:769-783.

20. Duncavage JA, Aly A, Halter S, et al. Laser surgery of the larynx. In: Ford CN, Bless DM, eds. *Phonosurgery: Assessment and Surgical Management of Voice Disorders.* New York, NY: Raven; 1991:167-181.

21. Karlan MS, Ossoff RH. Laser surgery for benign laryngeal disease; conversation and ergonomics. *Symp Laser Surg.* 1984;64:981-993.

22. Ossoff RH, Werkhaven JA, Raif J, et al. Advanced microspot microslad for the CO_2 laser. *Otolaryngol Head Neck Surg.* 1991;105(3):411-414.

23. Kotby MN, Nassar AM, Seif EI, et al. Ultrastructural features of vocal fold nodules and polyp. *Acta Otolaryngol (Stockh).* 1988;105(5-6):477-482.

24. Courey MS, Garrett CG, Ossoff RH. Medial microflap for excision of benign vocal fold lesions. *Laryngoscope.* 1987;107:340-344.

25. Sataloff RT, Spiegel JR, Heuer RJ, et al. Laryngeal mini-microflap: a new technique and reassessment of the microflap saga. *J Voice.* 1995;9(2):198-204.

26. Courey MS, Gardner GM, Stone RE, Ossoff RH. Endoscopic vocal fold microflap: a three-year experience. *Ann Otol Rhinol Laryngol.* 1995;104(4):267-273.

27. Kleinsasser O. *Microlaryngoscopy and Endolaryngeal Microsurgery.* Philadelphia, PA; Hanley & Belfus; 1991:34.

28. Postma GN, Courey MS, Ossoff RH. Microvascular lesions of the true vocal fold. *Ann Otol Rhinol Laryngol.* 1998;107(6):472-476.

29. Courey MS, Postma GN. Microvascular lesions of the true vocal folds. *Curr Op Otol.* 1996;4:134-137.

30. Hochman I, Sataloff RT, Hillman RE, Zeitels SM. Ectasias and varices of the vocal fold: clearing the striking zone. *Ann Otol Rhinol Layrngol.* 1999;108(1):10-16.

31. Lin PT, Stern JC, Gould WJ. Risk factors and management of vocal cord hemorrhages: an experience with 44 cases. *Voice.* 1991;5(1)74-77.

32. Merati AL, Andrews RJ, Courey MS, Garrett CG, Ossoff RH. Phonomicrosurgical management of intracordal cysts. *Op Tech Otol.* 1998;9(4):230-237.

33. Shohet JA, Courey MS, Ossoff RH. The value of videostroboscopic parameters in differentiating benign true vocal fold cysts, nodules and polyps. *Laryngoscope.* 1996;106:19-26.

34. Bouchayer M, Cornut G. Microsurgical treatment of benign vocal fold lesions: indications, technique, results. *Folia Phoniatr (Basel).* 1992;44:155-184.

35. Lumpkin SM, Bishop S, Bennett S. Comparison of surgical techniques in the treatment of laryngeal polypoid degeneration. *Ann Otol Rhinol Laryngol.* 1987;96:254-257.

36. Pontes P, Behlau M. Treatment of sulcus vocalis: auditory perceptual and acoustical analysis of the slicing mucosa surgical technique. *J Voice.* 1993;7(4):365-376.

37. Ford CN, Inagi K, Khidr A, Bless DM, Gilchrist KW. Sulcus vocalis: a rational analytical approach to diagnosis and management. *Ann Otol Rhinol Laryngol.* 1996;105(3):189-200.

38. Gray SD, Bielamowicz SA, Titze IR, Dove H, Ludlow C. Experimental approaches to vocal fold alteration: introduction to the minithyrotomy. *Ann Otol Rhinol Laryngol.* 1999;108(1):1-9.

39. Emerich KA, Spiegel JR, Sataloff RT. Phonomicrosurgery III: pre- and postoperative care. *Otolaryngol Clin North Am.* 2000;33(5):1071-1080.

CHAPTER 37

Laryngeal Framework Surgery

Steven M. Zeitels, MD, FACS

Ramon A. Franco, Jr., MD

Restoration of vocal function with laryngeal framework surgery (laryngoplastic phonosurgery) was introduced at the beginning of the 20th century. Today, these procedures have emerged as the dominant surgical management approach for the treatment of the aerodynamic incompetence and acoustic deterioration associated with vocal fold paralysis/paresis. Other indications include cancer defects, vocal fold scar, sulcus vocalis, bowing associated with vocal fold atrophy, laryngeal trauma, and neuromuscular disorders including abductor spasmodic dysphonia and parkinsonism. Laryngeal framework surgery has also been employed to alter pitch for gender reassignment; however, this is not discussed in this chapter.

Although medialization of the musculomembranous vocal fold by means of rearranging the laryngeal cartilage framework was described by Payr[1] in 1915, and others in the middle 20th century,[2,3] Isshiki[4-6] championed the systematic analysis and laryngoplastic treatment of glottal incompetence in the 1970s. He designed his medialization procedure of the musculomembranous vocal fold with the use of a synthetic implant in 1974.[4] Gore-Tex has become the authors' implant choice for medialization laryngoplasty; the unique characteristics of this bioimplant are delineated below. In 1978, Isshiki designed the arytenoid adduction[5] procedure to treat patients with large glottal gaps secondary to a malpositioned arytenoid. One of his outstanding contributions is that he taught sur-

geons that laryngeal framework procedures could be done with facility utilizing local anesthesia with sedation. The concept that the cricoarytenoid joint could be dissected and manipulated under local anesthesia to allow for phonatory feedback was revolutionary. Based on this seminal work, the adduction arytenopexy[2,7,8] and cricothyroid subluxation[7-9] procedures were introduced to further enhance phonatory reconstruction.

PRINCIPLES AND THEORY OF LARYNGEAL FRAMEWORK SURGERY

The ideal procedure(s) to treat aerodynamic glottal incompetence that is associated with paralytic/paretic dysphonia should attempt to simulate the normal vocal fold position during phonation with regard to the following interdependent parameters: (1) Position of the musculomembranous region in the axial plane, (2) position of the arytenoid in the axial plane, (3) height of the vocal fold, (4) length of the vocal fold, (5) contour of the vocal fold edge in the musculomembranous region, (6) contour of the vocal fold edge in the arytenoid region, and (7) mass and viscoelasticity of the vocal fold.

Furthermore, the procedure(s) should ideally be easy to perform, associated with few complications, reliable, reversible, and not threatening to the airway.[10] Although not reversible, the adduction arytenopexy procedure[2] more closely models the synchronous agonist-antagonist function of the lateral cricoarytenoid, interarytenoid, lateral thyroarytenoid, and posterior cricoarytenoid muscles during phonatory adduction. Cricothyroid subluxation[7,9] is a phonosurgical procedure for recurrent nerve-induced paralytic/paretic dysphonia. This technique is designed to primarily increase unilateral length and tension of the vocal fold by simulating cricothyroid muscle function. Gore-Tex medialization[7,11] has a number of unique qualities, but like many prior innovations, it is a modification of Isshiki's conventional implant approach.

TRADITIONAL APPROACHES

Surgical interventions for support or placement of the true vocal folds can be divided into injection thyroplasty techniques and laryngeal framework surgical techniques. A brief review of the traditional approaches serves to highlight the recent innovations in surgical technique. As this is an overview, the reader is referred to surgical atlases and surgical manuscripts to obtain detailed descriptions of these procedures.

Injection Thyroplasty

Many materials have been used for injection thyroplasty, each with its own indications, advantages, and disadvantages. These materials are typically injected deep within the paraglottic space to effect a change in the contour and medialize the edge of the paralyzed true vocal fold.

Teflon

Although popularized in the 1960s,[12] vocal fold augmentation with Teflon has fallen into disfavor because of its irreversibility, propensity to extrude and form granulomas, its imprecise placement, and the stiffness which can occur if it is injected superficially. Today Teflon is best used in those patients with terminal diseases who require a one-time, quick procedure, which will decrease aspiration caused by glottal incompetence. A disadvantage, which is common to all injected materials, is their inability to effect a change in the position of the arytenoid and height of the vocal fold. If there is not favorable synkinetic reinnervation, misalignment of the vocal folds remains with resultant air escape. In an effort to avoid the sequelae caused by Teflon, other materials have been used for medialization including autologous fat, collagen, and gelfoam.

Autologous Fat Injection Thyroplasty

Autologous fat injection thyroplasty requires the harvesting of a small amount of fat (axillary or abdominal) and some preparation (washing, drying of excess moisture and dicing into small pieces) prior to injection. A Brunings syringe is used to introduce the fat into the true vocal fold. The vocal fold is over-injected by up to 50% with fat as there is a variable loss of tissue during the first 6 weeks. Several studies have reported good long-term results with persistent glottal closure.[13,14] The obvious disadvantages include the imprecision of the final result because of limitations in quantifying the injection and unpredictable variable resorption.

Collagen

When collagen is used it is injected into the superficial lamina propria (SLP) allowing for precise placement where it is needed most. Collagen's main disadvantages include variable resorption and relative high cost for the material. In an effort to decrease the resorption of collagen, autologous collagen has been introduced to eliminate the antigenicity associated with bovine collagen.[15] However, autologous collagen requires a donor site of resected skin from the patient.

Gelfoam

Gelfoam is injected into the paraglottic region in a fashion similar to Teflon injection. It is a temporary procedure introduced in 1978 by Schramm,[16] which is easy to perform with a very low complication rate. Gelfoam is prepared prior to injection by mixing a gelatin powder with saline to form a gelfoam paste, which is injected into the lateral paraglottic region. It is a very effective way to medialize the musculomembranous vocal fold in those who may have spontaneous return of activity for two to three months; other procedures, including medialization thyroplasty and arytenoid procedures, can be performed subsequent to gelfoam injections.

Laryngeal Framework Surgery

The foundation of laryngeal framework surgery was established by Isshiki et al during the early 1970s.[4-6] They demonstrated improvement in hoarseness by direct manipulation and rearrangement of the laryngeal framework to achieve closure of the glottal gap and restore competence to the glottal valve. Isshiki described four basic surgical procedures, which he termed thyroplasty types I-IV[6] for altering the conformation of the thyroid cartilage, and the arytenoid adduction, which attempts to close the posterior (cartilaginous) glottis.

Thyroplasty Type I

Thyroplasty type I (Figure 37-1) is the most widely used of Isshiki's original thyroplasty techniques. It involves creating a rectangular cartilaginous window at the level of the true vocal fold and using cartilage, silas-

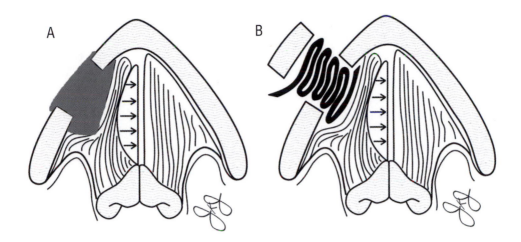

FIGURE 37-1. *Illustration of a thyroplasty type I procedure using (A) a solid or (B) Gore-Tex implant to achieve medialization of the vocal fold.*

tic, Gore-Tex, or other implant material to medialize the true vocal fold. This procedure achieves closure of the musculomembranous vocal fold only; arytenoid position is not appreciably altered by the implant. Thyroplasty type I is a relatively simple and reversible procedure which is ideally performed with local anesthesia to facilitate fine tuning of the voice with precise placement of the implant material. There have been a large number of manuscripts describing a multitude of variations of the original procedure, primarily introducing different implant materials and their placement. As thyroplasty type I does not primarily influence arytenoid position, this procedure is often coupled with an arytenoid adduction or arytenopexy to close both the anterior (musculomembranous) and posterior (cartilaginous) glottis.

Isshiki's Other Thyroplasty Classifications

Thyroplasty type II is a procedure in which the posterolateral thyroid lamina is lateralized; there are few indications for its use.[6] Thyroplasty type III is used to lower the vocal pitch by shortening the anteroposterior (A-P) dimension of the glottis. The primary function is to release vocal fold tension to lower pitch. Conversely, thyroplasty type IV increases the A-P dimension of the glottis, thereby increasing the tension on the vocal folds and raising the vocal pitch. Thyroplasty types III and IV have been used in gender reassignment surgery to bring the fundamental frequency into the normal range for the newly assigned sex.[6]

Arytenoid Adduction

Arytenoid adduction was described by Isshiki[5] as a way of mimicking the medializing effect of the lateral cricoarytenoid muscle on the vocal process. A paralyzed arytenoid will tend to fall forward and laterally on the cricoid facet, shortening the A-P length of the vocal fold and moving the arytenoid away from the midline. The classic arytenoid adduction procedure is performed under local anesthesia with sedation by exposing the posterior aspect of the thyroid lamina. The cricoarytenoid joint is identified, and a suture is placed through the muscular process of the arytenoid and passed anteriorly through the thyroid lamina, thereby rotating the vocal process medially to meet the opposite vocal process during phonation. Prior to the conclusion of the surgical procedure the position is visually verified by means of a flexible fiberoptic laryngoscope.

SURGICAL INNOVATIONS

Adduction Arytenopexy

Patients who require repositioning of the arytenoid secondary to paralysis-induced displacement typically have minimal or unfavorable synkinetic reinnervation of the intrinsic laryngeal musculature. Therefore, the arytenoid is malpositioned anteriorly, inferiorly, and laterally, resulting in a flaccid foreshortened vocal fold. Isshiki's classical arytenoid adduction procedure mimics contraction of the lateral cricoarytenoid muscle and achieves rotation of the arytenoid by means of a suture that is placed through its muscular process and directed anteriorly through the thyroid lamina. However, the agonist-antagonistic adductor function of the other intrinsic muscles (lateral thyroarytenoid, interarytenoid, and posterior cricoarytenoid) is not simulated.

The adduction arytenopexy procedure was designed to model the synchronous function of the aforementioned musculature.[2] In this technique, the arytenoid is positioned on the medial aspect of the cricoid facet, simulating normal adduction of the arytenoid during phonation. In addition, an implant is placed lateral to the paraglottic muscles (inner thyroid perichondrium) to avoid wide excursion of the glottal tissues during entrained oscillation. The dennervated musculature of the paraglottic region is highly susceptible to the potential closing forces secondary to Bernoulli's effect. This fact is utilized to counter-balance the loss in normal elastic-recoil closing forces from the denervation. Placing the arytenoid in appropriate position posteriorly, prior to the placement of an implant, achieves most of the medialization that is necessary for the edge of the musculomembranous vocal fold.[2,7,8]

Adduction arytenopexy procedure results in a slightly longer vocal fold, which is appropriately aligned in all three dimensions with a well-conformed medial edge of the glottal aperture. This clinical observation was confirmed in a cadaver study.[2] In contradistinction to the classical arytenoid adduction in which an anterolateral directed suture is used, the adduction arytenopexy procedure achieves a longer vocal fold by posteromedially displacing the arytenoid and maintaining its position with a posteriorly based suture. In the same study, the adduction arytenopexy procedure was more effective than was the classical arytenoid adduction in closing interarytenoid gaps. Furthermore, the adduction arytenopexy does not result in excessive hyper-rotation of the vocal process.

During adduction arytenopexy, the body of the arytenoid is medialized to the limit of the medial cricoarytenoid joint capsule in a normal gliding fashion along the cricoid facet. It is clear from the convex contour of the cricoid facet and the precisely accommodating concave contour of the arytenoid base that hyper-rotation (simulating the lateral cricoarytenoid muscle) based on an axial plane does not simulate normal arytenoid adduction. Furthermore, pathologic hyper-rotation of the arytenoid and hyperfunction of the lateral cricoarytenoid are typically observed in patients who present with arytenoid granulomas.[17] Both Koufman's diagrammatic depiction of a typical arytenoid adduction[18] as well as Neuman and Woodson et al's[19] cadaver study reveal an abnormally contoured medial arytenoid that results in an abnormal interarytenoid chink. In many patients, the clinical significance of this chink may be minimized by redundant interarytenoid and periarytenoid soft tissue.

The adduction-arytenopexy dissection method[2,7,8] of the cricoarytenoid joint can be performed without complication and is simpler than other techniques. Additionally, using the anatomic configuration of the cricoid facet to select the ideal position of the arytenoid has not been reported previously. These factors lead to placement of the arytenoid in a more normal adduction position, and, therefore, more effective glottal closure during laryngeal sound production.

Despite ideal positioning of the arytenoid from the arytenopexy procedure, intraoperative observations revealed that optimal vocal quality required an accompanying medialization laryngoplasty. This is because of the flaccidity of the denervated glottis, which results in valvular incompetence. The denervated glottal tissues have impaired elastic-recoil closing forces caused by atrophy and fibrosis. On stroboscopy, this is revealed as an abnormally wide excursion of the vocal edge and as a long open-phase quotient during vibratory cycles.

A well-positioned arytenoid obviates the need for complex implant shapes that are intended to close the posterior glottis from an anteriorly positioned thyroid-lamina window. Additionally, there are a number of technical advantages to performing medialization laryngoplasty with adduction arytenopexy rather than with arytenoid adduction. As there is not an anterior thyroid-lamina suture, the implant is unencumbered by the adduction of the arytenoid. Furthermore, the adduction arytenopexy is done prior to the medialization so that the implant can be sized more accurately with the structural positioning of the posterior glottis already established. Finally, complex implant shapes that violate the thyroid-lamina inner perichondrium are unnecessary.

The adduction arytenopexy, which positions the arytenoid for normal phonation, can allow for a simple smaller implant shape to be placed lateral to the thyroid perichondrium because posterior glottic tissues are already aligned. *The primary goal of the implant with arytenopexy is to prevent lateral excursion of the flaccid paraglottic tissue during oscillatory cycles rather than to medialize the vocal edge, which is accomplished mostly by the adduction arytenopexy.* The technique for implant medialization becomes similar to what is required for patients with vocal-muscle atrophy, which is easy to correct.

Observations made from the vocal-outcome data in the patients who underwent adduction arytenopexy and medialization laryngoplasty revealed that fairly normal conversational level phonation was achieved.[2] However, there were remarkable limitations of maximal range capabilities, especially frequency variation and maximal phonation time. This was thought to be secondary to suboptimal viscoelastic tension in the denervated vocal fold soft tissues despite the aforementioned improvements in three-dimensional repositioning of the vocal edge. The need to increase viscoelastic tension in the denervated vocal fold, and thereby improve aerodynamically efficient entrained oscillation, catalyzed the development of the cricothyroid [C-T] subluxation procedure.[7,9]

In summary, repositioning the arytenoid should primarily be done when the malpositioned cartilage leads to phonatory aerodynamic glottal incompetence. Adduction arytenopexy[2] is the first modification of Isshiki's arytenoid adduction procedure, which was designed over 20 years ago. The arytenoid adduction procedure only simulates the lateral cricoarytenoid muscle, while the adduction arytenopexy models the synchronous adductor contraction of all the intrinsic musculature.

Gore-Tex Medialization Thyroplasty

The use of Gore-Tex as a medialization implant for the musculomembranous vocal fold was introduced by Hoffman and McCulloch[20] and has been employed by the senior author for three years.[7,8,11] The primary advantages of Gore-Tex are its ease of handling, placement, and adjustability, all of which enhance the speed and precision with which the operation can be performed. The position of the Gore-Tex can even be adjusted and fine-tuned extensively while the implant remains within the patient rather than removing it for modification as is done with silastic. This is unlike virtually all other implant approaches. Furthermore, precise positioning of the thyroid-lamina window is less critical because Gore-Tex can be placed into appropriate position despite a slightly malpositioned window.

Because of these characteristics, Gore-Tex is also well suited to restore aerodynamic glottal competence in scenarios in which there are complex anatomic defects such as those encountered with trauma and cancer resections. Even subtle contour changes from the loss of superficial lamina propria associated with sulcus vergeture can be reconformed to treat a small glottal gap. The versatility of Gore-Tex is demonstrated by its ease of use in the treatment of these varied irregular tissue abnormalities. In a current review there have been minimal complications in over 90 cases.[11]

To facilitate placement of the implant, an inferiorly based thyroid perichondrial flap is developed and a window is made in the thyroid lamina lateral to the musculomembranous vocal fold. The inner perichondrium of the thyroid lamina is preserved at the perimeter of the window. A small implant is then fashioned from a thin sheet of Gore-Tex so that it can be layered lateral to the inner perichondrium of the thyroid lamina. The Gore-Tex can be stabilized with a 4-0 Prolene suture. The thyroid lamina cartilage that was removed to make the window can be repositioned in its original site.

Cricothyroid Subluxation

Once the adduction arytenopexy and medialization laryngoplasty are completed, a cricothyroid subluxation is performed to further enhance vocal quality. The newly described cricothyroid subluxation is accomplished by placing a 2-0 Prolene suture around the inferior cornu of the thyroid lamina on the denervated side.[9] It is then passed in a submucosal fashion underneath the cricoid anteriorly. The suture is pulled taut, which increases the distance between the cricoid facet and the attachment of the anterior commissure ligament. This ultimately increases the tension and length of the musculomembranous vocal fold on the paralyzed side. The tension on this suture is adjusted by using a slipknot while the patient performs phonatory tasks. These include maximal-range tasks such as use of pulse-register (vocal fry) through a falsetto register and glissando sliding scales.

This cricothyroid subluxation suture simulates cricothyroid muscle contraction for counter-tension on the thyroarytenoid muscle and for increasing length of the musculomembranous vocal fold. Once this is completed, the strap muscles are reattached with 3-0 Vicryl suture in a running fashion. The wound is irrigated and a Penrose drain is placed. The platysma is approximated in a running fashion with Vicryl suture as well, and then the skin is closed with 4-0 nylon suture. A pressure dressing is applied and the drain is removed on the first postoperative morning. The patient is started on a liquid diet on the first postoperative morning and is advanced to a normal diet as tolerated. Fiberoptic laryngoscopy is performed prior to discharge to ensure that there is not an excessive amount of edema that would warrant further observation. Typically, patients can be discharged on the first postoperative day.

Clinical Experience with Cricothyroid Subluxation

The cricothyroid subluxation (C-T sub) procedure[7,9] has further enhanced postoperative vocal quality as it is an easily adjustable method of increasing and varying tension and length of the paralyzed and denervated musculomembranous vocal fold. This is unlike all prior operations, which were designed primarily to treat paralytic dysphonia by repositioning the vocal fold edge.[2,4-6,18,21] Those procedures that alter tension and length of the vocal fold were conceived to modify pitch rather than to treat paralytic dysphonia.[22-25] The cricothyroid subluxation suture: (1) models cricothyroid muscle contraction, (2) produces counter-tension on the thyroarytenoid muscle, and (3) increases the length of the musculomembranous vocal fold.[7] C-T subluxation is easy to perform, has been free from complications, and improves the acoustic outcome of other laryngoplastic phonosurgical procedures.

The modified biomechanical properties of vocal fold vibration that occurred subsequent to C-T sub resulted in improved vocal outcome in all patients[9] and was most remarkable in maximal range capabilities. C-T sub enhanced the postoperative voice of patients, regardless of whether they required medialization laryngoplasty alone or with adduction arytenopexy. Unlike stretching/lengthening procedures associated with gender reassignment, voice results in denervated patients have not deteriorated with follow-up >1 year. *Because of the decreased elasticity of denervated vocal folds, the optimal length (for vibration) is longer than that of normal vocal folds. Denervated vocal fold tissue has a different resonant frequency than if it is innervated.*

Although the adduction arytenopexy had been shown to result in improvements in a number of objective measures of vocal function[2] by simulating normal glottal closure and reproducing the synchronous adductor contractile characteristics of all the intrinsic muscles, vocal outcome measures revealed limitations in maximal range tasks, especially dynamic frequency range.[2] This finding was most likely caused by persistent flaccidity of the denervated thyroarytenoid musculature. Both Isshiki's[5,6] and Zeitels'[2] adducting arytenoid techniques separate the cricothyroid joint to expose the cricoarytenoid joint. During a collaborative cadaver dissection, R. Sataloff (personal communication) observed that separation and destabilization of the ipsilateral cricothyroid joint impairs the function of the contralateral cricothyroid muscle. Based on a similar observation, other authors have exposed the cricoarytenoid joint during arytenoid adduction by removing a posterior window of the thyroid lamina and leaving the cricothyroid joint intact.[26]

Clinical observations revealed that after the cricothyroid joint was opened, the inferior cornu of the thyroid lamina became retro-displaced with relation to the cricoid. This meant that the previously fixed vocal fold length was shortened, and the tension of flaccid denervated thyroarytenoid muscle was reduced further. Essentially, there was a decrease in the normal distance between the cricoarytenoid joint and the insertion of the anterior commissure tendon into the thyroid lamina.

Foreshortening of the paralyzed vocal fold, induced by separating the cricothyroid joint, probably led to compensatory hyperfunctional foreshortening of the normal vocal fold. This hyperfunctional adaptation occurs to align the vocal processes, which is a prerequi-

site for normal entrained oscillation during phonation. The decreased phonatory length of both vocal folds and the decreased viscoelastic tension of the paralyzed vocal fold resulted in limitations in acoustic maximal-range capabilities. Despite the fact that the paralyzed vocal fold was surgically placed under higher tension (than its preoperative state) after C-T subluxation,[7-9] almost all patients could reach a frequency lower than in their preoperative state. This paradox is probably explained by the fact that the post-subluxation lengthened vocal fold results in reduced hyperfunction of the entire laryngeal complex.

The cricothyroid subluxation procedure was designed to rectify the mechanical impediments that were partially precipitated by disruption of the cricothyroid joint during cricoarytenoid joint dissection. However, C-T subluxation also improved the vocal outcome of those patients who did not require an arytenoid procedure (because of somewhat-favorable synkinesis). In both scenarios, the objective measures of vocal function reveal that C-T subluxation improved the aerodynamic efficiency of the glottal valve with a commensurate enhancement of the maximal-range acoustic characteristics of the voice. Subjective perceptions revealed that most patients demonstrated a register transition between modal and falsetto, an observation not previously reported.

OPERATIVE TECHNIQUE

Adduction Arytenopexy

Unless contraindicated, patients are given 0.2 mg/kg of Decadron one hour prior to the procedure. This helps to minimize intraoperative swelling, which can alter judgment regarding the implant size and to reduce postoperative airway swelling. A horizontal incision is made in a natural neck crease overlying the region of the cricothyroid space. Subplatysmal flaps are raised to expose the infrahyoid strap musculature, and Gelpi retractors are placed to maintain the flaps. A transverse incision is made through the strap muscles to expose the thyroid lamina. A double-pronged skin hook is placed lateral to the edge of the thyroid lamina and it is rotated anteromedially. This defines the edge of the thyroid lamina and inferior cornu of the thyroid cartilage. A needle-tipped electrocautery knife is used to separate the inferior constrictor from the thyroid lamina (Figure 37-2). The inferior cornu is identified and isolated so that the cricothyroid joint can be separated with a Mayo scissors (Figure 37-3). Separating the cricothyroid joint and associated inferior constrictor muscle from the thyroid cartilage allows for further anteromedial rotation of

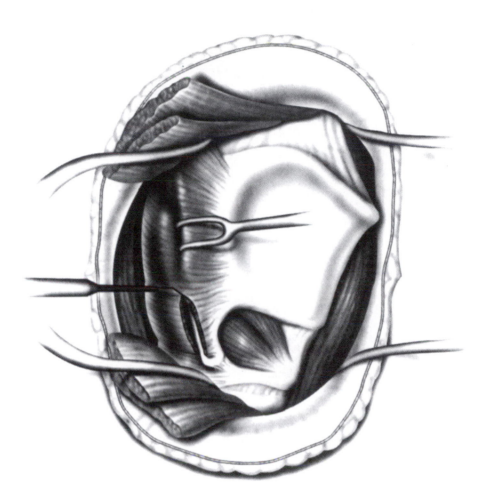

FIGURE 37-2. *A needle-tipped electrocautery knife is used to separate the inferior constrictor from the thyroid lamina. (From Operative Techniques in Otolaryngology—Head and Neck Surgery. 1999;10(1):9-16)*

the thyroid lamina (Figure 37-4). Blunt dissection is performed in a cephalad and slightly anterior direction from the cricothyroid facet along the cricoid cartilage until the superior rim of the cricoid is encountered (Figure 37-4). In performing these maneuvers, the lateral aspect of the pyriform mucosa has been bluntly dissected from the inner aspect of the thyroid lamina and the medial aspect of the pyriform mucosa has been separated from the posterolateral aspect of the cricoid (Figure 37-4). Posterior superior dissection along the top of the cricoid results in separation of the lateral cricoarytenoid muscle from the muscular process and ensures that the cricoarytenoid joint will be identified easily (Figure 37-5). The dissection along the superior rim of the cricoid leads to the muscular process of the arytenoid. The lateral cricoarytenoid muscle is severed from its attachment to the arytenoid. The posterior cricoarytenoid muscle is then separated from the muscular process of the arytenoid (Figure 37-5). The cricoarytenoid joint is opened widely with a Steven's

scissors, and the curved, glistening white surface of the cricoid facet is identified (Figure 37-6). The posterior cricoarytenoid muscle is separated from the posterior plate of the cricoid so that the posterior aspect of the cricoarytenoid joint is seen well and there is room to place a suture through this region (Figure 37-6). A 4-0 Prolene suture on a cutting needle is placed through the posterior plate of the cricoid just medial to the facet, and the needle is brought out through the medial aspect of the cricoarytenoid joint (Figure 37-7). The needle is then passed through the body of the arytenoid, followed by the inner aspect of the cricoid. The needle is then advanced under the cricoid facet and through the posterior plate of the cricoid, where a slipknot is placed (Figure 37-7). The arytenoid is positioned so that its body is subluxed medially, just off the facet, and so that it is rocked internally in the natural plane of the curved joint. Once the arytenoid is secured, the thyroid lamina is replaced into its natural anatomic position. The arytenoid is visualized by means of a flexible fiberoptic

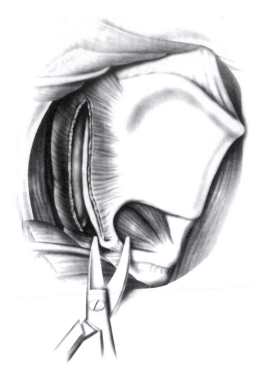

FIGURE 37-3. *The inferior cornu is identified and isolated so that the cricothyroid joint can be separated with Mayo scissors. (From Operative Techniques in Otolaryngology—Head and Neck Surgery. 1999;10(1):9-16).*

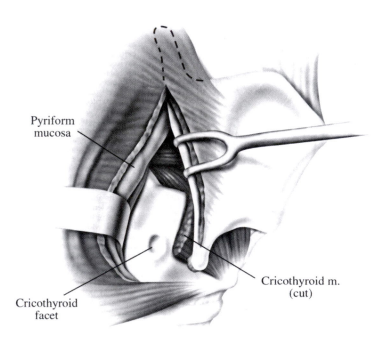

FIGURE 37-4. *Separating the cricothyroid joint and associated inferior constrictor muscle from the thyroid cartilage allows for further anteromedial rotation of the thyroid lamina. Blunt dissection is performed in a cephalad and slightly anterior direction from the cricothyroid facet along the cricoid cartilage until the superior rim of the cricoid is encountered. The lateral aspect of the pyriform mucosa is bluntly dissected from the inner aspect of the thyroid lamina, and the medial aspect of the pyriform mucosa is separated from the posterolateral aspect of the cricoid. (From Operative Techniques in Otolaryngology—Head and Neck Surgery. 1999;10(1):9-16)*

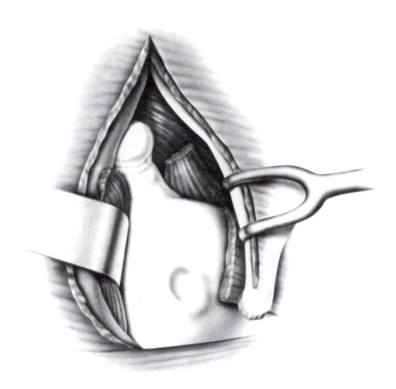

FIGURE 37-5. *The posterior cricoarytenoid muscle is then separated from the muscular process of the arytenoid. (From* Operative Techniques in Otolaryngology—Head and Neck Surgery. *1999;10(1):9-16)*

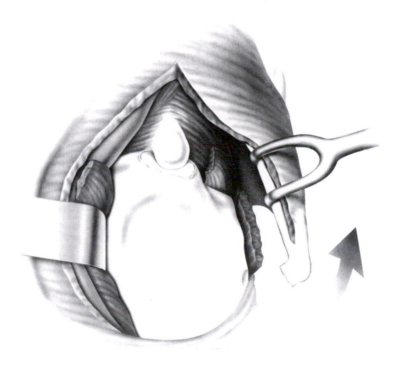

FIGURE 37-6. *The posterior cricoarytenoid muscle is separated from the posterior plate of the cricoid so that the posterior aspect of the cricoarytenoid joint is well seen and there is room to place a suture through this region. (From* Operative Techniques in Otolaryngology—Head and Neck Surgery. *1999;10(1):9-16)*

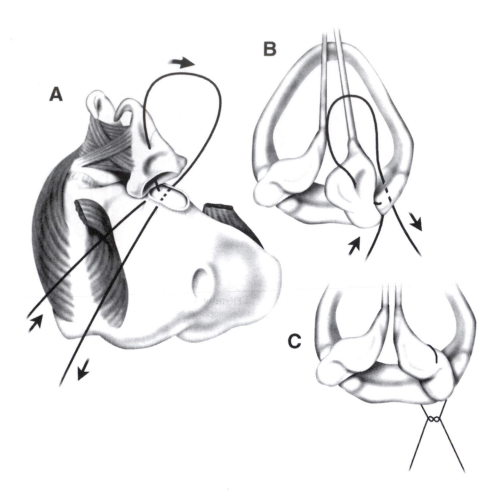

FIGURE 37-7. *A 4-0 Prolene suture on a cutting needle is placed through the posterior plate of the cricoid just medial to the facet and the needle is brought out through the medial aspect of the cricoarytenoid joint (A). The needle is passed through the body of the arytenoid and then through the inner aspect of the cricoid (B). The needle is advanced under the cricoid facet and through the posterior plate of the cricoid, where a slipknot is placed (C). (From* Operative Techniques in Otolaryngology—Head and Neck Surgery. *1999;10(1):9-16)*

laryngoscope to check position during a number of phonatory tasks. If the arytenoid is in good position, the arytenoid suture is affixed permanently. The voice is typically still dysphonic until the implant is placed to support the paraglottic musculature.[2]

Subsequently, an inferiorly based thyroid perichondrial flap is developed and a standard window is made in the thyroid lamina lateral to the musculomembranous vocal fold as previously described by Isshiki (Figure 37-8). The inner perichondrium of the thyroid lamina is preserved at the perimeter of the window. A small implant is then fashioned from a thin sheet of Gore-Tex so that it can be layered lateral to the inner perichondrium of the thyroid lamina. The Gore-Tex can be stabilized with a 4-0 Prolene suture and the thyroid-lamina window can be reposi-

tioned. The external perichondrium (Figure 37-9) can be preserved and closed over the thyroid-lamina window.

Once the adduction arytenopexy and medialization laryngoplasty are completed, a cricothyroid subluxation is performed to further enhance vocal quality. The newly described cricothyroid subluxation is accomplished by placing a 2-0 Prolene suture around the inferior cornu of the thyroid lamina. It is then passed in a submucosal fashion underneath the cricoid anteriorly (Figure 37-10). The suture is pulled taut (Figure 37-11), which increases the distance between the cricoid facet and the attachment of the anterior commissure ligament. This ultimately increases the tension and length of the musculomembranous vocal fold on the paralyzed side. The tension on this suture is adjusted by using a slipknot

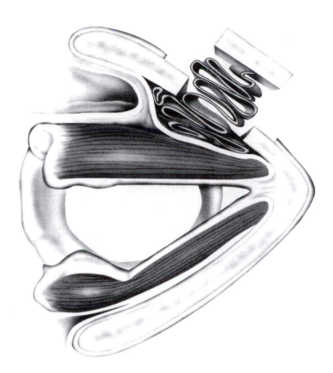

FIGURE 37-8. *If a thin sheet of Gore-Tex is used, it is layered in position and can be stabilized with a 4-0 Prolene suture. (From* Operative Techniques in Otolaryngology—Head and Neck Surgery. *1999;10(1):9-16)*

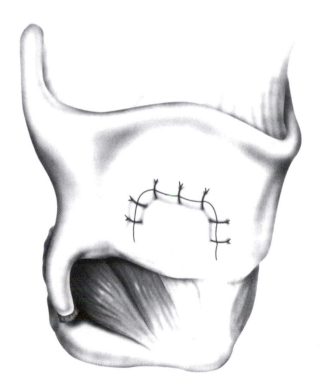

FIGURE 37-9. *The thyroid cartilage window can be replaced and stabilized with either a Prolene suture or with its external perichondrium. (From* Operative Techniques in Otolaryngology—Head and Neck Surgery. *1999;10(1):9-16)*

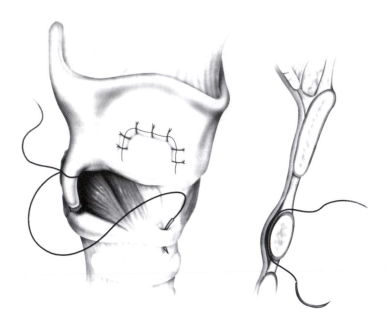

FIGURE 37-10. *The C-T subluxation is accomplished by placing a 2-0 Prolene suture around the inferior cornu of the thyroid lamina. It is then passed in a submucosal fashion underneath the cricoid anteriorly. (From* Operative Techniques in Otolaryngology—Head and Neck Surgery. *1999;10(1):9-16)*

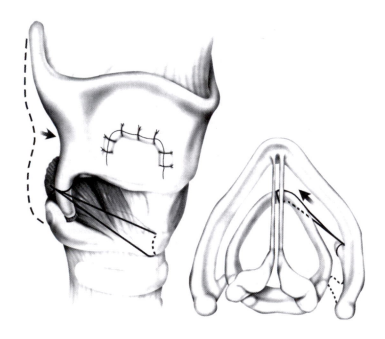

FIGURE 37-11. *The suture is pulled taut, increasing the distance between the cricoid facet and the attachment of the anterior commissure ligament. (From* Operative Techniques in Otolaryngology—Head and Neck Surgery. *1999;10(1):9-16)*

while the patient performs a number of phonatory tasks. This includes maximal-range tasks such as use of pulse-register (vocal fry) through a falsetto register and glissando sliding scales.

This cricothyroid subluxation suture simulates cricothyroid muscle contraction for counter-tension on the thyroarytenoid muscle and for increasing length of the musculomembranous vocal fold. Once this is completed, the strap muscles are reattached with 3-0 Vicryl suture in a running fashion. The wound is irrigated and a Penrose drain is placed. The platysma is approximated in a running fashion with Vicryl suture as well, and then the skin is closed with 4-0 nylon suture. A pressure dressing is applied and the drain is removed on the first postoperative morning. The patient is started on a liquid diet on the first postoperative morning and is advanced to a normal diet as tolerated. Fiberoptic laryngoscopy is performed prior to discharge to ensure that there is not an excessive amount of edema that would warrant further observation. Typically, patients can be discharged on the first postoperative day.

Anterior Commissure Laryngoplasty

The anterior commissure tendon is composed of a coalescence of the fibers of the vocal ligament, inner perichondrium of the thyroid laminae, and the thyroepiglottic ligament[27] (Figure 37-12). Blunt trauma to the neck can result in a fracture of the thyroid cartilage and retro-displacement of the anterior commissure tendon. This is typically encountered in motor vehicle accidents (ie, steering wheel) and contact sports such as hockey, rugby, martial arts, football, as well as basketball. After mobilization of the segment of cartilage with its underlying tendon, a mini-plate (Figure 37-13) can be used to reposition the tendon to reestablish vocal fold tension. This approach can also be used to elevate pitch for gender reassignment.

With the advancement of techniques for more extensive endoscopic glottic cancer excisions, a portion of the anterior commissure tendon may be resected. The associated dysphonia is the result of the persistent keyhole aperture anteriorly as well as the stiffness of the epithelium of the neocord. Implant medialization will not correct this defect. An anterior laryngoplasty procedure was designed recently to solve this problem by employing a laryngofissure to infracture one thyroid ala inside the other[28] (Figures 37-14 to 37-17).

SUMMARY

Laryngeal framework surgery has evolved to be a dominant treatment modality for dysphonia associated with a malpositioned vocal fold. The knowledge acquired from the management of paralytic/paretic dysphonia has catalyzed approaches for the reconstruction of glottic cancer defects. Gore-Tex implant medialization has been shown to be efficacious, especially when there is a tissue defect in the muscle or the layered microstructure of the vocal fold. Gore-Tex is easy to shape, position, and adjust, even in vivo, and is positioned lateral to the inner

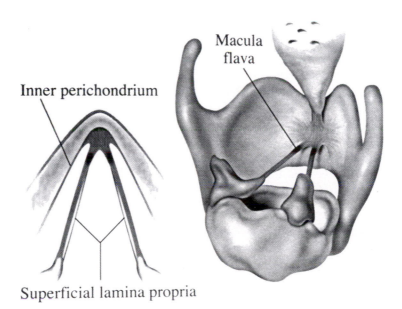

FIGURE 37-12. *The anterior commissure tendon is composed of fibers from the vocal ligament, inner perichondrium of the thyroid laminae, and the thyroepiglottic ligament.*

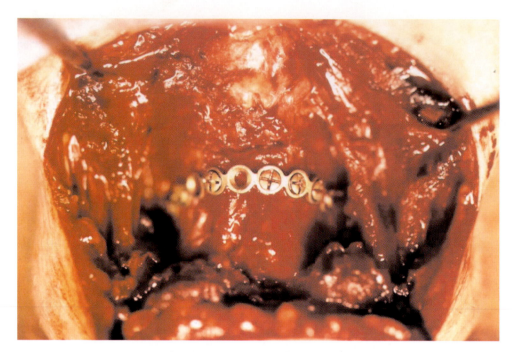

FIGURE 37-13. *A mini-plate is used to affix the repositioned tendon and cartilage to reestablish vocal fold tension.*

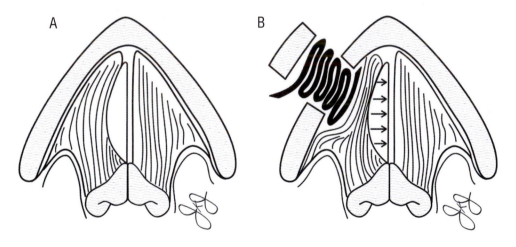

FIGURE 37-14. *(A) Diagrammatic representation of an endoscopic partial laryngectomy defect which does not allow for glottal closure. This results in excessive air escape with loss of vocal power and dysphonia. (B) Gore-Tex is used to medialize the neocord to allow for entrained oscillation of the opposite vocal fold and closure of the defect.*

perichondrium of the thyroid lamina. However, silastic implants and other materials are still viable options and are still used widely by phonosurgeons.

Paralytic dysphonia is the most common indication for static reconstruction of the larynx. Prior procedures have addressed primarily the position of the vocal fold in the axial and vertical planes. However, dynamic pitch range capabilities and vocal flexibility have been limited secondary to the flaccid, denervated vocal fold tissue. Novel procedures have been designed to address these issues by optimally positioning the arytenoid and restoring tension in the flaccid vocal fold. The new adduction arytenopexy procedure more closely models the biomechanics underlying normal cricoarytenoid adduction than the classic arytenoid adduction does. It should be done when there is a malpositioned arytenoid, which

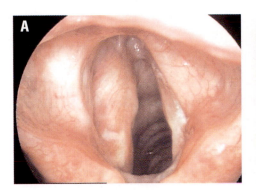
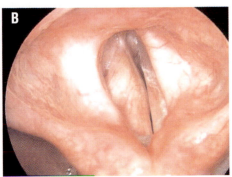

FIGURE 37-15. *(A) Videostroboscopic assessment after endoscopic partial laryngectomy (left) and reconstruction with fat. Part of the left anterior commissure tendon was resected for complete removal of the cancer. (B) Despite fat augmentation there is a persistent keyhole aperture anteriorly through which the air is preferentially shunted, decreasing glottal efficiency and vocal power.*

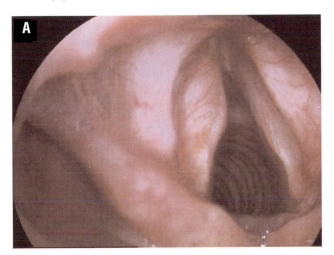
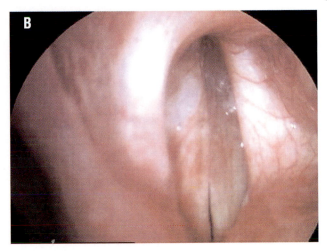

FIGURE 37-16. *(A) Anterior commissure laryngoplasty was performed to close the anterior keyhole aperture. (B) There is complete closure anteriorly.*

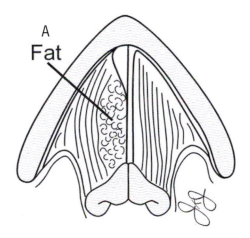
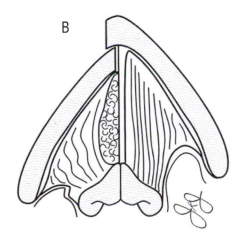

FIGURE 37-17. *(A) Diagram representing the anterior keyhole aperture, which remains after partial resection of the anterior commissure tendon. The fat augmentation did not allow for complete closure. (B) The left thyroid lamina is subluxed into the right to close the persistent aperture.*

leads to aerodynamic incompetence during phonation. This procedure allows for gliding, rocking, and rotating of the arytenoid on the cricoid facet, thereby simulating simultaneous agonist-antagonist function of the interarytenoid, lateral cricoarytenoid, lateral thyroarytenoid, and posterior cricoarytenoid muscles.

Cricothyroid subluxation was designed as a technique to increase the distance between the cricoid facet and the insertion of the anterior commissure ligament. This results in an increased length and tension of the denervated thyroarytenoid musculature so that there is improved oscillation, and in turn, phonatory function. Cricothyroid subluxation enhances the postoperative voice of patients, regardless of whether they required medialization laryngoplasty alone or with adduction arytenopexy.

The postoperative vocal outcome from the combined use of adduction arytenopexy, Gore-Tex medialization laryngoplasty, and cricothyroid subluxation for paralytic dysphonia is such that in the authors' hands, most patients will have a normal phonation time and >2 octaves of dynamic range with minimal acoustical perturbation.[9] Older surgical approaches are still viable in selected cases but have not generally produced outcomes comparable to those obtained from these newer approaches. With the addition of the adduction arytenopexy and cricothyroid subluxation procedures to the armamentarium of the phonosurgeon, all parameters for static reconstruction of the paralyzed vocal fold appear to have been addressed. These new procedures have all been performed reliably for over three years with minimal complications. The future should lie primarily in dynamic reconstruction (reinnervation and electrical pacing) of the intrinsic laryngeal musculature.

REFERENCES

1. Payr E. Plastik am schildknorpel zur Behebung der Folgen einseitiger Stimmbandlahmung. *Dtsch Med Wochensch.* 1915;43:1265-1270.

2. Zeitels SM, Hochman I, Hillman RE. Adduction arytenopexy: a new procedure for paralytic dysphonia and the implications for medialization laryngoplasty. *Ann Otol Rhinol Laryngol.* 1998;107(suppl 173):1-24.

3. Zeitels SM. The evolution of the assessment and treatment of paralytic dysphonia. *Otolaryngol Clin North Am.* 2000;33:803-816.

4. Isshiki N, Morita H, Okamura H, Hiramoto M. Thyroplasty as a new phonosurgical technique. *Acta Otolaryngol (Stockh).* 1974;78:451-457.

5. Isshiki N, Tanabe M, Sawada M. Arytenoid adduction for unilateral vocal cord paralysis. *Arch Otolaryngol.* 1978;104:555-558.

6. Isshiki N. *Phonosurgery: Theory and Practice.* Tokyo: Springer-Verlag; 1989.

7. Zeitels SM. Adduction arytenopexy with medialization laryngoplasty and crico-thyroid subluxation: a new approach to paralytic dysphonia. *Oper Tech Otolaryngol Head Neck Surg.* 1999;10:9-16.

8. Zeitels SM. New procedures for paralytic dysphonia: adduction arytenopexy, goretex medialization, and cricothyroid subluxation. *Otolaryngol Clin North Am.* 2000;33:841-854.

9. Zeitels SM, Hillman RE. Cricothyroid subluxation for enhancing laryngoplastic phonosurgery. *Ann Otol Rhinol Laryngol.* 1999;108:1126-1131.

10. Zeitels SM. Phonosurgery. *Comprehensive Therapy.* 1996;22:222-230.

11. Zeitels SM, Jarboe J, Hillman RE. *Medialization Laryngoplasty with Gore-Tex for Voice Restoration Secondary Glottal Incompetence.* Presented at the Voice Symposium, Philadelphia; 2000.

12. Arnold GE. Vocal rehabilitation of paralytic dysphonia. IX. Technique of intracordal injection. *Arch Otolaryngol Head Neck Surg.* 1962;76:358.

13. Mikaelian DO, Lowry LD, Sataloff RT. Lipoinjection for unilateral vocal cord paralysis. *Laryngoscope.* 1991;101:465-468.

14. Shaw GY, Szewczyk MA, Searle J, Woodroof J. Autologous fat injection into the vocal folds: technical considerations and long-term follow-up. *Laryngoscope.* 1997;107:177-186.

15. Ford CN, Bless DM, Autologous collagen vocal fold injection: a preliminary clinical study. *Laryngoscope.* 1995;105:944-948.

16. Schramm VL, May M, Lavorato AS. Gelfoam paste injection for vocal cord paralysis: temporary rehabilitation of glottic incompetence. *Laryngoscope.* 1978;88:1268-1273.

17. Zeitels SM, Hillman RE, Radu A. *Salient Characteristics of Patients With Posterior Laryngeal Granulomas and Ulcerations.* Presented at the Voice Symposium; 1997. Philadelphia, PA.

18. Koufman JA, Isaacson GL. Laryngoplastic phonosurgery. *Otolaryngol Clin North Am.* 1991;24:1151-1177.

19. Neuman TR, Hengesteg A, Lepage MS, Kaufman KR, Woodson GE. Three-dimensional motion of the arytenoid adduction procedure in cadaver larynges. *Ann Otol Rhinol Laryngol.* 1994;103:265-270.

20. Hoffman HH, McCulloch TM. Medialization laryn-goplasty with expanded polytetrafluoroethylene: surgical technique and preliminary results. *Ann Otol Rhinol Laryngol.* 1998;07:427-432.

21. Koufman JA. Laryngoplasty for vocal cord medial-ization: an alternative to teflon. *Laryngoscope.* 1986.96:726-731.

22. Isshiki N. Recent advances in phonosurgery. *Folia Phoniatr.* 1980;32:119-154.

23. Isshiki N. Surgery to Elevate Vocal Pitch, in *Phonosurgery: Theory and Practice.* Tokyo: Springer-Verlag; 1989:141-155.

24. LeJeune FE, Guice CE, Samuels PM. Early experi-ences with vocal ligament tightening. *Ann Otol Rhinol Laryngol.* 1983;92:475-477.

25. Tucker H.M. Anterior commissure laryngoplasty for adjustment of vocal fold tension. *Ann Otol Rhinol Laryngol.* 1985;94:547-549.

26. Miller FR, Bryant GL, Netterville JL. Arytenoid adduction in vocal fold paralysis. *Oper Tech Otolaryngol Head Neck Surgery.* 1999;10:36-41.

27. Hartig G, Zeitels SM, Optimizing voice in conser-vation surgery for glottic cancer. *Oper Tech Otolaryngol Head Neck Surg. (Phonosurgery Part 1).* 1998;9:214-223.

28. Jarboe J, Zeitels SM, Hillman RE. *Phonosurgical Reconstruction of Glottic Cancer Defects.* Presented at the Voice Symposium, Philadelphia; 2000.

CHAPTER 38

Laryngeal Reinnervation

Harvey M. Tucker, MD, FACS

The larynx is subject to a number of disease processes and potential injuries that can result in paralysis or paresis of one or both vocal folds. Moreover, ankylosis or fixation of the cricoarytenoid joint(s) may immobilize vocal folds more often than has been appreciated in the past.[1] Bilateral vocal fold immobility usually entails significant airway restriction but relatively little effect upon the voice; therefore, it will be considered in only limited fashion in this chapter. Because it is now possible to deal with unrecovered vocal compromise caused by unilateral vocal fold immobility by several approaches, it is essential that the physician who would care for such patients have a clear understanding of what can be accomplished with each of them.

DIAGNOSIS

When a patient presents with unilateral vocal fold immobility with no obvious cause, systematic evaluation should be performed to identify the underlying disease process. Table 38-1 suggests a series of screening tests that can identify such cause(s) in approximately 60% of patients with apparently idiopathic paralysis. The cause will never be found in the remaining 40%.[2] In cases in which history or appearance of the larynx under videostroboscopy suggests that ankylosis may have produced limitation of motion, EMG or direct palpation under paralytic anesthesia may be necessary to correct-

1. Otolaryngologic examination usually including fiberoptic or videoscopic endoscopy.

2. CT of chest

3. CT scan of the skull base and neck, with contrast

4. Panendoscopy

5. Glucose tolerance test

6. Serology for syphillis and Lyme disease

TABLE 38-1. *Suggested Evaluation of Idiopathic Vocal Fold Paralysis (Adapted from Tucker HM.* The Larynx, *2nd ed. New York, NY: Thieme Medical; 1993:chap 12.)*

ly identify the cause. Once the cause is determined and does not require further intervention or no cause is found, the treating physician can begin to consider the best approach to management.

MANAGEMENT

Because approximately 60% of patients with idiopathic unilateral vocal fold paralysis will spontaneously recover recurrent laryngeal nerve function within one year of onset (80% of these within 6 months) and many of the remaining 40% can compensate to satisfactory voice levels, no *irreversible* intervention should be undertaken to restore voice before a year has elapsed, unless 1) the cause is known and is not expected to recover, or 2) the patient cannot delay restoration of voice for physical, social, occupational, or psychologic reasons.

There are three general ways in which unrecovered or uncompensated unilateral vocal fold paralysis can be managed.

Speech Therapy

Although at least some degree of compensation is to be expected in all patients as they attempt to speak over time, they often arrive at strategies for voice production that are functional, but potentially damaging to the larynx (ie, contact ulcers). These undesirable vocal habits can be avoided and compensation can be accelerated under the supervision of an experienced speech-language pathologist. Moreover, the voicing strategies learned in this process will be advantageous to the patient's further improvement if surgical intervention becomes necessary. Therefore, all patients with unilateral vocal fold paralysis should be managed in consultation with a voice professional. (See also Chapter 31)

Vocal Fold Medialization

Loudness, durability, sustainability, and projection can be improved by any of several techniques designed to force the paralyzed vocal fold toward the midline so that the remaining mobile vocal fold can meet it more efficiently. These procedures include injection techniques (Teflon, Gelfoam, cross-linked collagen, fat, and so forth), surgical medialization with implantation of various alloplastic or autogenous tissues, and arytenoid adduction. (See also Chapter 37.) Although these techniques are usually successful in correcting the incompetence of the laryngeal valve, they cannot address the issue of poor voice quality, as they cannot restore muscular activity and the ability to change tension in the vocal fold. As a result, many patients whose strength of voice has been restored by one of these techniques continue to be hoarse, diplophonic, or experience frequent "breaks." Furthermore, it is not unusual for a patient with initially good restoration of vocal strength to notice gradual deterioration of this improvement after several months or years because of further wasting of the unreinnervated vocal fold musculature.

Reinnervation

Reinnervation of paralyzed vocal fold musculature is the only currently available approach that can restore the ability to change tension in the vocalis muscle. This is essential to good voice quality and can provide sufficient resting muscle tonus to prevent later deterioration because of further wasting. There are several techniques to accomplish this, but all of them suffer from a delay of weeks to months between surgery and beginning restoration of function because of the time required for degeneration and regeneration of nerve fibers and subsequent strengthening of the shrunken vocal fold musculature once reinnervation has occurred. Nevertheless, if the physician managing such a patient wishes to restore as normal a voice as is possible, reinnervation should be at least a part of the process.

Reinnervation may be accomplished by 1) muscle onlay technique, 2) nerve anastomosis techniques, and 3) nerve-muscle pedicle technique.

Muscle Onlay Technique

This technique is primarily of historic interest.[3,4] It assumes that if an innervated muscle (ie, sternothyroideus) is partially detached and sutured to a denervated muscle (ie, posterior cricoarytenoideus) sprouting of nerves from the donor muscle will colonize empty motor endplate sites in the recipient muscle. Although this concept has been confirmed in the laboratory, clinical use has been sparse, largely because of technical difficulties and the bulk of the donor muscle.

Nerve Anastomosis/Implantation Technique

This approach to reinnervation is both the oldest[5,6] and most varied of the techniques now available. It can be used to restore nerve supply from the ipsilateral recurrent laryngeal nerve (when this source is available), or from the vagus, the phrenic, or branches of the ansa hypoglossi nerves, any of which can be a suitable donor nerve.

When the recurrent laryngeal nerve has been injured, but is still available in sufficient length close to the larynx, direct *end-to-end anastomosis* is possible.[7-10] The vagus nerve can be split and a portion of it used to anastomose to the distal remnant of a cut recurrent laryngeal nerve when the proximal recurrent nerve itself is not available. Both of these methods seek to redirect appropriate ipsilateral vagus nerve fibers to the distal recurrent laryngeal nerve remnant and, thus, to the muscles of the larynx. This approach is not often clinically useful because of the loss of regenerating nerve fiber population, scarring at the anastomotic site, and narrowing of the neural tubules in the distal nerve segment, all of which conspire to severely limit the success of reinnervation. Moreover, it has been recognized that when successful reinnervation *does* occur, only tonic adduction is to be expected, which might be useful in cases of unilateral paralysis, but would worsen the airway problem in bilateral paralysis. In the unlikely event that the recurrent laryngeal nerve were discovered to have been transected on one side during surgery and sufficient length remained, anastomosis would be worth a try in hopes of regaining tonus and adduction of the reinnervated vocal fold. However, such an approach is not warranted if the paralysis is discovered after surgery and when it is not certain that the nerve has been transected.

The cut end of the recurrent laryngeal nerve or split vagus nerve can be *implanted directly into laryngeal muscles* (ie, posterior cricoarytenoideus[11,12]) and produce useful return of function. This approach avoids some of the drawbacks of anastomotic techniques, but is most often suitable when bilateral paralysis requires return of abduction rather than for restoration of voice.

Other nerves can serve as sources of reinnervation when the vagus and its branches are not available. The phrenic nerve[13-17] and branches of the ansa hypoglossi[18,19] or the XIIth cranial nerve itself[20] are most commonly used. For the most part, such approaches have been intended to produce abduction rather than adduction and voice, but vocal fold tightening as a result of cricothyroideus muscle activity would be improved if the arytenoid cartilage were stabilized by reinnervation of an antagonist like the posterior cricoarytenoid muscle.

Selective reinnervation of adductor muscles is feasible to restore tonus, adduction, and tensing capability of a paralyzed vocal fold, whether it is achieved by end-to-end anastomosis or by implantation. When restoration of voice is at issue, reinnervation of only the adductors and tensors of the vocal fold is both sufficient and advantageous, as simultaneous restoration of abductor function can limit ability to bring the vocal folds together. *Intralaryngeal anastomosis* of donor nerves to adductor divisions of the recurrent laryngeal nerve can effectively restore active adduction and with it, improved voice.[21]

Nerve-Muscle Pedicle Reinnervation

Surgical techniques that require transection and anastomosis/implantation of nerves to achieve reinnervation (see above) all suffer from certain disadvantages:

1. Time must be allowed for retrograde and antegrade degeneration of the donor nerve after it has been sectioned;

2. More time is needed for eventual regeneration of the donor nerve from the next highest node of Ranvier or from the nerve cell body itself to the anastomotic site; and

3. This delay allows time for scarring at the anastomosis and for shrinkage of neural tubules dis-

tal to the anastomosis, with potential for loss of some of the regenerating fibers.

A technique that can permit reinnervation of motor endplate sites in a selected recipient muscle and which does not require either anastomosis or inordinate delay while retrograde degeneration and regeneration of cut nerve fibers take place should be more successful and efficient than those discussed above.

Selective reinnervation of adductor musculature is not only possible, but has been shown to restore improved strength and quality of the voice in properly selected cases.[22-27]

Technique

Surgery can be carried out under local or general anesthesia. Via a skin crease incision at the level of the lower border of the thyroid cartilage, the anterior border of the sternocleidomastoid muscle is mobilized posteriorly to expose the jugular vein. If care is taken with hemostasis, the ansa hypoglossi nerve is often visible through the loose areolar tissue overlying the vein. If not, the nerve can be identified by mobilizing the anterior belly of the omohyoid muscle. The motor branch of the ansa hypoglossi to this muscle belly will be seen entering its undersurface from posterosuperior (Figure 38-1). It can then be traced back to the main loop of the descendens hypoglossi division of the ansa.

A nerve-muscle pedicle is designed around the point of entry of the nerve into the muscle's undersurface, but it should be noted that the nerve often travels several millimeters between the muscle fibers before it arborizes. The true point of entry can best be visualized by separating the muscle bundles adjacent to the appar-

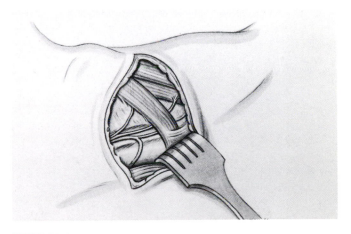

FIGURE 38-1. *Exposure of the ansa hypoglossi and its branches beneath the fascia of the jugular vein. (Courtesy of H.M. Tucker, MD, FACS)*

ent point of entry of the nerve (Figure 38-2). The muscle pedicle should measure only 2-3 mm on a side, as about 60% of the motor endplates subtended by the nerve are within this distance from its point of entry and because the transferred muscle mass should be as small as possible to avoid necrosis and scarring around its periphery that might interfere with eventual neurotization of the recipient muscle. The nerve-muscle pedicle may be obtained from any available branches of the ansa hypoglossi to the strap muscles, but the omohyoid muscle is usually well situated for easy access and is essentially vestigial in humans, so that it is the most common source chosen for reinnervation (Figure 38-3).

The lateral aspect of the thyroid cartilage is exposed by retracting the strap muscles. A window of cartilage is removed after reflecting the perichondrium overlying the lower half of the thyroid ala to expose the inner perichondrium. This is incised to reveal the lateral-most fibers of the lateral thyroarytenoideus muscle, which is the major adductor of the vocal fold. The nerve-muscle pedicle is sutured to the raw surface of this muscle using two 5-0 nylon sutures. The sutures are intended only to retain an onlay approximation of the muscle fibers in the pedicle to those of the underlying recipient muscle (Figure 38-4). The strap muscles are approximated with 3-0 chromic sutures and the skin is closed after placement of a Penrose drain.

Although voice results have been very good with this technique,[25] there is a delay of from two to six months before return of function begins. Therefore, selective

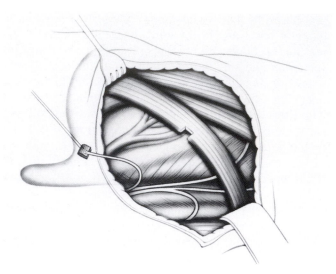

FIGURE 38-3. *Development of nerve-muscle pedicle from anterior belly of omohyoid muscle. (Courtesy of H.M. Tucker, MD, FACS)*

nerve-muscle pedicle reinnervation is now most often combined with surgical medialization of the paralyzed vocal fold in patients not suffering from cricoarytenoid joint fixation in addition to recurrent nerve paralysis (Figure 38-5).[26] In this manner, almost immediate improvement in strength and durability of the voice is achieved with medialization and further improvement in voice quality is noted weeks or months later when nerve-muscle pedicle reinnervation begins.[27]

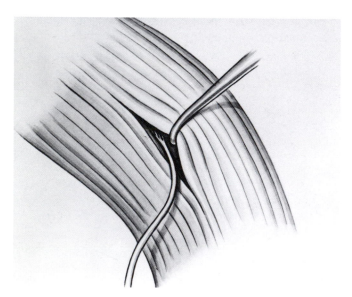

FIGURE 38-2. *Exposure of nerve branch between muscle bundles. Note that the nerve travels for 2 or 3 mm between the muscle fibers before it begins to arborize. (Courtesy of H.M. Tucker, MD, FACS)*

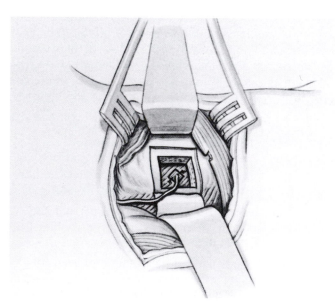

FIGURE 38-4. *Nerve-muscle pedicle sutured to exposed surface of lateral thyroarytenoideus muscle. (Courtesy of H.M. Tucker, MD, FACS)*

REINNERVATION FOR LARYNGEAL TRANSPLANTATION

In 1974, at the Centennial Conference on Laryngeal Cancer held in Toronto, Canada, a panel discussion was held on the subject of laryngeal transplantation. As a result of this conference, it was agreed that the necessary techniques for reestablishment of blood supply, and for reinnervation of a laryngeal transplant were already available. The one problem yet to be solved was the need for immunosuppression in a recipient who had recently been treated for a malignancy. It was felt that unless the

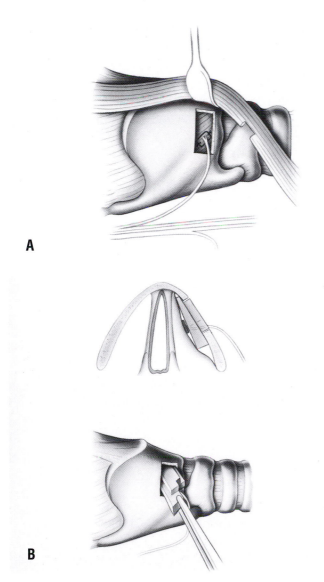

FIGURE 38-5. *(A) Nerve-muscle pedicle rotated and sutured to exposed muscle. (B) Silastic prosthesis is inserted without disturbing pedicle. Note posterior-inferior corner has been removed to provide space for free passage of the nerve-muscle pedicle. (Courtesy of H.M. Tucker, MD, FACS)*

donor larynx could be rendered non-antigenic or that means of immunosuppression that would not potentiate malignancy could be found, the risks of laryngeal transplantation would not be justified.[28]

The first reported human laryngeal transplantation was accomplished[29] at the Cleveland Clinic on January 4, 1998 in a patient whose larynx had been crushed and in whom reconstruction for voice and airway had been unsuccessful. Although the transplanted larynx has survived and the patient is now able to maintain nutrition by mouth, he still requires a "permanent" tracheostomy stoma for adequate airway. According to personal communications, the larynx transplant has not been successfully reinnervated (M. Strome, MD, personal communication, 2000).

Any of several means of reinnervation could theoretically be applied in cases of laryngeal transplant. Nerve-muscle pedicle technique was reported to have been successful after reimplantation of totally excised canine larynges.[29] Any anastomotic technique should also succeed, but it will probably be necessary to selectively reinnervate only the abductor divisions in order to restore adequate airway capability. Many studies have shown that if both the adductor and abductor divisions are reinnervated, adduction usually overpowers any abductor function that may be restored, thus interfering in ability to eventually extubate the airway. Since the position assumed by bilaterally denervated vocal folds is usually appropriate for reasonable voice production, unopposed abductor function can be achieved more easily than when both divisions of the recurrent laryngeal nerve are reinnervated.

Which, if any, of the currently available reinnervation techniques might be successful in restoring adequate voice and airway in a transplanted larynx will have to wait for further experience. As the problem of immunosuppression is as yet unsolved, it seems unlikely that any such experience will be available in the near future.

ELECTRONIC PACING FOR VOCAL FOLD PARALYSIS

Several attempts to devise electronic pacemakers that could adduct or abduct paralyzed vocal folds have been reported.[30,31] Those researchers who have reported direct implantation of wire electrodes into denervated laryngeal muscles have generally succeeded in an acute laboratory setting, but it seems unlikely that such an arrangement would be adequate in the long-term. To begin with, laryngeal muscles denervated for several months are known to lose bulk, making direct implantation and the necessary fixation of the wires extremely difficult in an active person, whose laryngotracheal complex can be expected to move vigorously during swallowing, coughing, and even with necessary head and neck movements. Second, experience with direct implantation of wire electrodes into cardiac muscle shows that chemical changes and scarring around the tips eventually results in increasing electrical resistance. Finally, direct electrical stimulation does not seem to prevent deterioration and wasting of skeletal muscle, even though it may succeed in causing depolarization. Only restored neurohumoral depolarization appears to prevent further muscle deterioration.

Broniatowski et al have published several reports using perineural electrodes with a previously placed nerve-muscle pedicle.[32-36] This approach would appear more likely to succeed than direct implantation techniques in an actual clinical setting. The electrode contact with the nerve-muscle pedicle can be at some distance from the larynx itself, thus permitting more stable placement around the nerve (as opposed to implantation) and much less movement in an active patient. Moreover, this technique results in neurohumoral depolarization at the subtended motor endplate sites in the recipient muscle, thus preventing further deterioration of the reinnervated muscle. Finally, nerve-muscle pedical electronic pacing lends itself to *selective* reinnervation so that the pacing efforts can be directed to those precise muscle groups that are needed, rather than gross reinnervation of all the muscles in the organ.

SUMMARY

Loss of vocal capability because of immobility of one vocal fold can be corrected by any of several means, but only reinnervation can restore tensing capability and thus optimize voice quality. Anastomosis techniques have been successful, but require availability of sufficient length of donor nerve, as well as a distal nerve segment with patent neural tubules to which it can be attached. Direct implantation of a cut donor nerve may be difficult because of insufficient length. Nerve-muscle pedicle technique avoids most of these problems and can be combined with surgical medialization so that improvement in vocal strength can be achieved immediately, while the patient awaits onset of reinnervation from the nerve-muscle pedicle. This approach to voice rehabilitation offers the patient restoration of function as close to normal as is possible with existing techniques.

REFERENCES

1. Tucker HM. Vocal cord paralysis—1979: etiology and management. *Laryngoscope.* 1980;90:585.

2. Tucker HM, Lavertu P. Paralysis and paresis of the vocal folds. In: Blitzer A, et al, eds. *Neurologic Disorders of the Larynx.* New York, NY: Thieme Medical Publishers; 1992:chap 17.

3. Evoy M. Experimental activation of paralyzed vocal cords. *Arch Otolaryngol.* 1968;87:155.

4. King BT, Gregg RL. An anatomical reason for the various behaviors of paralyzed vocal cords. *Ann Otol Rhinol Laryngol.* 1948;57:925.

5. Exner S. Notiz zu der Frage von der Faservertheilung mehrerer Nerven in einem Muskel. *Pflugers Arch Ges Physiol.* 1885;36:572.

6. Horsley JA. Suture of the recurrent laryngeal nerve with report of a case. *Trans S Surg Gynecol Assoc.* 1909;22:161.

7. Lahey FH. Suture of the recurrent laryngeal nerve for bilateral abductory paralysis. *Ann Surg.* 1928;87:481.

8. Colledge L. On the possibility of restoring movements to a paralyzed vocal cord by nerve anastomosis. *Br Med J.* 1925;2:547.

9. Frazier CH, Mosser WB. Treatment of recurrent laryngeal nerve injury. *Surg Gynecol Obstet.* 1926;43:134.

10. Ballance C. Some experiments on nerve anastomosis. *Mayo Clin Proc.* 1928;3:317.

11. Doyle PJ. Surgical treatment of bilateral adductor laryngeal paralysis. *Proc Can Otol Soc.* 1964;18.

12. Miglets AW. Functional laryngeal abduction following reimplantation of the recurrent laryngeal nerves. *Laryngoscope.* 1974;84:1996.

13. Ballance C. Results obtained in some experiments in which the facial and recurrent laryngeal nerves were anastomosed with other nerves. *Br Med J.* 1924;2:349.

14. Taggart JP. Laryngeal reinnervation by phrenic nerve implantation in dogs. *Laryngoscope.* 1971;81:1330.

15. Crumley RL. Experiments in laryngeal reinnervation. *Laryngoscope.* 1982;92(suppl 30):1.

16. Crumley RL. Update of laryngeal reinnervation concepts and options. In: Bailey R, Biller H, eds. *Surgery of the Larynx.* Philadelphia, PA: WB Saunders; 1988:135-147.

17. Crumley RL, Izdebski K, McMicken B. Nerve transfer versus Teflon injection for vocal cord paralysis: a comparison. *Laryngoscope.* 1988;98:1200-1204.

18. Crumley RL, Izdebski K. Voice quality following laryngeal reinnervation by ansa hypoglossi transfer. *Laryngoscope.* 1986;96:611-616.

19. Olsen DEL, Goding GS, Michael DD. Acoustic and perceptual evaluation of laryngeal reinnervation by ansa cervicalis transfer. *Laryngoscope.* 1998;108:1767-1772.

20. Paniello RC. Laryngeal reinnervation with the hypoglossal nerve: II. Clinical evaluation and early patient experience. *Laryngoscope.* 2000;110:739-748.

21. Iwamura S. Functioning remobilization of the paralyzed vocal cord in dogs. *Arch Otolaryngol.* 1974;100:122.

22. Tucker HM. Reinnervation of the unilaterally paralyzed larynx. *Ann Otol Rhinol Laryngol.* 1977;86:789.

23. Applebaum EL, Allen GW, Sisson GA. Human laryngeal reinnervation: the Northwestern experience. *Laryngoscope.* 1979;89:1784-1787.

24. May M, Beery Q. Muscle-nerve pedicle laryngeal reinnervation. *Laryngoscope.* 1986;96:1196.

25. Tucker HM. Neurologic disorders. In: *The Larynx.* New York, NY: Thieme Medical Publishers; 1987:chap 11.

26. Tucker HM. Combined laryngeal framework medialization and reinnervation for unilateral vocal fold paralysis. *Ann Otol Rhinol Laryngol.* 1990;99:778.

27. Tucker HM. Phonosurgery for voice disorders. In: *The Larynx.* 2nd ed. New York, NY: Thieme Medical Publishers; 1993:chap 13.

28. Tucker HM. Laryngeal transplantation: current status 1974. *Laryngoscope.* 1975;85:787-796.

29. Tucker HM. Selective reinnervation of paralyzed musculature in the head and neck: functioning autotransplantation of the canine larynx. *Laryngoscope.* 1978;88:162-171.

30. Obert PM, Young KA, Tobey DN. Use of direct posterior cricoarytenoid stimulation in laryngeal paralysis. *Arch Otolaryngol.* 1984;110:88-92.

31. Bergman K, Wartzel H, Eckhardt HU, Gerhardt HJ. Respiratory rhythmically regulated electrical stimulation of paralyzed laryngeal muscles. *Laryngoscope.* 1984;94:1376-1380.

32. Broniatowski M, Tucker HM, Kaneko S, Jacobs GJ, Nose Y. Entrainement Electronique du Larynx: Etudes Preliminaires—Principes de Base Appliques Aux Muscles Sous-hyoidiens Reinnerves Chez le Chien: *81 Congres Francais. Paris. September 25, 1984.*

33. Broniatowski M, Kaneko S, Nose Y, Jacobs GJ, Tucker HM. Laryneal pacemaker, II. Electronic pacing of reinnervated posterior cricoarytenoid muscles in the canine. *Laryngoscope.* 1985; 95(10):1194-1198.

34. Broniatowski, M, Tucker HM, Kaneko S, Jacobs G, Nose Y. Laryngeal pacemaker. Part 5. I. Electronic pacing of reinnervated strap muscles in the dog. *Otolaryngol Head Neck Surg.* 1986;94(1):41-44.

35. Broniatowski M, Tucker HM, Nose Y. Laryngeal biostimulators: rational, clinical applications and future perspectives. *Otorhinolaryngol Head Neck Surg.* 1990.

36. Broniatowski M, Davies CR, Jacobs GB, et al. Artificial restoration of voice. I: Experiments in phonatory control of the reinnervated canine larynx. *Laryngoscope.* 1990;100(11).

CHAPTER 39

Premalignant Lesions of the Larynx

Carole M. Dean, MD, FRCS(C)

Joseph R. Spiegel, MD, FACS

Robert T. Sataloff, MD, DMA, FACS

Accurate diagnosis and management of premalignant lesions of the larynx can prevent the development of laryngeal carcinoma or allow control of malignancy in an early stage. When laryngeal examination reveals an epithelial abnormality suspicious for malignancy, biopsy is indicated to provide a histologic diagnosis. Irregular masses and ulcerations of the mucosa are most suspicious, but more subtle surface changes are often the earliest manifestations of malignancy. Suspicion of cancerous change is greatly increased when the patient has a history of known etiologic risk factors such as cigarette smoking, alcohol use, asbestos exposure, and chemical or dust exposure. After biopsy, the laryngologist must work with the pathologist, radiation oncologist, medical oncologist, and the patient to develop a management strategy based on clinical and histologic findings.

TERMINOLOGY

Clinical Terms

Leukoplakia describes any white lesion of a mucous membrane (Figures 39-1, 39-2, 39-3). According to Wenig,[1] it is not necessarily indicative of an underlying malignant tumor. *Erythroplakia*, a red lesion of a mucous membrane, is more often indicative of an underlying malignant tumor. *Erythroleukoplakia*,[2] refers to a mix of red and white changes of the mucous membrane (Figure 39-4). *Pachydermia* describes abnormal thickening of the mucous membrane with or without leukoplakia (Figure 39-5).

Histologic Terms

Hyperplasia is the thickening of the epithelial surface as a result of an absolute increase in the number of

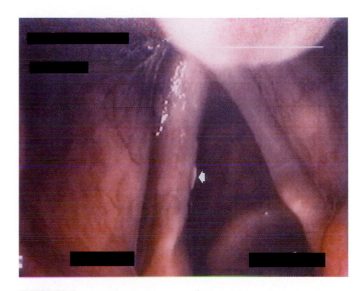

FIGURE 39-1. *Mild leukoplakia of the left vocal fold (arrow)*

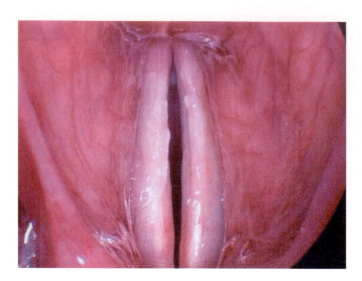

FIGURE 39-2. *Moderate leukoplakia, worse on the left*

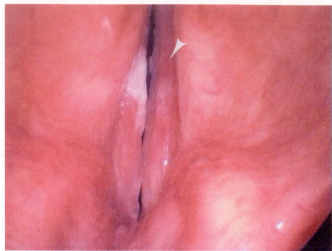

FIGURE 39-4. *Left prominent leukoplakia with mild erythema. Right erythroplakia (arrowhead) with adjacent patchy white areas of leukoplakia*

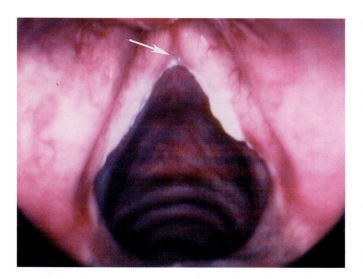

FIGURE 39-3. *More severe leukoplakia involving both vocal folds and an anterior web (arrow)*

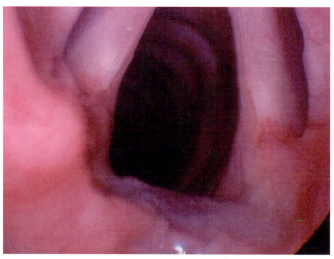

FIGURE 39-5. *Pachydermia of the posterior larynx, most commonly associated with chronic laryngopharyngeal reflux*

cells. *Pseudoepitheliomatous hyperplasia* is an exuberant reactive or reparative overgrowth of squamous epithelium (hyperplasia) displaying no cytologic evidence of malignancy. This lesion may be mistaken for an invasive carcinoma. *Keratosis* is the presence of keratin on the epithelial surface. *Parakeratosis* refers to the presence of nuclei in the keratin layer and *dyskeratosis* is abnormal keratinization of individual cells. *Metaplasia* is a change from one histologic tissue type to another. For example, squamous metaplasia denotes the replacement of respiratory epithelium by stratified squamous epithelium; it generally occurs as a result of tissue injury. *Koilocytosis* is cytoplasmic vacuolization of a squamous cell suggestive of viral infection such as human papilloma virus (HPV). *Dysplasia* is a qualitative alteration toward malignancy in the appearance of cells, consisting of cellular aberrations and abnormal maturation. Cellular aberrations include nuclear enlargement, irregularity, and hyperchromatism; increased nuclear/cytoplasmic ratios; dyskeratosis; crowding of cells; loss of polarity; and increased mitotic activity. Dysplasia is graded mild if the changes are within the inner third of the surface epithelium, moderate if it involves one-third to two-thirds, and severe if it is found from two-thirds to just short of full thickness. Severe dysplasia is differentiated from *carcinoma in situ* (CIS) by normal maturation in the most superficial layers of epithelium and from *invasive carcinoma* (Figure 39-6) by the integrity of the basement membrane.

Many classifications have been used to describe laryngeal epithelial changes. Many of them are similar; some are more or less identical. However, none of the proposed classification systems is perfect. Friedman's classification[3] is modeled on gynecologic pathology for lesions of the uterine cervix. They use the term *laryngeal intraepithelial neoplasm* (LIN) to include both dysplasia and CIS. Their classification is as follows: LIN-I corresponds to mild or minimal dysplasia; LIN-II corresponds to moderate dysplasia; and LIN-III corresponds to severe dysplasia and CIS. Unlike cancer of the uterine cervix, many carcinomas of the larynx do not go through the stage of CIS and are invasive from the start.[4] Hellqvist's classification system is also divided into three groups.[5] Group I is squamous cell hyperplasia with or without keratosis and/or mild dysplasia; Group II is squamous cell hyperplasia with moderate dysplasia; Group III is squamous cell hyperplasia with severe dysplasia or classical CIS with full thickness atypia.[6-12]

In Europe, a classification system was designed by Kleinsasser and has been widely applied throughout the world. His classification has three groups that include:

Class I = Simple Squamous Cell Hyperplasia

Class II = Squamous Cell Hyperplasia with Atypia

Class III is CIS.

EPIDEMIOLOGY AND ETIOLOGIC FACTORS

Laryngeal cancer is primarily a disease of middle age with a peak incidence in the sixth and seventh decades. In the United States, in the year 2000, its incidence was much higher in men than in women with a 4:1 ratio. However, this ratio was 20:1 just twenty years prior; the trend reflects the changing pattern of tobacco use in society. This decrease in the male to female ratio has also been observed worldwide.[13] The incidence is also higher among black people when compared to Caucasians.[13,14]

The major etiologic factor in the development of laryngeal cancer is tobacco use. Numerous studies have shown a dose dependent relationship between cigarette use and the development of cancer.[15,16] Smoking cigarettes has a strong association with cancer of the larynx while smoking cigars and pipes has a weaker association.[15,16] Most studies have shown that smoking cessation reduces the risk of laryngeal cancer. The importance of smoking cessation must be emphasized to patients with either premalignant or malignant lesions. One study showed that patients who continued to smoke after the diagnosis of head and neck cancer had a four-fold increase in the recurrence rate over those who never smoked, and a doubled increase for those who stopped smoking.[17]

Heavy alcohol use is also a factor in the development of laryngeal cancer and the relative risk is higher for supraglottic cancer than glottic cancer.[18] There has been a consistent finding of an interaction between cigarette smoking and alcohol consumption on laryngeal cancer risk. Yet, while studies have demonstrated that the combined effect of both cigarette smoking and alco-

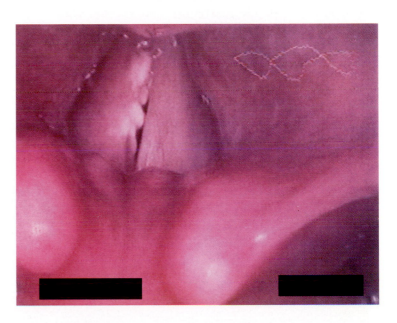

FIGURE 39-6. *Leukoplakia associated with T1 invasive carcinoma of the left true vocal fold. From gross appearance alone, it is not distinguishable from benign leukoplakia.*

hol consumption is greater than the sum of the individual effects, the biologic basis of this synergistic effect is still not clear. It has been reported that alcohol and tobacco account for over 80% of the squamous cell carcinomas of the mouth, pharynx, larynx, and esophagus in the United States.[19] The presence of this kind of interaction stresses the importance of eliminating at least one factor for subjects engaged in both habits.

There is increasing evidence that reflux laryngitis may be a carcinogenic cofactor in the development of laryngeal cancer. The association of reflux, Barrett's esophagus, and esophageal carcinoma is well established and can be used as an analogous model for the larynx.[20,21] Reflux of gastric acid causes acute and chronic inflammation of the larynx; that inflammation may (as in Barrett's esophagus) cause malignant transformation. Ward et al reported 19 cases of laryngeal carcinoma in lifetime nonsmokers who had moderate to severe reflux.[22] Freije et al[23] also proposed that laryngopharyngeal reflux (LPR) plays a role in the development of laryngeal carcinoma in patients without the typical risk factors.

Diet is being increasingly studied as an etiologic factor in the development of laryngeal carcinoma, and its role in the causal pathway has gained importance. It has been suggested that a high intake of fruit, salads, and dairy products may help reduce the risk of laryngeal cancer.[18] There is also evidence that deficiencies in vitamins A, C, E, beta-carotene, riboflavin, iron, zinc, and selenium have been associated with an increased risk of laryngeal cancer. The relationship between dietary factors and the occurrence of laryngeal cancer continues to be studied, as does an individual's dietary habits related to cancers elsewhere in the body.

Radiation exposure and/or avocational or occupational exposure to hazardous materials such as nickel, mustard gas, wood products, wood stove emissions, coal mines, insecticides, silica, and dry-cleaning chemicals have been implicated as etiologic factors as well.[24-27] The etiologic effect of asbestos on laryngeal cancer is still controversial, but it appears to be limited to active smokers.[16] In a study by Maier et al,[18] 92% of laryngeal squamous cell carcinoma patients were labeled as "blue-collar" workers. The risk ratio for those workers having no specialist training or higher education, compared to those with occupational training or higher educational level, was a 3.8:1 ratio. This means that subjects with low occupational training levels have a significantly increased risk of developing laryngeal cancer (after adjustment for alcohol and tobacco consumption).

The role of human papilloma virus and its relationship to the development of laryngeal cancer is discussed in detail later in this chapter.

The goal of treatment for premalignant laryngeal lesions is the prevention of malignant transformation, or the early diagnosis and treatment of laryngeal cancer. Control of potential etiologic factors, especially tobacco use, is necessary for this treatment to be complete and effective.

MALIGNANT TRANSFORMATION

Inconsistent use of terminology in reporting laryngeal cancer has hampered the collection of data that could be used to create a prognostic classification system. A clinical term such as keratosis can describe a lesion that has normal underlying epithelium or it can describe the surface of an invasive carcinoma.[28,29] There is poor consistency among pathologists in the histologic diagnoses as well. Goldman[30] studied 28 patients retrospectively with epithelial hyperplastic lesions of the larynx. Fifty-two operative biopsies were performed. Evaluation by 11 pathologists in 4 different laboratories yielded 21 different histologic diagnoses exclusive of invasive cancer. The grading of dysplasia is subjective. Blackwell et al[31] reported that one pathologist performed a blinded review of 148 laryngeal biopsies and only agreed with the original pathologic interpretation in 54% of the cases reviewed. However, the majority of cases differed by only one grade level (ie, mild vs moderate).

Although the rate of malignancy associated with a pathologic diagnosis of dysplasia varies widely, the pattern of increasing risk of malignancy with a worsening dysplasia grade is consistent. Fiorella et al[6] reported an incidence of 6% malignant transformation in keratosis without atypia and 17% when atypia was present. Kambivc et al[28] reported a rate of malignant change of 0.3% for keratosis and 9.5% for keratosis with atypia. Blackwell et al[31] retrospectively reviewed 65 patients with long-term follow-up after laryngeal biopsy and found the following cancer rates: 0% (0/6) for keratosis without atypia, 12% (3/26) for mild dysplasia, 33% (5/15) for moderate dysplasia, 44% (4/9) for severe dysplasia, and 11% (1/9) for carcinoma in situ.

While the presence and grade of dysplasia certainly have prognostic implications, the presence of keratosis has almost no predictive value. Frangeuz et al[29] reviewed 4,291 cases and reported that surface keratosis was present in simple and atypical hyperplasia in 68.8% and 85.5%, respectively. Follow-up of these patients showed malignant transformation to be 0.8% of cases with simple hyperplasia and 8.6% of those with atypical hyperplasia. Keratosis can mask epithelial changes and is not a predictor of underlying atypia. However, dyskeratosis is an important morphologic feature in the process of carcinogenesis[29] One study revealed a transformation rate of 50% (6/12) in patients with dyskeratosis.[7]

Blackwell et al[8,31] identified five histologic parameters that were found to be significantly different when comparing dysplastic lesions that resolved or remained stable to those that progressed to invasive carcinoma. These were abnormal mitotic figures, mitotic activity, stromal inflammation, maturation level, and nuclear pleomorphism. The five factors were not statistically different when comparing severe dysplasia and carcinoma in situ. Surface morphology, nuclear prominence, and koilocytosis were not significantly different in the two groups.

Histologic examination remains the basis of diagnosis in mucosal lesions of the larynx; however, the prognostic value of the morphologic criteria is limited. Quantification of histologic parameters may become an important supplement to the traditional grading of dysplasia. Proliferation associated changes such as a count of mitotic figures, or Ki67- or PCNA-labeling index gives additional hard data which are correlated to histologic grade.[9-11] DNA histograms are being utilized as an addition to microscopic evaluation. There is evidence that lesions with abnormal DNA content are more likely to persist or progress to intraepithelial or invasive carcinoma. However, it is important to note that the same studies show that the lack of abnormal DNA content does not exclude malignant transformation and that some cancers have so few chromosomal abnormalities that they are below the threshold sensitivity of image analysis or flow cytometry.[12] The prognostic value of p53 immunohistochemistry is controversial[3] and many studies have not found any significant association between p53 immunoreactivity and the evolution of carcinoma.[3,11,32-34]

All patients found to have dysplastic lesions of the laryngeal mucosa need to be followed closely for many years. Progression to invasive carcinoma often is a slow process allowing for early diagnosis, which should yield improved cure rates. Blackwell et al[31] reported that the average interval between the first biopsy and the diagnosis of invasive carcinoma was 3.9 years, suggesting that a 5-10-year follow-up plan is reasonable. Velasko et al[7] also suggested a more strict follow-up of patients with dyskeratosis as a result of a 50% (6/12) malignant transformation rate. Their report was based on a retrospective study in which all pathologies were reviewed by one pathologist. The period of follow-up ranged from one year to 130 months with a mean of 73 months follow-up. Their conclusion was that there is a longer interval between biopsy and malignant changes when you compare with patients having invasive carcinoma, the majority of whom will relapse within two years. The ability to provide dedicated long-term care for patients at risk for head and neck cancer is now limited by the financial constraints of managed care[30] in addition to all the other factors that have resulted in delayed diagnosis and treatment. The value of clinical examination, including strobovideolaryngoscopy, at regular intervals cannot be overstated. The senior authors (JRS, RTS) follow their patients every one to three months for cancer surveillance with videostrobscopy performed at each office evaluation. Such practice allows for early diagnosis of small invasive carcinomas and use of surgical options that yield greater laryngeal preservation and better voice quality postoperatively.

The strategy of biopsy differs if there is a single area of suspicion versus broad or multifocal lesions. Single, small lesions should be excised with a small mucosal margin. This will be sufficient treatment for many dysplastic lesions and intraepithelial neoplasms. When excision requires the removal of a large area of the true vocal fold, or a critical site such as the anterior commissure or medial margin, a small incisional biopsy may be more appropriate to allow for treatment planning with optimal voice preservation. In patients with broad-based or multifocal lesions, accurate microscopic biopsy at multiple sites is required. While it is always possible for biopsy sampling to miss areas of invasive carcinomas, these techniques are usually sufficient. However, if invasion is suspected clinically and not confirmed pathologically, the surgeon and patient must be prepared to proceed with additional biopsies. The availability of high resolution microscopic guidance with suspension laryngoscopy permits both aggressive diagnostic biopsy and mucosal preservation. Contact endoscopy may be helpful in guiding biopsy location. Vocal fold stripping is no longer indicated in the treatment of mucosal lesions of the vocal folds.

Carcinoma in Situ (CIS)

CIS is defined as cellular dysplasia involving the entire thickness of the mucosa without compromise of the basement membrane. The dysplasia may extend into adjacent mucous glands and is still considered an in situ lesion, as long as the lesion is confined to the duct and does not extend in the periductal lamina propia.[1,35] In other words, it is a malignant epithelial neoplasm which has all the characteristics of a true carcinoma except invasiveness and the ability to metastasize.[36] It may exist as an isolated lesion, but it is frequently associated with an invasive squamous cell carcinoma (SCCa), lying either adjacent to or remote from it.[1] Unlike cervical intraepithelial neoplasia, laryngeal CIS is not a required precursor to SCCa. Pathologically, the difference between CIS and severe dysplasia may be very difficult to determine with absolute certainty and is in many ways subjective, resulting in wide differences in the reported incidence and prevalence. However, in practice, the difference between these two lesions is not critical, as both indicate a significant risk for the future development of invasive cancer.

CIS must be evaluated carefully and invasive carcinoma must be ruled out. This is even more significant in the face of CIS of the supraglottis and subglottis than on the vocal folds,[1] as those two sites are considered the "silent area" that usually presents at a later stage of disease. Thus, CIS generally is present in association with an invasive carcinoma.[37] If a small biopsy reveals CIS, then there must be a high suspicion that an adjacent invasive cancer was missed, as reported by Ferlito.[36]

The incidence of CIS ranges from 1%-15% of all malignant laryngeal tumors.[36] There is a distinct male predominance, and it is most frequently seen in the sixth and seventh decades of life.[1] Although it can occur anywhere in the larynx, it most often involves the anterior portion of one or both vocal folds.[1,36,38] It may appear as leukoplakia, erythroplakia, or hyperkeratosis. CIS is a microscopic diagnosis, and its presenting signs, symptoms, and appearance are indistinguishable from other lesions of dysplasia or hyperkeratosis.[36]

The biologic behavior of this tumor is unknown. However, the main pathologic issue is whether or not all CIS will eventually develop into invasive carcinoma. Auerbach[15] presents indirect evidence that some cases of laryngeal CIS may be reversible in an autopsy study that showed lower rates of CIS in ex-smokers than in active smokers. Stenersen et al[4] observed 41 patients with the diagnosis of CIS or severe dysplasia, but who did not develop invasive carcinoma in the first year following their initial biopsy. The average observation time was 100 months. 46 percent (19/41) developed invasive SCCa after a mean interval of 50 months and 54% (22/41) returned to normal mucosa following biopsy. In a literature review, Bouquot and Gnepp[39] found that an average of 29% of cases of laryngeal CIS eventually resulted in invasive carcinoma with a reported range in the different studies of 3.5% to 90%. Untreated cases of CIS were associated with higher rates of transformation: 33.3%-90%. When considering all these data, it appears that some cases of CIS are cured by excisional biopsy and some lesions are reversible if the patient controls tobacco use. Yet, despite close observation and treatment, many CIS lesions will progress to invasive carcinoma.

There are some prognostic factors that can be utilized to guide treatment of patients with CIS. Myssiorek

et al[37] studied 41 patients with CIS retrospectively and found a much higher rate of transformation in lesions of the anterior commissure (92%) (11/12), than of lesions on the membranous vocal fold (17%) (5/29). This may reflect understaging caused by inadequate biopsy at the anterior commissure. This study also found no association of epidermal growth factor receptors (EGFR) in predicting lesions that will progress to invasive cancer. Epidermal growth factor (EGF) may play a role in the regulation of the growth of cancer of the larynx. Some in vitro studies have shown that cancer cells are stimulated by EGF/EGFR (immunohistochemical analysis of overexpression), while others evaluated if it had any prognostic value in determining which premalignant lesion or CIS would progress to invasive carcinoma. Results concerning its usefulness are inconsistent in the literature.[3,32] In another study, 37% (7/19) of patients with CIS who developed invasive laryngeal carcinoma were found to have had the carcinoma arise at a different anatomic site from the original CIS.[4] The authors concluded that there should be a high clinical suspicion of a lesion that arises separately from the site of known CIS.

Treatment of CIS has included surgery and radiation therapy. A recent review of primary surgical treatment with microscopic laser excision showed a local recurrence rate of 8% and an ultimate control of 100%. Small's[40] et al literature review revealed that radiotherapy as the primary treatment of CIS yielded an overall recurrence rate of 20% and an ultimate local control rate of 96%, following salvage treatment. They offered two explanations for the discrepancies found in the published data. First, there may be understaging of CIS (false CIS) and second, the total doses of radiation given were inadequate. Most CIS lesions are treated surgically because the biopsy itself provides the opportunity for complete excision and because of the limitations of primary radiation therapy. Most importantly, patients with CIS are at increased risk for development of an epithelial malignancy at other laryngeal and head and/or neck sites, the mucosa field effect. Dedicating a large portion of the lifetime radiation dose to the treatment of an early premalignant lesion or superficially malignant lesion may limit severely future treatment options if an invasive malignancy arises at another site. Additionally, radiation therapy requires an extended course of treatment[41,42] and its secondary effects on the local mucosa can mask recurrent tumors.[41] Yet, radiation therapy still plays a major role in the treatment of CIS and microinvasive carcinoma. Radiation therapy is indicated in patients who are poor risks for general anesthesia, those who have recurrent lesions after previous surgical excision, lesions that cannot be adequately exposed or resected endoscopically, and patients with recurrent lesions who cannot be adequately followed.[37,40-44]

LARYNGEAL PAPILLOMAS

Human Papilloma Virus: Epidemiology and Molecular Biology

Human papilloma virus (HPV) is a small, non-enveloped DNA virus. More than 70 HPV types have been identified. Based on studies of cervical cancer, different HPV[16,18,31,33,35] types have been graded as high risk oncogenic viruses because they are associated with high grade dysplasia or invasive carcinoma. The low risk HPV types[6,11,13,32,34,40,42-46] are usually associated with benign lesions such as uterine cervical condylomas. HPV 6 and HPV 11 are commonly associated with genital lesions as well as with laryngeal papillomas.[45] HPV types 16 and 18 also occur in the larynx.[46]

There is a high correlation of the risk of malignant transformation of infected cells in the presence of high-risk virus types. The viral genome of the HPV includes the E6 and E7 oncogene that is responsible for the viral proteins E6 and E7, respectively. The properties of these two oncoproteins have been reported extensively. High-risk types of HPV encode E6 and E7 oncoprotein that bind the Rb-related proteins and p53 with as much as 10-fold higher affinity, than the low risk HPV types.[47] For example, the E6 oncoprotein of HPV 16, can complex with the host cell p53 tumor suppressor protein thereby inducing p53 degradation.[45,46] Loss of p53 function leads to deregulation of the cell cycle and promotes mutation, chromosomal instability, and carcinogenesis of the host genome. Nevertheless, it has been reported that p53 can still preserve the tumor suppressor activity in the presence of HPV types 6 and 11, which are the predominant types in laryngeal papillomatosis.[46]

The relationship between HPV, p53, and other cellular control genes in SCCa of the head and neck is potentially complex. Molecular epidemiologic research is needed to evaluate the independent and joint effects of tobacco, HPV, and alterations of other genes involved in carcinogenesis.

Estimates of the prevalence of HPV types in normal tissue, benign papillomas, and cancers of the larynx are inconsistent because of the ongoing evolution in typing methods. Polymerase chain reaction (PCR) is a method of amplifying target sequences from a DNA specimen thus providing a higher degree of sensitivity than traditional hybridization methodologies. A high interlaboratory agreement has been achieved on sample acquisition and processing methods, leading to concordant results.

McKaig et al[45] reviewed the literature to determine HPV prevalence in head and neck cancer. Using PCR, HPV was found in 34.5% (416/1205). 40 percent contained HPV 16, 11.9% contained HPV 18, and 7% contained both types. In addition, 3.8% were positive for HPV 6, 7.4% for HPV 11, and 10.9% for both HPV 6 and HPV 11. Prevalence was also reported by site with 33% of laryngeal carcinomas found to be positive. Of those, 46% contained HPV 16 and 15.9% contained HPV 16 and HPV 18. Despite the prevalences reported, no correlation between virus infection and disease course or prognosis could be made.

The precise mechanism of malignant transformation in laryngeal papillomatosis is still unknown. In a retrospective study of 24 cases of laryngeal papillomatosis, Luzar et al[46] tried to determine any prognostic markers which might reflect the biologic behavior of the infected epithelium; they found that 23 of the 24 cases were HPV positive using PCR. All sections were immunostained for p53 protein and for c-erbB-2 oncogene product. The authors concluded that further molecular studies are needed to investigate whether increased p53 truly represents p53 overexpression or only stabilized wild type p53 gene product, and whether this possible overexpression may be a marker of malignant transformation. The staining pattern for the c-erbB-2 oncogene changed from membranous to cytoplasmic in cells demonstrating atypical hyperplasia. The real impact of this change also requires further study.

Majoros et al[48] published a pathologic review of 101 patients with juvenile laryngeal papillomatosis treated at the Mayo Clinic between 1914 and 1960 and noted greater cellular activity from the beginning of the disease process in the 6 patients who underwent malignant transformation. This may also reflect the difficulty in histologically diagnosing malignant transformation in benign papillomas.[49-51] Majoros'[48] retrospective study of 101 patients with the juvenile form of the disease revealed no carcinoma in the 58 patients treated only with surgery and a malignancy rate of 14% (6/43) in the irradiated patients. The interval between the XRT and the diagnosis of carcinoma ranged from 6 to 21 years except in one patient with an interval of only one year.

Clinical data regarding the association of laryngeal papillomas and carcinoma are variable. The incidence of cancer is higher in patients with papillomas who have received radiation therapy (XRT). Lindeberg[52] found that XRT produced a 16-fold increased risk of developing subsequent carcinoma compared to nonirradiated patients. These results support the commonly accepted view that cofactors play an important role in human papilloma virus (HPV)-related cancer. Rabbett's[53] statement that the only cases of juvenile laryngeal papillomatosis at risk for malignancy are those with a history of XRT has been proven wrong in the recent literature. Shapiro[54] reported a case of cancer in a juvenile laryngeal papilloma (JLP) patient without a history of XRT, but with a history of heavy cigarette and alcohol use. There were three other similar cases from the literature also described in that review. In 1982, Bewtra[55] reported one patient with malignant transformation of JLP without any history of XRT, smoking, or alcohol use. This report also reviewed four other cases of malignant transformation in patients with longstanding diffuse papillomatosis involving the trachea and bronchi as well as the larynx. Keim[51] also reported a single case of malignant change in a patient with JLP without any history of XRT. Assessing all these reports, it is apparent that while uncommon, it is certainly possible for benign laryngeal papillomas to undergo malignant transformation without the stimulus of radiation. The possible effects of treatment of papillomas (such as repeated laser excision) on the development of malignancy are unknown, but we believe that they warrant study.

Lie et al[56] presented a retrospective study of 102 patients with laryngeal papillomas treated between 1950 and 1979 with follow-up ranging from 4 to 58 years. Eight patients developed carcinoma, seven laryngeal and one bronchial. The intervals between diagnosis of the benign papillomas and diagnosis of cancer were 4 to 55 years. Three patients had the juvenile form of disease and five had the adult type. The male to female ratio was 1:1. Two patients had received XRT, four were smokers, and one patient had received bleomycin and interferon. The authors concluded that HPV played a role in carcinogenesis, but that cofactors may also have played an important role. Klozar et al[57] reported a retrospective study of 179 HPV infected patients with a 1.7% incidence of cancer. These patients underwent 668 operations from 1982-1995. When he separated the patients by their clinical presentation, he found the incidence of malignancy to be 3% (3/102) in patients with the adult form and 0% (0/77) in those with the juvenile form (Table 39-1).

The concept of a possible cofactor in malignant transformation was supported by Koufman.[21] He found 21% (14/88) of patients with adult onset papillomatosis developed SCCa of the aerodigestive tract either at the site of the known papilloma or at another site after a 10-year follow-up. All the patients who developed cancer were smokers or had documented gastroesophageal reflux disease (GERD). Franceshi et al[47] reviewed HPV and cancer of the upper aerodigestive tract and found that the association of smoking, drinking, and betel nut chewing was too pervasive to permit judgment about HPV as a carcinogenic factor.

Rabkin et al[58] studied the incidence of second primary cancer in over 25,000 women with cervical cancer reported from 9 US cancer registries. There was a significantly increased risk of cancer of the oral cavity (relative risk 2.2) and of the larynx (relative risk 3.4). As HPV is a well-established risk factor for development of cervical cancer, this suggests that the cervical cancer and second primaries may share HPV as a causal agent.

Malignant transformation of laryngeal papillomas is diagnosed as a result of clinical observation, assessment of etiologic risk factors and careful preparation and examination of biopsy specimens. Majaros[48] stated that as all his patients had been hoarse from the time of their original presentation with papillomas, there were no early clinical signs of malignancy. Consequently, presenting signs and symptoms are superimposed on the underlying papillomatosis and may include airway obstruction, throat pain, referred otalgia, and hemoptysis. Both Keim[51] and Fechner et al[49] report patients with progressive symptoms of malignancy but benign histology on early biopsies before invasive cancer was diagnosed. When the clinical suspicion is justified, repeated biopsy, deep biopsy, and even laryngectomy may be necessary to establish an accurate diagnosis. It is essential for the patient to be informed informed fully in such challenging clinical circumstances. Singh et al[50] reviewed three of seventeen papilloma patients who developed cancer that revealed yet a different potential problem: simultaneous presentation of benign and malignant exophytic laryngeal lesions. All 3 cancer patients were diagnosed less than one year after their diagnosis of papillomas. Singh et al concluded that clinical indicators for carcinoma in patients with papillomas include gross laryngeal edema, airway obstruction, reduced vocal fold mobility, dysphagia, subglottic extension, and cervical adenopathy. When malignant transformation of laryngeal papillomas is suspected, a benign biopsy result may be misleading. Atypia can be found in both adult and juvenile papillomas and is not predictive of malignant transformation.[45] Clinical suspicion based on presenting signs and symptoms and a complete history of risk factors should guide patient management.

In conclusion, it is important for laryngologists to be familiar with the broad spectrum of benign premalignant and malignant disease that may afflict the larynx. Premalignant lesions must be assessed histologically for malignancy and the entire larynx must be fully evaluated because of the risk of multifocal abnormalities. Adequate preoperative examination, meticulous surgical

Study	Number of Patients	Incidence of Malignant Transformation	Presence of Cocarcinogens	Interval Between Diagnosis of Papilloma and Malignant Transformation
Majoros et al[48] (1914-1960	101 Juvenile 101 Adult 0	6%	Radiation 6 (14%; 6 of 43 who received XRT; 0%; of 58 patients not treated by XRT)	6-21 years; except 1 case (1 year)
Lie et al[56] (1950-1979)	102 Juvenile 53 Adult 49	8% (8/102) 6% (3/53) 10% (5/49)	2 previous XRT 2 Bleomycin +/- interferon 4 smokers	4-55 years
Klozar et al[57] (1982-1995)	179 Juvenile 77 Adult 102	1.7% (3/179) 0% 3%	2 smokers 1 nonsmoker	2-8 years

TABLE 39-1. *Papilloma to Malignant Transformation*

technique, and long-term surveillance are necessary in every case. While early detection of carcinoma must be our primary goal, diagnostic and treatment strategies should be individualized with functional considerations in mind.

REFERENCES

1. Wenig BM. *Atlas of Head and Neck Pathology.* Philadelphia, PA: W.B. Saunders; 1993:221-239.

2. Silver CE, Ferlito A. *Surgery for Cancer of the Larynx and Related Structures.* 2nd ed. Philadelphia, PA: W.B. Saunders; 1996:29-31.

3. Friedman I. Precurors of squamous cell carcinoma. In: Ferlito A, ed. *Surgical Pathology of Laryngeal Neoplasms.* London, UK: Chapman and Hall Medical 2-6 Boundary Row; 1996:108-121.

4. Stenersen TC, Hoel PS, Boysen M. Carcinoma in-situ of the larynx: an evaluation of its natural clinical cause. *Clin Otolaryngol.* 1991;16(4):358-363.

5. Hellqvist H, Lundgren J, Olofson J. Hyperplasia, dysplasia and CIS of the vocal cords: a follow-up study. *Clin Otolaryngol.* 1982;7:11-27.

6. Fiorella R, DiNicola V, Resta L. Epidemiological and clinical relief on hyperplastic lesions of the larynx. *Acta Otolaryngol (Stockh).* 1997;527 (suppl):77-87.

7. Velasko JRR, Niero CS. DeBustos CP, Marcos CA. Premalignant lesions of the larynx: pathological prognostic factors. *J Otolaryngol.* 1987;16(6):367-370.

8. Blackwell KE, Fu YS, Calcaterra TC. Laryngeal dysplasia. A clinicopathologic study. *Cancer.* 1995;75(2):457-463.

9. Burkhardt A. Morphological assessment of malignant potential of epithelial hyperplastic lesions. *Acta Otolaryngol (Stockh).* 1997;527(suppl):12-16.

10. Zhao R, Hirano M, Kurita S. Expression of proliferating cell nuclear antigen in premalignant lesion of the larynx. *Am J Otolaryngol.* 1996;17(1):36-40.

11. Pignataro L, Capaccio P, Pruneri G, et al. The predictive value of p53, MDM-2, cyclin D1, and Ki67 in the progression from low-grade dysplasia towards carcinoma of the larynx. *J Laryngol Otol.* 1998;112(5):455-459.

12. Bracko M. Evaluation of DNA content in epithelial hyperplastic lesion in the larynx. *Acta Otolaryngol. (Stockh).* 1997;527(suppl);62-65.

13. Cattaruzza MS, Maisonneuve P, Boyle P. Epidemiology of laryngeal cancer. *Oral Oncol Eur J Cancer.* 1996;32(5):293-305.

14. Wasfie T, Newman R. Laryngeal carcinoma in black patients. *Cancer.* 1988;61(1):167-172.

15. Auerbach O, Hannond EC, Garfinkel L. Histologic changes in the larynx in relation to smoking habits. *Cancer.* 1970;25(1):92-104.

16. Burch JD, Howe GR, Miller AB, Semenciw R. Tobacco, alcohol, asbestos, and nickel in the etiology of cancer of the larynx: a case-control study. *J Natl Cancer Inst.* 1981;67(6):1219-1224.

17. Stevens M, Gardner JW, Parkin JL, Johnson LP. Head and neck cancer survival and life-style change. *Arch Otolaryngol.* 1983;109(11):746-749.

18. Maier H, Gewelke U, Pietz A, Heller WD. Risk factors of cancer of the larynx: results of the Heidelberg case-control study. *Otolaryngol Head Neck Surg.* 1992;107(4):577-582.

19. Thomas DB. Alcohol as a cause of cancer. *Environ Health Perspect.* 1995;103(8);153-160.

20. Sataloff RT, Castell DO, Katz, PO, Sataloff DM. *Reflux Laryngitis and Related Disorders.* San Diego, CA: Singular Publishing Group; 1999.

21. Koufman JA, Burke AJ, The etiology and pathogenesis of laryngeal carcinoma. *Otolaryngol Clin North Am.* 1997;30(1):1-19.

22. Ward PH, Hanson DG. Reflux as an etiological factor of carcinoma of the laryngopharynx. *Laryngoscope.* 1988;98:1195-1199.

23. Freije JE, Beatty TW, Campbell BH, Woodson BT, Schultz CJ, Toohill RJ. Carcinoma of the larynx in patients with gastroesophageal reflux. *Am J Otolaryngol.* 1996;17(6):386-390.

24. Pinros J, Franco EL, Kolwalski LP, Oliveira BV, Curado MP. Use of wood stoves and risk of cancer of the upper aero-digestive tract: a case control study. *Int J Epidemiol.* 1998;27(6):936-940.

25. Haguenoer JM, Cordier S, Morel C, Lefebvre JL, Hemon D. Occupational risk factor for upper respiratory tract and upper digestive tract cancers. *Br J Ind Med.* 1990;47:380-383.

26. Bravo MP, Espinosa J, del Rey Calero J. Occupational risk factors for cancer of the larynx in Spain. *Neoplasma.* 1990;37(4):477-487.

27. Vaughan TL, Stewart PA, Davis S, Thomas DB. Work in dry cleaning and the incidence of cancer of the oral cavity, larynx, and esophagus. *Occup Environ Med.* 1997;54:692-695.

28. Kambivc V. Epithelial hyperplastic lesions—a challenging topic in laryngology. *Acta Otolaryngol (Stockh).* 1997;527(suppl):7-11.

29. Frangeuz I, Gale N, Luzar B. The interpretation of leukoplakia in laryngeal pathology. *Acta Otolaryngol (Stockh).* 1997;527(suppl):142-144

30. Goldman NC. Problems in outpatients with laryngeal hyperplastic lesions. *Acta Otolaryngol (Stockh).* 1997;527(suppl):70-73.

31. Blackwell KE, Calcatura TC, Fu YS. Laryngeal dysplasia: epidemiology and treatment outcomes. *Ann Otol Rhinol Laryngol.* 1995;104:596-602.

32. Gale N, Zidar N, Kambic V, Poljak M, Cor A. Epidermal growth factor receptor, c-erbB-2 and p53 overexpression in epithelial hyperplastic lesion of the larynx. *Acta Otolaryngol (Stockh).* 1997;527(suppl);105-110.

33. Krecicki T, Jelen M, Zalesska-Krecicka M, Szkudlarek T, Szajowski K. Immunohistochemically stained markers (p53, PCNA, bcl-2) in dysplastic lesion of the larynx. *Cancer Lett.* 1999;143:23-28.

34. Ioachim E, Assimakopoulos D, Peschos D, Zissi A, Skervas A, Agnantis NJ. Immunohistochemical expression of metallothionein in benign premalignances and malignant epithelium of the larynx: correlation with p53 and proliferative cell nuclear antigen. *Pathol Res Pract.* 1999;195:809-814.

35. Fried MP. *The Larynx: A Multidisciplinary Approach.* 2nd ed. St. Louis, MO: Mosby Year Book; 1995:470-473.

36. Ferlito A, Polidoro F, Rossi M. Pathological basis and clinical aspects of treatment policy in carcinoma-in-situ of the larynx. *J Laryngol Otol.* 1982;95(2):141-154.

37. Myssiorek D, Vambutas A, Abramson AL. Carcinoma in situ of the glottic larynx. *Laryngoscope.* 1994;104(4):463-467.

38. Myers EN, Sven JY. *Cancer of the Head and Neck.* 3rd ed. Philadelphia, PA: W.B. Saunders; 1996:381-421.

39. Bouquot JE, Gnepp DR. Laryngeal precancer: a review of the literature, commentary, and comparison with oral leukoplakia. *Head Neck.* 1991;13(6):488-497.

40. Small W, Mittal BB, Brand WN, et al. Role of radiation therapy in the management of carcinoma in situ of the larynx. *Laryngoscope.* 1993;103(6):663-667.

41. Maran AGD, Mackenzie IJ, Stanley RE. Carcinoma in situ of the larynx. *Head Neck Surg.* 1984;(7):28-31.

42. Nguyen C, Naghibzadeh B, Black MJ, Rochon L, Shenouba G. Carcinoma in situ of the glottic larynx: excision or irradiation? *Head Neck Surg.* 1996;18(3):225-228.

43. Rothfield RE, Myers EN, Johnson JT. Carcinoma in situ and microinvasive squamous cell carcinoma of the vocal cords. *Ann Otol Rhinol Laryngol.* 1991;100(10):793-796.

44. Medini E, Medini I, Lee CKK, Grapany M, Levitt SH. The role of radiotherapy in the management of carcinoma in situ of the glottic larynx. *Am J Clin Oncol.* 1998;21(3):298-301.

45. McKaig RG, Baric RS, Olshan AF. Human papillomavirus and head and neck cancer: epidemiology and molecular biology. *Head Neck.* 1998;20(3):250-265.

46. Luzar B, Gale N, Kambivc V, Poljak M, Zidar N, Voobvnik A. Human papillomavirus infection and expression of p53 and c-erbB-2 protein in laryngeal papillomas. *Acta Otolaryngol (Stockh).* 1997;527(suppl):120-124.

47. Franceshi S, Munoz N, Bosch XF, Snijders PJF, Walboomers JMM. Human papillomavirus and cancers of the upper aerodigestive tract: a review of epidemiological and experimental evidence. *Cancer Epidemiology, Biomarkers Prev.* 1996;5(7):567-575.

48. Majoros M, Devine KD, Parkhill EM. Malignant transformation of benign laryngeal papilloma in children after radiation therapy. *Surg Clin North Am.* 1963;43(4):1049-1061.

49. Fechner RE, Goepfert H, Alford BR. Invasive laryngeal papillomatosis. *Arch Otolaryngol.* 1974;99(2):147-151.

50. Singh B, Ramsaroop R. Clinical features of malignant transformation in benign laryngeal papillomata. *J Laryngol Otol.* 1994;108(8)642-648.

51. Keim RJ. Malignant change of laryngeal papilloma: a case report. *Otolaryngol Head Neck Surg.* 1980;88(6):773-777.

52. Lindeberg H, Elbrond O. Malignant tumors in patients with a history of multiple laryngeal papillomas: the significance of irradiation. *Clin Otolaryngol.* 1991;16:149-151.

53 Rabbett WF. Juvenile laryngeal papillomatosis: the relation of irradiation to malignant degeneration in this disease. *Ann Otol Rhinol Laryngol.* 1965;74(4):1149-1163.

54. Shapiro RS, Marlowe FI, Butcher J. Malignant degeneration of nonirradiated juvenile laryngeal papillomatosis. *Ann Otol.* 1976;85(1):101-103.

55. Bewtra C, Krishnan R, Lee SS. Malignant change in non-irradiated juvenile laryngotracheal papillomatosis. *Arch Otolaryngol.* 1982;108(2):114-116.

56. Lie ES, Engh V, Boysen M, et al. Squamous cell carcinoma of the respiratory tract following laryngeal papillomatosis. *Acta Otolaryngol (Stockh).* 1994;114(2):209-212.

57. Klozar J, Taudy M, Betka J, Kana R. Laryngeal papilloma-precanerous condition? *Acta Otolaryngol (Stockh).* 1997;527(suppl):100-102.

58. Rabkin CS, Biggar RJ, Melbye M, Curtis RE. Second primary cancers following anal and cervical carcinoma: evidence of shared etiologic factors. *Am J Epidemiol.* 1992;136(1):54-58.

CHAPTER 40

Surgery for Laryngeal Cancer

Ramon A. Franco, Jr., MD

Steven M. Zeitels, MD, FACS

GLOTTIC CARCINOMA—DISEASE PRESENTATION AND PHILOSOPHY OF MANAGEMENT

Hoarseness is the most frequent symptom associated with glottic cancer; however, patients may also complain of throat clearing and pain, as well as hemoptysis, airway obstruction, and otalgia (at advanced stages). Tobacco smoking is the most frequently associated factor influencing the pathogenesis of laryngeal cancer, of which 95% are of the squamous cell type.[1] Because of the relative paucity of lymphatics at the level of the true vocal folds, nearly 75% of patients with glottic carcinoma will have localized disease at presentation (ie, no regional nodal or distant spread).[2] The majority of vocal fold cancers present in the musculomembranous region so that very small lesions (1 mm) can cause a functional change (dysphonia). This characteristic of disease presentation allows for highly favorable treatment outcomes as compared with other sites of the upper aerodigestive tract.

Laryngeal cancer is staged using the standard TNM classification system (Table 40-1) based on the subsite affected (supraglottic, glottic, or subglottic). As with other cancers, the TNM system provides some prognostic value for survival and at times may assist with the selection of treatment modalities.

The two main treatment modalities for glottic carcinoma are radiation therapy (XRT) and surgery.

Successful transcervical (1869)[3] and transoral (1886)[4] resection of early glottic cancer predated the use of radiotherapy by several decades. Despite the fact that endolaryngeal surgery[5-10] and XRT[11,12] are equally successful in curing early disease, radiotherapy became the dominant treatment method in the 20th century. Endoscopic management[5,6] was considered difficult and open surgery was deemed to be excessively morbid because of the associated vocal dysfunction and the frequent need for a temporary tracheotomy.

RADIOTHERAPY FOR GLOTTIC CANCER

Early Disease

Patients whose larynx cannot be adequately exposed during staging endoscopy are ideal candidates for radiotherapy. The optimal clinical scenario for using XRT in early glottic cancer is diffuse superficial disease (T1b) in which surgical intervention would disrupt the basic architecture of both vocal folds, the anterior commissure tendon, and/or the laminae propria. The disadvantages of XRT include treatment of noncancerous vocal-fold tissue (T1a, T2a), which frequently results in scarring of the mucosa of the normal vocal fold with associated dysphonia.[13] There is a relative contraindication for using XRT in early glottic cancer in young people as it is a one-time treatment and there is a significant risk for metachronous lesions. In addition, there is the theoretic risk for radiation-induced cancer.[14] Finally, radiation is more expensive than endoscopic resection.

More Advanced Disease (T3, T4)

Radiotherapy is used when patients are not surgical candidates. Retrospective studies suggest that XRT as a single modality treatment for more advanced lesions results in diminished control rates as compared to surgery. Furthermore, morbid complications from XRT may include acute odynophagia and dysphagia necessitating gastrostomy tube placement. Severe dysphonia and dryness may be permanent as is chondroradionecrosis.[15]

Radiation therapy is typically administered over 6 weeks to a total dosage of 5,600 to 7,600 centi-Gray. Investigations with neoadjuvant chemotherapy[16] (cis-

---

Supraglottic

Tis:

T1: Tumor confined to site of origin with normal mobility

T2: Tumor involving adjacent supraglottic site(s) or glottis without fixation

T3: Tumor limited to larynx with fixation or extension or both to involve the postcricoid area, medial wall of pyriform sinus, or pre-epiglottic space

T4: Massive tumor extending beyond larynx to involve oropharynx, soft tissues of neck, or destruction of thyroid cartilage

Glottis

Tis:

T1: confined to vocal cords with normal mobility (includes involvement of anterior or posterior commissure)

T1a: unilateral involvement

T1b: bilateral involvement

T2: supraglottic or subglottic extension of tumor or both with normal or impaired cord mobility

T3: tumor confined to larynx with cord fixation

T4: massive tumor with thyroid cartilage destruction or extension beyond confines of larynx or both

Subglottis

Tis:

T1: tumor confined to the subglottic region

T2: tumor extension to vocal cords with normal or impaired cord mobility

T3: tumor confined to larynx with cord fixation

T4: massive tumor with cartilage destruction or extension beyond confines of larynx or both

N0: no regional LN metastasis

N1: <3 cm, single ipsilateral LN

N2: 3 cm-6 cm

    N2a: single ipsilateral 3-6 cm

    N2b: multiple ipsilateral <6 cm

    N2c: bilateral or contralateral all <6 cm

N3: >6 cm

Staging

Stage I: T1, N0, M0

Stage II: T2, N0, M0

Stage III: T3, N0, M0, T1, T2 or T3, N1, M0

Stage IV: T4, Nx, Mx

    Tx, N2 or N3, M0

    Tx, Nx, M1

TABLE 40-1. *TNM Staging of Laryngeal Cancer. Used with the permission of the American Joint Committee on Cancer (AJCC®), Chicago, Illinois. The original source for this material is the AJCC® Cancer Staging Handbook 5th edition (1998) published by Lippincott-Raven Publishers, Philadelphia.*

platin and 5-fluorouracil) suggest that there is a sub-population of individuals in whom this approach constitutes ideal management. However, this patient cohort has yet to be clearly delineated and it is difficult to determine whether induction chemotherapy provides a therapeutic advantage over advanced single-modality radiotherapy (ie, BID treatment).

SURGERY FOR GLOTTIC CANCER

Surgery has long been a mainstay of treatment for glottic cancer. If the correct procedure is selected and executed appropriately, local control is >90% regardless of the disease stage. Effective management comprises: (1) oncologically sound margins that minimize loss of non-involved tissue,[10,17-21] and (2) creative reconstruction[20-22] that optimizes the postoperative airway, voice, and deglutition. Surgery is typically less expensive than radiotherapy[23] and unlike XRT, there is immediate oncologic eradication without intercurrent disease during the treatment course. Surgical resection of glottic cancer can be done transorally or transcervically.

Endoscopic Treatment of Early Glottic Cancer

The goal of endoscopic treatment of an isolated T1 lesion of the musculomembranous vocal fold is eradication of the disease with maximal preservation of the normal layered microstructure (epithelium and laminae propria). This approach results in the optimal postoperative voice without compromising oncologic cure. The universal modular glottiscope was designed specifically to perform endolaryngeal resection of glottic cancer.[24,25] It has a number of advantages for exposing the tumor as well as for instrumenting the tissue.

There are four basic procedures that are based on the depth of excision (Figures 40-1)[10,20,21]: (1) dissection just deep to the epithelial basement membrane and superficial to the superficial lamina propria for epithelial atypia and microinvasive cancer, (2) dissection within the superficial lamina propria for microinvasive cancer that is not attached to the vocal ligament, (3) dissection between the deep lamina propria (vocal ligament) and the vocalis muscle for lesions that are attached to the ligament but not through it, and (4) dissection within the thyroarytenoid muscle for lesions penetrating the vocal ligament and invading the vocalis. This approach can be fine-tuned further by performing partial resections of any of the layered microstructure. The specimen is always oriented for whole-mount histologic analysis and frozen-section margin assessment is employed selectively to verify a complete excision.

If dissection is performed in the SLP, cold instruments facilitate precise tangential dissection around the curving vocal fold (Figures 40-2 through 40-4).[10,17,20] This allows for maximal preservation of the superficial lamina propria and for pliability of the regenerating epithelium. Dissection between the vocal ligament and the vocalis muscle can be performed equally well with cold instruments alone or with assistance by the laser. Dissection within the muscle is performed most precise-

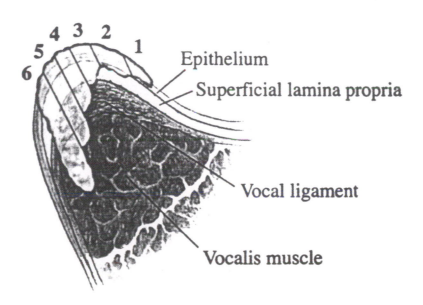

FIGURE 40-1. *This diagram describes how a surface vocal fold lesion may harbor a variety of invasion patterns. (Courtesy of* Operative Techniques in Otolaryngology—Head and Neck Surgery[21])

ly with the CO_2 laser, which allows for improved visualization because of its hemostatic cutting properties.

Subepithelial saline-epinephrine infusion into Reinke's space[19,20,26] (Figures 40-5 and 40-6) improves pre-excisional assessment of lesion depth. If the tumor has invaded the vocal ligament, the SLP at the perimeter of the lesion will distend creating a contour depression in the region of the cancer. Assessment of depth of invasion is also enhanced by palpation of the cancer. The subepithelial infusion assists with the surgeon's technical execution of the surgery in a number of other ways: (1) the infusion facilitates mucosal incisions by improving visualization of the lateral border of the lesion and by distending the SLP so that the overlying epithelium is under tension; (2) the infusion also increases the depth of the superficial lamina propria, which facilitates less traumatic dissection in this layer and leads to regenerated epithelium that is more flexible; (3) the epinephrine and hydrostatic pressure of the infusion vasoconstrict the microvasculature in the SLP and this improves visualization and a precise dissection; and (4) if the laser is used, the saline acts as a heat sink, which decreases thermal trauma to the normal vocal fold tissue.

Endoscopic Vertical Partial Laryngectomy

If adequate endoscopic exposure can be achieved, transoral partial laryngectomy is usually feasible if the disease is confined to the glottis. Subglottic and supra-glottic extension can dramatically compound the difficulty in performing an oncologically sound resection. As impaired mobility implies deep invasion in the musculature of the paraglottic space and/or the cricoarytenoid joint, detailed radiographic imaging (CT, MRI) is often helpful toward procedure planning.

As with all endoscopic procedures, exposure is of paramount importance for the successful completion of the surgery. The largest laryngoscope that can be inserted into the patient with a suitable suspension device is used. The universal modular glottiscope[24] is designed to facilitate the resection of the anterior and lateral glottis because its shape simulates the contours of the inner thyroid laminae. After obtaining adequate endoscopic exposure, the tumor is inspected under high magnification to determine the limits of the resection prior to distortion of the specimen. This three-dimensional perspective is often enhanced by the use of telescopes.

Subsequent to histologic confirmation of cancer, the CO_2 laser is used with a microspot (0.3 mm) to outline the area of excision. Typically, the vestibular folds and infrapetiole region of the supraglottis must be resected prior to the cancer removal to facilitate adequate exposure of the antero-lateral limits of the lesion.[20,27] Laryngeal forceps are used to retract the true vocal fold medially while the CO_2 laser is used in a repeated pulsed mode (~0.1 second interval and duration) at approximately 2.5 watts. The counter-traction provided by the forceps is invaluable in completing the dissection

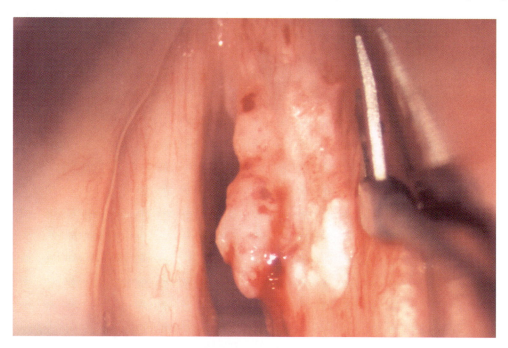

FIGURE 40-2. *(7X) An upturned scissors is used to perform an epithelial cordotomy, which serves as a perimeter margin.*

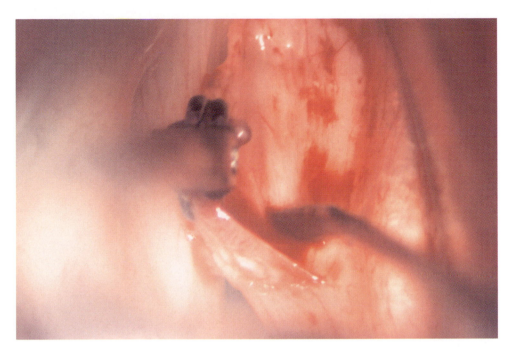

FIGURE 40-3. *(7X) The edge of the microflap is retracted medially with an angled forceps, which reveals normal superficial lamina propria. A left curved dissector is used to easily dissect the lesion from the residual normal SLP.*

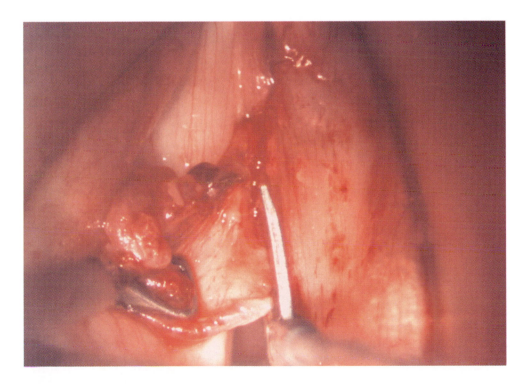

FIGURE 40-4. *(7X) The dissection is completed to the inferior margin of the lesion. The lesion is retracted and an upturned scissors is used to complete the resection.*

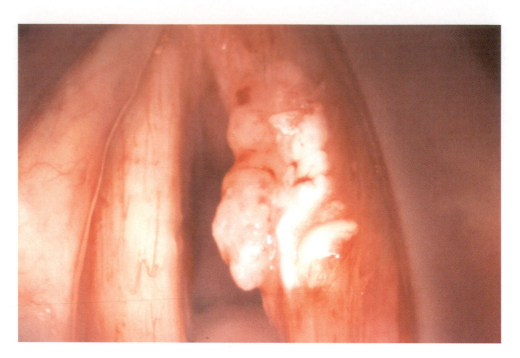

FIGURE 40-5. *(7X) A T1 Carcinoma of the true vocal fold.*

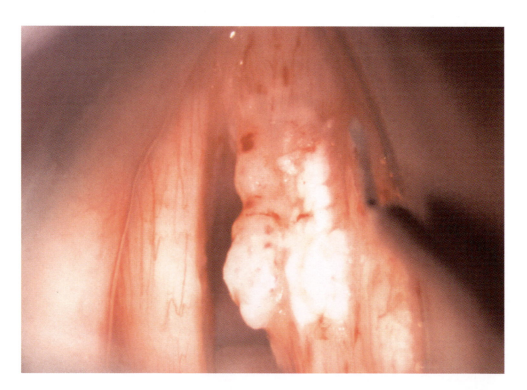

FIGURE 40-6. *(7X) A subepithelial infusion is done; the specially designed needle is seen on the superior surface of the vocal fold.*

accurately and expeditiously. Removal of the entire vocal fold including the anterior commissure and arytenoid can be done as is necessary.

Endoscopic Treatment of Glottic Carcinoma in the Anterior Commissure[20,27,28]

The anterior commissure tendon, or Broyle's ligament, is a confluence of the vocal ligament, the thyroepiglottic ligament, the conus elasticus, and the internal perichondrium of the thyroid ala (Figure 40-7). There is a misconception that T1 cancers at the anterior commissure have a great predilection for understaging and that many of these lesions have occult invasion of the thyroid cartilage (T4 stage). This is based upon the misunderstanding that the anatomy of the dense anterior-commissure ligament is a less resilient tumor barrier than the adjacent thin thyroid perichondrium (Figure 40-7). Kirchner[29,30] has made clear that T1a and T1b carcinomas rarely erode through Broyle's ligament to invade thyroid cartilage. Anterior commissure tumors that have thyroid cartilage invasion typically display cephalad surface invasion of the infrapetiole region of the supraglottis or caudal surface invasion of the subglottis (both T2 by surface staging criteria) (Figure 40-8).

There has been divergent opinion as to whether cancer can be endoscopically eradicated from the anterior commissure. The proscriptions imposed by some are based primarily on the difficulty in obtaining adequate surgical exposure in this area.[31] The rate-limiting fac-

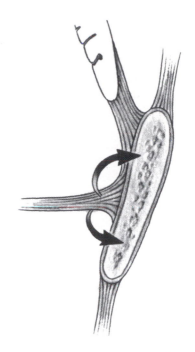

FIGURE 40-8. *Diagrammatic representation of how cancer spreads around the anterior commissure tendon to invade the thyroid cartilage. (Courtesy of* Operative Techniques in Otolaryngology—Head and Neck Surgery[21])

tors for resection of early cancer in the anterior commissure are the true extent of the disease (is it invading cartilage?) and the endoscopic exposure required to

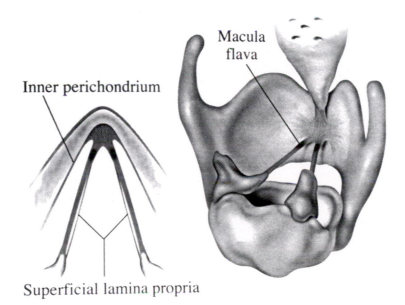

FIGURE 40-7. *Diagrammatic representation of the anterior commissure tendon. (Courtesy of* Operative Techniques in Otolaryngology—Head and Neck Surgery[21])

encompass the lesion. Davis[32] and the Boston University group and later Koufman et al[33] demonstrated that cancer could be removed from the anterior commissure; however, it required great skill to excise the lesion without vaporizing the specimen. Vaporizing cancer without obtaining clear resection margins is inadequate surgical oncologic technique. This factor, as well as underestimating the extent of disease, probably led to the reported failures by a number of investigators.[31,34-36]

If one accepts Kirchner's histopathologic data regarding the invasion pattern of T1 glottic cancer, there is no reason to believe that an adequate soft-tissue resection of small-volume soft-tissue disease is not adequate treatment. This premise is further substantiated by a number of reports that did not find a correlation between anterior commissure involvement with T1 glottic cancer and failure of radiotherapy as a curative modality.[15,37]

The extensive European experience reported by Steiner,[38] Eckel and Thumfart,[39] and Rudert[40] substantiates that glottic cancer in the anterior commissure can be removed transorally. The problem with any surgical approach to the anterior commissure (for true T1a, T1b, and T2 lesions) is that these procedures disturb the structural integrity of the anterior commissure and result in a poor voice. Lesions that are invading cartilage are T4 by stage, require open partial (or total) laryngectomy, and are not suitable for endoscopic excision. An endoscopic exploration of the infrapetiole region of the supraglottis allows for definitive determination about whether a presumed T1 lesion has cartilage invasion (T4).[27] This procedure facilitates precise staging (without disarticulating Broyle's ligament), commensurate management, and optimal post-treatment voice quality.

Glottic Reconstruction Subsequent to Endolaryngeal Cancer Resection

If there is an excavated neocord subsequent to epithelialization, various reconstructive procedures can be done, including lipoinjection and/or Gore-Tex medialization (Figure 40-9). As necessary, a laryngofissure can be performed to sublux one thyroid lamina within the other to close anterior defects that result from resection of the anterior commissure tendon. The midline straight neocord provides a surface for the normal vocal fold to vibrate against during phonation. Normal conversational-level voicing is usually achieved if aerodynamic competence is reestablished.

OPEN GLOTTIC CANCER SURGERY

The first curative transcervical resection of glottic cancer was done by Solis-Cohen[3] in 1869. He performed

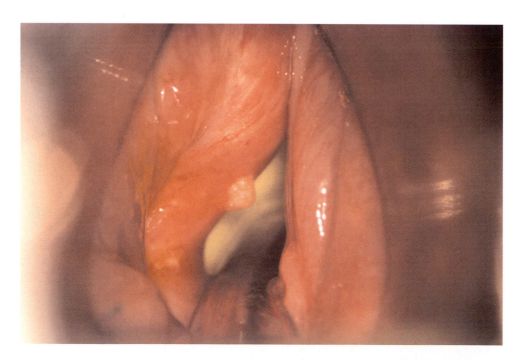

FIGURE 40-9. *(4X) The vocal fold has been augmented with fat. A small amount of the graft is extruding from the puncture site and should be removed with cold instruments to avoid a granuloma. Note the convexity of the vocal fold.*

a vertical partial laryngectomy having never seen the procedure. Shortly thereafter, Billroth[41] performed the first total laryngectomy for cancer. His patients, as well as those of others, typically died of aspiration because the reconstruction of the soft tissues had not been worked out. This procedure was perfected by Solis-Cohen[42,43] and Gluck as they effectively separated the airway from the digestive tract. In the 20th century, a variety of techniques for open laryngectomy were designed. While some details of these procedures are presented in this chapter, the reader is encouraged to seek primary resources for a more comprehensive discussion of this subject matter.[44,45]

Laryngofissure and Cordectomy

Transcervical cordectomy can be used for patients with T1 and selected T2 lesions of the true vocal fold who are not candidates for laser resection. Patients with larynges not well visualized on suspension laryngoscopy, those who have failed primary radiotherapy, those with lesions approaching the anterior commissure, and those with lesions extending onto the anterior vocal process are poor candidates for the endoscopic approach. The last two indications can now often be approached transorally because of improvements in endoscopic instrumentation (laryngoscopes, hand instruments, microspot lasers). In this procedure, one should plan on a temporary tracheotomy in most patients. Generally, these patients will have a delayed recovery secondary to the laryngofissure and, for many, tracheotomy as compared to an endoscopic resection.

Technique

After accomplishing adequate exposure of the larynx, the thyroid cartilage perichondrium is divided in the midline and the cartilage is similarly divided without entering the airway. Next, the cricothyroid membrane is entered from below and a straight cut is made through the anterior commissure taking care not to violate the cancer. If the procedure is being used for tumors of the middle third of the fold, this will still allow an adequate anterior margin and better preserve the anterior attachment of the contralateral cord. Next, cuts are made at the level of the subglottis and at the apex of the laryngeal ventricle. The deep extent of the resection can preserve or include the thyroid perichondrium. In lesions that are more anterior, it is advisable to take the perichondrium to provide a more substantial margin. The posterior aspect of the resection is dictated by the tumor extent. When performing an open cordectomy without a tracheotomy one can simply retract the endotracheal tube to the non-involved side of the larynx. Reconstruction of the cordectomy defect is best accom-

plished by mobilizing the false-fold mucosa and suturing over the cordectomy defect with absorbable (chromic gut or polyglycolic acid) suture. During closure, careful re-approximation of the anterior commissure will be an important component in optimizing voice. When the remaining vocal folds meet at different vertical levels, the voice is usually breathy and weak. This can result in vibration occurring between the normal vocal fold and the false fold of the operated side. Brasnu et al[46] reported their voice results of 151 patients with and without false-fold flap reconstruction. The incidence of moderate and severe voice alteration was significantly higher in the non-reconstructed group.[46] Without reconstruction, the patient typically has a persistent glottic gap during phonatory tasks. Although other methods of glottic reconstruction are available,[47] we feel that this technique is simple and results in consistently good voice.

Open Partial Vertical Laryngectomy

Using the same laryngofissure approach described for cordectomy, one can address selected T1 and T2 lesions of the glottic larynx. Routine partial vertical laryngectomy is contraindicated if there is fixation of the vocal fold (>T3 lesions), as this implies significant involvement of paraglottic musculature or the cricoarytenoid joint and/or escape through the cricothyroid membrane. Impaired mobility caused by tumor bulk or localized anterior paraglottic involvement is not a contraindication, but should be viewed with caution to be assured that the tumor is not more extensive than suspected; preoperative radiographic imaging can be very helpful in this regard. This procedure is contraindicated in tumors that invade thyroid cartilage, extend across the ventricle onto the false fold, or involve the interarytenoid mucosa.

Technique

With regard to thyroid cartilage resection, the classic procedure of removing all but a thin posterior strut of thyroid lamina cartilage is rarely necessary. In many cases, cartilage resection can be limited to removal of a rectangular block of cartilage anteriorly. Because the vocal fold is closer to the cartilage anteriorly, cartilage resection is more important in this location. If a patient has a tumor that comes close to the cartilage posteriorly, he/she could have deep paraglottic involvement and should not be a candidate for a routine partial vertical laryngectomy procedure. The soft tissue cuts made are also variable. The superior extent of the resection is usually above the false vocal fold and the inferior cut in the subglottis. For tumors that involve the infraglottic surface of the true vocal fold, one must be cautious of submucosal involvement down to the level of the cricoid cartilage along the conus elasticus. If this is suspected intraoperatively, a rim of cricoid cartilage should also be taken to maintain oncologic safety. The posterior extent of the resection is the variable that has the most significant impact on the person's functional outcome. In those patients who lose the entire arytenoid, the likelihood of aspiration is significantly higher. Often those who have a portion of the arytenoid removed do better. Even though the residual arytenoid may become fixed, the bulk provided to approximate the contralateral arytenoid helps complete the protective sphincteric action occurring during swallowing. With regard to voice after partial vertical laryngectomy procedures, the goal should be to provide adequate long-term bulk to approximate the contralateral normal true vocal fold. A number of reconstructive techniques have been described. Those that fill the void with healthy viable tissue are most successful and are discussed below. Leaving as much thyroid cartilage as is safely possible is also important in reconstruction, particularly with muscle flap techniques as the cartilage keeps the flap in a medial position.

After resection, the base of the epiglottis is pulled inferiorly and can be rotated and sewn to the subglottic margin of resection, which will cover the entire defect with healthy mucosalized tissue. The entire epiglottis need not be used; instead, the epiglottis can be divided at the midline and the ipsilateral half utilized. Other reconstructive techniques include the use of strap muscle flaps and pharyngeal mucosa. Closure of the laryngofissure is then performed. In patients who have had an arytenoid removed, recovery is more protracted and swallowing rehabilitation to avoid aspiration becomes a greater concern. The contralateral mobile arytenoid must extend further medially, and consequently the remaining normal half of the larynx will become hypertrophic in an effort to produce an adequate sphincter. When this happens, the likelihood of supraglottic voicing is increased. When vibration and phonation occur in supraglottic, rather than glottic tissues, increased roughness and a lower fundamental frequency result.

Open Frontolateral Hemilaryngectomy

Patients with lesions which cross the anterior commissure to involve 1/3 or less of the contralateral vocal fold are candidates for frontolateral procedures (T1b and T2b glottic lesions) (Figure 40-10). Vocal fold fixation or thyroid cartilage involvement are contraindications. Early disease seldomly invades the cartilage unless there is surface extension subglottically or to the infrapetiole region of the supraglottis.[29,30] This in turn makes a site where no clean plane exists between the anterior commissure and the thyroid cartilage. However, it is not usu-

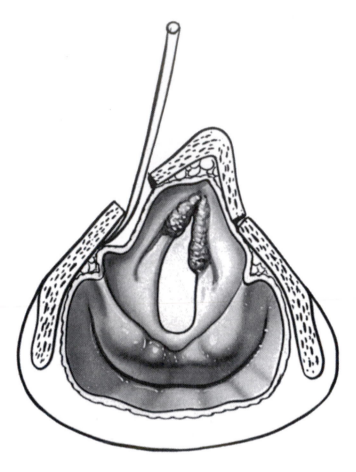

FIGURE 40-10. *Anterior frontal partial laryngectomy, a transverse section demonstrating subperichondrial elevation of the soft tissues off the thyroid lamina, in a tumor crossing the anterior commissure. From: Silver CE, Rubin JS.* Atlas of Head and Neck Surgery. *2nd ed. New York, NY: Churchill Livingstone; 1999:200. Reproduced with permission.*

ally necessary to take the thyroid cartilage more than one cm to either side of the midline. Although tumor may extend along the true fold posterior to this point, it will be far enough from the cartilage to allow an adequate margin without taking cartilage. The amount of remaining cartilage becomes important in reconstruction and in the avoidance of laryngeal foreshortening.

Exposure of the thyroid cartilage is the same as that in other open vertical procedures. The difficult portion of the resection is in making the first cut from the cricothyroid membrane up through the vocal fold on the less involved side of the larynx. In order to make the cut at the proper position, one can make a "marker" cut in the leading edge of the vocal fold at a point 5 mm behind the posterior aspect of the tumor at the beginning of the operation. This can be performed on direct laryngoscopy, creating the incision with a microscissors. This marker can then be visualized from below and followed from the subglottis up through the vocal fold. The contralateral cut will be made under direct visualization and is easy to make accurately. Reconstruction may be of two types: primary closure or flap closure. For resections where only a very small amount of vocal fold and anterior thyroid cartilage is removed, primary re-approximation of the vocal ligaments anteriorly and re-approximation of the thyroid cartilages to one another will produce a functional but slightly foreshortened larynx. Depending on the magnitude of cartilage resection, the thyroid lamina can be sutured together primarily (wire or Prolene) or a T-shaped keel can be used to stent open the larynx (Figure 40-11). This allows for decannulation and resumption of an oral diet. The T-shaped keel will prevent webbing at the new anterior commissure. These patients are discharged home after several days, and the keel is removed as a separate open outpatient procedure 6-8 weeks later.

In situations where a greater amount of the anterior larynx has been removed, primary closure is not possible. The goal becomes the creation of a neoglottic airway, which has adequate dimensions for respiration and preserves the sphincteric action of mobile arytenoids. Phonation occurs through approximation of the arytenoids with one another or remaining supraglottic soft tissue. This will produce a hoarse but serviceable voice without significant range of pitch.

Reconstruction in patients who have lost significant amounts of anterior soft tissue and cartilage is accomplished with a full epiglottic mobilization, bilateral strap muscle/perichondrial flaps, or both. These tissues are brought over an intralaryngeal stent, which is maintained for 6-8 weeks before endoscopic removal. The stent used must function as an adequate lumen-keeper without producing necrosis of the flap or non-operated laryngeal tissues. Molded silastic laryngeal stents work well.

SUPRAGLOTTIC CARCINOMA

In striking contrast to glottic cancer, nearly 70% of supraglottic cancer patients present with advanced stage disease (Stages III and IV). In fact, a palpable neck node is often the first sign of a supraglottic carcinoma. The supraglottic region is rich in lymphatics, in contrast to the lymphatic-poor glottis. This harks back to the embryology of the region where the supraglottis and glottis are derived from separate tissues. Because of the higher propensity to metastasize early, the nodal status of the neck is carefully evaluated in each patient.

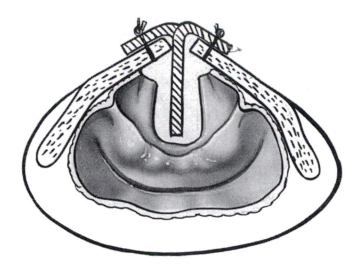

FIGURE 40-11. *Transverse section demonstrating relation of the keel to the laryngeal structures after placement. From: Silver CE, Rubin JS.* Atlas of Head and Neck Surgery. *2nd ed. New York, NY: Churchill Livingstone; 1999:202. Reproduced with permission.*

Selective neck dissection (bilateral) is included as part of the surgical therapy in either a diagnostic or therapeutic capacity.

Endoscopic Supraglottic Resection

Endolaryngeal laser cancer resections were first designed and done by Vaughan.[48] A number of other investigators have subsequently established the efficacy of this approach.[49-55] The supraglottic region is typically well-visualized with the use of the bivalved laryngoscope and the microscope. Supraglottic endoscopic surgery is performed with the use of the CO_2 laser. The decision to treat the neck should not be altered by the choice of endoscopic excision.

As with other endoscopic approaches, exposure is paramount. Lesions of the epiglottic tip (suprahyoid epiglottis) are easily managed by grasping the epiglottis with a forceps and using the CO_2 laser at 2 watts to amputate the tip with a 1 cm margin of normal tissue. Lesions involving the false vocal folds can be addressed by splitting the epiglottis vertically. The hyoid bone and thyroid cartilage are identified and the false vocal fold is dissected away from the inner aspect of the thyroid cartilage to the level of the ventricle. The pre-epiglottic space can be resected if needed via the endoscopic approach. The hemostatic effect of the CO_2 laser allows the surgeon to work in the richly vascular supraglottic region with adequate visualization of the involved tissues.

Open Horizontal Supraglottic Laryngectomy (Supraglottic Laryngectomy)

The horizontal partial laryngectomy (HPL) procedure was devised for T1 and T2 carcinomas involving the infrahyoid and suprahyoid epiglottis, ventricular folds, and aryepiglottic folds. Lesions staged as T3 because of pre-epiglottic space involvement are also adequately treated with a horizontal partial laryngectomy. Lesions within 5 mm of the anterior commissure, those with impairment or fixation of vocal fold motion, and those with thyroid cartilage involvement are excluded. As aspiration and pneumonia are the most common complications, patients must have good pulmonary reserve and the capacity, and will, to work with a speech-language pathologist postoperatively for swallowing rehabilitation, to be considered for the HPL.

Technique

A local tracheotomy is performed and after the induction of general anesthesia, bilateral selective neck dissection is carried out via an apron incision. After skeletonizing the hyoid bone, the infrahyoid muscles are detached. The neurovascular bundle of the involved side is ligated, while care is taken to preserve it on the uninvolved side. Perichondrial incisions are made along the superior border of the thyroid cartilage and the perichondrium is carefully elevated inferiorly to the midlevel of the thyroid cartilage. The cartilage cuts are now made using an oscillating saw. On the involved side the cut is made at the level of the middle of the thyroid cartilage, while on the uninvolved side, the cartilage cut sweeps upward toward the superior edge of the thyroid cartilage between the superior horn and thyroid notch (Figure 40-12).

The pharyngotomy can be performed either through the pyriform sinus of the uninvolved side or through the vallecula. The epiglottic involvement is inspected by grasping it with an Allis clamp and moving it around to inspect its laryngeal and lingual surfaces. Mucosal cuts are made under direct vision across the vallecula, along the aryepiglottic fold and into the laryngeal ventricle. Using a curved scissors, mucosal cuts are made from the ventricle on the uninvolved side along the cartilage cuts present. This allows greater access to the area of resection. The incision on the involved side is carried along the aryepiglottic fold and posterior part of the false vocal fold and into the ventricle. This is extended anteriorly to the thyroid cartilage allowing the removal of the supraglottic specimen (Figure 40-13). A cricopharyngeal myotomy is performed and a nasogastric tube is inserted prior to closure of the larynx.

While a mucosa-to-mucosa closure is not usually achievable, some tongue base mucosa is approximated with that of the pyriform sinus. The remainder of the closure is achieved by suturing the base of the tongue to the perichondrium of the thyroid cartilage (Figure 40-14). The sutures are first placed and then tied together. A suction drainage device is placed, the skin closed in two layers, and a cuffed tracheotomy tube is placed.

Supracricoid Laryngectomy With Cricohyoidopexy (CHP)

Patients with T1 or T2 lesions of the glottis who have good pulmonary function (similar to horizontal partial laryngectomy patients) are candidates for this type of laryngectomy. The supracricoid laryngectomy with CHP can address lesions that extend into the paraglottic space and pre-epiglottic space because the entire thyroid cartilage and paraglottic space is excised. As all glottic tissue from the arytenoid forward is removed, bilateral true-vocal fold involvement and anterior commissure involvement is not a contraindication. The thyrohyoid membrane is sutured to the cricoid cartilage for reconstruction (Figure 40-15). Postoperative aspiration is common, as in horizontal partial laryngectomy patients. Arytenoid mobility allows for some protective effects, as does the shelving effect of the base of tongue over the remaining larynx. As the cricoid and arytenoid cartilages are left intact, conditions that would allow cancer to spread onto the cricoid or arytenoids are contraindications to the supracricoid laryngectomy (arytenoid fixation, posterior commissure involvement, cricothyroid membrane involvement). With education and therapy, most patients are decannulated and are able to eat by mouth. Disease control rates are excellent and patients retain the ability to phonate in a "natural" way.

Near-Total Laryngectomy

The near-total laryngectomy is a procedure for lateral cancers of the larynx and pyriform sinus that cause limitation of vocal fold movement. It is also used for lateral supraglottic or aryepiglottic fold cancers with impairment or fixation of the true vocal fold or glottic extension. The larynx is removed except for a narrow posterolateral column of uninvolved subglottic, arytenoid, and pyriform tissue from the uninvolved side. A dynamic tracheopharyngeal myomucosal shunt is used for generating a voice using pulmonary air. This shunt is composed of a column of innervated soft tissues from the larynx and a small, local rotation flap from the ipsilateral pharynx (Figure 40-16). Primary subglottic cancers and postcricoid cancers as well as bilateral anterior transglottic tumors are contraindication to this procedure.

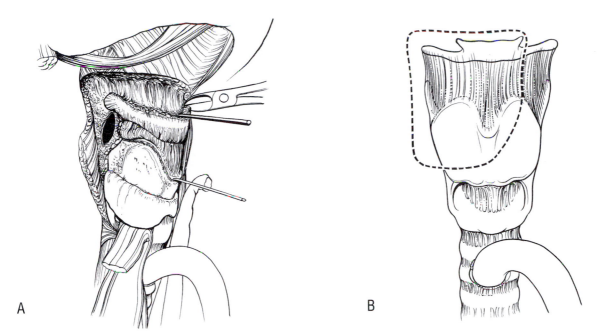

FIGURE 40-12. *Supraglottic subtotal laryngectomy. (A) The larynx has been skeletonized. The perichondrial flap is reflected, exposing the portion of thyroid cartilage to be resected. (B) The bone and cartilage cuts are shown. Resection will include the body and right greater cornu of the hyoid bone, the upper half of the right thyroid ala, and an oblique portion of the left thyroid ala. From: Silver CE, Rubin JS.* Atlas of Head and Neck Surgery. *2nd ed. New York, NY: Churchill Livingstone; 1999:210. Reproduced with permission.*

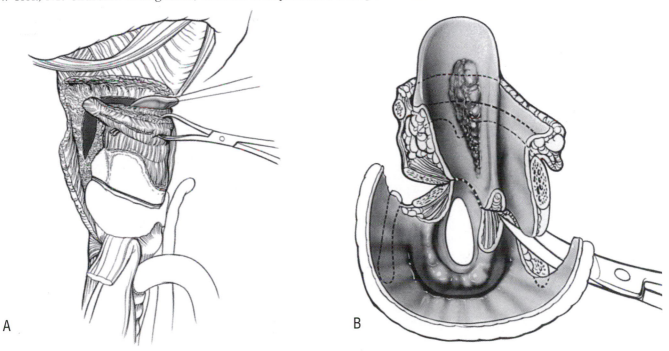

FIGURE 40-13. *(A) The hypopharynx is entered through the pyriform sinus and the incision is extended through the valleculae. Careful inspection is required. The epiglottis is delivered through the mucosal incision. (B) The incision has been carried through the posterior part of the false vocal fold into the ventricle and continued anteriorly through the ventricle to the anterior midline. As wide a margin of normal mucosa as possible is maintained, although inferiorly this may be no more than a few millimeters. From: Silver CE, Rubin JS.* Atlas of Head and Neck Surgery. *2nd ed. New York, NY: Churchill Livingstone; 1999:210,211. Reproduced with permission.*

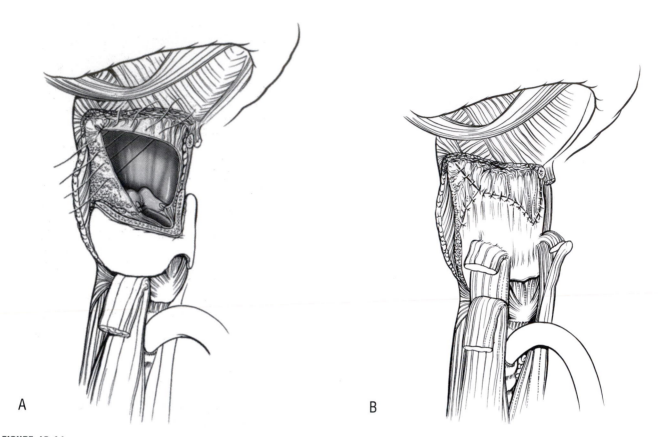

A

B

FIGURE 40-14. *(A) The mucosal defect is seen from the external aspect. Starting posteriorly, the hypopharyngeal mucosa is sutured directly as far as approximation without tension will allow. (B) The remaining defect is closed by suturing the perichondrial flap to the base of the tongue. Resultant nonmucosal surfaces will reepithelialize spontaneously. From: Silver CE, Rubin JS.* Atlas of Head and Neck Surgery. *2nd ed. New York, NY: Churchill Livingstone; 1999:213,214. Reproduced with permission.*

Total Laryngectomy

In this age of conservation surgery for laryngeal cancer, there continues to be a role for the wide-field total laryngectomy. Locally advanced carcinomas with thyroid cartilage invasion and extension into the surrounding neck, bilateral bulky transglottic lesions, and recurrent carcinomas unsuitable for partial procedures make up the majority of indications for this procedure. An advantage of the exposure that is afforded by the total laryngectomy is the ability to easily include any adjacent structure that is involved with the cancer.

Technique

A horizontal cervical incision is created, which courses over the thyrohyoid membrane from the anterior border of the trapezius muscles. The tracheostoma is outlined at the start of the case for development later. The suprahyoid muscles are detached from the hyoid. The

neurovascular pedicle is identified as it pierces the thyrohyoid membrane and ligated. The infrahyoid muscles are detached low in the neck and the larynx is elevated. The thyroid gland isthmus is ligated to allow access to the trachea for creation of the tracheostoma. The outlined skin is removed and the trachea is cut obliquely leaving a longer posterior wall. This is then sutured to the skin at the site of the proposed tracheostoma and the endotracheal tube transferred to the stoma (Figure 40-17).

The larynx is retracted cephalad and the plane between the larynx and esophageal mucosa is developed. After all external attachments to the larynx are severed (constrictors), the pharynx is entered and the mucosal incision is continued along the edge of the larynx, allowing for clear margins around the tumor. Care is taken not to resect more mucosa than is necessary as this will have an impact on the closure, which should be tension-free (Figure 40-18). The pharynx is closed using interrupted 2-0 chromic sutures from the mucosa of the

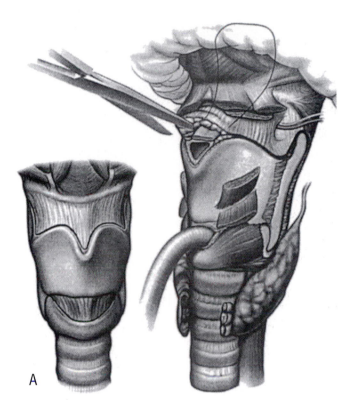

A

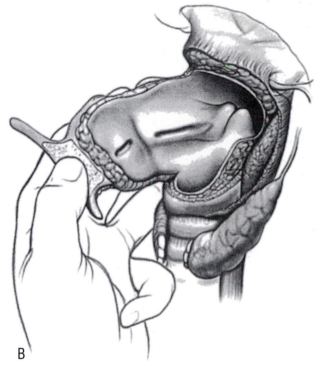

B

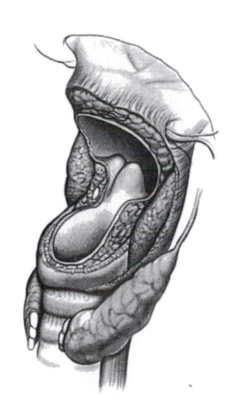

C

FIGURE 40-15. *Supracricoid laryngectomy. (A) The inferior constrictors have already been incised along the posterior border of the thyroid cartilage and the pyriform sinus dissected from the internal aspect of the thyroid alae. The cricothyroid joint has been separated, being aware of the location of the recurrent laryngeal nerve. The larynx has been entered through the cricothyroid membrane and the incision extended posterolaterally. An incision has been made through the thyrohyoid membrane and the epiglottis sharply transected at the petiole, thereby allowing the larynx to be entered into. The incision is now extended posteriorly on either side. It follows the contour of the thyroid cartilage and will transect the aryepiglottic fold. (B) The glottic structures are retracted posteriorly and the tumor visualized and assessed. A vertical incision is made through the aryepiglottic fold, anterior to the arytenoid on the contralateral side and carried forward. The surgeon now fractures the larynx along its midline, opening it "like a book" and now allowing for complete removal of the tumor under direct visualization. (C) Remaining structures after resection include both arytenoids, cricoid, epiglottis above the petiole (in this case), and both pyriform sinuses. From: Silver CE, Rubin JS. Atlas of Head and Neck Surgery. 2nd ed. New York, NY: Churchill Livingstone; 1999:218-220. Reproduced with permission.*

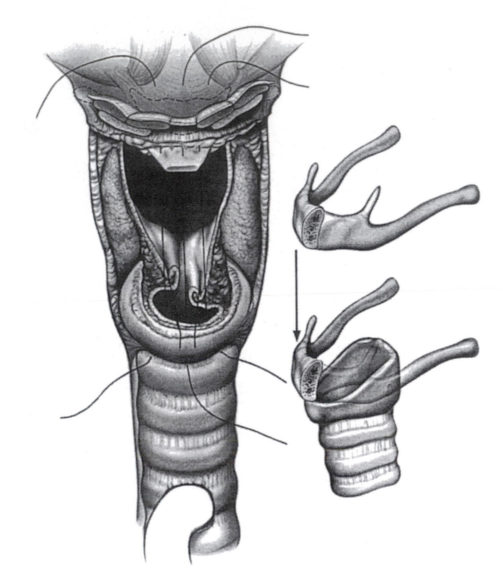

D

FIGURE 40-15. *(D) Reconstruction commences, with the hyoid bone and anterior cricoid brought together. From: Silver CE, Rubin JS.* Atlas of Head and Neck Surgery. *2nd ed. New York, NY: Churchill Livingstone; 1999:218-220. Reproduced with permission.*

tongue base and the hypopharyngeal mucosa. At least one more layer is usually closed above this first closure. Suction drains are placed and the skin is closed.

SUMMARY

Surgery for laryngeal cancer has now been an ongoing process for well over a century. Technical advances in reconstruction and improved understanding of laryngeal anatomy and physiology have led to laryngeal framework procedures with improved functional outcomes over the past 30 years. During the last decade, there have been further advances. As in many surgical paradigms, these advances have centered around the evolution of techniques for minimally invasive resection and phonosurgical reconstruction. The modern oncologic surgeon needs to be firmly based in physiology and anatomy of the larynx, and to have, at his or her command, the flexibility to approach laryngeal tumors on a case by case basis. In each instance, the physiologic outcome must be considered. Effective management dictates oncologically sound margins with minimal loss of non-involved tissues, and reconstruction that optimizes postoperative airway, voice, and deglutition.

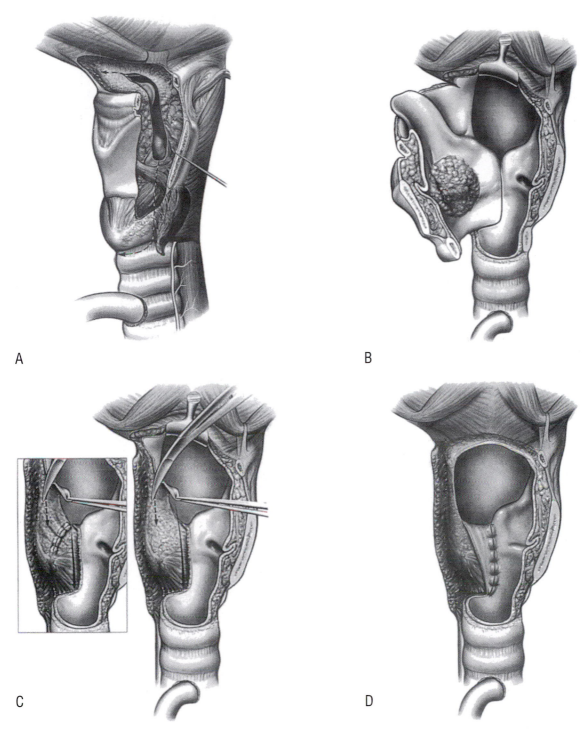

A

B

C

D

FIGURE 40-16. *Near-total laryngectomy. (A) Removal of a vertical portion of mid-lateral thyroid ala has exposed the soft tissues overlying the ventricle, through which the larynx is entered, at the level of the ventricle, the incision then being carried up into the vallecula. The larynx is inspected. (B) The incision is carried down through the cricoid, around under the cricoid, and then vertically up between the arytenoids, posteriorly. The cricoid is fractured posteriorly in midline and deeper structures incised, care being taken to preserve the underlying hypopharyngeal mucosa. (C) The specimen is then removed and the reconstructive phase begun. This consists of creating a phonatory shunt from myomucosal tissues, augmented by a rotation flap of pyriform sinus mucosa. (D) The flap is sewn to itself. (Continues)*

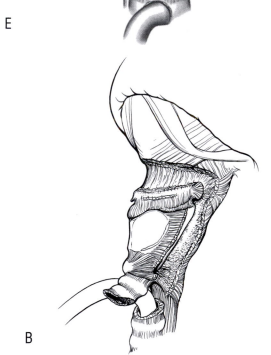

FIGURE 40-16. *(E) The myomucosal segment is now tubed, using a small catheter as a template. From Silver CE, Rubin JS.* Atlas of Head and Neck Surgery. *2nd ed. New York, NY: Churchill Livingstone; 1999:241-245. Reproduced with permission. (Continued)*

E

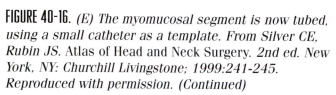

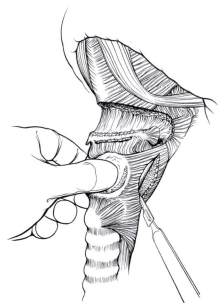

A

B

FIGURE 40-17. *Total laryngectomy. (A) The strap muscles have already been transected low in the neck, and the ipsilateral thyroid lobe mobilized to be included in the specimen. Paratracheal tissues have been mobilized and the surface of the trachea dissected free along the proposed line of resection. The mobilization has proceeded superiorly, the superior thyroid artery ligated, and the suprahyoid musculature freed along the body and greater cornu of the hyoid bone. On the contralateral side the thyroid gland is preserved, and separated from the trachea. The superior thyroid artery is ligated on this side as well and the inferior constrictor fibers sharply freed off the posterior thyroid lamina. (B) The larynx is now completely mobilized, the trachea transected and a cuffed endotracheal tube inserted. The trachea should be divided at least 2 cm below the tumor, and beveled upwards, posteriorly, to increase the size of the tracheostoma. From: Silver CE, Rubin JS.* Atlas of Head and Neck Surgery. *2nd ed. New York, NY: Churchill Livingstone; 1999:228,230. Reproduced with permission.*

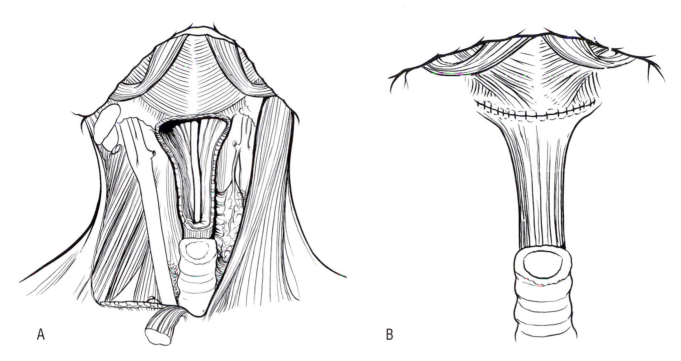

A   B

FIGURE 40-18. *Total laryngectomy continued. (A) The larynx has now been entered away from the tumor, in this instance in the pyriform sinus, and the incision carried up into the vallecula, allowing for better visualization of the tumor. The ipsilateral pyriform will be resected widely around the tumor. The resection has been completed. Before closure, it is prudent to obtain frozen sections. A nasogastric tube is inserted and secured to the nasal columella. (B) Reconstruction commences. Closure is frequently performed with interrupted sutures with the knots tied on the inside. Generally a transverse closure, without tension, can be attained; occasionally a "t" shape closure is required. The closure is reinforced by approximating the cut edges of the inferior constrictor muscles. From: Silver CE, Rubin JS, Atlas of Head and Neck Surgery. 2nd ed. New York, NY: Churchill Livingstone; 1999:231,232. Reproduced with permission.*

REFERENCES

1. Batsakis JG. *Tumors of the Head and Neck Clinical and Pathological Considerations.* 2nd ed. Baltimore, MD: Williams & Wilkins; 1984.

2. Lindberg R. Distribution of cervical lymph node metastases from squamous cell carcinoma of the upper respiratory and digestive tracts. *Cancer.* 1972;29:1446-1449.

3. Solis-Cohen J. Clinical history of surgical affections of the larynx. *The Medical Record.* 1869;4:244-247.

4. Fraenkel B. First healing of a laryngeal cancer taken out through the natural passages. *Archiv fur Klinische Chirurgie.* 1886;12:283-286.

5. Lynch RC. Intrinsic carcinoma of the larynx, with a second report of the cases operated on by suspension and dissection. *Trans Am Laryngol Assoc.* 1920;40:119-126.

6. LeJeune FE. Intralaryngeal operation for cancer of the vocal cord. *Ann Otol Rhinol Laryngol.* 1946;55:531-536.

7. Lillie JC, DeSanto LW. Transoral surgery of early cordal carcinoma. *Trans Am Acad Ophthalmol Otolaryngol.* 1973;77:92-96.

8. Vaughan CW, Strong MS, Jako GJ. Laryngeal carcinoma: transoral treatment using the CO_2 laser. *Am J Surg.* 1978. 136:490-493.

9. Blakeslee D, Vaughan CW, Shapshay SM, Simpson GT, Strong SM. Excisional biopsy in the selective management of T1 glottic cancer: a three year follow-up study. *Laryngoscope.* 1984;94:488-494.

10. Zeitels SM. Phonomicrosurgical treatment of early glottic cancer and carcinoma in situ. *Am J Surg.* 1996;172:704-709.

11. Kanonier G, Rainer T, Fritsch E. Radiotherapy in early glottic carcinoma. *Ann Otol Rhinol Laryngol.* 1996;105:759-763.

12. Cragle SP, Brandenburg JH. Laser cordectomy or radiotherapy: Cure rates, communication, and cost. *Otolaryngol Head Neck Surg.* 1993;108:648-653.

13. Lehman JJ, Bless DM, Brandenburg JH. An objective assessment of voice production after radiation therapy for stage I squamous cell carcinoma of the glottis. *Otolaryngol Head Neck Surg.* 1988;98:121-129.

14. DeSanto LW, ed. Selection of treatment for in situ and early invasive carcinoma of the glottis. In: Alberti PW, Bryce DB, eds. *Workshops from the Centennial Conference on Laryngeal Cancer.* New York, NY: Appleton-Century-Crofts; 1976:146-150.

15. Mendenhall W, Parsons JT, Stringer SP, Cassissi NJ. Management of Tis, T1, T2 squamous cell carcinoma of the glottic larynx. *Am J Otolaryngol.* 1994;15:250-257.

16. Wolf GT, Hong WK, Fisher HG, et al. Induction chemotherapy plus radiation compared with surgery plus radiation in patients with advanced laryngeal cancer. *N Engl J Med.* 1991;324:1685-1690.

17. Zeitels SM. Microflap excisional biopsy for atypia and microinvasive glottic cancer. *Oper Tech Otolaryngol Head Neck Surg (Phonosurgery Part I).* 1993;4:218-222.

18. Zeitels SM, ed. Transoral treatment of early glottic cancer. *Laryngeal Cancer: Proceedings of the 2nd World Congress on Laryngeal Cancer.* Smee R, Bridger P, eds. Amsterdam: Elsevier; 1994:373-383.

19. Zeitels SM. Premalignant epithelium and microinvasive cancer of the vocal fold: the evolution of phonomicrosurgical management. *Laryngoscope.* 1995;67(suppl):1-51.

20. Zeitels SM. *Atlas of Phonomicrosurgery and Other Endolaryngeal Procedures for Benign and Malignant Disease.* Delmar: Clifton Park, NY. In press.

21. Hartig G, Zeitels SM. Optimizing voice in conservation surgery for glottic cancer. *Oper Tech Otolaryngol Head Neck Surg. (Phonosurgery Part 1).* 1998;9:214-223.

22. Zeitels SM, Jarboe J, Hillman RE. *Phonosurgical Reconstruction of Glottic Cancer Defects.* Presented at the Voice Symposium; 2000.

23. Myers EN, Wagner RL, Johnson JT. Microlaryngoscopic surgery for T1 glottic lesion: a cost-effective option. *Ann Otol Rhinol Laryngol.* 1994;103:28-30.

24. Zeitels SM. A universal modular glottiscope system: the evolution of a century of design and technique for direct laryngoscopy. *Ann Otol Rhinol Laryngol.* 1999;108(suppl 179):1-24.

25. Zeitels SM. inventor *Universal Modular Laryngoscope/Glottiscope System.* US patent 5 893 830.1999.

26. Zeitels SM, Vaughan CW. A submucosal vocal fold infusion needle. *Otolaryngol Head Neck Surg.* 1991;105:478-479.

27. Zeitels SM. Infrapetiole exploration of the supraglottis for exposure of the anterior glottal commissure. *J Voice.* 1998;12:117-122.

28. Desloge RB, Zeitels SM. Microsurgery at the anterior glottal commissure: controversies and observations. *Ann Otol Rhinol Laryngol.* 2000;109:385-392.

29. Kirchner JA, Carter D. Intralaryngeal barriers to the spread of cancer. *Acta Otolaryngol (Stockh).* 1987;103:503-513.

30. Kirchner JA. What have whole organ sections contributed to the treatment of laryngeal cancer? *Ann Otol Rhinol Laryngol.* 1989;98:661-667.

31. Wolfensberger M, Dort JC. Endoscopic laser surgery for early glottic carcinoma: a clinical and experimental study. *Laryngoscope.* 1990;100:1100-1105.

32. Davis K, Jako GJ, Hyams VJ, Shapshay SM. The anatomic limitations of CO_2 laser cordectomy. *Laryngoscope.* 1982;92:980-984.

33. Koufman JA. The endoscopic management of early squamous carcinoma of the vocal cord with the carbon dioxide surgical laser: clinical experience and a proposed subclassification. *Otolaryngol Head Neck Surg.* 1986;95:531-537.

34. Wetmore SJ, Key M, Suen JY. Laser therapy for T1 glottic carcinoma of the larynx. *Arch Otolaryngol Head Neck Surg.* 1986;112:853-855.

35. Krespi Y, Meltzer CJ. Laser surgery for vocal cord carcinoma involving the anterior commissure. *Ann Otol Rhinol Laryngol.* 1989;98:105-109.

36. Casiano R, Cooper JD, Lundy DS, Chandler JR. Laser cordectomy for T1 glottic carcinoma: a 10-year experience and videostroboscopic findings. *Otolaryngol Head Neck Surg.* 1991;104:831-837.

37. Benninger M, Gillen J, Thieme P, Jacobson B, Dragovich J. Factors associated with recurrence and voice quality following radiation therapy for T1 and T2 glottic carcinomas. *Laryngoscope.* 1994;104:294-298.

38. Steiner W. Results of curative laser microsurgery of laryngeal carcinomas. *Am J Otolaryngol.* 1993;14:116-121.

39. Eckel H, Thumfart WF. Laser surgery for the treatment of larynx carcinomas: indications, techniques, and preliminary results. *Ann Otol Rhinol Laryngol.* 1992;101:113-118.

40. Rudert HH, ed. Transoral CO_2-laser surgery of early glottic cancer (CIS-T2). In: Smee R, Bridger P, eds. *Laryngeal Cancer: Proceedings of the 2nd World Congress on Laryngeal Cancer.* Amsterdam: Elsevier; 1994:389-392.

41. Gussenbauer C. Ueber die erste durch Th. Billroth am Menschen, Ausgerfuhrte Kehlkopf Exstirpation und die Anwendungeines kunstlichen Kehlkopfes. *Archiv fur Klinische Chirurgie.* 1874;17:343-356.

42. Solis-Cohen J. Two cases of laryngectomy for adeno-carcinoma of the larynx. *Trans Am Laryngol Assoc.* 1892;14:60-67.

43. Solis-Cohen J. Pharyngeal voice: illustrated by presentation of a patient who phonates without a larynx and without the use of the lungs. *Trans Am Laryngol Assoc.* 1893;15:114-116.

44. Silver CE. *Conservation Surgery for Glottic Carcinoma. Surgery for Cancer of the Larynx.* New York, NY: Churchill Livingstone; 1981;83-121.

45. Weinstein G, Laccourreye O. Vertical partial laryngectomies. In: Weinstein G, Laccourreye O, Brasnu D, Laccourreye H, eds. *Organ Preservation Surgery for Laryngeal Cancer.* San Diego, CA: Singular; 2000;59-71.

46. Brasnu D, Laccourreye O, Weinstein G, Fligny I, Chabardes E. False vocal cord reconstruction of the glottis following vertical partial laryngectomy: a preliminary analysis. *Laryngoscope.* 1992;102:717-719.

47. Milutinovic Z. Composite myo-mucosal reconstruction of the vocal fold. *Eur Arch Oto-Rhino-Laryngol.* 1995;252:119-122.

48. Vaughan CW. Transoral laryngeal surgery using the CO_2 laser. Laboratory experiments and clinical experience. *Laryngoscope.* 1978;88:1399-1420.

49. Davis RK, Shapshay SM, Strong SM, Hyams V. Transoral partial supraglottic resection using the CO_2 laser. *Laryngoscope.* 1983;93:429-432.

50. Steiner W, ed. Transoral microsurgical CO_2 laser resection of laryngeal carcinoma. *Functional Partial Laryngectomy.* Berlin: Springer-Verlag; 1984;121-125.

51. Steiner W. Experience in endoscopic laser surgery of malignant tumours of the upper aerodigestive tract. *Adv Otorhinolaryngol.* 1988;39:135-144.

52. Zeitels SM, Vaughan CW, Domanowski GF, Fuleihan NF, Simpson GT. Laser epiglottectomy: endoscopic technique and indications. *Otolaryngol Head Neck Surg.* 1990;103:337-343.

53. Zeitels SM, Vaughan CW, Domanowski GF. Endoscopic management of early supraglottic cancer. *Ann Otol Rhinol Laryngol.* 1990;99:951-956.

54. Davis RK, Kelley SM, Hayes J. Endoscopic CO_2 laser excisional biopsy of early supraglottic cancer. *Laryngoscope.* 1991;100:680-683.

55. Zeitels SM, Davis RK, eds. Cancer of the supraglottis: endoscopic laser management. In: Smee R, Bridger P, eds. *Laryngeal Cancer: Proceedings of the 2nd World Congress on Laryngeal Cancer.* Amsterdam: Elsevier; 1994;444-456.

CHAPTER 41

Diagnosis and Management of Postoperative Dysphonia

Peak Woo, MD

Persistent dysphonia and recurrent dysphonia after endoscopic laryngeal surgery are clinical problems that have confronted all laryngologists. An unsatisfactory postoperative voice, as perceived by the patient, can be a particularly vexing problem. On the one hand, the patient's expectation of an improved and long-lasting postoperative voice may not have been met. On the other hand, the surgeon is faced with a new set of diagnostic and therapeutic dilemmas imposed by surgical trauma superimposed on existing impairments caused by the initial lesion.

The literature on this topic is sparse. As the problem of voice impairment is traditionally largely one of patient perception, residual dysphonia may be neglected by the clinician if no obvious masses are present. If the patient failed to improve in function, rehabilitation by referral to a speech-language pathologist is commonly the only recommendation. The impetus to "find" a better voice is a result of patient dissatisfaction; to satisfy the patient's request for a better voice. The laryngologist has several therapeutic options, which include further surgery,[1,2] evaluation and treatment by speech-language pathologists,[3-5] and patient counseling with therapeutic assurance. Brodnitz, in his large series of patients undergoing speech therapy for a variety of organic and functional disorders,[3] mentions several situations in which speech therapy resulted in a successful return of the voice following surgical treatment of laryngeal webs. He also cited the poor results with speech therapy in several patients with intubation-related injury to the larynx.

Spectrographic analysis and vocal measurements after surgical treatment show a variety of residual postoperative dysphonias ranging from mild to severe.[5] Baker et al[4] studied a small series of patients with persistent dysphonia after vocal fold surgery and correlated persistent dysphonias with other medical illnesses such as allergies, sinus infections, and chronic respiratory tract infections. Renowned endolaryngeal surgeons have noted variable voice results after microlaryngeal surgery for benign disease.[6-8] From their writings, one gathers that voice results may be variable depending on the size and type of lesion involved. More recently, vocal measurements after laser cordectomy, partial laryngectomy, and microlaryngeal surgery have provided evidence of residual disabilities in voice varying between slight dysphonia and aphonia.[9-12]

The optimal treatment of patients with postoperative dysphonia is not established; clearly, there is no consistently effective and corrective surgical treatment. Ford and Bless reported use of collagen for a variety of vocal fold defects.[1] Other autologous implants and thyroplastic phonosurgical treatments are being investigated, including autologous fat implanted in the vibratory margin of the vocal fold.[13]

At the Voice Clinic at SUNY Health Science Center at Syracuse, a multidisciplinary approach to the persistently dysphonic postsurgical patient gave us a perspective not easily obtained by one physician. By combining the referral base from otolaryngology, speech-language pathology, and speech and voice science, the medical, surgical, and speech rehabilitation needs of the persistently dysphonic patient can be better appreciated. Increasingly, patients who are persistently dysphonic after prior endolaryngeal microsurgery are being referred or are referring themselves for evaluation. This makes one suspect that the true incidence and scope of persistent dysphonia after laryngeal surgery are significant.

This chapter will (1) highlight etiologic factors that contribute to persistent postoperative dysphonia, (2) discuss the differential diagnostic evaluations of patients with persistent dysphonia—as an accurate diagnosis is critical to the selection of patients who may benefit from medical, surgical, or speech therapy, the diagnostic aspects of the workup will be emphasized—and (3) discuss medical, surgical, and speech therapy options for patients with postsurgical dysphonia.

DIAGNOSIS OF POSTSURGICAL DYSPHONIA

It is often not clear which component of persistent postoperative dysphonia is caused by which lesion: intrinsic disease, residual disease, or hyperfunctional voice disorder. Postoperative dysphonia is not one entity. It occurs in patients with recurrent contact granulomas shortly after removal, poor voice results after PTFE (Teflon) injection, poor voice results after vocal fold stripping for benign and neoplastic lesions, and poor voice results after endomicrolaryngeal surgery. One should also include those patients with poor voice after hemilaryngectomy, subtotal laryngectomy, laryngeal fracture, and prolonged intubation; however, such inclusion would make this discussion overly expansive. Thus, although many of the diagnostic and therapeutic treatments may be applicable to these "more severe" problems, this discussion will be limited to patients with persistent dysphonia after endolaryngeal surgery. These surgical procedures include (1) microlaryngeal surgery with and without CO_2 laser for benign vocal fold lesions (polyps, webs, microangiomas, papillomas, cysts, nodules), (2) microlaryngeal surgery with and without CO_2 laser for dysplastic, hyperplastic, or neoplastic disorders of the vocal fold cover (eg, carcinoma in situ (CIS), sulcus vocalis, hyperplastic laryngitis, hyperkeratosis of the vocal folds), (3) endoscopic treatment of vocal fold paralysis (PTFE injection, PTFE granuloma), (4) endoscopic treatment of contact granuloma, and (5) diagnostic endoscopy and biopsy.

SCOPE OF PROBLEM

In a review of 1,380 stroboscopies performed in our clinic from 1987 to 1992, 62 patients sought consultation for improved vocal function after endolaryngoscopic surgery. The numbers would be larger if patients with dysphonia after surgical intubation and dysphonia after open laryngeal surgery were included. Prior surgical treatment included microlaryngoscopy with surgical excision (N = 44), direct laryngoscopy and excision (N = 13), and PTFE injection (N = 5). Women outnumbered men by a 2:1 margin. This may be related to sociocultural aspects of voice perception in women compared with those in men.

These patients present difficult management problems. The average number of otolaryngologists visited by these patients was 2.4. The actual number of visits to their otolaryngologists was far higher. Many had had their complaints dismissed or trivialized or were told the cause of their dysphonia was psychogenic or functional. Diagnostic examination carried out to reach these conclusions had consisted of mirror examination or flexible laryngoscope examination. Many patients had tried multiple courses of empirical therapy that included watchful waiting, antibiotic therapy, speech therapy, or a combination of these. The mean duration between the initial surgery and consultation with us was 3.4 months, with a range of 1 month to 18 years.

CLINICAL PRESENTATION

One common situation at the voice clinic is the referral of a postsurgically dysphonic patient for speech therapy to reverse functional ventricular dysphonia. Figure 41-1 shows an example of ventricular phonation viewed by endoscopy.

In view of the clinical presentation, it is not surprising how many patients with persistent dysphonia are told by well-meaning physicians to seek psychological or speech therapy help. When viewed by indirect mirror or flexible laryngoscopy, the vocal folds often appear straight and free of organic disease. Yet when the patient is asked to phonate, the larynx takes on a tight, squeezed appearance. The ventricles adduct, the arytenoids may roll forward, and a raspy rough sound quality is produced (Figure 41-1). This has the appearance of ventricular dysphonia or dysphonia plica ventricularis (DPV). Ventricular dysphonia in the absence of vocal fold abnormality is often thought to have a functional or psychogenic cause, thus the reason for referral to speech therapy. What is not clear from observations using direct light is the vibratory function of the vocal folds. Vocal fold

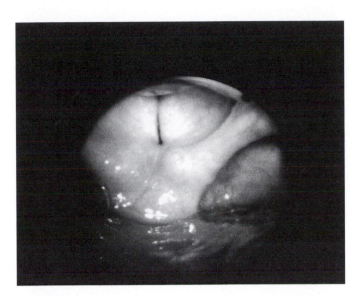

FIGURE 41-1. *Ventricular phonation after prior laryngeal surgical intervention. The patient was referred for reversal of ventricular hyperfunction. The undiagnosed problem of poor vibratory fold function is the most common cause of this finding.*

vibratory function is a dynamic process that cannot be evaluated adequately by mirror examination. The presentation of persistent dysphonia after microlaryngeal surgery is one indication for stroboscopic examination of vocal fold vibratory function as it is now known that DPV is often a compensatory effort (rather than psychogenic) to overcome vocal fold pathology.

A second pattern of failure occurs in the patient who undergoes microlaryngeal surgery with good initial restoration of vocal function. This good voice, unfortunately, lasts for only a brief period and is followed by progressive deterioration of function or renewal of symptoms.

A third pattern of failure occurs in the patient noted to have some improvement of vocal function, but the degree of improvement does not meet the patient's expectations. This prompts revisits to the physician or self-referral for a second opinion.

DIFFERENTIAL DIAGNOSIS OF POSTOPERATIVE DYSPHONIA

The history and examination of clinical voice disorders have been covered in Chapter 11. In addition to a careful history, it is important for the laryngologist to review the clinical voice history after surgical treatment. With a good history, the clinician should be able to distinguish persistent dysphonia after surgery from recurrent dysphonia after surgery. The degree of clinical improvement and/or lack of improvement after surgery should be documented by specific examples. This helps the clinician to (1) gauge the extent of patient expectations, (2) assess the efficacy of the previous laryngeal surgery, and (3) direct the search for contributing causes of dysphonia. If the patient had a good voice after surgery followed by voice deterioration, one suspects a recurrent lesion (ie, recurrent vocal fold nodules, contact granuloma). If the patient always had a poor voice after surgery, the cause may be the results of healing (hypertrophic scarring) or the surgery (adynamic segment). If the voice remained the same or improved marginally, comorbid causes such as chronic laryngitis, reflux laryngitis, habitual hyperfunctional voice disorder, and residual disease should be considered. Table 41-1 lists the varieties of clinical failure and their possible causes. This should be considered only a partial list of likely causes, as a new unrelated vocal fold lesion could present with a similar history and symptomatology.

The severity of the patient's complaints may not be well-correlated with the examiner's perception of the

1. Residual disease
   (ie, papilloma on the undersurface of the vocal fold, contralateral cyst or scar)

2. Unrecognized comorbidity
   Scar and prior vocal fold injury
   Inflammatory laryngitis

3. Recurrent disease
   Recurrent vocal nodules
   Recurrent polypoid degeneration
   Recurrent contact granuloma

4. Poor surgical result
   Hypertrophic scar
   Nonvibrating segment
   Overinjection of the vocal fold with PTFE (Teflon)
   PTFE granuloma

5. Surgical scar caused by repeated surgery or injury
   Repeated papilloma surgery
   Postradiation scarring
   Scarring after repeated vocal fold stripping

6. Patient expectations not met

7. Functional and hyperfunctional dysphonia

TABLE 41-1. *Possible Causes of Poor Voice After Surgery*

severity of dysphonia. Some patients with severe to moderate dysphonia after surgery only want to be reassured that recurrent lesion or neoplasm is absent. Others have dysfunctional voices that interfere with activities of daily living. Still others have subtle dysphonia that affects only a small range of their phonation, and the patients seek help because of professional voice needs. True psychogenic dysphonia caused by conversion reaction and functional dysphonia for purposes of secondary gain are rare.

Without adequate preoperative documentation of the severity of dysphonia, the preoperative state cannot be appreciated. In almost all patients with postoperative complaints, vocal characteristics that can be readily identified by the examiner as a "hoarse" voice are generally present. The voice qualities are usually rough, husky, strident, or combinations thereof. Further questioning usually reveals a voice that is decreased in loudness and pitch range. The onset of phonation may require more effort. The duration of voicing per breath may be reduced. Speaking or singing effort is often increased. In some, a loss of clarity, brilliance, and timbre after surgery is the main complaint. For the experienced clinician, these are typical vocal characteristics of scarred vocal folds, of immobile vocal folds caused by inflammation, or of residual mass lesions. these vocal qualities should spur the clinician to examine the vibratory capabilities of vocal folds and reach a clearer diagnosis.

PHYSICAL EXAMINATION

Examination of the larynx should include videolaryngostroboscopy. Stroboscopy offers the clinician the most practical way to observe vibratory function of the vocal folds. Without direct observation of vibratory function, much of laryngoscopic diagnosis is guesswork. With direct observation, the interpretation of the pathophysiology of dysphonia can be made much clearer. For example, one common diagnosis made by referring physicians is hyperfunctional voice disorder with ventricular adduction. When laryngostroboscopy examination is carried out, a nonvibratory segment or diffuse edema with poor mucosal amplitude or mass differences between the vocal folds is often detected. When these factors are corrected medically or surgically, the ventricular hyperadduction often clears spontaneously. Thus, one can conclude that ventricular hyperadduction is very often a compensatory gesture of the larynx to attempt phonation at higher pressures. In our series of 62 postoperative dysphonic patients seen in the clinic, 33 were found on flexible laryngoscope to exhibit features of ventricular adduction. When stroboscopic examination was used to further examine vocal fold vibratory function in these 33 patients, 26 had poor vibration of the true vocal folds (TVFs). This suggests that ventricular adduction is a compensatory gesture in these patients. In this series, only 7 of 33 patients had the diagnosis of hyperfunctional voice disorder without vibratory anomaly.

Stroboscopy helps the clinician to distinguish between the various differential diagnoses. For the patients with persistent dysphonia, the differential diagnosis groupings can be separated into (1) scar and localized stiffness, (2) a residual mass lesion, (3) diffuse inflammation with bilaterally poor vibratory function, (4) lesion recurrence, and (5) hyperfunctional voice disorder. Table 41-2 lists the relative incidence in our series of 62 patients.

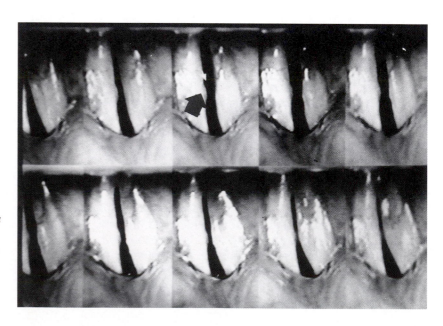

FIGURE 41-2. *A series of stroboscopic images of a nonvibrating vocal fold after microsurgery. The vocal fold that vibrates is the one with the translucent jelly layer. The nonvibrating vocal fold is whiter and stiffer and has a residual nodule (arrow).*

Diagnosis	No. of Patients
Scar and stiffness	27
Diffuse inflammation	13
Residual mass	8
Hyperfunction	7
Recurrent lesion	4
Unclear	3
Total	62

TABLE 41-2. *Stroboscopic Diagnosis of 62 Patients With Persistent Postoperative Dysphonia*

Scar and Stiffness

Localized scar with stiffness is the most common cause of persistent dysphonia after surgery (Table 41-2). This can be differentiated easily from the other causes as a diminution of mucosal amplitude and mucosal wave on stroboscopy. The site of involvement may be localized to a small area over the vocal fold or it may involve the entire fold. Grossly, the affected vocal fold is usually whiter or pinker than the uninvolved vocal fold. When viewed by magnifying laryngoscope, the translucent, clear Reinke's layer is often absent. Figure 41-2 shows some typical stroboscopic findings, including one vocal fold with a translucent layer that vibrates. The contralateral fold is white and stiff (arrow). If these patients were re-examined under anesthesia, palpation of the vocal folds would show them to be stiff and lacking resilience and pliability, although stroboscopy may be better at detecting such problems. Compared with the contralateral vocal fold, the affected vocal fold may seem atrophic and bowed. A vocal fold that is pink or rose-colored may also be increased in size and have prominent vascular ectasias. This appearance suggests the presence of a hypertrophic scar (Figure 41-3).

DIFFUSE INFLAMMATION OR EDEMA

Poor mucosal hygiene is often present in patients developing benign laryngeal lesions. Infectious laryngitis, chronic nonspecific laryngitis, hyperplastic laryngitis, chronic allergic laryngitis, and reflux laryngitis all contribute to make phonation more of an effort. The changed rheology of mucous membranes caused by poor mucosal hygiene contributes to the development of polypoid corditis and hyperplastic laryngitis. If these factors are not carefully corrected preoperatively and persist or

recur after phonosurgery, they will contribute to persistent dysphonia that will disappoint both the surgeon and the patient. Inflammatory edema that affects vibration can be identified by visual means. By mirror examination, the vocal folds appear thick and have increased mucus production or stranding. The arytenoids are often erythematous from chronic throat clearing. The superior surfaces of the vocal folds often have a salt-and-pepper appearance (Figure 41-4). The stroboscopic examination

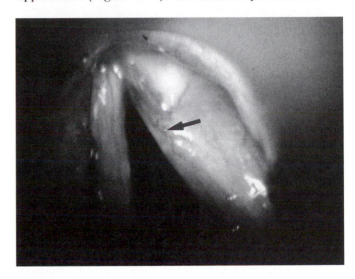

FIGURE 41-3. *Hypertrophic scar of the right vocal folds with telangiectasia after previous microlaryngoscopy. Notice the neovascular changes originating from the center of the scar (arrow).*

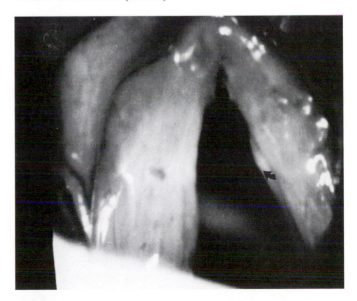

FIGURE 41-4. *Hyperemia, edema, and salt-and-pepper appearance of the vocal folds in a patient with excessive inflammation and small right sulcus vocalis (arrow).*

shows a symmetrically decreased amplitude and a decreased mucosal wave. Vocal characteristics of chronic laryngitis are characterized by a reduced dynamic range in both loudness and frequency. Many patients have a reduced ability to phonate a soft, easy low tone.

Mass Lesions

Residual mass lesions such as a small subglottic papilloma or intracordal cyst can be difficult to see (Figure 41-5). This is especially so if they are small enough to cause only intermittent dysphonia at certain frequencies. By mirror examination, the vocal fold edge usually appears linear. Mirror examination may show a small area of mucus stranding that is confused with a nodule. Stroboscopy helps to isolate the effects caused by residual masses from other problems. One method to assist in the visualization of the vocal folds is to request loud phonation during stroboscopy. With loud phonation, the phase shift is accentuated and a subtle subglottic mass often becomes obvious. Another technique that is useful is to view the vocal folds at an angle using rigid or flexible laryngoscopy. When the videolaryngoscopy is being reviewed, particular attention should be paid to the abduction during deep inspiration. This maneuver helps to flatten the vocal folds laterally and accentuates any subglottic asymmetry. Figure 41-5 is an example of residual mass lesion after prior microlaryngeal surgery. Notice that the superior edge of the vocal fold is linear and shows good vibration, but the inferior lip is irregular and has small areas of papilloma.

In a small percentage of patients, recurrence of the original lesion can occur. Lesions prone to recurrence are (1) contact granulomas, (2) recurrent benign keratosis, and (3) recurrent vocal fold nodules. These lesions present with features similar to their original presentation.

HYPERFUNCTIONAL VOICE DISORDER

In a select group of patients, postoperative healing occurs uneventfully, but residual dysphonia persists. Flexible examination and stroboscopic examination demonstrate good vibratory function of both vocal folds, yet the patient continues to be dysphonic. Flexible laryngoscopy of these patients may reveal the larynx to phonate in unusual supraglottic and glottic configurations. These patterns can be systematically evaluated by a review of the flexible laryngoscopy tape. In the absence of vibratory abnormalities of vocal folds, these patients are classified as having hyperfunctional or functional voice disorders. The possible causes of hyperfunctional dysphonia may be (1) poor vocal habits developed before surgery, (2) an intrinsic hyperfunctional voice disorder that predates the laryngeal lesion, or (3) psychogenic posturing of vocal folds.

Laryngoscopic findings in patients with functional dysphonia are best appreciated by flexible laryngoscopy using connected speech. The speech-language pathologist is particularly valuable during this portion of the examination. When hyperfunction is suspected, the speech-language pathologist should be present to help in the diagnosis and try therapeutic maneuvers while the flexible laryngoscope is in place.

On flexible laryngoscopy, the features that are relevant to the diagnosis of hyperfunction include the obser-

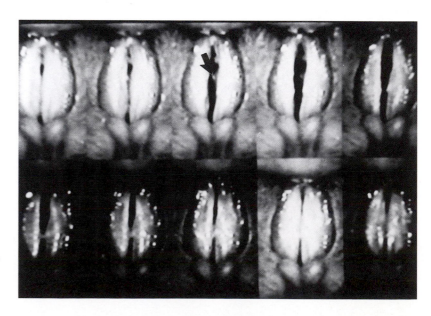

FIGURE 41-5. *Residual subglottic papilloma (arrow) in a patient after recent microlaryngoscopy. The voice was improved but not perfect.*

vation of pharyngeal and laryngeal squeeze during speech. Some features of hyperfunction are

1. Pharynx squeezing during speech

2. Inappropriate elevation of the larynx during phonation

3. Shortened anteroposterior diameter of the vocal folds

4. Ventricular hyperadduction (Figure 41-6)

5. Excessive arytenoid approximation and anterior displacement of the arytenoids

6. Myasthenia larynges with poor closure

7. Coup de glotte with harsh glottal attack during onset of phonation.

Stroboscopic features of hyperfunction are characteristic but are not critical to the diagnosis. These include

1. Abnormally shortened vocal folds suggestive of thyroarytenoid muscle (TA) hyperfunction (Figure 41-7)

2. A shortened or prolonged closed phase during the glottal cycle

3. A shortened closing time

4. A phase shift difference between vocal folds

5. Habitually too loud or too soft phonation during comfortable phonation

Figure 41-8 shows a patient with residual nodular diathesis after previous surgery. The vocal folds show

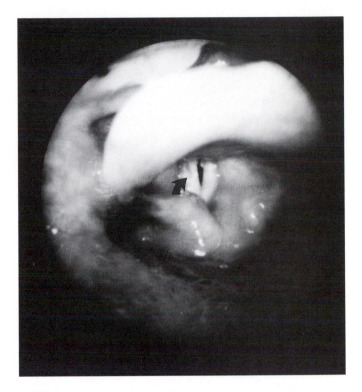

FIGURE 41-7. *Excessive shortening of the posteroanterior diameter of the vocal folds during phonation in a patient with benign keratosis after prior resection. This gesture may be indicative of TA hyperfunction. Speech therapy is useful to correct this after lesion removal. However, if there is excessive scarring, the prognosis for voice is guarded.*

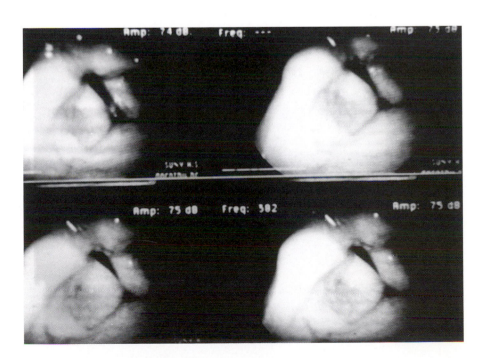

FIGURE 41-6. *Ventricular hyperadduction in a patient with incomplete closure of the folds after lesion removal. The series of stroboscopic pictures shows the false folds to oscillate with an open glottis below.*

preferential midfold contact. There is an hourglass appearance to the vocal folds, and there is only brief vocal fold contact with large posterior chink (Figure 41-8).

Interdisciplinary evaluation is often a critical part of the evaluation of postsurgical dysphonia. Our preference is to perform the history and examination together so that discussions of the pathophysiology can be done immediately. When the speech-language pathologist is present, therapeutic speech therapy probes can be done at the same time as fiberoptic laryngoscopy. This often provides clues about which interventional maneuvers to try during subsequent speech therapy sessions. The speech-language pathologist should, in most cases, independently verify the validity of the diagnosis prior to instituting a course of therapy. Since many patients may already have tried speech therapy, the validation of the diagnosis is a critical step before a recommendation for further speech therapy. Both the laryngologist and speech-language pathologist must have confidence in the accuracy of the diagnosis.

OBJECTIVE EVALUATIONS

The objective evaluation of vocal function is a useful adjunct to understanding changes in vocal function. As a research tool, it helps to identify specific acoustic, aerodynamic, and visual features that correlate with improved voice and vocal function. As a clinical tool, it helps to document the condition before and after treatment.

Of the various instruments, the recording of the voice and videostroboscopy appears to be the most useful. Aerodynamic measures, electroglottography (EGG),

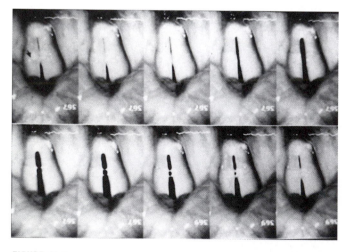

FIGURE 41-8. *Nodular diathesis after previous laryngeal polypectomy. The patient had an excellent postoperative voice initially but returned to her previous vocal habits.*

and acoustic waveforms help to identify relevant parameters that can be compared among treatment groups.

Measures such as glottal efficiency (AC/DC ratio), mean airflow, phonation time, and maximal loudness and pitch range give some objective "feel" for the patient's phonatory ability. Other acoustic measures such as jitter, shimmer, signal/noise ratio, and ratio of spectral energy of high frequency to low frequency energy help to simplify and document the complex acoustic signal.

TREATMENT

Avoidance of Complications

The best way to treat postoperative dysphonia is by prevention. This comes in the form of realistic patient counseling, accurate diagnosis, and careful preoperative, operative, and postoperative management. However, even in the best of hands, complications sometimes occur.

Preoperative Evaluation and Counseling

If a hyperfunctional voice disorder is present and surgery is unavoidable, speech therapy consultation before and after the surgery should be incorporated into the treatment plan. The patient should meet with the speech-language pathologist before surgery in an attempt to reverse the hyperfunctional habits before surgery. In these patients, the surgical treatment and speech rehabilitation of voice should be discussed as a unified treatment.

If there is significant inflammation of the laryngeal structures, reversal of the causative factors before surgery usually means a less turbulent postoperative course. This includes corrective measures for factors such as hydration, voice abuse, smoking, sinobronchial infections, and reflux laryngitis. If such factors cannot be reversed, their implication for return of "normal" vocal function should be honestly discussed and documented. Occasionally, preoperative treatment with systemic antibiotics and steroids for 72 hours before surgery and carried through the postoperative period may be useful to reduce postoperative inflammation.

Because the most common cause of postsurgical dysphonia is a nonvibratory segment, the surgeon should use the smallest microinstruments—laser or nonlaser—to achieve the most precise treatment of tissue lesions. Conservation of normal mucosa and preservation of the layered structure is the best insurance against a nonvibratory segment.

The scarred and immobile vocal fold that is free of residual mass lesions does not participate functionally in modulating airflow. All steps should be taken to avoid such results. In general, successful rehabilitation of voice by surgery or speech therapy is accompanied by the restoration of mucosal vibration and mucosal wave. This feature is often more important than a fine linear vocal edge. Failure to achieve good vibratory function may be related to a host of factors, including (1) the type and extent of the lesion, (2) the amount of fibrosis and scar involving Reinke's layer, (3) the amount of surgical dissection, and (4) the extent of epithelial resection and the resultant secondary healing. Several authors have stressed the importance of preserving the delicate layered structure of the vocal folds.[14,15] Loss of the layered structure of the vocal folds coupled with inflammation, fibrosis, and secondary re-epithelialization all contribute to produce a scarred, stiffened vocal fold. Such scarred vocal folds will not vibrate with ease, creating a crippled phonatory layer and a poor functional result.

The excision of large surface epithelial lesions contributes to the production of reduced amplitude of vibration. To avoid excessive injury, the dissection should be limited to within the layer of pathologic involvement. When the lesion is intraepithelial, the histologic specimen should stop at the basement membrane. The glistening gelatinous structures deep to the vocal fold epithelium should be left undisturbed. This helps ensure a vocal fold that is not tethered to the vocal ligament. When in doubt, it is often preferable to leave an irregular vocal fold edge that vibrates rather than a vocal fold that is straight yet stiff. Likewise, when the lesion spares the epithelium, normal epithelium should be left and preserved. The cordotomy procedures, in which an incision is made on the superior surface followed by microdissection, spares the normal epithelium better than cup forceps and scissor excision. In the management of intracordal masses, cysts, and polypoid degeneration, cordotomy followed by careful gentle evacuation of the subepithelial lesion may give the best chance for the restoration of normal vibratory function. Figure 41-9 illustrates this concept diagrammatically. Figure 41-10 illustrates a typical lesion evacuated without excessive epithelial removal. To help reduce the size of the epithelial defect, a small 6-0 plain gut suture can be placed endoscopically to approximate the vocal fold edge. This seems to help reduce the amount of secondary healing.

One problem of postsurgical care that can result in poor function is excessive perioperative and postoperative inflammation. Patients at risk are smokers with polypoid corditis who have chronically thick mucus. Patients having a large amount of tissue resection are also at risk for prolonged inflammation after surgery as are patients who use their voices excessively in the

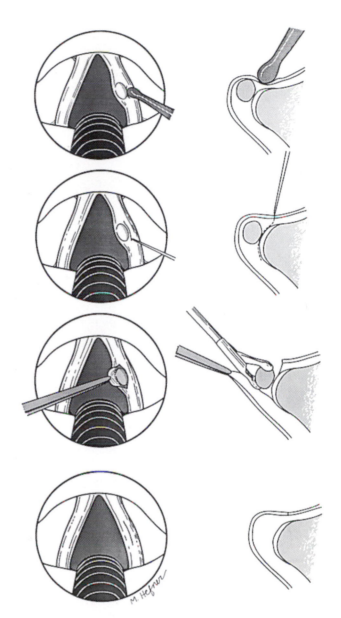

FIGURE 41-9. *Schematic diagram of cordotomy incision and evacuation of a subepithelial lesion. The mucosa is spared using this approach.*

immediate postoperative period. Evaluation of vocal fold vibration 1 week after surgery helps to assess the healing progress. If there is excessive edema and inflammation, aggressive retreatment by broad-spectrum antibiotics, mucolytics, and systemic steroids may be indicated as well as relative voice rest and voice therapy. Factors that contribute to laryngeal irritation should be considered and ruled out. These factors include smoking, excessive throat clearing, coughing, reflux laryngitis, allergic laryngitis, and voice abuse. Antitussives are used liberally in the postoperative

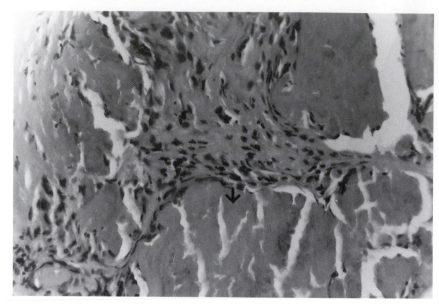

FIGURE 41-10. *Histopathology of a subcordal mass lesion. Notice the absence of epithelium in the specimen evacuated by cordotomy. Arrow points to hyaline material seen in a pseudocyst of the subcordal space.*

patient to reduce chronic irritation and cough. Hydration, mucolytics, and antitussives coupled with careful monitoring of abusive behavior often can reverse the prolonged healing process and allow vibration to begin.

MANAGEMENT

Some patients with persistent dysphonia after laryngeal surgery do not need further treatment. Each patient has his or her own needs and motivations. Some are seeking to be reassured that there is no evidence of neoplasia, while others seek improvements in vocal function even at the expense of a great deal of time and money. The degree of motivation to follow treatment suggestions is a key factor in determining whether further treatment should be suggested. An accurate assessment of patient needs and whether these needs can be met by further treatment is the first step in treatment planning.

Appropriate pretreatment discussions should provide the patients with an in-depth review of their pathophysiology and of what can and cannot be done realistically to improve the situation. The surgeon and speech-language pathologist should not be overly optimistic about the hoped-for results. In deciding to undergo another treatment course, the patient may indeed risk being "disappointed" again. In general, the patients the laryngologist can reasonably expect to help are those with realistic expectations in whom the objective evidence of vibratory abnormality can be directly related to their dysphonic complaints. For example, the evacuation of a small residual intracordal cyst can be reasonably expected to improve vocal fold mass and symmetry and improve the voice if the mass is causing

the dysphonia. A small subglottic papilloma that interferes with speaking can be removed by CO_2 laser bounced off a subglottic mirror. Other clinical problems are more challenging. For example, the patient with stiff vocal folds after PTFE injection is especially challenging. If there is no evidence of granuloma formation or airway obstruction, what is the role of speech therapy or surgery? Indeed, it is doubtful that repeat endolaryngeal surgery in the face of massively stiffened vocal folds will improve the voice. At worst, voice results may even suffer. One example of carefully limiting further surgery is in the patient with benign keratosis and a poor voice. If the diagnosis of benign keratosis is certain from prior biopsies, repeated stripping of an offending lesion that recurs can lead to worsening of vocal fold function. In these patients, selective biopsies based on supravital staining may be more appropriate than repeated strippings that leave the patient further disabled. In patients with benign keratosis, close follow-up is essential; selected biopsies may prolong vocal function with little increased risk.

In the absence of an obvious residual or recurrent mass lesion, a graduated approach of treatment planning seems appropriate. Generally, aggressive medical therapy and mucosal hygiene are instituted. This includes the restriction of caffeine and nicotine in the diet. Mucosal hygiene and hydration alone yield benefits in many patients. If such an approach fails, all drugs taken by the patient are reviewed with an eye toward side effects of mucositis and drying. If such drugs are identified, they are replaced by an alternative medication. The third step in medical management consists of careful environmental and dietary control and review.

Avoidance of heavy coughing, throat clearing, and shouting is stressed and reviewed by the voice care team. Medications that have been found useful to restore vibratory function include steroidal and nonsteroidal anti-inflammatory agents, mucolytics, and broad-spectrum antibiotics. A steroid given in systemic form is much preferable to topical sprays. Longer-term steroid use can be managed with less endocrine suppression using an alternate-day dosing. If the introduction of mucolytics, anti-inflammatory medication, and antibiotics fails to bring about less erythema and edema, further treatment is instituted. This includes an antitussive and nonmedical anti-reflux regimen and nasal irrigations to remove offending thick secretions. The possibility of reflux laryngitis, sinobronchial infection, and allergic laryngitis should be considered, and, if tests are positive, medical treatment for these problems should be begun.

Once maximal medical treatment has been achieved, a course of voice therapy is instituted to reverse hyperfunction and improve vocal fold flexibility. Despite moderate to severe functional loss of vocal fold vibration, many patients with isolated nonvibratory segments can have their vibratory function restored using a regimen of vocal fold exercises.

If the patient is motivated, the speech-language pathologist meets with the patient in six to eight 1-hour sessions. Instruction on proper vocal care and usage is given along with vocal fold exercises and a voice practice regimen designed to increase vocal fold flexibility. In our center, these therapeutic exercises include:

1. Lip and tongue trills at an ascending and descending scale and loudness

2. Vocal range and loudness exercises

3. Easy-onset phonation and tone focus exercises

4. The use of aspirate voice

Using such an approach, some patients show dramatic improvements in vocal fold vibratory function and better voice results in 6 to 8 weeks. If improvements are not present at the end of 8 weeks, further speech therapy is not advocated in most cases.

Surgical re-exploration is indicated for recurrent or residual masses that fail to respond to conservative measures. In the patient with poor closure and a nonlinear edge, re-operation to improve closure has a good chance of improving function. If the scarring is localized, surgical re-excision with lysis of the tethered scar band, followed by steroid injection, can lead to an improvement in voice. The number of patients undergoing such treatments is too small for any definitive conclusions regarding long-term efficacy.

Table 41-3 shows the initial diagnosis and the primary treatment rendered in our patient series. The equal distribution of patients undergoing primary treatments by medical, surgical, speech rehabilitation, and no therapy supports the equal role each treatment has in the management of these patients.

CASE HISTORIES

Some clinical case histories help to illustrate the management issues.

Case A

Patient A was a 36-year-old male science teacher with intermittent voice breaks and easy vocal fatigue. He underwent a direct laryngoscopy and biopsy for a "polyp" at another hospital. Postoperatively, his voice failed to return to its preoperative function. He began to experience persistent and continuous dysphonia and pain with speaking. He was unable to return to his teaching. After 6 months of persistent dysphonia he presented to our voice clinic. His voice had a rough, breathy, and diplophonic quality with frequent voice breaks. Strobovideolaryngoscopy showed a stiff immobile segment on the left vocal fold with poor vibratory function (Figure 41-11). He was diagnosed to have a stiff vocal fold segment caused by surgical scarring. He underwent 6 weeks of voice therapy consisting of exercises designed specifically to increase vocal fold flexibility, such as trill exercises and vocal range exercises. Re-examination at the end of 8 weeks of voice therapy showed a remarkably improved voice. Repeat strobovideolaryngoscopy showed

Initial Diagnosis	Primary Treatment[a]
Polyps, nodules, cysts N = 22	Surgery N = 14
Epithelial lesion N = 15	Speech therapy N = 15
Sulcus vocalis N = 4	Medical therapy N = 17
Contact granuloma N = 3	None N = 16
Cancer N = 4	
Paralysis N = 5	
Unknown N = 6	

[a] The treatment plan may include combinations of surgery, speech therapy, medical therapy, and therapeutic assurance.

TABLE 41-3. *Initial Diagnosis and Treatment Given in 59 Patients with Postsurgical Dysphonia*

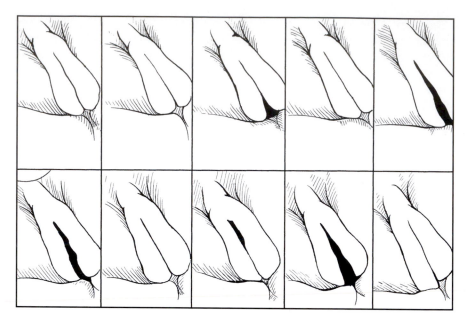

FIGURE 41-11. *Case A, before speech therapy. This series of stroboscopic illustrations shows irregular vocal fold opening from aperiodic vocal fold oscillation caused by a scarred and stiff vocal fold. There is an irregular posterior chink and an absence of a discrete open and closed phase.*

a mobile, less stiff vocal fold with excellent amplitude and mucosal wave (Figure 41-12).

This case demonstrates the value of speech therapy in restoring vibratory function in a stiffened vocal fold caused by microlaryngoscopy. It is unlikely that the return of vocal vibratory function came about through continued spontaneous postoperative healing as the therapy was given 6 months after his surgery.

Case B

Patient B was a 45-year-old female smoker who had a "polyp" removed from the left vocal fold 1 $1/2$ years ago. She stated that her voice never became normal

after her surgery. Her voice was inappropriately low and continued to be mistaken for a man's. On examination, she was found to have a fundamental frequency of 180 Hz. Her voice was slightly rough with a veiled, husky quality. Strobovideolaryngoscopy revealed a mass difference between the right and the left vocal folds. Her previously operated side vibrated well with good amplitude and mucosal wave. On the right side there was evidence of Reinke's edema with polypoid degeneration. After a course of mucolytics and aggressive vocal hygiene failed, she was taken to the operating room, where a right subcordal evacuation of mucoid material was done by microdissection. Postoperatively, her voice was

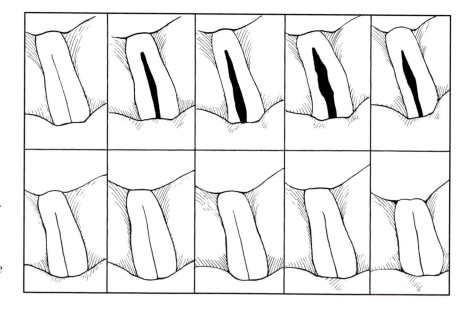

FIGURE 41-12. *Case A, after speech therapy. With improved voice the videostroboscopy shows a regular opening and closing phase, good amplitude, and increased vibration of the side with the vocal fold scar.*

immediately improved. Her fundamental frequency was restored to 205 Hz with increased loudness and clarity of voice. Her laryngostroboscopy from the preoperative and postoperative examination is shown in Figures 41-13 and 41-14.

This case illustrates the added role of strobovideo-laryngoscopy in detecting subtle mass differences between the vocal folds that could not be appreciated by nonstroboscopic means. The repeat operation restored vocal fold vibration and symmetry, resulting in a more normal vibratory pattern of vocal fold function. This correlated well with improved vocal function.

Case C

Patient C was a 58-year-old female smoker who worked in a noisy, smoky environment. She developed

large bilateral laryngeal polyps with polypoid degeneration of the vocal folds. These were removed by microlaryngoscopy. She failed to experience voice improvement after surgery and brief voice rest. Examination 4 weeks after surgery revealed a diffusely reddened larynx with little vibratory amplitude or mucosal wave on either vocal fold. Further questioning revealed that the patient worked in a hot, noisy environment that required her to shout dietary orders. She also continued to smoke and cough. She was given a course of antibiotics, systemic steroids, and mucolytics and put on further voice rest for 2 weeks. Re-examination at the end of 2 weeks revealed an improved voice with good vocal function.

The diagnosis was inflammatory laryngitis exacerbated by her work environment and smoking. She was excused from her work environment and has continued

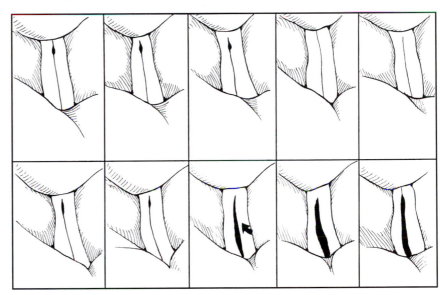

FIGURE 41-13. *Case B, before surgery. A fullness of the right side is appreciated by stroboscopic examination. The fullness failed to oscillate (arrow), thereby indicating a residual mass lesion.*

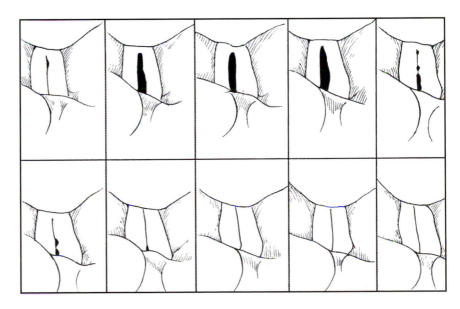

FIGURE 41-14. *Case B, after surgery. Improved vocal fold oscillation of both vocal folds is apparent.*

to function well. Figure 41-15 shows vocal folds that are swollen and fail to vibrate. The ventricular folds are adducted with a posterior glottic chink. After medical therapy, the vocal folds show much less erythema with good vibratory function (Figure 41-16).

This case illustrates the impact of medical and environmental factors that prevented the return of vocal function. Optimizing her work environment, improving vocal hygiene, and medical treatment resulted in a more functional voice.

RESULTS

The results of treatment using such an approach can be good. In our experience, patients who are motivated and follow through on a diagnostic and treatment voice therapy program have a good chance of improved function using a combined approach. Table 41-3 shows the primary diagnosis and the various primary treatments rendered. Table 41-4 lists the results broken down by the types of problems. Patients with lesion recurrence, residual mass lesions, and hyperfunctional voice disorders did better than patients with localized scar with stiffness and inflammation. But despite the high rates of no improvement in the latter groups, improved vibratory function and voice were achieved in a significant percentage of patients.

The objective measures of vocal function help to lend support to stroboscopic observations of improved vibratory function. Table 41-5 lists some acoustic measures in 30 individuals undergoing treatment, while Table 41-6 lists the aerodynamic measures in 41 patients undergoing treatment. The acoustic measures show trends toward decreased perturbation, decreased shimmer, improved signal/noise ratio, and improved average SPL and pitch range. The mean flow was reduced from 160 ml/s to a more normal 120 ml/s, while glottal efficiency as defined by the AC/DC ratio has increased. The maximum loudness was slightly decreased. This may be because of less stridency and fewer harsh glottal attacks noted in the majority of patients.

In summary, using a multidisciplinary approach to the diagnosis of postsurgical dysphonia, management issues in these difficult patients can be made easier. Moreover, treatment of these patients, utilizing the skills

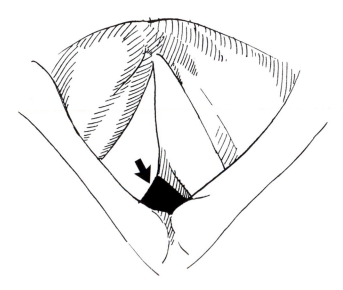

FIGURE 41-15. *Case C, swollen and edematous vocal folds after microlaryngeal surgery. The patient's attempt at phonation results in a large posterior chink without vocal fold oscillation (arrow on posterior chink).*

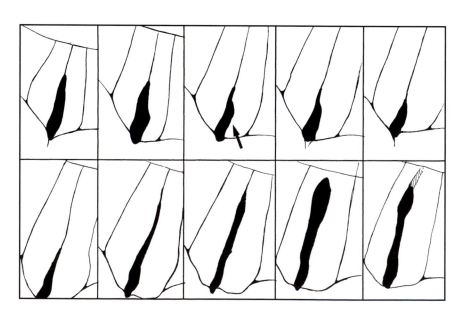

FIGURE 41-16. *Case C, after medical therapy with steroids and antibiotics. Vocal folds now oscillate. There is still a sizable posterior chink (arrow).*

	Diagnosis					
Results	Scar With Stiffness	Residual Mass	Inflammation	Hyperfunction	Recurrence	Unknown
Excellent	7	5	6	2	2	0
Improved	3	2	2	3	1	0
No improvement	8	1	3	0	0	0
No Follow-up	4	0	2	2	1	3
Total	22	8	13	7	4	3

TABLE 41-4. *Results in the Series Treated by Combined Approach*

	Pre (N = 30)	Post (N = 30)
Mean speaking F$_o$ (Hz)	179	219
Dynamic range (db)	25.7	25.2
Pitch range (semitones)	26.0	27.1
Average SPL (dB)	74.6	77.8
Signal/noise ratio (dB)	25.6	26.9
Shimmer (%)	1.7	0.25
Perturbation (ms)	0.015	0.01

TABLE 41-5. *Acoustic Measures in 30 Patients Undergoing Combined Treatment for Postsurgical Dysphonia*

	Pre (N = 41)	Post (N = 39)
Mean flow rate (ml/s)	160	120
AC/DC ratio	0.23	0.30
Maximum loudness (dB)	85	84

TABLE 41-6. *Selected Phonatory Function Measures in 41 Patients Before and 39 Patients After Combined Speech, Medical, and Surgical Treatment*

of the otolaryngologist, speech scientist, and speech-language pathologist, can be combined to improve vocal function in a large percentage of patients. Careful observation and understanding of vibratory function before and after phonosurgery should assist the phonosurgeon in avoiding pitfalls that result in persistent postoperative dysphonia.

REFERENCES

1. Ford C, Bless D. Collagen injection in the scarred vocal fold. *J Voice.* 1987;1:116-118.

2. Dedo HH. Injection and removal of Teflon for unilateral vocal cord paralysis. *Ann Otol Rhinol Laryngol.* 1992;101:81-86.

3. Brodnitz FS. Results and limitations of vocal rehabilitation. *Arch Otol.* 1963;77:148-156.

4. Baker et al. Persistent hoarseness after surgical removal of vocal cord lesions. *Arch Otol.* 1981; 107:148-151.

5. Wolfe VI, Ratsunik DL. Vocal symptomatology of postoperative dysphonia. *Laryngoscope.* 1981;91: 635-643.

6. Andrews AH. Surgery of benign tumors of the larynx. *Otolaryngol Clin North Am.* 1970;3:517-527.

7. Strong MS, Vaughn CW. Vocal cord nodule and polyps—the role of surgical treatment. *Laryngoscope.* 1971;81:911-923.

8. Kleinsasser O, Glanz H, Kimmich T. Endoscopic surgery of vocal cord cancers. *HNO.* 1988;26:412-416.

9. Leeper HA, Heeneman H, Reynolds C. Vocal function following vertical hemilaryngectomy. A preliminary investigation. *J Otolaryngol.* 1990;19: 62-70.

10. Casiano RR, Cooper JD, Lundy DS, et al. Laser cordectomy for T$_1$ glottic carcinoma: a 10 year experience and videostroboscopic findings. *Otolaryngol Head Neck Surg.* 1991;104:831-837.

11. Watterson T, McFarlane SC, Menicacci AL. Vibratory characteristics of Teflon injected and noninjected paralyzed vocal folds. *J Speech Hear Dis.* 1990;55:61-66.

12. McGuirt WF, Blalock D, Koufman JA, et al. Voice analysis of patients with endoscopically treated early laryngeal carcinoma. *Ann Otol Rhinol Laryngol.* 1992;101:142-146.

13. Sataloff RT, Spiegel JR, Hawkshaw M, et al. Autologous fat implantation for vocal fold scar: a preliminary report. *J Voice.* 1996;11(2):238-246.

14. Bouchayer M, Cornut G, Witzig E. Microsurgery for benign lesions of the vocal folds. *Ear Nose Throat J.* 1988;67:446.

15. Kleinsasser O. Restoration of the voice in benign lesions of the vocal folds by endolaryngeal microsurgery. *J Voice.* 1991;5:257-263.

INDEX

postnatal critical periods, 11-12

precursors, 4-7

primordia, 3

segmental organization, 3-4

spatial organization, 7-11

Laryngeal transplantation, 132

reinnervation, 663

Laryngeal webs, 328-329, 328i, 329i, 347, 347i

and congenital heart disease, 337t

Laryngitis

corticosteroid use for, 517-518

and GERD, 73

nonspecific, 73

with serious vocal fold injury, 304

without serious damage, 304-305

Laryngoceles, 331, 346-347

Laryngofissure and cordectomy, 687

Laryngology, research issues, 131-133

Laryngomalacia, 321-324, 322i, 324i

types, 322t

Laryngopharyngeal reflux (LPR), 73, 381-382, 590

and associated conditions, 384t

and cancer, 670

diagnosis, 385-386

medications for, 518-519

pediatric, 389-390

symptoms, 383t

treatment, 386-389

Laryngospasm, 109

Laryngotracheal bronchitis, 395

Laryngotracheal re-anastomosis, 611

Laryngotracheal stenosis, 133

Laryngotracheoesophageal cleft (LTEC), 329-330, 330i, 348

Laryngotracheoesophageal, type 4 cleft, 25

Laryngoplastic phonosurgery, 641

Larynx, 3

adult framework injuries, 597-598

amyloidosis, 401-402

anatomy and radiography, 259-260

biomechanics of, 561, 567

blood supply, 35-36

blunt injury to, 597

carcinoma in situ (CIS), 671-673

chemoreflexes, 109

clinical subdivisions, 36

coronal section, 30

CT scan reconstructions, 270i-273i

development, 17, 18i, 20i, 345

dynamic aspects, 260

early development theories, 17

framework, 27-28, 27i, 28i, 273i

functions, 27

fungal infections of, 399-400

gender effects, 132-133

geriatric, 38, 47

glands, 47

as hormonal target, 356

human papilloma virus (HPV), 673-675

immune diseases, 400

infectious disorders of, 394-399

injury, 72-73

innervation, 34-35, 34i, 49-50, 50i

lesions, 74-82, 346

lymphatic drainage, 36

manipulation, 561, 571-572

mucosa, 30-31

muscles, 31-34, 32i, 33i, 34i

neuroanatomy, 107-110

neuromuscular anatomy, 50-60

pediatric, 37, 45, 346, 601-602

phonation, 60-66, 87-99

premalignant lesions, 667-670

proprioreceptors, 110

research studies, 18-19

soft tissue injuries, 602

spaces, 36

surgery, 315-316

taste buds, 35

transplantation, 132

vocal fold anatomy, 70-72

vocal fold histology, 36-37, 37i

Larynx-nasopharynx interlocking, 12

Lateral cricoarytenoid muscle, innervation, 52-53, 53i